D0035249

Helping Health Workers Learn

A book of methods, aids, and ideas for instructors at the village level

David Werner and Bill Bower

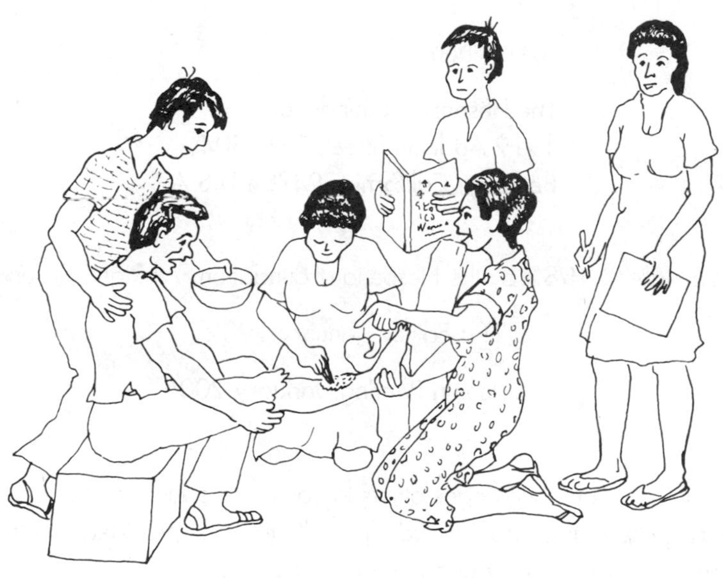

drawings by

David Werner Pablo Chavez
Regina Faul-Jansen Marie Ducruy

Library of Congress Cataloging-in-Publication Data

Catalog Card No.: 81-85010

Werner, David Bradford and Bower, Bill Larned
Helping Health Workers Learn

Palo Alto, CA: Hesperian Foundation

632 p.

8111 811015

ISBN: 0-942364-10-4

PUBLISHED BY:

The Hesperian Foundation
1919 Addison Street, Suite 304
Berkeley, California 94704 U.S.A.

First Edition, January 1982

Thirteenth Printing, January 2005

This book is dedicated to the village health team of Ajoya, Mexico, from whom we have learned a great deal...

and to health workers everywhere who side with the poor.

REQUEST FOR YOUR COMMENTS, CRITICISMS, AND IDEAS:

This book is only a beginning. We want to improve it—with your help.

If you have any ideas, teaching methods, visual aids, or ways of exploring or learning that you feel might be put into this book, please send them to us.

Also let us know which parts of the book you find most useful, and which parts, pages, or paragraphs you find confusing, badly written, least useful, incorrect, or unfair. We think the book is too long, and ask your help in deciding what to leave out.

WE ARE ESPECIALLY INTERESTED IN GETTING SUGGESTIONS FROM VILLAGE AND COMMUNITY HEALTH WORKERS WHO HAVE BECOME INSTRUCTORS.

Please write to:

The Hesperian Foundation
1919 Addison Street, Suite 304
Berkeley, California 94704 U.S.A.

Thank you.

THANKS

The creation of this book has been a long, cooperative effort. We have borrowed ideas from many sources. Included in these pages are methods and suggestions from health and development programs in 35 countries on 5 continents. Often we mention the programs or countries from which particular ideas have come as we discuss them in the text. Here, however, we give our warm thanks to all programs, groups, and persons whose ideas, suggestions, and financial assistance have contributed to this book.

Our heartfelt appreciation goes to the village health team in Ajoya, Mexico, especially to Martín Reyes, Miguel Angel Manjarrez, Roberto Fajardo, Miguel Angel Alvarez, Pablo Chávez, Jesús Vega Castro, Rosa Salcido, Guadalupe Aragón, Alejandro Alvarez, Teresa Torres, Anacleto Arana, and Marcelo Acevedo. It is from working with the Ajoya team for many years that we have come to understand the meaning of community-based health care.

We would also like to renew our thanks to the dedicated persons who helped put the first edition of this book together back in 1982: Myra Polinger, Lynn Gordon, Mary Klein, Michael Blake, Hal Lockwood, Christine Taylor, Richard Friedman, Susan Klein, Andy Browne, Ken Tull of World Neighbors, Meg Granito, and Emily Goldfarb. Trude Bock generously provided her home and all-round assistance during the three years it took to give birth to this book

Our special thanks to B.A. Laris for undertaking the editing, layout, **and paste-up for the** tenth printing. Her efforts make this printing easier to use with the 1992 revision of *Where There Is No Doctor*. Davida Coady updated the **antibiotic learning game** found in Chapter 19 and Martín Lamarque provided current information on organizations that make practical teaching materials available.

For their outstanding drawings, we thank Regina Faul-Jansen, Marie Ducruy, and Pablo Chávez of the village health team in Ajoya. Pablo also invented and helped develop several of the most imaginative teaching aids shown in this book. For many of the drawings and most of the photographs, credit also goes to David Werner.

David Morley, Murray and Gerri Dickson, Fred Abbatt, Pia Moriarity, Sunil Mehra, Laura Goldman, and Esther de Gally reviewed early drafts of this book. We remain grateful for their valuable suggestions and encouragement.

Early drafts of **Helping Health Workers Learn** were field tested in Latin America, Africa, and the Philippines. From these various field trials we received many helpful ideas and suggestions. We are deeply thankful to all those health workers, instructors, volunteers, and health officers who contributed.

For many years our books have been packaged and mailed by a dedicated group of volunteers who contribute their labor to support the Foundation's efforts to make health information available. Without their commitment, far fewer copies of our publications would now be available to people throughout the world. Our thanks to Barbara and Herb Hultgren, Tom Beckett, Paul Chandler, Bob and Kay Schauer, Marge West, and Betsy Wallace.

Over the years we have received financial assistance from many sources for the development and distribution of this book. We are grateful to the Ella Lyman Cabot Trust, the Public Welfare Foundation, Brot für die Welt, OXFAM England, the Sunflower Foundation, Misereor, Helmut and Brigitte Gollwitzer, and Reinhart Freudenberg. We also thank the Carnegie Corporation of New York for funding gratis distribution of this, and other Hesperian publications, in Africa. We wish to thank the many generous friends of the Hesperian Foundation who have donated their time and resources to support the struggle for better health and a better world.

CONTENTS

INTRODUCTION

Health for all by the year 2000 has become the goal of the World Health Organization (WHO) and most countries around the earth.

Such a world-wide goal is very worthy. But in some ways it is dangerous. For there is a risk of trying to reach that goal in ways that become so standardized, so impersonal, so controlled by those in power, that many of the human qualities essential to health—and to health care— are lost.

There is already evidence of this happening. In the last 10 or 15 years, a great many attempts have been made to bring basic health care to poor communities. Billions have been spent on large national or regional programs planned by highly trained experts. But the results have often been disappointing. In most countries, the number of persons suffering from preventable or easily curable illness continues to grow.

On the other hand, certain community health programs have been more or less successful in helping the poor meet their health-related needs. Studies by independent observers* have shown that **programs generally recognized as successful, whether large or small, often have the following things in common:**

1. **Small, local beginnings and slow, decentralized growth.** Even the more successful large programs usually have begun as small projects that gradually developed and evolved in response to the needs of particular communities. As these programs have grown, they have remained *decentralized.* This means that important planning and decision making still take place at the village or neighborhood level.

2. **Involvement of local people—especially the poor—in each phase of the program.** Effective programs recognize and try to deal with the conflicts of interest that often exist between the strong and the weak, even in a small community. Not just local leaders, but the most disadvantaged members of society, play a leading role in selecting their own health workers and determining program priorities. A conscious aim of such programs is to help strengthen the position and bargaining power of the poor.

3. **An approach that views planning as a 'learning process'.** The planning of program content and health worker training does not follow a predetermined 'blueprint'. Instead, planning goes on continually as a part of a learning process. Participants at every level (instructors, student health workers, and members of the community) are invited to help shape, change, and criticize the plans. This allows the program to constantly evolve and adapt, so as to better meet people's changing needs. Planning is both local and flexible.

---

*See, for example, David Korten's analysis of successful programs in Asia, "Community Organization and Rural Development: A Learning Process Approach," ***Public Administration Review,*** September/October, 1980, p. 480-510.

4. **Leaders whose first responsibility is to the poor.** Programs recognized as effective usually have leaders who are strongly committed to a just society. Often they have had intense personal experience working with the poor in community efforts to help solve critical needs. Even as their programs have grown and expanded, these program leaders have kept up their close relations with the poor working people in individual communities.

5. **A recognition that good health can only be attained through helping the poor improve the entire situation in which they live.** Successful programs link health activities with other aspects of social development. Health is seen as a state of wholeness and well-being in which persons are able to work together to meet their needs in a self-reliant, responsible way. This means that to become fully healthy, each person needs a clear understanding of himself or herself in relation to others and to the factors that influence all people's well-being. In many of the most effective health programs, activities that help people to develop a more critical awareness have become a key part of training and community work.

In view of these features common to success, the failure of many national and regional 'community health' programs is not surprising. Most are carried out in quite the opposite way. Although their top planners speak proudly of "decision making by the community," seldom do the people have much say about what their health workers are taught and told to do. 'Community participation' too often has come to mean "getting ***those people*** to do what ***we*** decide." Rather than helping the poor become more self-reliant, many national health and development programs end up increasing poor people's dependency on outside services, aid, and authority.

One of the biggest obstacles to 'health by the people' has been the unwillingness of experts, professionals, and health authorities to let go of their control. As a result, community health workers are made to feel that their first responsibility is to the health system rather than to the poor. Usually they are taught only a very limited range of skills. They become the servants or 'auxiliaries' to visiting doctors and nurses, rather than spirited leaders for change. They learn to follow orders and fill out forms, instead of to take initiative or to help people solve their problems on their own terms. Such health workers win little respect and have almost no influence on overall community health. Many of them get discouraged, grow careless, become corrupt, or quit. Results have been so disappointing that some experts, even within WHO, have begun to feel that the goal of 'health for all through community involvement' is like the pot of gold at the end of the rainbow—a dream that has been tried, but failed.

In spite of the failure of most large, centrally controlled programs to achieve effective community participation, in many countries there are outstanding examples of enthusiastic community involvement in health. This is especially true in small, non-government programs that take what we call a ***people-centered*** or ***community-strengthening*** approach to health care.

Within these community-based programs, there is a wealth of variety in terms of innovation and adaptation to local conditions. But at the same time, there is a striking similarity in their social and political objectives in many parts of the world—Pakistan, India, Mozambique, the Philippines, Mexico, Nicaragua, Honduras, El Salvador, and Guatemala.

In these community-based programs, a new kind of health worker has begun to play a leading role. These health workers speak out for the 'voiceless' poor. Their goal is health for all—but health that is founded on human dignity, loving care, and fairer distribution of land, wealth, and power.

To us, one of the most exciting aspects of this new world-wide community-based movement, decentralized and uncoordinated as it may be, is that it goes far beyond any rigid religious or political doctrine. Most of the leaders in these programs recognize the dangers to ordinary people in any large, centrally controlled system, be it capitalist or communist. They have far greater faith in small, self-directed groups of working people. Rather than accept any established dogma, they are asking searching questions. They welcome criticism, and encourage others to observe for themselves and form their own conclusions. They believe in helping the powerless to gain strength through a greater understanding of the factors that shape their health and their lives.

Around this practical human vision has gradually grown a whole new approach to the training, role, and responsibilities of community health workers. Ideas and methods are being shared and further developed through a series of informal networks around the world.

Many of the ideas in this book have been gathered from these networks of community-based health programs, and especially from Project Piaxtla, a small, villager-run program based in Ajoya, Sinaloa, Mexico.

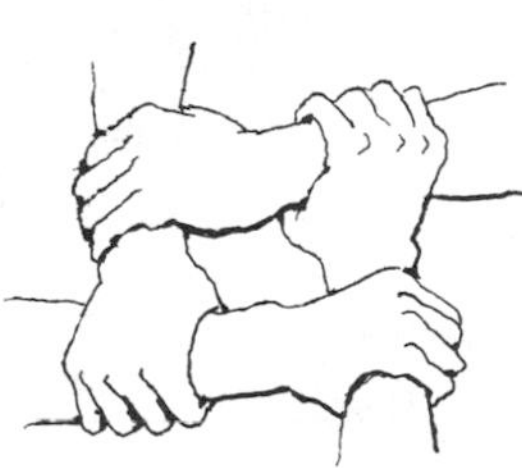

WARNING

This is not a 'recipe book' of how to plan and conduct a training course for health workers. Experience has taught us that such a book could easily do more harm than good. Instead, this is a collection of examples and ideas, of group experiences and outrageous opinions, of 'triggers to the imagination'. It is an invitation to adventure and discovery.

Part of the value and excitement of learning is in finding out 'how to do it' for yourself and with others. It lies in looking at the ways things have been done before, then improving and adapting them to suit your own circumstances. This sort of open-ended, creative learning process is as important for instructors of health workers as for the health workers themselves. After all, finding ways to do things better is the key to improving health. The instructor can set the example.

To be fully alive and meaningful, a training course cannot be either pre-packaged or 'replicable' (able to be copied). It needs to be redesigned not only for each area and set of conditions where it is taught, but each time it is taught.

A training program, like a person, ceases to be interesting when it ceases to grow or be unique!

So rather than being a 'blueprint' on how to build a training program, this book is a craftsman's kit of nuts and bolts and tools. Many of the methods and suggestions come from our personal experience, which has been mostly in Latin America. So pick and choose from them critically. Use and adapt what you can, in order to create—and continually re-create—your own very special, unique, and always-new program. Try to make planning a continuous learning process for everyone concerned: instructors, students, and members of the community.

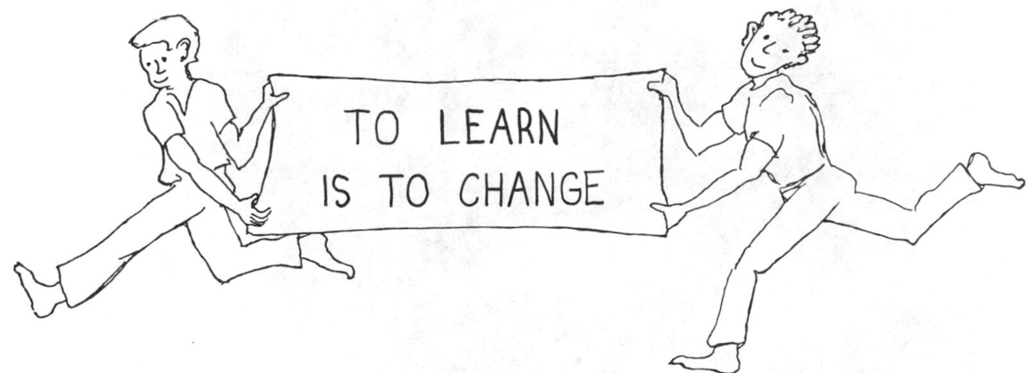

Many of the ideas and suggestions in this book are controversial and will not apply to all areas. We do not ask anyone simply to accept and use them. Instead, we ask you to challenge them, adapt them, criticize them—and use only what makes sense for the people and needs in your own area.

We ask you to consider—and urge you to doubt and question—everything we say.

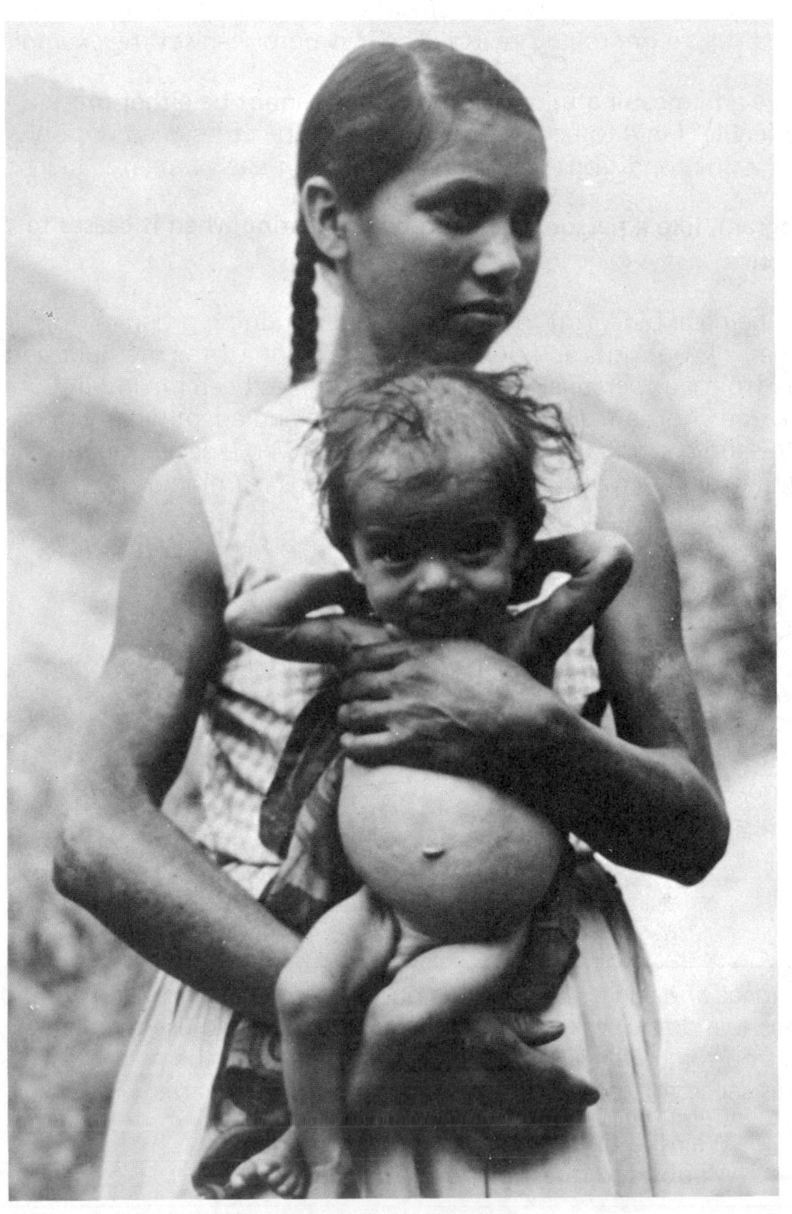

from ***Where There Is No Doctor,*** p. 114

WHY THIS BOOK IS SO POLITICAL

When, 17 years ago, I (David Werner) first began working for improvements in health with villagers in western Mexico, I did not look far beyond the immediate causes of ill health. As I saw it, worms and diarrhea were caused by poor hygiene and contaminated water. Malnutrition was mainly caused by scarcity of food in a remote, mountainous area where drought, floods, and violent winds made farming difficult and harvests uncertain. The high death rate in children (34%) resulted from the combination of infection, poor nutrition, and the long distance to the closest health centers.

In short, I saw people's needs in physical terms, as determined by their physical surroundings. This short-sightedness on my part was understandable, for my training had been in life sciences. I had little social or political awareness.

I might have remained that way, as do many health workers, except that I came so close to the mountain people. I knew from the first that they had strengths, skills, and endurance that I lacked. And so I was able to let them teach me about the human—and inhuman—side of their needs and their lives. They did not sit down and spell things out for me; rather they shared with me their homes, their hardships, and their dreams. Many times I have struggled with a family, against odds, to prevent the loss of a child, a cornfield, or hope. Sometimes we won; sometimes we lost.

Little by little, I became aware that many of their losses—of children, of land, or of hope—not only have immediate physical causes, but also underlying social causes. That is to say, they result from the way some people treat or affect the lives of others. Time and again, I have experienced occasions where death and suffering of children and other persons I have to come to love have been the direct or indirect result of human greed.

On page 114 of ***Where There Is No Doctor*** there is a photograph of a very thin little boy in the arms of his malnourished mother. The boy eventually died—of hunger. The family was—and still is—very poor. Each year the father had to borrow maize from one of the big landholders in the area. For every liter of maize borrowed at planting time, he had to pay back 3 liters at harvest time. With these high interest rates, the family went further and further into debt. No matter how hard the father worked, each year more of his harvest went to pay what he owed to the landholder. Each year he had to borrow more, and pay back 3 times as much. Eventually, the family had to sell their few chickens and pigs, and finally even the beans they had grown on the steep mountain slopes, to buy enough corn to survive.

With no eggs or beans to eat, the mother became increasingly malnourished. Her breasts failed to produce milk for her baby. So she fed him the only food they had—cornmeal and water. In time the child died.

Part of the problem may also have been that the father occasionally drinks with the other men. When he gets drunk, he loses his judgement and sometimes, to buy rounds of drinks, sells a part of the family's precious supply of corn.

This is sad. But look at the father's life. The hard work he does only to go deeper into debt. The death of a child he loved and whom he feels he failed. The apparent hopelessness of his situation. And frequently his own hunger—not only for food, but for a fair chance to benefit from his own hard work. We cannot blame him if he occasionally drinks too much!

Perhaps no one is really to blame. Or perhaps we all are—all of us, at least, who live with more than we need while others hunger. In any case, it is not right, it is not kind, it is not human, to remain silent in a world that permits some persons to grow fat from the hard work of others who go hungry.

The child in the photograph who died is not alone. In the mountain villages I know, there are hundreds of similar children—some dead and some waiting. In the world there are millions. One fourth of the world's children are undernourished, most for reasons similar to those I have just described. Their problems will not be solved by medicines or latrines or nutrition centers or birth control (although all of these, if approached decently, may help). What their families need is a fair chance to live from their own labor, a fair share of what the earth provides.

Do I make myself clear? Let me tell you about Chelo and his family, whom I have become close to over the years. Chelo has advanced tuberculosis. Before the villager-run health center was started in his village, he received no treatment. He knew he had tuberculosis. He wanted treatment. But he could not afford the medicines. (Basic tuberculosis medicines are not expensive to produce. But in Mexican pharmacies, they are sold at up to ten times their generic price in the United States and other developed countries.) Although the government's tuberculosis control program does give free medication, it requires that patients go often to one of its city health centers for tests and medication. For Chelo, this would have meant 250 kilometers of travel every two weeks. He simply could not afford it.

For years, Chelo had worked for the richest landholder in the village. The landholder is an unhappy, overweight man who, apart from his enormous landholdings, owns thousands of cattle. When Chelo began to grow weak from his illness and could not work as hard as before, the landholder fired him, and told him to move out of the house he had been lending him.

Chelo, his wife, Soledad, and his stepson, Raul,* built a mud-brick hut and moved into it. By that time Chelo was coughing blood.

Around the same time, the community-based health program was getting started in the area, but as yet no health worker had been trained in Chelo's village. So a visiting health worker taught Chelo's 11-year-old stepson, Raul, to inject him with streptomycin. Raul also learned to keep records to be sure Chelo took his other medicines correctly. The boy did a good job, and soon was injecting and doing follow-up on several persons with tuberculosis in the village. By age 13, Raul had become one of the central team of health workers in the area. At the same time, he was still attending school.

*These are real persons, but I have changed their names.

Meanwhile, Chelo's family had cleaned up a small weed patch and garbage area at the lower edge of town. With much hard work they had constructed a simple irrigation system using ditches and grooved logs. At last they had a successful vegetable plot, which brought in a small income. Chelo's health had improved, but he would never be strong. Treatment had begun too late.

Economically, Chelo had one setback after another. Just when he was beginning to get out of debt to the storekeepers and landholders, he fell ill with appendicitis. He needed hospital surgery, so health workers and neighbors carried him 23 kilometers on a stretcher to the road, and from there took him to the city by truck. The surgery (in spite of the fact that the doctor lowered his fee) cost as much as the average farmworker earns in a year. The family was reduced to begging.

The only valuable possession the family had was a donkey. When Chelo returned from the hospital, his donkey had disappeared. Two months later, a neighbor spotted it in the grazing area of one of the wealthier families. A new brand—still fresh—had been put right on top of Chelo's old one.

Chelo went to the village authorities, who investigated. They decided in favor of the wealthy thief, and fined Chelo. To me, the most disturbing thing about this is that when he told me about it, Chelo did not even seem angry—just sad. He laughed weakly and shrugged, as if to say, "That's life. Nothing can be done."

His stepson, Raul, however, took all these abuses very hard. He had been a gentle and caring child, but stubborn, with an enormous need for love. As he got older, he seemed to grow angrier. His anger was often not directed at anything in particular.

An incident with the school was the last straw. Raul had worked very hard to complete secondary school in a neighboring town. Shortly before he was to graduate, the headmaster told him in front of the class that he could not be given a certificate since he was an illegitimate child—unless his parents got married. (This happened at a time when the national government had decided to improve its statistics. The president's wife had launched a campaign to have all unwed couples with children get married. The headmaster's refusal to give graduation certificates to children of unwed parents was one of the pressures used.) Chelo and his wife did get married—which cost more money—and Raul did get his certificate. But the damage to his pride remains.

Young Raul began to drink. When he was sober, he could usually control himself. But he had a hard time working with the local health team because he took even the friendliest criticism as a personal attack. When he was drunk, his anger often exploded. He managed to get hold of a high-powered pistol, which he would shoot into the air when he was drinking. One night he got so drunk that he fell down unconscious on the street. Some of the young toughs in town, who also had been drinking, took his pistol and his pants, cut off his hair, and left him naked in the street. Chelo heard about it and carried Raul home.

After this, Raul hid in shame for two weeks. For a while he did not even visit his friends at the health post. He was afraid they would laugh. They did not. But Raul had sworn revenge—he was never quite sure against whom. A few months later, when drunk, he shot and killed a young man who had just arrived from another village. The two had never seen each other before.

This, to me, is a tragedy because Raul was fighting forces bigger than himself. As a boy of 12, he had taken on the responsibilities of a man. He had shown care and concern for other people. He had always had a quick temper, but he was a good person. And, I happen to know, he still is.

Who, then, is to blame? Again, perhaps no one. Or perhaps all of us. Something needs to be changed.

After the shooting, Raul fled. That night, the State Police came looking for him. They burst into Chelo's home and demanded to know where Raul was. Chelo said Raul had gone. He didn't know where. The police dragged Chelo into a field outside town and beat him with their pistols and rifles. Later, his wife found him still lying on the ground, coughing blood and struggling to breathe.

It was more than a year before Chelo recovered enough to work much in his garden. His tuberculosis had started up again after the beating by the police. Raul was gone and could not help with the work. The family was so poor that, again, they had to go begging. Often they went hungry.

After a few months, Chelo's wife, Soledad, also developed signs of tuberculosis and started treatment at the village health post. The local health workers did not charge for her treatment or Chelo's, even though the health post had economic difficulties of its own. However, Chelo's wife helped out when she could by washing the health post linens at the river. (This work may not have been the best thing for her TB, but it did wonders for her dignity. She felt good about giving something in return.)

About 4 years have passed since these last incidents. Chelo and his wife are now somewhat healthier, but are still so poor that life is a struggle.

Then, about a year ago, a new problem arose. The landholder for whom Chelo had worked before he became ill decided to take away the small plot of land where Chelo grew his vegetables. When the land had been a useless weed patch and garbage dump, Chelo had been granted the rights to it by the village authorities. Now that the parcel had been developed into a fertile and irrigated vegetable plot, the landholder wanted it for himself. He applied to the village authorities, who wrote a document granting the rights to him. Of course, this was unlawful because the rights had already been given to Chelo.

Chelo took the matter over the heads of the village authorities to the Municipal Presidency, located in a neighboring town. He did not manage to see the President, but the President's spokesman told Chelo, in no uncertain terms, that he should stop trying to cause trouble. Chelo returned to his village in despair.

Chelo would have lost his land, which was his one means of survival, if the village health team had not then taken action. The health workers had struggled too many times—often at the cost of their own earnings—to pull Chelo through and keep him alive. They knew what the loss of his land would mean to him.

At an all-village meeting, the health workers explained to the people about the threat to Chelo's land, and what losing it would mean to his health. They produced proof that the town authorities had given the land rights to Chelo first, and they asked for justice. Although the poor farm people usually remain silent in village meetings, and never vote against the wishes of the village authorities, this time they spoke up and decided in Chelo's favor.

The village authorities were furious, and so was the landholder.

The health team had taken what could be called political action. But the health workers did not think of themselves as 'political'. Nor did they consider themselves capitalists, communists, or even socialists. (Such terms have little meaning for them.) They simply thought of themselves as village health workers—but in the larger sense. They saw the health, and indeed the life, of a helpless person threatened by the unfairness of those in positions of power. And they had the courage to speak out, to take action in his defense.

Through this and many similar experiences, the village health team has come to realize that the health of the poor often depends on questions of social justice. They have found that the changes that are most needed are not likely to come from those who hold more than their share of land, wealth, or authority. Instead, they will come through cooperative effort by those who earn their bread by the sweat of their brows. From themselves!

More and more, the village team in Ajoya has looked for ways to get their fellow villagers thinking and talking about their situation, and taking group action to deal with some of the underlying causes of poor health.

Some of the methods they have developed and community actions they have led are described in several parts of this book. For example, three of the village theater skits described in Chapter 27 show ways in which the health team has helped the poor look at their needs and organize to meet them.

These 3 skits are:

SMALL FARMERS JOIN TOGETHER TO OVERCOME EXPLOITATION (page **27**-27),

USELESS MEDICINES THAT SOMETIMES KILL (page **27**-14), and

THE WOMEN JOIN TOGETHER TO OVERCOME DRUNKENNESS (page **27**-19).

These popular theater skits had, and are still having, a marked social influence. Villagers participate with new pride in the cooperative maize bank set up to overcome high interest on loans. Women have organized to prevent the opening of a public bar. And storekeepers no longer carry some of the expensive and dangerous medicines that they sold before. In general, people seem more alert about things they had simply accepted.

On the other hand, new difficulties have arisen. Some of the health workers have been thrown out of their rented homes. Others have been arrested on false charges. Threats have been made to close down the villager-run program.

But in spite of the obstacles, the health team and the people have stood their ground. The village team knows the road ahead will not be easy. They also know that they must be careful and alert. Yet they have chosen to stand by their people, by the poor and the powerless.

They have had the courage to look the whole problem in the eye—and to look for a whole answer.

The story of Chelo and his family is true, though I have not told the half of it. It is typical, in some ways, of most poor families. Persons in several parts of the world who are poor or know the poor, on reading Chelo's story have commented, "It could have been written here!"

I have told you Chelo's story so that you might understand the events that have moved us to include in this book ideas and methods that might be called 'political'.

What I have tried to say here has been said even better by a group of peasant school boys from Barbiana, Italy. These boys were flunked out of public school and were helped, by a remarkable priest, to learn how to teach each other.*

The Italian peasant boys write:

Whoever is fond of the comfortable and the fortunate stays out of politics. He does not want anything to change.

But these school boys also realize that:

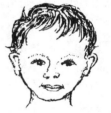

To get to know the children of the poor and to love politics are one and the same thing. You cannot love human beings who were marked by unjust laws and not work for other laws.

Letter to a Teacher,* by the school boys of Barbiana. For more ideas of these school boys, see p. **16-16.

PART ONE

APPROACHES AND PLANS

In **Part One** of this book, we look at approaches to planning and carrying out a training program for community health workers.

But before getting into different aspects of planning, in **Chapter 1** we explore alternative approaches to learning and teaching. We do this because the educational methods instructors decide to use will in part determine how the training course is designed and who takes part in the planning. In health education, the methods are as important as the message.

Chapter 2 is about the selection of both health workers and instructors. We consider the reasons why persons selected from and by their own communities usually make the best leaders for change. We also discuss why experienced village health workers often make the best instructors of new health workers.

In **Chapter 3,** we consider steps in planning a training course, and in **Chapter 4,** how to get the course off to a good start.

Chapters 5, 6, 7, and 8 explore activities in the 3 main places of learning in a training course: the classroom (Chapter 5), the community (Chapters 6 and 7), and the clinic or health center (Chapter 8). We point out that in each of these places, the classroom included, the most effective form of learning is through actual practice in solving common problems.

Chapter 9 discusses ways of finding out how well people are teaching, learning, and meeting local needs. Here we look for ways in which tests, exams, and evaluation can be organized to strengthen the position of the weak and help everyone reach a better understanding of the training program as a whole.

In **Chapter 10,** we consider what happens after the initial training course is completed and health workers are back in their own communities. This includes supportive follow-up and continued opportunities to learn.

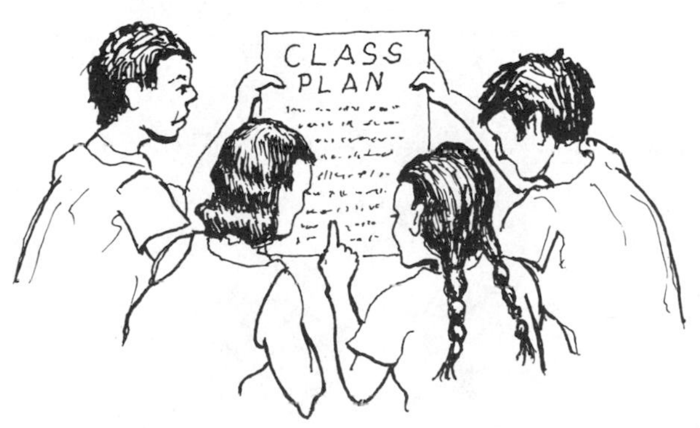

Chapter 2 [illegible] [illegible] We also discuss [illegible] [illegible] best [illegible]

Chapters 5, 6, 7, and 8 [illegible] activities in the [illegible] (Chapter [illegible]) [illegible] (Chapter [illegible]) [illegible] (Chapter 8), we point out that [illegible] [illegible] included, but most [illegible] [illegible] [illegible]

Chapter 9 [illegible] [illegible] [illegible]

CHAPTER 1

Looking at Learning and Teaching

A health worker's most important job is to teach—to encourage sharing of knowledge, skills, experiences, and ideas. The health worker's activities as an 'educator' can have a more far-reaching effect than all his or her preventive and curative activities combined.

But depending on how it is approached, and by whom, health education can have either a beneficial or harmful effect on people's well-being. It can help increase people's ability and confidence to solve their own problems. Or, in some ways, it can do just the opposite.

Consider, for example, a village health worker who calls together a group of mothers and gives them a 'health talk' like this:

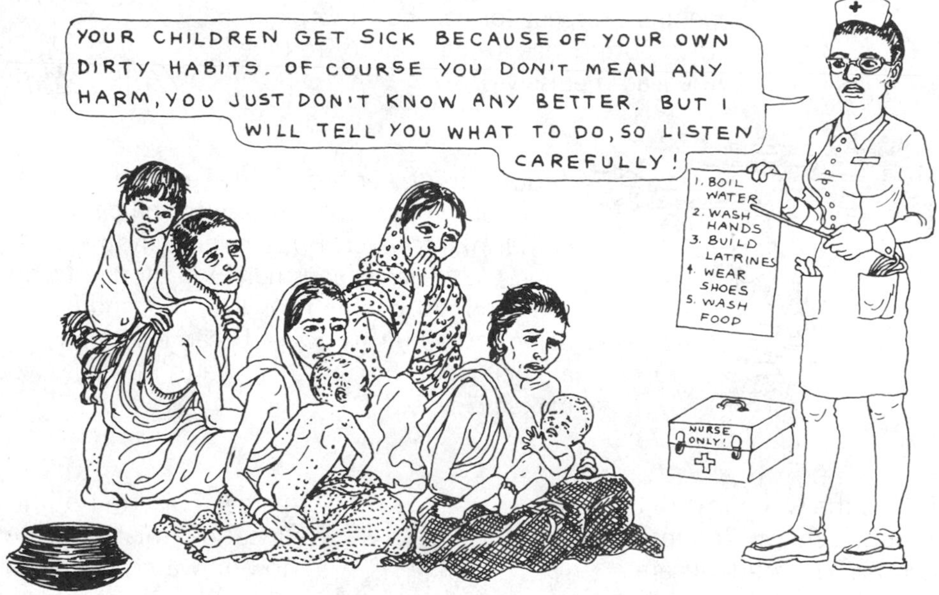
YOUR CHILDREN GET SICK BECAUSE OF YOUR OWN DIRTY HABITS. OF COURSE YOU DON'T MEAN ANY HARM, YOU JUST DON'T KNOW ANY BETTER. BUT I WILL TELL YOU WHAT TO DO, SO LISTEN CAREFULLY!
1. BOIL WATER
2. WASH HANDS
3. BUILD LATRINES
4. WEAR SHOES
5. WASH FOOD
NURSE ONLY!

What effect does this kind of teaching have on people?

You can discuss this question with your fellow instructors or with the health workers you are training. Or health workers can discuss it with people in their villages. You (or the learning group) may come up with answers something like these:

"It's the same old message everybody's heard a hundred times! But what good does it do?"

"It goes in one ear and out the other!"

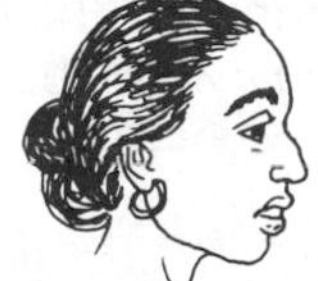

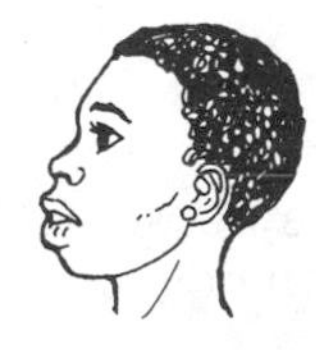

"The mothers just sit and listen. They don't take part."

The more deeply your group explores this example of 'health education', the clearer the picture will become. Encourage the group to notice ways in which this kind of teaching affects how people view themselves, their abilities, and their needs. Persons may observe that:

"That kind of teaching makes the mothers feel ashamed and useless—as if their own carelessness and backwardness were to blame for their children's ill health."

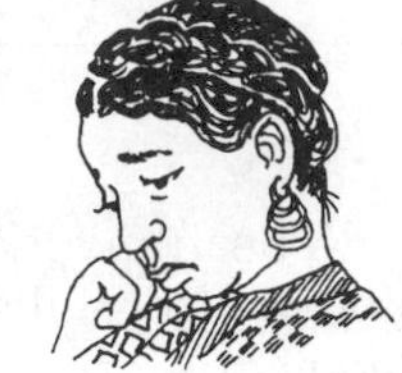

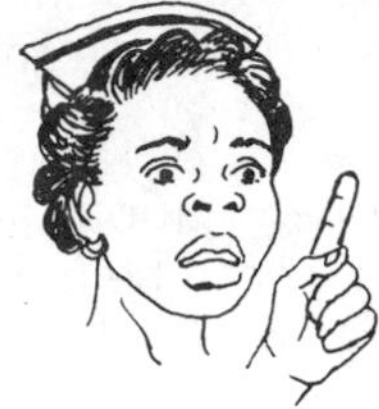

"The health worker acts like she is God Almighty! She thinks she knows it all and the mothers know nothing!"

"Her uniform separates her from the mothers and makes her seem superior. It gives her outside authority. This may strengthen people's respect for her, but it weakens their confidence in their ability to take the lead themselves."

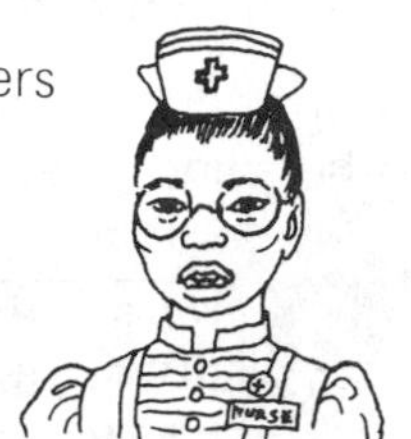

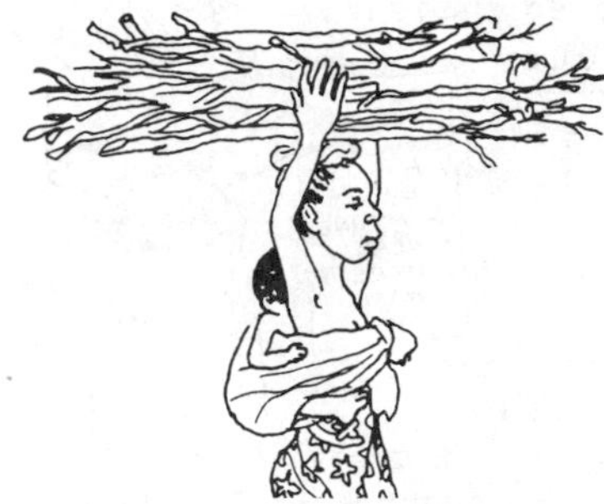

"I don't think her health advice is realistic. Not for the poor in our area! It's easy to tell people to boil drinking water. But what if a mother with hungry children spends her food money to buy firewood? Also, where we live, the land is already being turned into a desert because so many trees are being cut. For us, this 'health message' would make no sense."*

"This is the way most of us were taught in school. The teacher is the boss. The students are considered to 'know nothing'. They are expected simply to repeat what they're told. But isn't this just another way of keeping the poor on the bottom?"

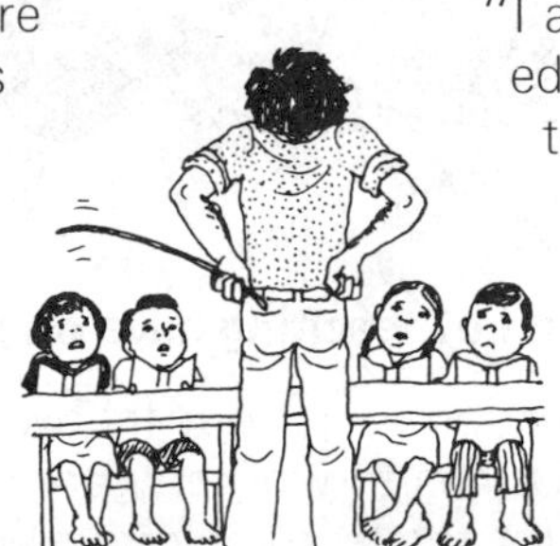

"I agree! This kind of 'health education' might get mothers to boil water, wash their hands, and use latrines. But in the long run **it may do more to prevent than to promote the changes we need for lasting improvements in our health."**

The instructors, health workers, or villagers who discuss this question may arrive at answers similar to or very different from those suggested above. Their responses will depend, in part, on the local situation. But in part they will depend on how carefully the group ***looks at, thinks about,*** and ***'analyzes'*** the issues involved.

---

*For more discussion about boiling drinking water, see p. **15**-3.

Now consider another example. Here, a health worker gets together with a group of mothers and discusses their problems with them. She starts by asking questions like these:

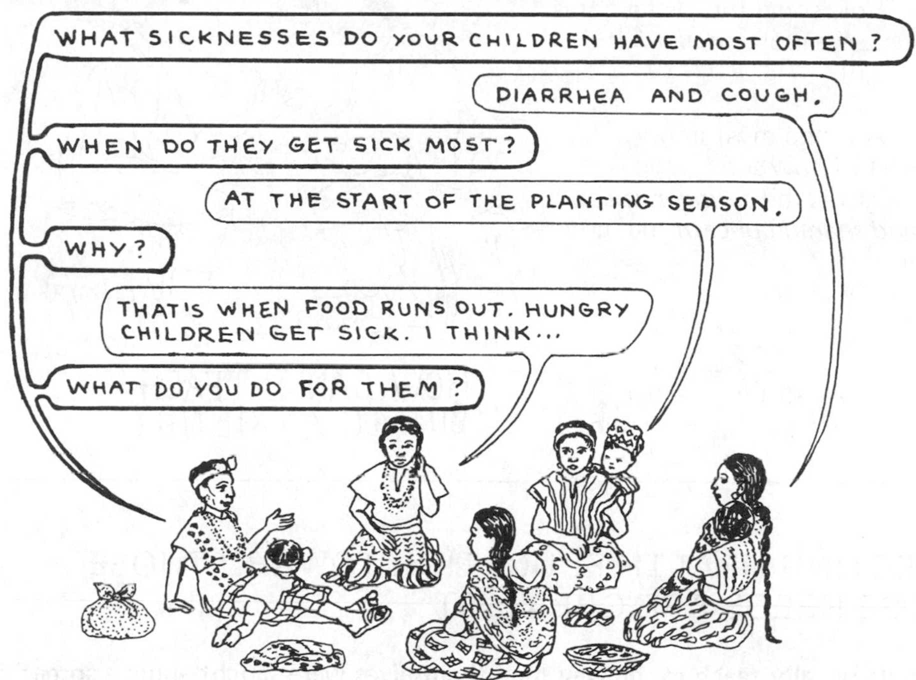

WHAT SICKNESSES DO YOUR CHILDREN HAVE MOST OFTEN ?
DIARRHEA AND COUGH.
WHEN DO THEY GET SICK MOST ?
AT THE START OF THE PLANTING SEASON.
WHY ?
THAT'S WHEN FOOD RUNS OUT. HUNGRY CHILDREN GET SICK. I THINK...
WHAT DO YOU DO FOR THEM ?

What effect does this kind of teaching have on people? In discussing this question with your group, you may hear answers like these:

"Everybody takes part. It gets the group of mothers thinking and talking about their own problems."

"The health worker doesn't just tell them the answers. Everyone looks for answers together."

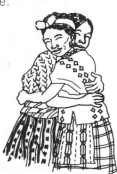

"The health worker dresses like the other mothers and puts herself on their level. She is their friend, not their 'master'. It makes everyone feel equal."

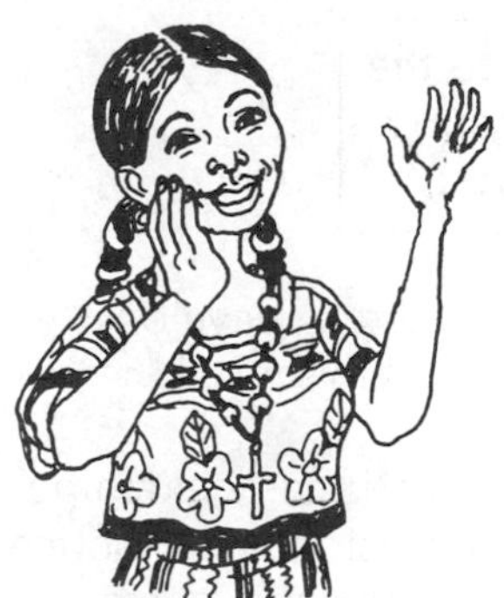

"This sort of teaching certainly isn't like what we got in school! It lets people feel their ideas are worth something. It helps people figure out their problems and work toward solving them themselves."

"I'll bet the mothers will want to keep working and learning together, because they are respected as thoughtful, capable human beings. It makes learning fun!"

Once again, when you discuss this teaching example with fellow instructors, health workers, or villagers, their answers may be very different from the ones shown here—or from your own. But if the group discusses the issues in depth, relating them to their own concerns and experiences, they will make many valuable observations. You will all learn from each other.

How something is taught is just as important as *what* is taught.

And the most important part of *how* something is taught is the *caring, respect, and shared concern* that go into it.

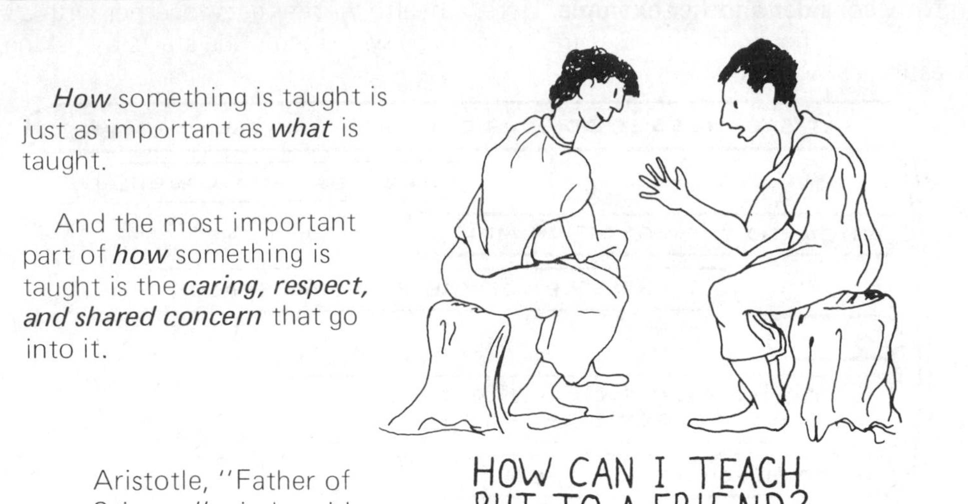
HOW CAN I TEACH
BUT TO A FRIEND?

Aristotle, "Father of Science," wisely said . . .

DIRECTING HEALTH EDUCATION TOWARD THOSE WHOSE NEEDS ARE GREATEST

People usually teach in the way they themselves were taught—unless something either alarming or loving happens to change the way they view things and do things. This is true for health workers. And it is true for those of us who are instructors of health workers. Most of us teach as we were taught in school.

Unfortunately, the purposes and methods of public schools are not always in the best interests of those whose needs are greatest. As we shall discuss, schools tend to reward the stronger students and leave the weak behind.

But the aim of 'people-centered' learning is just the opposite. It is to help those who are weakest become stronger and more self-reliant.

Community health education is appropriate to the extent that it helps the poor and powerless gain greater control over their health and their lives.

To become effective community educators, health workers need to develop approaches very different from what most of us have experienced in school.

For this to happen, it is essential that student health workers critically examine different ways of teaching during their training. They need to develop and practice teaching methods that can help ordinary working people to gain the awareness and courage needed to improve their situation.

In this chapter, we will look at the educational roles of both health workers and their teachers. Then we will consider some ways of helping health workers explore alternative approaches for teaching and learning with people.

THE TEACHING ROLE OF HEALTH WORKERS

Early during training, be sure to **have health workers think about the range of opportunities they will have for sharing and exchanging ideas in their communities.** After discussing the many possibilities, they might post them on a wall as a reminder:

OPPORTUNITIES FOR SHARING AND EXCHANGING IDEAS WITH PEOPLE IN OUR VILLAGES

We health workers can look for ways to . . .

Help families of sick persons find ways to care for them better and to prevent similar sickness in the future.

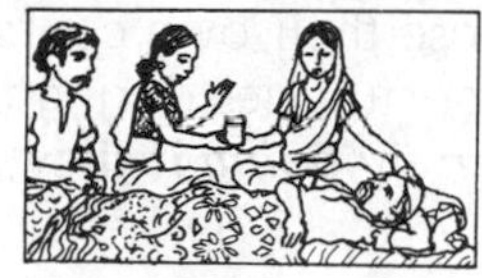

Help organize village meetings to discuss local problems. Encourage others to become 'health leaders'.

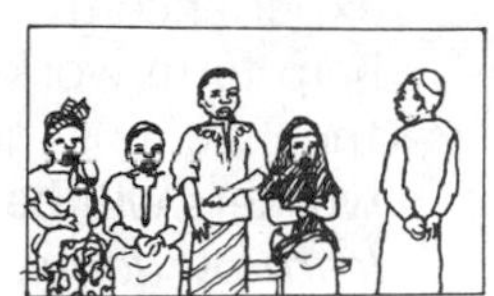

Help mothers find ways to protect their own health and that of their children.

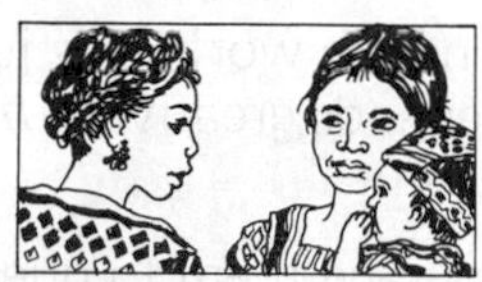

Exchange ideas and information with local midwives, bone setters, and traditional healers.

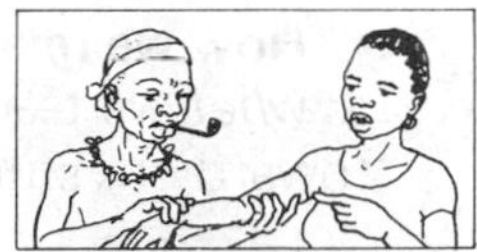

Interest school children (and those who do not go to school) in learning to meet the health needs of their younger brothers and sisters.

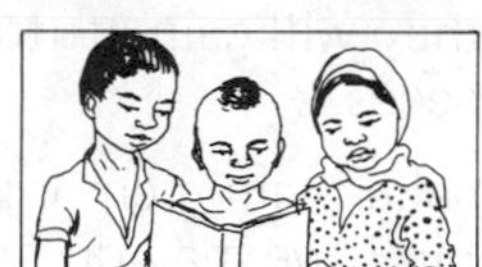

Talk with youth groups and farmers about possible ways to improve their crops or to defend their land and rights.

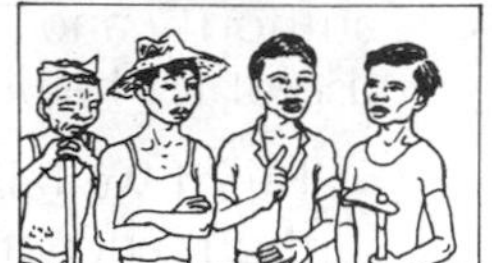

This list is only a beginning. Your group may think of many other possibilities.

Also, try to get the group thinking about the different ways people learn. In their village, there may be many people who have never gone to school. They may not be used to classes, lectures, or 'health talks'. Traditionally, people learn from stories and play, by watching, copying, and helping others work, and through practical experience. **Ask your students what are the customary ways of learning in their villages.**

Encourage your students to think of ways that they might adapt health education to people's local forms of learning. Here are some possibilities, which we discuss in the chapters indicated.

- story telling, Ch. 13
- songs, p. **1**-26 and **15**-15
- play (learning games), Ch. 11, 19, and 24
- make-believe (learning by imitating), Ch. 24
- role playing (acting out problems and situations), Ch. 14
- popular theater and puppet shows, Ch. 27
- apprenticeship (learning by helping someone more skilled), Ch. 8
- practical experience, Ch. 6 and 8
- small group discussions, Ch. 4 and 26
- solving real problems, Ch. 8, 10, 14, 17, 25, 26, and 27
- trial and error (finding things out for oneself), Ch. 11, 17, and 24
- building on the knowledge, skills, customs, and experience that people already have, Ch. 7 and 13

We health workers need to adapt our teaching to people's traditional ways of learning—ways they are already used to and enjoy.

THE ROLE OF HEALTH WORKER INSTRUCTORS

It is not enough to explain to health workers about 'people-centered' education. We teachers must set an example. This means we must carefully and frequently examine our own teaching habits, in terms of both **the methods we use** and **the way we relate to our students.**

- **The methods we use.** If we would like health workers to use stories when teaching village mothers, then we, too, need to use stories for helping health workers learn. If we would like them to help children learn through puppet shows, games, and discovering things for themselves, we must let them experience the excitement of learning in these ways. If health workers are to help farm workers discuss problems and choose their own courses of action, then we must give health workers similar opportunities during training. **Health workers will be more able to help others *learn by doing* if they, themselves,** *learn by doing.*

- **How we relate.** *How* we instructors teach health workers is just as important as ***what*** we teach them. But ***how we teach*** depends greatly on ***how we feel*** toward our students.

  If we respect our students' ideas, and encourage them to question our authority and to think for themselves, then they will gain attitudes and skills useful for helping people meet their biggest needs.

  But if we fail to respect our students, or make them memorize lessons without encouraging them to question and think, we may do more harm than good. Our experience has shown us that health workers trained in this way make poor teachers and bossy leaders. Rather than helping people gain the understanding and confidence to change their situation, they can even stand in the way.

To set a good example for health workers, we instructors need to:

- Treat the health workers as our equals—and as friends.
- Respect their ideas and build on their experiences.
- Invite cooperation; encourage helping those who are behind.
- Make it clear that we do not have all the answers.
- Welcome criticism, questioning, initiative, and trust.
- Live and dress modestly; accept only modest pay.
- Defend the interests of those in greatest need.
- Live and work in the community. Learn together with the people, and share their dreams.

These ideas are beautifully expressed in this old Chinese verse:

Go in search of Your People:
Love Them;
Learn from Them;
Plan with Them;
Serve Them;
Begin with what They have;
Build on what They know.

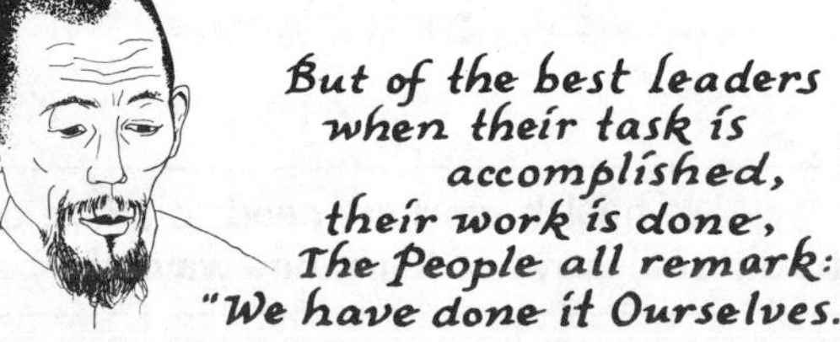

But of the best leaders
when their task is
accomplished,
their work is done,
The People all remark:
"We have done it Ourselves."

The rest of this chapter concerns methods for helping people look at the strengths and weaknesses of different educational approaches, **especially as they affect the lives and well-being of the poor.** We try to do this by using the same methods we recommend. We include examples of stories, role plays, and discussions that various groups have found useful in health worker training.

We ask you to use these materials not as they are, but as sparks for ideas. Think about them. Criticize them. Tear them to pieces. If you find any parts useful, adapt them to fit the people and needs in your own area.

We encourage you to tear our ideas to pieces. Save only what you can use or adapt to your area.

BEGINNING WITH YOUR OWN TRUE STORY

Helping people begin to look at things in new ways is a teacher's chief job. This is easier if we **look at ideas, not in terms of general theories, but through real-life examples.** It is better still when the examples come from the lives and experiences of the learning group.

As the instructor, why not start by setting the example? Tell a story from your own experience, one that brings out certain points or problems that need to be considered. The group can then discuss the story, adding to it from their own ideas and experiences.

Stories can bring learning closer to life—
especially true stories told from personal experience.

It is important that, as group leader, you 'expose' yourself by telling personal experiences that matter deeply, or that somehow changed the way you look at things. This will help others to open up and speak of things that really matter to them.

The following story is both true and personal. We have used it to start groups of health workers and instructors thinking about some of the human factors related to teaching and learning. But we do not provide any follow-up discussion here. We leave that up to you and your group.

You can try using this story 'as is' with your students and your group. Or even better, tell a story from your own experience. Let your students know you as a person!

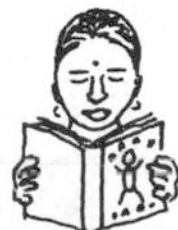
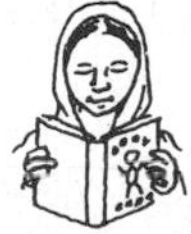

A suggestion for reading stories:
If a story like that which follows is read in a group, take turns reading. Let each person read a paragraph.

A true story: THE IMPORTANCE OF NOT KNOWING IT ALL

A teacher of village health workers who had a college degree was working as a volunteer in the mountains of western Mexico. One day he arrived at a small village on muleback. A father approached him and asked if he could heal his son. The health worker followed the father to his hut.

The boy, whose name was Pepe, was sitting on the floor. His legs were crippled by polio ***(infantile paralysis).*** The disease had struck him as a baby. Now he was 13 years old. Pepe smiled and reached up a friendly hand.

The health worker examined the boy. "Have you ever tried to walk with crutches?" he asked. Pepe shook his head.

"We live so far away from the city," his father explained apologetically.

"Then why don't we try to make some crutches?" asked the health worker.

The next morning the health worker got up at dawn. He borrowed a ***machete*** (long curved knife) and went into the forest. He hunted until he found two forked branches.

He took the branches back to the home of the crippled boy and began to make them into crutches, like this. ⟶

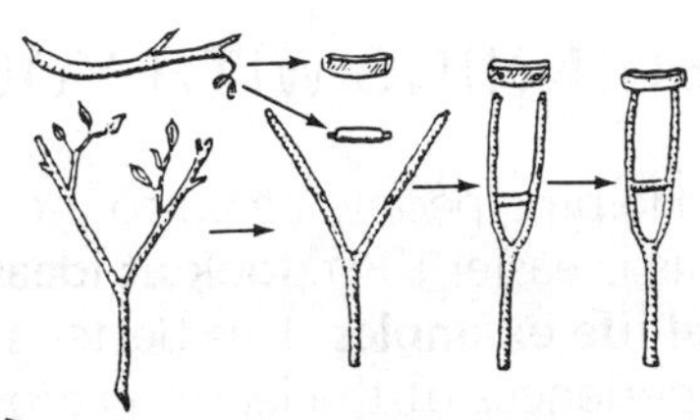

The father came up and the health worker showed him the crutches he was making. The father examined them for a moment and said, "They won't work!"

The health worker frowned. "Wait and see!" he said.

When both crutches were finished, they showed them to Pepe, who was eager to try them out. His father lifted him into a standing position and the health worker placed the crutches under the boy's arms.

But as soon as Pepe tried to put his weight on the crutches, they doubled and broke.

"I tried to tell you they wouldn't work," said the father. "It's the wrong kind of tree. Wood's weak as water! But now I see what you have in mind. I'll go cut some branches of ***jutamo.*** Wood's tough as iron, but light! Don't want the crutches to be too heavy."

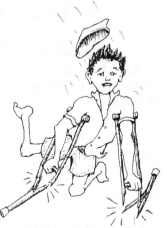

He took the ***machete*** and trotted into the forest. Fifteen minutes later he was back with two forked sticks of ***jutamo.*** At once he set about making the crutches, his strong hands working rapidly. The health worker and Pepe assisted him.

When the new crutches were finished, Pepe's father tested them by putting his full weight on them. They held him easily, yet were lightweight. Next the boy tried them. He had trouble balancing at first, but soon was able to hold himself upright. By afternoon, he was actually walking with the crutches. But they rubbed him under the arms.

"I have an idea," said Pepe's father. He went across the clearing to a ***pochote,*** or wild kapok tree, and picked several of the large, ripe fruits. He gathered the downy cotton from the pods, and put a soft cushion of kapok onto the top crosspiece of each crutch. Then he wrapped the kapok in place with strips of cloth. Pepe tried the crutches again and found them comfortable.

"Gosh, Dad, you really fixed them great!" cried the boy, smiling at his father with pride. "Look how well I can walk now!" He bounded about the dusty patio on his new crutches.

"I'm proud of you, son!" said his father, smiling too.

As the health worker was saddling his mule to leave, the whole family came to say good-bye.

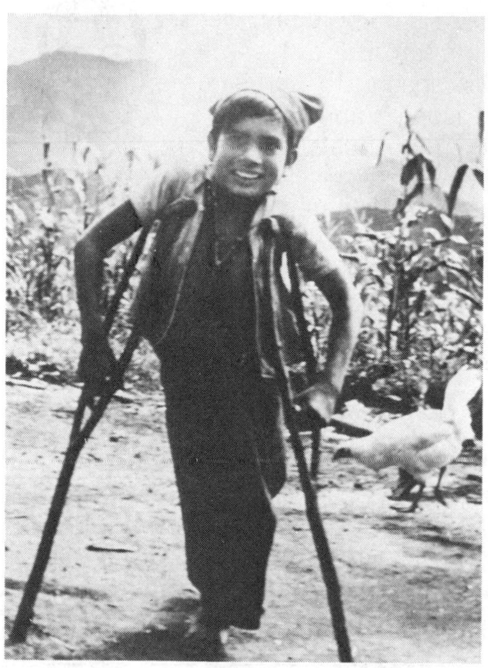

"I can't thank you enough," said the father. "It's so wonderful to see my son able to walk upright. I don't know why I never thought of making crutches before . . ."

"It's I who must thank you," said the health worker. "You have taught me a great deal."

As the health worker rode down the trail he smiled to himself. "How foolish of me," he thought, "not to have asked the father's advice in the first place. He knows the trees better than I do. And he is a better craftsman.

"But how fortunate it is that the crutches that I made broke. The idea for making the crutches was mine, and the father felt bad for not having thought of it himself. When my crutches broke, he made much better ones. That made us equal again!"

So the health worker learned many things from the father of the crippled boy—things that he had never learned in college. He learned what kind of wood is best for making crutches. But he also learned how important it is to use the skills and knowledge of the local people—important because a better job can be done, and because it helps maintain people's dignity. People feel more equal when each learns from the other.

It was a lesson the health worker will always remember. I know. I was the health worker.

David Werner

IDEAS FOR A DISCUSSION ABOUT SHARING AND SELF-RELIANCE

People's health depends on many things—on food, on water, on cleanliness, on safety. But above all, it depends on sharing—on letting everyone have a fair share of land, opportunity, resources—and knowledge.

Unfortunately, many doctors (and many traditional healers) tend to carefully guard their knowledge rather than to share it openly. Too often they use their special knowledge to gain power or privilege, or to charge more for their services than is fair.

Health workers can easily fall into these same unhealthy habits. So their training must help them guard against this. It should help them realize that to share their knowledge and skills freely is important to people's health. Sharing of knowledge helps people become more self-reliant.

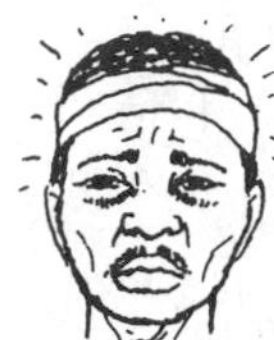

Self-reliance as a measure of health: A person who is very sick needs to be cared for completely. He can do almost nothing for himself. But as his health improves, so does his capacity for self-care. Health is closely related to people's ability to care for themselves and each other—as equals.

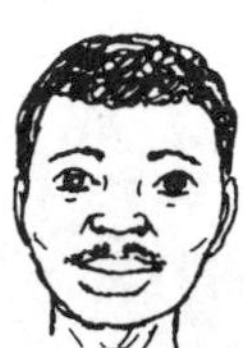

These may be important ideas. But at present they are just ***our*** ideas. How is it possible to get a group of health workers thinking about and reacting to ideas like these? And forming their own ideas? Lecturing will do little good. A better way is to help people discover things through thoughtful discussion.

To start, you might find it helpful to ask questions like these:

- How are persons who are sick different from persons who are healthy?
- Which are better able to care for themselves? Who needs to be taken care of?
- Who have more health problems, the rich or the poor? Why?
- What do health and well-being have to do with self-reliance? Of a person? Of a family? Of a village or community? Of a nation?
- Can you give examples from your own experience?

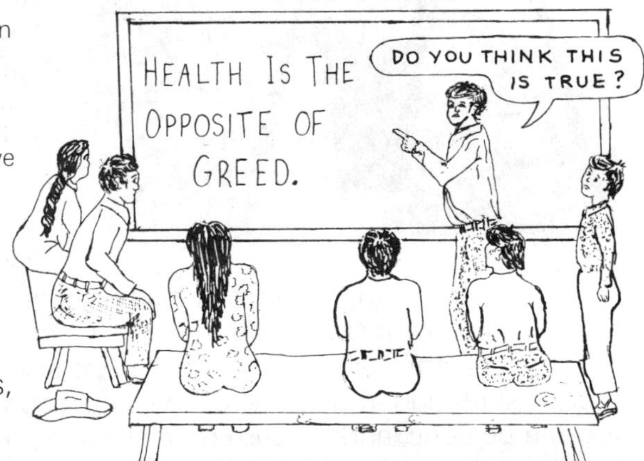
HEALTH IS THE OPPOSITE OF GREED.
DO YOU THINK THIS IS TRUE?

STARTING A DISCUSSION

After discussing these questions, you might ask:

- What should be the main goal of health education?
- What should be your responsibilities as a health worker?

Guide the students in discussing these things, but let them come up with their own answers.

A PUZZLE TO GET PEOPLE THINKING IN NEW WAYS

All of us, teachers and students alike, get into 'ruts'. And like horses with blinders, we often tend to look at things from a narrow point of view. We keep on trying to solve problems in the same old way.

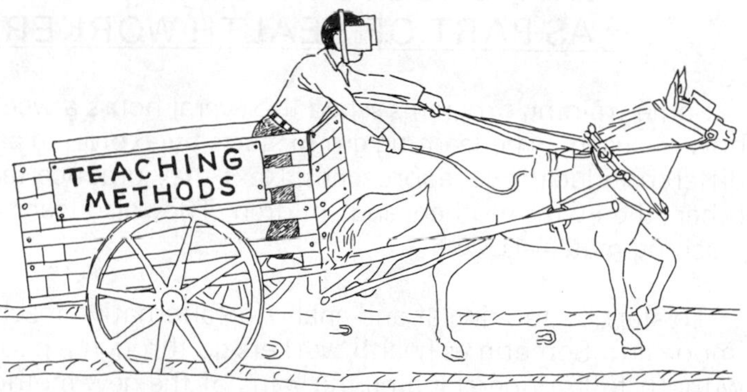

New approaches to health care require new approaches to teaching and learning. This means tearing off the conventional 'blinders' that limit our vision and imagination. It means going beyond the walls of the standard classroom and exploring afresh the world in which we live and learn.

A number of 'tricks' or puzzles can be used to help planners, instructors, or students realize the importance of looking at things in new ways—of going beyond the limits their own minds have set. Here is an example:

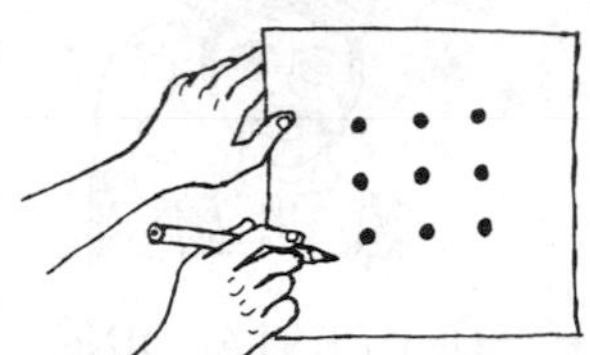

Draw 9 dots on a paper, on the blackboard, or in the dust, like this:

Ask everyone to try to figure out a way to connect all the dots with 4 straight lines joined together (drawn without lifting the pencil from the paper).

You will find that most persons will try to draw lines that do not go outside the imaginary square or 'box' formed by the dots.

no

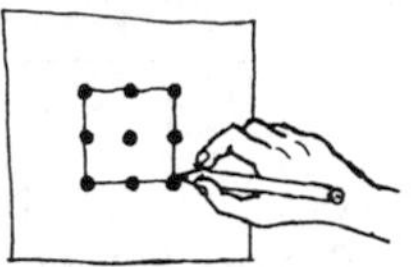

Some may even conclude that it is impossible to join all the dots with only 4 lines. You can give them a clue by saying that, **to solve the puzzle, they must go beyond the limits they set for themselves.**

no

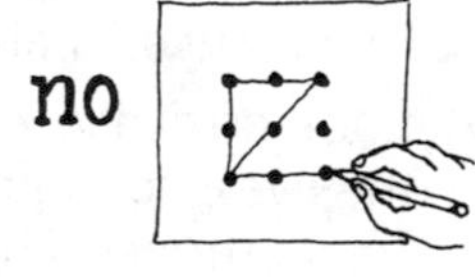

At last, someone will probably figure out how to do it. The lines must extend beyond the 'box' formed by the dots. (Be careful not to shame the students or make them feel stupid if they cannot solve the puzzle. Explain that many doctors and professors also have trouble with it.)

yes!

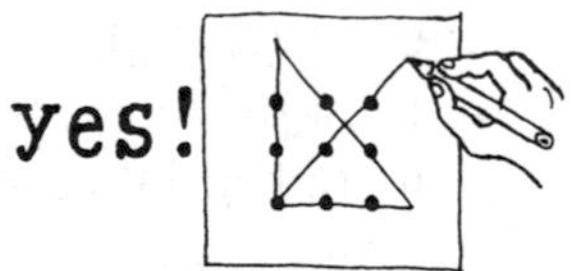

After the group has seen how to solve the puzzle, ask some questions that help them consider its larger significance. You might begin with questions like these:

- In what way is a classroom like the box formed by the dots?
- How does the idea that 'education belongs in a classroom' affect the way we look at learning? At health? At each other?

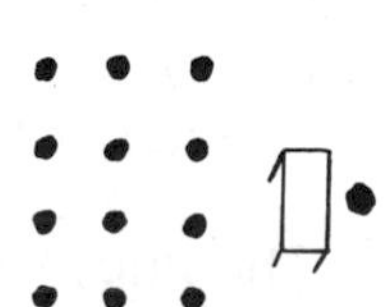

And end with questions like these:

- What can we do to help each other climb out of the mental 'boxes' or 'ruts' that confine our thinking, so we can explore new ways with open minds? Is this important to people's health? How so?

'CRITICAL STUDY OF TEACHING METHODS' AS PART OF HEALTH WORKER TRAINING

Some training programs schedule several hours a week for the study of 'learning how to teach'. The learning group starts by exploring and critically analyzing different educational approaches. Next they practice teaching—first with each other, then with mothers and children. They also learn to develop their own teaching materials.

To start by looking at and analyzing alternative teaching methods is especially important. Sometimes health workers go through a people-centered course without fully understanding the value of the new methods used. They may not realize that **the way they teach can either break down or build up people's self-confidence and community strength.** Without such understanding, they may later slip back into the more conventional 'teacher as boss' style of teaching. We have often seen this happen.

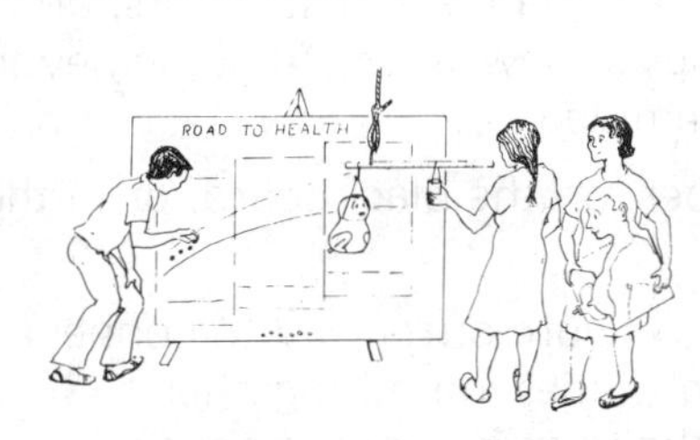

PRACTICE

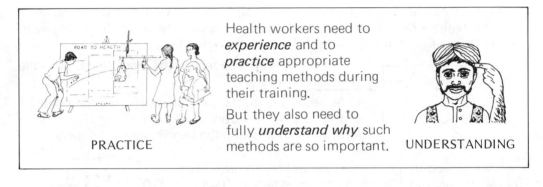

Health workers need to *experience* and to *practice* appropriate teaching methods during their training.

But they also need to fully *understand why* such methods are so important.

UNDERSTANDING

To assist health workers in developing this understanding, be sure to **allow time for the critical study of alternative approaches to learning.** Help the group to:

- Experience, analyze, and compare contrasting educational methods.
- Look critically at the existing school system in your area and how it affects the lives, economy, social position, and health of the poor. Discuss how conventional schooling influences the values and job performance of health officers, civil servants, teachers, and others.
- Look for ways that they (the health workers) can begin to change unfair or inappropriate social structures, especially the school system. This would mean to . . .
- Explore possibilities of working with school children, non-school children, and teachers in ways that relate learning to the lives and needs of the children. (See Chapter 24.)
- Try using more appropriate, friendlier teaching methods. And help others discover for themselves the value and excitement of people-centered learning.

The study of these issues will, of course, be more effective if you **use the same methods you want your students to learn** (see p. **1**-6). Students can conduct their own investigation of different educational methods. Your role as instructor is to help the learning group ask searching questions, look critically at alternatives, and try out more people-centered teaching methods during training.

IDEAS FOR DISCUSSION ABOUT THE PURPOSE OF SCHOOLING

Whose needs is schooling designed to meet?

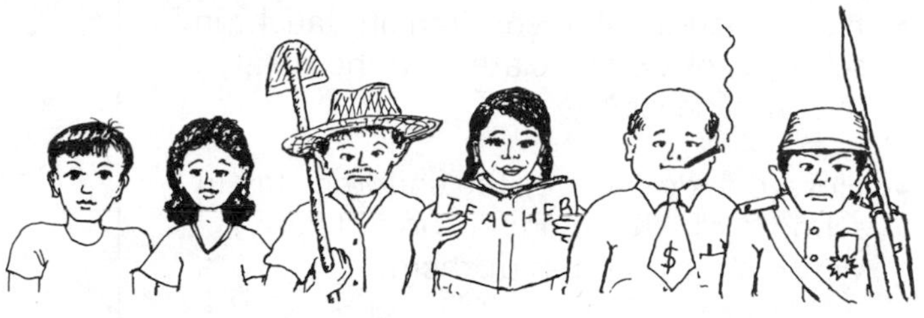

Many educators agree that **the primary purpose of education should be to help persons gain the knowledge, skills, and awareness necessary to meet life's needs.**

But do the schools that most children—or health workers— attend really do this?

To answer this question, you and your group of teachers or health workers may first want to consider carefully: ***What are the biggest problems or needs of most people in your village or community?*** To do this, you probably do not have to conduct a survey or 'community diagnosis'—at least not at first. You may already have a good idea of how most people in your area live, whether they have enough to eat, what they suffer from most, and why.

What is necessary is to openly and honestly **discuss the people's needs, why they exist, and what might be the biggest obstacles to overcoming them.**

If you live in a village or poor community—as do most of the people in the world—your local situation may be something like this:

A TYPICAL VILLAGE (How does it compare with your own?)

PROBLEMS OR NEEDS	CAUSES	OBSTACLES TO IMPROVEMENT
Poor health, unnecessary suffering	**Poverty, too much in the hands of too few**	**Selfishness of some, hopelessness of others**
• many children are thin, small, big bellied, often sick; many die • mothers are often pale, weak, and tired; many die, especially during or after childbirth • many fathers cannot find work, are not paid enough, or do not have enough land to meet the family's needs for food, water, housing, health care, and education; many get drunk or lose hope; violence is the main cause of death in young men (between ages 15 and 40)	• poor food, sweets and 'junk food', poor sanitation, inadequate health care; poor nutrition lowers resistance to infectious disease • large families because of economic necessity (children provide low-cost labor) • most of the land, wealth, and power are in the hands of a few; the rich underpay and exploit the poor • government (local, national, and international) favors the rich	• greed and corruption of those in control • people's lack of self-confidence; no hope that things can be changed *(fatalism)* • lack of organization and effective leadership among the poor • increasing dependency of the poor on outside services, giveaways, resources, entertainment, and authority • inadequate and inappropriate education (for rich and poor alike)

After discussing the needs in your village, ask questions about the local schools and whose needs they are designed to serve.

Examples of questions to get people thinking and talking about the purpose of schooling:

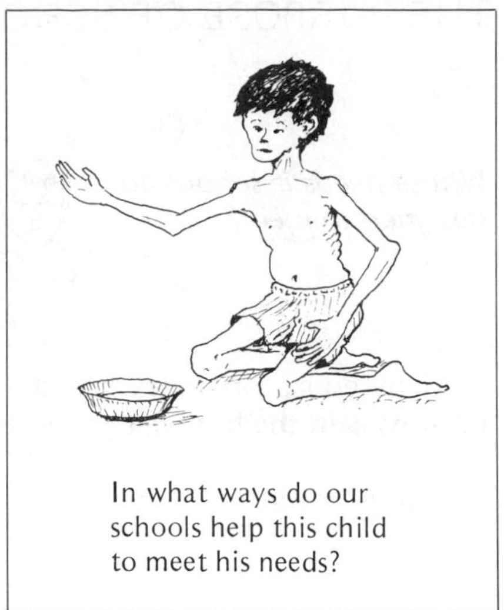

In what ways do our schools help this child to meet his needs?

- How much of what children are taught in school is ***relevant*** (related) to their daily lives and needs?
- How long do most of the children stay in school? Which children drop out early? Why? What becomes of them?
- Which children continue with their schooling? Why? Do they usually return to serve the community? Why or why not?
- In what ways does the teacher set a good example or a bad example for the students? How does he or she relate to them? As a friend? As an equal? As their master?
- Who does the work that makes money available for schooling?
- Who decides what is taught in the schools and how? Should the people in a village or community have some say as to what their children are taught? Should the opinions of the children be listened to?* (See footnote.)
- In what ways do schools shape children's values? How does this affect their families? Their community? The poor?
- Are children taught to question those in positions of authority, or to obey them? Why? How does this affect those who are powerless?
- Whose needs does schooling serve the most, the weak or the strong? In what ways?
- In what ways does schooling benefit or harm people in villages? In slums?
- What changes have been taking place in recent years in the content or approach to schooling? Why? What changes would be needed for the schools to better serve the interests of the poor?

---

*For those who believe that children are too unwise or too inexperienced to make intelligent judgements about their educational needs, we suggest you read ***Letter to a Teacher,*** by the school boys of Barbiana, Italy (see p. **16**-16).

These school boys from poor farming communities make remarkably sound and challenging suggestions for changing the school system to better meet the needs of the poor majority. Recognizing that many children of the poor leave school after only a few years, they insist that, "If schooling has to be so brief, then it should be planned according to the most urgent needs." They question the usefulness of each major subject. They ask, "How much math does one have to know for his immediate needs at home and at work?" History as taught in schools, they insist, is "no history at all," but "one-sided tales passed down to the peasants by the conqueror. There is talk only of kings, generals, and stupid wars among nations. The sufferings and struggles of the workers are either ignored or stuck into a corner."

These boys also criticize the fact that most schools encourage competition among students. It would be better, they say, if schools helped each child to feel that "Others' problems are like mine. To come out of them together is good politics. To come out alone is stinginess."

Schooling as a form of social control

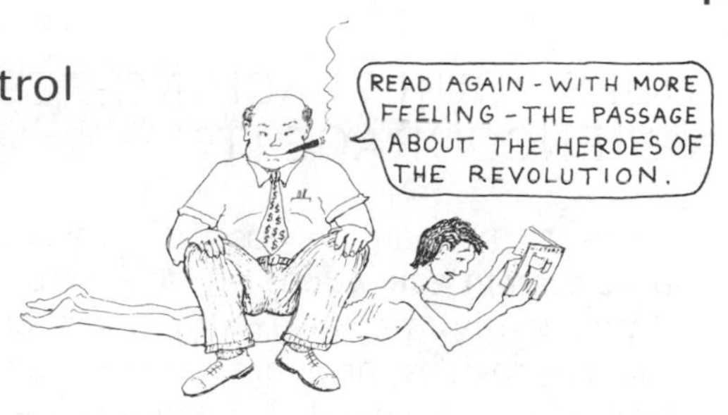
READ AGAIN - WITH MORE FEELING - THE PASSAGE ABOUT THE HEROES OF THE REVOLUTION.

Whose needs does your school system serve?

Government schools tend to serve government purposes. Only to the extent that government is truly by and for the people, is schooling likely to prepare students to work toward meeting the needs of the majority of citizens in effective and lasting ways.

In the world today, most governments do not represent all their people equally. Many governments are controlled by a powerful minority of politicians, businessmen, wealthy landholders, military leaders, and professionals (especially lawyers and doctors). These persons often care more about protecting their own interests than about looking for ways to improve the well-being of the poor majority. When they do consider doing something to help the poor, they are usually careful to do so in ways that do not threaten their own interests and authority.

Schooling, from the viewpoint of those in power, involves a risk. When the poor learn to read and write, they can communicate and organize in new ways, in greater numbers, over larger distances. They can read things that help them discover their legal and human rights. They may ask themselves if it is really 'God's will' that a few persons have far more than they need, while others do not have enough to eat. They may even begin to realize that they can do something to change their situation.

This means that, for the few to keep their control, schools must teach poor people to obey authority as well as to read and write. So most schools teach students to fit into the existing social order rather than to question or try to change it.

How is this done? By putting emphasis on following rules, being on time, and 'behaving'. Students are encouraged to compete more than cooperate, to memorize rather than think. School books paint the present government as completely good and just, with leaders who always have the interests of all the people at heart.

But perhaps the most powerful means the schools have for teaching children to 'listen and obey' are the teaching methods themselves. Students are led to believe that the only way to learn is to be taught—by someone who knows more than they do. The teacher is set up as the 'master', an authority whose statements must not be questioned.

This kind of education is called ***authoritarian,*** because its purpose is to strengthen the authority of those in control. It is education designed to keep things as they are—***education that resists change.***

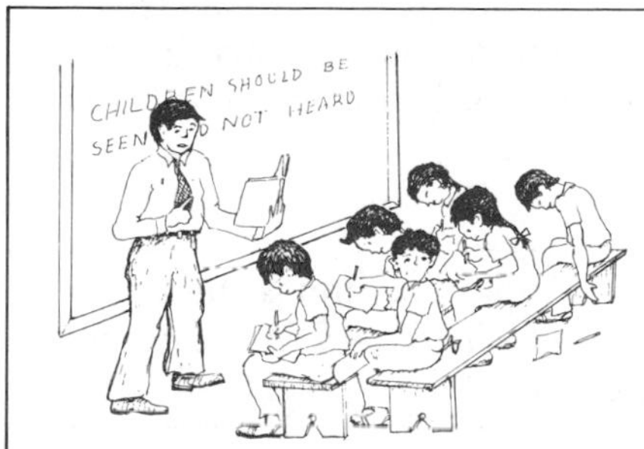
CHILDREN SHOULD BE SEEN AND NOT HEARD

"The lecture method of teaching is the best way to transfer the teacher's notes to the students' notebooks without ever passing through their minds."

DOES YOUR TEACHING RESIST CHANGE, OR ENCOURAGE IT?

One of the main purposes of conventional or ***authoritarian*** education is to teach students to fit obediently into the existing social order. The teacher provides the approved knowledge, and the students receive it. The emptier the student's head to begin with, the better a student he is—according to the teacher and the system.

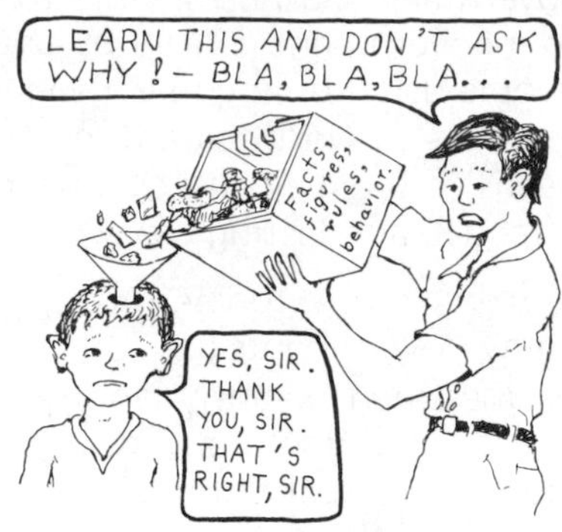
LEARN THIS AND DON'T ASK WHY! – BLA, BLA, BLA. . .
Facts, figures, rules, behavior.
YES, SIR. THANK YOU, SIR. THAT'S RIGHT, SIR.

EDUCATION OF AUTHORITY:
putting ideas in

Unfortunately, many training programs for village or community health workers use this same kind of authoritarian approach. Students are taught to follow, not to explore; to memorize, not to think. They are taught to believe that their first responsibility is to the health system rather than to the poor.

Usually instructors teach this way, not because they mean any harm, but simply because they themselves grew up in an authoritarian school system. They may not know any other way to teach.

EDUCATION THAT ENCOURAGES CHANGE:

But there are other ways—ways that build the students' confidence in their capacity to observe, criticize, analyze, and figure things out for themselves. These ways let the students discover that they are just as good as their teachers and everyone else. They learn to cooperate rather than compete in order to gain approval. They are encouraged to consider the whole social context of their people's needs, and to look for imaginative and courageous ways of meeting them.

> *Teaching suggestion*
>
> *Rather than tell the members of your group these things, help them to recall their own experiences and to figure things out for themselves.*

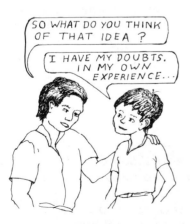

This we will call ***education for change.*** Emphasis is more on learning than on teaching. Students are encouraged to voice their own ideas. They figure things out for themselves, and explore ways to help people free themselves from the causes of poverty and poor health.

If a health worker is to be a 'leader for change', helping people find ways to solve their biggest problems, then it is important that his training itself set an example.

EDUCATION OF CHANGE:
drawing ideas out

> **Good teaching is the art,**
> **not of *PUTTING IDEAS INTO* people's heads,**
> **but of *DRAWING IDEAS OUT.***

ROLE PLAYS THAT HELP PEOPLE EXPLORE TWO KINDS OF TEACHING

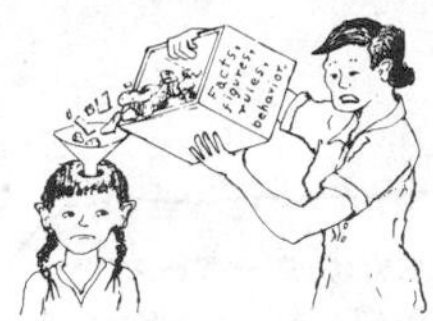
The bossy teacher

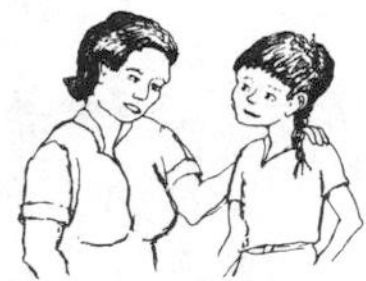
The friendly group leader

For health workers to appreciate the importance of appropriate teaching, it helps if they experience two kinds of teaching and then compare them.

A good way to do this is through 'role playing' (see Chapter 14). Here we give ideas for two role plays to compare the ***bossy teacher*** with the ***good group leader.***

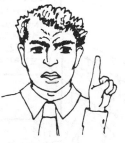

These role plays are most effective if they take the students by surprise. Although the whole class participates, at first students will not realize that the instructor is 'acting'— and that they are actors, too!

In the role plays, the instructor (or two different instructors) will **teach the same health topic in two very different ways.** Then the students compare their reactions to the two lessons. They discuss how each of the classes affects the learners personally, and how each prepares them to meet important needs in their communities.

The two role plays we present here deal with dental care. They have been used effectively in Latin America and Africa. But of course you can choose any health topic you want.

The first role play: THE BOSSY TEACHER in a conventional classroom

Suggestions to the instructor:

- Before the students arrive, put chairs or benches in neat rows, with a desk or podium at the front.
- When the students arrive, greet them stiffly and ask them to sit down. Make sure they are quiet and orderly.
- Begin the lecture exactly on time. Talk rapidly in a dull voice. Walk back and forth behind the desk. If some students come late, scold them! Use big words the students cannot understand. Do not give them a chance to ask questions. (It helps if you prepare in advance a few long, complicated sentences that use difficult medical terminology. Look in a medical dictionary, or copy phrases out of any professional textbook.)
- If any student does not pay attention, or whispers to a neighbor, or begins to go to sleep, ***BANG*** on the table, call the student by his last name, and scold him angrily. Then continue your lecture.
- From time to time, scribble something on the blackboard. Be sure it is difficult to see and understand.
- Act as if you know it all, as if you think the students are stupid, lazy, rude, and worthless. Take both yourself and your teaching very seriously. Permit no laughter or interruptions. But be careful not to exaggerate too much! Try not to let the students know you are acting.

The first role play: THE BOSSY TEACHER

The teacher talks over the heads of the bored and confused students, like this:

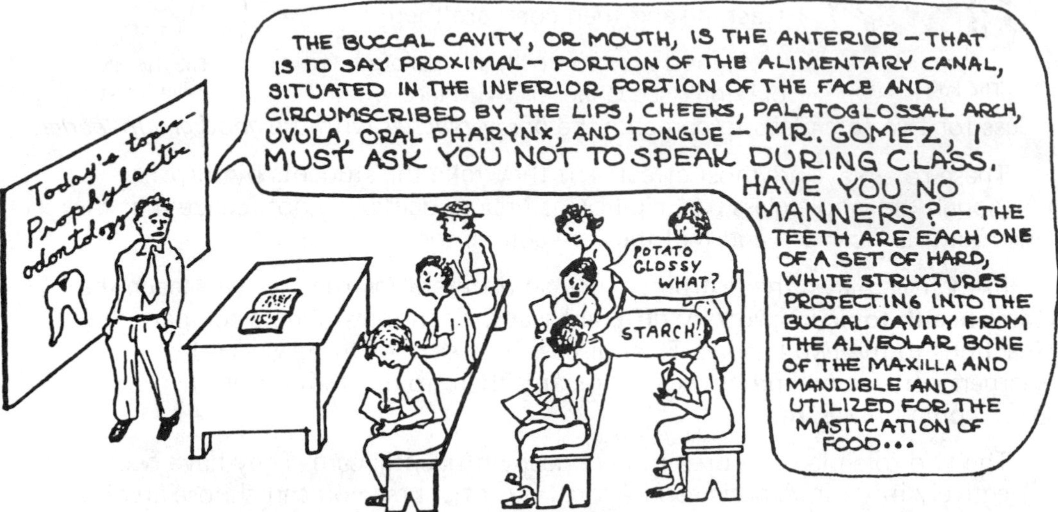
Today's topic - Prophylactic odontology
THE BUCCAL CAVITY, OR MOUTH, IS THE ANTERIOR - THAT IS TO SAY PROXIMAL - PORTION OF THE ALIMENTARY CANAL, SITUATED IN THE INFERIOR PORTION OF THE FACE AND CIRCUMSCRIBED BY THE LIPS, CHEEKS, PALATOGLOSSAL ARCH, UVULA, ORAL PHARYNX, AND TONGUE - MR. GOMEZ, I MUST ASK YOU NOT TO SPEAK DURING CLASS. HAVE YOU NO MANNERS? - THE TEETH ARE EACH ONE OF A SET OF HARD, WHITE STRUCTURES PROJECTING INTO THE BUCCAL CAVITY FROM THE ALVEOLAR BONE OF THE MAXILLA AND MANDIBLE AND UTILIZED FOR THE MASTICATION OF FOOD...
POTATO GLOSSY WHAT?
STARCH!

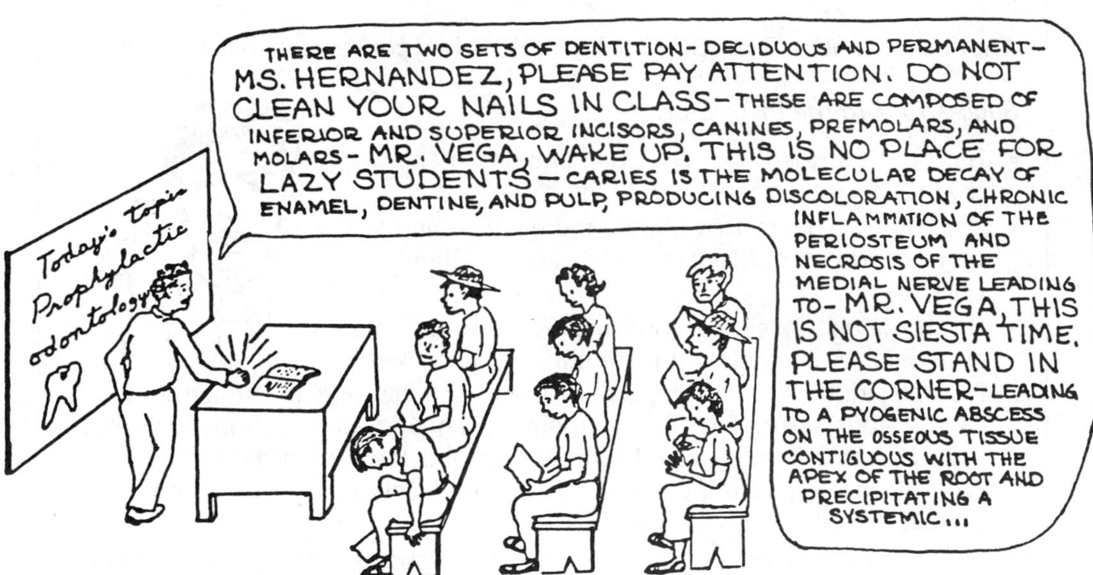
Today's topic Prophylactic odontology
THERE ARE TWO SETS OF DENTITION - DECIDUOUS AND PERMANENT - MS. HERNANDEZ, PLEASE PAY ATTENTION. DO NOT CLEAN YOUR NAILS IN CLASS - THESE ARE COMPOSED OF INFERIOR AND SUPERIOR INCISORS, CANINES, PREMOLARS, AND MOLARS - MR. VEGA, WAKE UP. THIS IS NO PLACE FOR LAZY STUDENTS - CARIES IS THE MOLECULAR DECAY OF ENAMEL, DENTINE, AND PULP, PRODUCING DISCOLORATION, CHRONIC INFLAMMATION OF THE PERIOSTEUM AND NECROSIS OF THE MEDIAL NERVE LEADING TO - MR. VEGA, THIS IS NOT SIESTA TIME. PLEASE STAND IN THE CORNER - LEADING TO A PYOGENIC ABSCESS ON THE OSSEOUS TISSUE CONTIGUOUS WITH THE APEX OF THE ROOT AND PRECIPITATING A SYSTEMIC...

The lecture goes on and on—all very serious. At the end of the class, the teacher may simply walk out. Or he may ask a few questions like, "MR. REYES, WILL YOU GIVE US THE DEFINITION OF CARIES?" And when he gets no answer, scold him by shouting, "SO, YOU WERE SLEEPING, TOO! THIS GROUP HAS THE ATTENTION SPAN OF 5-YEAR-OLDS!" And so on.

The second role play: THE GOOD GROUP LEADER or 'facilitator'

This time, the instructor treats the students in a friendly, relaxed way—as equals. (This role can be played by the same instructor or a different one. Or perhaps a student could prepare for it in advance.)

Suggestions to the group leader:

- At the beginning of class, suggest that people **sit in a circle** so they can see each others' faces. Join the circle yourself as one of the group.
- As a group leader, you 'teach' the same subject as the instructor in the first role play. But whenever possible, try to **draw information out of the students from their own experience.**
- Be careful to **use words the students understand.** Check now and then to be sure they *do* understand.
- **Ask a lot of questions.** Encourage students to think critically and figure things out for themselves.
- **Emphasize the most useful ideas and information** (in this case, what the students can do in their communities to prevent tooth decay).
- **Use teaching aids that are available locally** and are as close to real life as possible. For example, you might invite a young child to the class so students can see for themselves the difference between baby teeth and permanent teeth.
- Do not waste a lot of time discussing detailed anatomy. Instead, include such information when it is needed for understanding specific problems.
- Have students look in each others' mouths for cavities. Then pass around some rotten teeth that were pulled at the health center. Let students smash the teeth open with a hammer or rock, so they can see the different layers (hard and soft) and how decay spreads inside a tooth. Ask someone to draw the inside of a tooth on the blackboard.
- **Encourage students to relate what they have seen and learned to real needs and problems** in their own communities. Discuss what action they might take.

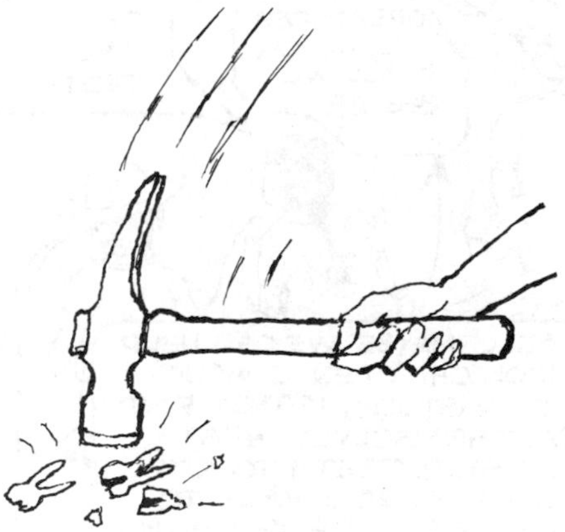

Students can break open teeth that have been pulled to see for themselves what the inside of a tooth looks like and what damage a cavity can cause.

The second role play: THE GOOD GROUP LEADER

The teacher or leader tries to get a discussion started—then stays in the background as much as possible, like this:

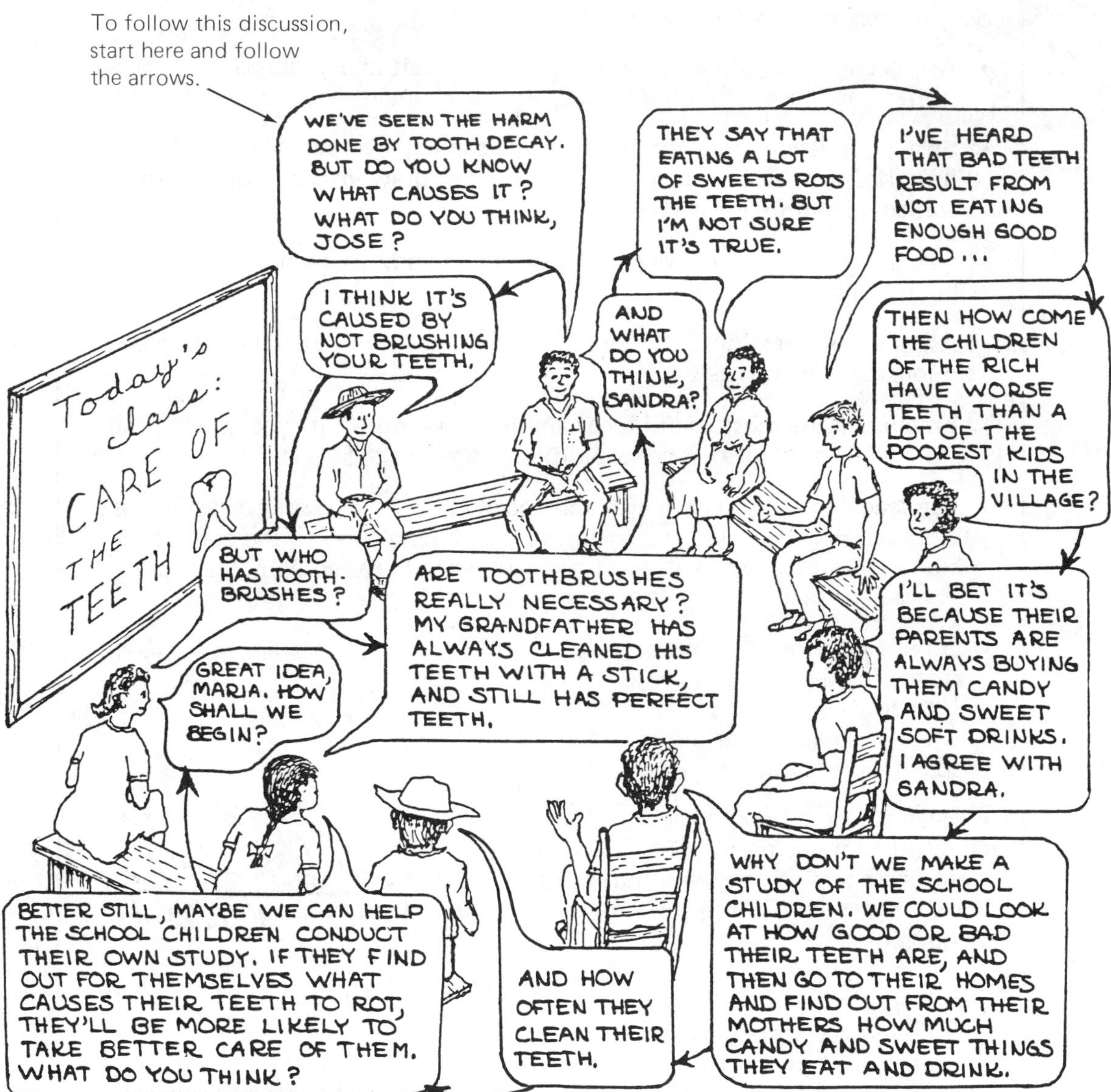
To follow this discussion, start here and follow the arrows.
WE'VE SEEN THE HARM DONE BY TOOTH DECAY. BUT DO YOU KNOW WHAT CAUSES IT? WHAT DO YOU THINK, JOSE?
I THINK IT'S CAUSED BY NOT BRUSHING YOUR TEETH.
BUT WHO HAS TOOTH-BRUSHES?
ARE TOOTHBRUSHES REALLY NECESSARY? MY GRANDFATHER HAS ALWAYS CLEANED HIS TEETH WITH A STICK, AND STILL HAS PERFECT TEETH.
AND WHAT DO YOU THINK, SANDRA?
THEY SAY THAT EATING A LOT OF SWEETS ROTS THE TEETH. BUT I'M NOT SURE IT'S TRUE.
I'VE HEARD THAT BAD TEETH RESULT FROM NOT EATING ENOUGH GOOD FOOD . . .
THEN HOW COME THE CHILDREN OF THE RICH HAVE WORSE TEETH THAN A LOT OF THE POOREST KIDS IN THE VILLAGE?
I'LL BET IT'S BECAUSE THEIR PARENTS ARE ALWAYS BUYING THEM CANDY AND SWEET SOFT DRINKS. I AGREE WITH SANDRA.
WHY DON'T WE MAKE A STUDY OF THE SCHOOL CHILDREN. WE COULD LOOK AT HOW GOOD OR BAD THEIR TEETH ARE, AND THEN GO TO THEIR HOMES AND FIND OUT FROM THEIR MOTHERS HOW MUCH CANDY AND SWEET THINGS THEY EAT AND DRINK.
AND HOW OFTEN THEY CLEAN THEIR TEETH.
BETTER STILL, MAYBE WE CAN HELP THE SCHOOL CHILDREN CONDUCT THEIR OWN STUDY. IF THEY FIND OUT FOR THEMSELVES WHAT CAUSES THEIR TEETH TO ROT, THEY'LL BE MORE LIKELY TO TAKE BETTER CARE OF THEM. WHAT DO YOU THINK?
GREAT IDEA, MARIA. HOW SHALL WE BEGIN?
Today's class: CARE OF THE TEETH

At the end of class, the leader asks the group what they have learned and what they plan to do with what they have learned. He helps them realize that the ideas raised in class need not end in the classroom, but can be carried out into the real world—into the communities where the health workers live and work.

Group discussion following the two role plays

You may want to discuss what the students think about the first role play as soon as it is over. Or you may want to wait until both role plays have been presented, so the students can compare them.

Good questions to start a discussion might be:

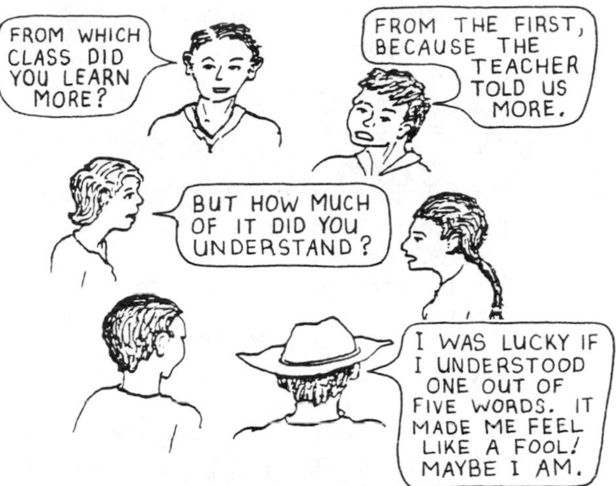
FROM WHICH CLASS DID YOU LEARN MORE?
FROM THE FIRST, BECAUSE THE TEACHER TOLD US MORE.
BUT HOW MUCH OF IT DID YOU UNDERSTAND?
I WAS LUCKY IF I UNDERSTOOD ONE OUT OF FIVE WORDS. IT MADE ME FEEL LIKE A FOOL! MAYBE I AM.

- What did you think of the two classes (on dental care)?
- From which class did you learn more?
- Which did you like better? Why?
- Who do you think was the better teacher? Why?

You may be surprised at some of the answers you get! Here are a few answers we have heard students give:

"I learned more from the first class, because the teacher told us more. I learned a lot of new words. Of course, I didn't understand them all . . ."

"The first class was much better organized."

"I liked the second class better, but the first one was better taught."

"The second class was too disorderly. You could scarcely tell the teacher from the students."

"The first teacher wasn't as nice, but he had better control of the class."

"The first teacher was by far the best. He told us something. The second one didn't tell us anything we didn't already know!"

"I felt more comfortable in the first class—I don't know why. I guess I knew that as long as I kept my mouth shut, I'd be all right. It was more like real school!"

"The second class was more fun. I forgot it was a class!"

By asking still more questions, you may be able to get the students to look more closely at what they learned—and have yet to learn—from the two classes. Follow through with questions like these:

- In which class did you **understand** more of what was said? Does this matter?
- From which class can you **remember** more? Does this matter?

- Do you remember something better when you are told the answer, or when you have to figure out the answer for yourself?
- In which class did students seem more interested? More bored?

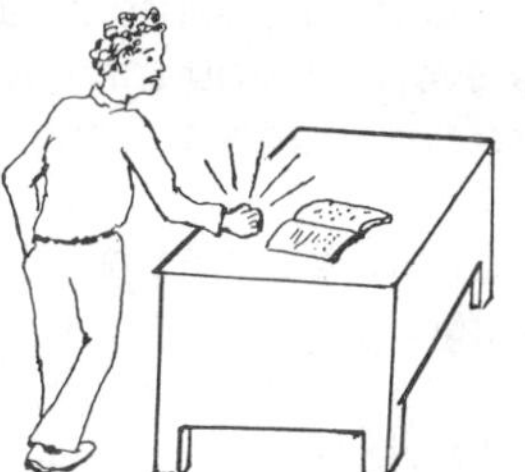
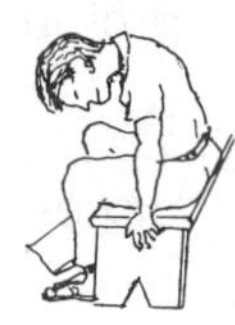

- In which class did you feel freer to speak up and say what you think?
- Which class had more to do with your own lives and experience?
- From which class did you get more ideas about ways to involve people in their own health care?
- Which class seemed to bring the group closer together? Why? Does this matter?
- Which teacher treated the students more as his equals? Could this affect the way the students will relate to sick persons and to those they teach?
- Which is the better teacher—one who has to be 'tough' in order to keep the students' attention? Or one who keeps their attention by getting them interested and involved?

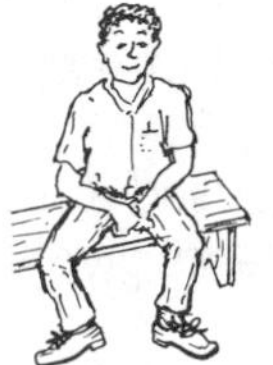
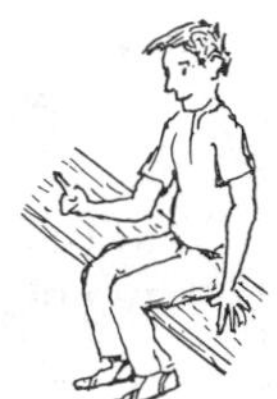

- Did you learn anything useful from these classes, apart from dental care? What?
- In what ways are the relations between each teacher and the students similar to relations between different people in your village? For example, between landholders and sharecroppers? Between friends?

With questions like these, you can **help the students to look critically at their own situation.** As much as you can, **let them find their own answers, even if they are different from yours.** The less you tell them, the better.

If the discussion goes well, most of the questions listed above will be asked—and answered—by the students themselves. Each answer, if approached critically, leads to the next question—or to even better ones!

If the students do not think things over as carefully as you would like, do not worry. And whatever you do, **do not push them.** Your answers have value only for yourself. Each person must come up with his or her own. There will be many other opportunities during the training to help students discover how education relates to life. In the last analysis, **your example will say far more than your words**—for better or for worse.

If you want lasting results:
POINT . . . . but don't *PUSH.*

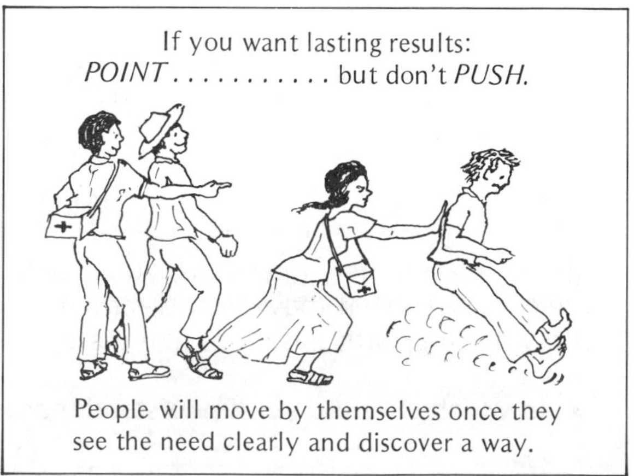

People will move by themselves once they see the need clearly and discover a way.

Analysis of the two role plays

After discussing the differences between the two approaches to teaching, it helps to summarize them in writing. (Or you may want to do this during, rather than after, the discussion.) One of the students can write the group's ideas on a blackboard or large sheet of paper.

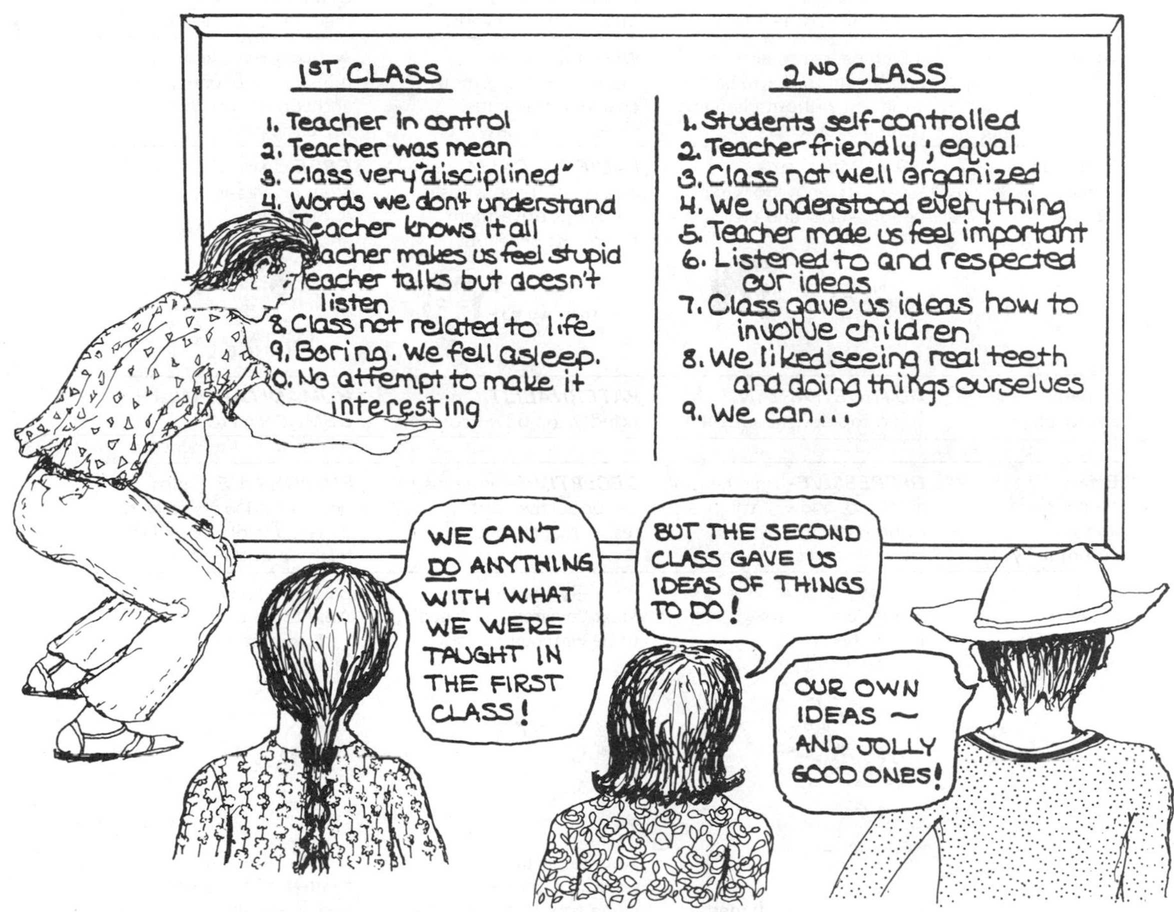
1ST CLASS
1. Teacher in control
2. Teacher was mean
3. Class very "disciplined"
4. Words we don't understand
Teacher knows it all
acher makes us feel stupid
Teacher talks but doesn't listen
8. Class not related to life.
9. Boring. We fell asleep.
0. No attempt to make it interesting
2ND CLASS
1. Students self-controlled
2. Teacher friendly; equal
3. Class not well organized
4. We understood everything
5. Teacher made us feel important
6. Listened to and respected our ideas
7. Class gave us ideas how to involve children
8. We liked seeing real teeth and doing things ourselves
9. We can...
WE CAN'T DO ANYTHING WITH WHAT WE WERE TAUGHT IN THE FIRST CLASS!
BUT THE SECOND CLASS GAVE US IDEAS OF THINGS TO DO!
OUR OWN IDEAS ~ AND JOLLY GOOD ONES!

As everyone is leaving the classroom, perhaps one of the students will put his hand on your shoulder and say:

"You know, I don't really think those two classes were to teach us about teeth. I think they were to help us learn about ourselves."

"They were to do both at once. That's the secret of education," you will reply. But you will want to hug him.

If no one says anything, however, don't worry. It takes time. You and your students will learn from each other.

THREE APPROACHES TO EDUCATION

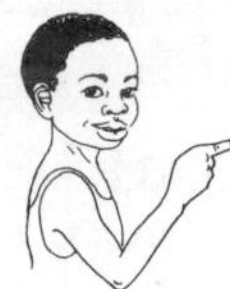

This chart gives a summary of 3 approaches to teaching. It may help instructors to evaluate their own teaching approach. But we do not recommend that this analysis be given to health workers. Analyzing stories and role plays will work better. So pass by this chart if you want.

Function	**CONVENTIONAL** to ***CONFORM***	**PROGRESSIVE** to ***REFORM***	**LIBERATING** to ***TRANSFORM***
Aim	Resist change. Keep social order stable.	Change people to meet society's needs.	Change society to meet people's needs.
Strategy	Teach people to accept and 'fit in' to the social situation without changing its unjust aspects.	Work for certain improvements without changing the unjust aspects of society.	Actively oppose social injustice, inequality, and corruption. Work for basic change.
Intention toward people	***CONTROL*** them—especially poor working people—farm and city. NO CHANGE	***PACIFY*** or ***CALM*** them—especially those whose hardships drive them to protest or revolt. BEHAVIOR CHANGE	***FREE*** them from oppression, exploitation, and corruption. SOCIAL CHANGE
General approach	***AUTHORITARIAN*** (rigid top-down control)	***PATERNALISTIC*** (kindly top-down control)	***HUMANITARIAN*** and ***DEMOCRATIC*** (control by the people)
Effect on people and the community	***OPPRESSIVE***—rigid central authority allows little or no participation by students and community.	***DECEPTIVE***—pretends to be supportive, but resists real change.	***SUPPORTIVE***—helps people find ways to gain more control over their health and their lives.
How students (and people generally) are viewed	Basically passive. Empty containers to be filled with standard knowledge. Can and must be tamed.	Basically irresponsible. Must be cared for. Need to be watched closely. Able to participate in specific activities when spoon fed.	Basically active. Able to take charge and become self-reliant. Responsible when treated with respect and as equals.
What the students feel about the teacher	***FEAR***—Teacher is an absolute, all-knowing boss who stands apart from and above the students.	***GRATITUDE***—Teacher is a friendly, parent-like authority who knows what is best for the students.	***TRUST***—Teacher is a 'facilitator' who helps everyone look for answers together.
Who decides what should be learned	The Ministry of Education (or Health) in the capital.	The Ministry, but with some local decisions.	The students and instructors together with the community.
Teaching method	• Teacher lectures. • Students ask few questions. • Often boring.	• Teacher educates and entertains students. • Dialogue and group discussions, but the teacher decides which are the 'right' answers.	• Open-ended dialogue, in which many answers come from people's experience. • Everyone educates each other.
Main way of learning	***PASSIVE***—students receive knowledge. Memorization of facts.	More or less active. Memorization still basic.	***ACTIVE***—everyone contributes. Learning through doing and discussing.

	CONVENTIONAL	PROGRESSIVE	LIBERATING
Important subjects or concepts covered	• the strengths and rightness of the present social order • national history (distorted to make 'our side' all heroes) • rules and regulations • obedience • anatomy and physiology • much that is not practical or relevant—it is taught because it always has been • unnecessary learning of big words and boring information	• integrated approach to development • how to make good use of government and professional services • filling out forms • desirable behavior • simple practical skills (often of little use—such as learning 20 bandages and their Latin names). 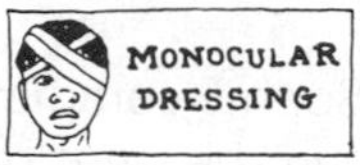 MONOCULAR DRESSING	• critical analysis • social awareness • communication skills • teaching skills • organization skills • innovation • self-reliance • use of local resources • local customs • confidence building • abilities of women and children • human dignity • methods that help the weak grow stronger
Flow of knowledge and ideas	school or health system → teacher → students 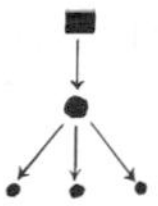 all one way	school or health system → teacher → students 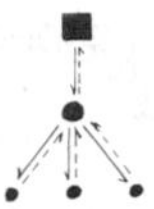 mostly one way	students ⇄ group leader ⇄ school or health system 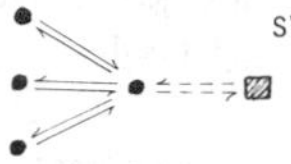 both ways
Area for studying	The classroom.	The classroom and other controlled situations.	Life—the classroom is life itself.
How does the class sit?	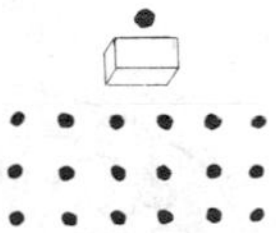	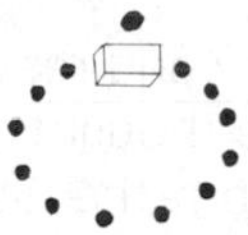	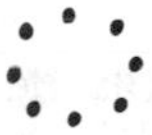
Class size	Often ***LARGE.*** Emphasis on quantity, not quality, of education.	Often fairly small, to encourage participation.	Often ***SMALL,*** to encourage communication and apprenticeship learning.
Attendance	Students ***have to*** attend. 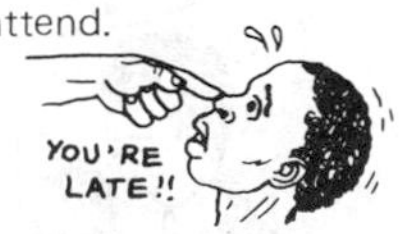 YOU'RE LATE!!	Students often ***want to*** attend because classes are entertaining and they will earn more if they graduate. 'Incentives' are given.	Students ***want to*** attend because the learning relates to their lives and needs, and because they are listened to and respected.
Group interaction	Competitive (cooperation between students on tests is called cheating).	Organized and directed by teacher. Many games and techniques used to bring people together.	Cooperative—students help each other. Those who are quicker assist others.
Purpose of exams	Primarily to 'weed out' slower students; grades emphasized. Some students pass. Others fail. PASS FAIL 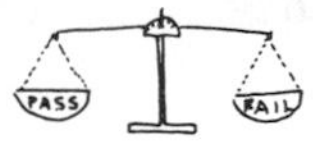	Variable, but generally tests are used to pass some and fail others.	Primarily to see if ideas are clearly expressed and if teaching methods work well. No grades. Faster students help slower ones.
Evaluation	Often ***superficial***—by education or health system. Students and community are the objects of study.	Often ***over-elaborate***—by education or health 'experts'. Community and students participate in limited ways.	***Simple*** and ***continual***—by community, students, and staff. Students and teachers evaluate each others' work and attitudes.
At end of training, students are given . . .	• diplomas • irregular, police-like supervision 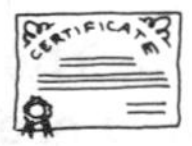 CERTIFICATE	• diplomas • uniforms • salaries • 'supportive' supervision 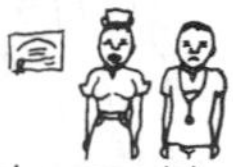	• encouragement to work hard and keep learning • supportive assistance when asked for
After training, a health worker is accountable to . . .	his supervisor, the health authorities, the government	mainly to the health authorities, less so to local authorities and the community	mainly to the community—especially the poor, whose interests he defends

APPROPRIATE AND INAPPROPRIATE TEACHING: TWO STORIES

In addition to role plays, you may want to use stories to help students and other instructors see the value of the new teaching methods. Telling stories often takes less preparation than role plays, and if the stories are imaginary or from another area, no one will be blamed for the mistakes that are described. Here are 2 stories comparing different teaching approaches and their results.

STORY 1*

A health worker named Sophie completed her training and passed all the exams at the end of the course. Then she went back to her village. It was a long journey because the village was far away. When Sophie arrived everybody was pleased to see her again. Her mother was especially pleased and proud that her daughter had done so well.

After the first greetings, Sophie's mother said, "It's good that you're back, because your baby cousin is ill with diarrhea and doesn't look well at all. Do you think you could help?"

Sophie went to see the baby and realized that he was badly dehydrated. She thought the baby should go to a health center, but the journey was too long. So she thought about what she had been taught. She could remember the anatomy of the gastro-intestinal tract, and all about electrolyte balance. And she remembered that a mixture of salt and sugar in water would help. But she could not remember how much sugar and how much salt to put in the water.

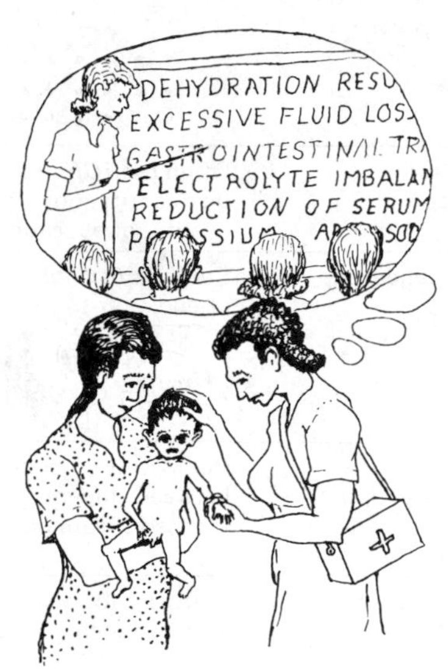

Sophie was very worried that the amounts would be wrong. She did not know whether to send for help or to guess how much to use. She thought that the baby was so sick she would have to do something. In the end, she made up the sugar and salt solution in the wrong proportions, and the baby died.

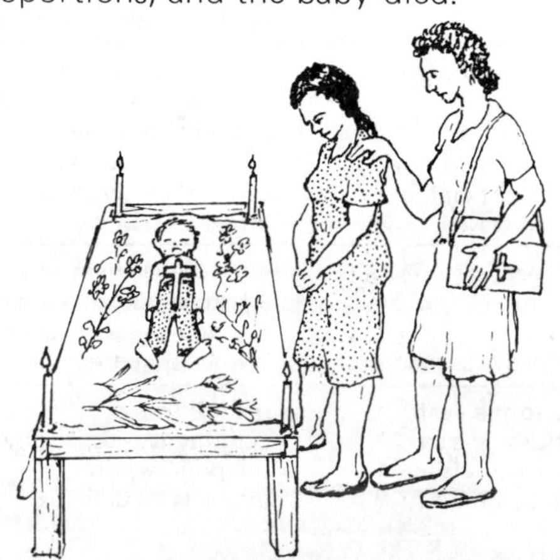

Moral of the story: Some training courses spend too much time on detailed facts, many of which have little importance. As a result, the most important things are not learned well. **The most important facts are those needed for solving common problems in the community.**

---

*Adapted from ***Teaching for Better Learning,*** by Fred Abbatt, WHO, Geneva, 1980.

STORY 2

In a short training program for village health workers, students decided that one of the most serious problems in their villages was diarrhea in children. They learned that the main danger with diarrhea is dehydration. They discussed ***Oral Rehydration Solution,*** and agreed that teaching mothers and children how to make and use it should be one of their first responsibilities.

"It won't be easy," said one of the students, herself a mother. "People don't understand funny words like ***oral, rehydration,*** or ***solution."*** So the group decided it would be better to speak of ***Special Drink***—even among themselves, so they would not be tempted to use fancy words in their villages.

"What if the mothers put in too much salt?" asked a student whose uncle was a doctor. "Wouldn't that be dangerous?"

"Yes," said the instructor. "We need to find ways of teaching that will help parents and children remember the right amounts. How do people remember things best in your villages?"

"We all remember songs," said one of the health workers. "People are always singing and learning new ones. We remember every word!"

So the group decided to write a song about diarrhea and Special Drink. They all worked on it together. But they got into an argument over what to call the baby's ***stool.*** For most people, a stool was something to sit on. Nobody understood words like ***feces*** and ***excrement.*** The word ***shit*** some people considered dirty. "But it's the word everyone understands—even children," argued one health worker. "Especially children!" said the mother. Finally they agreed that ***shit*** was the most appropriate word—at least in their area.

The song they wrote is shown below. (It can be sung to "Twinkle, Twinkle, Little Star" or another simple tune. With children, have them SHOUT the words printed in CAPITAL LETTERS.)

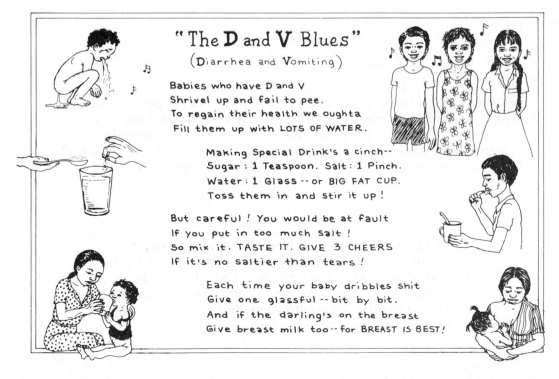

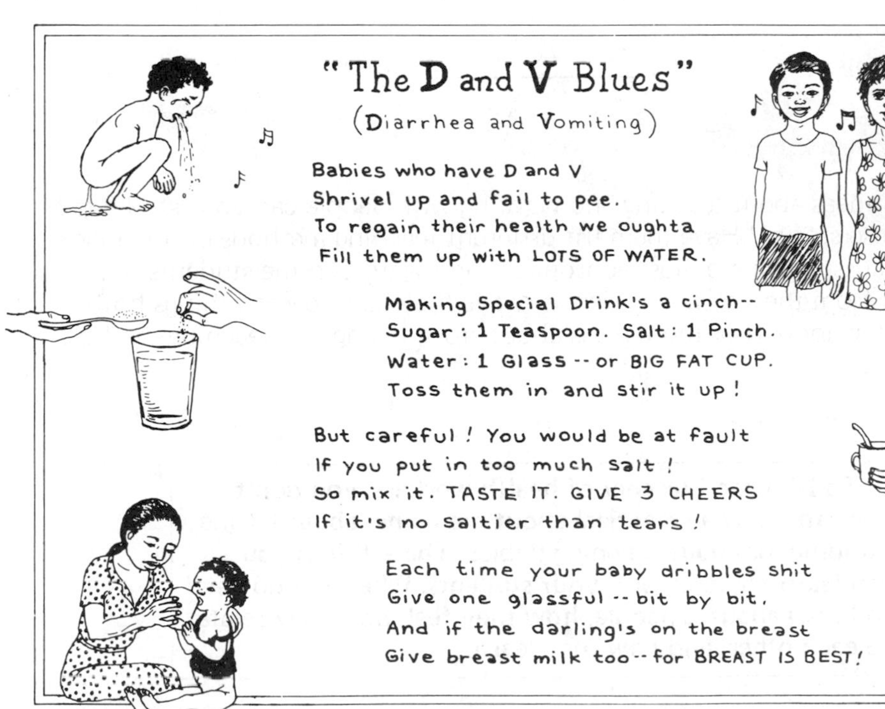

"The D and V Blues"
(Diarrhea and Vomiting)
Babies who have D and V
Shrivel up and fail to pee.
To regain their health we oughta
Fill them up with LOTS OF WATER.
Making Special Drink's a cinch--
Sugar : 1 Teaspoon. Salt : 1 Pinch.
Water : 1 Glass -- or BIG FAT CUP.
Toss them in and stir it up!
But careful! You would be at fault
If you put in too much salt!
So mix it. TASTE IT. GIVE 3 CHEERS
If it's no saltier than tears!
Each time your baby dribbles shit
Give one glassful -- bit by bit.
And if the darling's on the breast
Give breast milk too -- for BREAST IS BEST!

Several months later, after the course was over and the students were back in their villages, one of the health workers, named Rosa, was met in the street by a mother. The mother gave her 7 eggs wrapped in a leaf.

"Thank you," said Rosa with surprise. "But why . . .?"

"You saved my baby's life!" said the mother, hugging the health worker so hard she broke 3 eggs.

"But I didn't even see your baby!" said Rosa.

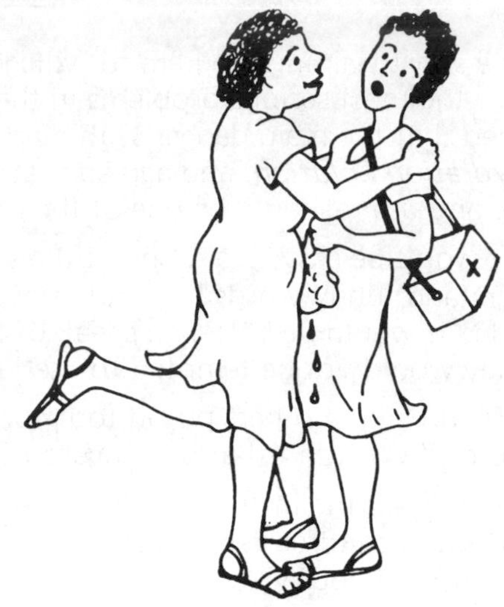

She hugged the health worker so hard she broke 3 eggs!

"I know," said the mother. "You see, my baby had diarrhea, but the river was flooded so I couldn't bring him to the health post. He was all shriveled up and couldn't pee. He was dying and I didn't know what to do! Then I remembered a song you had taught the children in school. My daughter's always singing it. So I made up the Special Drink, tasted it, and gave it to my baby, just like the song says. And he got well!"

Moral of the story: Training gives better results if it keeps language simple, focuses on what is most important, and uses learning methods people are used to and enjoy.

What other ideas about teaching and working with people can your students draw from these stories? Have them list different teaching methods on the blackboard and discuss which are most appropriate and why. Can the students tell similar stories from their own experience—ways they have learned things both in and outside of school? (For more ideas about story telling as a teaching method, see Chapter 13.)

To be a good teacher of health workers, you don't need to know a great deal about medicine, about latrine building, or about weighing babies. These things you can learn together with your students. What you do need to know about is people, how they feel, how they relate to each other, and how they learn.

ON CHANGING HABITS AND ATTITUDES

Many experts now tell us that the principal goal of health education should be to change people's habits and attitudes.

Unfortunately, such a goal points the finger at ***what people do wrong,*** rather than building on ***what they do right.*** It is based on the paternalistic view that the 'ignorance' of poor people is the main cause of their ill health, and that it is society's job to correct their bad habits and attitudes.

A people-centered approach to health education takes the opposite position. It recognizes that the ill health of the poor is, in large part, the result of a social order that favors the strong at the expense of the weak. Its main goal is not to change the poor, but to help them gain the understanding and skills needed to change the conditions that cause poverty and poor health.

THE AIMS OF HEALTH EDUCATION

BEHAVIOR CHANGE or SOCIAL CHANGE

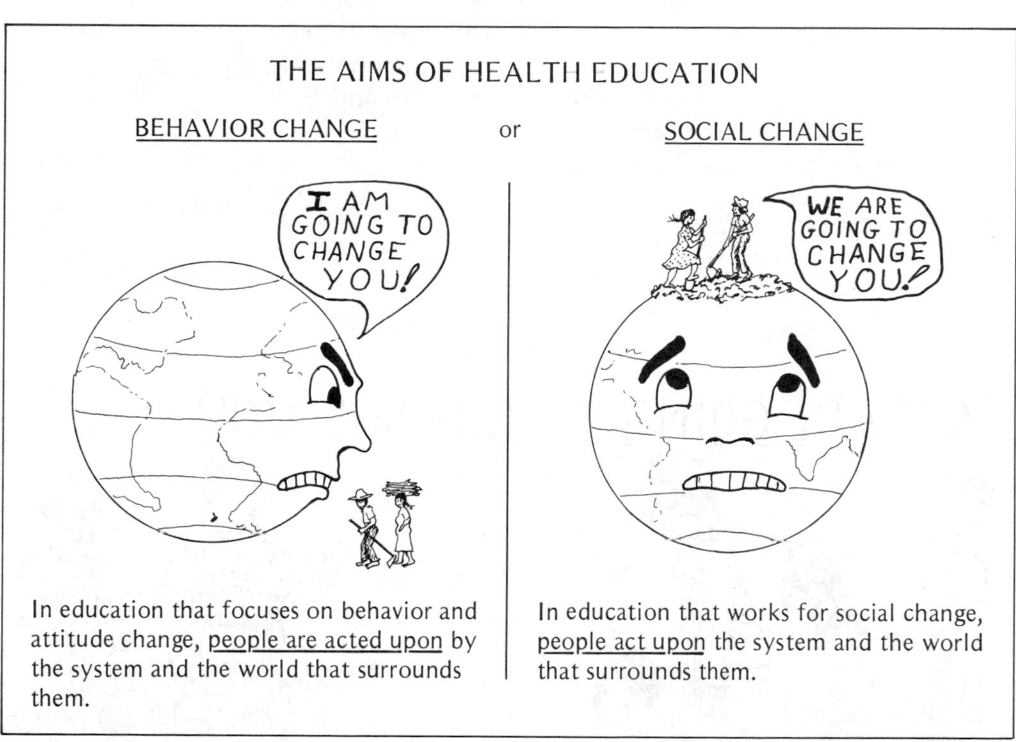

I AM GOING TO CHANGE YOU!
WE ARE GOING TO CHANGE YOU!

In education that focuses on behavior and attitude change, people are acted upon by the system and the world that surrounds them.

In education that works for social change, people act upon the system and the world that surrounds them.

In making these points, we are not saying that there is no need for changes in personal attitudes and behavior. But whose attitudes need changing the most? Whose attitudes and habits cause more human suffering—those of the poor or those of the 'well-educated' dominating classes?

The unhealthy behavior of both rich and poor results partly from the unfair social situation in which we live. So rather than trying to reform people, **health education needs to focus on helping people learn how to change their situation.**

As people become more sure of themselves and their capacity for effective action, their attitudes and behavior may change. But lasting changes will come from inside, from the people themselves.

When considering your effectiveness as a health educator, ask yourself: "How much does what I do help the poor gain more control over their health and their lives?"

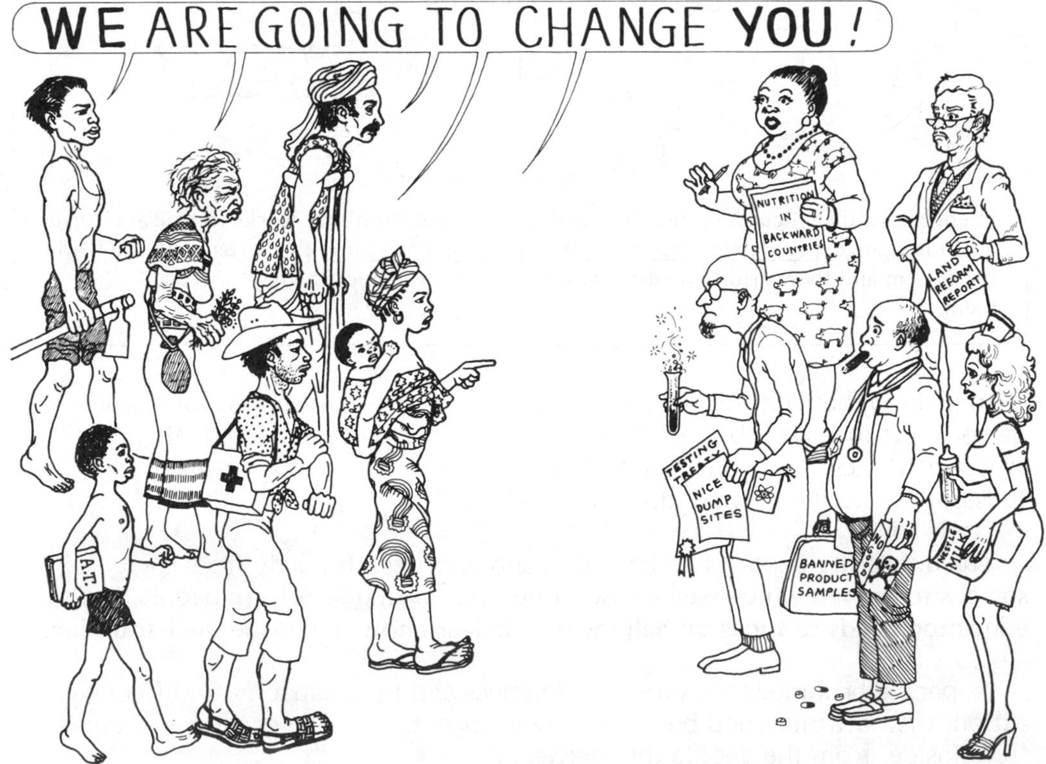

Selecting Health Workers, Instructors, and Advisers

CHAPTER 2

WHO MAKE THE BEST HEALTH WORKERS?

SHOULD HEALTH WORKERS BE FROM THE VILLAGE OR COMMUNITY WHERE THEY WORK?

Many health programs, large and small, agree that it is important for health workers to be selected from the communities where they will work. But their reasons differ:

TWO EXPLANATIONS FOR WHY IT IS BETTER THAT HEALTH WORKERS BE FROM THE COMMUNITIES WHERE THEY WORK

The 'expert' with little community experience:

GUESS WHO?
PEOPLE ARE QUICKER TO TRUST AND LISTEN TO SOMEONE FROM THEIR OWN COMMUNITY WHO SPEAKS IN THEIR TERMS AND KNOWS THEIR CUSTOMS AND PROBLEMS.

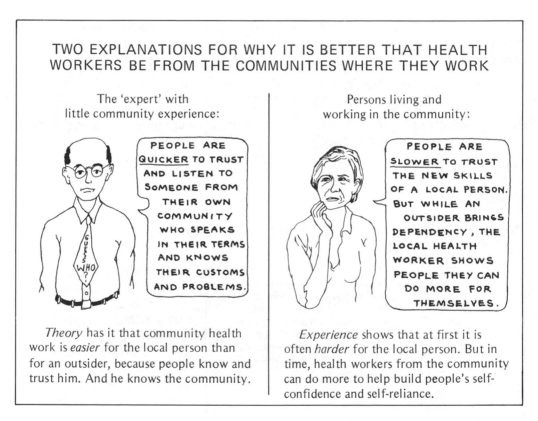

Theory has it that community health work is *easier* for the local person than for an outsider, because people know and trust him. And he knows the community.

Persons living and working in the community:

PEOPLE ARE SLOWER TO TRUST THE NEW SKILLS OF A LOCAL PERSON. BUT WHILE AN OUTSIDER BRINGS DEPENDENCY, THE LOCAL HEALTH WORKER SHOWS PEOPLE THEY CAN DO MORE FOR THEMSELVES.

Experience shows that at first it is often *harder* for the local person. But in time, health workers from the community can do more to help build people's self-confidence and self-reliance.

There is an old saying: ***No one is a prophet in his own land.*** A villager complains, "What does Mary, the health worker, know? I remember her as a skinny little girl!"

Such distrust in their own health worker reflects people's lack of confidence in themselves: "How could one of **us** understand new ideas or master new skills?" This lack of self-confidence is especially great when it comes to health care. Most people believe that modern medicine requires mysterious knowledge that only "strangers better than ourselves" can master.

Some American Indian health workers in Arizona found it so hard to win the trust of people in their own villages that they traded jobs with health workers in distant villages. They found that as 'outsiders' they could command more immediate authority. People were quicker to follow their advice without question.

Similar 'swaps' have been made by health workers in several countries. And some of the larger health programs make it a point **not** to send health workers to work in their own communities.

We feel this is a mistake. A stranger to a community, no matter how well he works, perpetuates dependency on outside help. **Only when a health worker is from the community can his example show "what we people in this village can do for ourselves."**

WHO SELECTS HEALTH WORKERS AND HOW?

Many programs feel that health workers should not only be **from the community** where they work, but that they should also be **selected by the community.** These are the reasons:

- If everyone takes part in the selection, chances are greater that the health worker will be well accepted.
- Participation in the selection process is a step toward greater responsibility and control by people over factors that affect their health.
- A health worker chosen by the community is more likely to feel that his or her first responsibility is to the community.

Problems with selection by the community

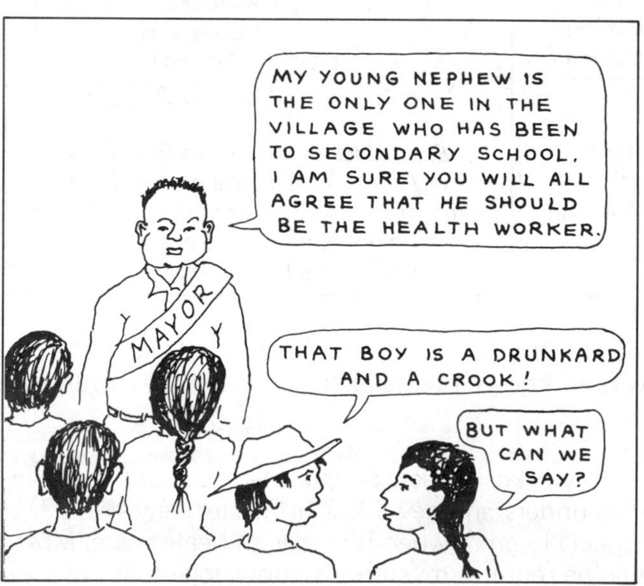

MY YOUNG NEPHEW IS THE ONLY ONE IN THE VILLAGE WHO HAS BEEN TO SECONDARY SCHOOL. I AM SURE YOU WILL ALL AGREE THAT HE SHOULD BE THE HEALTH WORKER.
MAYOR
THAT BOY IS A DRUNKARD AND A CROOK!
BUT WHAT CAN WE SAY?

Problem: In many villages, the local headman, mayor, or a powerful landowner insists that one of his children or family members be chosen as health worker. Even if a public vote is taken, the poorer people may be afraid to suggest or vote for someone else. As a result, the health workers selected may represent the interests of those with land and power rather than those with greatest need. This is a problem reported from many countries.

Another problem: Sometimes villagers select a person who is very young, inexperienced, or irresponsible. This may be because people feel that "study is for the young." Also, older persons frequently have too many other responsibilities.

Part of the reason for poor choice of health workers, however, is that often the selection is made in a hurry, without enough critical discussion. Somebody suggests a friend, or someone he likes. Someone else suggests another friend, and a vote is taken. More often than not, the winner is the person for whom the first show of hands is called.

Still another problem: Many programs find that health workers with more than a primary school education are likely to leave their villages for better-paying jobs in the cities.

To avoid these and other problems, some community-based programs in the Philippines do not accept the following persons for health worker training:

- close relatives of village leaders or officials
- young people and those likely to marry soon
- those with more than a primary school education
- those with many other responsibilities or official positions

In a similar way, a health program in Iran decided to exclude from health worker selection, family members of any village authority or large landholder. After this decision was made, villagers chose health workers who were more representative of the poor and more concerned with their needs.

Ways to help communities select wisely

Rather than deciding for the community what kinds of persons it should or should not select, it is often better to help the community decide wisely for itself. But this takes time and care.

For example, instructors from the villager-run health program in Ajoya, Mexico ride on muleback to mountain villages, spending a few days in each. Often they will make several visits, getting to know the people better. Then an all-village meeting is held. Women and children are encouraged to attend (instead of only men, as is customary). The instructors try to get an active discussion going: *What are our health needs? Do we need our own health worker? What qualities should this person have?* As the people make suggestions, these are written on large sheets of paper or a blackboard, and discussed further.

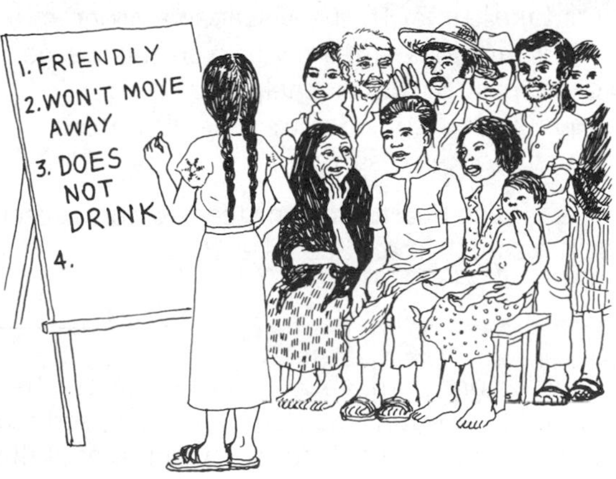

The people's list might include any combination of the following.

THIS LIST CONTAINS SUGGESTIONS FROM SEVERAL PROGRAMS.

We want a health worker who:

- is kind
- is responsible
- is honest and shows good judgement
- has a mature personality
- is interested in health and community work
- is humble; feels equal to and not superior to others
- will probably stay in the village (not move away)
- is accepted and respected by all the people, or at least by the poor
- has the full agreement and cooperation of his or her family
- can read and write (preferably)
- does not have more than a primary school education
- is eager to learn; open to new ideas
- is a good leader and organizer
- has healthy habits (does not smoke, does not drink too much)
- can draw, or is a good storyteller
- works well with mothers, children, and working people
- has a good record of taking part in or leading community activities
- has some experience in health care or healing (preferably)
- understands and respects people's beliefs and traditional practices
- identifies with and defends the interests of those in greatest need

The team in Ajoya feels it is important for the villagers to develop the list of qualities themselves, rather than to have a list handed to them. If, however, the people forget certain important qualities, the instructors may ask questions that help the people consider those points.

Only after the list of qualities has been developed and thoroughly discussed, are the people asked to suggest names of persons who might make good health workers. **If certain persons are known to dominate discussions or decisions, they are asked, politely, to remain silent** so that those who seldom speak can make their suggestions first. When necessary, the vote is taken by secret ballot.

In this way, selection of a health worker is the beginning of a process in which the poor find a voice and fairer representation. But all this takes time. In the Makapawa program in the Philippines, a team works in the village for at least 3 months, helping the poor organize and consider their needs before a health worker is selected.

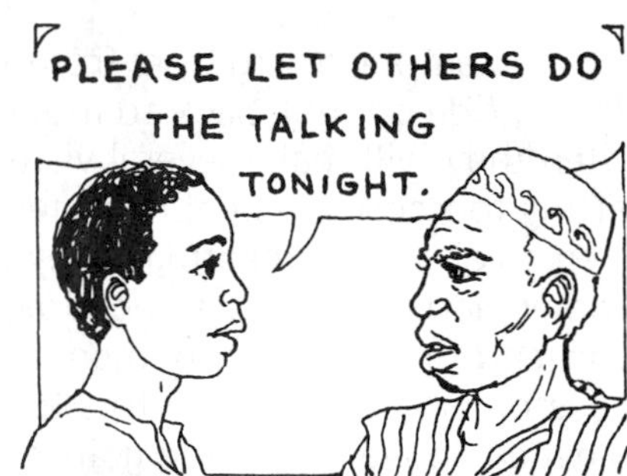
PLEASE LET OTHERS DO THE TALKING TONIGHT.

A village health committee is often chosen at the same time. (See page **10**-3).

Other programs take different approaches to the selection of health workers. Some have requirements for age, sex, schooling, physical health, etc. Some give simple tests to check for such things as skill with one's hands. Generally, the more distant the headquarters, the more requirements are set in advance.

Joint selection by the community and program leaders

Some programs feel the best selection of health workers results from combining **the community's knowledge** of its people with **the program leaders' experience.** The village is asked to pick 3 or 4 'candidates'. From these, the instructors choose the one they think most suited—perhaps after testing their skills and attitudes.

HANDICAPPED PERSONS AS HEALTH WORKERS

Some programs require that health workers be in "excellent physical health." Clearly, health workers should be free of contagious diseases such as untreated tuberculosis, and healthy enough to handle their responsibilities.

We have found, however, that **some of the best health workers are persons with serious physical handicaps;** polio, for instance, or an amputated arm or leg. Unable to do hard physical labor, they may find more time for health work and greater satisfaction in doing it. Because of their own problems, they also have more understanding for others who are ill or handicapped. In some ways, their weakness becomes their strength. As health workers serving their community, they set an example for others who are handicapped.

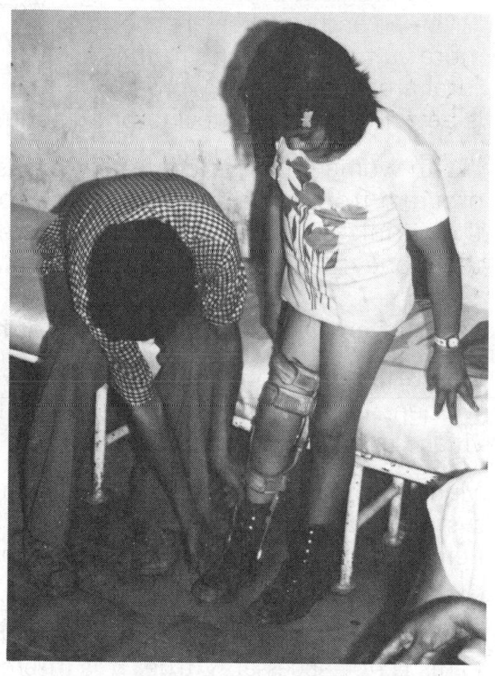

Handicapped persons often make excellent health workers. Here a young man, himself crippled by juvenile arthritis, repairs braces for a child with polio. (Mexico—Project Piaxtla)

WHO MAKE BETTER HEALTH WORKERS—MEN OR WOMEN?

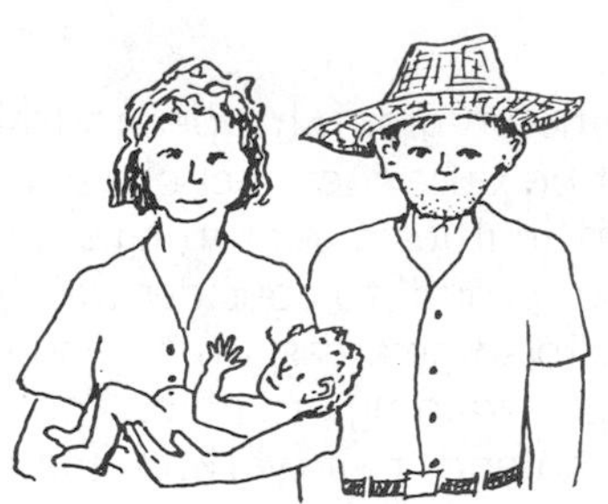

Some programs train only men as health workers. Others only women. Others train both.

Reasons often given for selecting <u>women</u> as health workers:

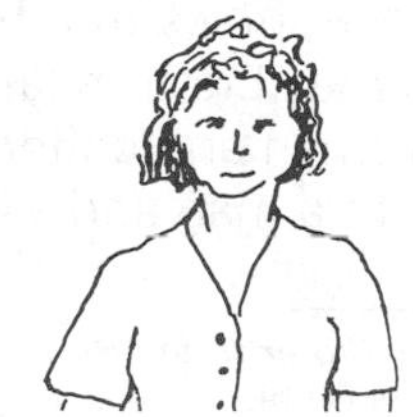

- Women and children make up ¾ of the population. Their health needs are especially great. And women usually prefer health workers who are women.
- Women have more experience in caring for children, and may be more tender.

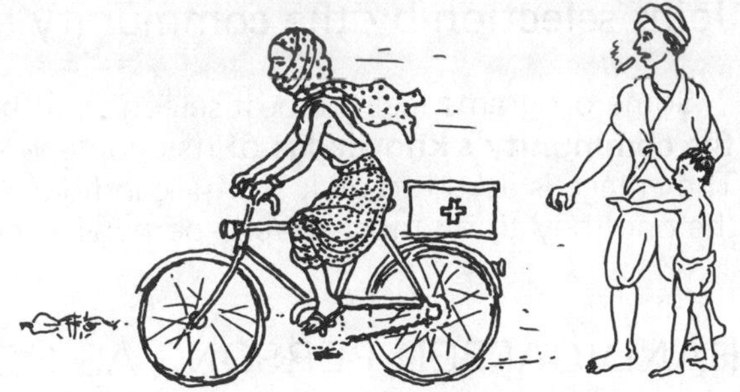

Women health workers in Bangladesh ride bicycles, which only the men used to do. This is helping women gain more equal rights.

- Women usually stay closer to the village, and so are more available when needed.
- Women often are more exploited and abused than men. Therefore their sympathies are more likely to lie with those who have less power and greater need. A health program in India states: "Women and children are the more vulnerable groups in the rural area, therefore a woman is best able to motivate and bring about change."*
- "With women there is less fear of misuse or malpractice," states the same program from India. In many areas, women tend to be more responsible, and they drink less. They may also be more willing to work for the people, not the money.

Reasons often given for selecting <u>men</u> as health workers:

- Men often can move about more safely and freely than women. They can go alone or at night to a distant house or village to attend an emergency.
- Much of the work to improve health involves farming, water systems, latrine building, and other activities for which the help of men is needed. Men can perhaps be better led by a male leader.
- Where part of the health worker's job is to work toward social change, men are more likely to take action and to organize the people than are women. (This is not necessarily true. It is interesting to note, however, that in some countries where human rights are often violated, government-run health programs train mostly women health workers. In those same countries, community-based programs working for land rights and social change often train mostly men health workers.)

Some programs happen to train mostly men, others mostly women. Usually this is **not** because they feel one sex makes better health workers. In some places there are difficulties in recruiting either men or women. Men (especially young men) may be too 'proud' to consider training for 'nursing' work—especially if on a volunteer basis. In some areas, unmarried women may not be permitted to leave home to attend a training program. And married women may be unable to leave their children and their work, or their husbands may not let them.

Experience shows that **both women and men can make good health workers.** Often men are able to relate better to the health needs of men, and women to the needs of women and children. Some health programs resolve this difference by training both a man and a woman (sometimes a married couple) from each village.

---

*From ***Moving Closer to the Rural Poor,*** by the Mobile Orientation and Training Team, Indian Social Institute, New Delhi.

YOUNGER OR OLDER HEALTH WORKERS—WHICH WORK OUT BEST?

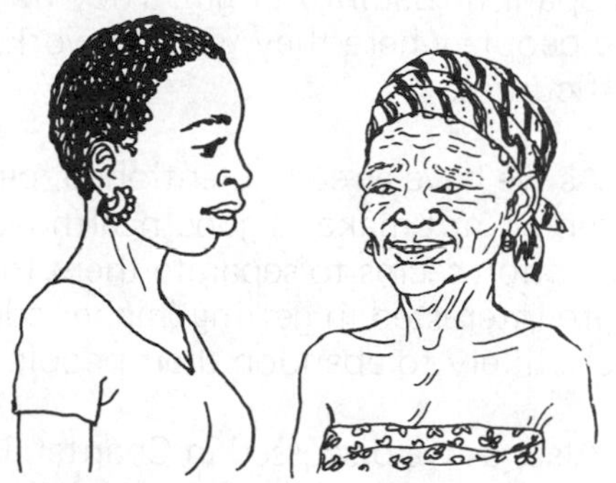

Although most health programs train health workers who are quite young, many find that **somewhat older or middle-aged persons often work out better.** Young people sometimes have more open minds (and may be easier to recruit), but they have more difficulty in winning people's confidence and cooperation. Also, younger persons may be less likely to stay in the village. Some programs find that unmarried girls are likely to get married and move away. Other programs find that young men often move to the cities or to migrant farm-working camps.

Older persons are usually more likely to remain in their communities, and to work with great dedication and responsibility. Also, people are more likely to respect and listen to them. But they may be more fixed, or even rigid, in their ideas. This can be both a strength and a problem.

In the experience of many programs, the most reliable age group is from about 25 to 40. When health workers are younger or older than that, more difficulties seem to arise. There are, of course, many exceptions. In Ajoya, Mexico, the present leaders of the program began as 'junior health workers' when they were 13 to 16 years old.

EDUCATIONAL LEVEL

Capable health workers have been trained from every educational level, from persons who cannot read to those with university or medical degrees. Each level presents special strengths and special problems.

Persons who cannot read and write often have unusually well-developed memories—sometimes far better than those of us who depend on writing things down. But to train health workers who cannot read and write calls for somewhat different educational methods. Few instructors have been taught these methods, but they can learn them with the help of the students.

In most programs, the average education level of community health workers is from 3 to 6 years of primary school. Yet some programs make 6 years of primary school a minimum requirement. Others require completion of secondary school.

Education requirements sometimes give rise to problems. For example, in Guatemala, a government training program for 'health technicians' in the highland Indian communities started with two requirements: 1) Applicants must speak a native Indian language as well as Spanish. 2) They must have completed secondary school. However, it turned out that very few native language speakers had finished secondary school. One of the two requirements had to be dropped.

Unfortunately, the language requirement was dropped and the education requirement kept. This meant that almost all the health technicians trained were of Spanish *(Ladino)* origin. They neither spoke the local languages nor represented the people where they were to work. As a result, the program has had many difficulties.

As we have already mentioned, persons who have completed secondary school often do not make as good health workers as those with less schooling. Their education seems to separate them from the majority of their people. Many are more interested in getting 'higher education' or 'better jobs' in the city. They are more likely to abandon their people.

Also, as we discussed in Chapter 1, persons with much formal education may have an extra burden of unhealthy values. They need to unlearn and relearn a great deal in order to become effective community health workers.

By contrast, persons with less formal education tend to feel themselves more in harmony with, and equal to, the poor majority. They may be more ready to commit themselves to community health work.

Persons with only a few years of schooling often make more reliable, more community-strengthening health workers than those who have had more formal education.

Once again, of course, there are exceptions.

TRADITIONAL HEALERS AND MIDWIVES AS HEALTH WORKERS

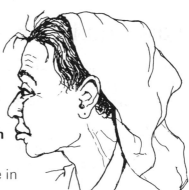

Many programs have trained traditional healers, herbalists, bone setters, and traditional midwives as village health workers—often with good results.

Advantages to training traditional healers as health workers:

- They already have the confidence of the people in their own special area of health care.
- They have a strong grounding in traditional and spiritual forms of care and healing. To these they can add concepts of modern health care and medicine. Often the combination of the old and the new, unique to the area, is better than either way by itself.
- They are usually persons with great experience and strong beliefs. So they may be more able to defend their people's culture and resist the use of foreign ideas and technologies not suited to local needs.
- They are often persons firmly rooted in their communities and deeply committed to serving people in need. (But be careful. Some traditional healers use their special knowledge to exploit or gain power over others.)

Difficulties in training traditional healers as health workers:

Traditional healers often are **very set in their ways.** Like modern medicine, traditional medicine includes many practices that are helpful, others that are useless, and some that are harmful. Traditional healers, like many modern doctors, may be reluctant to examine critically the practices they have always followed. They may be unwilling to omit or change harmful but profitable practices. (These may include the misuse or overuse of certain modern medicines, sometimes combined with herbal medicines.)

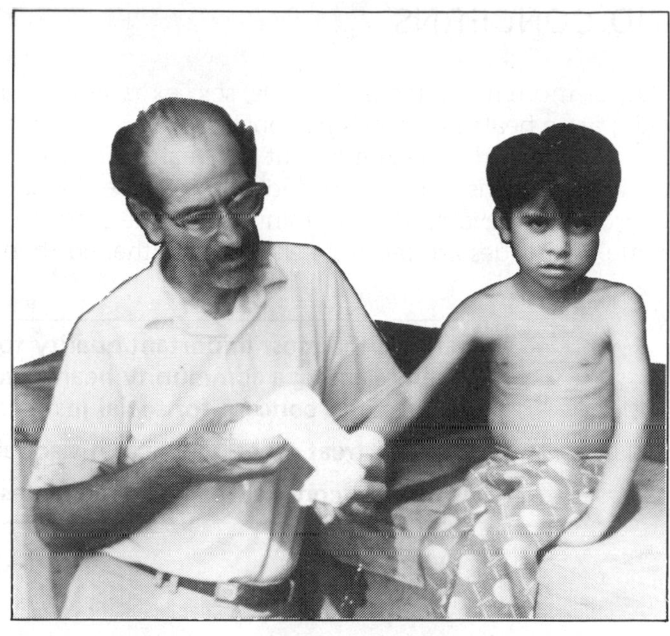

This 'herb doctor' was chosen by his village to train as a health worker. His art of healing adds much to the science of health care. Today, he combines aspects of modern and folk medicine. (Mexico)

A common difficulty with traditional healers relates to their approach to problem solving. **Most traditional healers rely, to a large extent, on the psychological 'power of suggestion'.** This is a very important part of the healing process as they know it. The traditional healer convinces the sick person and his family that he or she knows immediately just what the illness is, what caused it, and how to treat it. This immediate and absolute certainty is a key to traditional healing.

But the science of modern medicine calls for just the opposite approach. **The scientific healer begins with doubt, not certainty.** He starts by asking questions, collecting related information, and systematically considering and testing possibilities (see Ch. 17).

It is often difficult for persons used to traditional healing to learn the more scientific approach. As established healers, they may find it especially difficult to ask for advice or suggestions, or to admit when they have trouble diagnosing an illness.

An instructor who is unaware of all this, may treat these persons as if they were ignorant or dishonest. This makes it more difficult for both to admit their doubts or mistakes. In our own experience, however, we have found that when an instructor understands and appreciates the local forms of healing, most misunderstandings with traditional healers can be avoided. When this is so . . .

Traditional healers can become some of the most capable and dedicated primary care workers.

PERSONAL QUALITIES, ATTITUDES, AND CONCERNS

Of far more importance than age, sex, experience, education, and even place of origin, are a health worker's personal qualities—his or her understanding of people and their needs. It is essential that the health worker identify with the poor and have a strong sense of fairness and social justice. To some extent, these attitudes can grow and develop during training. But the seeds need to be there already. People's attitudes are far more easily strengthened than changed.

Perhaps the most important quality to look for when selecting a community health worker is the person's concern for social justice.

Does he treat other people as his equals?

Is his first concern for those in greatest need?

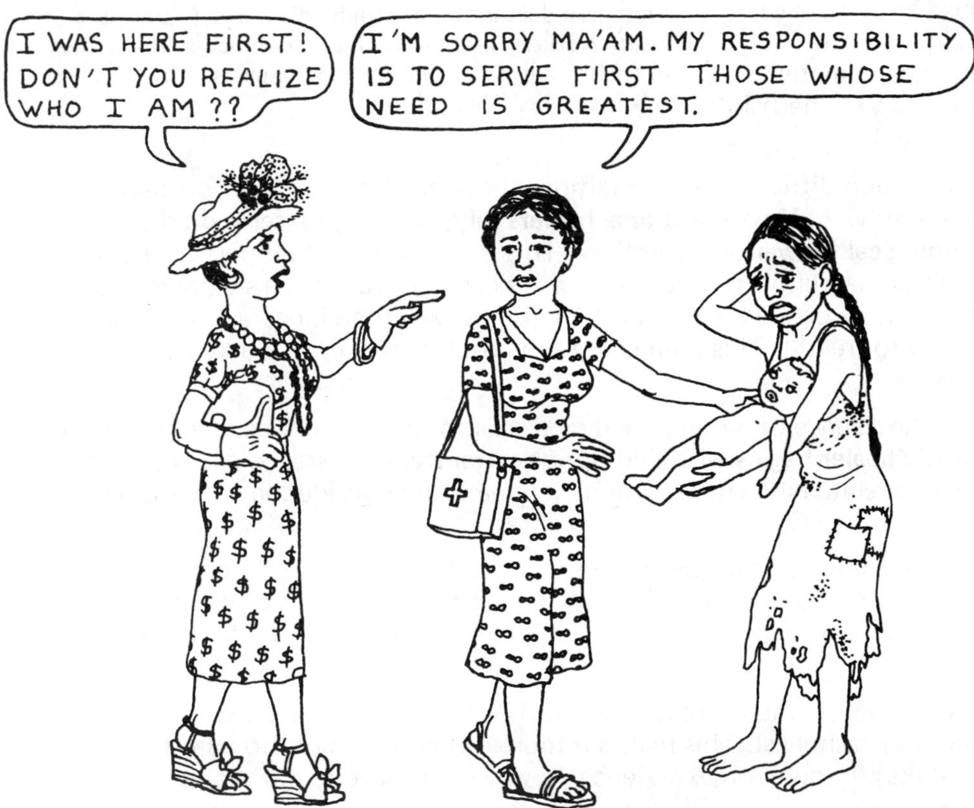
I WAS HERE FIRST! DON'T YOU REALIZE WHO I AM??
I'M SORRY MA'AM. MY RESPONSIBILITY IS TO SERVE FIRST THOSE WHOSE NEED IS GREATEST.

This is a scene from a 'Farmworkers' Theater' production in Ajoya, Mexico. It was presented to help villagers recognize the differences between a good health worker and the typical doctor.

WHO MAKE THE BEST TEACHERS OF VILLAGE HEALTH WORKERS?

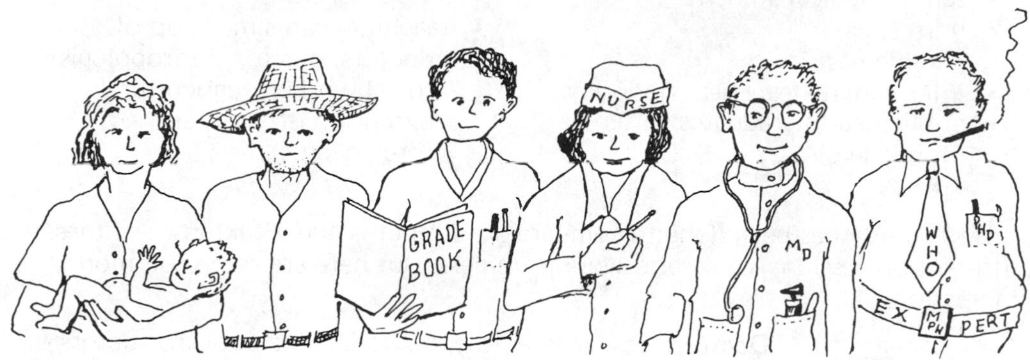

Selection of appropriate instructors is just as important as selection of the health workers themselves. **Instructors provide the example or 'role model' for teaching and learning** that health workers follow when they return to their communities.

If the instructor bosses and 'talks down' to students, the students, in turn, will be more likely to 'talk down' and act superior to others when they become village health workers. But if the instructor relates to the students as his equals, building on strengths and knowledge that they already have, then the health workers will be more likely to work with their people in a similar way.

THE EDUCATION GAP

A common problem: Instructors often have a very different social and educational background from that of the health workers they teach. They may be doctors, nurses, social workers, or health officers who have grown up in cities and have had far more formal education. They can easily lose touch—if they ever were in touch—with the wisdom, hardships, strengths, and weaknesses of people who still live close to the land, the seasons, and physical work.

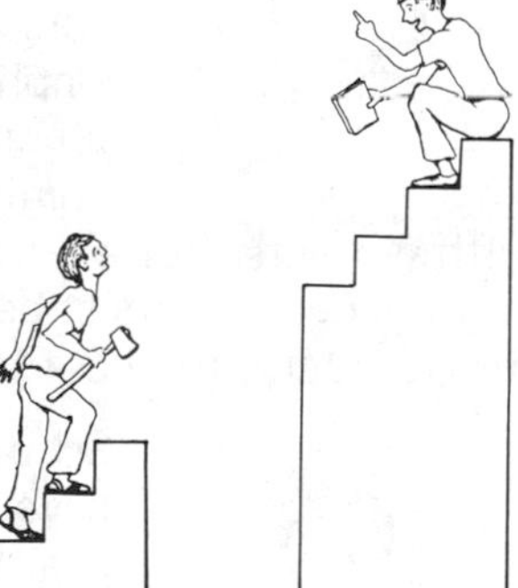

The knowledge of highly educated persons is not necessarily ***better*** than that of most of us, but it is ***different.*** It is as difficult for the doctor to speak in the basic, clear, colorful language of the villager, as it is for the villager to understand the long Latin words of the doctor.

This wide separation between instructor and students is called an 'education gap'. When the 'gap' is too wide, it is often difficult to bridge. So teacher and students never really come to know, appreciate, or learn very much from each other.

Many kinds of professionals have served as trainers of health workers:

- doctors
- senior medical students
- nurses
- paramedics
- intermediate-level health workers
- public health graduates (often foreigners)
- social workers
- school teachers
- teaching teams made up of doctors, nurses, anthropologists, social workers, agricultural extension officers, and foreign experts

Little study has been done to compare the strengths and weaknesses of these different professionals as health worker trainers. But here are some common impressions:

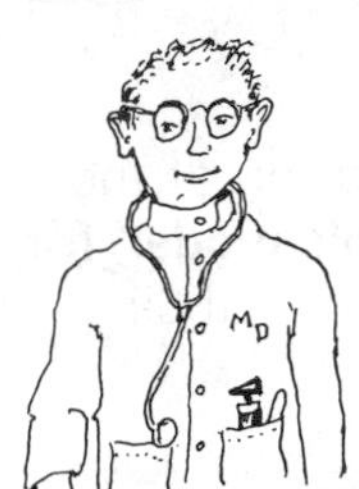

Doctors. As a general rule, doctors make poor instructors of health workers. Their curative, hospital-based training does not prepare them to look at the needs of a whole community. Attitudes are also a problem. Doctors have a tendency to take charge, to regard themselves as decision-makers even in areas they know little about. Feeling that even simple diagnosis and treatment are 'risky' without years of medical school, they often limit teaching of curative medicine to a few minor chores. This severely weakens the role of health workers in the community. Yet the courses doctors teach usually include a deadly overdose of anatomy, with countless Latin names. This gives the health worker a magic vocabulary with which to confuse and impress the people in his community.

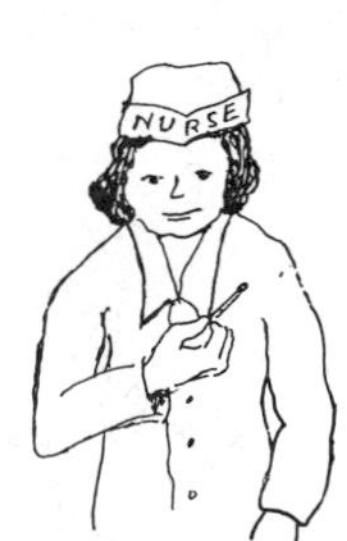

Nurses. Some nurses make excellent instructors of health workers. But such nurses are exceptional. The nurses' job has traditionally been to take orders without question, and to clean up after the doctors. They are given little decision-making responsibility. So it is not surprising that, when nurses instruct village health workers, they place strong emphasis on unquestioning obedience, filling out forms, and functioning as errand boys or girls. As they have been dominated and undervalued, they tend to do the same with health workers. For a nurse to effectively prepare health workers as leaders of social change, she must be a true rebel. Fortunately, many such nurses exist! Unfortunately, they are rarely chosen as instructors.

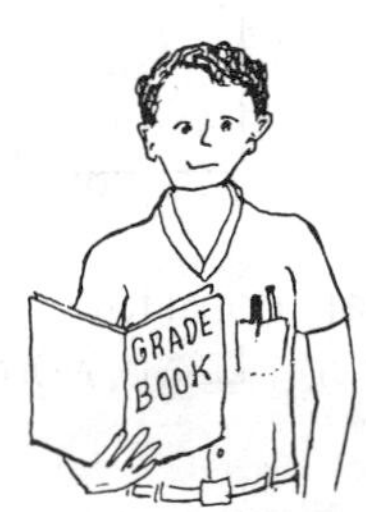

School teachers. In Honduras, some young school teachers have proved to be surprisingly good instructors of village health workers. These teachers are given 2 or 3 months of special training in community development and primary care activities. Then they are sent to teach and work with village health workers. The young teachers are far more willing to go to remote villages than are nurses or doctors. They also are able to relate well to the health workers and local people. Having a limited background in health, they do not set themselves up as 'authorities'. Rather, they explore and learn with others about approaches to solving different health problems. This puts them on a more equal footing with students and villagers. It seems that, in some circumstances at least, **teaching skills may be more important than an extensive background in medicine and health care.**

Bridging the education gap

If, as an instructor, you find you are separated from your students by a wide social and educational gap, there are things you may be able to do to help bridge it:

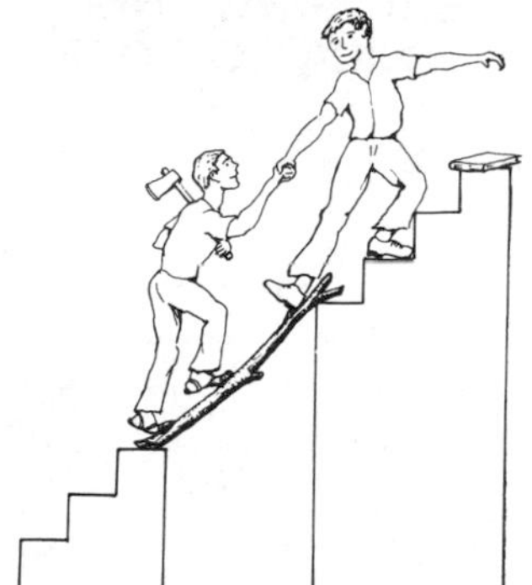

1. **Admit openly to your students that the gap exists**—and that the shortcoming is yours as much as theirs. Invite your students to discuss and look for ways of bridging the gap together.

2. Do whatever you can to **understand in a personal way the life, language, customs, and needs of your students and their communities.** Live, if you can, with one of the poorer families in the community (paying your way). Eat their food. Drink their water. Help each day with some of the physical or farm work. Accept no more income than an average member of the community earns. (This is only a suggestion—but a good one.)

3. If you are from out of the area, or are specialized in a narrow field of health care (like medicine), **try not to be the main teacher,** but rather a teaching assistant or auxiliary. (The main teacher will need a wide range of skills and knowledge, including, above all, teaching skills and inside knowledge of the local people. He or she needs personal understanding of what it is like to approach learning new things without much formal education.)

4. When teaching, make every effort to **always begin with the knowledge and skills the health workers already have, and help them build on these.** You are the stranger, so try to adapt your language to theirs; don't make them adapt to yours. If they are used to learning from stories or from actually doing things, rather than from lectures and books, try to adapt to their way of learning—even if this means exploring forms of teaching and learning that are new to you.

5. Most important! **Make yourself as unnecessary as possible, as soon as possible.** Look for local persons who are socially more qualified (less schooled, more in harmony with the people) to take over the training. Work toward having more experienced village health workers become the teachers of new village health workers as soon as possible. Every chance you get, move one step further into the background. Become the teacher of teachers. Then, just an adviser or 'person with ideas'. Then leave.

BRIDGING THE EDUCATION GAP

If the student is at this level

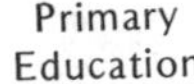

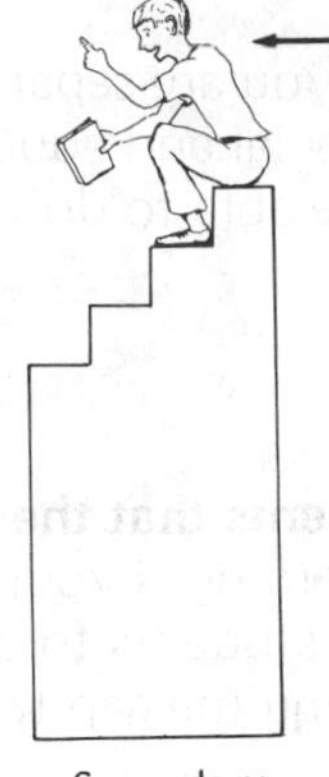

Primary Education

Secondary Education (or more)

and you try to teach him from this level, you will be talking over his head. You will bore him and, in time, lose him. You will make him feel stupid and he may hate you for it—because he is not stupid. There are probably many things he can do much better than you can, and many important things he knows that you do not.

If you try to **learn from him,** and to make good use of the language, knowledge, and skills he already has, often you can help him bridge the gap to learning new skills.

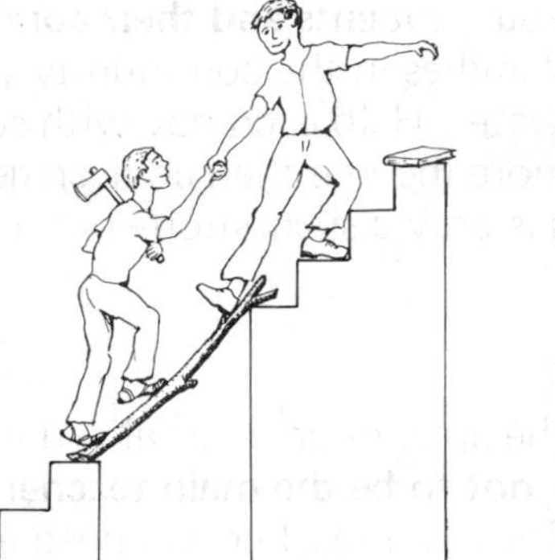

There are many shortcuts to increasing the student's skill and understanding: teaching aids, problem solving, role playing, learning by doing, etc. But it is important to begin with the skills and understanding the person already has.

Go more than halfway to meet him.

Start with the knowledge and skills a person already has—and help him build on these.

CLOSING THE GAP

If the educational gap is wide, better than trying to bridge it is to close it. Work toward training community persons who are closer to the educational level of the students, so they can take over most or all of the teaching.

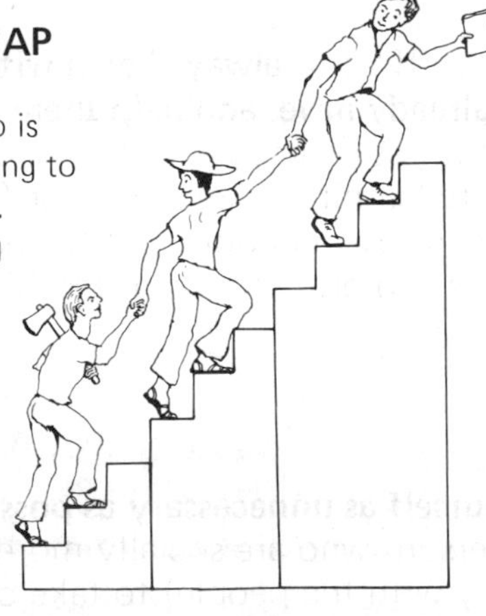

The sooner a local health worker can be trained to take over the teaching of new health workers, the better. Then training is more likely to be appropriate and helpful.

If you are an outsider, **work toward making yourself as unnecessary as possible, as soon as possible.**

Closing the education gap: community persons as instructors

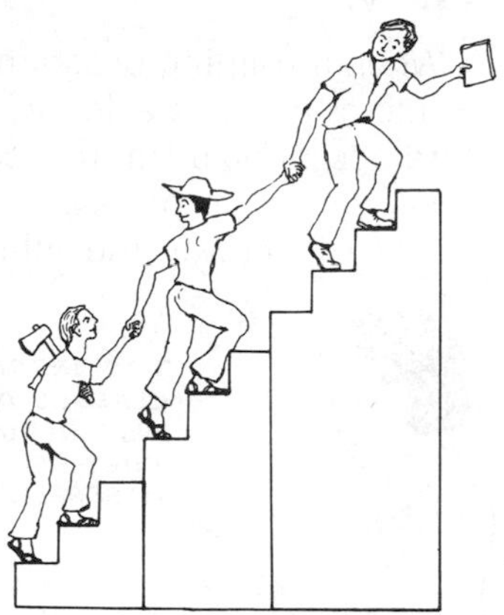

When there is a wide 'education gap' between instructor and students, try, instead of bridging it, to close it or avoid it. This means trying to find or prepare instructors who:

- are from the same immediate area as the health workers-in-training
- speak the local language
- have the same cultural and social background (a farmer, worker, father, mother, etc.)
- have had more or less the same amount of formal education as those they teach (although they may have had far more experience or training in health care at the community level)
- dress, act, speak, and feel as equals to the students and villagers

It is important that instructors be culturally close to the students. But they also need enough basic knowledge and skills (in health care, in problem solving, and in teaching) to help students learn effectively. At first it may be difficult to find local persons with this combination of culture and skills. During the first few years, 'outside' instructors may be needed. But their first responsibility should be to **prepare local people to take over most or all of the instruction.** The more outstanding and experienced health workers are often the best ones for the job.

CAN LOCAL PERSONS BECOME EFFECTIVE INSTRUCTORS OF HEALTH WORKERS?

Health professionals may be skeptical (doubtful) about whether villagers can make effective instructors. But community-based programs in many countries have found that:

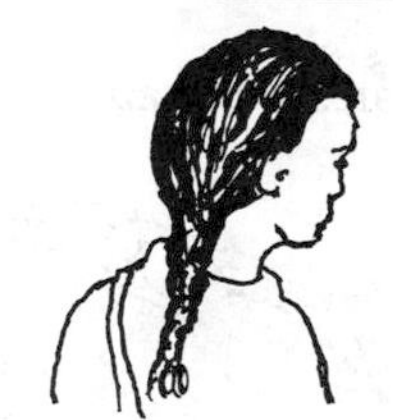

Experienced village health workers—with appropriate preparation, back-up, and friendly criticism from the learning group—can make excellent instructors.

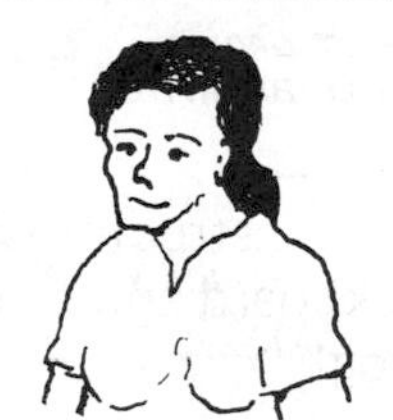

Just as with doctors and nurses, villagers who make good instructors are exceptional. The challenge is to find persons with the right combination of attitudes, interests, and talents, and then to create the situation that permits and helps them to grow.

STRENGTHS AND WEAKNESSES OF VILLAGE-LEVEL INSTRUCTORS

A story:

When a training program is taught and run by village-level instructors, certain problems and obstacles are avoided. But others commonly arise. Once, when we were observing a training course taught by villagers, a visiting nurse was present. Herself a trainer of health auxiliaries in a neighboring program, she was highly critical of the way the village-level instructors conducted the course:

TOO INFORMAL.
CLASSES DO NOT BEGIN ON TIME.
INSTRUCTORS SLOPPILY DRESSED.
THEY USE VULGAR EXPRESSIONS.
MISSPELLED WORDS.
INCOMPLETE COVERAGE OF MATERIAL.
FREQUENT STRAYING FROM THE TOPIC BEING TAUGHT.
TOO MUCH NOISE AND LAUGHTER.
INACCURATE INFORMATION.

After listening to her many complaints, the village instructors invited the nurse to give a class to show them how to do it better. They suggested a class on "The Human Body and How It Works."

So the visiting nurse presented a class on "Anatomy and Physiology." It was carefully timed: 40 minutes of lecture with 10 minutes for questions at the end. She briefly and expertly covered each of the body systems, naming the major organs and stating their functions. When she finished, she asked one of the health workers if he had understood. He slowly shook his head. "I didn't understand beans!" She called on student after student to see what they had learned. But with the exception of two who had studied in secondary school, her lecture had gone completely over their heads. One of the village instructors had made a list of over 60 words she had used, which no one understood. He asked her to explain some of the words. But each time she tried, she used 2 or 3 more words that nobody understood.

The students then asked if the nurse would be willing to give the class over again, but more simply. The nurse admitted she didn't think she could. She asked one of the village instructors to do it for her.

The next day, one of the local instructors led a discussion about "The Body and How it Works" (not "Anatomy and Physiology"). Rather than lecturing, he started by holding up a box. He challenged the students to ask as many questions as they could in order to find out whether the box contained something living or not. They asked questions like:

DOES IT GROW?
DOES IT BREATHE?
DOES IT MOVE BY ITSELF?
DOES IT NEED WATER AND FOOD?
DOES IT PEE AND SHIT?
CAN IT MAKE BABIES OR SEEDS?

The instructor wrote the questions on the blackboard and then opened the box. Out jumped a frog!

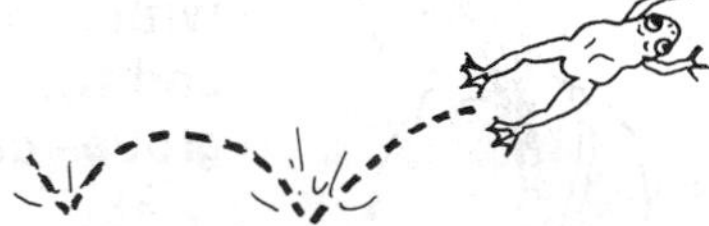

Next, the instructor asked how we, as people, also do each of the things listed on the blackboard. He started with what the class knew about the body, and built on that, asking questions like:

WHAT BECOMES OF THE FOOD WE EAT?

WHAT HAPPENS TO US WHEN WE DON'T GET ENOUGH FOOD?

At one point, he asked two of the students to run fast around the building, and had the group observe them and take their pulse. Then he asked:

WHY DO WE SWEAT, BREATHE HARD, AND HAVE A FAST PULSE WHEN WE RUN OR DO HARD WORK?

WHAT IS THE PURPOSE OF THE HEART AND LUNGS?

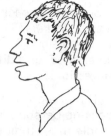

After the group had given their ideas (which were mostly correct), he asked:

WHY DO PEOPLE WHO ARE VERY PALE GET TIRED MORE QUICKLY?

WHAT IS THE PURPOSE OF BLOOD?

He spoke in the people's language, using the village names for different parts of the body: 'guts' for intestines and 'belly' for abdomen.

In this way, the students themselves were able to piece together many of the different systems of the body and their functions. It was like solving a mystery or putting together a puzzle. The students loved it. And everyone understood. The class was noisy and went overtime, but no one objected—this time not even the nurse!

Of course, some of the body systems were forgotten, and others were barely mentioned.

"There is a lot more to the body than we have talked about today," explained the group leader at the close of the class. "But we will talk about other parts of the body and how they work when we need to, to understand about particular health problems as they come up." (See p. **5**-11.)

By the time the visiting nurse left, she had changed her mind—and said so. She had seen that, in spite of certain inaccuracies and shortcomings of the teaching, the students had learned more and taken a more active part in the classes taught by their fellow villagers!

Not all the credit is due, of course, to the fact that the instructors were villagers themselves. Much of the difference was in the teaching methods they used. But **the technique of building on the students' own knowledge and experience is often easier for a local person who shares a common background.**

In Project Piaxtla in Mexico, we (the authors) and other outsiders used to do most of the teaching for the health worker training courses. Then, several years ago, the local health team (made up entirely of experienced village health workers) took charge of the training. The first year that the course was taught by the village team only, 3 students were present who had taken previous courses taught by outsiders. When asked which course they thought better and more appropriate, all 3 agreed, "This one, taught by the village health workers." Their reasons:

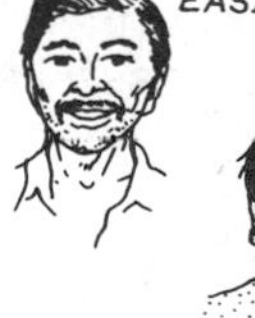

EASIER TO UNDERSTAND.

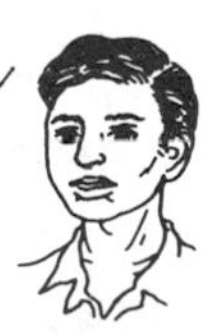

THE INSTRUCTORS SEEM TO KNOW JUST HOW SLOW OR FAST TO GO TO BE SURE WE UNDERSTAND BUT DON'T GET BORED.
WE FEEL MORE COMFORTABLE WITH THE TEACHERS WHO ARE OUR OWN PEOPLE. IT MAKES LEARNING EASIER. IF THEY CAN UNDERSTAND SOMETHING, WE KNOW WE CAN, TOO!

'TRAINING ORGANIZERS' OR 'BACK-UP PERSONS'

Supportive back-up (supervision) can be as important for instructors as for health workers. This is true for instructors who are doctors and nurses, as well as for village-level instructors. **We all can benefit when someone with more experience, or a different perspective, observes our teaching and makes helpful suggestions.**

The person who provides this sort of support and suggestions can be called a 'back-up person', 'advisor', or 'training organizer'. Since her main goal is to help people meet their needs, the training adviser should not only be an experienced health worker, but should also sympathize and identify with the poor.

The role of the training organizer in a health worker training program in Bangladesh has been described as follows:*

"The 'Training Organizer' will sit in the class, quietly and discreetly at the back, and then review the class with the teacher afterwards, with emphasis on points like:

- Did the message get across clearly?
- Did the trainees have an active or passive role in the class?
- Were visual aids used effectively?
- How many of the trainees fell asleep before the end of the class?

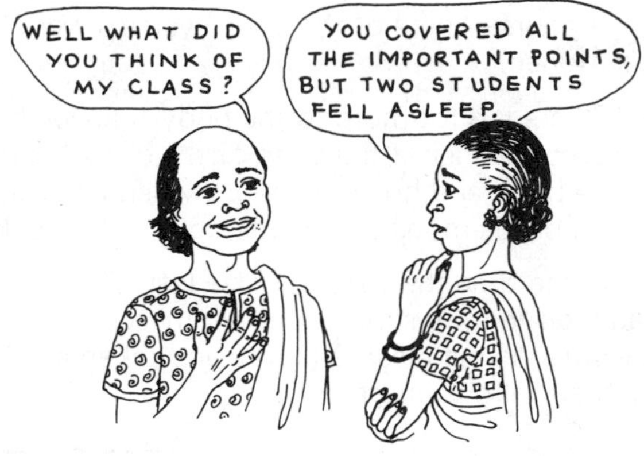
WELL WHAT DID YOU THINK OF MY CLASS?
YOU COVERED ALL THE IMPORTANT POINTS, BUT TWO STUDENTS FELL ASLEEP.

"The 'Training Organizer' will review some of the above points with the trainees as well as the teacher."

Village health workers can make excellent instructors. But at first they often lack basic teaching skills and experience in course planning. It is here that the training organizer can help. But it is essential that he or she be willing to stay in the background and let the community-based instructors assume full responsibility. Once again:

Advise, don't boss!

To emphasize the secondary role of this advisor, 'training assistant' might be a better term than 'training organizer'. To move into this back-up role is a natural step for the outside professional or foreigner who has been active as an instructor early in the program. It allows the outside person to begin phasing herself out, to pass teaching and organizing responsibilities to local workers. In time, outstanding local instructors (who started off as community health workers) may likewise be able to take over the role of 'training assistant'. In this way, the outsider moves one more step into the background. The sooner she is not needed, the more successful she has been.

* From a personal communication with Martin Schweiger, Medical Adviser/Administrator, Rangput Dinajpur Rehabilitation Service Program, Lalmanirhat-Rangpur, Bangladesh.

CHAPTER 3

Planning a Training Program

The primary aim of this book is to look at ways of learning, not to discuss the details of a training program. But the way a training course is planned, and by whom, can greatly affect how teaching and learning take place.

Many approaches are possible. But two things are of key importance: 1) **Each training program should be designed according to the special needs and circumstances of the area it serves.** 2) **Each course should be adapted to the experiences and needs of each new group of students.**

We have reasons for placing this chapter on planning after those on approaches to learning and selection of health workers, instructors, and advisers. The educational approach and the persons involved can affect how course content is decided. For if a 'community-strengthening' approach is taken, **some of the course planning is best done by the participants.**

THE TRAINING COURSE AS PART OF A LARGER LEARNING PROCESS

In this chapter we focus on training courses for health workers. But keep in mind that 'training' takes place in many ways and on many levels.

The training course is—or should be—closely linked with a vital network of continuous learning and teaching that takes place in the community. The diagram below shows some of the possibilities.

THE NETWORK OF LEARNING FOR COMMUNITY HEALTH

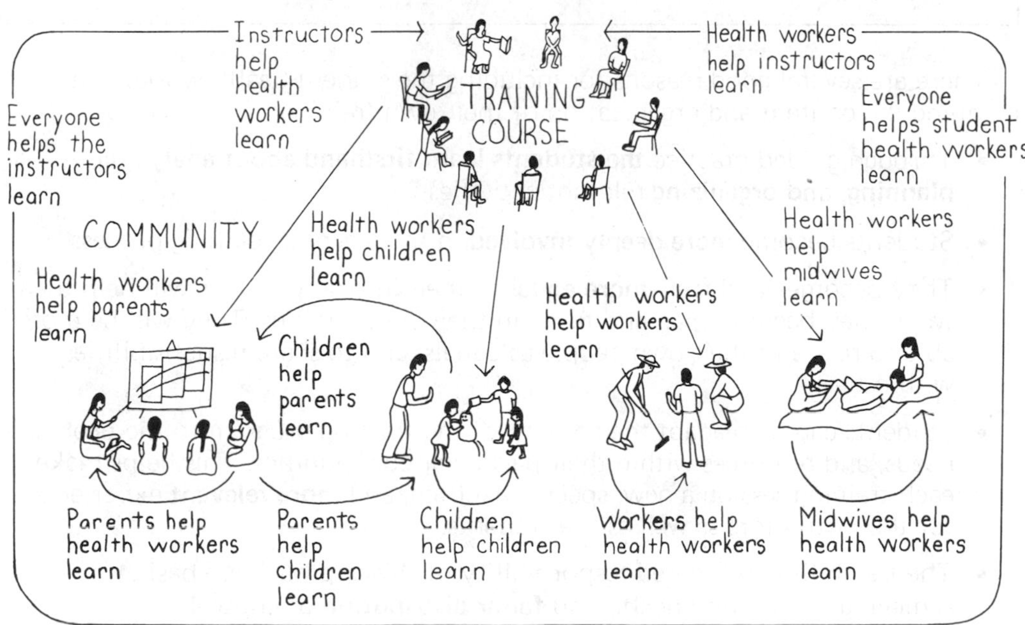
Instructors help health workers learn
Health workers help instructors learn
TRAINING COURSE
Everyone helps the instructors learn
Everyone helps student health workers learn
COMMUNITY
Health workers help children learn
Health workers help midwives learn
Health workers help parents learn
Health workers help workers learn
Children help parents learn
Parents help health workers learn
Parents help children learn
Children help children learn
Workers help health workers learn
Midwives help health workers learn

THE IMPORTANCE OF HAVING STUDENTS TAKE PART IN THE PLANNING

The ability to **plan effectively**—to **analyze** and **organize** what needs to be done—is basic to the self-reliance of every individual, family, and community. Planning skills are especially important for health workers who are to become leaders, teachers, and organizers in their communities.

This does not mean that a training program must include special classes on 'planning and management'. Instead, it points to the value of **including the student group in the planning process.**

LESS APPROPRIATE
MORE APPROPRIATE
TODAY WE ARE GOING TO STUDY ABOUT PLANNING AND MANAGEMENT!
LET'S PLAN THIS PROGRAM TOGETHER, BASED ON YOUR VILLAGES' NEEDS!

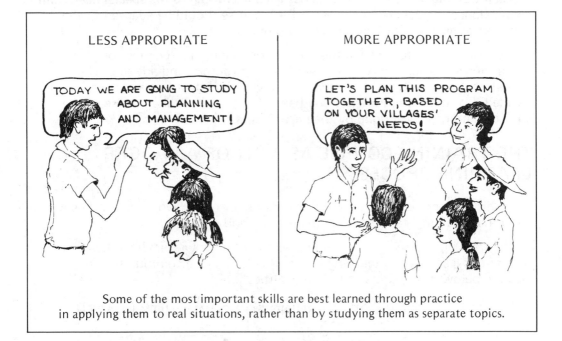

Some of the most important skills are best learned through practice in applying them to real situations, rather than by studying them as separate topics.

There are several good reasons for including the student health workers in planning the content and organization of their own training:

- Through guided practice **the students learn firsthand about analyzing, planning, and organizing** relevant activities.
- Students become **more deeply involved** in the teaching-learning process.
- They become—and feel—**more equal** to their instructors. This will help them when they begin to plan and teach in their communities. They will be more able to relate to their own people as equals, and to share responsibilities with others.
- Students can help adapt the content of the training program to the problems, needs, and resources within their particular communities. This helps make each training session a new, special, exciting, and **more relevant** experience—for the instructors as well as the students.
- The flexibility and shared responsibility of this approach are basic to achieving community health and **fairer distribution of control.**

A COMMON PROBLEM: PLANNING THINGS BACKWARDS

- Why are so many health worker training courses taught by persons who have no community experience?
- Why do so many instructors give more class time to the study of anatomy and filling out forms than to child diarrhea, nutrition, and teaching methods?
- Why do so many courses fail to prepare health workers to solve many of the basic problems they will face?

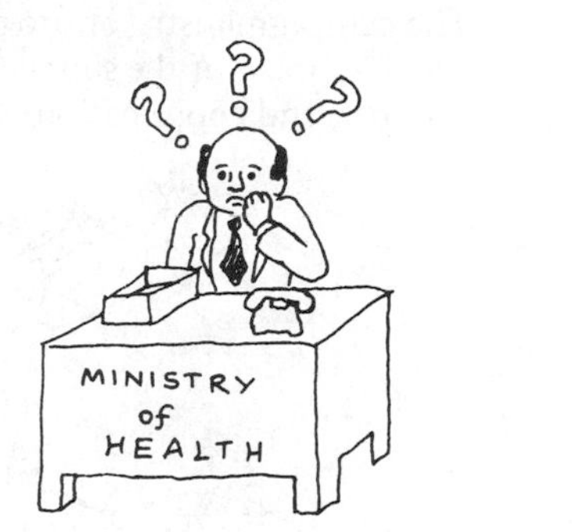
MINISTRY
of
HEALTH

The answers to these questions lie in the fact that training programs too often are planned backwards. The time and place are fixed, instructors chosen, and course content decided *before* planners consider the special difficulties, resources, customs, and strengths of the people involved. As a result, what is taught does not match either the community's needs or the students' abilities.

Many training programs today teach too much of what matters little—and too little of what matters most. To make things worse, the *way they teach* is often as unrelated to people's needs as is the *subject matter.*

If training is to be appropriate (adapted to people's needs, resources, customs, and abilities), things need to be done the other way around:

1st: Invite the people from the communities that the program will affect to determine and make known their needs.

2nd: Let the people's needs, resources, and abilities determine what should be taught, and to whom.

3rd: Let **what** should be taught, **how,** and to **whom,** determine **who** should teach, **where,** for **how long,** and in **what way.**

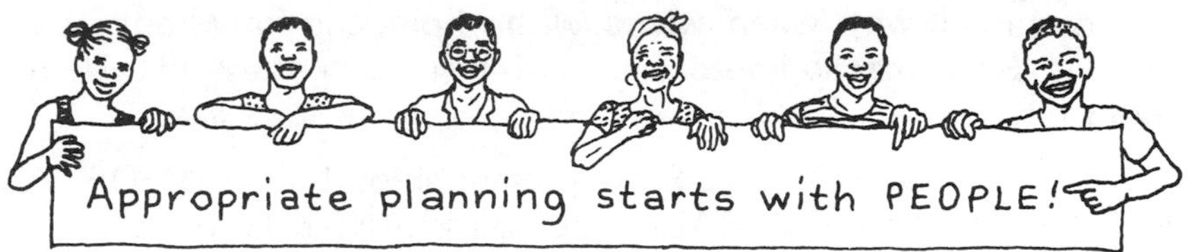
Appropriate planning starts with PEOPLE!

This people-centered or 'decentralized' approach to planning can be relatively easy for small programs that are community based. But it may be extremely difficult for a large, regional program. An appropriate approach may still be possible, however, if those in positions of central authority are willing to:

- Permit planning and basic decisions to take place at the community level.
- Act not as a controlling body, but as a center for communications, advice, support, and supply.

} the decentralized or people-centered approach

THE DECENTRALIZED APPROACH TO PLANNING

(the solid arrows show the main direction of flow)

The central ministry or program provides most of the supplies, support, and coordination.

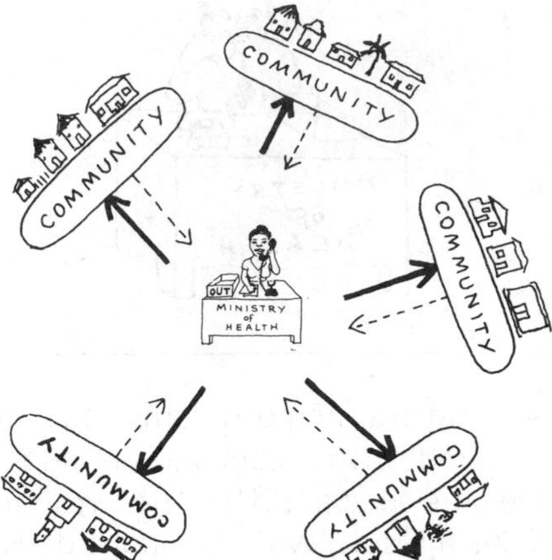

The communities provide most of the advice, planning, and control.

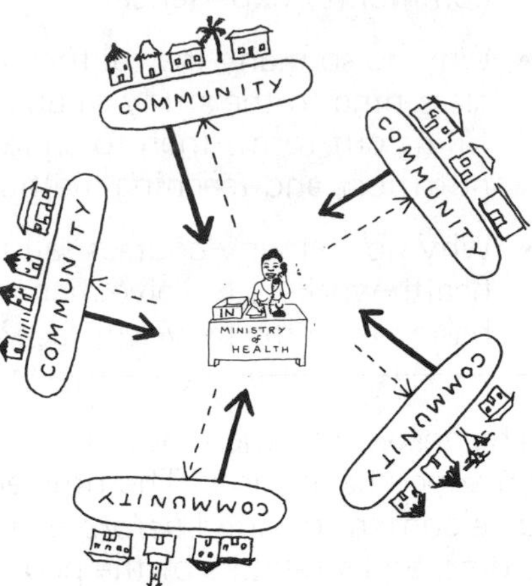

When groups are very large, central planning-and-control very easily becomes rigid, bureaucratic, change resistant, and corrupt. **Planning-and-control has more chance of being appropriate, flexible, and responsive to human needs when it takes place in groups that are small enough for everyone to know each other.**

DECIDING HOW MUCH TO PLAN IN ADVANCE AND HOW MUCH TO PLAN DURING THE COURSE

As we have noted, it is advisable to leave some of the planning of a training course until after it begins. This allows the course content to be planned or modified according to the students' interests, experiences, needs, and capabilities.

Clearly, however, some planning must be done in advance. Someone has to make decisions about **why, when, where, with whom,** and **for whom** the training will take place. **Resources** and **needs** must also be considered. And certain **preparations** need to be made.

On the next four pages (**3**-5 to **3**-8) we present an outline of IMPORTANT CONSIDERATIONS FOR OVERALL COURSE PLANNING. It includes:

Section A: Planning to be done before the training course begins
Section B: Continued planning after the training course begins
Section C: Planning and programming after the course is completed

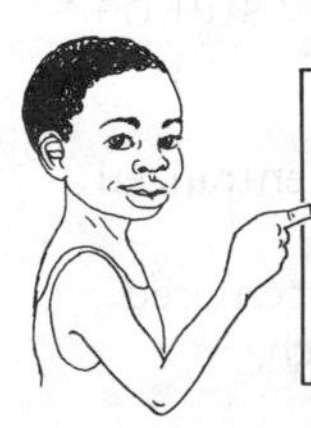

Note: The outline to follow is intended as a sort of checklist and question raiser. You do not have to read it in detail as you read through this chapter. Refer to it as you need to when planning a course.

IMPORTANT CONSIDERATIONS FOR OVERALL COURSE PLANNING

A. Planning to be done before the training course begins:

1. FIRST CONSIDERATIONS— PURPOSES AND QUESTIONS

- Whose needs will the training program be primarily designed to meet?
- Will it only **extend** the existing health system, or will it help to **change** it?
- How much will it prepare the health worker to understand and deal with the social (economic, cultural, political) causes of ill health?
- Will it make the poor more **dependent,** or help them to be more **self-reliant?** Will it promote or resist social change?
- What are the general goals and objectives of the program? (To express goals in terms of numbers and dates is probably unwise at this stage. Why?)
- Who is (or should be) involved in all these decisions?

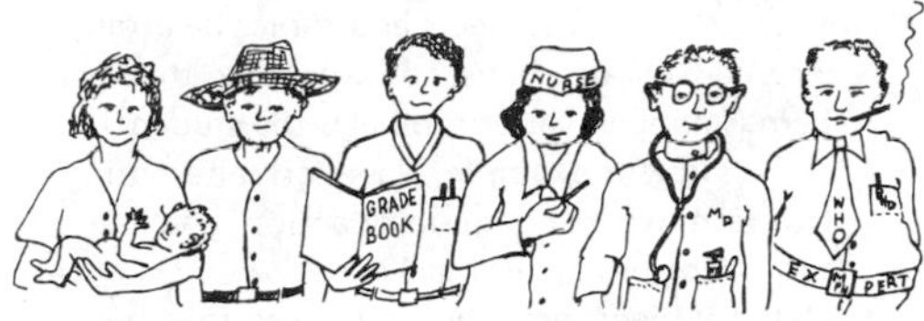

2. OBSERVATION OF NEEDS AND RESOURCES

(Talking with a few observant persons from the area can often provide more useful information than a census or elaborate 'community diagnosis', at far lower cost, more quickly, and with less abuse.)

Information worth considering:

- Common health problems: how frequent and how serious?
- Causes of main problems: physical and social, coming from inside and outside the community.
- People's attitudes, traditions, and concerns.
- Resources: human, physical, economic, from inside and outside the area.
- Characteristics of possible health workers: age, experience, education, interest, etc.
- Possible choices of instructors and training organizers.
- Possible sources of funding and assistance. (Which are more appropriate?)
- Reports and experiences of other programs.
- Obstacles: certain, likely, and possible.

3. EARLY DECISIONS— Who? Where? How many? When?

- **Selection of health workers:** by the community, by the health program, or by both? (How can selection of a health worker be a learning experience for the community?)
- **Selection of instructors and advisers:**
  - How much understanding and respect do they have for village people? Do they treat them as equals?
  - How committed are they to working toward social change?
  - Do they have the necessary knowledge and skills (public health, education, group dynamics, community organization, medicine, etc.) or are they willing to learn?

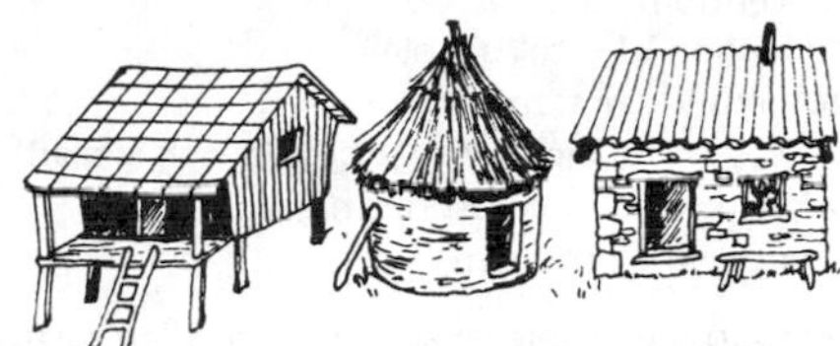

- **Location:**
  - Where will the training take place? Near or far? Village or city? Why?
  - Where will everyone eat and sleep? In hotels? In special facilities? With village families?

  (How can these decisions influence what they will learn?)
- **Numbers:** How many students will take part in the training course? (Beyond 12 or 15, quality of training usually decreases. This must be weighed against the need to train more health workers.)
- **Timing:**
  - How long will the training course last?
  - What time of year is best? (Consider how these decisions may affect who can take part in the course.)
  - Will the training be done in one continuous stretch, or be divided into short blocks so that students can return home (and practice what they have learned) between sessions?

  (Whose needs and opinions should be considered in answering these questions?)
- **Funding:**
  - From where? How much money should come from outside the local area?
  - What are the interests of possible funding groups?
  - What are the advantages and disadvantages of asking communities to pay part of the cost of training their health worker?
  - How can costs be kept low? How much is needed?
- **Follow-up and support:**
  - What opportunities may there be for continued learning or training after the course is over?
  - What kind of support or supervision will the health workers receive?

  (Why is it important to consider follow-up before the training program begins?)

4. ANALYSIS OF PRIORITIES
(deciding what is most important)

Problems can be compared by considering the following:
- How common are they?
- How serious are they?
- How contagious are they?
- How much concern do people feel about them?
- How much do they affect other problems?
- How much could a community health worker do about them in terms of . . .
  - diagnosis and treatment?
  - referral, when needed?
  - prevention?
  - education of local people?
  - community action?
- How easy or difficult will it be to teach a health worker to take safe, responsible action with respect to the problem?

Then group the problems according to their relative importance, or ***priority,*** and decide which ones to include in the course. (Be sure to include common social problems that affect health—such as drinking, overuse and misuse of medicines, local forms of exploitation of the poor, and misuse of resources—as well as physical diseases.)

5. RE-EXAMINING OBJECTIVES
- In view of the information you have gathered and analyzed, how can the training program be best designed . . .
  - so that it prepares health workers to help the people in their villages solve their problems and needs?
  - so that it is adapted to fit the particular strengths and weaknesses of the students?

6. ORGANIZING STUDY MATERIAL FOR APPROPRIATE LEARNING
- What general subject areas and specific topics might be taught in order to prepare students to act upon the important problems and needs in their communities?
- How many hours of organized study time will there be during the course?
- How much time is needed to adequately cover each topic?
- How can the time available be best divided among the different topics, according to their priority?
- Which topics are best approached through classroom learning, through practice (in clinic, community, or field), or a combination?

(At this point, some program planners make a list for each subject area, stating exactly what the health workers should know and be able to do. What are the strengths and weaknesses of this approach? See Chapter 5.)

7. PLANNING FOR BALANCE
- How can the subject matter be approached so as to maintain an appropriate balance between . . .
  - classwork and practical experience?
  - learning in the training center and learning in the community?
  - preventive and curative health care?
  - physical and social causes of ill health?
  - the needs of the poor and the requirements of those in positions of control?
  - caution and innovation?
  - health skills, teaching skills, and leadership skills?
  - work and play?

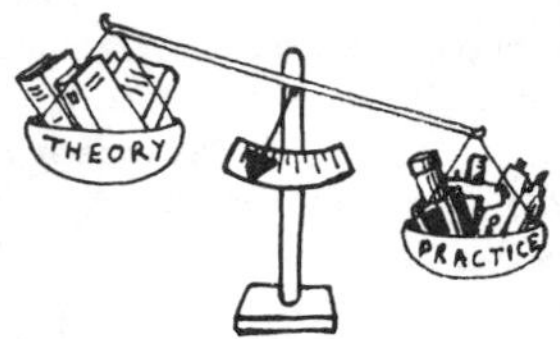

8. PREPARING A ROUGH TIMETABLE OR CLASS SCHEDULE
(without details, to be changed later)
- How can different subjects and topics be arranged, according to hours, days, and weeks, so that . . .
  - there is enough variety to keep the students interested (for example, classwork alternating with farm work, community action, and learning of practical skills)?
  - related subjects are scheduled close together or in a logical order?
  - more difficult subjects come early in the day, and more fun subjects later (when people are tired)?
  - all key subject matter is included?
  - high-priority subjects are given more emphasis in the training course?
  - skills and knowledge needed for immediate use and practice are learned early (for example, learning about medical history, physical exams, preventive advice, Road to Health charts)?
- How can study time and free time be best arranged to meet students' and instructors' needs?
- How can the schedule be kept open and flexible enough to allow for unplanned learning opportunities and special needs as they arise? (It helps to leave the last week of the course unscheduled, to allow for review and for making up 'displaced classes'.)
- How can the schedule be presented in a clear, simple form that can be easily seen and understood by students and instructors?

WEEKLY PLAN

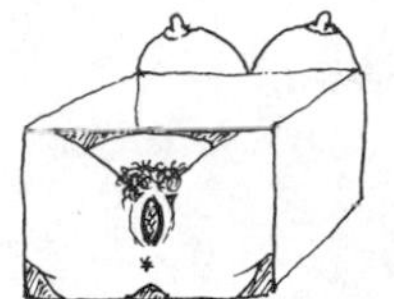
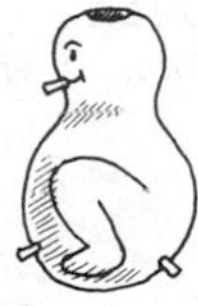
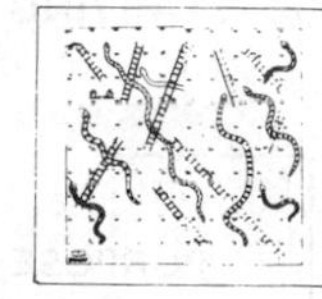

9. PLANNING APPROPRIATE TEACHING METHODS AND AIDS

- What teaching approach is best suited to persons who are more used to learning from experience than from lectures and books?
- What approaches to learning will help the health worker be an effective teacher in his community?
- What attitudes on the part of the teacher will encourage the health worker to share knowledge gladly and treat others as equals?
- What teaching methods might aid the health worker in helping community people to become more confident and self-reliant?
- What teaching aids can be used that will lead the health worker to make and invent teaching aids after returning to his village?
- What approach to learning will best prepare the health worker to help his people understand and work together to solve their biggest problems?
- What approach to health problems will enable the health worker to learn how to approach the solving of other community problems?
- What can be done to ensure that all learning is related to important needs?
- How can classwork be made more friendly and fun?
- How can tests and exams be presented so that students use them to help each other rather than to compete? How can tests and exams be used to judge the instructor as well as the students?

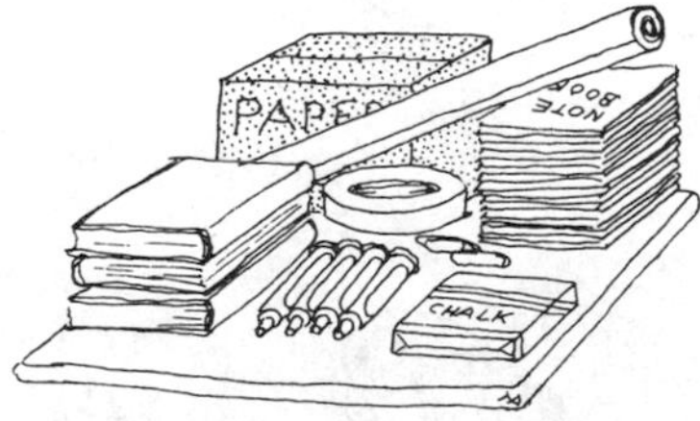

10. GETTING READY AND OBTAINING SUPPLIES

- What preparations are needed before the course begins? (transportation, eating and sleeping arrangements, study area, wash area, etc.)
- What furnishings and teaching materials are needed to begin? (benches, blackboard, etc.)
- What can be done if some of these are not ready on time?

11. DETAILED PLANNING OF ACTIVITIES AND CLASSES FOR THE BEGINNING OF THE COURSE

- How many days of classes and activities should be planned in detail before the course begins?
- Why is it important that the details of all the classes and activities ***not*** be planned in advance?

B. Continued planning after the training course begins:

12. INVOLVING STUDENTS IN PLANNING THE COURSE CONTENT (based on their experience and the needs in their communities)

- Why is it important that the students take part in planning the course?
- How can the students' participation in planning help them to learn about . . .
  - examining and analyzing the needs in their communities?
  - recognizing both the strengths and the weaknesses of their people's customs?
  - ways to plan and organize a learning group?
  - the value of learning by doing, and of respecting and building on their own experiences?
  - shared decision making?

13. REVISING THE PLAN OF STUDIES (COURSE CONTENT) ACCORDING TO STUDENT SUGGESTIONS

- To what extent do the priorities determined by the students, according to problems and needs in their own villages, correspond to those already considered by the instructors and planners? (How do you explain the similarities and differences?)
- How important is it to revise the course plans in order to better meet the concerns and expressed needs of the student group?

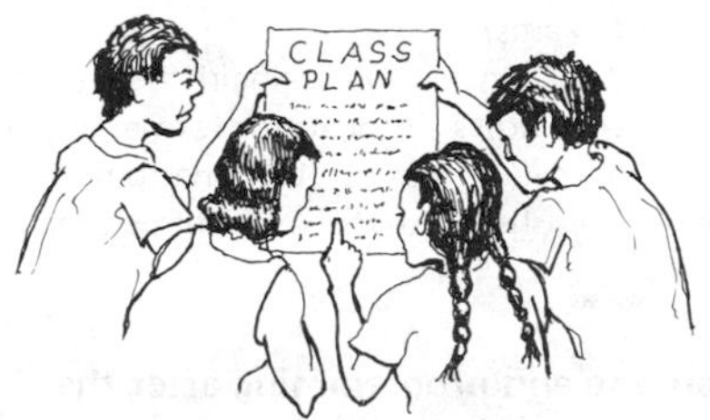

14. PREPARING INDIVIDUAL CLASSES AND ACTIVITIES

- How detailed should class plans be?
- How far in advance should a class or activity be planned? Why?
- Is it helpful to use a particular outline or formula for preparing a class? If so, what should it include?
- Can each class or activity be planned to include . . .
  - all of the basic points to be learned or considered?
  - active student participation and interaction?
  - use of appropriate learning aids?
  - opportunities for the students to explore questions and discover answers for themselves?
  - practice in solving problems similar to those health workers will meet in their work?
  - a chance for students to summarize what they have learned and to ask questions?
- To what extent can students take part in the preparation of classes and of teaching aids? (Is this important? Why?)

15. CONTINUED REVISION OF THE SCHEDULE—to make room for new ideas, learning opportunities, needs, and problems as they arise

- What are the advantages and disadvantages to keeping the program open and flexible? (How might this influence a health worker's ability to work toward, or tolerate, change in his or her community?)

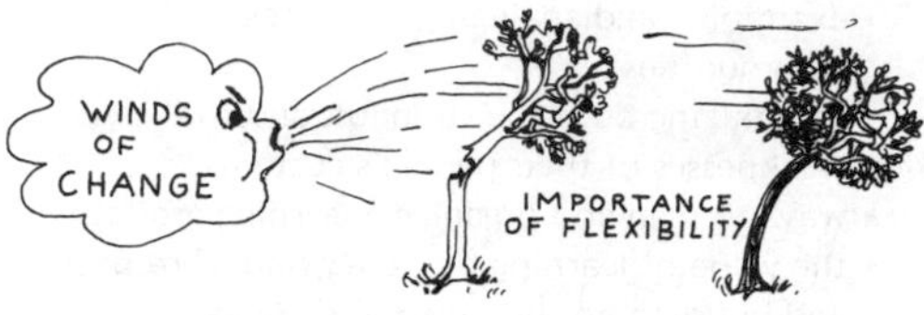

16. EVALUATION DURING THE TRAINING PROGRAM—to consider how it might be improved (see Chapter 9)

- In what ways can this be done?
- Who should be involved?
- What is the value of . . .
  - round-table discussions in which all students and staff have a chance to express their feelings about the program and each other?
  - similar discussions with members of the community where the training program takes place?
  - tests and exams?
  - setting specific goals and seeing if they are met?
- If evaluation studies (informal or formal, ongoing or final) are made, what can be done to help assure that results are useful and will be used?

C. Planning and programming after the course is completed:

17. FOLLOW-UP AND *FEEDBACK** (see Chapter 10)

- How can a supportive learning situation be continued between instructors and students, and among the students themselves, once the training course is completed?
- How can the following be involved in supporting the health worker:
  - members of the community (a health committee)?
  - other health workers?
  - program instructors, leaders, and advisers?
  - other support groups and referral centers?
- How can the experiences, successes, and difficulties of the health workers in their communities be recorded and used to make the next training course better than the last? (Can this be done so that health workers know they are contributing, rather than being judged?)

18. STARTING OVER

The whole process is repeated:

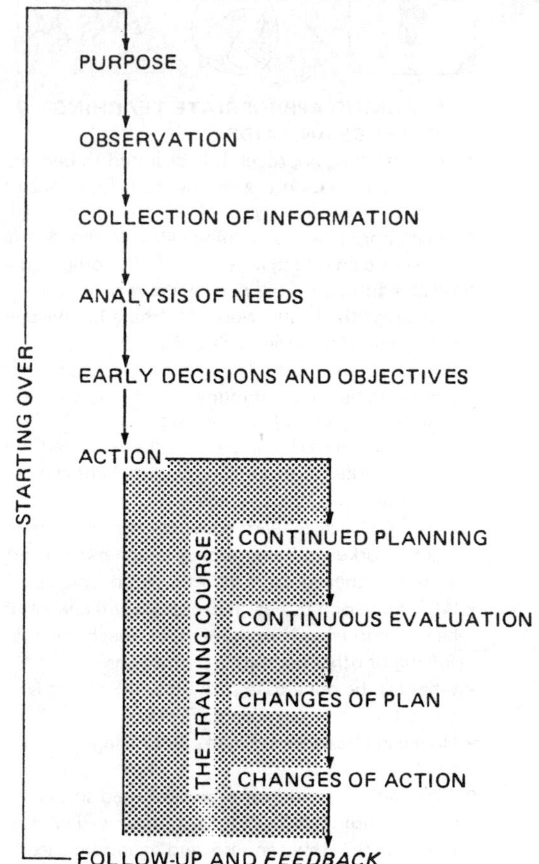

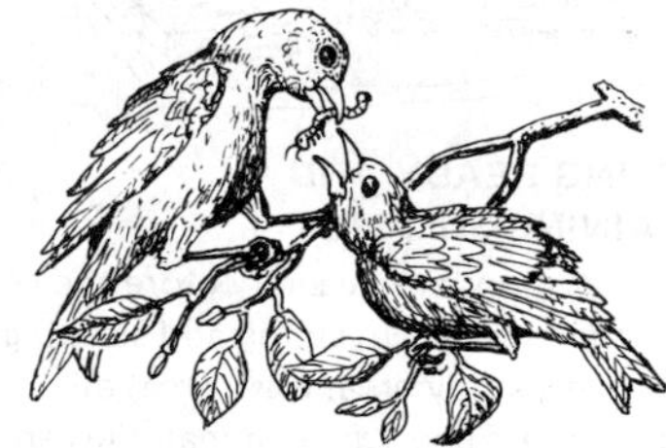

**FEEDBACK:* helpful ideas and suggestions sent back to planners or instructors by health workers.

EARLY DECISIONS

Location of training

It is best if training takes place in a situation close to that where health workers will work. Closeness in distance is convenient. But closeness in terms of community setting is essential. **Village health workers are best trained in a village.** That way, they can practice solving problems and carrying out activities under conditions much like those in their own communities.

If possible, training should take place in a village with a health center where students can gain clinical experience. It helps if the health center is run by experienced local health workers, and has strong community participation. **A small community-based health center is usually far more appropriate for training villagers than a large clinic or hospital** (see page 8-4). The closer the situation of learning to the situation in which health workers will later work, the better.

For the same reasons, it is important that the building in which training takes place—and even the furniture, if any—be similar to those in the villages of the health workers.

In this book and in *Where There Is No Doctor,* we often show drawings of health workers-in-training sitting on chairs or benches. That is because people customarily make and use such furniture in the villages of Latin America where we work. But in areas where people traditionally sit on the ground during meetings and discussions, it makes sense that the same traditions be observed in the training course.

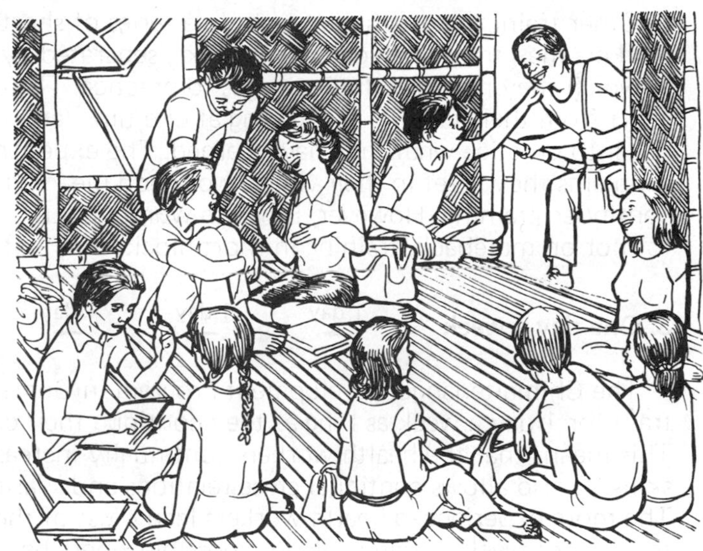

In places where villagers traditionally sit on the floor, it is appropriate that the training course follow the same custom. This drawing is from *Ang Maayong Lawas Maagum,* a Philippine equivalent of *Where There Is No Doctor.*

In the same way, there are advantages to having health workers live with families in the community rather than staying in a separate 'dormitory'. This is discussed further in Chapter 6.

Numbers

LESS APPROPRIATE

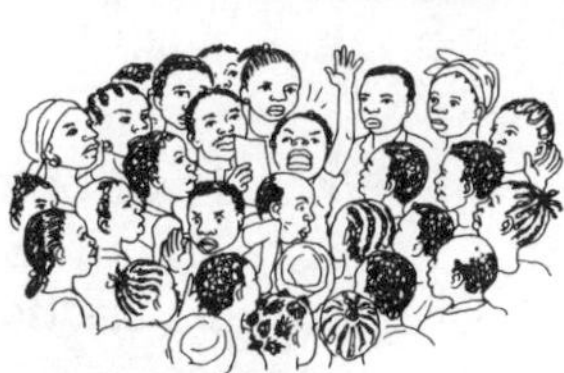

MORE APPROPRIATE

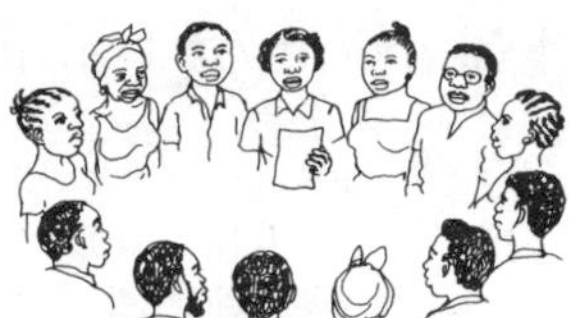

Many programs have found that from 12 to 15 is a good number of students for a course. A group this size is large enough for discussions to be exciting, but small enough so that everyone can take part.

Timing

1. Continuous 2 to 3 months →

Some training courses are taught in one continuous block of time. Two to three months is the average length of such a course. This is usually long enough for health workers to learn the basic skills needed for primary care. Yet it is short enough so that villagers with families and responsibilities at home can (sometimes) afford the time away.

2. Short blocks of training alternating with practice 2 weeks → 2 weeks → 2 weeks →

Other training courses are taught in a series of shorter blocks of time. Health workers may train for blocks of 2 weeks, separated by periods of 1 or 2 months in which they return to their villages to practice. This way health workers are not apart from their families for so long at one time, and they have a chance to put into practice what they have learned. The experience they gain and the problems they meet in their village work add meaning and direction to their continued training. However, if health workers must come a long distance by foot or on muleback, training in short blocks may not be practical.

3. One day a week 1 day → 1 day → 1 day → 1 day → 1 day → etc.

The Chimaltenango Development Program in Guatemala has health workers train for 1 day a week as long as they continue their community health work. This means that the health workers continually increase their knowledge and skills. It also allows continual close relations and sharing of ideas within the group. The more experienced health workers lead most of the training sessions. Clearly, this sort of weekly training is only possible where health workers live nearby or where public transportation is adequate.

Combination: Any combination of these plans is possible—for example, a 2-week initial course followed by training one day a week, or a 1-month course with follow-up training every 3 months.

Time of year: For health workers who are also farmers, certain times of year will be convenient for training, while others will be impossible. It is important that villagers be consulted about what time of year to have the training course, and whether training would be more convenient in one continuous period or in shorter blocks of time.

Funding

Most training courses we know about depend on funding from sources outside the area being served. The amount of outside funding varies greatly from program to program. As a general rule, **the more modest the funding, the more appropriate the training.**

The struggle to manage with very limited outside funding can be a valuable learning experience for those involved in a training program. It helps bring the program closer to the reality of the people it serves, and closer to the community as a whole.

For example, a community-based training program in Nuevo Leon, Mexico was begun with very little money. The students and instructors started by building their own mud-brick training center with the help of local villagers.

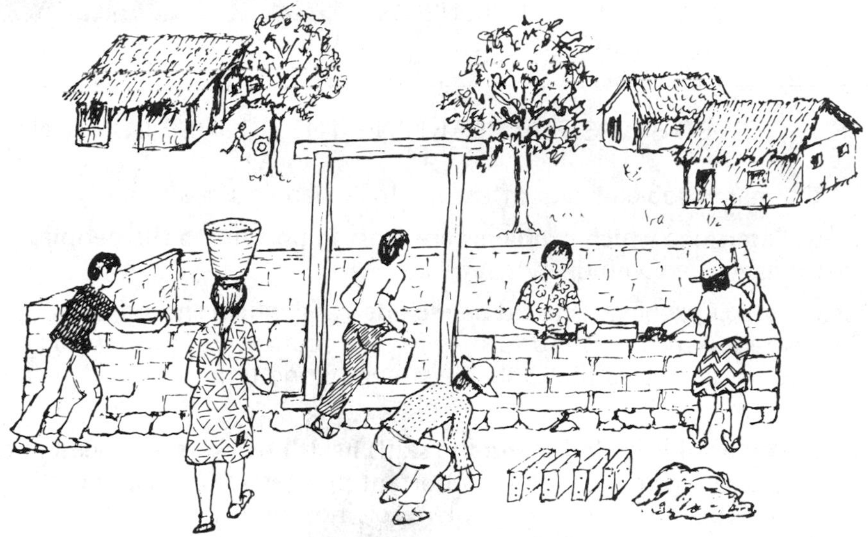

Later, when outside funding was stopped, the staff and students began raising goats and other animals, and opened a small butcher shop. Their struggle to survive economically brought the community and the health program closer together. When we visited, we were struck by the close, caring relationships between people in the village and participants in the training program.

Outside funding often means outside control. Therefore, it is usually wise to **allow no more than half the funding for a health or development activity to come from outside the area served.** If at least half the funding is provided locally, there is more of a chance that control of the program will also be local. Then, in a very real way, the program will belong to the people.

In Project Piaxtla, Mexico, each village that sends a student to the training course is encouraged to pay half of his or her living expenses during training. Other programs in Central America organize villagers to help with their health worker's farming or other work while he is away at training. This helps the village feel more responsibility for its health worker. And it helps the health worker feel more responsible to his village.

MAKING A ROUGH PLAN OF COURSE CONTENT

Before the training course begins, it helps to make a rough plan of what the course might cover—even though this may later be changed with help from the student group. As much as possible, the plan should be based on the needs of both the communities and the students. But the strengths, talents, and resources of the students and their communities also need to be taken into account.

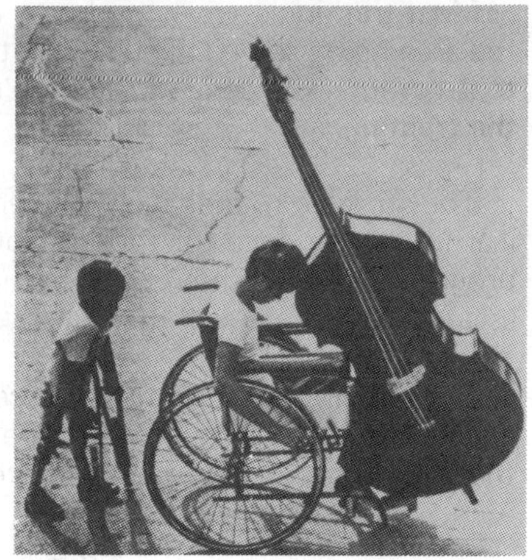

CONSIDER PEOPLE'S STRENGTHS AS WELL AS THEIR NEEDS.

SUGGESTED STEPS FOR PLANNING THE COURSE CONTENT

1. **List the main problems** that affect the local people's health and well-being.
2. Try to **determine which problems are most important to the people** (priorities in the community).
3. **Decide which problems should be included and which should be emphasized in the course** (priorities for the course). To do this, consider local factors as well as the probable strengths and limitations of the health workers.
4. **List the areas of knowledge and the skills health workers will need** in order to help people solve their more important problems. Arrange these into groups or subjects for active, problem-solving study.
5. Given the length of the course, **consider how much time may be needed** for each subject or study area.
6. For each subject, try to **balance discussion-type learning (classes) with learning by doing (practice).** Also seek a balance between curative, preventive, and teaching skills, physical work, and play.
7. **Make up a rough course plan,** including timetables for each week (but not in great detail, as these will probably be changed with the students' help).
8. **Prepare detailed plans for at least the first few days.**

In the rest of this chapter, we discuss these steps in greater detail. You may find these planning suggestions useful at 3 stages:

- before the course, to help instructors draw up a general course plan,
- during the course, to help the instructors and students adapt the course according to needs in their communities, and
- after the course, to help health workers and people in their communities plan activities according to their needs.

Step 1. Looking at and listing needs

To help a group of health workers (or villagers) plan a course of study or action according to their needs, the first step is to have them look carefully at their recent problems.

Ask each person to speak of his own problems and needs, both big and small. Someone can write the list on the blackboard or a large sheet of paper.

Ask questions that call for specific answers, so that people discuss problems from their own experiences.

LESS APPROPRIATE— too vague	MORE APPROPRIATE— specific
What are the worst problems of people in your village?	*What is the worst problem your family had this year?*

Although the focus will be on health problems, encourage people to mention other problems and concerns that also relate to health or well-being:

"Our chickens died."

"The crops failed."

"We had to sell our land to pay our debts."

"My neighbor let his cows loose in my cornfield."

Before deciding which health problems to begin discussing in class, one training program in the Philippines has the health workers visit different homes in the village. During these visits, they ask people what they feel to be their biggest problems and needs. This way the community's wishes are brought into the training and planning from the start.

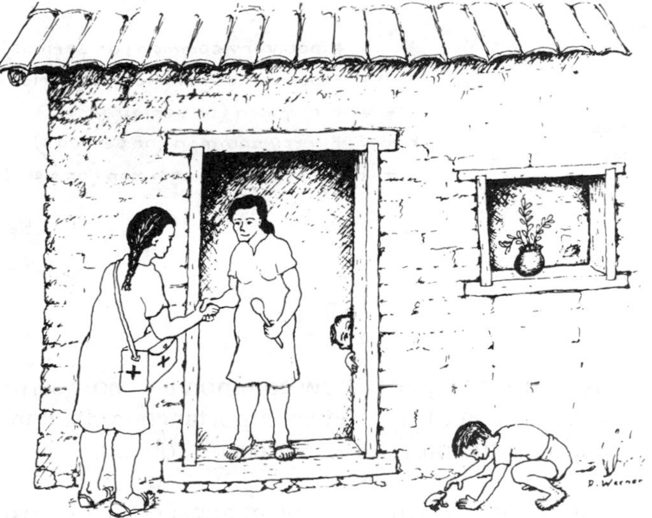

Talk to people about their problems and needs from the very start of training.

Step 2. Considering the relative importance of the different problems the group has listed

This can be done in several ways, some simpler, some more complete.

One way is to make a chart on a blackboard or a large piece of paper. Have the group discuss **how common** and **how serious** they feel each problem to be. Then mark from 1 plus (+) to 5 pluses (+++++) in each column, like this:

PROBLEM	HOW COMMON	HOW SERIOUS	HOW IMPORTANT
Babies have diarrhea	+ + + + +	+ + + +	9
Children have worms	+ + + +	+ +	6
Children very thin	+ + + +	+ + +	7
Skin sores	+ + + + +	+	6
Toothaches	+ +	+ + +	5
Chickens died	+ + +	+ + +	6
Too far to water	+ + + + +	+ +	7
Fever and chills	+ + +	+ + + +	7
Fathers often drunk	+ + +	+ + + +	
Crops failed	+ + +	+ + + + +	
Food in store too costly	+ + + +	+ + + +	
Heart attacks	+	+ + + +	
Women pale and weak	+ + +	+ + +	
Problems after birth	+ +	+ + + +	
Measles	+ +	+ + +	
Common colds	+ + + + +	+	

\+ not very common (or serious)
\+ + somewhat common (or serious)
\+ + + common (or serious)
\+ + + + very common (or serious)
\+ + + + + extremely common (or serious)

By considering both **how common** and **how serious** a problem is, the students can get an idea of its **relative importance in the community.** To help in this, they can add up the plus marks for each problem.

Ask the group which problem appears to be most important. (In this case it is diarrhea, with 9 pluses.) Then, which are next in importance? (Those with 8 pluses. Which are they?) And so on.

A more complete way to look at the relative importance of problems is to consider the following 4 questions for each problem:

1. How **COMMON** is the problem in the community?

2. How **SERIOUS** are the effects on individuals, families, communities?

3. Is it **CONTAGIOUS?** (Does it spread to other people?)

4. Is it **CHRONIC?** (Does it last a long time?)

Again, plus marks can be used to add up the results. But a more fun way that gets everyone involved is to use cut-out symbols:

SKULLS mean SERIOUS.

big skulls: EXTREMELY SERIOUS (deadly)

middle-sized skulls: VERY SERIOUS

small skulls: SERIOUS

SAD FACES  mean COMMON. The more common a problem is, the more faces you put next to it.

FACES WITH ARROWS  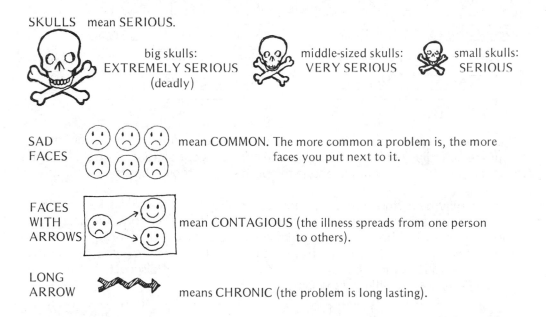 mean CONTAGIOUS (the illness spreads from one person to others).

LONG ARROW  means CHRONIC (the problem is long lasting).

These symbols can be made of flannel or soft cloth, to be used on a 'flannel-board' (see p. **11**-16). First, have the group members draw them and cut them out. They will need at least:

100 sad faces
15 skulls
15 faces with arrows
10 long arrows

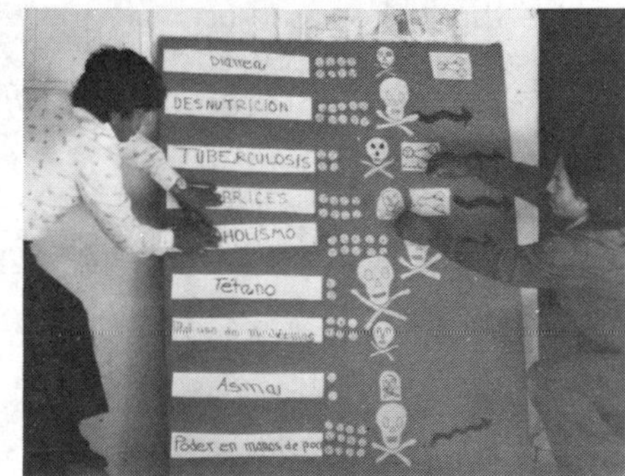

Use a different color for each symbol.

Now write the name of each problem on a strip of paper or cloth. Attach these strips to the flannel-board.

Then discuss the problems one by one. Have students come forward and place the symbols they think fit each problem.

When they are done, the flannel-board could look something like this:

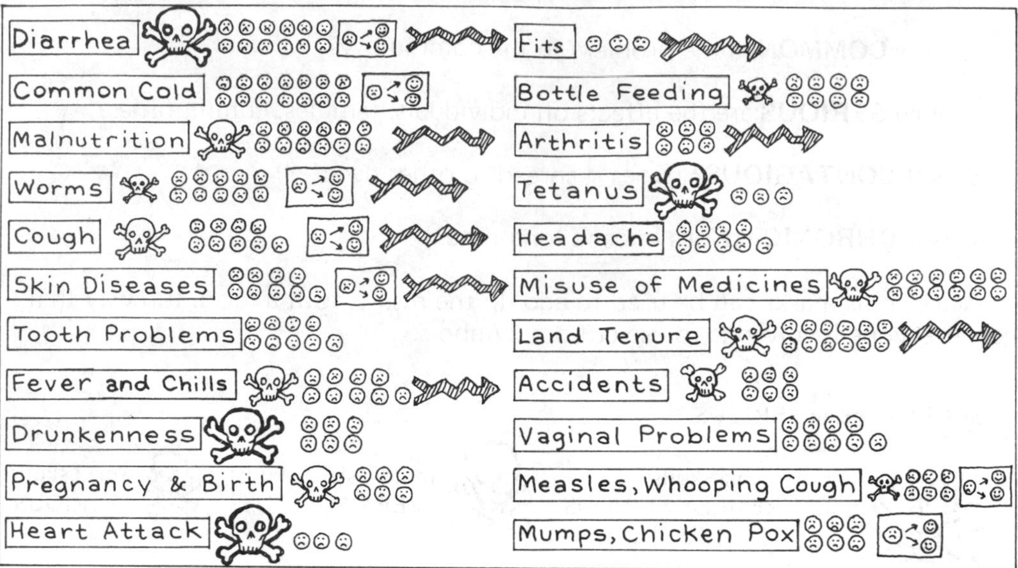

Let the students argue about how many sad faces to put up for 'cough' as compared to 'diarrhea', or whether 'drunkenness' is contagious or not. This will get them thinking and talking about the problems in their villages.

There may be differences of opinion, especially if the health workers come from different areas. For example, in Project Piaxtla in Mexico, some health workers come from hot, lowland villages where diarrhea, hookworm, and typhoid are more common. Others come from mountain villages where colds, bronchitis, and pneumonia are more common. So health workers will discover that problems and needs vary from village to village.

For those who cannot read:

Health workers can use these same methods with persons who cannot read. To show the problems, they can use simple drawings instead of words. Once the drawings are explained, people rarely forget what they represent.

Here is an example: ⟶

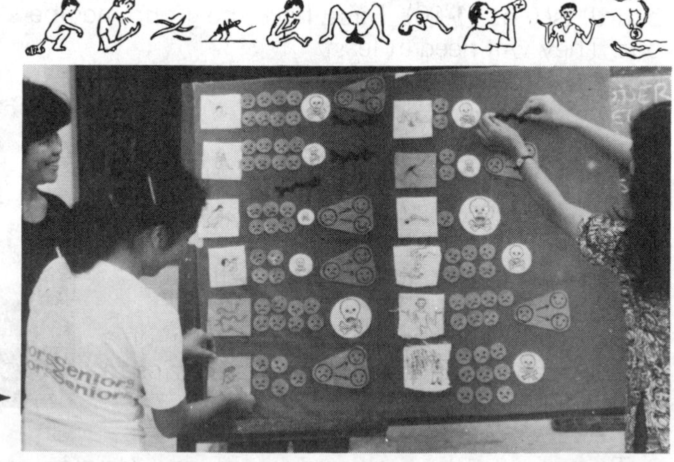

Can you identify each problem?

Step 3. Determining priorities for what to cover in the course

After looking at the relative importance, or priority, of the different problems found in the students' communities, the instructors need to consider how much emphasis, or priority, should be given to each of these problems in the course.

To do this, you can again make a chart. But this time ask some additional questions about each problem. For example:

- Are local people concerned about the problem?
- How much does it affect other health problems?
- What is the possibility for teaching effectively about the problem?
- How much would community health workers be likely to do to correct the problem, if taught?

Mark your answers with pluses (+++++) on a blackboard or a sheet of paper.

PROBLEM	HOW COMMON	HOW SERIOUS	PEOPLE'S CONCERN	HOW MUCH IT AFFECTS OTHER HEALTH PROBLEMS	POSSIBILITY FOR TEACHING PREVENTION OR TREATMENT	HOW MUCH CHW COULD OR WOULD DO ABOUT IT IF TAUGHT	IMPORTANCE TO BE GIVEN IN COURSE
Diarrhea	++++	++++	+++	++	++++	++++	21
Malnutrition	++++	+++	++	++++	++++	++++	21
Worms	++++	++	++++	++	++++	++++	20
Cough							
Common Cold	++++	+	++++	+	++	++	14
Pneumonia	++	+++	++	++	+++	++++	16
Tuberculosis	++	++++	+++	+++	++++	++++	20
Skin Diseases	+++	+	+++	+	+++	++++	15
Stomach ache	+++	++	+++	+	++	+++	14
Tooth problems	+++	+	+	+++	+++	++++	15
Fever	+++	++	+++	+++	++++	++++	19
Drunkenness	++	+++	++++	++++	+	+	15
Pregnancy & Birth	++	++	++	++++	+++	++++	17
Heart Attack	+	++	++	+	++	+	9
Epilepsy	+	++	+	+	++	+	8
Bottle Feeding	+++	+++	+	++++	++++	+++	18
Tetanus	+	++++	+++	+	++++	++	15
Headache	+++	+	+	+	++	+	9
Misuse of medicine	++++	+++	0	+++	++++	++	16
Land tenure	++++	++++	++++	++++	++++	+?	21
Accidents	++	+++	+++	++	+++	+++	16
Vaginal Problems	+++	+	++	++	+++	+++	14
Measles	++	++++	++	+++	+++	+++	17
Whooping Cough	++	+++	+++	++	+++	+++	16

Add up the plus marks for each problem to judge its relative importance for inclusion or emphasis in the course.

Suggestion: When working with a group of health workers you may **not** want to use this chart. It may be too complicated. Perhaps you will want to just discuss the 6 questions it considers.

Step 4. Listing appropriate areas of study

After looking carefully at the problems you want to cover in the course (based on people's needs), the next step is to consider:

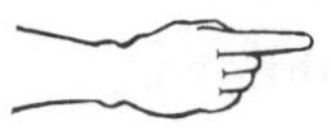

What skills, knowledge, and practice will health workers need to help people solve these problems?

The skills and knowledge health workers need to learn should be carefully analyzed (see Task Analysis, pages **5**-7 to **5**-9). Skills in both curative and preventive medicine will be important. But so will skills—and practice—in community organizing, teaching (of both adults and children), problem analysis, record keeping, and so on. Some programs include certain agricultural skills, veterinary skills, and even basic dentistry.

One of the most important areas of study for health workers concerns the way people relate to each other: Why people act and do things as they do! So health worker training should include learning about 'group dynamics', and even 'consciousness raising' or 'building social awareness'.

One community-based program in the Philippines spends more than half of training time helping health workers to gain an understanding of 'what makes people tick'.

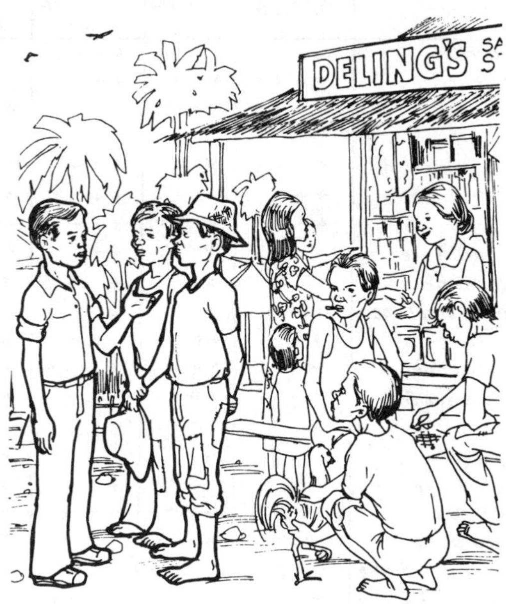

Drawing by Lino C. Montebon in ***Ang Maayong Lawas Maagum,*** a Philippine equivalent of ***Where There Is No Doctor.***

Based on the priorities of local problems, **list all the different areas of learning** or activity you think should be covered in the course. The subjects chosen must be realistic in terms of needs, resources, and time available for training. Then **arrange these subjects in sensible groups or 'areas of study'.** It will help if you organize these into 3 general categories:

- PREVENTIVE
- CURATIVE
- COMMUNITY OR SOCIAL

On the next page is an example of a blank **worksheet for planning the content of a training course.** This kind of sheet has been used by Project Piaxtla in Mexico. Following the blank worksheet is a copy of the same sheet with a list of possible study areas for health worker training. You are welcome to use this as a checklist. But probably you will want to omit some items and add others, according to your local situation.

Cut out and use as needed.

WORKSHEET FOR PLANNING THE CONTENT OF A TRAINING COURSE

estimated hours: ______
hours available: ______

estimate must be lowered by: ______ hours

Total hours of course time available: ___ hours per day x ___ days = ______ hours

SUBJECT UNDER CONSIDERATION	ESTIMATED HOURS NEEDED	RELATIVE PRIORITY (+ to +++++)	ADJUSTED NUMBER OF HOURS	CLASSROOM STUDY	PRACTICAL ACTIVITY	NOTES:

WORKSHEET FOR PLANNING THE CONTENT OF A TRAINING COURSE

estimated hours: ______
hours available: ______
estimate must be lowered by: ______ hours

Total hours of course time available: ___ hours per day x ___ days = ______ hours

SUBJECT UNDER CONSIDERATION	ESTIMATED HOURS NEEDED	RELATIVE PRIORITY (+ to +++++)	ADJUSTED NUMBER OF HOURS	CLASSROOM STUDY	PRACTICAL ACTIVITY	NOTES:
PREVENTION						
Mother/child health						
Nutrition						
Agricultural work						
Hygiene and sanitation						
Vaccines						
Prenatal care & childbirth						
Family Planning						
DIAGNOSIS AND TREATMENT						
History & physical exam						
Care of the sick						
(Anatomy and physiology)						
Diagnosis, treatment,						
and prevention						
Medical emergencies						
Clinical practice						
Use & misuse of medicines						
Use of book(s)						
Limits and referral						
Record keeping						
Treatment techniques						
COMMUNITY AND SOCIAL						
Awareness raising						
Community development						
and health						
Group dynamics						
(Role plays)						
Teaching methods and aids						
Teaching practice						
Leadership						
(Planning and management)						
Home visits						
Finding out needs						
Village theater, etc.						
Round-table discussion						
Games and sports						
Tests and evaluation						
Review and make-up time						

Step 5. Consider how much time to allow for each area of study

This can be done using the same worksheet. As an example of how to do it, see the next page.

- First, figure out the total number of hours of study time for the whole course. Write the sum at the top of the sheet, beside "total hours of course time available." (A two-month intensive course at 8 hours a day, 6 days a week, would have 384 hours available.)

- Then, in the column for ESTIMATED HOURS NEEDED, write the number of hours you think will be needed to cover each subject. Keep in mind the total hours of course time.

- When you have filled in the estimated hours for each subject, add them up and compare your total with the "total hours available." (See the upper right corner of the chart.) Subtract to find the difference. This lets you know how many hours you need to add or subtract from different subjects. But before making these adjustments . . .

- Fill in the third column, RELATIVE PRIORITY, using information from your previous studies (steps 2 and 3). This will help you to make study time adjustments according to priority of needs.

- Now adjust the hours for different subjects until the total equals the number of hours available. (Be sure to allow time for review and missed classes.)

Note: Not all of the subjects for study will require separate class time. Some can be included within other subjects. For example, we suggest that 'anatomy' not be taught as a separate subject, but that it be included as needed when studying specific health problems. Subjects that do not require separate hours can be written in parentheses (like this).

Some subjects with scheduled hours can also, in part, be covered in classes on related subjects. For example, preventive measures like hygiene and sanitation can be reviewed during classes covering specific illnesses. Physical exam, history taking, and the correct use of medicines can be reinforced during the daily clinical practice.

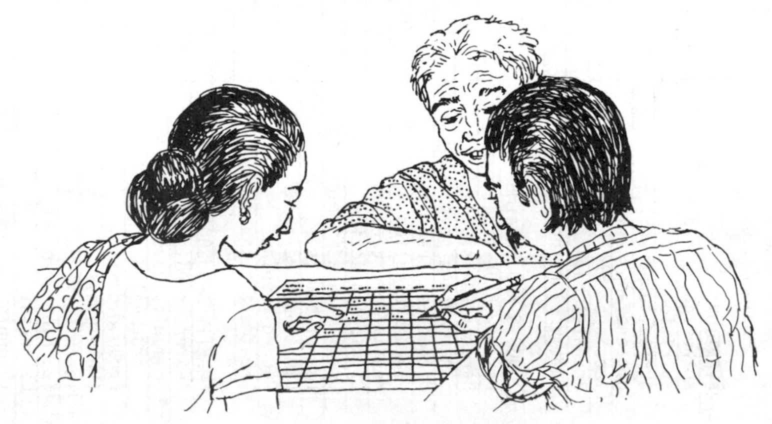

WORKSHEET FOR PLANNING THE CONTENT OF A TRAINING COURSE

estimated hours: 537
hours available: 384

estimate must be lowered by: 153 hours

Total hours of course time available: 8 hours per day x 48 days = 384 hours

SUBJECT UNDER CONSIDERATION	ESTIMATED HOURS NEEDED	RELATIVE PRIORITY (+ to +++++)	ADJUSTED NUMBER OF HOURS	CLASSROOM STUDY	PRACTICAL ACTIVITY	NOTES:
PREVENTION						
Mother/child health	10 +	+++++	8 +			
Nutrition	10 +	+++++	7 +			
Agricultural work	24	+++	12			
Hygiene and sanitation	10	+++++	8 +			
Vaccines	5	++++	4			
Prenatal care & childbirth	5	+++	3			
Family Planning	3	++	2			
DIAGNOSIS AND TREATMENT						
History & physical exam	6 +	+++++	5 +			
Care of the sick	3 +	++++	2 ++			
(Anatomy and physiology)	0 +	+	0 +			
Diagnosis, treatment, and prevention	100	+++++	70 +			
Medical emergencies	10	++++	6 +			
Clinical practice	100	+++++	80 +			
Use & misuse of medicines	5 +	+++++	4 +			
Use of book(s)	16 +	+++++	14 +			
Limits and referral	2	++++	1 +			
Record keeping	3	++	1 +			
Treatment techniques	3	++++	3 +			
COMMUNITY AND SOCIAL						
Awareness raising	10 +	+++++	8 +			
Community development and health	10	+++++	8 +			
Group dynamics	2 +	++++	1 +			
(Role plays)	0 +	++++	0 +			
Teaching methods and aids	6 +	+++++	8 +			
Teaching practice	10	+++++	8 +			
Leadership	2	+++	1 +			
(Planning and management)	0 +	+++	0 +			
Home visits	24	+++++	16 +			
Finding out needs	6 +	++++	4 +			
Village theater, etc.	20	+++	12 +			
Round-table discussion	16	++++	8			
Games and sports	48	+++	12 ++			
Tests and evaluation	12	++++	12 +			
Review and make-up time	56	+++++	56			
	537		384			

Step 6. Balancing the course content

A training course needs to be balanced in both content and learning methods.

- **Try for a balance between preventive, curative, and community or social aspects of health care.** Add up the hours in each of these 3 areas. Consider if the balance is appropriate in terms of the people's needs and concerns. Adjust the hours if necessary.

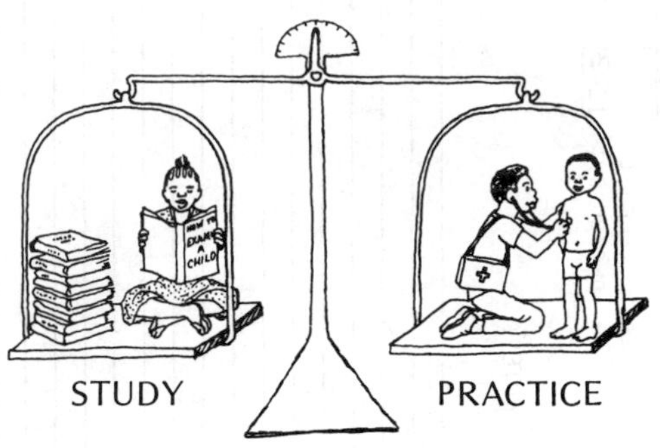

- **Balance discussion-type learning (classwork) with learning by doing (practice), physical work, and play.**

More and more programs are realizing the importance of learning by doing. Increasing emphasis is being placed on activities in the community, in the clinic, in schools, and in the fields as a part of health worker training. Even classwork—some of which remains necessary—can involve a great deal of active practice in using skills and solving problems.

Many programs also are recognizing the importance of physical work and play as a part of health worker training. Physical work serves many purposes—especially if it is health related (gardening, digging latrines, building equipment). It provides a change of pace. It keeps health workers close to the land and the working people. It helps them learn new agricultural or building skills. And in some projects, the health workers' daily farm work produces food that helps make the training program self-sufficient.

Learning through games and play is especially important for occasions when health workers work with children.

To plan a balance between classroom study and practical activity, you can use the same worksheet as before. Go down the list of subjects, marking the balance you think is appropriate for each one. You can do it this way:

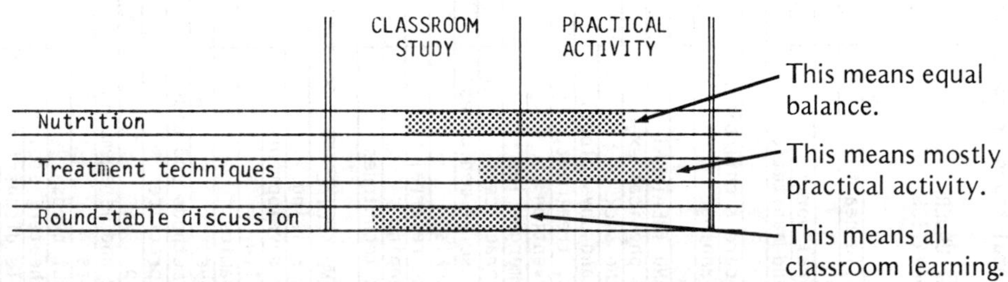

After marking each subject, look at the overall balance. If too much time is given to classwork, try to think of ways more learning can take place through practice and experience.

WORKSHEET FOR PLANNING THE CONTENT OF A TRAINING COURSE

estimated hours: 537
hours available: 384
estimate must be lowered by: 153 hours

Total hours of course time available: 8 hours per day x 48 days = 384 hours

SUBJECT UNDER CONSIDERATION	ESTIMATED HOURS NEEDED	RELATIVE PRIORITY (+ to +++++)	ADJUSTED NUMBER OF HOURS	CLASSROOM STUDY	PRACTICAL ACTIVITY	NOTES:
PREVENTION						
Mother/child health	10 +	+++++	8 +			includes monthly baby-weighing
Nutrition	10 +	+++++	7 +			includes some practice cooking
Agricultural work	24	+++	12			plus early morning before class
Hygiene and sanitation	10	+++++	8 +			plus time for building latrines and wells
Vaccines	5	++++	4			includes vaccinating children
Prenatal care & childbirth	5	+++	3			also attend births with midwives
Family Planning	3	++	2			
DIAGNOSIS AND TREATMENT						
History & physical exam	6 +	+++++	5 +			
Care of the sick	3 +	++++	2 ++			also attend emergencies
(Anatomy and physiology)	0 +	+	0 +			to be integrated with other classes
Diagnosis, treatment, and prevention	100	+++++	70 +			details on other sheet
Medical emergencies	10	++++	6 +			
Clinical practice	100	+++++	80 +			
Use & misuse of medicines	5 +	+++++	4 +			
Use of book(s)	16 +	+++++	14 +			twice each week
Limits and referral	2	++++	1 +			
Record keeping	3	++	1 +			
Treatment techniques	3	++++	3 +			
COMMUNITY AND SOCIAL						
Awareness raising	10 +	+++++	8 +			
Community development and health	10	+++++	8 +			
Group dynamics	2 +	++++	1 +			
(Role plays)	0 +	++++	0 +			on many subjects
Teaching methods and aids	6 +	+++++	8 +			
Teaching practice	10	+++++	8 +			with schoolchildren and adults
Leadership	2	+++	1 +			
(Planning and management)	0 +	+++	0 +			
Home visits	24	+++++	16 +			every Saturday morning
Finding out needs	6 +	++++	4 +			
Village theater, etc.	20	+++	12 +			planning and practice time
Round-table discussion	16	++++	8			
Games and sports	48	+++	12 ++			include more outside of class time
Tests and evaluation	12	++++	12 +			every Friday morning
Review and make-up time	56	+++++	56			one hour a week plus the last week
	537		384			

PLANNING A BALANCE OF LEARNING ACTIVITIES

From the first day of the course, it is a good idea to have a balance of different learning activities.

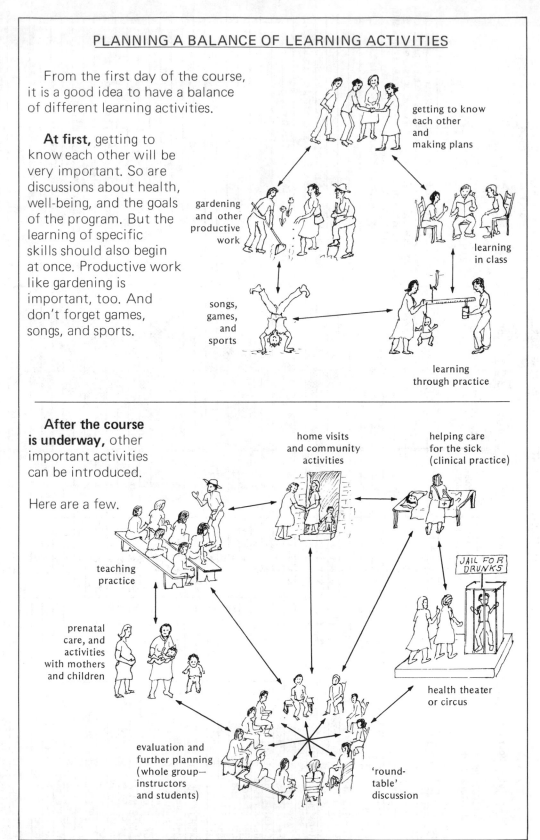

At first, getting to know each other will be very important. So are discussions about health, well-being, and the goals of the program. But the learning of specific skills should also begin at once. Productive work like gardening is important, too. And don't forget games, songs, and sports.

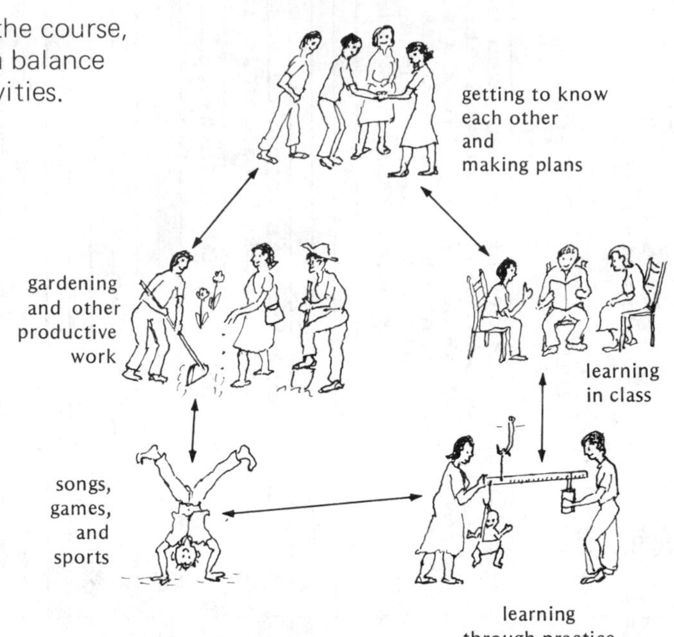

After the course is underway, other important activities can be introduced.

Here are a few.

home visits and community activities

helping care for the sick (clinical practice)

teaching practice

JAIL FOR DRUNKS

prenatal care, and activities with mothers and children

health theater or circus

evaluation and further planning (whole group—instructors and students)

'round-table' discussion

Step 7. Preparing a timetable and making the weekly schedules

Once the overall content for the course is decided, you can plan the classes and other activities on a week-by-week basis. It helps if you mimeograph blank planning sheets similar to the one on page **3**-29, but adapted to your needs. The larger the planning sheet, the more details can be written in later. You can make a large one by joining 2 sheets together. Each week the plan can be posted for students to see. Following the blank weekly schedule is an example of one that was filled out and used during a training course in Project Piaxtla, Mexico.

In preparing a weekly timetable, think about how to best use the hours of the day. Plan your schedule according to the local rhythm of life: the hours when people usually wake up, work, eat meals, rest, and so on. Try to include a variety of activities during each day, to avoid doing the same kind of thing for too long. You may also want to allow a few minutes between classes for relaxing or quick games. When planning times, be sure to get the suggestions and agreement of the students and the families with whom they are staying.

Now consider **which** subjects should be taught **when.** Here are some ideas based on our own experience:

Be sure afternoon classes have plenty of action.

NOT APPROPRIATE

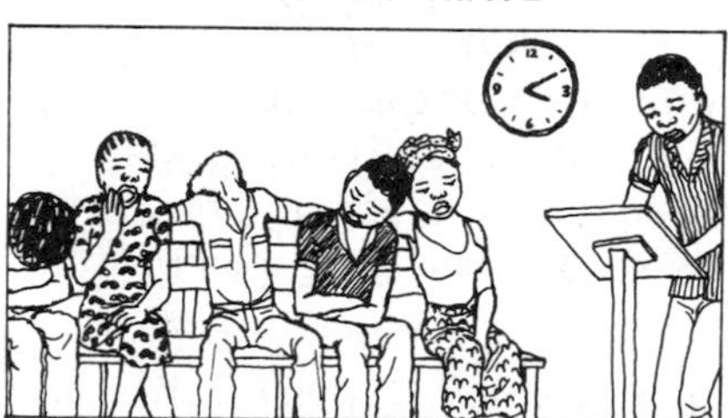

APPROPRIATE

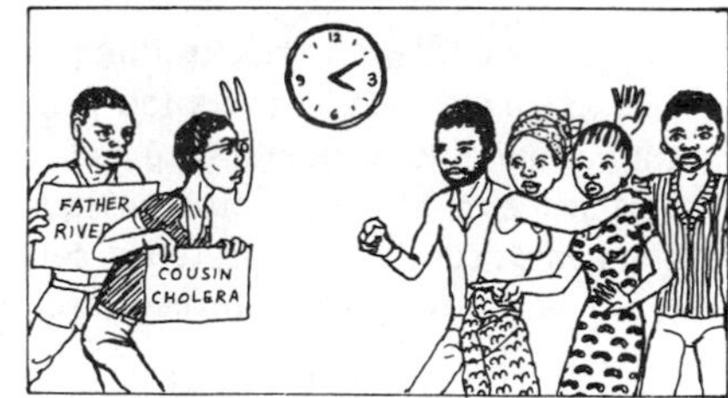

Which time of day is best for what?

- Early morning hours, before the day is hot, are good for gardening and physical work.
- The morning is also a good time for classes on serious subjects that require thoughtful study. Everyone is fresh and eager to learn at this hour.
- The afternoon, when students are tired, is a good time for active discussions, role playing, and projects like making teaching materials.
- Evenings are best for slide and filmstrip presentations, and for meetings with community persons who may be busy all day.

Every day? Or once or twice a week?

- Subjects such as curative-and-preventive medicine and clinical practice, which cover a great deal of material and require a lot of time, are best included every day.
- Skills such as using a reference book ***(Where There Is No Doctor)*** or using medicines correctly are best taught once or twice a week—in such a way that they reinforce other subjects the students are learning.
- Review sessions should follow consultations or exams as soon as possible.
- Community visits should be scheduled for times when people are likely to be at home—a couple of evenings each week or on a weekend morning.

At the beginning of the training course? Or near the end?

- Knowledge and skills needed to examine, care for, and give advice to people who are sick should be covered at the beginning of the course. See page **8**-5.
- Teaching in the community and putting on village theater shows are good activities for later in the course, when students have more knowledge and self-confidence. But be sure to plan and practice for these well in advance.

Before the course begins (or shortly after, so as to include student suggestions), **make rough weekly plans for the whole course.** This helps ensure that you allow time for everything you intend to include. It is easy to run out of time before all the important material has been covered!

When making an early plan of the whole course, you do not need to fill in many details. Later, during the course, the instructors can meet with the student planning committee (see p. **4**-14) each week to prepare a more detailed plan for the following week. Be sure you schedule a regular time for this planning, too.

WEEKLY PLANNING SHEET -- HEALTH WORKER'S TRAINING COURSE

AJOYA CLINIC, AJOYA, SINALOA, MEXICO

WEEK NUMBER 2 DATES January 25 to January 31, [illegible]

TIME	MONDAY	TUESDAY	WEDNESDAY	THURSDAY	FRIDAY	SATURDAY	SUNDAY
7:00	WORK	IN THE	VEGETABLE	GARDEN			
8:00	BREAKFAST	BREAKFAST	BREAKFAST	BREAKFAST	BREAKFAST	BREAKFAST	BREAKFAST
8:00–10:00	CURATIVE MEDICINE: DIARRHEA AND DEHYDRATION; USE OF MEDICINES [illegible]	CURATIVE MEDICINE: CAUSES AND TREATMENT OF DEHYDRATION; USE OF THE BOOK (WTND) [illegible]	CURATIVE MEDICINE: STOMACH ULCERS; USE OF MEDICINES [illegible]	CURATIVE MEDICINE: [illegible]; USE OF THE BOOK (WTND)	WEEKLY TEST	[illegible] COMMUNITY VISITS; COMMUNITY VISITS (REMIND MOTHERS ABOUT BABY WEIGHING ON MONDAY)	
10:00–12:00	PRACTICE IN	CLINICAL	HEALTH CARE	(MEDICAL AND	DENTAL)		
12:00–1:00	REVIEW CONSULTATIONS; CURATIVE MEDICINE: [illegible] METHOD	REVIEW CONSULTATIONS; CURATIVE MEDICINE: MEDICAL HISTORY	REVIEW CONSULTATIONS; CURATIVE MEDICINE: INTRODUCTION TO PHYSICAL EXAM	REVIEW CONSULTATIONS; CURATIVE MEDICINE: VITAL SIGNS	REVIEW CONSULTATIONS; CURATIVE MEDICINE: VITAL SIGNS		
2:00	LUNCH	LUNCH	LUNCH	LUNCH	LUNCH; MEET WITH SCHOOL CHILDREN TO PLAN PUPPET SHOW	LUNCH	LUNCH
3:00–5:00	PREVENTIVE MEDICINE: HOW TO PREVENT DIFFERENT KINDS OF DISEASE; ROUND-TABLE DISCUSSION	PREVENTIVE MEDICINE: SPREAD OF INFECTIOUS DISEASES; HEALTH EDUCATION: [illegible] POSTERS	PREVENTIVE MEDICINE: PREVENTION OF [illegible] DISEASES; HEALTH EDUCATION: MAKING POSTERS	PREVENTIVE MEDICINE: IMPORTANCE OF SANITATION AND NUTRITION; HEALTH EDUCATION: PLAN MEETING WITH SCHOOL CHILDREN	REVIEW OF TEST AND WEEK'S CLASSES; OPEN DISCUSSION	[illegible] PUPPETS WITH SCHOOL CHILDREN	
6:00	DINNER	DINNER	DINNER	DINNER	DINNER	DINNER	DINNER
7:00–8:00	CLINIC WEEKLY BUSINESS MEETING		SLIDE SHOW AND DISCUSSION ABOUT CHILD-TO-CHILD PROGRAM	STUDENTS' SELF EVALUATION MEETING	MEETING TO PLAN NEXT WEEK'S SCHEDULE		

An important suggestion: MAKE YOUR TIMETABLE FLEXIBLE

It often happens that some classes or subjects take longer than planned. Others are poorly or even wrongly taught, or prove especially difficult for students to understand. Such classes may need to be repeated. For this reason, it is wise to leave plenty of extra time for review: about 1 or 2 hours of 'open' time each week, plus several unplanned days at the end of the course.

This open time also allows you to adjust the schedule when classes are missed or postponed. Especially if training takes place in a real-life setting (like a village), **medical emergencies and other unplanned learning opportunities are bound to come up.**

For example, during a training course in Ajoya, Mexico, a class was interrupted when news arrived that a man had broken his leg on a mountain trail. The students and instructor carried the man to the health center on a stretcher, set the broken bone, and put a cast on his leg (see photo).

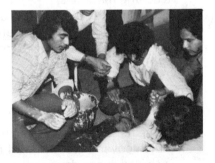

The interrupted class was given later. This was easy to manage because extra time had been allowed in the schedule.

Do not be afraid to change your plans.

Step 8. Preparing detailed plans for the first few days of the course

This will be discussed in the next chapter.

WEEKLY PLANNING SHEET -- HEALTH WORKER'S TRAINING COURSE

WEEK NUMBER ____ DATES ________ to ________, ____

TIME	MONDAY	TUESDAY	WEDNESDAY	THURSDAY	FRIDAY	SATURDAY	SUNDAY
7:00-							
-							
8:00-							
-							
9:00-							
-							
10:00-							
-							
11:00-							
-							
12:00-							
-							
1:00-							
-							
2:00-							
-							
3:00-							
-							
4:00-							
-							
5:00-							
-							
6:00-							
-							
7:00-							
-							
8:00-							

AJOYA CLINIC
AJOYA, SINALOA
MEXICO

WEEKLY PLANNING SHEET -- HEALTH WORKER'S TRAINING COURSE

WEEK NUMBER 2 DATES January 25 to January 31, 1979

TIME	MONDAY	TUESDAY	WEDNESDAY	THURSDAY	FRIDAY	SATURDAY	SUNDAY
7:00–	WORK IN THE VEGETABLE GARDEN						
	BREAKFAST	BREAKFAST	BREAKFAST	BREAKFAST	BREAKFAST	BREAKFAST	BREAKFAST
8:00–	CURATIVE MEDICINE: DIARRHEA AND DEHYDRATION	CURATIVE MEDICINE: CAUSES AND TREATMENT OF DEHYDRATION	CURATIVE MEDICINE: STOMACH ULCERS	CURATIVE MEDICINE: OTHER GUT PROBLEMS	WEEKLY TEST	PREPARE FOR COMMUNITY VISITS	
9:00–	USE OF MEDICINES: RISKS AND PRECAUTIONS WITH MEDICINES	USE OF THE BOOK (WTND) KINDS OF DIARRHEA	USE OF MEDICINES: HOW TO MEASURE AND GIVE MEDICINES	USE OF THE BOOK (WTND)		COMMUNITY VISITS (REMIND MOTHERS ABOUT BABY WEIGHING ON MONDAY)	
10:00–11:00	PRACTICE IN CLINICAL HEALTH CARE (MEDICAL AND DENTAL)						
	REVIEW CONSULTATIONS	REVIEW CONSULTATIONS	REVIEW CONSULTATIONS	REVIEW CONSULTATIONS	REVIEW CONSULTATIONS		
12:00–	CURATIVE MEDICINE: SCIENTIFIC METHOD	CURATIVE MEDICINE: MEDICAL HISTORY	CURATIVE MEDICINE: INTRODUCTION TO PHYSICAL EXAM	CURATIVE MEDICINE: VITAL SIGNS	CURATIVE MEDICINE: VITAL SIGNS		
1:00–	LUNCH	LUNCH	LUNCH	LUNCH	LUNCH	LUNCH	LUNCH
2:00–					MEET WITH SCHOOL CHILDREN TO PLAN PUPPET SHOW		
3:00–	PREVENTIVE MEDICINE: HOW TO PREVENT DIFFERENT KINDS OF DISEASES	PREVENTIVE MEDICINE: SPREAD OF INFECTIOUS DISEASES	PREVENTIVE MEDICINE: PREVENTION OF OTHER DISEASES	PREVENTIVE MEDICINE: IMPORTANCE OF SANITATION AND NUTRITION	REVIEW OF TEST AND WEEK'S CLASSES	CONTINUE MAKING POSTERS AND PUPPETS WITH SCHOOL CHILDREN	
4:00–	ROUND-TABLE DISCUSSION	HEALTH EDUCATION: LEARNING TO DRAW MAKING POSTERS	HEALTH EDUCATION: MAKING POSTERS	HEALTH EDUCATION: PLAN MEETING WITH SCHOOL CHILDREN	OPEN DISCUSSION		
5:00–6:00–	DINNER	DINNER	DINNER	DINNER	DINNER	DINNER	DINNER
7:00–8:00–	CLINIC WEEKLY BUSINESS MEETING		SLIDE SHOW AND DISCUSSION ABOUT CHILD-TO-CHILD PROGRAM	STUDENTS' SELF-EVALUATION MEETING	MEETING TO PLAN NEXT WEEK'S SCHEDULE		

HOW MUCH CURATIVE MEDICINE SHOULD A TRAINING PROGRAM INCLUDE?

If health workers are to win people's confidence and cooperation, they need to START WHERE THE PEOPLE ARE AND BUILD ON THAT.

Prevention may be more important than cure. But not to a mother whose child is sick! Most people feel far more need for curative than preventive medicine. If health workers are to respond to what people want, they must be able to diagnose and treat a wide range of common health problems.

To teach health workers to start out by focusing on prevention can be a big mistake. People do not immediately see the results of preventive work. They will respond more eagerly if health workers begin with curative medicine and use that as a doorway to prevention.

In a community-based program, curative care cannot be separated from prevention. The first leads to the second.

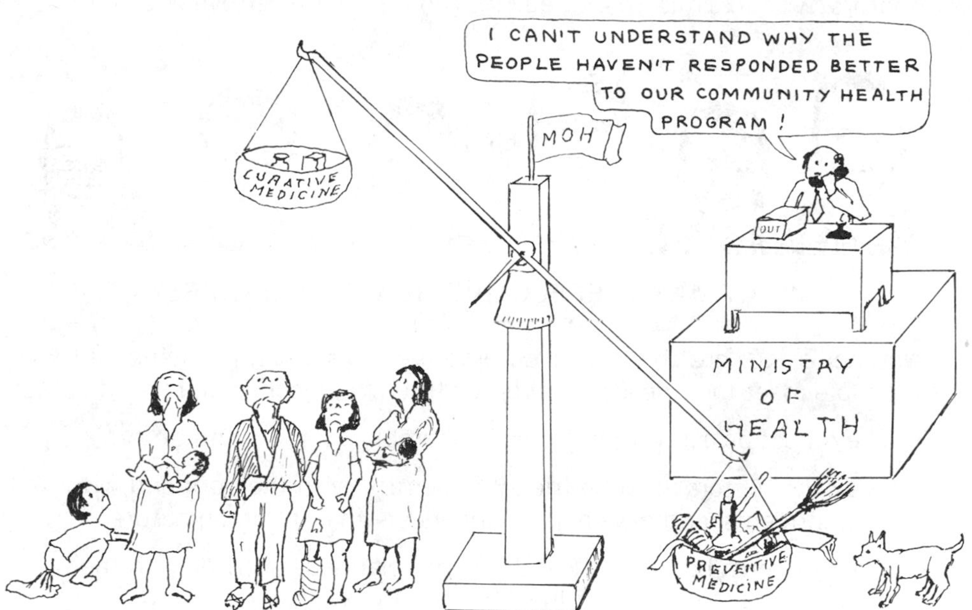
I CAN'T UNDERSTAND WHY THE PEOPLE HAVEN'T RESPONDED BETTER TO OUR COMMUNITY HEALTH PROGRAM!
MOH
CURATIVE MEDICINE
OUT
MINISTRY OF HEALTH
PREVENTIVE MEDICINE

A HEALTHY BALANCE BETWEEN PREVENTIVE AND CURATIVE MEDICINE MUST TAKE INTO CONSIDERATION WHAT THE PEOPLE WANT.

Unfortunately, many programs provide training only in preventive measures and 'health education'. Curative care, if taught, is limited to the treatment of a few 'basic symptoms', using 5 or 6 harmless or unnecessary medicines (see p. **18**-2). Sometimes health workers end up learning less about diagnosis, treatment, and the use of modern medicines than many villagers already know. This so reduces the community's confidence in the health workers that they become less effective even in their preventive work.

A common argument against preparing health workers adequately in curative care is that "It would be dangerous! There is just too much material to cover in a short course."

This is true if training focuses on making the students memorize a lot of detailed facts and information. But if training helps them learn basic skills through role playing and actual practice, it is amazing how quickly they can become effective in a wide range of curative skills. To develop reliable curative ability, training needs to focus on 4 areas of learning:

1. Step-by-step **problem solving** (scientific method).
2. **History taking** and **physical examination** of a sick person.
3. **Practice in using a handbook** to diagnose, treat, and advise people about common problems.
4. **Learning to recognize one's own limits,** and to judge which problems to refer to more highly trained workers.

In our experience in Latin America, **village health workers can, in 2 months of practical training, learn to effectively attend 80 to 90% of the sick people they see.** In time, as they gain experience and receive good follow-up training, they can effectively attend up to 95%. The best health workers learn to work as capably as most doctors, with less misuse of medicines and more preventive education.

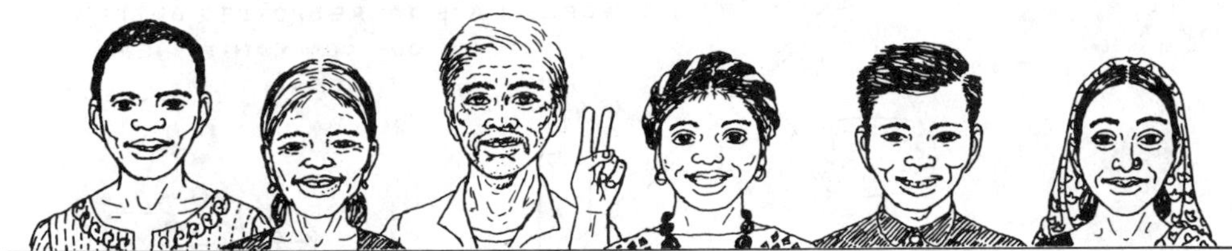

WHAT MAKES EFFECTIVE HEALTH WORKERS?

Whether or not health workers develop the skills and understanding to help people meet their needs, on their own terms, depends on many factors:

- They must be carefully selected, preferably by the community.
- Their instructors must be friendly, identify with the poor and with their students, and have a good understanding of human nature.
- Training must be carefully and flexibly planned—according to the needs of the students and their communities.
- Teaching must be appropriate and effective—built around problem solving and practice.
- Follow-up after the training course must be supportive and reliable.

In Chapters 2 and 3, we have looked at the first three factors on the list above. In the next chapters, we will look at others.

But first, it is important to get off to a good start.

CHAPTER **4**

Getting Off to a Good Start

BE PREPARED—EVEN WHEN YOU ARE NOT

The first days of a training program are often the most difficult—especially if the instructors are not very experienced. It is important to **have as much as possible ready ahead of time,** including:

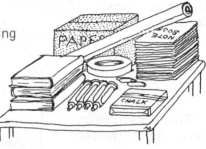

- living and eating arrangements for students
- study area with places to sit and good lighting
- blackboard and chalk (white and colors)
- plenty of wrapping paper or poster paper
- crayons, pencils, and marking pens
- notebooks and textbooks for students
- whatever tools or supplies may be needed for building things, making teaching aids, agricultural work, and any other activities that may be planned with the students at the start of the course
- timetable and class plans for at least the first few days (see next page)

Students can help get things ready

Sometimes not all the materials and furniture are ready by the time the course begins, or the students may not all arrive the same day. In this case, you may want to spend a part of the first day or two with students, helping to make benches, blackboards, flannel-boards, and other preparations. By doing these things together, the group gets off to an active start. People get to know each other through working together.

It is important that the instructors work together with the students, not just doing it for them and not just telling them what to do. By doing the job together as equals, a good learning relationship, as well as a friendship, begins.

But if you are going to start by making benches, blackboards, or other items, be sure you have the necessary supplies ready.

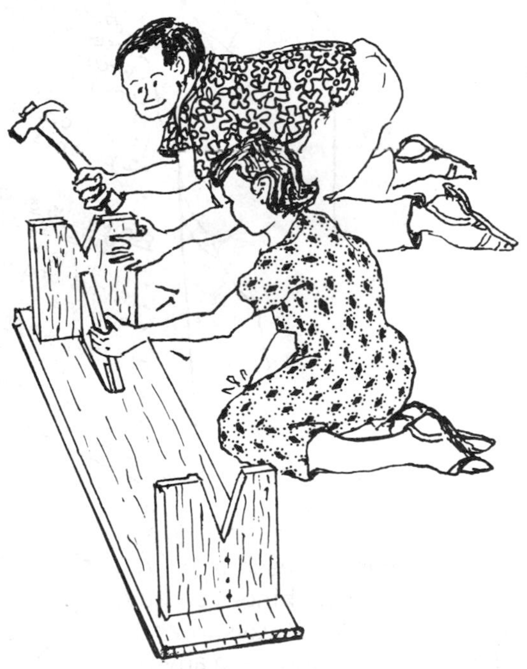

Making equipment or supplies for the course is a practical way to start. It helps people get to know each other.

CHECKLISTS

To help yourself remember and plan what to get ready, you may want to make lists of:

1. SUPPLIES THAT ARE NEEDED

2. THINGS TO BE DONE in time for the course

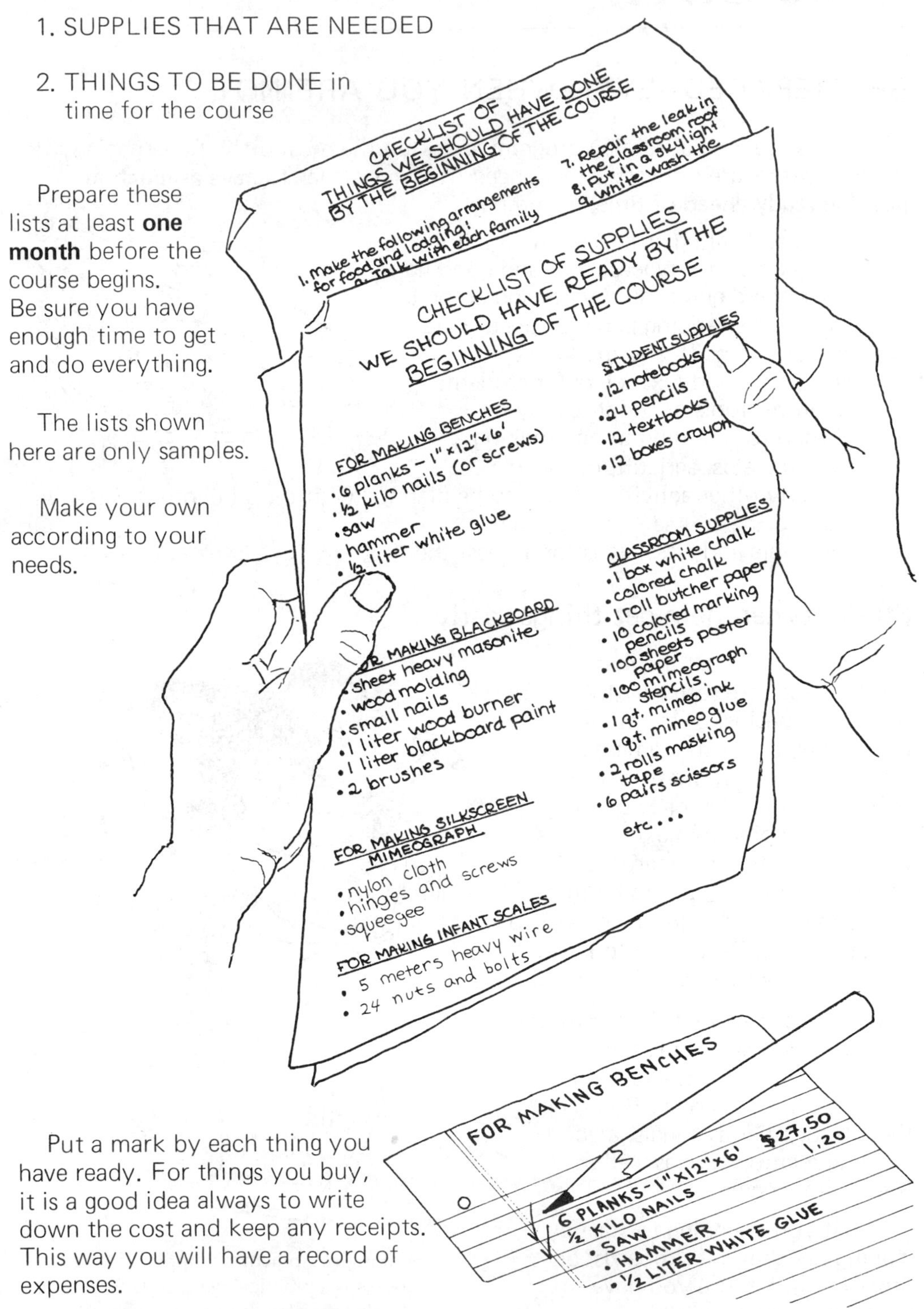

CHECKLIST OF THINGS WE SHOULD HAVE DONE BY THE BEGINNING OF THE COURSE
1. Make the following arrangements for food and lodging:
Talk with each family
7. Repair the leak in the classroom roof
8. Put in a skylight
9. White wash the
CHECKLIST OF SUPPLIES WE SHOULD HAVE READY BY THE BEGINNING OF THE COURSE
FOR MAKING BENCHES
• 6 planks – 1" x 12" x 6'
• ½ kilo nails (or screws)
• saw
• hammer
• ½ liter white glue
R MAKING BLACKBOARD
sheet heavy masonite
• wood molding
• small nails
• 1 liter wood burner
• 1 liter blackboard paint
• 2 brushes
FOR MAKING SILKSCREEN MIMEOGRAPH
• nylon cloth
• hinges and screws
• squeegee
FOR MAKING INFANT SCALES
• 5 meters heavy wire
• 24 nuts and bolts
STUDENT SUPPLIES
• 12 notebooks
• 24 pencils
• 12 textbooks
• 12 boxes crayon
CLASSROOM SUPPLIES
• 1 box white chalk
• colored chalk
• 1 roll butcher paper
• 10 colored marking pencils
• 100 sheets poster paper
• 100 mimeograph stencils
• 1 qt. mimeo ink
• 1 qt. mimeo glue
• 2 rolls masking tape
• 6 pairs scissors
etc. . .
FOR MAKING BENCHES
6 PLANKS - 1" x 12" x 6' $27.50
½ KILO NAILS 1.20
• SAW
• HAMMER
• ½ LITER WHITE GLUE

Prepare these lists at least **one month** before the course begins. Be sure you have enough time to get and do everything.

The lists shown here are only samples.

Make your own according to your needs.

Put a mark by each thing you have ready. For things you buy, it is a good idea always to write down the cost and keep any receipts. This way you will have a record of expenses.

A POSSIBLE TIMETABLE FOR THE FIRST WEEK

Here is a sample timetable showing classes and activities that might be plannec for the first few days of a two-month training program. Of course, you will want to plan each activity or class in more careful detail. (See Chapter 5 for suggestions.) In our experience, these first classes often run overtime, so many in this example are scheduled for 1½ to 2 hours, instead of only 1 hour.

WEEKLY PLANNING SHEET -- HEALTH WORKER'S TRAINING COURSE

AJOYA CLI
AJOYA, SIN
MEXICO

WEEK NUMBER 1 DATES JANUARY 18 to JANUARY 24, 1979

TIME	MONDAY	TUESDAY	WEDNESDAY	THURSDAY	FRIDAY	SATURDAY	SUND
7:00-			WORK IN	COMMUNITY	GARDEN		
8:00-		BREAKFAST	BREAKFAST	BREAKFAST	BREAKFAST	BREAKFAST	BREAK
8:00–9:00		WELCOME: Introduce students and instructors	HOPES AND DOUBTS small groups / large group	CLINICAL ETHICS: Discussion and Role Plays	DISCUSSION: Abuses of medicines	PREPARE FOR COMMUNITY VISITS	
9:00-		BREAKING THE ICE			ROLE PLAY: Balance between prevention and treatment	FIRST COMMUNITY VISITS	
10:00-		Explain schedule; answer questions; show them garden, clinic, etc.	GAMES	Importance of Clinical History			
10:00–11:00			USE OF BOOK: index, contents, vocabulary	OBSERVE CLINICAL AND DENTAL PRACTICE	OBSERVE CLINICAL AND DENTAL PRACTICE	(Introduction: explain why and for how long)	SWIM IN T RIVER
11:00-		GETTING THINGS READY	DISCUSSION: What are the main problems in our communities? (priorities)	REVIEW CONSULTATIONS	REVIEW CONSULTATIONS		
12:00-		1. whitewash walls 2. repair benches 3. paint blackboard	STORIES: appropriate and inappropriate teaching	CLINICAL HISTORY: Practice and role plays	HEALING WITHOUT MEDICINES: discussion/practice		TANN CLIN
1:00–3:00		LUNCH	LUNCH	LUNCH	LUNCH	LUNCH	*LUN
3:00-	MOST STUDENTS ARRIVE	Discussion: students' experiences with home remedies	DISCUSSION: What causes disease?	ROLE PLAYS: BOSSY TEACHER AND GOOD GROUP LEADER	DISCUSSION: What makes a good health worker or instructor?	REVIEW FOR LATECOMERS	
4:00-		HAND OUT BOOKS	STORYTELLING: "Not Knowing It All" Stories from students	Analysis			
5:00-	Informal welcome; Show them living arrangements	GAMES	VOLLEYBALL	GAMES	FOOTBALL	VOLLEYBALL WITH SCHOOLTEACHERS	
6:00-		DINNER	DINNER	DINNER	DINNER	DINNER	DIN
7:00-		TOWN MEETING: Introduce students to Community	FORM STUDENT COMMITTEES		MEETING TO PLAN NEXT WEEK'S SCHEDULE		
8:00-							

...AND ACTIVITIES IN THE FIRST FEW DAYS

... days are not only the most difficult, they are also among the most ... is the time when the members of the learning group meet and ... to know each other.

Getting to know each other in a friendly, open way is perhaps the most important thing that can happen in these first days. There are a number of things you can do to help this happen. (See 'Breaking the Ice', page **4**-6.)

During the first days there is lots of talking. People are getting acquainted. Many things need to be explained and discussed. On page **4**-11, we look at some of the important things to discuss.

But there is also a danger of talking and discussing things too much! **Students come to learn specific skills.** They may not yet know that the art of listening and of sharing ideas openly in a group is one of the most valuable skills a health worker can master. They want to get on with more exciting things—like using a stethoscope and giving injections.

There are, of course, good reasons **not** to start by teaching how to inject or use a stethoscope. (See the next page.)

Nevertheless, new health workers-in-training are eager to start learning useful skills. Too much talk will discourage them. So from the first day of the course, include activities that help students master practical skills—skills they can put to use as soon as the need arises.

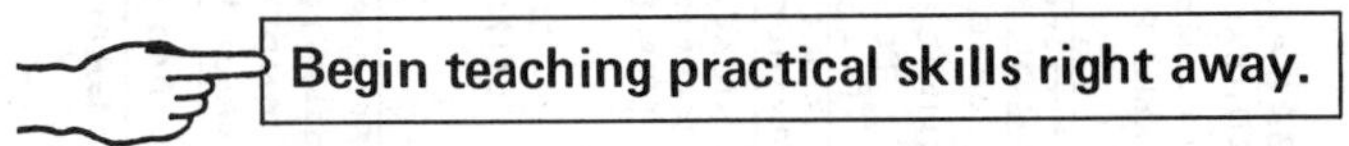

Begin teaching practical skills right away.

Taking student interest into account

In the beginning, health workers—like most people—are more interested in treatment than in prevention. During the course, the importance of prevention and of health education should become clear. But at first—and often to the last, if secretly—the biggest interest of most health workers is in curative medicine. After all, the health worker wants to be appreciated. He therefore wants to help meet people's felt needs. And this we must respect.

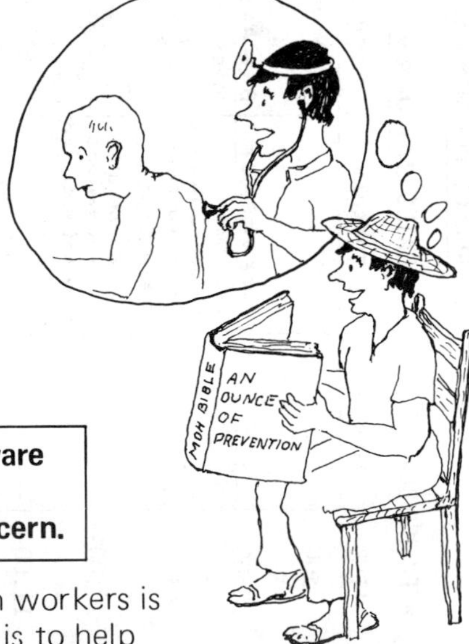

THE DREAM AND THE REALITY (WHICH IS WHICH?)

Only when the whole community becomes aware of the need for preventive action is the health worker likely to make prevention his first concern.

The challenge for both instructors and health workers is not simply to respond to people's felt needs. It is to help people look at and understand their needs more clearly. But the process cannot be forced or hurried. People need to discover the reasons and decide to take steps themselves.

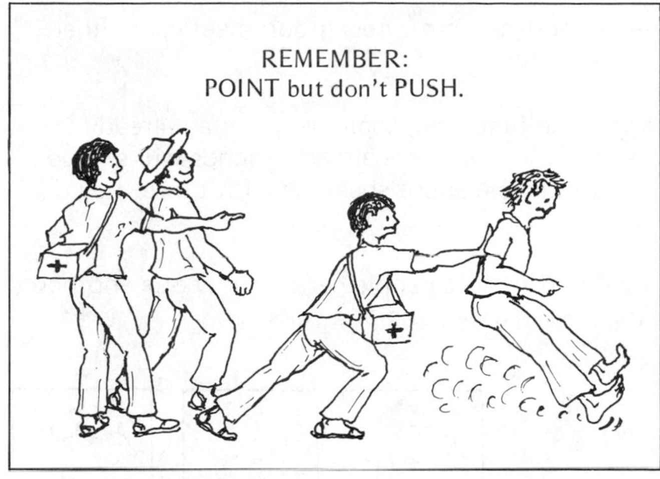

The health worker can point the way, but must not push—not if he or she wants lasting results.

The same thing is true for instructors.

Whenever possible, **start where the students' interests lie. But be selective. Try to direct their interests toward meeting important community needs.**

If the students' first interest is curative medicine, start with that. But take care **not** to start by teaching frequently misused skills, such as how to give injections or use a stethoscope. Too often, doctors and health workers use the needle and the stethoscope as signs of prestige and power. The people see these instruments as magic. To reduce this problem, some programs do not teach how to inject until late in the course. This is probably wise. Consider beginning the study of curative medicine by looking at **useful home remedies** (see *WTND,* Chapter 1). Or start with ways of **healing without medicines** *(WTND,* Chapter 5). This is more appropriate because:

- It places emphasis on local traditions and resources.
- It encourages self-reliance.
- It lets students begin by speaking from their own experience.
- It helps take some of the mystery out of both traditional and modern remedies.
- It can help awaken students to the problems of overuse and over-dependence on modern medicines.

As you can see, this approach is partly preventive, even though it deals mainly with treatment.

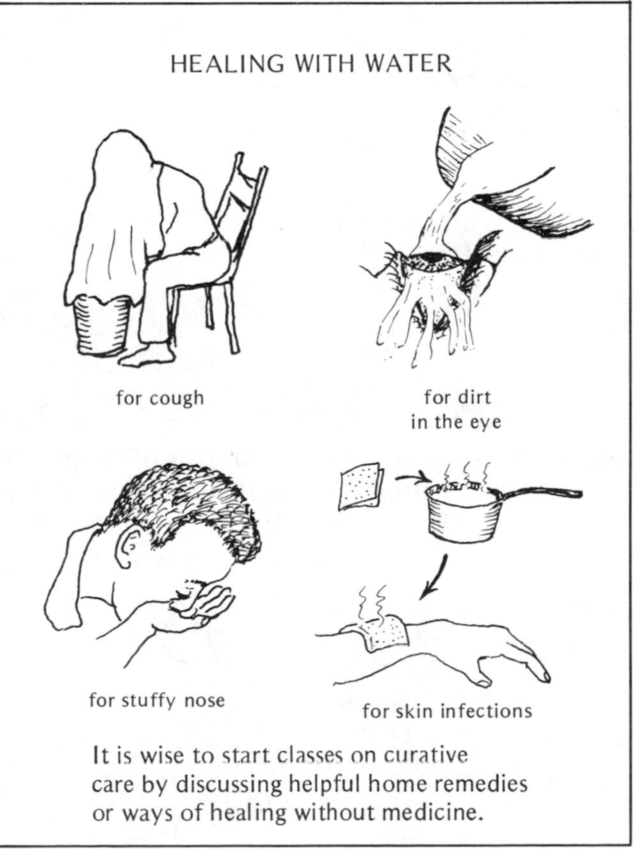

It is wise to start classes on curative care by discussing helpful home remedies or ways of healing without medicine.

'BREAKING THE ICE'—methods to help a new group meet each other, relax, and start talking

When a group comes together for the first time, some people may already know each other, but many may not. Often those who are already friends will sit and talk with each other, but feel uncomfortable about speaking with those they do not yet know.

Various games or 'tricks' can be used to help people get to know one another and feel comfortable about taking part in a meeting or a class:

1. PAIRING OFF FOR INTRODUCTIONS

Draw hearts, animals, or other figures on slips of paper. (Draw one figure for every 2 people.)

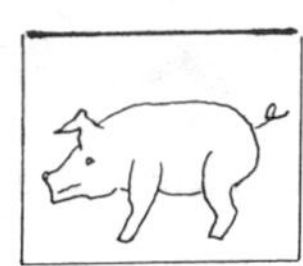
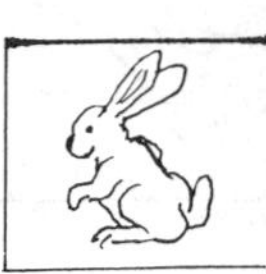
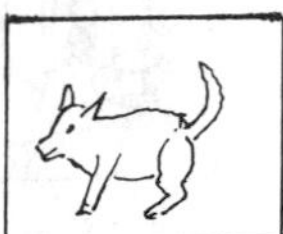
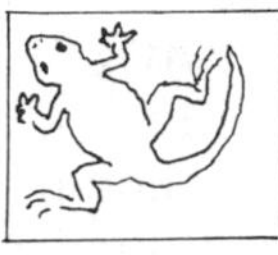
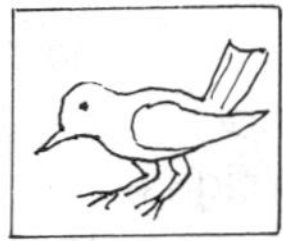
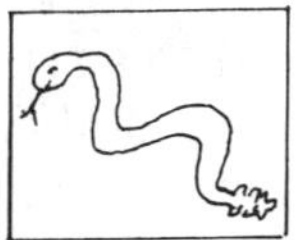

Tear each slip in two.

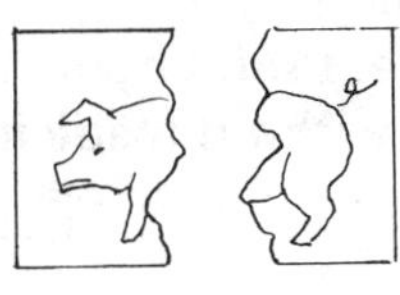
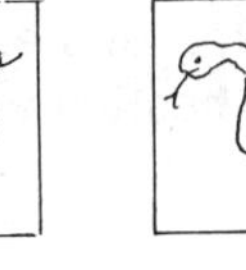
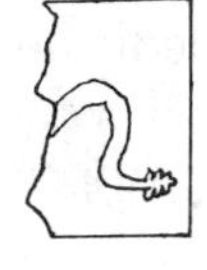

Crumple the pieces into balls.

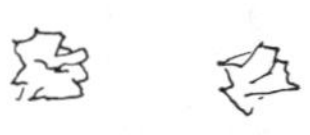
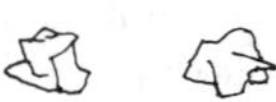

Put them into a hat and let each person pick one.

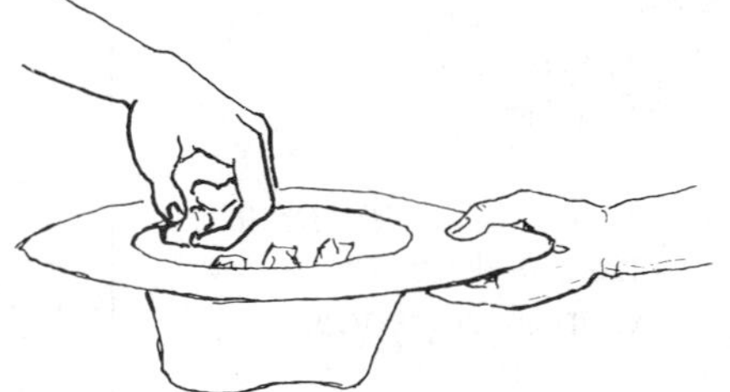

Now each person tries to find his 'other half'.

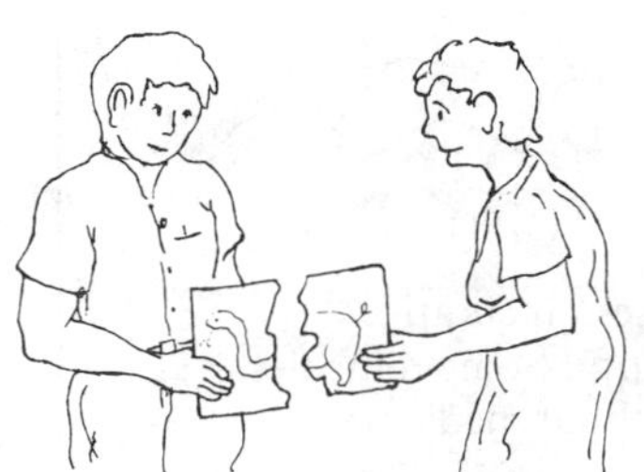

Each pair of people with matching halves spends 10 or 15 minutes getting to know each other.

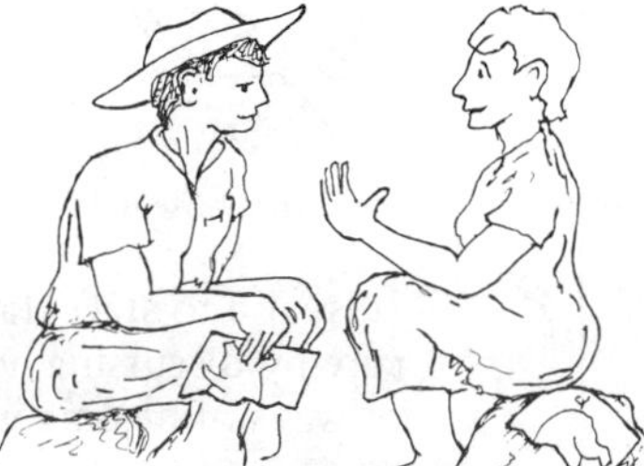

At last the group meets again, and everyone takes turns introducing his partner to the group.

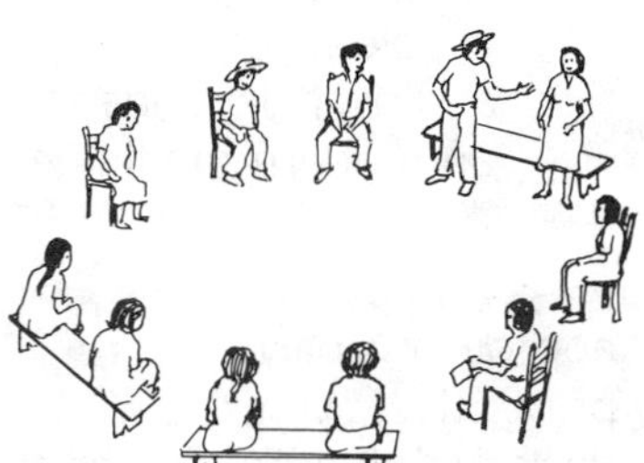

2. MERRY-GO-ROUND OR 'TRAINS'

The group divides into two halves by counting off—ONE, TWO, ONE, TWO—around the circle.

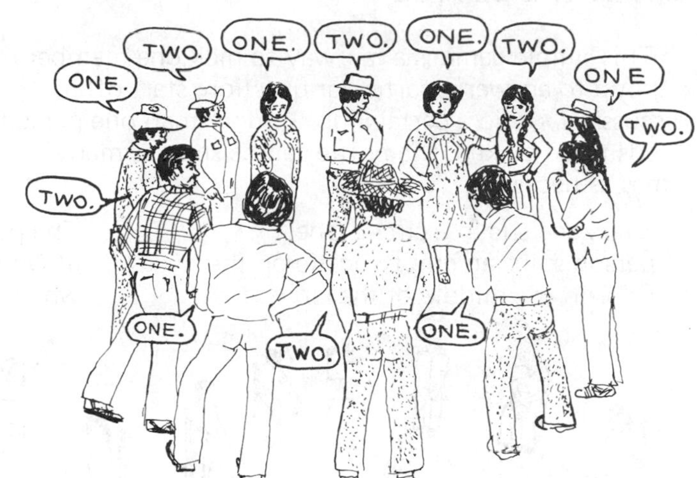

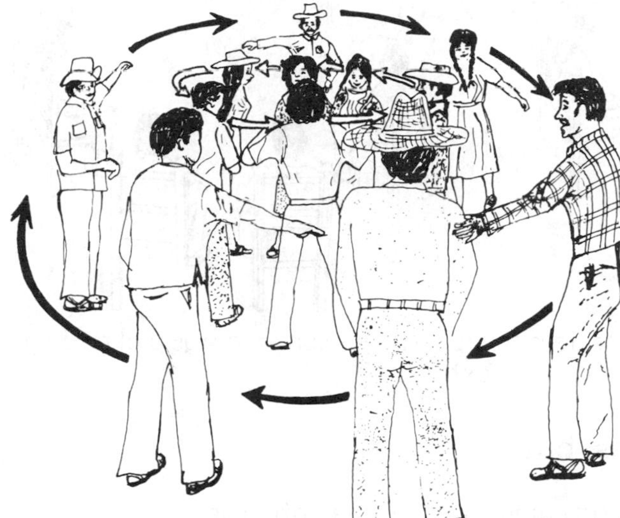

Then all the ONE's form a circle, and all the TWO's form another circle around them.

When the leader says "GO," circle ONE runs in one direction and circle TWO runs in the other—whistling and puffing like trains.

When the leader shouts "STOP," each person turns to the nearest person in the other circle and introduces himself or herself. Each pair talks together about a topic the leader or someone else has suggested.

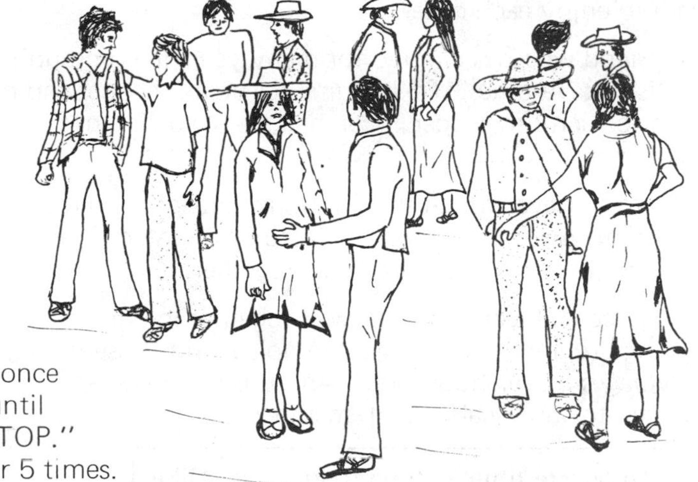

After a minute or two, the leader shouts "GO" again, and each circle at once begins to run as before until the leader again cries "STOP." This can be repeated 4 or 5 times.

Afterwards the whole group can meet to discuss what they learned.

3. SPIN THE BOTTLE

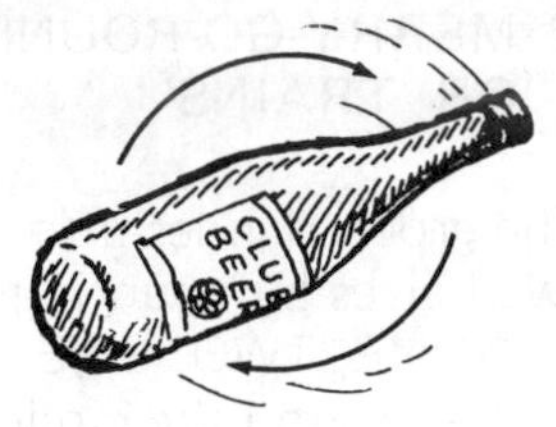

This simple game is a fair way to pick one member of a group to answer a particular question, start off a discussion, or do a certain job. If more than one person needs to be picked, the bottle can be spun as many times as necessary.

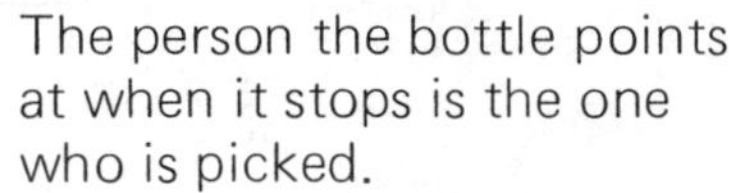

Everyone sits in a circle. One person spins an empty bottle on the floor in the middle of the circle.

The person the bottle points at when it stops is the one who is picked.

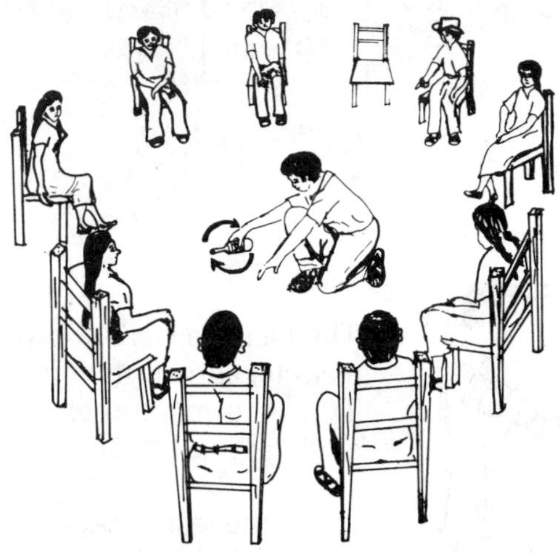

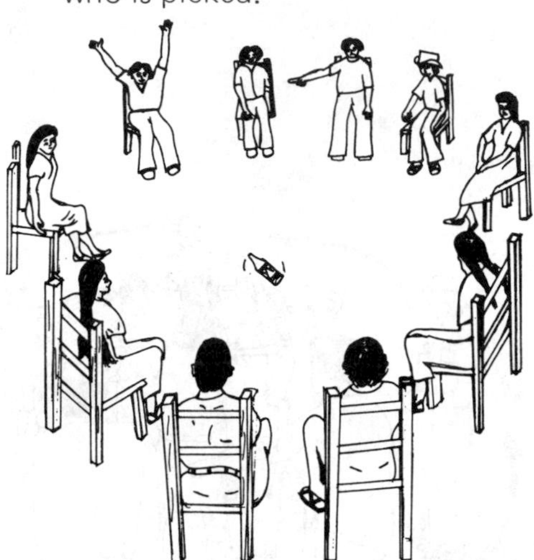

After he answers the question or does the job, the person who was picked spins the bottle again to see who will be picked next.

Silly? A waste of time? Yes, but . . .

'Ice-breaking' games may seem ridiculous. In fact, they often are. Some people may not like them or may feel they are a waste of time. Sometimes they are. But sometimes they can help a group that is too serious or stiff, to loosen up and begin to enjoy each other.

A friend who has worked for many years in community health says: "To waste time is to save time." Taking time to 'break the ice' and help people begin to relate to each other openly can make a big difference in what people learn from the course.

We must never forget that, although latrines and medicines and vaccines are important, the most important factor that determines human health is how people work and live and share and learn together.

If we can all learn to work well together in our training program, perhaps we can do so with those in our villages or neighborhoods. And this would be a real step toward health! So remember . . .

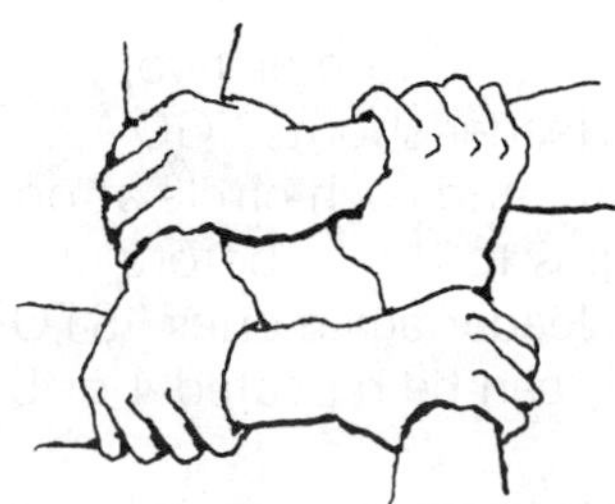

To 'waste time' getting to know and like each other may save time later.

THE WORKINGS OF A GROUP (group dynamics)

When a group of persons from different villages comes together for a training program, at first it is usually hard for everyone to share his thoughts openly with the others.

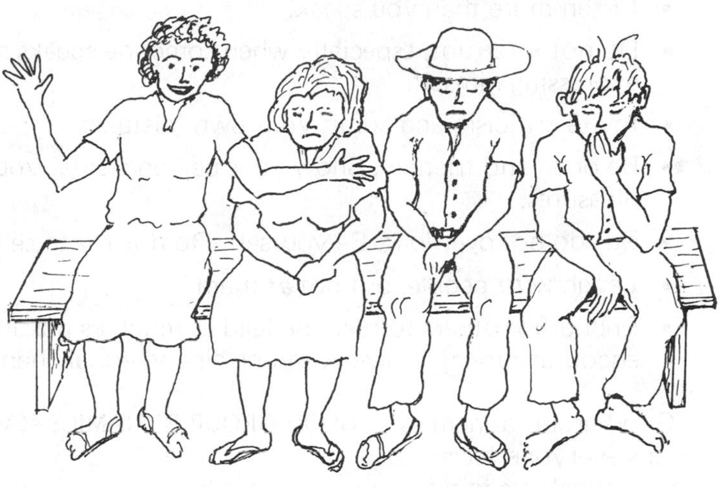

POOR GROUP DYNAMICS—
ONE PERSON TALKS, MOSTLY TO HERSELF.

Many people at first find it easier to listen than to talk, while a few find it easier to talk than to listen. **A good group leader looks for ways to help those who are silent to speak out. At the same time, he helps show those who are quick to speak how important it is to give others a chance.**

Above all else, an effective group leader learns how to keep silent—and when he does speak, to limit himself to asking questions that help draw ideas out of others, especially those who say the least.

Getting the members of a group to talk openly with each other as equals is not easy. It is especially hard when people come from villages or communities where public meetings are controlled by officials or rich persons who have power. In such meetings, only certain individuals are expected to talk. Usually they make a speech, or just give orders. Lies may be told, facts covered up, laws violated, and the people listen silently. Often they feel they have no choice. Even when a vote is taken, most persons will not raise their hands until they see the man who owns the house they rent or the land they plant raise his. Long experience has taught them the cost of not remaining silent. (Silence can be enforced in many ways.)

In addition, because the group has come together to begin a training program or 'class', many persons will at first think of it as 'school'. As we discussed in Chapter 1, for most of us school is a place where the teacher, or schoolmaster, is boss. When the student is asked a question, the 'right' answer is not what he thinks or deeply believes, but rather what the teacher reads from the textbook. What the student thinks or feels is of small importance. In fact, the less he manages to think or feel, the better he is likely to get along in the classroom.

The experiences of many of the group's members, then, both in village meetings and in school, often make them reluctant or afraid to speak freely and openly—especially in the presence of a leader with authority. It therefore helps if the group leader, or instructor, is himself a villager from the area. From the very first, **the leader needs to do all he can to show he considers himself on the same level with all the others.**

As group leader, your actions say more than your words. It helps if you:

- Sit in the circle with everyone else, not apart or behind a desk.
- Dress simply in local style (especially if you are local).
- Listen more than you speak.
- Do not interrupt, especially when someone speaks slowly or has trouble expressing himself.
- Invite criticism and admit your own mistakes.
- Be open and friendly. Show your personal side: your fears, weaknesses, and pleasures.
- But do not overdo it. Be yourself. Do not try to sell yourself.
- Laugh ***with*** people, but not ***at*** them.
- Encourage others to take the lead as much as possible, and at the same time encourage them to give everyone else an equal chance.

Good group dynamics means everyone feels free to speak his mind, but is ready to listen earnestly to others. It is essential for effective learning and community well-being.

Help health workers understand this process, so they can work toward good group dynamics with people in their communities.

GOOD GROUP DYNAMICS—EVERYONE INVOLVED

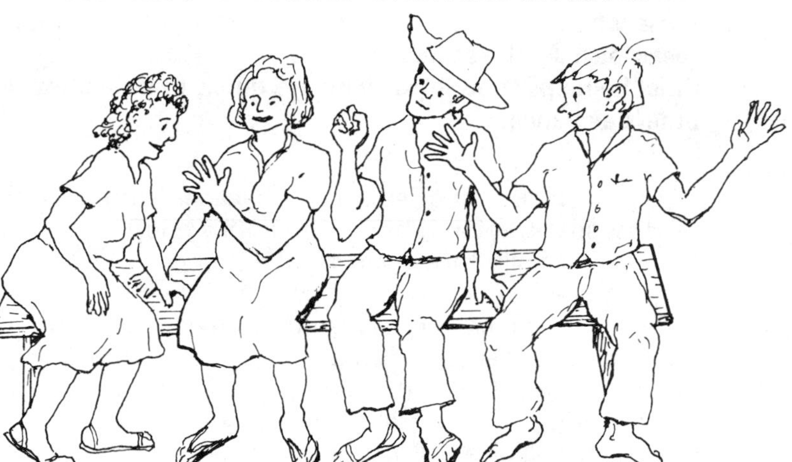

TEACHING 'GROUP DYNAMICS'

At an 'educational exchange' for village instructors of health workers in Mexico, the group leader helped people look at group dynamics in this way: Without telling anyone why, he led two discussions on vague subjects like "the meaning of community health."

In the first discussion, he allowed those who tended to talk more to dominate the discussion. He even encouraged this by asking the same persons to explain things further. By the end, one person talked for 15 minutes straight. Her ideas were good, but the other people were falling asleep or beginning to talk among themselves.

The second discussion was led in a way that got everybody taking part, with no one dominating. The discussion became lively and the group was enthusiastic.

No one realized until afterwards that the two discussions had been set up to study group dynamics. Then the leader asked the group to compare the two discussions, including the role of the leader and the responses of the group.

Everyone learned a lot, especially the person who had talked so much. But she took it well, and took care not to dominate the discussion again.

IMPORTANT THINGS TO START DISCUSSING IN THE FIRST FEW DAYS

To start a training course in a positive way, and to avoid misunderstandings, certain things need to be discussed or made clear during the first few days. You may want to consider scheduling group discussions in the following areas:

- **Hopes and doubts** (of both students and instructors) concerning the course
- **Sharing of responsibilities** and planning (students and instructors together)
- What are the **characteristics of a good health worker?** Of a good instructor?
- Different ways of looking at **health, illness, and being human**
- Goals, objectives, and **the larger vision** of the program
- **Precautions, warnings,** and recognizing our own **limits**
- **Students' experiences** of needs and problems in their communities
- **Need for balance** between prevention, treatment, education, and community action

CAUTION: Although all of the above topics are of key importance and can lead to exciting discussion, they involve a lot of very serious talking. Also, some people may not be used to thinking about these ideas or may be afraid to discuss some of them openly. So in leading these discussions, **try to be sensitive to the feelings, fears, and needs of each member of the group.**

Also, because these are all 'heavy' subjects, it is wise not to weigh people down with too much at once. Space these discussions between classes and activities that are practical, have easier answers, and in which students learn by handling, making, and doing things.

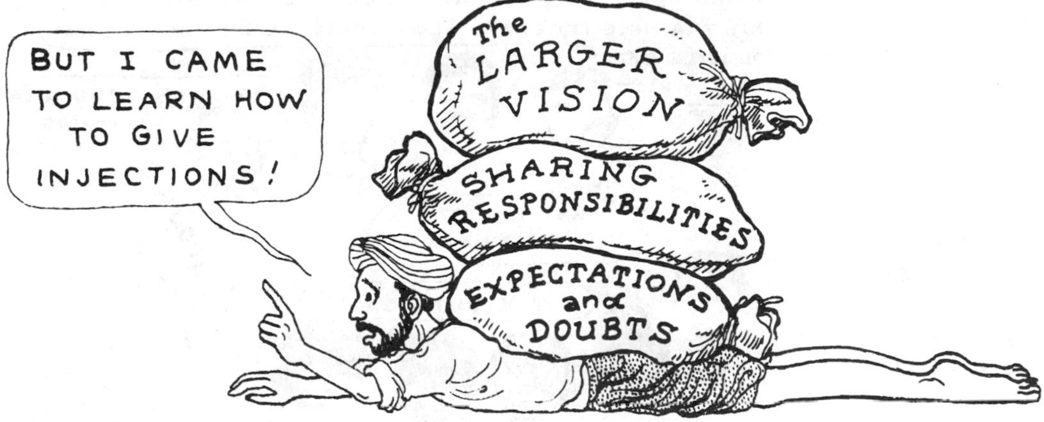

Try not to burden students at first with too many heavy discussions.
Balance discussions with learning of practical skills.

Hopes and doubts

Many training programs find it helpful to spend one of the first discussion periods giving everyone a chance to express his hopes and doubts about the course. Each student and instructor is asked:

- "What do you hope to learn from or get out of the training program?"
- "What fears, doubts, or uncertainties do you have about the program?"

Giving everyone a chance to express his expectations and doubts has three advantages:

- It starts people talking with each other about things that really matter to them.
- It helps students realize that their ideas and concerns are important, and will be taken into consideration in planning the course.
- It gives instructors ideas for adapting the course to better meet the students' desires and needs.

All this sounds good on paper, but will it work? Will new students, mostly strangers to each other, speak openly about their hopes and doubts?

Often they will not—at least not if asked in front of the whole group.

But if they split up into small groups of 2 or 3 persons, they usually will feel more comfortable about expressing their feelings. One person in each group can be chosen to take notes during these discussions, and later report to the whole group. It can be surprising how many important concerns come to the surface.

GETTING PEOPLE TO EXPRESS THEIR DOUBTS

(the advantage of starting discussion in very small groups)

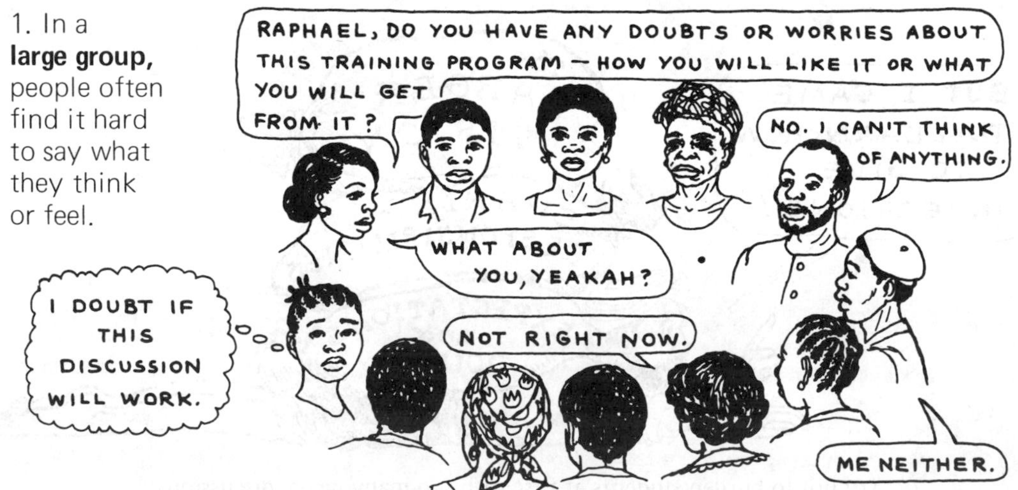
RAPHAEL, DO YOU HAVE ANY DOUBTS OR WORRIES ABOUT THIS TRAINING PROGRAM — HOW YOU WILL LIKE IT OR WHAT YOU WILL GET FROM IT?
NO. I CAN'T THINK OF ANYTHING.
WHAT ABOUT YOU, YEAKAH?
I DOUBT IF THIS DISCUSSION WILL WORK.
NOT RIGHT NOW.
ME NEITHER.

1. In a **large group,** people often find it hard to say what they think or feel.

2. But in very **small groups** they can speak out more easily.

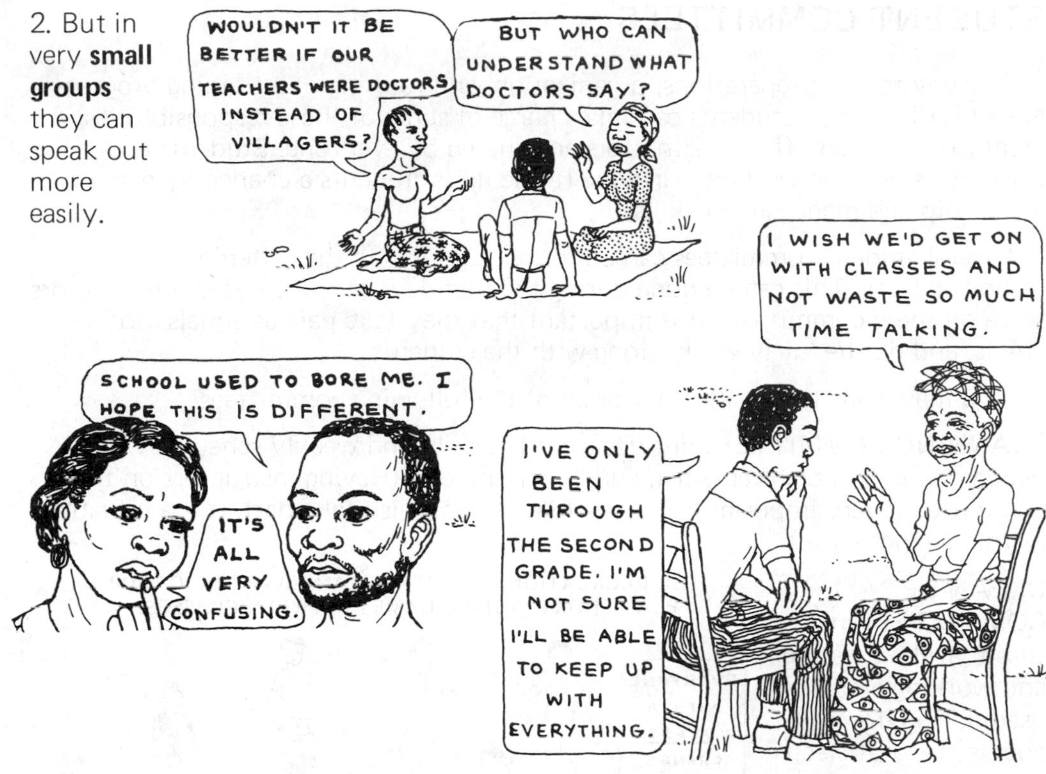
WOULDN'T IT BE BETTER IF OUR TEACHERS WERE DOCTORS INSTEAD OF VILLAGERS?
BUT WHO CAN UNDERSTAND WHAT DOCTORS SAY?
I WISH WE'D GET ON WITH CLASSES AND NOT WASTE SO MUCH TIME TALKING.
SCHOOL USED TO BORE ME. I HOPE THIS IS DIFFERENT.
IT'S ALL VERY CONFUSING.
I'VE ONLY BEEN THROUGH THE SECOND GRADE. I'M NOT SURE I'LL BE ABLE TO KEEP UP WITH EVERYTHING.

3. So it makes sense first to get people saying what they think in small groups. They can then go back and report to the big group.

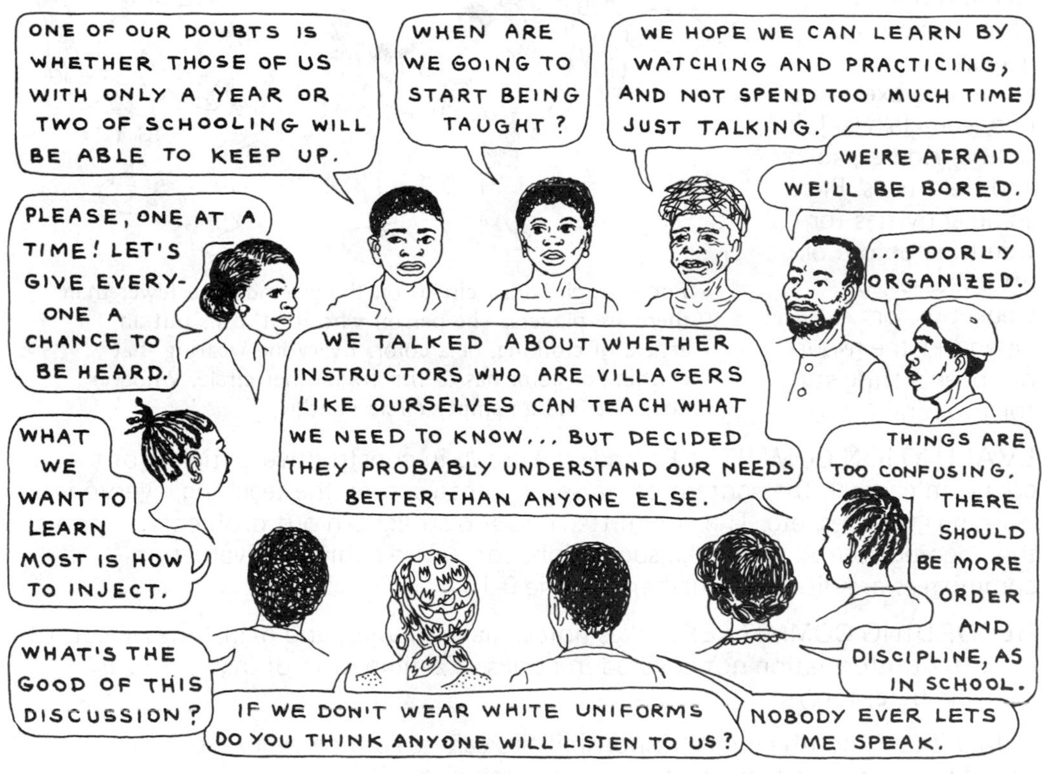

STUDENT COMMITTEES

The day-to-day preparations, organization, and running of a training program are a lot of work. If students can take charge of some of these responsibilities, a great load is taken off the instructors and shared by everyone. Students and instructors become working partners. It also gives students a chance to learn leadership and management skills.

Several student committees can be formed to take on the different responsibilities. This can be done during the first days of the course. If instructors serve on these committees, it is important that they take part as equals, not chiefs, and do the 'dirty work' along with the students.

You may want to consider any or all of the following committees:

PLANNING COMMITTEE: decides what the daily and weekly schedule will be, which classes will be given when and by whom, etc. (Having instructors on this committee is very important. But if a few students also take part, it is a valuable learning experience.)

CLEAN-UP COMMITTEE: makes sure that the meeting and working areas used during the course are kept clean and neat.

RECREATION COMMITTEE: organizes group games, short stretching exercises between classes, joke telling, riddles, songs, and field trips. Plan some activities for free time before or after classes, on weekends, or whenever the group has been sitting still for too long.

THE RECREATION COMMITTEE CAN HAVE THE GROUP PLAY SHORT, ACTIVE GAMES BETWEEN CLASSES.

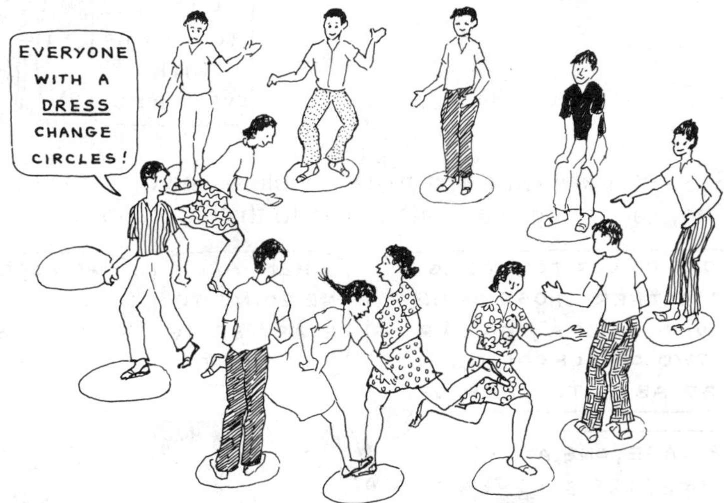

For example, draw circles on the ground—one fewer than there are players. The person who is 'it' calls out an article of clothing, or a color. Everyone wearing that clothing or color has to run to another circle. Whoever does not find an empty circle is 'it'.

EVALUATION COMMITTEE: leads the group in constructive criticism of the course in general, the content of classes, the instructors, the teaching, everyone's learning attitudes, etc. The committee helps to straighten out problems, improve the ongoing course, and make suggestions for future courses. (Evaluation committees are discussed further on page **9**-15.)

RECORDING COMMITTEE: takes notes, makes copies, and distributes sheets of important information not covered in books. (Participation of instructors is valuable here, too.)

In a 2 to 3 month course, responsibilities can be rotated every week or so. This gives everyone a chance to work on each committee.

CHAPTER 5

Planning a Class

TWO APPROACHES—CLOSED AND OPEN

Some instructors follow a standard or 'closed' outline in planning their classes. Others use a more 'open-ended' approach, and feel free to change or adapt the class plan to meet specific needs as they arise. On the following pages we give examples of 2 quite different class plans.

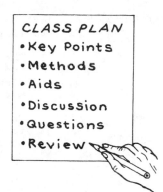

CLASS PLAN
• Key Points
• Methods
• Aids
• Discussion
• Questions
• Review

1. **The first class plan** is taken from a manual for teaching village mothers. It is very specific in telling exactly what the listeners will know and be able to do by the end of the class.

Notice that the writer of the manual has decided in advance exactly what will be taught, and what the students will know, without even knowing who the students will be. According to this kind of class plan, the 'all-knowing' instructor (who really only needs to know how to follow instructions) funnels pre-packaged knowledge into the heads of 'unknowing' receivers. The students 'parrot back' the knowledge provided.

2. **The second class plan** shows a more open approach. In this case, the experience of the students has value. Importance is given not only to the subject of the class, but also to the less clearly defined learning that happens along the way. Such learning includes:

- experimenting with new teaching methods
- showing quick learners ways to assist those who learn more slowly
- observing and respecting each other's traditions and beliefs, strengths and uncertainties

The first class plan, with its tone of authority and more rigid instructions, makes us feel it should be followed obediently and exactly. The second class plan is quite the opposite. It invites the students and instructor to evaluate the class together, and to make recommendations for improving it the next time around. The difference between the 2 plans lies in the question of growth and change:

- The first class plan is structured so that the same teaching pattern can be repeated or 'replicated' time after time, in program after program. Just follow the instructions!
- With the second class plan, each time the class is taught it is original. The ideas and assistance of the learning group make it better each time.

The second approach is designed for change. The first, to resist it.

FIRST EXAMPLE OF A CLASS PLAN*

(using the 'resistant to change' approach)

LESSON 8A: CONJUNCTIVITIS :

Symptoms and treatment of conjunctivitis.

GOAL: To make listeners aware of the symptoms of conjunctivitis and how it can be treated.

OBJECTIVES: At the end of this lesson, listeners will be able to list the following:

1. The symptoms of conjunctivitis are: red eyes and swollen eyelids, slight itching and a discharge when waking up in the morning; eyelids are sometimes stuck together with pus.

2. To avoid serious complications, it is advisable to seek medical attention. Before going, you should wash your eyes with boiled, slightly salted water after allowing it to cool a bit. The warm salty water will help remove the pus so the medicine you are given can be more effective.

3. Until conjunctivitis is completely cured, you should wash your eyes three times a day with salt water.

VISUAL AIDS:
- Child with conjunctivitis (red, puffy eyes with a discharge).
- Mother washing her child's eyes.
- Mother bringing child to health center.
- A clean piece of cloth.
- Warm salt water.
- Water and soap.
- Bowl.

PRESENTATION:
- Has your child already had conjunctivitis?

- What do your eyes look like when you have conjunctivitis?

Show poster of child with conjunctivitis.

- Look at Abdulie. What is wrong with him?

- If your child has conjunctivitis like Abdulie, what should you do?

Show poster of woman washing her child's eyes and poster of woman bringing her child to a health centre as they answer the previous question.

- How should you wash his eyes?

---

*Copied from *Health and Sanitation Lessons (Africa),* No. 27, Appropriate Technologies for Development, Action/Peace Corps, Washington, D.C. Publication not dated.

SECOND EXAMPLE OF A CLASS PLAN
(using the 'education of change' approach)

Subject: *Common Health Problems* Date: *Nov. 10* Time: *3 PM*

Topic: *Fever* Instructor: *Pablo*

Main ideas, information skills, or activities	Teaching methods	Materials and preparation needed	Pages in book
1. Review of use of thermometer	- questions and practice	- 6 thermometers - alcohol - cotton	WTND, p. 31
2. What fever is, and how to treat it	- role playing - use of book	- 2 baby dolls - student actors - play thermometers - bucket, rags, and water	75-76
3. Dangerously high and dangerously low temperatures			31, 272

Related learning:

Use of book, role playing, teaching methods, understanding and respecting local beliefs and customs.

TIME	Class outline:	Points to be emphasized	How to emphasize
10 minutes	1. Review--Use of thermometer - "Who can show how to take a temperature?" (volunteers take temp. on each other, in mouth and under arm of same person)	- how to use thermometer, where and how long, how to read and clean	- demonstration - discussion - practice
5 minutes	- "How do mouth and arm temps. compare?" "And in anus?" "Any volunteers?" "Which way is best? On whom? Why?"	- understanding readings in arm, mouth, anus	- book, page 31
5 minutes	- Give students some real and some play thermometers to read. Have them check each other.		
15 minutes	2A. - Role play--High fever When review is almost completed, one of the woman students (prepared in advance) rushes in pretending she is the mother of a 'sick baby' (a large doll). The 'baby' is convulsing, and is all wrapped up. (Doll has been left in sun and is *very hot*.) Students try to figure out what to do, *fast*, using what they already know, and using their books. (Index? Contents?) Thermometer is used, under arm. "Why?" (Health worker shakes it down; mother sets it to 41º C.) Baby is *stripped naked*, bathed with *cold water*, given *water to drink* and *baby aspirin*.	- emergency problem solving: convulsions from fever - first things first - lower high fever first and fast: - take off clothes - bathe, cool water - cool drink - aspirin	- role play - book, p. 75-76 - practice - discussion

		Points to be emphasized	How to emphasize
	'Mother' at first objects to undressing and bathing the 'baby', but health worker explains why. When the 'baby' stops convulsing, she realizes these methods work.	- traditions and beliefs - how to deal with the human factor	- role play
10 minutes	2B. Reading aloud from book, p. 75-76 and discussion - "What did we do right?" - "What did we do wrong?" - "Do people in our villages wrap up babies when they have fever? Why?" - "What other beliefs or home treatments for fever do people have?" - "How did the mother feel about bathing the baby? How did we handle this?" - "Could we have done it better?"	- use of book - asking the right questions - evaluating our own actions - evaluating local ways of healing - being sensitive to the 'mother'	- read book - emphasize main points - ask questions to get people thinking about actual experiences
10 minutes	3A. Role play--Temperature too low Above discussion is interrupted by another student actor with a 'very sick baby' (a doll). The 'baby' is 2 weeks old, very cool, and naked. Health workers take temperature. Play thermometer says 34°C. Use books. (Index: Temperature, too low, p. 30 and 272. Have someone read these parts aloud.)	- recognizing low temperature as a danger sign - correct use of book and index	- role play - look up in book
5 minutes	3B. Discussion - "Low temperature in a newborn baby is usually a sign of what illness?" - "Should this baby be left naked or wrapped up? Why?" (It is important to keep this baby warm, but not too warm.) Put on blackboard:	- look out for dangerously low temperature, below 35°C. - feel child's body; put finger in his armpit to see if cool - warm a cold baby at once; put him next to mother's body	- discussion - blackboard

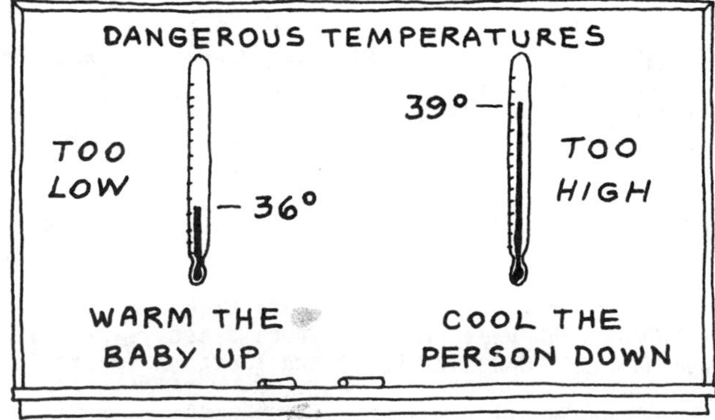

CAUTION: Take care not to get the class involved yet with the treatment of the infection causing the fever. (Explain that this will be covered in another class. Save time for review!)

	Points to be emphasized	How to emphasize
4. Review - Who can say briefly: - What do you do for someone with moderate fever? With high fever? - What do you do for a baby with too low a temperature? - Why is a high fever dangerous? - What else did you learn today? - about fever? - about customs and beliefs? - about ways to teach? - (role play, pretend thermometers, use of index, use of book) - What else? - Was anything in the class unclear? Did everyone take part? How could the class have been better? How can you use what you learned?	- all of above - check temp. first; if too high or low, correct at once - watch out for low temp. in newborn babies - treatment must respect customs - learning methods: - role play - practice - discussion - use of book - pretend thermometers - suggestions for improvement	- questions and discussion - make sure everyone gets to take part

Comments on how well the class went, and how it might be improved:

To be filled in after class.

Effectiveness:

- *Major points were all covered.*
- *Students enthusiastic: laughed, learned, no one slept.*
- *Students also expressed interest in teacher's methods; thought they would use them.*
- *Most students were involved, but some still kept very quiet while others talked more. In future will ask 'talkers' to find ways to help others participate more.*

Difficulties:

- *Class went overtime; 1 hour and 5 minutes. Perhaps I tried to put too much into it. Students took a long time to look things up in book. Also, discussion tended to wander, although there was a lot of valuable discussion about folk beliefs.*
- *One problem was that, although quicker students showed slower ones where to look in book, did not really help them learn how. Perhaps I can talk with the quicker students so that they try to guide, but not show the others where to look.*

Recommendations for future class on this subject:

- *Just one role play, not two.*
- *More time to discuss traditional beliefs. This appears to be one of the biggest and most delicate problems the health workers may have to deal with. It is especially important to explore how to lower the fever of a baby when his mother fears that uncovering or bathing the child will kill him.*

Questions for test:

(Questions that can be used in a test to reinforce what students have learned, and to see if main ideas were adequately covered in class.)

THESE 3 TEMPERATURES WERE TAKEN IN 3 DIFFERENT PERSONS:

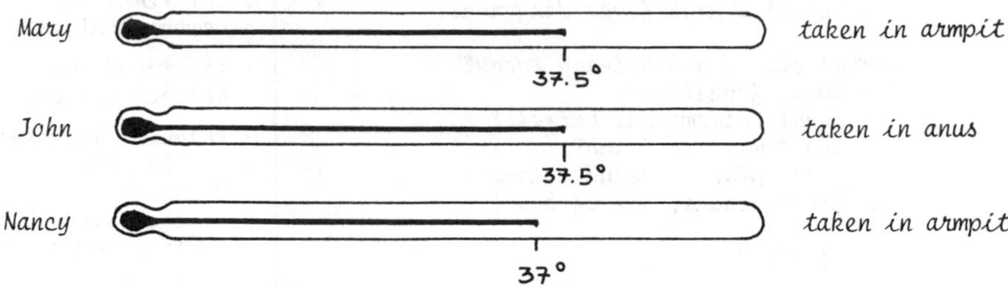

1. *Who has the highest fever?*
2. *Whose temperature is closest to normal?*
3. *What changes in temperature may occur when a newborn baby has an infection?*
4. *Name 4 steps to lower the temperature of a child with a very high fever.*
5. *What do you do if the temperature stays high in spite of measures taken to lower it?*
6. *What would you do if a baby has a very high fever, but his mother is afraid that undressing and bathing him will cause harm?*
7. *What would you do if you put your finger under a baby's arm and it feels cool?*

Note on this class plan:

This kind of plan may be longer than you have time to prepare for every class. However, complete plans like this are especially helpful if someone else will be preparing the class the next time. For your own use, you can write just enough to remind you of what to cover. You also can make class plans shorter by using abbreviations (**D** for discussion, **RP** for role play, etc.).

Do try to **list the main points** the health workers will need to learn in order to carry out their work in the community. Be sure all the important points are emphasized during the class, and briefly reviewed by the students at the end. Students can help you think of test questions, too.

TASK ANALYSIS—Finding out what is needed to do a job effectively

Story: Joe, a new instructor, led a series of classes and activities to help health workers learn about sanitation. He explained the importance of latrines, how deep to dig them, and how far they should be from houses and water sources. He showed drawings of different ways to make latrines, and took the students to see two 'model latrines' with cement platforms. He advised them about 'setting objectives' for the number of families they hoped would have latrines after one year.

At the end of the course, Joe gave the health workers an exam with many questions like: "How far should a latrine be from the river?" and "Why is a cement platform better than wood?" Everyone answered the questions correctly, and Joe was pleased.

But when the health workers tried to start latrine projects in their villages, they ran into difficulties.

Mary found that people simply were not interested in latrines because they "smell bad." She did not know how to deal with that.

Frank managed to get 7 people to build latrines—but then they did not use them.

John ran into construction problems. In his village, no one had ever made cement, so he did his best to cast the first platform himself. But John did not think to use reinforcing wire. And he did not know that cement will not harden well unless it is kept wet for 2 or 3 days after casting. So the platform was very weak.

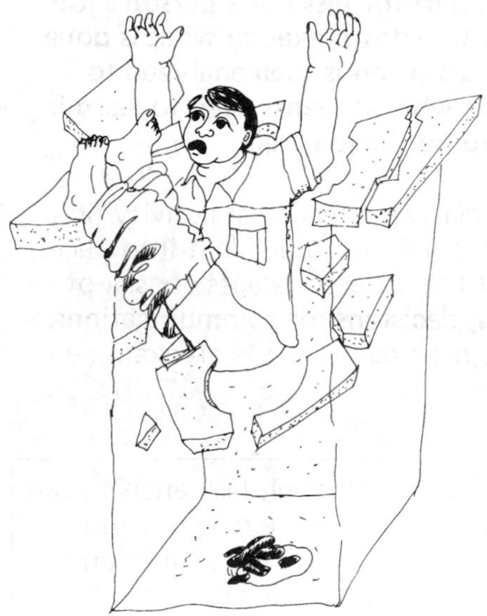

Unfortunately, John had convinced the village chief to build this first latrine. For several days the platform held together. But one evening the chief's brother, who was overweight, used the latrine and the platform broke to pieces.

Poor John learned a very important lesson!

Moral: When you teach something, be sure you cover all the points needed to do the job properly.

Clearly, Joe's teaching about latrines was not complete. Some of the most important factors and steps were left out. The training could have prepared the students to do their job more effectively . . .

- if they had learned about latrines by actually making them, not just talking about them and seeing them

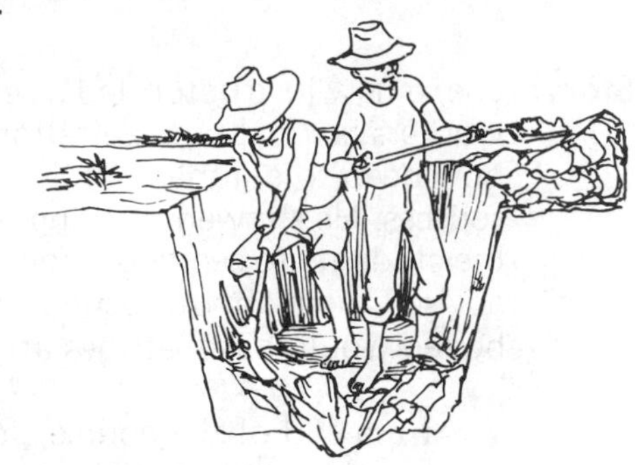

- if the instructor had invited some experienced health workers to talk about their own problems and experiences introducing latrines in their villages

- if the instructor had carefully analyzed each step or aspect of what health workers need to do and to know in order to successfully introduce and build latrines in their communities

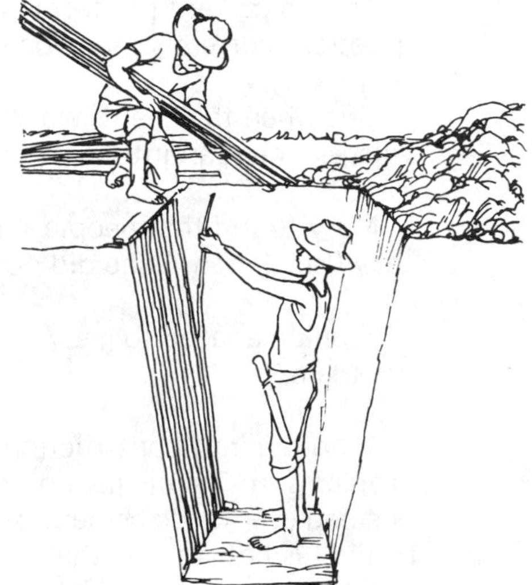

This last process is called *task analysis.* *

Task analysis is a method for looking at each part (or task) of a person's job and writing down exactly what is done. This description is then analyzed to find out what students need to learn in order to do the job well.

To analyze a particular activity or task, it is helpful to divide it into stages. Note if the different stages consist of **actions, decisions,** or **communications.** On the next page we give an example.

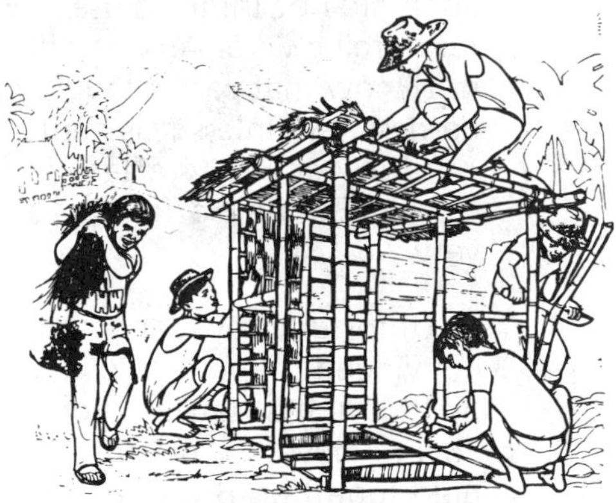

CAUTION: Although task analysis can be helpful, it must be remembered that each health worker's situation will be different. Flexibility, or readiness to adapt tasks to suit local conditions, should be built into the analysis.

The best way to be sure health workers know how to do each step of an activity is to have them actually do it during training. (drawings by Lino Montebon from *Ang Maayong Lawas Maagum,* the Philippines)

*These ideas for task analysis have been adapted from ***Teaching for Better Learning,*** by Fred Abbatt, WHO, Geneva, 1980.

The following is an example of a task analysis. It is not intended to apply to all communities. You will need to do your own.

TASK ANALYSIS SHEET The Task: Introducing latrines 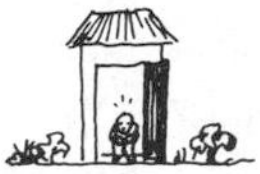		
Stages of the Task Actions (A) Decisions (D) Communications (C)	Knowledge and Skills Needed	Ways to Learn
1. Find out community interest. (C) 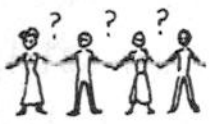	ability to explain and listen 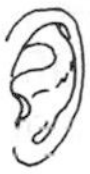	talk with experienced health workers; role plays; group dialogue
2. Decide if latrine project is possible at this time. (D)	understanding of people and customs 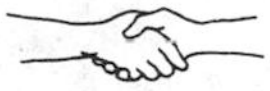	community dynamics; discussions about traditions & behavior
3. Help people learn importance of latrines to health. (C) 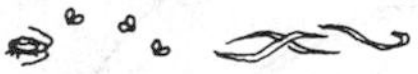	knowledge of how disease spreads; teaching skills 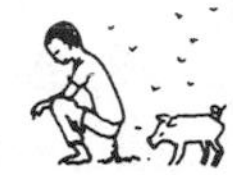	from observation, books, and discussions; practice teaching 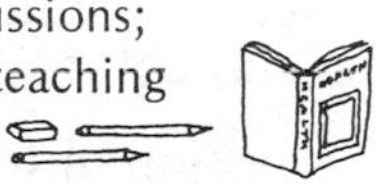
4. Decide where latrines will be built. (D)	knowledge of safety factors 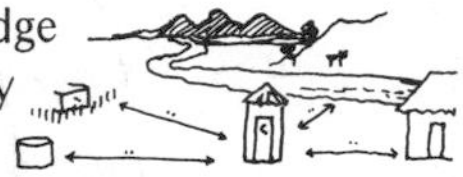	books and discussions; thinking it through with local people
5. Get materials needed. (A) 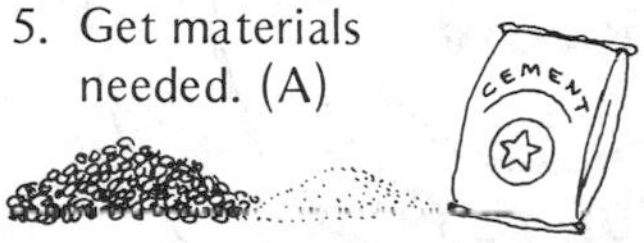	what local materials can be used; what else is needed; where to buy at low cost, etc.	talk with local mason; trip to market 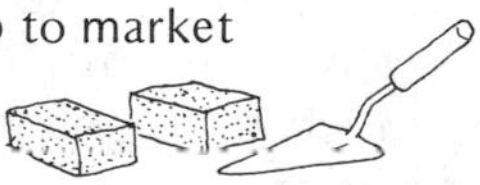
6. Help people build the latrines. (A) 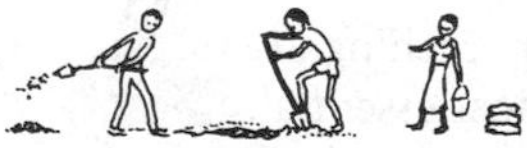	dimensions of pit and platform; how to mix, cast, reinforce, and cure cement; how to build outhouse & lid	have students take part in actually making latrines. 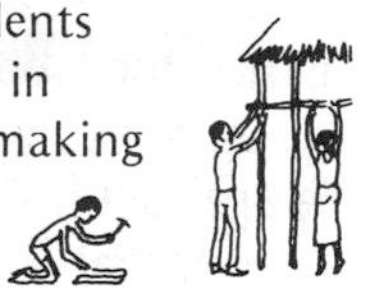
7. Encourage people to use latrines and to keep them covered and clean. (C)	home visits; art of giving suggestions in a friendly way 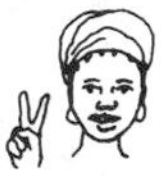	practice, role plays, and discussion 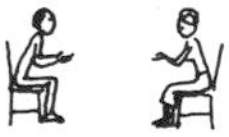

To collect the information you need to do a complete task analysis, you can use these sources:

- your own knowledge and experience
- books and information sheets
- observation of health workers in action
- discussion with other instructors or persons with the skills and experience required
- discussion with health workers

AIMING TEACHING AT WHAT IS MOST IMPORTANT

Many instructors waste a lot of time teaching relatively unnecessary knowledge and skills:

- Some devote long hours to anatomy and physiology.
- Others give long descriptions of diagnoses and treatments. (Time would be better spent helping health workers learn to look up the same information in their books during role plays and in clinical practice.)
- Still others spend days teaching minor skills, such as tying complicated bandages. (It would be more useful to help health workers think of what they might use when the bandage supply runs out!)

When teaching, it is easy to go into more detail than necessary, and in doing so, to lose sight of what is most important. Health workers cannot learn everything. Medicine, public health, teaching methods, understanding of traditions, and development of social awareness are all important. But to learn everything about these fields is impossible—even in a lifetime! Some form of selection is essential.

It may help, in deciding what to teach and what not to teach, to determine whether each aspect is . . .

- **essential to know,**
- useful to know, or
- nice to know.

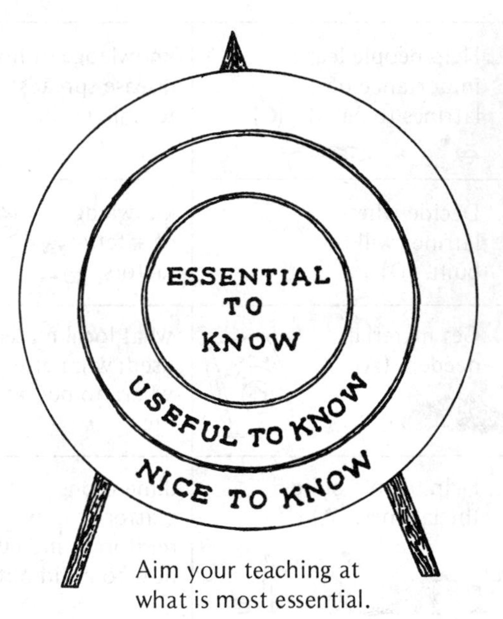

Aim your teaching at what is most essential.

Your main aim is to cover what is essential. Since time is limited, you need to aim carefully. Try not to spend too much time on what is less important.

But remember, the human and social aspects of health care are just as important as the technical information and skills.

TESTING OUR TEACHING:

For each subject, each class, and each point you teach, it helps to ask yourself:

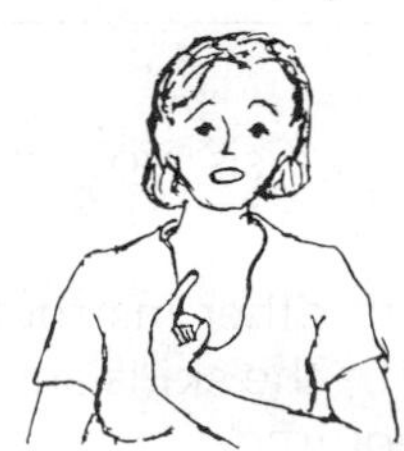

- Why am I teaching this?
- In what way does what I am teaching prepare health workers to perform a skill, or to work effectively in the community?
- Could this time be better used to teach something more important—or to teach the same thing more effectively?

For more ideas about evaluation of classes and teaching, see page **9**-14.

STARTING WITH WHAT IS ALREADY FAMILIAR TO STUDENTS

To have meaning, **learning must relate to life.** So to help health workers work effectively, their training needs to begin with ideas, situations, or problems already familiar to them. **Try to start with your students' own knowledge or experience—and build on that.**

STARTING WITH LIFE, NOT WITH ANATOMY:

Many instructors (especially some doctors) organize the teaching of health problems according to where they occur in the body, rather than how they occur in a community. To do this, they often start by teaching 'anatomy and physiology' (the parts of the body and how they work).

This approach has several disadvantages:

1. To start by studying people's ***insides*** is to start with something ***outside*** the experience of most students. It can make them feel lost or even stupid.

Here is an example:

It makes more sense (to students) to start discussing health problems in terms of what they have already experienced or seen. On this solid base new information can be added, in a way that relates more to the students' work.

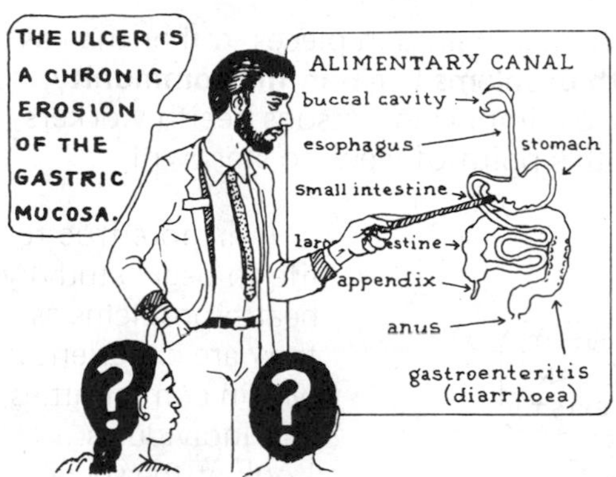

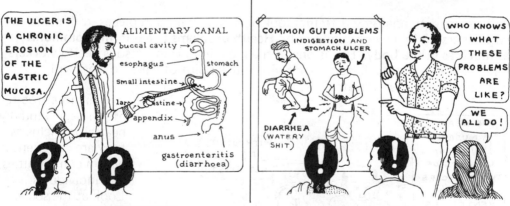

LESS APPROPRIATE

MORE APPROPRIATE

2. Starting with 'anatomy and physiology' usually means introducing a lot of big Latin words. The student is in danger of coming to believe that **big words,** rather than **health** and **problem solving,** are of first importance. When he returns to his community, he may try to impress and frighten others with his new words (just as he was at first frightened and impressed by them). Yet the health worker's job is to help people gain confidence in their own language and culture, to build on the knowledge and strengths they already have.

One of the most important skills that health workers and their instructors need to learn is to . . .

Discuss health problems in clear, simple language that everyone understands.

3. Organizing the study of common illnesses according to 'body systems' may make sense sometimes—but not always. For example, it may make sense to study different breathing (respiratory) problems as a group. Many of them have similar symptoms (cough) and they are sometimes confused. However, it is usually more practical to organize the study of diseases according to . . .

- how common or serious they are in the community,
- who they affect most (women, children, old people, the poor), or
- how (or if) they spread from person to person.

Under this last plan, whooping cough might be studied with 'contagious diseases of childhood'. (This does not, of course, prevent it being reviewed with other respiratory problems, for comparison and diagnosis.)

Unfortunately, some instructors are so rigid about teaching according to body systems that they lose sight of what comes first in a community. Thus they cover 'esophageal ulcers' before diarrhea, simply because the esophagus comes before the intestines in the digestive system. In terms of importance in most communities, diarrhea comes first—and should be studied first! As a general rule, it is more appropriate to . . .

Organize the study of different diseases according to their place in the community, not their place in the body.

4. To start with anatomy is to first look at human beings in pieces, rather than as whole persons in a living community. **Health problems begin in the community as much as in the body.** This is one of the most important lessons health workers (and their instructors) need to learn. From this point of view, to start with anatomy is the kiss of death.

It is more true to life to begin studying health problems as they are experienced within communities and individuals. Look at the social and physical causes, symptoms, and effects on people's health and lives. In this way, **the humanness of people can be kept alive.** It is easily lost when the body is first looked at in pieces.

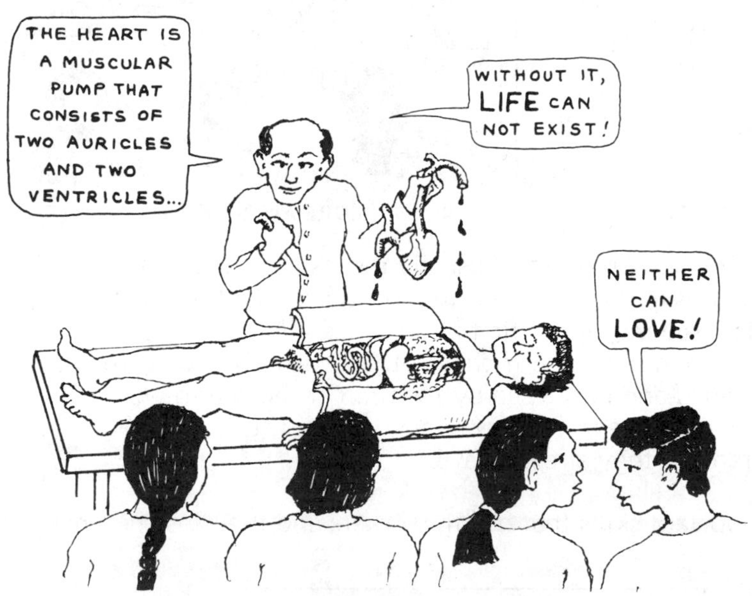

TWO WAYS OF LOOKING AT 'HEART'.
Which is more important to community health?

Start with community, not anatomy!

INTERESTING AND USEFUL WAYS OF TEACHING 'ANATOMY'

'Anatomy and physiology' can be deadly! Especially if taught as a separate subject early in a course. (See the story on page **2**-16.)

However, learning about 'parts of the body and how they work' can be useful—especially if taught, not separately, but as part of the study of familiar health problems.

People learn better and remember longer if they understand the reasons why things happen. If they discover the reasons for themselves, they remember even better. Therefore, 'anatomy and physiology' become more meaningful when students find out for themselves . . .

- why health problems they have seen affect the body as they do, and
- why certain measures are used to prevent or treat certain problems.

People remember better when they find things out for themselves and are not just told what to do.

For example, health workers may be taught to feel for a large spleen when they learn about physical examinations or about signs of malaria.

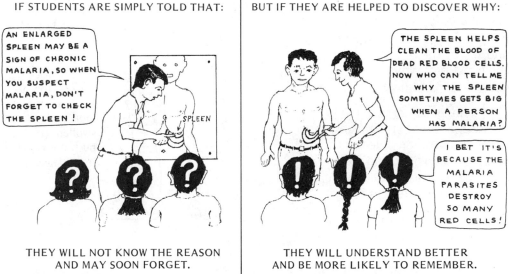

IF STUDENTS ARE SIMPLY TOLD THAT:

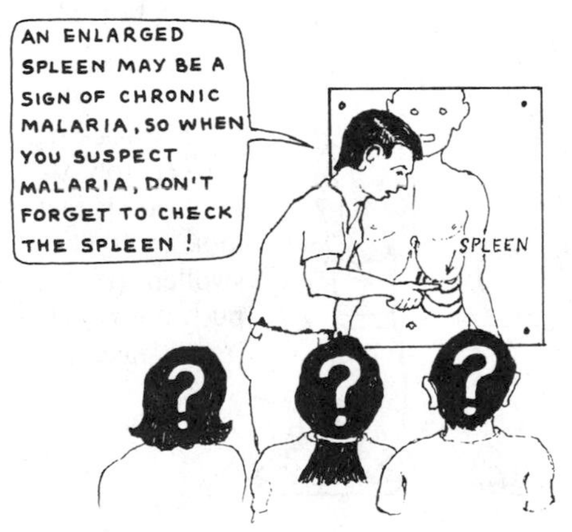

AN ENLARGED SPLEEN MAY BE A SIGN OF CHRONIC MALARIA, SO WHEN YOU SUSPECT MALARIA, DON'T FORGET TO CHECK THE SPLEEN!
SPLEEN

THEY WILL NOT KNOW THE REASON AND MAY SOON FORGET.

BUT IF THEY ARE HELPED TO DISCOVER WHY:

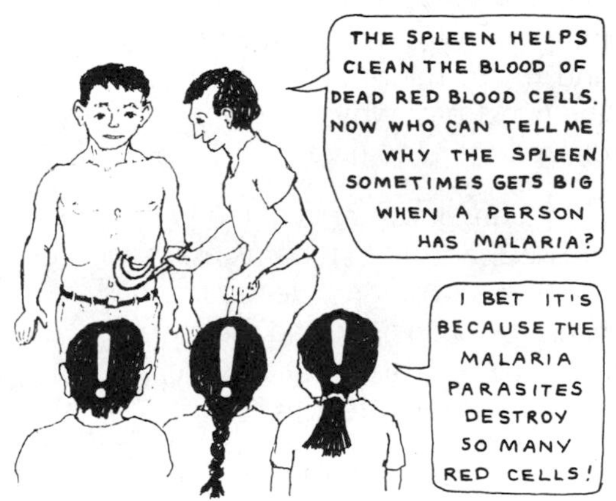

THE SPLEEN HELPS CLEAN THE BLOOD OF DEAD RED BLOOD CELLS. NOW WHO CAN TELL ME WHY THE SPLEEN SOMETIMES GETS BIG WHEN A PERSON HAS MALARIA?
I BET IT'S BECAUSE THE MALARIA PARASITES DESTROY SO MANY RED CELLS!

THEY WILL UNDERSTAND BETTER AND BE MORE LIKELY TO REMEMBER.

In this way, 'physiology' (how the body works) becomes useful immediately. It helps people discover the reasons for what happens and what needs to be done.

Notice also that, in the picture on the right, the instructor is drawing the anatomy on one of the students, not on paper. **Take every opportunity to bring anatomy to life and to keep it alive.** (See p. **11**-6.)

EXAMPLE OF ANATOMY BEING USED TO HELP EXPLAIN CERTAIN HEALTH PROBLEMS (RATHER THAN BEING TAUGHT SEPARATELY):

Topic: Diseases of the liver

Objective: To learn about common diseases of the liver—cirrhosis,* hepatitis, amebic abscess—and how to recognize, manage, and prevent them.

Instead of beginning the class with a description of the liver and its functions (which could be very dull), a common liver problem is 'brought to life' with a role play. For this, one of the students is prepared before the class:

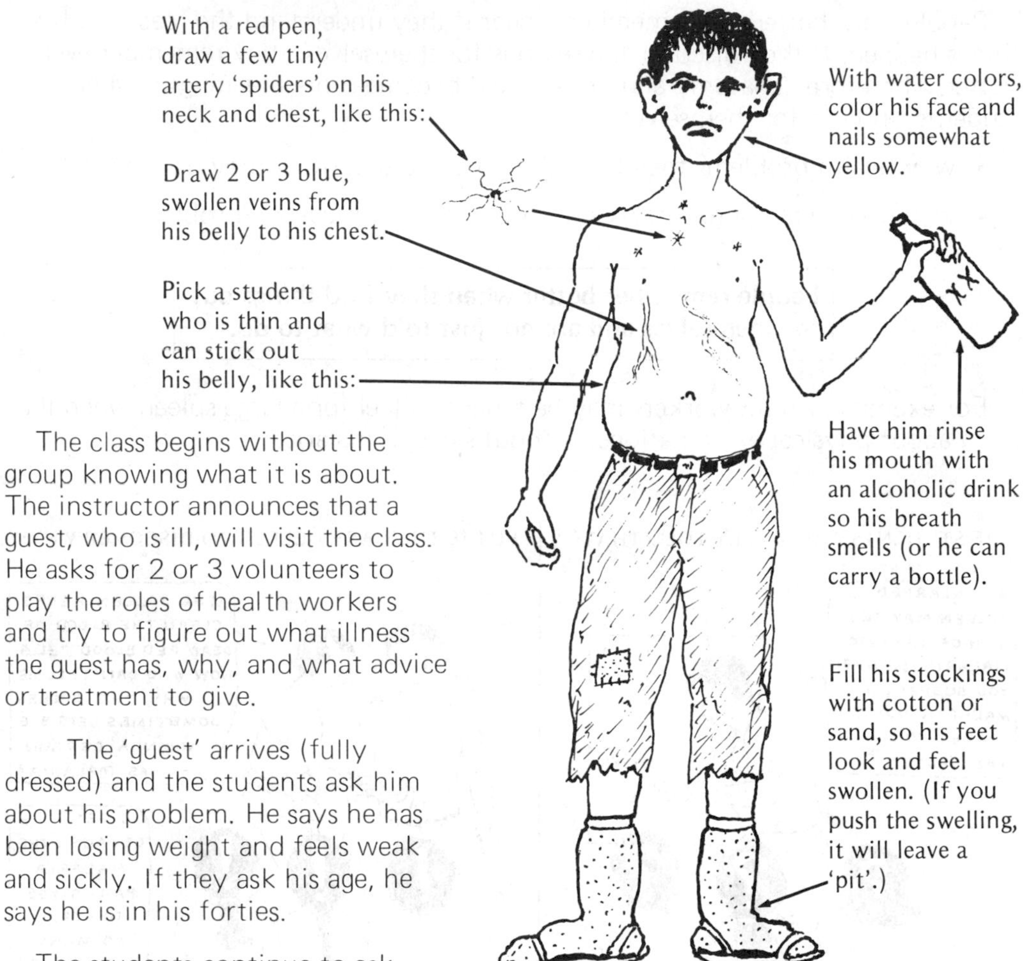

With a red pen, draw a few tiny artery 'spiders' on his neck and chest, like this:
Draw 2 or 3 blue, swollen veins from his belly to his chest.
Pick a student who is thin and can stick out his belly, like this:
With water colors, color his face and nails somewhat yellow.
XX
Have him rinse his mouth with an alcoholic drink so his breath smells (or he can carry a bottle).
Fill his stockings with cotton or sand, so his feet look and feel swollen. (If you push the swelling, it will leave a 'pit'.)

The class begins without the group knowing what it is about. The instructor announces that a guest, who is ill, will visit the class. He asks for 2 or 3 volunteers to play the roles of health workers and try to figure out what illness the guest has, why, and what advice or treatment to give.

The 'guest' arrives (fully dressed) and the students ask him about his problem. He says he has been losing weight and feels weak and sickly. If they ask his age, he says he is in his forties.

The students continue to ask questions and examine the guest. Using their books, they try to identify his problem. The guest (who has studied the signs and causes of cirrhosis before the class) answers the questions as a person with cirrhosis really might, but not always 'truthfully'. He might say, for example, that he has not had an alcoholic drink in years. Yet the smell on his breath will give him away—if the students are observant enough to notice.

The health workers decide that their guest probably has advanced cirrhosis of the liver.

---

*In some countries, cirrhosis of the liver is a leading cause of death in adults.

Some of the signs the students find, such as the artery 'spiders' and swollen veins on the stomach, are not mentioned in their book *(WTND)* and may puzzle them. The instructor can help them figure out how the different signs fit together, and why they occur. But for this, they need to learn something about the liver and how it works.

This learning can take place through questions and answers. The instructor provides some facts, but tries to encourage students to figure out the answers for themselves:

Facts (F): The liver serves, among other things, as a filter to clean poisons and waste material from the blood. Blood coming through veins from the gut passes through the liver before going back to the heart.

Question (Q): Now who can say why alcohol harms the liver?

Response to students' answers (R): Right! Alcohol is a poison. The liver works hard to remove it from the blood. If the person drinks a lot over many years, the liver itself becomes poisoned. The damage is greater if the person does not eat well.

F: The damaged liver is like a clogged filter. Blood cannot pass through it well, so it must find other ways to get back to the heart. Also, because the blood is dammed up by the liver, the pressure in the veins is higher. So clear liquid or 'serum' begins to leak out of the veins and smaller blood vessels (capillaries).

Q: Which of the signs of cirrhosis do these facts explain?

R: Swollen veins on the belly; swollen, fluid-filled belly. (The veins in the esophagus also swell, and sometimes burst, causing dangerous bleeding.)

F: The swollen feet (and, in part, the liquid in the belly) can be explained by looking at another job the liver performs. The liver builds new proteins from foods that have been digested. One of the functions of proteins in the blood is to prevent too much liquid (serum) from leaking out through the walls of the veins. This is why, when the damaged liver fails to produce protein normally, the feet often swell.

A picture like this will probably make sense to students only if they use it to help explain problems they actually see.

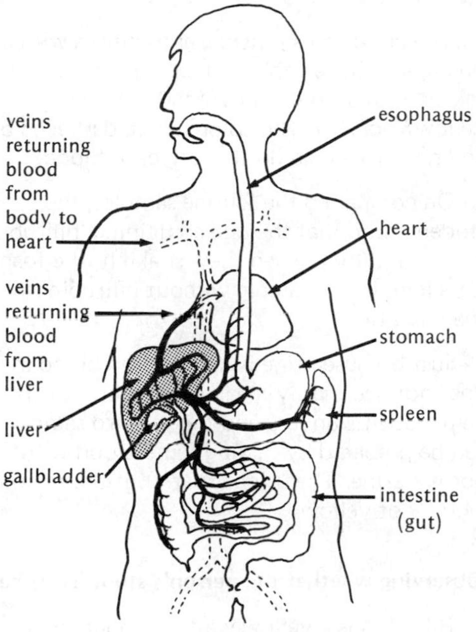

Q: Why do persons with cirrhosis often have such severe wasting (loss) of muscles and weight loss?
Clue: Muscles, like meat, are mostly protein.

F: One of the waste materials the liver removes from the blood is a yellow dye called bilirubin, which is left over when red blood cells die. (Red cells normally live only a few weeks.)

The waste materials collected by the liver become part of a green liquid called bile. Bile collects in the gallbladder and empties into the gut, where it helps digest fatty foods.

A sick or severely damaged liver cannot remove enough bilirubin from the blood.

Q: How does bilirubin affect the appearance of a person with severe liver damage? Why?

R: Yellow skin (and eyes)—'jaundice'.

F: When the sick liver does not remove bilirubin effectively or the bile cannot empty from the gallbladder, some bilirubin is removed by the kidneys.

Q: How do you suppose this affects the urine?

For a way to help the students find out, see the next page.

Test for bilirubin in the urine:

To find out if the urine has bilirubin in it, the students ask their 'guest with cirrhosis' to urinate in a bottle. For comparison, another student does the same.

The guest steps outside, and returns with a prepared urine sample containing normal urine mixed with a little yellow food coloring or yellow *Kool-Aid.* The color can be darkened by adding a little cola drink, coffee, or blood.

On comparing the 2 urine samples, the students find that the one containing 'bilirubin' is dark and that, when they shake it, the foam is yellow. In the sample without bilirubin, the foam is white.

Just because urine is dark, or has blood in it, does not necessarily mean it has bilirubin. To help students understand this, a third sample can be prepared by mixing some blood with normal urine. The urine is dark but the foam is white, not yellow.

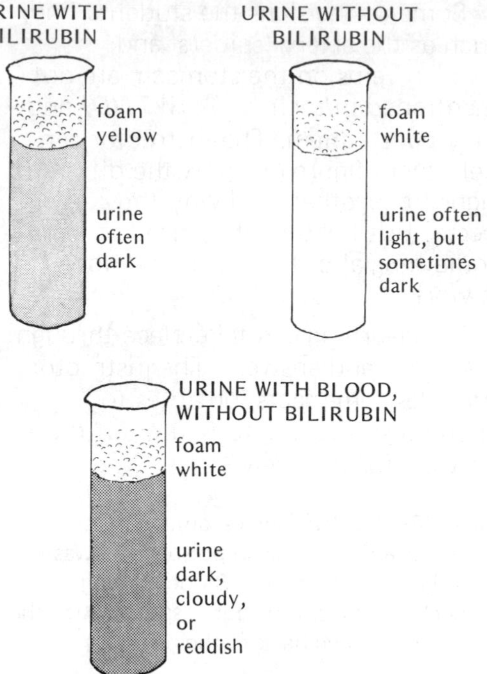

Observing whether the person's stool (shit) has bilirubin in it:

Bilirubin is a yellow waste product from broken-down hemoglobin, the red dye in red blood cells. When removed from the blood by the liver, it becomes part of the green bile. This slowly changes to brown in the gut, and gives the color to normal stools.

Have the students ask the 'guest with cirrhosis' (or one with gallbladder disease) for a 'stool sample'. The visitor returns with a pretend stool made of whitish clay, or old, sun-bleached dog shit. Ask students why it is whitish and why this is a sign of a liver or gallbladder problem.

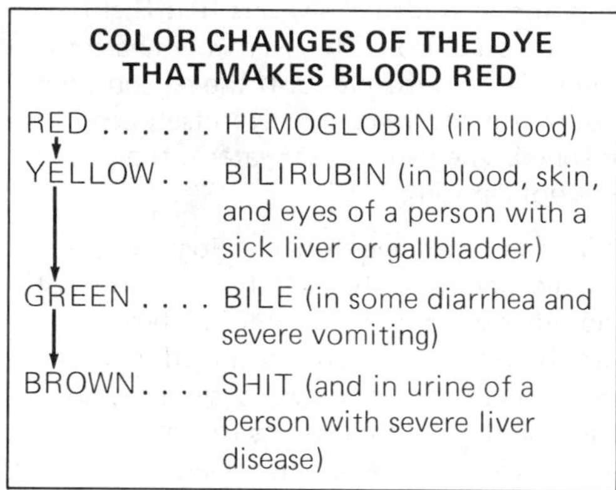

COLOR CHANGES OF THE DYE THAT MAKES BLOOD RED

RED	HEMOGLOBIN (in blood)
↓ YELLOW	BILIRUBIN (in blood, skin, and eyes of a person with a sick liver or gallbladder)
↓ GREEN	BILE (in some diarrhea and severe vomiting)
↓ BROWN	SHIT (and in urine of a person with severe liver disease)

Health Education:

After the students have diagnosed the 'cirrhosis', they can try to explain to their 'guest' what they have learned. They can tell him clearly and simply what his problem is, what it comes from, how the liver works, and the reason for each of his symptoms and signs.

To bring the class even closer to real life, students can also discuss among themselves what support they might be able to give their guest to help him stop drinking and eat better. They may decide to visit and talk with his family and friends.

They also may want to discuss the problem of heavy drinking or alcoholism in their communities, its causes, and possible steps to prevent it. This leads to questions of the social order, human dignity, and raising of people's awareness. Perhaps some of the ideas that are raised in this class can be explored further in classes on social awareness and preparation for home visits. (See Chapters 6 and 26.)

As can be seen from this class on cirrhosis, learning about the body and how it functions can be made interesting and meaningful. This is done by investigating a real person's problems in a lifelike and adventurous way.

We do not suggest that the instructor always include as much explanation of anatomy and body functions as we have done in this example. Your decision will depend on the students' interest, the time available, and the priorities of different subjects to be covered.

We do suggest, however, that **all coverage of anatomy and physiology be introduced in a way that helps students understand real problems within their lives and communities.** It should make sense to them!

Other examples of teaching anatomy and physiology in this book:

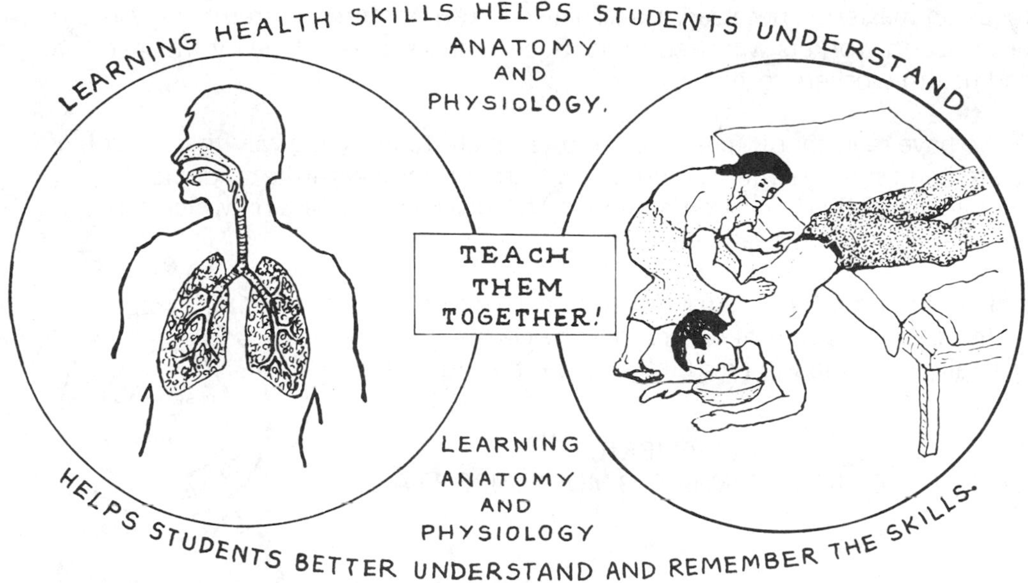

LEARNING HEALTH SKILLS HELPS STUDENTS UNDERSTAND
ANATOMY AND PHYSIOLOGY.
TEACH THEM TOGETHER!
LEARNING ANATOMY AND PHYSIOLOGY
HELPS STUDENTS BETTER UNDERSTAND AND REMEMBER THE SKILLS.

PRACTICE TEACHING

Practice makes perfect. Instructors need to practice teaching all year long so they will not lose their teaching skills. When not training health workers, they can lead classes with fellow instructors, groups of children, teenagers, or parents. This sets a good example, and can help prepare community groups for the students to practice teaching.

Teaching skills are as important for health workers as for their instructors. During training, new health workers can develop teaching skills in the following way:

STEPS IN LEARNING HOW TO TEACH A CLASS

1. Observe the instructors and discuss their teaching methods (see Ch. 1).
2. Take part in role plays to explore approaches to teaching (p. **1**-17).
3. Analyze teaching objectives and methods (Ch. 1, 3, and 5).
4. Practice task analysis (p. **5**-9) to be sure you cover all key points.
5. Discuss and make appropriate teaching aids (Ch. 11).
6. Take turns leading group discussions.
7. Plan classes and practice teaching the learning group (Ch. 5).
8. Begin teaching with community groups—mothers, children, teenagers.

At all stages of this teaching practice, it is important that the instructors and other students evaluate the teaching and class plans to give constructive suggestions. See Chapter 9 for evaluation ideas.

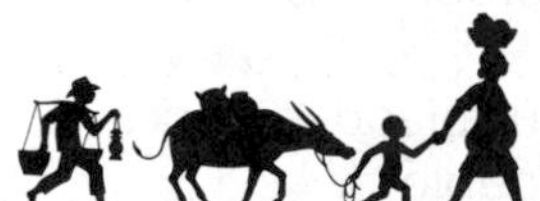

In this chapter we have looked at ways of teaching specific subjects. We have seen that, for health workers to do their job effectively, their training needs to focus on mastering necessary skills. This, in turn, requires a careful analysis of what health workers will need to do. Such analysis is best done by the instructor and health workers together.

We have seen that it makes sense to teach all subjects in a way that is problem related and skill oriented. Appropriate learning starts with the students' knowledge of their own communities. This provides the base on which new knowledge and skills can be built.

Training time is limited and precious. Therefore, the methods and content of classes must be constantly and critically examined to be sure they meet the students' needs.

REMEMBER:
AIM TEACHING AT WHAT IS MOST IMPORTANT.

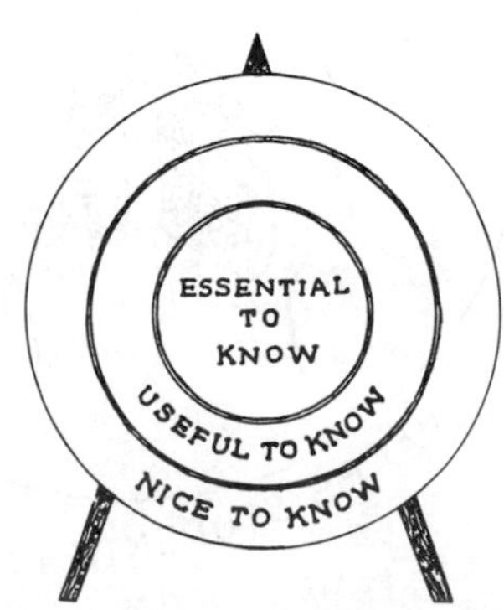

CHAPTER 6

Learning and Working with the Community

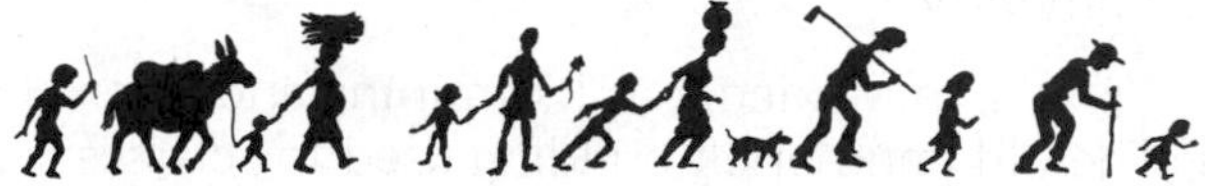

"In some ways, the village or community health worker has a far greater responsibility than does the average doctor. The doctor feels a responsibility for those sick or injured persons who come to him—those whom he sees as 'patients'. But the community health worker is responsible to the entire village or community where he lives and works. His concern is for the health and well-being of all the people. He does not wait for those in greatest need to come to him. He finds out who they are and goes to them."

How nice all this sounds! But in reality, many community health workers do little more than attend the sick who come to their health posts. They might as well be doctors!

If health workers are to develop a sense of responsibility to the whole community, they need these two things (at least) during their training.

- **Good role models:** Student health workers need the example of instructors who are themselves active members of the community. This does not simply mean instructors who make 'house calls'. It means instructors who are doing something to improve health in their village and who relate to the poor as their equals and friends.
- **Practice doing community work:** Health workers-in-training also need practice working with people in a village or neighborhood similar to their own. It is not enough to study in the classroom about 'community participation'. Theory is often far different from reality. If health workers are to work effectively with groups of villagers, mothers, and children, their training needs to provide first-hand community experience.

Community practice means more than discussions, flannel-boards, posters, and role plays (although all these can be useful if used imaginatively). It means finding ways for health workers-in-training to actually visit communities and carry out specific health-related activities with the people.

For many health programs, this will involve re-examining the course content, revising plans, and perhaps choosing different instructors.

Learning in and from the community is essential preparation for community work.

MAKING COMMUNITY EXPERIENCE A PART OF TRAINING

Some people-centered programs have found ways to make interaction with the community a key part of health worker training. These ways include:

1. **Locating the training center in a village or community similar to those where the health workers will be working.** This needs to be done in cooperation with members of the community.

Example: Project Piaxtla, in Mexico, has its training and referral center in a village of 950 people. The old, mud-brick building used for classes is actually the farm workers' meeting hall. The village permits its use when it is not needed for meetings. The fact that all the instructors are from that village, or nearby villages, also helps bring the community and the training program closer together.

2. **Arranging for health workers to live, eat, and sleep in local homes during training.** This has many advantages:

- It brings local families close to the training program. The people take responsibility for the health workers' well-being, not just the other way around.
- It spreads students out and mixes them in the community. This prevents them from becoming a group apart, as often happens when students live together.
- It gives the students a chance to exchange ideas every day with mothers, fathers, and children. They can observe the customs, attitudes, joys, and difficulties of the families. They experience the families' problems and their ways of solving them. At the same time, the families learn from and with the health workers, as they bring home new ideas from the training course.

When the course begins, it helps if instructors **hold a meeting with the host families.** Explain the purpose of the training and ask the families to take part in helping the health workers learn. That way, the local people may actually encourage the health workers to practice teaching them and their children, and may even offer suggestions and criticism. They will take pride in helping prepare health workers to serve other communities. So learning goes two ways.

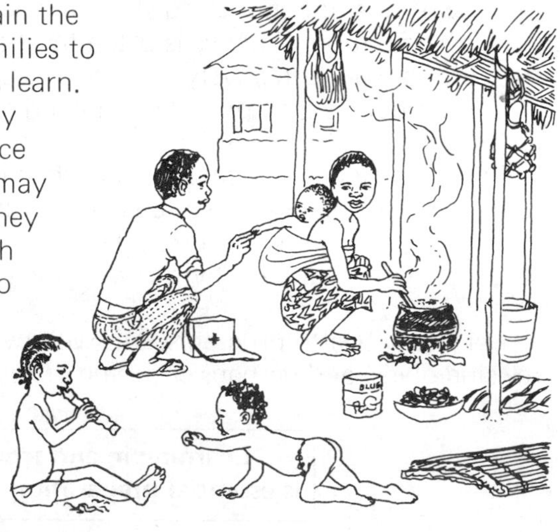

3. **Home visits.** Some programs make regular visits to homes (once or twice a week) an important part of health worker training.

Example: One program, located in a huge 'lost city' near the capital of Mexico, starts training by sending each student to visit 15 families in the poorest *colonias* (neighborhoods). The students try to help the families solve their health problems as best they can—through self-care when possible, or through public clinics and services. In this way, the students get to know the people and their hardships. They also discover the strengths and failings of the city's health and social services. **The content of the training course is planned by the students and instructors together, according to the needs and problems that they see during these home visits.**

Another example: Project Piaxtla also makes home visits a key part of health worker training. Each Saturday, the students plan what they hope to accomplish, then spend half the day visiting families. Each student always visits the same 8 or 10 homes. The main purpose of the visits is to listen to what people have to say. The students ask the families' opinions about community activities, and encourage their ideas and participation. They sometimes give suggestions about preventing or managing health problems. But they take care not to tell people what they ought to do. Perhaps for this reason, and because they rarely use formal questionnaires, in most homes the students are well received.

4. **Having student health workers carry out activities in local communities during their training.** In some training programs, students take part in some or all of the following:

- Under-fives and nutrition projects. Students visit nearby villages, hold meetings to plan activities, demonstrate ways of preparing food, conduct feeding programs for children, train mothers as nutrition volunteers, etc. (see p. **22**-12 and **25**-6,7,9, and 36).
- Cooperation with villagers in building latrines, garbage disposal areas, water systems, or rat-proof bins for grain storage.
- Vaccination campaigns in neighboring villages (with educational programs for parents and children).
- CHILD-to-child activities. Health workers meet with children in the local schools, or with groups of non-school children (see Ch. 24).
- Village clean-up campaigns with children and adults.
- Working with village people in family and community vegetable gardens.
- Helping to run a local cooperative or corn bank.
- Health festivals and circuses (see p. **27**-12).
- Theater and puppet shows with mothers and children (see Ch. 27).

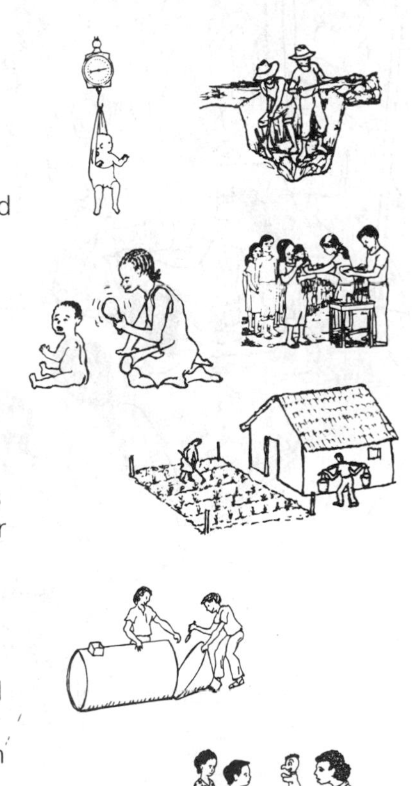

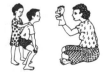

5. **Welcoming community participation in the training course.** People from the village or neighborhood can be involved not only in planned activities, but in a casual way, even in the classroom.

Here are some possibilities:

- **Open door policy.** Some community-based programs make a point of leaving classroom doors and windows open at all times to everyone. Mothers, fathers, farm workers, children, and especially teenagers often wander in or sit in windows to watch what is going on. The use of colorful, active teaching aids, role plays, and simple language to explore new ideas sparks the people's interest. Sometimes their opinions are asked, or they are invited to take part in role plays, games, or demonstrating teaching aids.

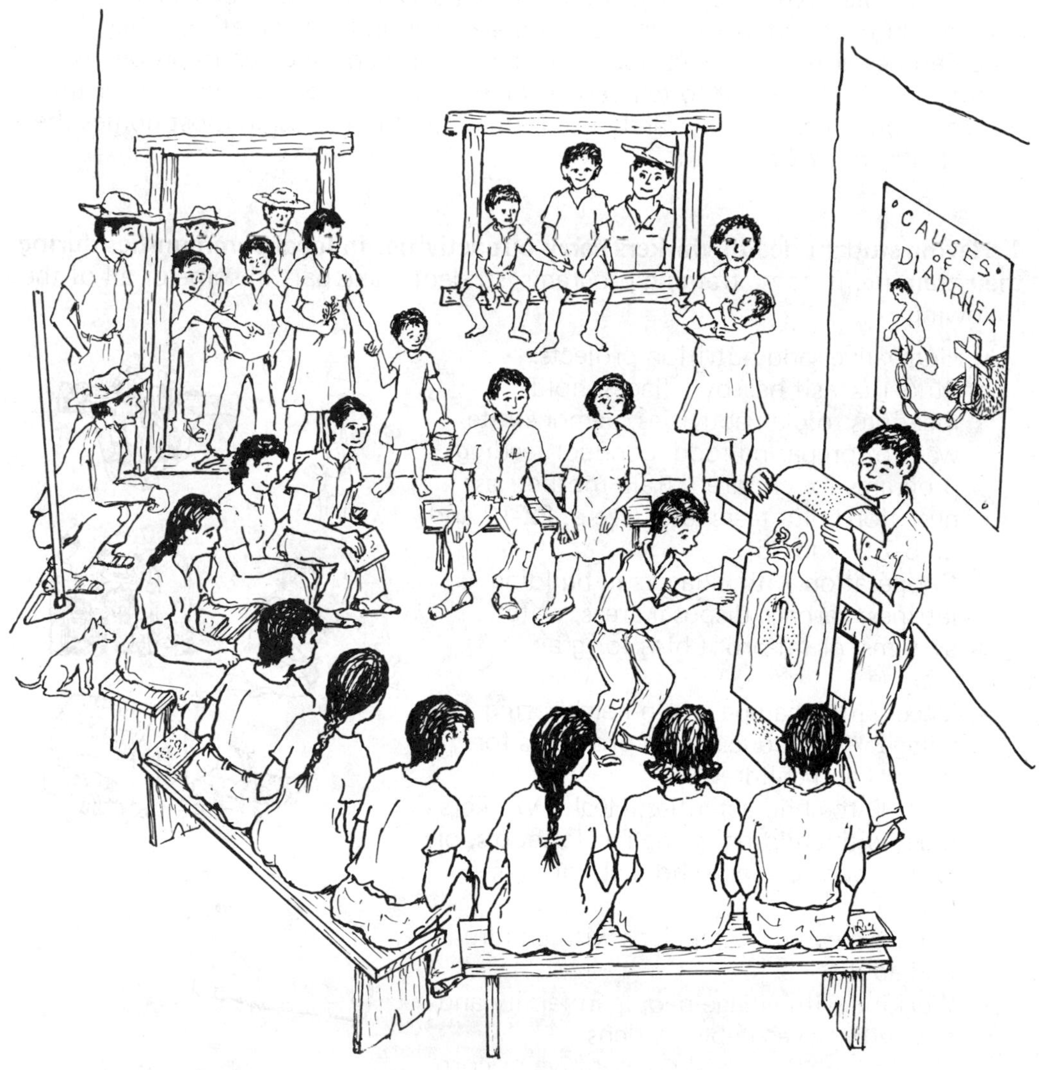

The 'open door' approach to classes for health workers can sometimes cause confusion, but it has many rewards. (For an explanation of the teaching aids shown here, see pages **11**-30 and **26**-6.)

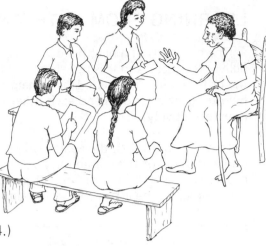

- **Inviting traditional healers, herb doctors, midwives, and other persons from the community to take part** in classes that deal with their special skills.

  One of the most memorable classes we have seen took place when a village midwife was invited to meet with a group of health workers-in-training. Together, they made lists of the specific information and skills that local midwives could share with health workers, and that health workers could share with midwives. (See p. **22**-4.)

- **Inviting mothers and children from the community to help with role plays and other activities.** Health workers need practice in dealing with the health needs of mothers and children. Role playing can help. But having health workers play the roles of babies is not very convincing. It is more realistic if village mothers can be persuaded to bring their small children to class, pretending they have certain health problems. (Real problems may be found as well.) This makes learning much more alive and exciting for everyone. See Chapter 14 for more ideas.

- **Inviting members of the community to slide shows or filmstrip presentations.** Most people love to see slides and films. When these are shown to health workers as part of their training, invite members of the community, too, and include them in the follow-up discussions. If health workers live with families, be sure they invite them.

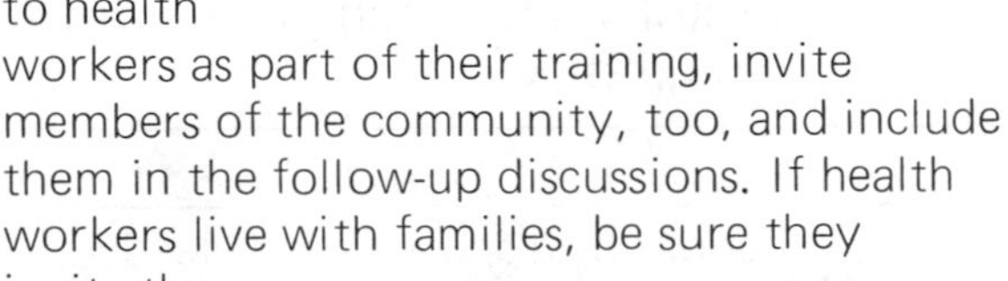

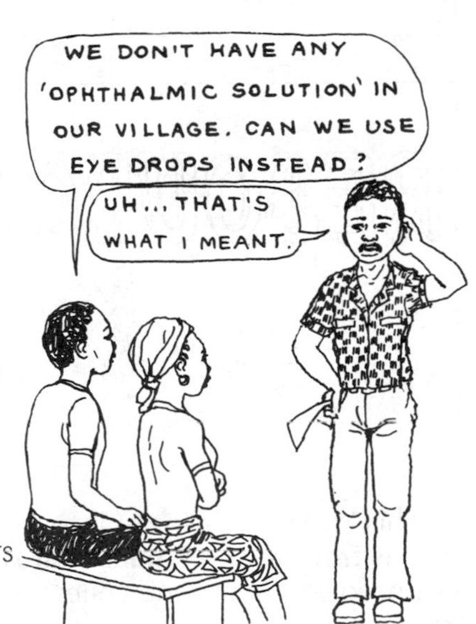

WE DON'T HAVE ANY 'OPHTHALMIC SOLUTION' IN OUR VILLAGE. CAN WE USE EYE DROPS INSTEAD?
UH... THAT'S WHAT I MEANT.

- **Use of clear, simple language, teaching aids, and methods that everyone can understand.** It is important for instructors to keep their language simple and clear, so that anyone can understand. This way, health workers will not have to 'translate' what they have learned in order to share it with villagers. If community people are present at some classes, encourage them to interrupt and ask for an explanation each time they do not understand a word. This helps both instructors and students to keep their language clear and simple. (See p. **2**-16.)

LEARNING FROM, WITH, AND ABOUT THE COMMUNITY

The main job of a health worker in a community-based program is not to deliver services. And it is not simply to act as a link between the community and the outside health system. It is to **help people learn how to meet their own and each other's health needs more effectively.**

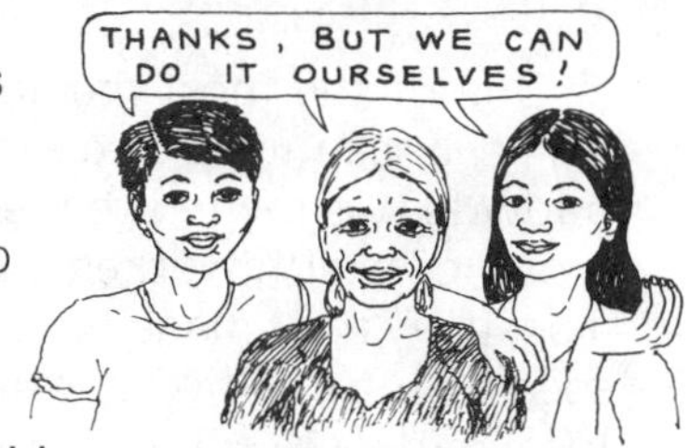
THANKS, BUT WE CAN DO IT OURSELVES!

In order to do this, the health worker needs a deep understanding of the community's strengths, problems, and special characteristics. Together with the people, the health worker will want to consider . . .

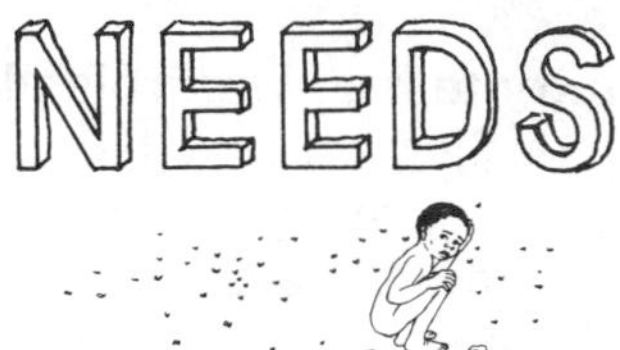
NEEDS

- local health problems and their causes
- other problems that affect people's well-being
- what people feel to be their biggest problems and needs

SOCIAL FACTORS

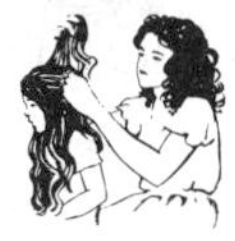

- beliefs, customs, and habits that affect health
- family and social structures
- traditional forms of healing and of problem solving
- ways people in the community relate to each other
- ways people learn (traditionally and in schools)
- who controls whom and what (distribution of land, power, and resources)

RESOURCES

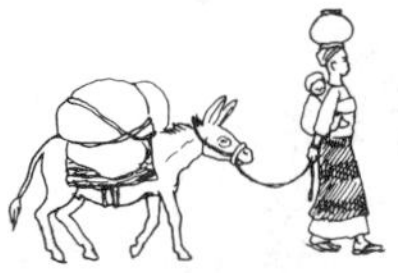

- people with special skills: leaders, healers, story tellers, artists, craftsmen, teachers
- land, crops, food sources, fuel sources (firewood, etc.), water
- building and clothing supplies
- markets, transportation, communication, tools
- availability of work; earnings in relation to cost of living

This looks like a lot of information. And it is! But fortunately, **a health worker who is from the community already knows most of the important facts.** He does not need to run around collecting a lot of data. All he needs to do is sit down with a group of people and look carefully at what they already know.

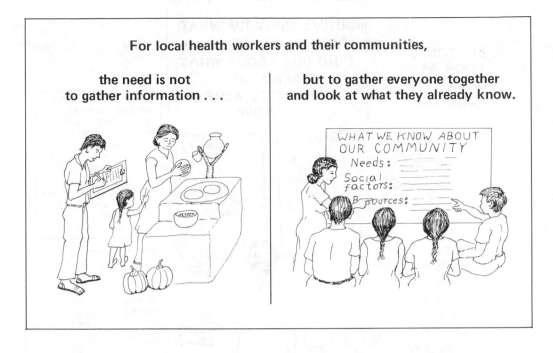

People in a village or community already know most of the essential facts from their own experience. (Not exact numbers, perhaps, but these are usually not needed.) What they need to do is ask themselves:

- How do the combined facts of our situation—needs, social factors, and resources—affect our health and well-being?

- How can we work with these facts—using some, changing or reorganizing others—to improve our health and well-being?

The process of looking at these questions in a community group is sometimes called ***community analysis*** or ***community diagnosis.*** At best, this means not only a diagnosis ***of*** the community, but a self-analysis ***by*** the community.

Community diagnosis—whom does it serve?

Ideally, a community diagnosis is a self-analysis by a community of the problems that concern people most. But watch out! The term ***community diagnosis*** is used quite differently by many of the larger health programs. To them it has come to mean a detailed survey, which health workers are required to conduct in their communities after training. Often the information collected through these surveys serves the needs of the health authorities, but means little to the people themselves.

To require a new health worker to conduct a long, complicated community survey can turn people against him from the first. Many people dislike or distrust surveys. This is especially true for the poorest of the poor, who are repeatedly studied but seldom see any real benefits.

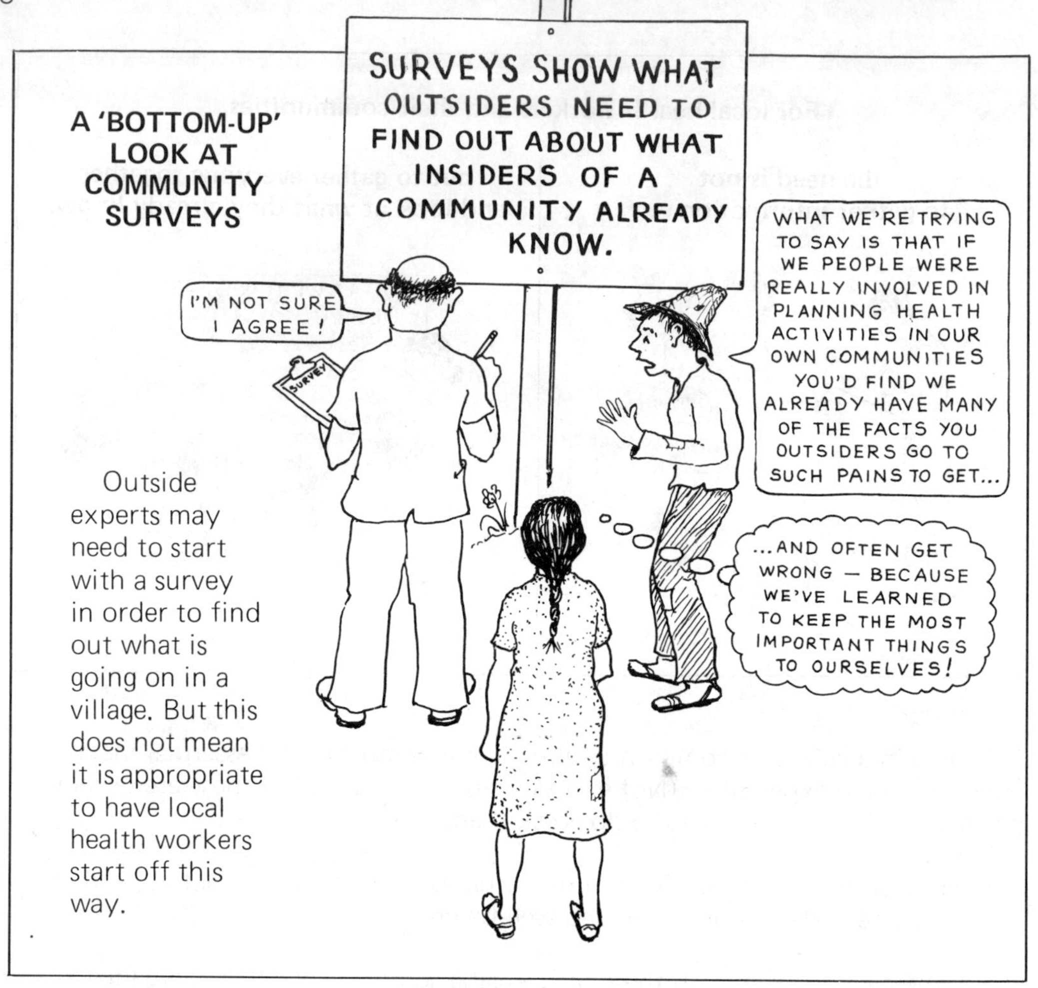

A 'BOTTOM-UP' LOOK AT COMMUNITY SURVEYS
SURVEYS SHOW WHAT OUTSIDERS NEED TO FIND OUT ABOUT WHAT INSIDERS OF A COMMUNITY ALREADY KNOW.
I'M NOT SURE I AGREE!
SURVEY
WHAT WE'RE TRYING TO SAY IS THAT IF WE PEOPLE WERE REALLY INVOLVED IN PLANNING HEALTH ACTIVITIES IN OUR OWN COMMUNITIES YOU'D FIND WE ALREADY HAVE MANY OF THE FACTS YOU OUTSIDERS GO TO SUCH PAINS TO GET...
...AND OFTEN GET WRONG — BECAUSE WE'VE LEARNED TO KEEP THE MOST IMPORTANT THINGS TO OURSELVES!
Outside experts may need to start with a survey in order to find out what is going on in a village. But this does not mean it is appropriate to have local health workers start off this way.

When does information gathering make sense?

Although starting off with a detailed community survey is often a mistake, there are times when a health worker and the people in his community may want to gather specific information. For example:

- People may want to see whether many children are underweight (poorly nourished) and therefore more likely to get sick. (See p. **25**-7.)
- They may want to find out if bottle-fed babies in their village get diarrhea more often than breast-fed babies. (See p. **24**-17.)
- They may want to see whether a particular health activity produces results. For example, a village may plan a campaign to control malaria. The people can take a survey before they begin, to find out how many persons have had fevers and chills. Then—after everyone has taken part by draining ditches, sleeping under mosquito nets, and getting early treatment—the villagers can take another survey and compare the results.

Because surveys often show results that would not otherwise be noticed, they can help to renew people's enthusiasm for continuing an activity (or to stop or change an activity that is not working). See Evaluation, Chapter 9, and On-the-spot Surveys, p. **7**-13.

Suggestions for gathering community information

There are no set rules or one 'right' approach for gathering needed information in a community. However, several people-centered programs have come up with the following ideas:

1. Go to people's homes and get to know them. But **do not start by taking a survey.** Information learned through friendly, casual visits is often truer and more useful. Put the needs and feelings of the people first.

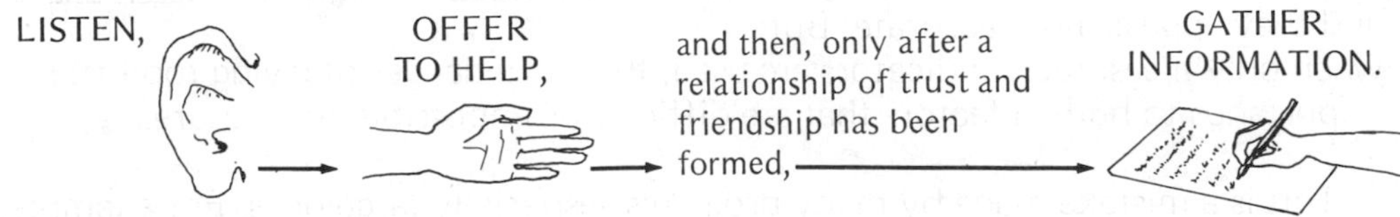

LISTEN,
OFFER TO HELP,
and then, only after a relationship of trust and friendship has been formed,
GATHER INFORMATION.

2. When gathering information, try to **find out what problems people feel are most important** or want to solve first. **Learn what ideas they have** for solving them.
3. **Ask only for information that makes sense** (and not simply because you were told to collect it). Be sure you and the people understand **why** the information is needed. For example, be sure parents understand why you weigh children **before** you do it.
4. **Involve local people in gathering the information.** Be sure studies are not *of* the people, but *by* the people. (For simple surveys in which children and non-literate people can take part, see p. **7**-13 and Chapters 24 and 25.)
5. When conducting a survey or community diagnosis, **try to avoid taking along written questionnaires.** Avoid writing notes while a person is talking to you. Listen carefully, remember what you can, and **write your notes later.** Always be honest and open about the purpose of your visit.
6. Look for ways of making the survey a learning, exploring experience for those being questioned. Try to ask questions that not only seek information, but that also get people thinking and looking at things in new ways.

   For example, instead of simply asking, "How many people in your family can read?" follow up by asking, "What good is it to know how to read and write?" "Does the school here teach your children what they most need to know?" "If not, who does?" (For more ideas about this type of question, see *Where There Is No Doctor,* p. w10 and w11.)
7. Observe people carefully. You can find out as much by watching the way people act and do things as you can by asking questions. Learn to look and listen.
8. **Go slowly when giving people advice,** especially when it concerns their attitudes and habits. It is often better to tell a story about how others solved a similar problem by trying a new way. And **set a good example yourself.**

Note: Where official records of births and deaths are fairly accurate, these can also provide important health information without bothering people in their homes. It is a good idea to compare the ***deaths in children under five*** with ***total deaths.*** For example, in one area of the Philippines, a rise in children's deaths from 35% to 70% of total deaths between 1975 and 1980 shows that conditions affecting health are getting worse!

Health indicators

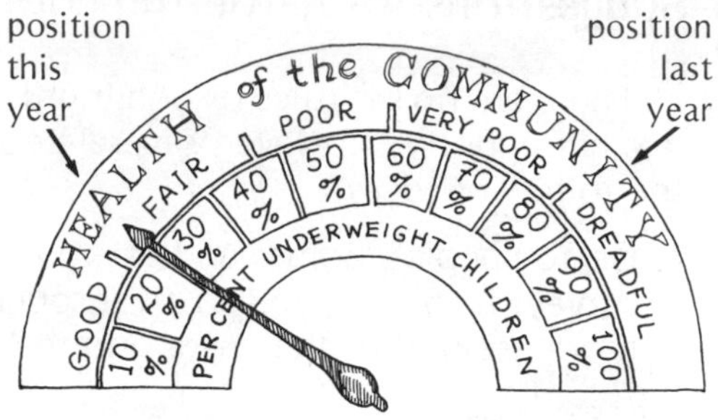

Health indicators are key facts or events that give an idea of the overall **level of health** in a community. Usually things that can be measured are chosen as indicators (see the list below). Measurable or 'numerical' indicators make comparisons and reporting easier, and they appear more accurate. But when only measurable indicators are used, there is a danger of giving too little importance to human factors that are difficult or impossible to measure.

This is a mistake made by many programs—especially large ones. For example, the success of family planning programs is often measured by indicators like: "How many new couples are recruited each month?" But such indicators ignore important human factors like: "To what extent are women pressured into accepting family planning?" or "How do people feel about programs that put more emphasis on birth control than on other aspects of health care?" Failure to consider these less measurable human indicators has resulted in some huge programs and development agencies being thrown out of countries.

In planning or evaluating community activities, it is important that health workers learn to look at the less measurable human indicators as well as the standard measurable ones.

Here is a list of some measurable and non-measurable health indicators. Add to it from your own experience.

Commonly used MEASURABLE INDICATORS of community health

Number or percent of:

- infant deaths
- deaths of children under 5, of adults, etc.
- well nourished or poorly nourished children
- children and pregnant women vaccinated
- children per family (family size)
- couples who plan their families
- families with piped water, latrines, etc.
- attendance at under-fives program
- cases of specific diseases

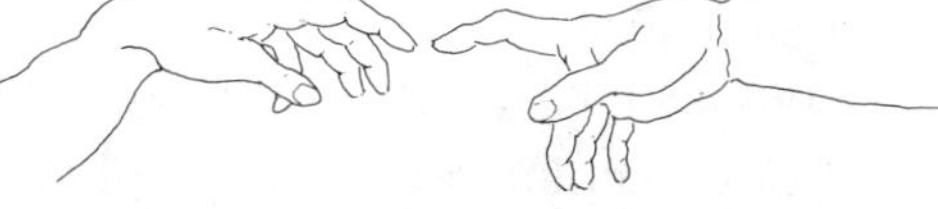

Less measurable, more HUMAN INDICATORS of community well-being

- attitudes of the people about themselves
- movement toward dependency or self-reliance
- examples of families helping each other (or fighting)
- how community decisions are made
- how well education relates to community needs
- fairness or corruptness of leaders
- extent to which leaders, health workers, and teachers serve as good role models, share their knowledge, and treat others as equals
- social awareness; ability of the poor to express and analyze their needs

COMMUNITY DYNAMICS AND PARTICIPATION

To do their work effectively, health workers need to be aware of many aspects of community life: people's customs, beliefs, health problems, and special abilities. But above all, they need to **understand the community power structure:** the ways in which different persons relate to, help, and harm each other. In the rest of this chapter we explore these aspects of ***community dynamics*** and what is meant by ***community participation.*** As we shall see, 'community' and 'participation' mean dangerously different things to different persons. In fact, the way we look at 'community' can strongly affect our approach to 'participation'.

It is essential that instructors and health workers together analyze the conflicting ideas, and draw conclusions based on their own experience.

What is a community?

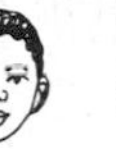

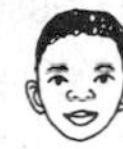
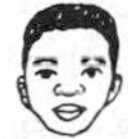
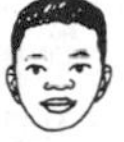

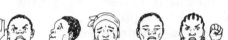

Many health planners think of a community as "a group of people living in a certain area (such as a village) who have common interests and live in a similar way." In this view, emphasis is placed on what people have in common. Relationships between members of a community are seen as basically agreeable, or harmonious.

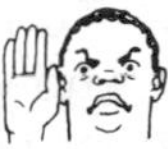
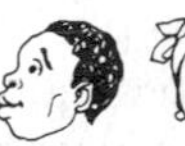
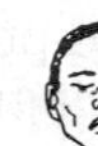
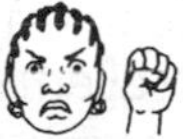

But in real life, **persons living in the same village or neighborhood do not always share the same interests or get along well with one another.** Some may lend money or grain on unfair terms. Others may have to borrow or beg. Some children may go to school. Other children may have to work or stay home to watch their younger sisters and brothers while their mothers work. Some persons may eat too much. Others may go hungry. Some may speak loudly in village meetings. Others may fear to open their mouths. Some give orders. Others follow orders. Some have power, influence, and self-confidence. Others have little or none.

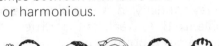

In a community, **even those who are poorest and have the least power are often divided among themselves.** Some defend the interests of those in power, in exchange for favors. Others survive by cheating and stealing. Some quietly accept their fate. And some join with others to defend their rights when they are threatened. Some families fight, feud, or refuse to speak to each other—sometimes for years. Others help each other, work together, and share in times of need. Many families do all these things at once.

> Most communities are not ***homogeneous*** (everybody the same). Often **a community is a small, local reflection of the larger society or country in which it exists.** It will have similar differences between the weak and the strong, similar patterns of justice and injustice, similar problems and power struggles. The idea that people will work well together simply because they live together is a myth!

Elements of harmony and shared interest exist in all communities, but so do elements of conflict. Both have a big effect on people's health and well-being. Both must be faced by the health worker who wishes to help the weak grow stronger.

What is participation?

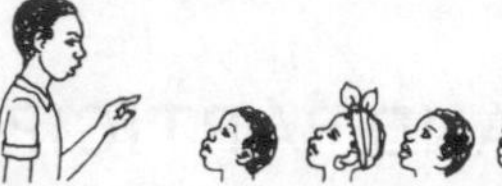

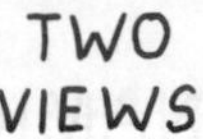

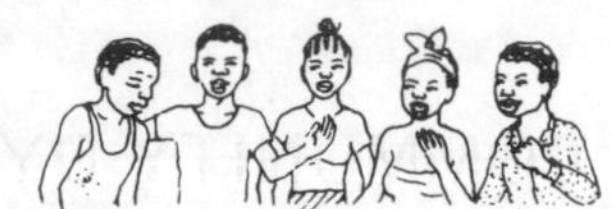

Two views have developed about people's participation in health:*

In the first, more conventional view, planners see participation as **a way to improve the delivery of standard services.** By getting local people to carry out pre-defined activities, health services can be extended further and will be better accepted.

In the second view, participation is seen as **a process in which the poor work together to overcome problems and gain more control** over their health and their lives.

The first view focuses on shared values and cooperation between persons at all levels of society. It assumes that **common interests** are the basis of community dynamics—that if everyone works together and cooperates with the health authorities, people's health will improve.

The second view recognizes **conflicts of interest** both inside and outside the community. It sees these conflicts as an important influence on people's health. It does not deny the value of people organizing and cooperating to solve common problems. But it realizes that different persons and social groups have different economic and political positions. Too much emphasis on common interests may prevent people from recognizing and working to resolve the conflicting interests underlying the social causes of poor health. This second view would suggest that:

Any community program should start by identifying the main conflicts of interest within the community.

It is also important to identify conflicts with forces outside the community and look at the way these relate to conflicts inside the community.

Which view of participation is taken by planners or program leaders will depend largely on what they believe is the cause of poverty and poor health:

Some believe that poverty results from the personal shortages or shortcomings of the poor. Therefore, their program's goal is to **change people to function more effectively in society.** They think that if the poor are provided with more services, greater benefits, and better habits, their standard of living will become healthier. The more the people accept and participate in this process, the better.

Others believe that poverty results from a social and economic system that favors the strong at the expense of the weak. Only by gaining political power can the poor face the wealthy as equals and act to change the rules that determine their well-being. Programs with this view work to **change society to more effectively meet the people's needs.** For this change to take place, people's participation is essential—but on their terms.

*Many of these ideas are taken from "On the Limitations of Community Health Programmes," by Marin das Merces G. Somarriba, reprinted in ***CONTACT—Special Series #3, Health: The Human Factor,*** Christian Medical Commission, June, 1980.

If we look at different health and development projects, we can see that their approaches to community participation range between two opposites:

Participation as a way to control people	Participation as a way for people to gain control

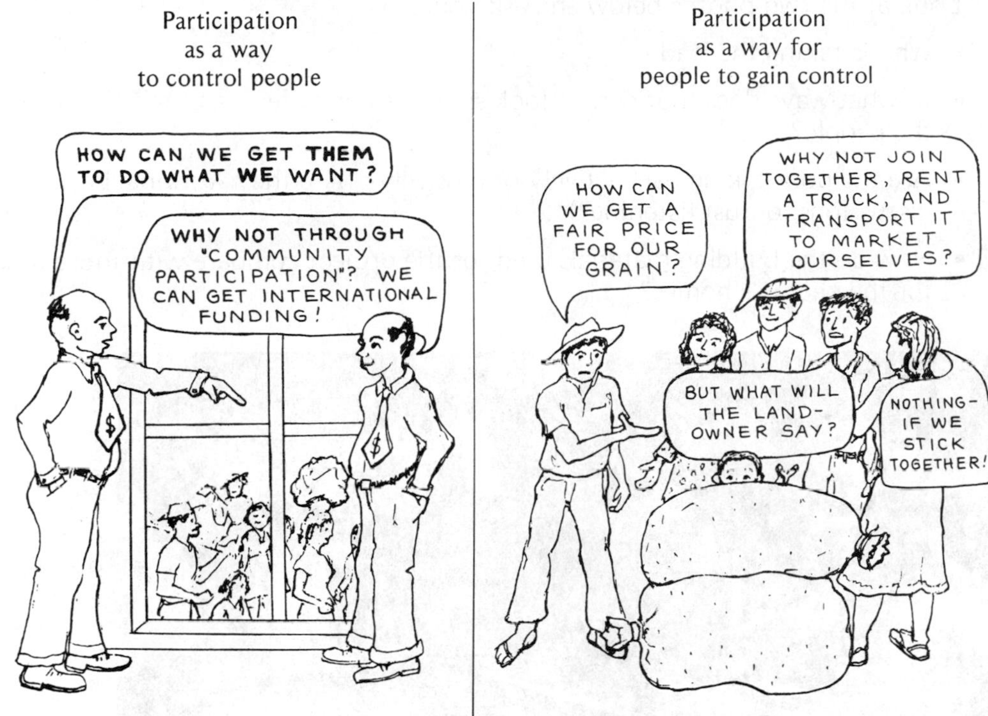
Participation
as a way
to control people
HOW CAN WE GET THEM TO DO WHAT WE WANT?
WHY NOT THROUGH "COMMUNITY PARTICIPATION"? WE CAN GET INTERNATIONAL FUNDING!
Participation
as a way for
people to gain control
HOW CAN WE GET A FAIR PRICE FOR OUR GRAIN?
WHY NOT JOIN TOGETHER, RENT A TRUCK, AND TRANSPORT IT TO MARKET OURSELVES?
BUT WHAT WILL THE LAND-OWNER SAY?
NOTHING— IF WE STICK TOGETHER!

Between these two opposites there are many intermediate stages. These vary according to . . .

(1) who really does the participating,

(2) the function of the participation, and

(3) the center of power.

We can get an idea of the degree to which participation is controlled by those at the top (the upper class) or by those on the bottom (the poor) by looking at the program's community-level participants—health workers, committee members, and others. We can ask:

- How were these community representatives selected?
- What is their social background? How wealthy are their families compared to the rest of the community?
- What are their links to those in positions of power or authority, both inside and outside the community?
- How physically big, fat, or well dressed are they compared to most of the people in the village or community?

Often it is easy to observe (even from photos or films) whether community participation is controlled by those on top or by the poor.

Look at the two photos below and ask yourself:

- Who is taking the lead?
- In what ways does that person look similar to or different from the rest of the people?
- Are the poor taking part actively or passively? (Are they working, having discussions, or just listening?)
- How do the building materials used for the project compare with those used for the people's homes?

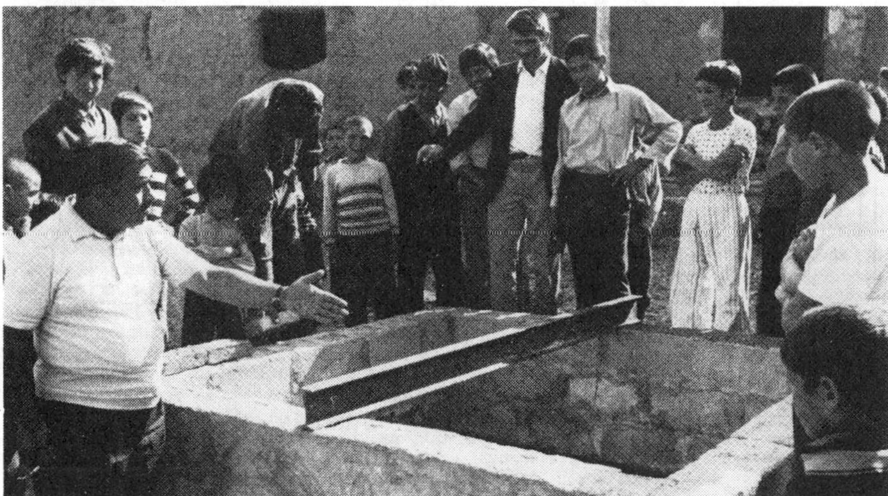

(Photo: D. Derias/WHO.)

In an Iranian village, a health worker gives instructions on how to cover a well to protect water from contamination.

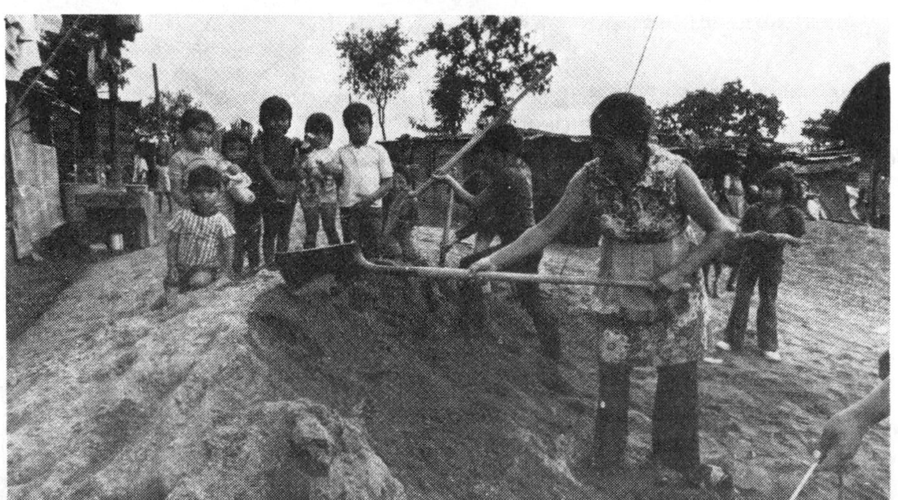

(Photo: Salgado/Christian Aid.)

Families do weekend work in a low-cost housing reconstruction project at Sakerty, on the fringe of Guatemala City.

LOOKING AT COMMUNITY LEADERSHIP

At the end of their training, when health workers return to their communities, they are often instructed:

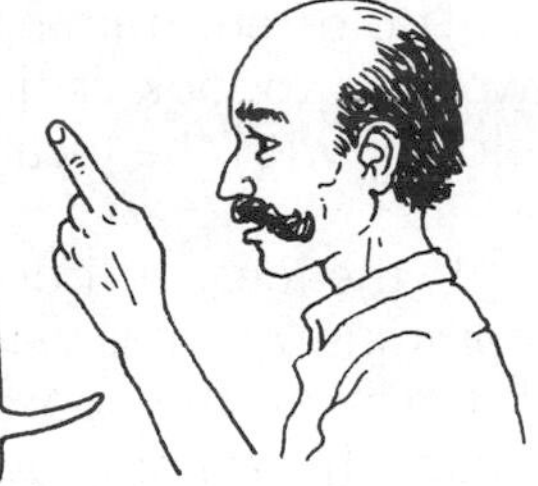

But which community leaders should health workers try to work with? Villages and neighborhoods usually have many kinds of leaders, including:

- local authorities (headmen, etc.)
- officials sent or appointed from the outside
- religious leaders
- traditional healers
- school teachers
- extension workers
- club, group, union, or cooperative leaders
- women's leaders
- children's and young people's leaders
- committees (health committee or local school committee)
- those who have powerful influence because of property or wealth
- opinion leaders among the poor
- opinion leaders of the rich

In nearly all communities there are some leaders whose first concern is for the people. But there may be others whose main concern is for themselves and their families and friends—often at the expense of the others in the community.

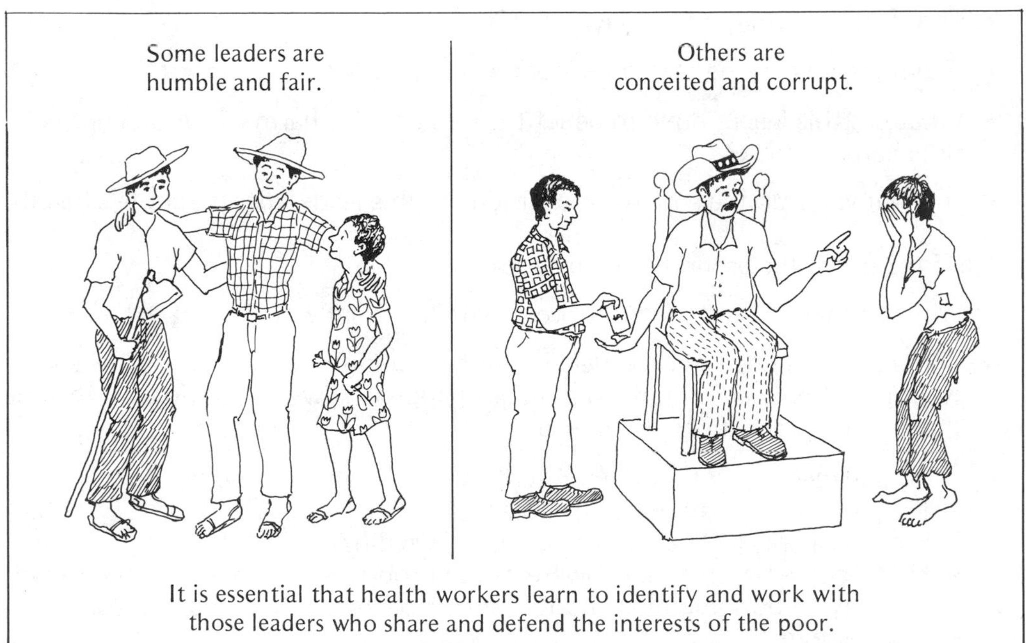

Some leaders are humble and fair.
Others are conceited and corrupt.

It is essential that health workers learn to identify and work with those leaders who share and defend the interests of the poor.

Too often, training programs (especially government ones) fail to advise health workers to look critically at leadership. They simply tell health workers to "work closely with the local authorities."

If the local authorities are honest and try to deal fairly with everyone in the community, all is well. But when the interests of those in power conflict with the interests of the poor, the health worker is faced with some difficult decisions. Unless his training prepares him for these, he may be at a loss. There is little doubt that . . .

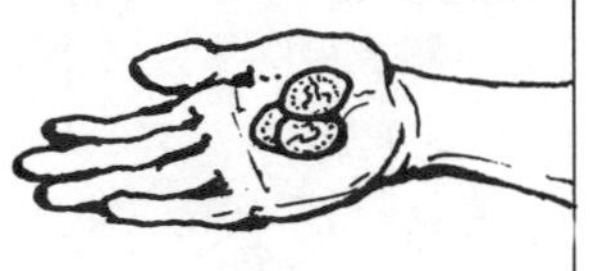

Corruption of local authorities, together with the frustration of health workers required to work with them, helps explain the lack of effectiveness of many health projects.

But frustration can be transformed, at least partly, into a challenge—if the health workers' training prepares them for it. Such preparation is of key importance in regions where corrupt leadership is common.

Learning to identify and work with leaders of the poor

You can start by having the group of health workers list the different types of leaders in their own villages or communities. Be sure they **include unofficial 'opinion leaders'** as well as local authorities.

Encourage the students to discuss each leader, using questions like these:

- How was this leader chosen, and by whom?
- Does this leader fairly represent the interests of everyone in the community?
- If not, for whom does he play favors?
- From whom does he take orders or advice?
- What has this leader done to benefit the village? To harm it? Who benefits or is harmed most?
- In what ways do the actions or decisions of this leader affect people's health?

Next try to get the group thinking about:

- Which leaders should we try to work with? In what ways?
- Should we include unfair leaders in our community health projects? If so, what might happen? If not, what might happen? If we do (or do not) include them, what precautions should we take?
- If local leaders do not fairly represent the poor, what should we do?
    - Keep quiet and stay out of trouble?
    - Protest openly? (What would happen if we did?)
    - Help people become more aware of the problems that exist and their own capacity to do something about them? If so, how? (See Chapter 26.)
    - What else might we do?

At first some students may find it difficult to look at these questions. Their thoughts may be deeply buried—especially if they come from families that have been taught to accept their situation and keep silent.

Other students may be eager to question established authority and work for fairer leadership. But they may be unaware of some of the problems that can arise. Caution is as essential as courage. To help get health workers thinking about both the possible courses of action and the difficulties that could arise, you might:

- Invite experienced health workers to talk with the group about their own successes and disappointments in working with different community leaders.
- Tell or read stories of experiences from other, but similar, areas. (The three stories on the next pages, about village water systems in different parts of the world, are examples. See also p. **26**-3 and **26**-36.)
- Use role playing to explore problems and possibilities in dealing with different leaders. (See Chapter 14, and also the Village Theater Show on p. **27**-19.)

It is important for health workers to remember that no leader is all good or all bad. One of their biggest challenges is to help bring out the best in any leaders they may work with.

WARNING: It is very important for people's health that health workers help the community look critically at local leadership. But it is important to the health workers' health that they do this with due caution and judgement. Both instructors and health workers need to weigh carefully the possible benefits and risks in their particular situation.

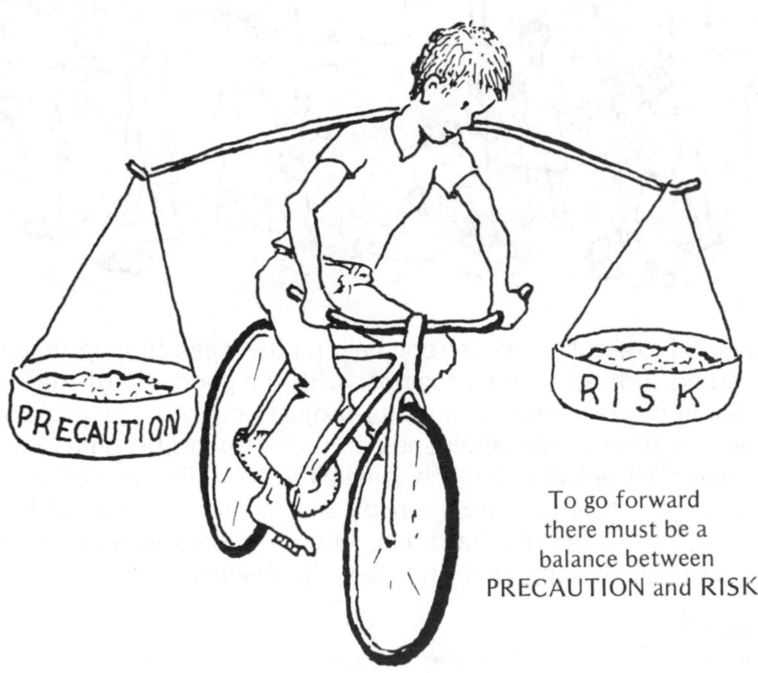

To go forward there must be a balance between PRECAUTION and RISK.

THREE STORIES ABOUT VILLAGE WATER SYSTEMS—for helping health workers look at questions of leadership and power structure

Should the strong help the weak, or the weak help each other—or both? Ideally, perhaps, the answer to this question is "both." The strong should help the weak to help each other. In some places this happens. Here is an example from Indonesia:*

"In the village of Losari, in Central Java, the people were helped by an outside volunteer agency (Oxfam) and an 'intermediate technology' agency (Yayasan Dian Desa) to put in a piped water supply. Looking ahead to the time when the pipes would rust, but outside assistance might no longer be available, a plan was made to raise money for eventually replacing the pipe. Each family along the water line has planted ten mahogany trees. In 15 or 20 years' time, these trees will be cut down and sold to raise money to replace the steel pipes.

"The village headman bought the mahogany seeds from the Agricultural Service and planted them on unused patches of his own land. After 12 months, he gave seedlings to the 85 families living near the water supply.

"If any young trees die, the people can ask the headman for replacements. He makes no charge for the seedlings and asks only that the people look after their trees well."

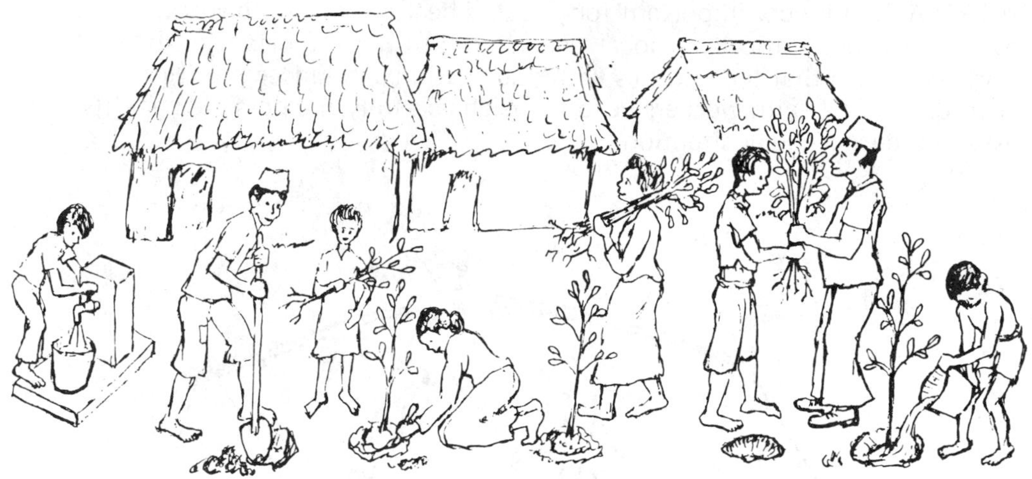

This is a good example of the strong helping the weak to help themselves. Outside funding and technology, together with the good will of the village headman, made this self-help community project possible. The project has double importance. It not only helps the people in the village to become more self-reliant through cooperative activity, but it also helps them to look ahead and actively plan for the future. What is more, it encourages the strong to share their resources with the weak. In this case the headman, who has more money and land than his neighbors, contributed some of each to benefit the project and the community.

---

*From the Indonesian Village Health Newsletter, ***Vibro,*** No. 22, p. 11, December, 1979.

Unfortunately, such harmony of interest between the strong and the weak does not always exist. Here is another example of an attempt by villagers to create their own water system:

> In the mountains of western Mexico, a village of 850 people decided to put in its own piped water supply. After considerable pressure from outside change agents, the richer landholders finally agreed that each family in the village should contribute to the costs in proportion to its wealth. Then one of the landholders, who is also ***cacique*** (headman), volunteered to be treasurer for the water program. Soon he took complete control. He arranged for water to be piped into the homes of the few big landholders before the public water supply was extended to the poorest parts of town. Then the ***cacique*** began to charge so much for the use of public taps that the poor could not afford to pay. So he turned off the public taps. The result was that the water system, built largely with the labor of the poor, was controlled and used exclusively by the rich.

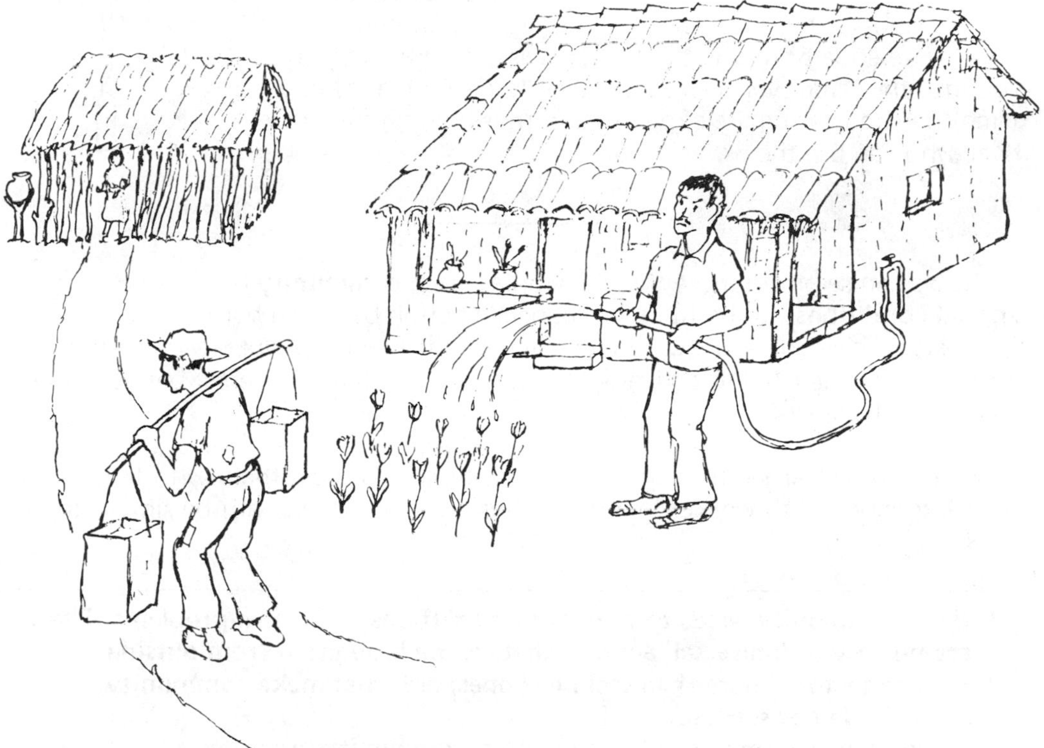

Unfortunately, situations like this exist in many parts of the world. Too often the strong within a village or community offer to help with development projects, and then take complete control or turn the benefits to their own advantage.

The lesson from such examples is clear:

Any program that would help the weak gain power must carefully consider how much help to accept from the strong, and under what conditions.

Some community-based projects have found that extra contributions, leadership, or even any participation at all by headmen or landholders should be avoided. An example comes from the Gonoshasthaya Kendra Project in Bangladesh. Their ***Progress Report*** (August, 1980) states:

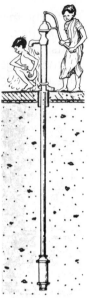

"In liaison with UNICEF, the government has given hand-pump tubewells to many villages. However, the majority have been situated on the rich men's property, resulting in limitation of their use . . .

"In our program, one tubewell is to serve 15 to 25 families (none of these having either private or government tubewells on their homesteads). The tubewell is donated by UNICEF, but the digging and platform expenses are borne by the families whom the well will serve. A committee made up of the various family members is responsible for seeing that 100 taka (local money) is deposited in either the bank or post office for the maintenance of the tubewell. All who use the tubewell must contribute equally to this fund. Otherwise, we are likely to run into the same system we are trying to overcome, of one (rich) person bearing the expenses and thus holding the power over who can use the water supply."

As we can see from these three examples, **each community has its own special conditions.** In the first village, participation based on harmony of interests succeeded. In the second, it failed. In the third, people learned (the hard way) of the need to actively deal with the conflict of interest between the weak and the strong.

What can be learned from these three examples? Discuss them with fellow instructors or health workers. Your conclusions may or may not be similar to ours:

1. **Each community needs to find its own solutions to its own problems. There are no easy or 'universal' answers that can be brought in from outside.**
2. **Human factors (more than technical ones) are what make community activities fail or succeed.**
3. **To serve those whose needs are greatest, community programs must make every effort to help the weak gain and keep control. (Sometimes this may mean refusing or limiting assistance from those in positions of power—whether inside or outside the community.)***
4. **To be healthy is to be self-reliant.**

---

*This is not an argument against government at any level. Rather it is an argument for sensible, flexible self-government at all levels—by individuals, by families, by communities, by nations, and by humankind. It is an argument for small, humane governmental units managed for and by the people. It is an argument for government that genuinely serves people rather than controls them; for government in which the weak are not only treated as human and as equals, but are fairly represented. Whether such government is possible, the world has yet to discover. But surely, the health of humankind rests on this.

CHAPTER 7

Helping People Look at Their Customs and Beliefs

LOOKING AT LOCAL CUSTOMS AND TRADITIONS

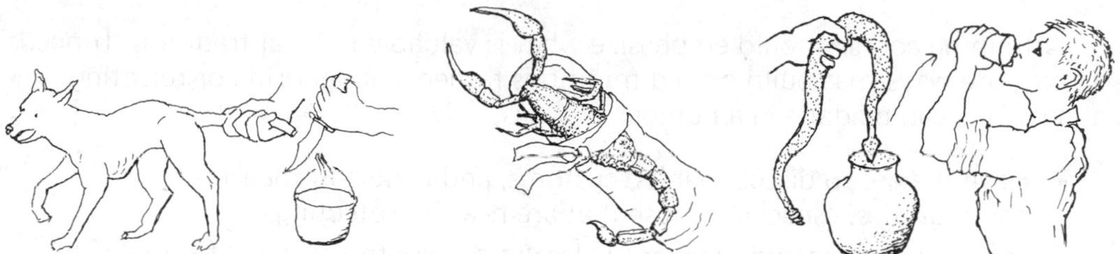

Training programs often make one of three common mistakes when helping health workers learn about people's customs and traditions.

- They *look down on* or 'scorn' local beliefs and traditional forms of healing as "old fashioned," "unscientific," and largely worthless.
- They *look up to* or 'romanticize' local customs and traditional medicine as completely admirable and beneficial.
- Or they *fail to look at all* at local traditions, customs, and forms of healing.

In reality, old ways, like new ways, have strengths and weaknesses. Health workers need to **help people look carefully and critically at both the old and the new, in order to avoid what is harmful and preserve what is best in each.**

But place greatest emphasis on what is best. Helping people rediscover the value of many of their traditional ways increases their confidence in their own knowledge, experience, and ability to meet their needs themselves.

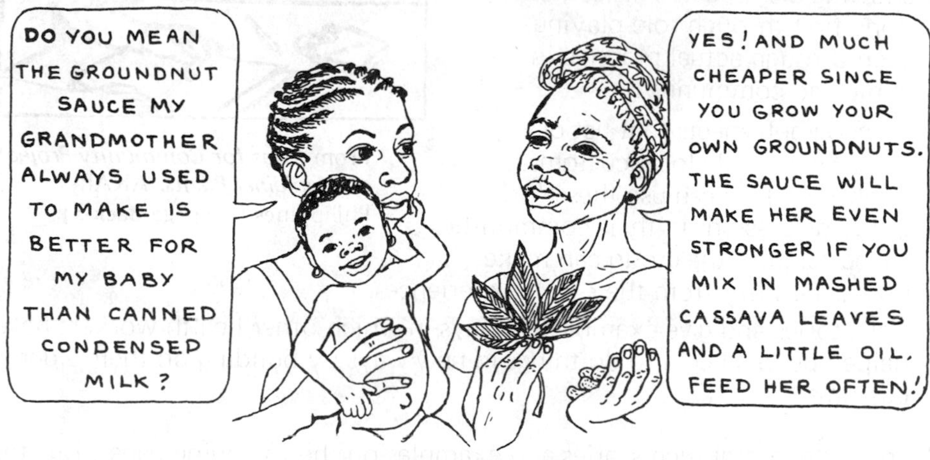

DO YOU MEAN THE GROUNDNUT SAUCE MY GRANDMOTHER ALWAYS USED TO MAKE IS BETTER FOR MY BABY THAN CANNED CONDENSED MILK?
YES! AND MUCH CHEAPER SINCE YOU GROW YOUR OWN GROUNDNUTS. THE SAUCE WILL MAKE HER EVEN STRONGER IF YOU MIX IN MASHED CASSAVA LEAVES AND A LITTLE OIL. FEED HER OFTEN!

Build on beneficial traditions.

HELPING PEOPLE RECOGNIZE THE STRENGTHS IN THEIR TRADITIONS

Of the 3 common mistakes in teaching about traditions (looking down on them, seeing no wrong in them, or ignoring them), the first is the worst. Even when health workers are villagers themselves, there is danger of their becoming so full of new ideas that they lose respect for the health-protecting traditions of the people. If this happens, they can easily make people feel small and ashamed, rather than more self-confident.

A training course should emphasize what is valuable in local tradition. It needs to explore ways that build on old traditions rather than ignoring or rejecting them. This can be done in a number of ways:

- Have the group discuss habits, customs, and beliefs in their own communities, especially those that are health protecting.
- Invite older men and women to class to discuss the origins of some of the old customs and beliefs.
- On home visits, students can observe and ask about traditional ways of doing things. Later they can discuss which seem most valuable, and which harmful. They can do this for both new customs and old.
- Encourage students to find out (through books, letters, and perhaps experiments) if and how some of the traditional ways of healing work. (Many countries have research groups investigating traditional medicine. You may want to contact and cooperate with these groups.)
- Explore ways of introducing new ideas by building on people's beliefs and traditions, rather than showing disrespect. This can be done first through role playing, then through actual practice in clinic and community.
- Mimeograph sheets that list or describe valuable local customs. Health workers can use these for group discussions in their communities. Or better still, the group can make up such a sheet from their own experiences.
- Tell stories and give examples of ways in which other health workers have helped people begin to do things in new ways by building on their older customs.

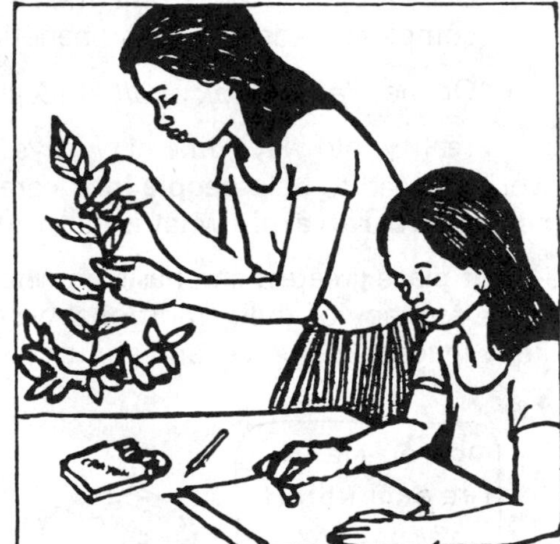

From *Ideas for Community Projects on Medicinal Plants.* AKAP—Philippines (see page **Back**-3)

We provide several such stories and examples on the following pages. But these are only 'examples of examples'. It will be far better if you choose mostly examples from your own area.

HEALTH PROBLEMS THAT RESULT WHEN OLD TRADITIONS ARE REPLACED BY NEW ONES

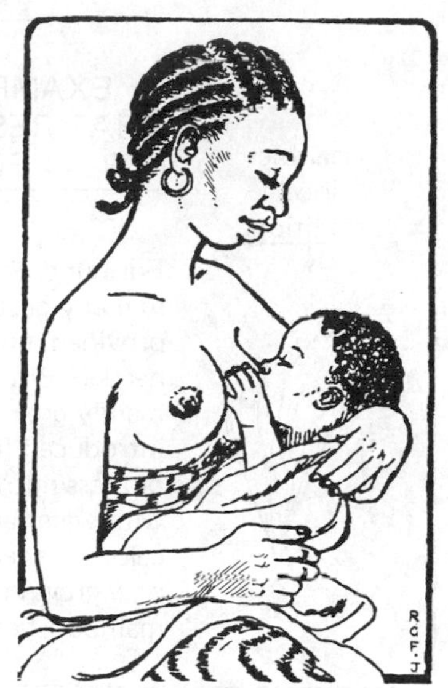

Many health problems in poor communities today have resulted partly because people have abandoned old customs for new ones. The coming of new habits, foods, religions, and laws from the outside—begun during colonization and still continuing today—has produced many cultural conflicts. It has broken down the traditional ways in which people used to meet their needs while keeping a fairly healthy balance with each other and with their natural surroundings. As a result, many new problems in child care, nutrition, land tenure, employment, family structure, and community politics have arisen.

AN EXAMPLE FROM LIBERIA, AFRICA:

In villages of Liberia, Africa, there are many more malnourished children today than in the past. Mothers bear more children now, and more mothers are anemic. Yet shortage of food and land does not seem to be a problem for most families.

What, then, is the cause of these recent health problems?

A health educator from the outside would be tempted to say, "The problem is ignorance. Mothers do not know how to use the foods available to feed their children adequately. Many prefer bottle feeding to breast feeding. They are slow to accept family planning. They are resistant to new ideas."

But if we look at these people's history, we find the opposite is true. The new health problems have resulted not because people have resisted, but because they have accepted new customs introduced by outsiders.

Liberia used to have the tradition of ***polygamy***—which means it was the custom for each man to have several wives. When a wife had a child, she went to live in her parents' compound for 3 or 4 years. During that time, she breast fed her baby. While breast feeding, she did not have sex because it was thought this would poison her milk. Yet she was not afraid of losing her husband to another woman. He already had other wives and it was culturally expected for her to return to him after weaning the child.

So the traditional society had a built-in process of child spacing (family planning). It guaranteed long breast feeding and allowed the mother to regain her strength before she became pregnant again.

With the coming of white men's ideas and religions, people were told that polygamy was 'bad'. Slowly, the new idea was accepted (enforced?) and polygamy was replaced by ***monogamy***—which means a man can have only one wife. But with monogamy, many of the old health-protecting traditions began to break down. Beliefs that had once been safeguards to health turned into obstacles.

After giving birth, a mother was now unwilling to move to her parents' compound for fear that her husband would abandon her for another wife (since he was now allowed only one). So she stayed and had sex with him. But since she feared sex would poison her milk, she tried to protect her child through another foreign custom: bottle feeding. She was also afraid to feed her child nutritious local foods because, traditionally, breast milk had been enough. Therefore, giving babies many of the local foods had been 'taboo' (against the old customs).

As a result of these changes in customs, women became pregnant more quickly, and turned from breast to bottle feeding. So today there are more large families, anemic mothers, and malnourished children than in the old days.

One thing seems clear in this example from Liberia: these villagers' health problems have, in some ways, increased because they have taken on ideas and customs from the outside. Their problem is not primarily one of ignorance, but of too much conflicting knowledge.

EXAMPLES OF HEALTH PROBLEMS THAT RESULT WHEN OLD CUSTOMS ARE REPLACED BY LESS HEALTHY NEW ONES

Healthier local tradition

Unhealthy new custom

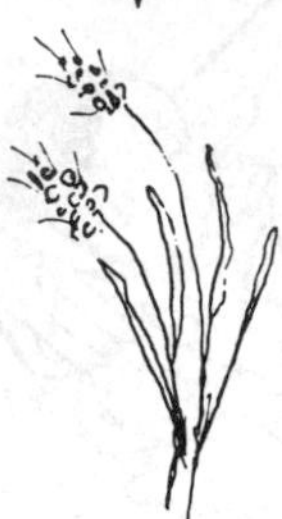

For hundreds of years, **millet** was the main food in many parts of Africa. As a whole grain it provided most of the vitamins and protein people needed. But today in much of Africa, people mainly grow and eat **cassava.** This new food, introduced from Latin America, is easier to grow but less nutritious than millet. It fills children with water and fiber before they get enough calories (energy). So in areas where cassava is now grown instead of millet, more children are malnourished.

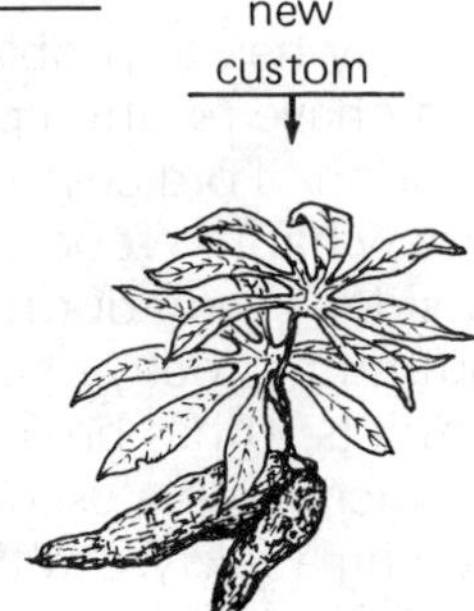

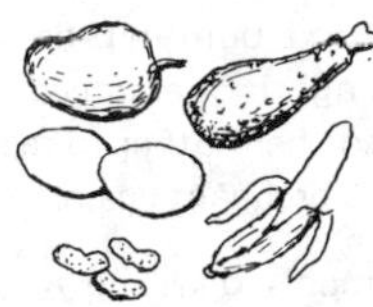

In many parts of the world, people spend money on expensive **junk foods** instead of eating **local fruit** and other nourishing foods. 'Junk foods' are pre-packaged snacks, sweets, and drinks that are high in sugar and low in nutrients. They cause poor nutrition, rotten teeth, diabetes, heart problems, and other ills. Around the world, people tend to have much worse teeth than their ancestors did—largely because of the sugar and junk foods people eat today.

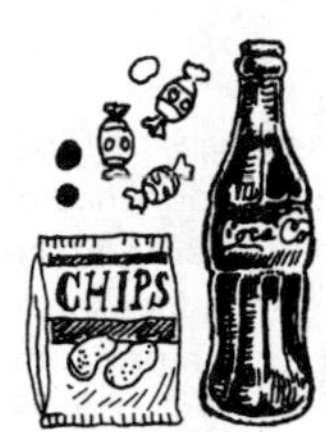

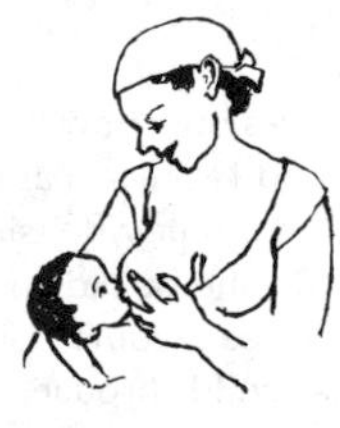

Bottle feeding and the use of **artificial, canned, and powdered milks** have become popular in many parts of the world, in spite of the fact that the old tradition of **breast feeding** is safer, better, and cheaper. (See ***WTND,*** p.120.) The popularity of bottle feeding is partly due to promotion by international companies, like Nestle's. They continue pushing their products with misleading advertising despite widespread protest. Some countries, such as Papua New Guinea, have forbidden the sale of baby bottles without a doctor's prescription.

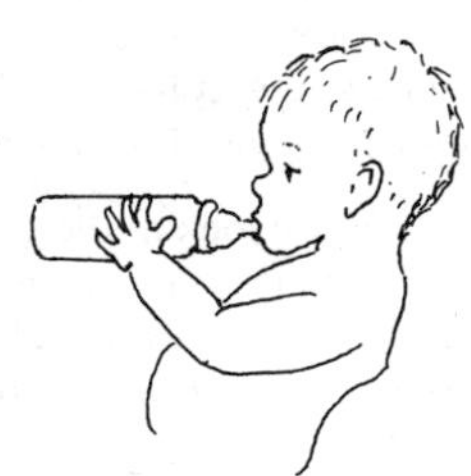

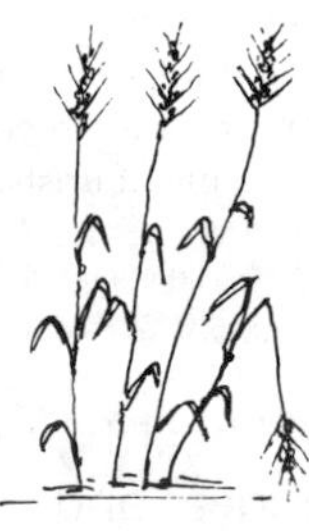

In many countries people no longer eat **whole-grain foods,** such as whole wheat or unpolished rice. They have grown used to the newer, whiter, **factory-milled flours and grains.** Because these are far less nutritious, health problems have developed. Even so, many people who used to grow and eat their own grain now sell their whole-grain crops to buy refined flour. In a similar way, a less nutritious white hybrid maize has replaced native yellow maize in much of Latin America. (See p. **15**-5.)

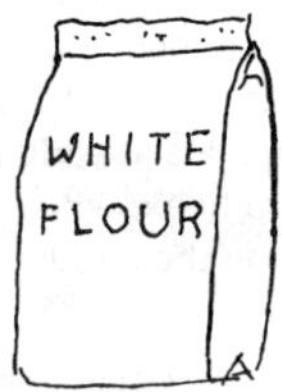

MORE EXAMPLES OF HEALTH PROBLEMS THAT RESULT WHEN OLD CUSTOMS ARE REPLACED BY LESS HEALTHY NEW ONES

Healthier local tradition

Unhealthy new custom

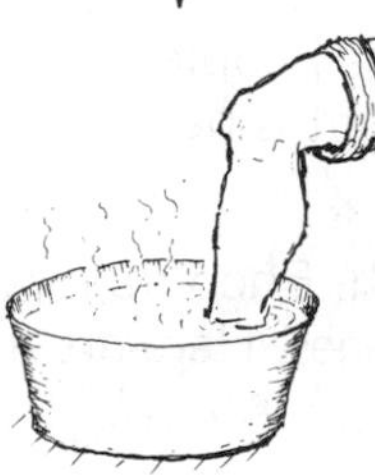

Modern medicines have replaced folk remedies and **traditional cures** in many areas. In some cases this has improved people's health. But in many cases traditional medicines are cheaper, safer, and just as effective as modern medicines. The overuse and misuse of modern medicines, due partly to promotion by international drug companies, has become a major economic and health problem in the world today.

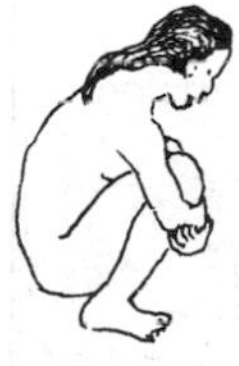

The traditional **squatting position for childbirth** is usually easier for the mother, because the weight of the baby helps her to push. The modern **lying-down position** is easier for the doctor, but not for the mother. This is only one of many examples of how modern medicine often puts the doctor's needs before the patient's.

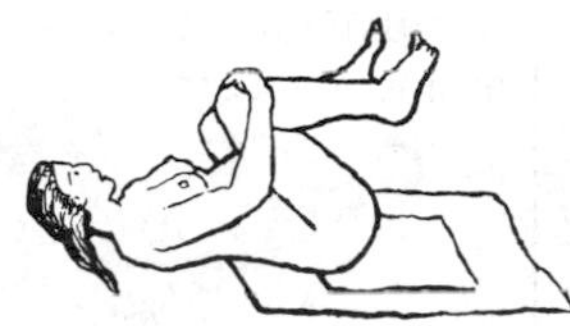

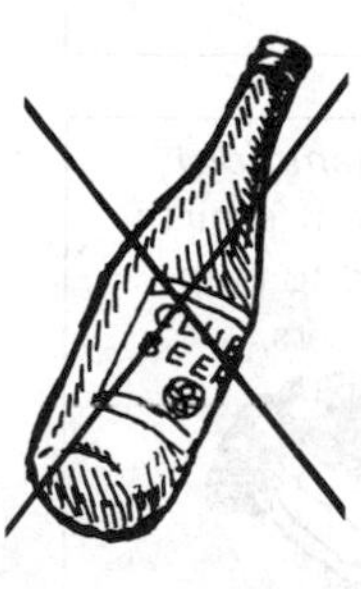

Most traditional cultures limited the **use of alcohol and other drugs** to special occasions and religious rites. As old traditions break down, drinking and drug abuse have become enormous problems in many societies. Alcoholism, with the resulting family problems and malnourished children, has become an especially big problem where Christianity has replaced religions that had strict 'taboos' (prohibitions) against drinking. In parts of Africa, for example, children are generally better nourished in Islamic villages, where drinking is prohibited, than in neighboring Christian villages where the men drink.

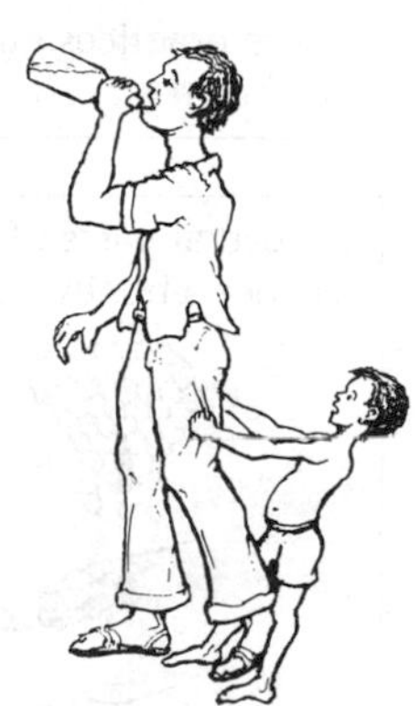

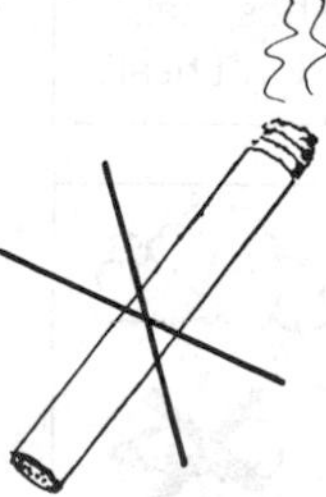

In most parts of the world, the **smoking of tobacco** is a relatively recent custom. Since it has been proved to cause lung cancer, harm unborn babies of women who smoke, and to be generally dangerous to health, people in rich countries now smoke less. As a result, the big tobacco companies have begun to push their products in poor countries, using massive advertising and sales campaigns. This is causing more people in poor countries, including women, to become smokers. The World Health Organization has called smoking "the biggest preventive health problem in the world today."

Problems follow when any group of people, regardless of how well intending, imposes or forces its ideas on another group of people.

IDENTIFYING HEALTH-PROTECTING CUSTOMS

The challenge for the health worker or educator is not to 'change people's behavior'. It is to help people understand, respect, and build on what is healthy in their own culture.

Every area has unique traditions and customs that protect health. Encourage health workers to identify the beneficial customs in their own villages. Here are a few examples from different parts of the world:

In Guatemala, village midwives put a hot coal against the freshly cut cord of a newborn baby. In other parts of the world, midwives press a red-hot knife against the cord.

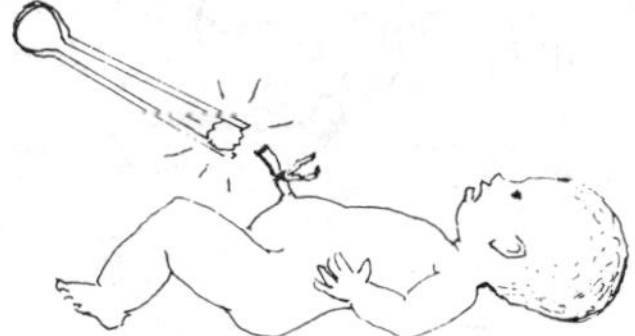

These practices kill germs and help dry out the cord, preventing tetanus.

In Mexico, long before penicillin had been discovered, villagers were treating women with 'childbed fever' by giving them a tea brewed from the underground fungus gardens of leaf-cutting ants.

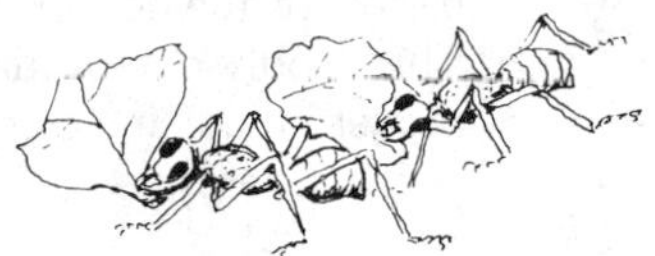

It is likely that this fungus is related to penicillin.

In several parts of the world, people use bee's honey to treat burns.

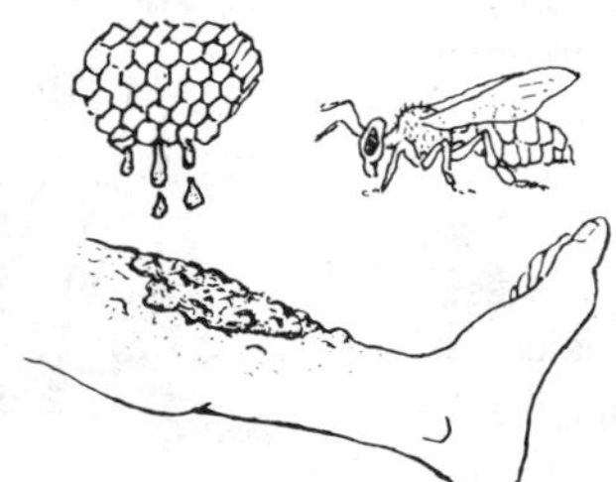

The concentrated sugar in honey prevents bacterial growth. Recently, doctors have been experimenting with similar treatment of burns.

The thin sac or membrane *(amnion)* attached to the placenta, or afterbirth, has long been used in Africa to help heal chronic wounds and ulcers.

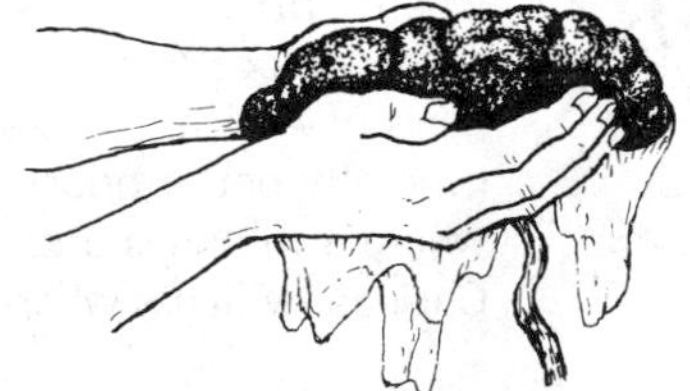

Recent studies have shown that the amnion has powerful healing properties. It is now being used in some hospitals for treatment of 'ulcers that don't heal'.

In West Africa, villagers eat yams during most of the year. But during the rainy harvest season, eating yams is 'taboo'. Scientists have found that this custom makes medical sense. Yams contain small amounts of a poison *(thiocyanate)* that helps control sickle cell anemia. This kind of anemia causes many problems and sometimes death. But it also helps protect people against malaria. So the tradition of eating yams only when malaria is less common (the dry season), helps protect people against both sickle cell anemia and malaria.

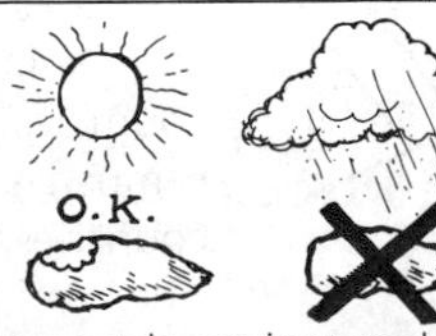

DISCOVERING WHICH HEALTH TRADITIONS ARE BENEFICIAL AND WHICH MAY BE HARMFUL

Helping people to look closely at their habits and customs is an important part of working toward a healthier community.

In every community there are some habits and traditions that are helpful. Others help little. And some probably are harmful. Often the people themselves are not sure which are truly helpful and which might be harmful.

A health worker can help people examine their traditional ways of meeting health needs. Perhaps together they can work out guidelines for deciding whether particular home remedies are helpful or might cause harm.

The following guidelines were developed with villagers in Mexico. How do they apply in your area? (For a fuller discussion, see *Where There Is No Doctor,* p. 10.)

Ways to tell if a home remedy is beneficial or harmful:

1. The more remedies there are for any one illness, the less likely it is that any of them works.
2. Foul or disgusting remedies are not likely to help—and are often harmful.
3. Remedies that use animal or human waste usually do no good, and can cause dangerous infections. Never use them.
4. The more a remedy resembles the sickness it is said to cure, the more likely that its benefits come only from the power of belief.

EXAMPLE OF A <u>HELPFUL</u> REMEDY

using cactus to control bleeding and as a clean bandage

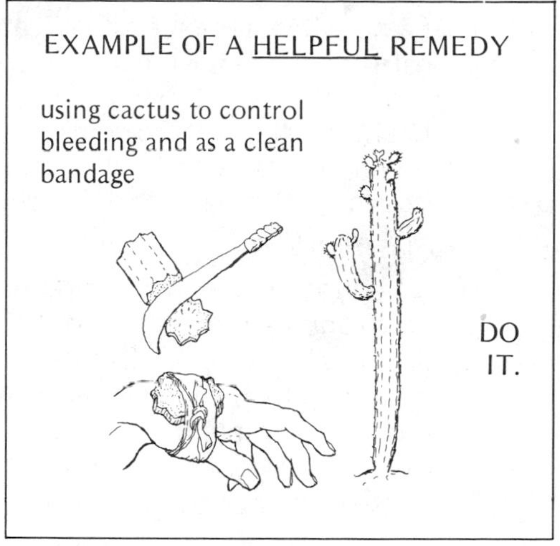

EXAMPLE OF A <u>HARMLESS</u> REMEDY (or not very helpful)

tying a crab to a goiter

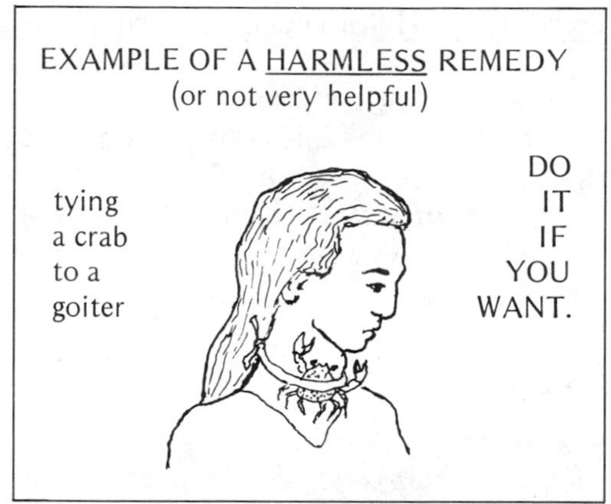

DO IT IF YOU WANT.

EXAMPLE OF A <u>HARMFUL</u> REMEDY

putting human shit around the eye to cure blurred vision

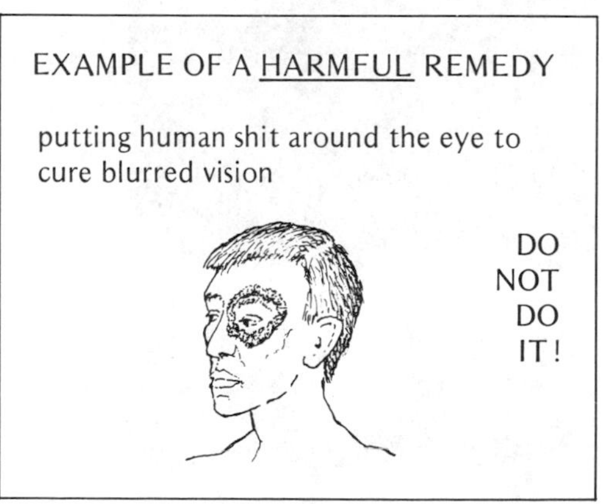

DO NOT DO IT!

When discussing the strengths and weaknesses of local traditions with people, be sure to **place more emphasis on the traditions that are helpful.** This will help people gain confidence in their own knowledge and abilities, rather than making them feel ashamed.

WAYS TO INTRODUCE NEW IDEAS BY BUILDING ON OLD ONES—Examples from Latin America

One of a health worker's most delicate jobs is to help people recognize and change health habits or customs that are harmful.

If the health worker says to someone, "What you do and believe is wrong," this usually will do more harm than good. How, then, can a health worker help people discover better ways of doing things without offending them, shaming them, or showing disrespect for their traditions? Here are some suggestions:

- Avoid telling people they are doing something wrong. Point out what they do right, and help them find out for themselves what they are doing wrong.
- Look for what is true or beneficial in a custom or belief that is partly harmful, and help people build new understanding around that.
- Help people explore the reasons, or even science, behind their beliefs and customs. Then help them realize the need to weigh the risks against the benefits—of both traditional and modern ways.

Example 1: Helping people learn a new way to treat diarrhea

In Mexico and much of Latin America, people believe that dangerous diarrhea results when a baby's soft spot, or ***fontanel,*** sinks in. They believe the baby's brains have fallen, causing the diarrhea.

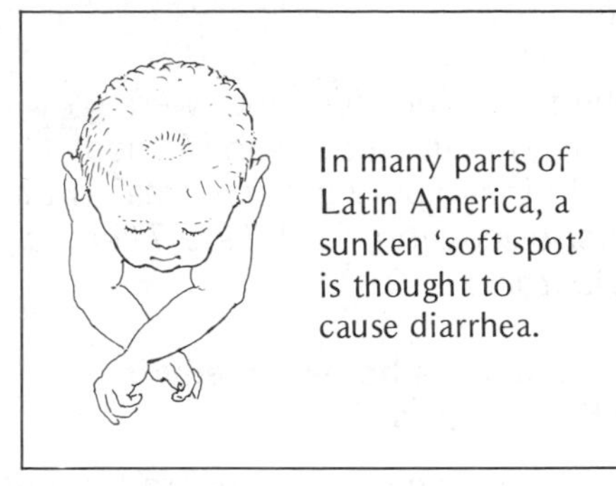

In many parts of Latin America, a sunken 'soft spot' is thought to cause diarrhea.

So when a baby with diarrhea has a sunken soft spot, they treat him by . . .

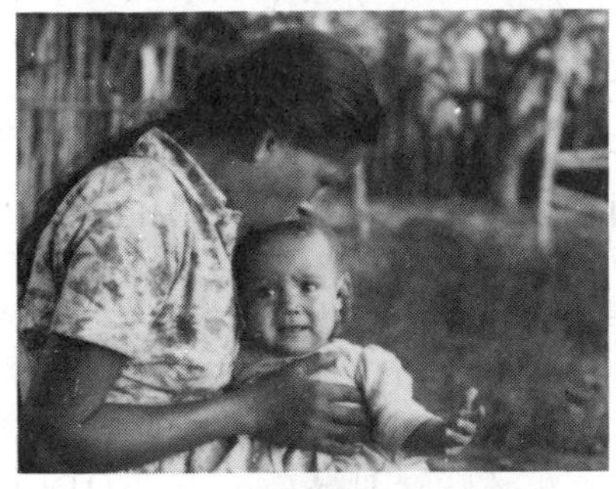

sucking on the soft spot,

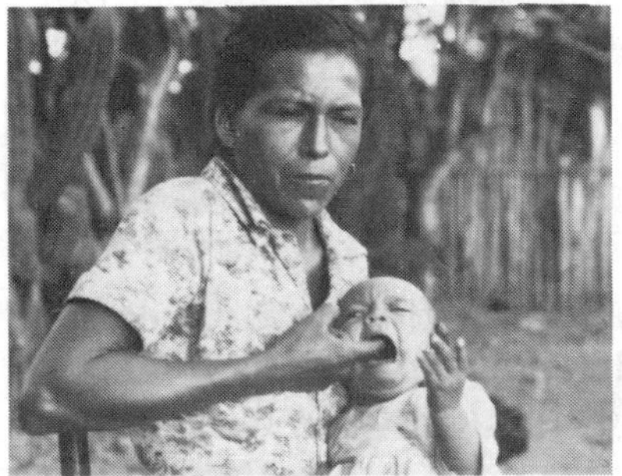

pushing upward on the roof of his mouth,

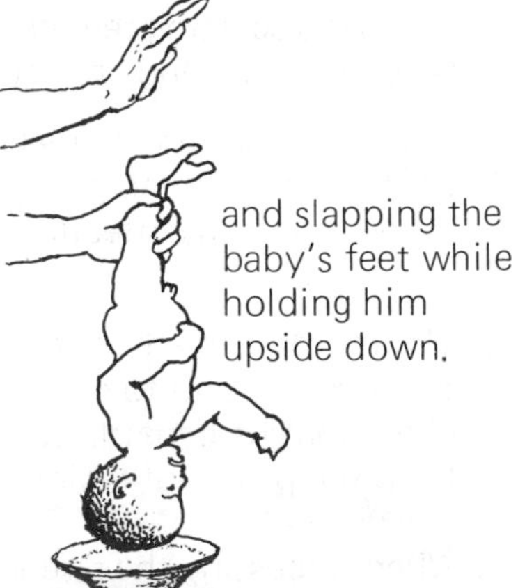

and slapping the baby's feet while holding him upside down.

How can health workers help a mother to realize that the sunken soft spot is not the cause of the diarrhea, but rather the result? That it sinks in because the baby has lost too much liquid?

Rather than say to the mother, "You're wrong!" the health workers **help her look for what is right in the tradition.** They say to the mother, "You are right that when your baby has diarrhea, a sunken soft spot is a sign of danger! Is anything else in your baby sunken in?"

"Well, yes!" says the mother. "His eyes!"

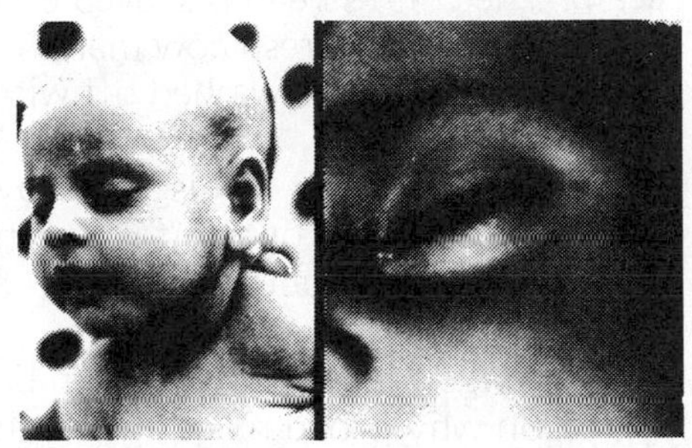

sunken eyes of a baby with dehydration

"Do you notice anything else different about the baby's eyes?"

"They look dry and dull. When he cries there aren't any tears."

"Does any other part of the body seem dry?"

"His mouth. It looks all pasty."

"When did he urinate last? When did he pee?"

"Now that you mention it, not since yesterday afternoon!"

"Why do you think the baby doesn't pee?"

In this way, the **health worker starts with what the mother already knows and observes.** She helps her discover for herself that the soft spot has sunk because the baby lacks liquid. The mother can then reason that this is the *result* of the baby's diarrhea—not the *cause.*

Now the health worker says, "Let's try a new way to bring the soft spot back up. We will give the baby lots of liquid . . ." She teaches the mother how to prepare Rehydration Drink and give it to her baby (see *Where There Is No Doctor,* p. 152).

Other ideas for helping mothers and school children learn about dehydration and rehydration are on pages **24**-17 to **24**-30.

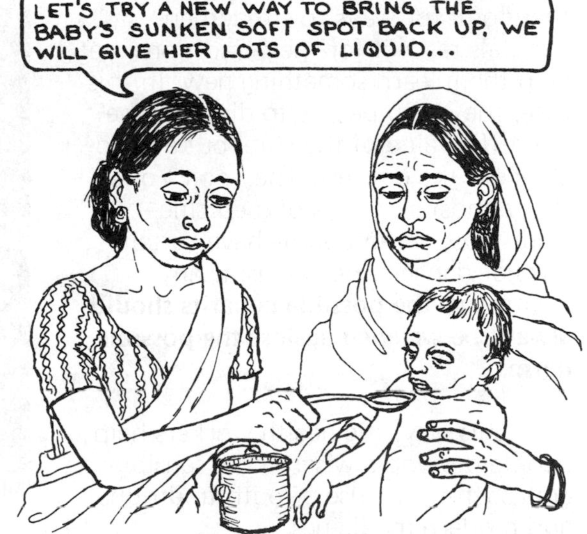
LET'S TRY A NEW WAY TO BRING THE BABY'S SUNKEN SOFT SPOT BACK UP. WE WILL GIVE HER LOTS OF LIQUID...

BUILDING ON PEOPLE'S TRADITIONS AND BELIEFS

Example 2: Helping people learn to weigh benefits against risks

Some home remedies—like some modern medicines—are relatively safe, while others are more dangerous. Health workers need to help people learn to always consider the possible risks or dangers of a treatment. **Never use a form of treatment that could prove more dangerous than the illness.**

In Mexico, villagers have an interesting home cure for deep fungus infections of the scalp. The child's head is shaved completely and covered with fresh cow manure. After 24 hours the manure is washed off with cow's urine.

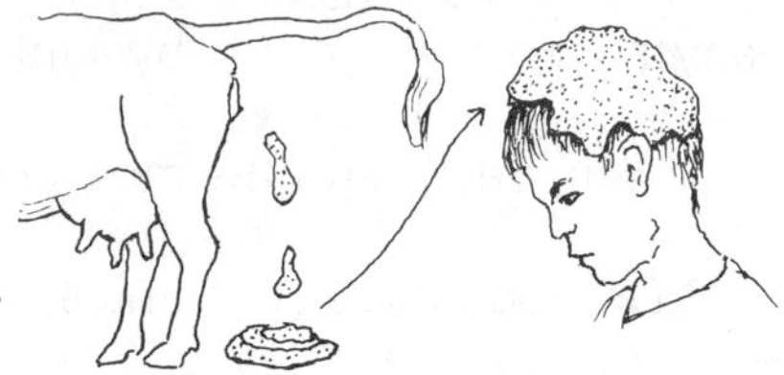

Many of us might be disgusted by this cow manure treatment, or say it is worthless. But stop to think about it; it may have some scientific value!

First, all feces (shit) contain bacteria that keep fungus from growing. (One reason why broad-range antibiotics sometimes cause diarrhea is that they kill the 'good' bacteria that prevent the growth of harmful fungus in the gut. See *WTND,* p. 58.)

Second, urine is a mild acid. Many modern anti-fungus medicines contain mild acids. So the urine as well as the manure has properties that help fight fungus infections.

On the negative side, however, this manure treatment has a high risk of causing tetanus or other serious bacterial infections. The cure could prove more dangerous than the illness.

The health workers in Ajoya therefore discourage this home treatment. But rather than tell people the cure is bad, they look for ways to strengthen people's respect for their traditions, yet help them learn something new. In this case, they help people to discover the scientific value of the cure, but also to consider the dangers. They point out that almost all forms of medicine—traditional and modern—have certain risks or dangers. Before using any treatment, **the possible benefits should always be weighed against the possible harm.**

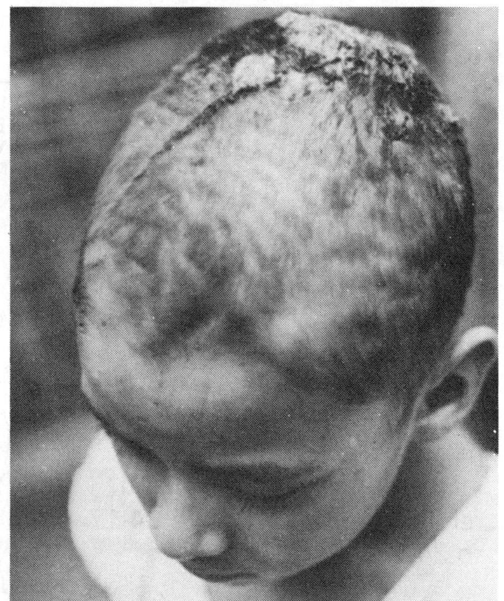

THE DEEP FUNGUS INFECTION OF THIS GIRL WAS TREATED WITH FRESH COW DUNG.

In this way, the health workers help people develop a wiser, more sensible approach to the use of both traditional and modern medicines.

For more ideas on the sensible use of medicines, see Chapter 18.

TEACHING METHODS FOR HELPING PEOPLE UNDERSTAND NEW IDEAS*

A village mother listens to a health worker explain the causes of her child's diarrhea and what she can do to prevent it. But she has a hard time believing that the flies in her home have anything to do with diarrhea. She has never seen the things called germs. She thanks the health worker for her advice—and does nothing about the flies.

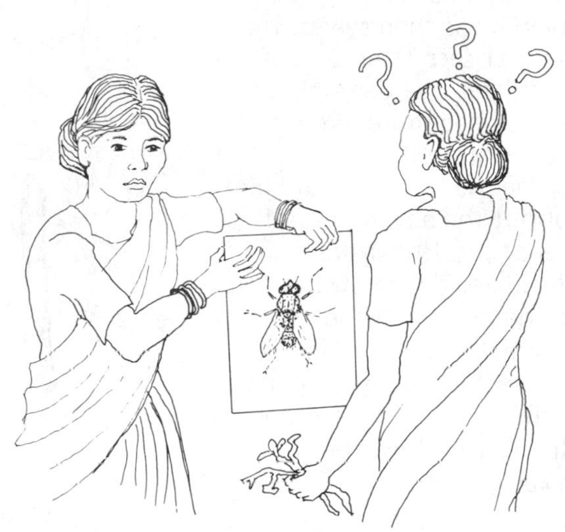

People, quite wisely, do not accept new ideas unless they understand them and how they relate to their lives. The following 4 teaching methods can **help people understand new ideas in terms of what is familiar to them.**

1. Association of ideas

People can often learn to understand a new idea if it is compared to something they already know about. This is an example:

"Do you have feet?" "Yes!" Feet are shown with laughter.

"If you step in cow shit, do you get some of it on your feet?" "Yes!"

"When you enter your house afterwards, does some of the shit get on the floor?" "Yes, if the shit was fresh and wet!"

"Do flies have feet?" "Oh, yes, 6 of them!"

"Do you think that in the same way you get cow shit on your feet, the fly gets human shit on its feet?" "Yes."

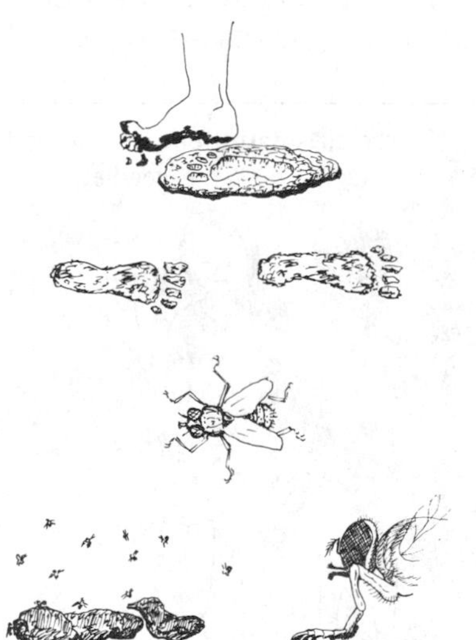

And so the discussion continues. An exchange like this gives new ideas greater meaning. It can also get people talking about them in relation to their own experience. Association of ideas can be used in many forms: in stories, role plays, puppet shows, and so on.

---

*Adapted from ***Vibro,*** an Indonesian newsletter on community development, which in turn borrowed ideas from Alan Holmes' book from rural Africa, ***Health Education in Developing Countries.***

2. Presenting ideas through real situations

People learn best through experience—by trying out new ideas themselves. If a farmer sees the result of fertilizer in a demonstration plot, he is more likely to try it for himself than if someone has only told him about the advantages of fertilizer. But if the fertilizer demonstration is done by one of the villagers on his own plot, and his harvest is greatly increased, others will be even more likely to follow the example.

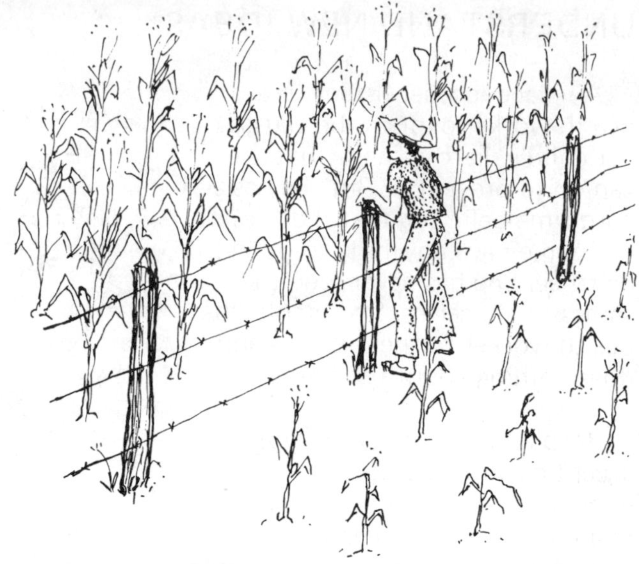

"If my neighbor can do it, so can I!"

3. Choosing an appropriate time

It helps to introduce new ideas as they relate to problems that arise in a family or community.

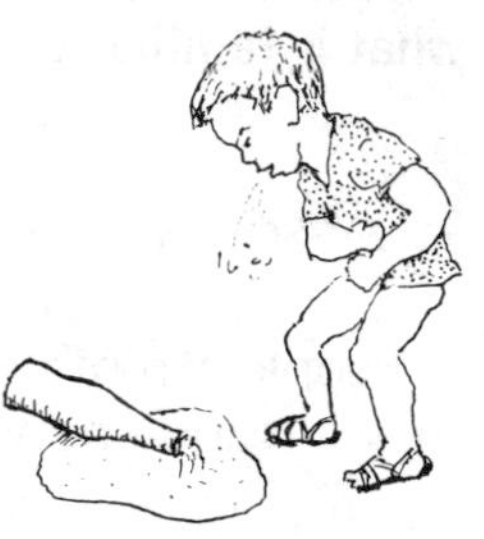

For example, if a local child has just died of kerosene poisoning, people will be more ready to consider advice about not keeping kerosene in old Coke or soft-drink bottles.

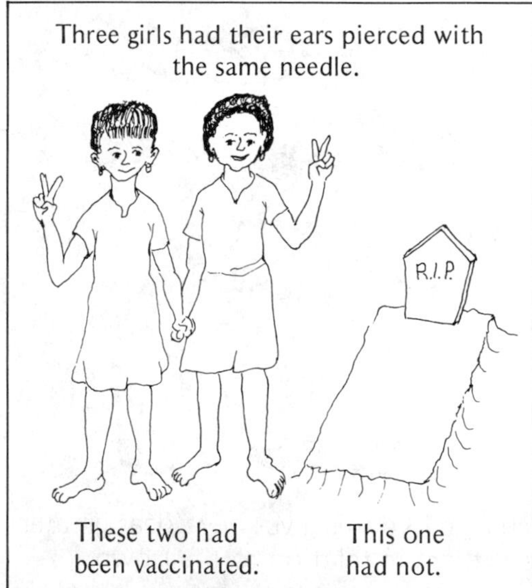
Three girls had their ears pierced with the same needle.
R.I.P.
These two had been vaccinated.
This one had not.

In one village, a health worker had a hard time convincing families to accept vaccinations. He succeeded in vaccinating only half the children.

Then a little girl named Cathy got tetanus and died. The health worker found out that a week before she fell ill, Cathy and two other girls had had their ears pierced with the same needle. The other two girls had been vaccinated against tetanus. But Cathy had not. The health worker helped the people understand that the vaccination had protected the two girls. Because Cathy had not been vaccinated, she lost her life. The next time the health worker vaccinated, not one child was missed!

In this way, the occasion of the death of one little girl was used by the health worker to educate his community and save many other lives. To do this effectively, great care and sensitivity are needed. Talk with your group about problems that might arise.

4. On-the-spot survey

To help people realize the effectiveness of new ways of doing things, it sometimes helps to take a simple 5-minute survey. This is based on the actual experiences of the participants in a meeting.

For example, a group of people who raise chickens might be uncertain about the value of vaccinating them. To see if vaccination has been worthwhile, each person can report the number of his chickens that have died in a certain time. The results are written on the blackboard and compared.

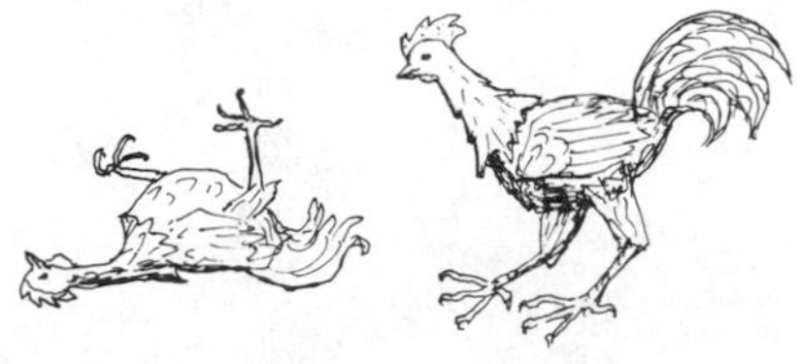

Chicken Owner	Number of birds in January	Number that died	Vaccinated ?
John	12	6	No
Maria	8	1	Yes
Alice	9	2	Yes
Joe	6	5	No
Sylvia	13		

This kind of on-the-spot survey lets people learn from the evidence of their own experience. The method can be used for various concerns, such as breast feeding instead of bottle feeding (see the children's census, p. **24**-18), or use of Rehydration Drink.

GOOD WILL, RESPECT, AND PRACTICE

In this chapter, we have given examples of ways in which health workers can help people look at things differently. These build on people's traditions or beliefs, and help them discover new ideas for themselves.

But to use these approaches successfully, good will, deep respect, and careful practice are needed. In the training program, students can help each other gain all of these.

Role playing can be a big help (see Ch. 14). Also, if students live in the homes of local families, they can try to share with them the new ideas that they have learned in class. When visiting homes in the community, they can do the same. Back in class, they can discuss their successes and difficulties.

Respect for people's beliefs, and tact or sensitivity in dealing with customs that may be harmful, are probably best taught through the good example the instructor sets for his or her students.

CHAPTER **8**

Practice in Attending the Sick

THE IMPORTANCE OF A SOLID BASE IN CURATIVE SKILLS

As we discussed in Chapter 3, ability to attend the sick is one of the most important skills a community health worker can learn. This is because:

- Curative medicinc answers a strong felt need. Most people show far more interest in curing their ills than in preventing them—at least at first.
- A health worker who is an effective healer will win people's confidence and cooperation more readily—even for preventive measures.
- Early, safe, low-cost treatment by people in their own homes is an essential part of prevention. It keeps many minor problems from becoming severe.
- Attending the sick provides a key opportunity for health education that relates to the family's immediate problems and concerns. (See the discussion below.)
- Only when health workers are well versed in curative medicine, including its risks and limitations, can they help people overcome common misunderstandings about modern medicine. (Training health workers only in 'prevention' can actually lead to greater misuse, overuse, and ***mystification**** of medicine!)

Appropriate curative medicine is a key part of prevention.

Treatment as a door to prevention

Many health workers have found that the 'clinical consultation', or occasion when a sick person seeks treatment, is one of the best opportunities to talk about preventive measures. Some find this more effective than organized health talks in small groups because . . .

- it is more immediate and personal,
- the sick person and her family are very much concerned with the illness in question, and
- many people come for treatment who might not come to health talks.

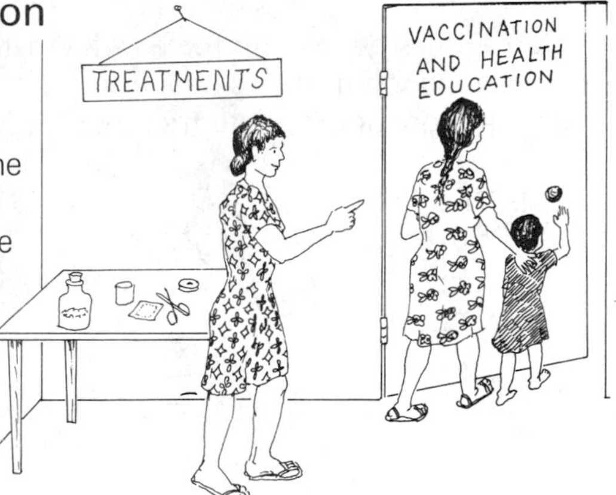

CURATIVE MEDICINE—
A DOORWAY TO PREVENTION

****Mystification:*** Making something seem magical or supernatural, beyond the understanding of ordinary people.

A health worker who can diagnose and treat, or help others to diagnose and treat many of their own health problems, has many more opportunities for health education.

Starting with what people want—then helping them explore what they need

The clinical consultation, or 'patient visit', offers an excellent opportunity for health education. It is a chance to talk about the causes, diagnosis, treatment, and prevention of the person's illness or injury.

However, when using the clinical consultation as a starting point for health education, it is wise to take certain precautions.

If you want people's good will and cooperation:

First **start with what people want** (their immediate or FELT needs).

Then help them to better understand and meet their underlying, long-term needs (REAL needs).

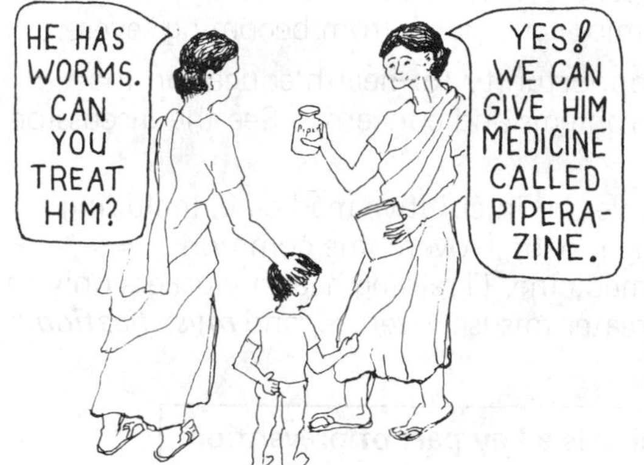
HE HAS WORMS. CAN YOU TREAT HIM?
YES! WE CAN GIVE HIM MEDICINE CALLED PIPERA-ZINE.

TREATMENT FIRST

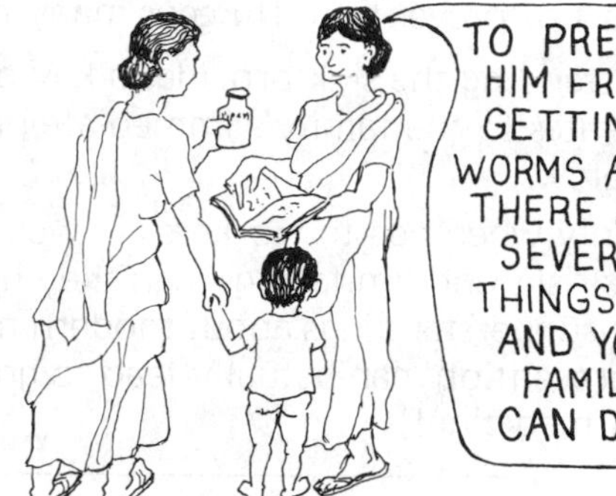
TO PREVENT HIM FROM GETTING WORMS AGAIN, THERE ARE SEVERAL THINGS YOU AND YOUR FAMILY CAN DO...

THEN PREVENTION

Sometimes people ask for treatment that is harmful, wasteful, or based on misunderstanding. If this happens, try to help them understand the situation and accept a more appropriate treatment. (See Chapter 18.)

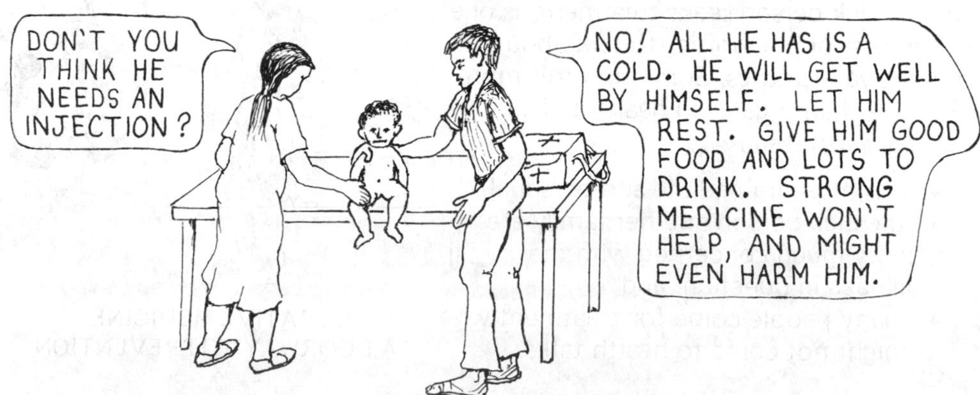
DON'T YOU THINK HE NEEDS AN INJECTION?
NO! ALL HE HAS IS A COLD. HE WILL GET WELL BY HIMSELF. LET HIM REST. GIVE HIM GOOD FOOD AND LOTS TO DRINK. STRONG MEDICINE WON'T HELP, AND MIGHT EVEN HARM HIM.

If medicines are not needed, take time to explain why.

LEARNING WHAT TO DO FOR THE SICK AND INJURED

Learning what to do for sick or injured people can be approached in a combination of ways:

- in the **classroom**—through study, reading, and discussion.
- through **role plays** (usually also in the classroom). Different illnesses are acted out, and students take turns diagnosing, treating, and giving advice.
- through **actual practice** in diagnosing, treating, advising, and caring for sick persons and their families.

The first two ways (classroom and role plays) are covered in Parts Two and Three of this book. In this chapter we will consider mostly the third way—which involves working directly with persons who are sick or injured.

Direct experience through 'clinical practice' is one of the most important parts of health worker training. It needs to be balanced with classroom learning and activities in the community. But be sure to allow plenty of time for clinical practice: perhaps 1½ to 2 hours a day. In addition, try to be flexible and interrupt class when there is a chance for students to observe and help treat emergencies or other important illnesses.

To follow are some ideas and suggestions that may help clinical practice during training to be more effective.

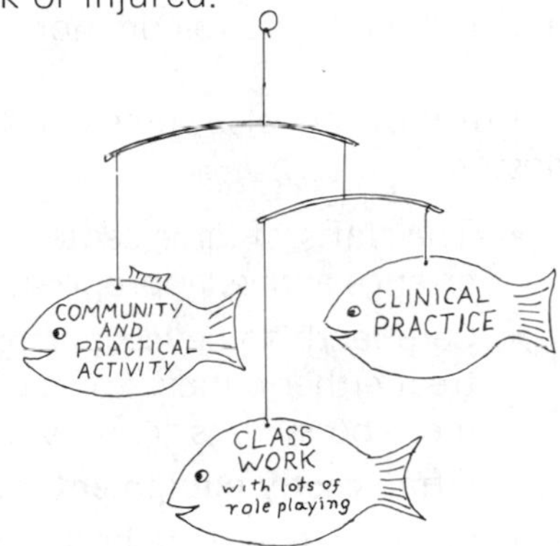

A GOOD BALANCE FOR A HEALTHY 'SCHOOL'

Clinical instructors

In some ways it is best for health workers-in-training to get clinical practice with experienced community health workers rather than with doctors. In any case, it is important that the clinical instructor be a person who makes clear his own limitations. He or she needs to set an example by referring sick persons with difficult or confusing problems to those who are more highly trained or specialized.

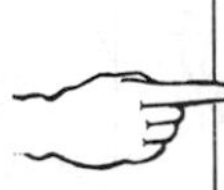

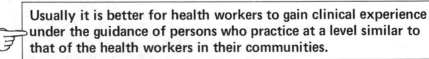

Usually it is better for health workers to gain clinical experience under the guidance of persons who practice at a level similar to that of the health workers in their communities.

It also helps if the clinical instructors are the same persons who work with the health workers in the rest of the training program. This way, classroom learning and community activities can be better related to clinical experience. **Classwork becomes more meaningful when it relates to real persons and problems recently seen in the clinic or community.**

The place and level (hospital, health center, or home)

The term 'clinical practice', as we use it, does not mean only activity in a clinic or health center. It includes visiting sick persons in their homes.

Many programs have found that health workers do not need a special, separate 'health post'. They can work well in their own homes, or by visiting the homes of the sick. The home is a more relaxed place for a consultation and puts the health worker and the sick person on more equal terms. It provides a more appropriate setting for talking about preventive measures. And it helps to 'demystify' or take the magic out of medical care.

There is, however, one big advantage to having students gain at least part of their clinical experience in a community clinic or health center. It gives them a chance to see a wider variety of health problems and to gain repeated experience in handling the more common problems.

But there are also some disadvantages to clinical practice in a large clinic or hospital:

- The staffs of large centers or hospitals tend to be **less flexible,** less able to arrange active, appropriate learning for health workers.
- Care tends to be **less personal** and more hurried. Staff may not have time to treat either patients or health workers as persons. Health workers may learn more bossy, less friendly attitudes and habits.
- Often **costly equipment** is used that will not be available in health posts.
- Students may take part in difficult diagnoses or treatments of problems that they would normally need to refer to a health center. This can lead to **confusion and temptation to go beyond their limits.**

LESS APPROPRIATE

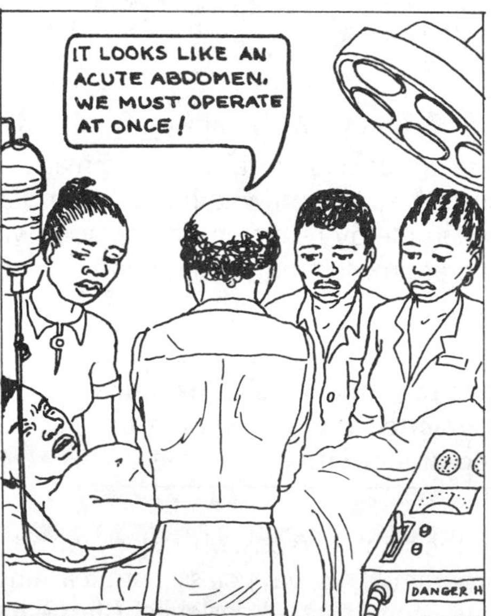
IT LOOKS LIKE AN ACUTE ABDOMEN. WE MUST OPERATE AT ONCE!
DANGER H

MORE APPROPRIATE

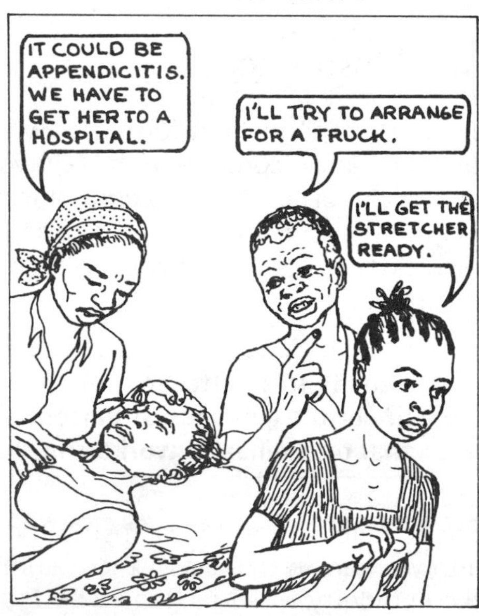

As much as possible, health workers should gain clinical experience in a situation similar to that in their own communities.

Generally it is wiser for health workers to gain clinical experience in a small community health center. Here things are more personal and more flexible. The staff, the sick and their families, and the health workers have more chance to learn about each other—not just as 'problems' and 'problem solvers', but as fellow human beings. They can all begin to care for and about each other.

In a small rural clinic, however, there may not be a wide enough range of problems for health workers to gain adequate experience.

Ideally, perhaps, students should have a chance to learn in both a small, unhurried village setting, and in a health center large and busy enough so that they can see a broad range of problems and persons.

A community-based program in Nuevo Leon, Mexico *(Tierra y Libertad),* has managed to do this. Training is based in a small village. But the students take turns spending time in a busy community health center in a poor neighborhood in the nearby city of Monterrey.

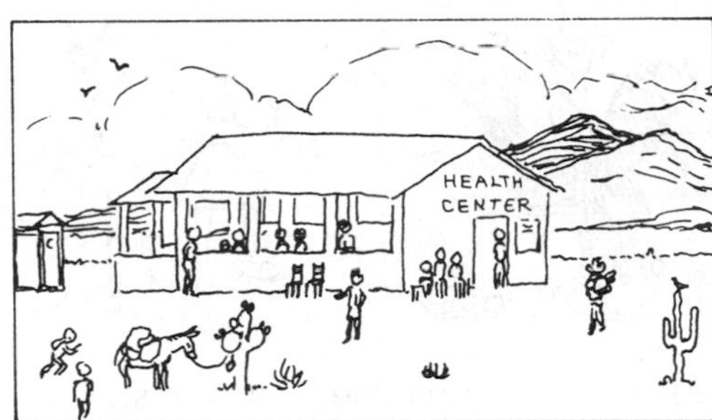

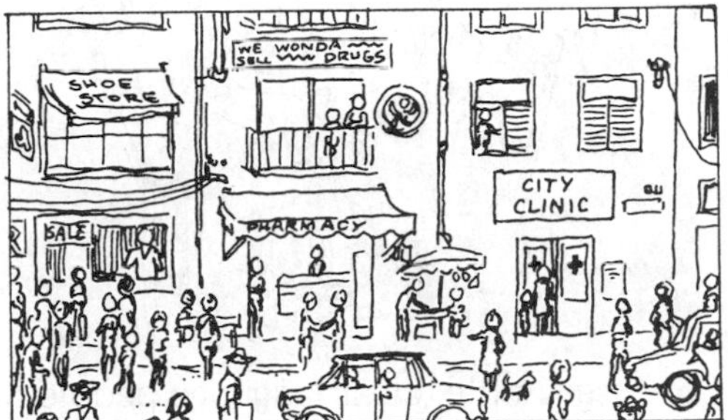

Classroom preparation

It is a good idea to begin clinical practice early in the course. So classroom preparation for this also needs to begin early. Classes might include:

- **clinical ethics** (relating to the sick as persons, not 'patients')
- **basic teaching and communicating skills** to help in understanding needs and explaining things clearly to a sick person and his family
- **how to examine a sick person** (see *Where There Is No Doctor,* Ch. 3)
- **how to take care of a sick person** (see *WTND,* Ch. 4)
- **practice in using record sheets** (see Ch. 22)
- **solving problems step by step** (scientific method, Ch. 17)
- **diagnosis, treatment, and prevention of common illnesses and injuries** (based on local needs and resources)
- **proper use and measurement of medicines** (see *WTND,* Ch. 5, 6, 7, and 8)
- **preventive measures** for specific health problems

In classroom study of these subjects, the closer the learning situation can be to the real-life situation, the better. Through role plays and sociodramas, students can practice all the above skills in a lifelike way. A **checklist,** or list of review questions, can be used to evaluate how well the students do (see page **8**-10).

ADVISING HEALTH WORKERS ABOUT 'CLINICAL ETHICS'

Before health workers begin clinical practice, it is a good idea to spend some time discussing guidelines for relating to the sick. These guidelines should be followed by the instructors, too, as they set the example for the health workers-in-training. You may want to include these points:*

Treat sick persons and their families as your friends and equals, not as 'patients' or 'cases'. For example:

- Make sure there are places for everyone to sit.
- Dress as they do, instead of wearing a uniform.
- Sit near them . . . . not behind a desk or table.

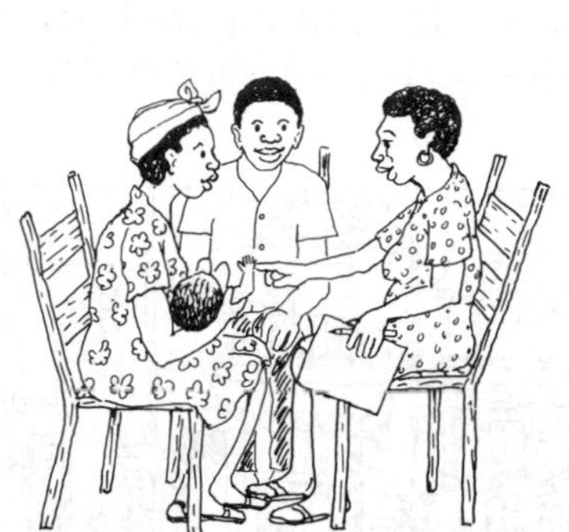

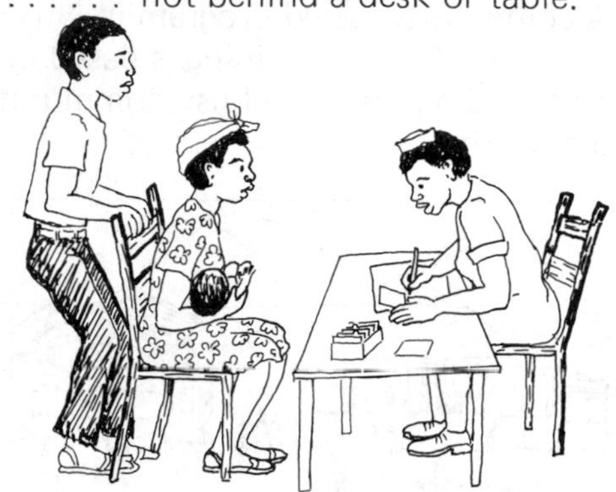

- Use simple, clear language people understand (avoid big medical terms).
- Ask about family and friends, not just about the health problem. Take interest in the life and ideas of the sick person and his family.
- Do not let record keeping interfere with communicating. Do not write while the person is talking.
- Respect people's traditions and beliefs.
- Learn how to listen. Be sympathetic to people's hopes and fears.

First serve those whose needs are greatest. When many persons are waiting to be seen, try to notice those who are especially sick or need immediate attention. Very sick persons need to be seen first. They should not have to 'wait their turn'.

If other workers at the training center (and people in the villages) can learn to recognize signs of serious illness, they can help to make sure that those who need attention immediately are seen first.

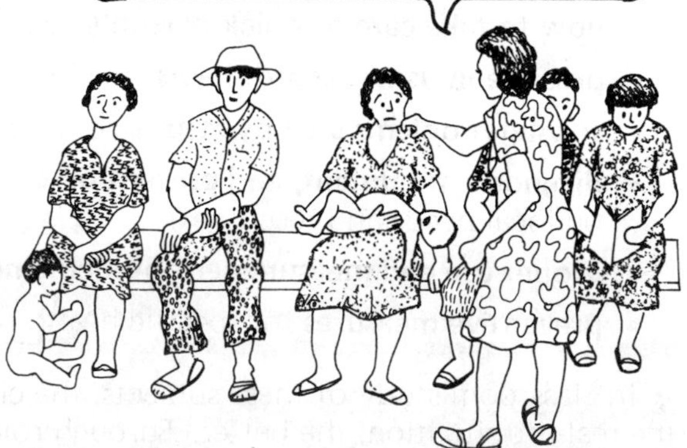

I KNOW IT'S NOT YOUR TURN. BUT YOUR BABY LOOKS SO ILL! I'M SURE NO ONE WILL MIND IF I SEE HIM FIRST.

*These guidelines are from a mimeographed sheet written by Project Piaxtla staff for village health worker trainees in Ajoya, Mexico.

Respect the confidence and privacy of the sick person. Do not discuss someone's health problems outside the clinic or classroom. This is especially important in a small village where gossip is a main form of entertainment.

If someone asks you, "What is wrong with Maria?" consider answering, "I'm sorry, I can't discuss a person's private problems except with members of the immediate family." This way, people will learn that they can trust you. They will then be willing to see you about problems they do not want others to know about.

Be honest with the sick person and his family—but also be kind. Sometimes when a person is very ill or dying, or has a frightening disease like leprosy or cancer, you may not be sure whether to tell him and his family the truth. But often both the sick person and his family already suspect the worst, and suffer because they try to hide their fears from each other. Each situation needs to be approached individually. But as a general rule, it is wise to **be as truthful as possible . . .** but in a way that is gentle and kind.

Help the sick person gain a better understanding of his illness. Explain the physical examination, diagnosis, causes of the illness, treatment, and prevention in clear, simple terms. Use your books or show pictures to help explain things. Help people take informed responsibility for their problems. Never use your knowledge of healing as a form of power over other people.

Use medicines only when needed, and help people understand why it is important to limit their use. In about 80% of illnesses, a person will get well without medical treatment.

On the average, a clinic should aim at giving medicines to only about half of the persons who come for treatment. But make every effort to see that those who go away without medicine are content with the advice or treatment given. One of the most important aspects of health education is to help people realize that **it is healthier, safer, and cheaper to manage many illnesses without medicines.** (See Ch. 18.)

Recognize your limits, and admit when you don't know something. No matter at what level a health worker is trained, there will be certain illnesses or problems she cannot diagnose or treat. This may be because the problem is not treatable, or because she lacks the skill, knowledge, medicine, or equipment to treat it. In any case, it is important that the health worker admit her limitations. When necessary, she should refer the sick person to where he is more likely to receive the attention he needs.

Also, when you have doubts or are unsure of how to do something, do not pretend to know. Admit your doubts and ask for assistance. This is as important for instructors as for students.

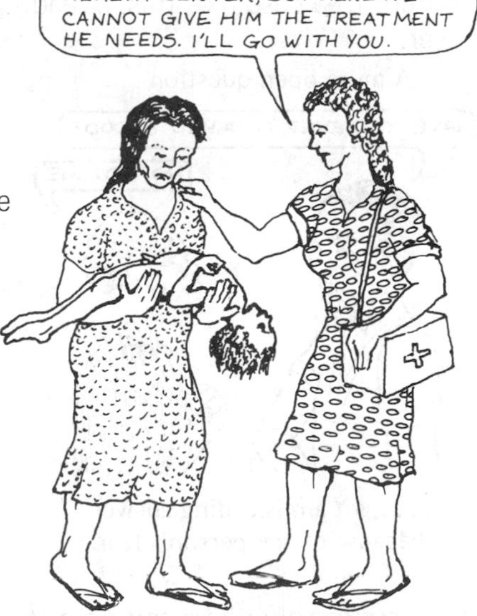

I KNOW IT'S A LONG WAY TO THE HEALTH CENTER, BUT HERE WE CANNOT GIVE HIM THE TREATMENT HE NEEDS. I'LL GO WITH YOU.

KNOW YOUR LIMITS

THE ART OF ASKING QUESTIONS

Sometimes a sick person will tell you what he thinks you want to hear, in hopes that you will treat him better if you are pleased with his answers.

Help students to be aware of this problem. Try to make sure that they ask questions carefully and get correct answers. They may have to ask about the same thing more than once. But have them take care not to insult the sick person by seeming to doubt his answers.

Usually it is a good idea to avoid asking questions that lead the person to answer in a certain way. For example, look at these questions and answers:

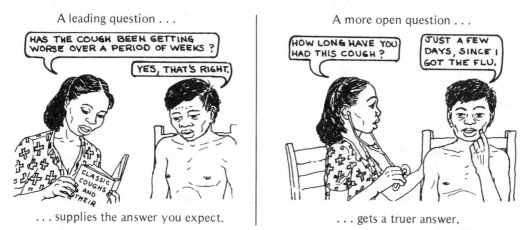

A leading question . . .

HAS THE COUGH BEEN GETTING WORSE OVER A PERIOD OF WEEKS ?
YES, THAT'S RIGHT.
CLASSIC COUGHS AND THEIR

. . . supplies the answer you expect.

A more open question . . .

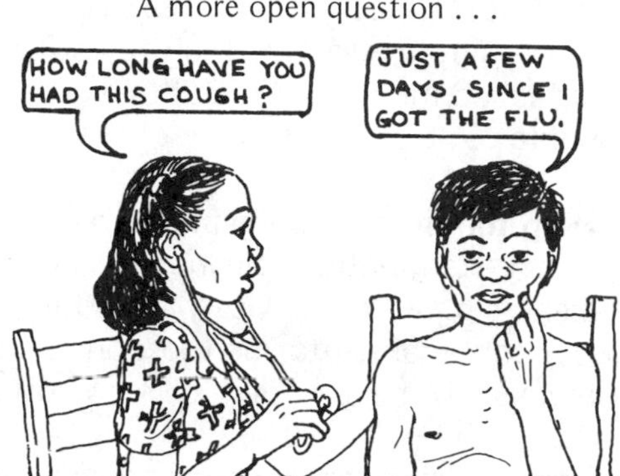
HOW LONG HAVE YOU HAD THIS COUGH ?
JUST A FEW DAYS, SINCE I GOT THE FLU.

. . . gets a truer answer.

In either case, the health worker will need to ask more questions in order to understand how and when the problem began.

A more open question is not always better. Often a sick person will be afraid to admit that he has signs of a disease such as tuberculosis or leprosy. These diseases are especially feared because many people still believe that they cannot be cured. In a case like this, a leading question will sometimes get a more revealing answer.

A more open question . . .

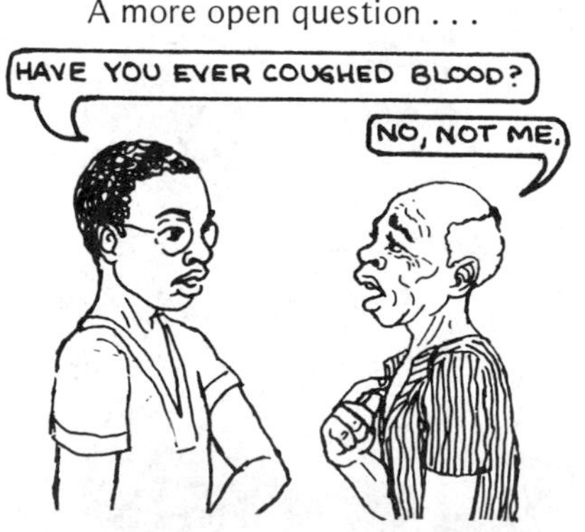
HAVE YOU EVER COUGHED BLOOD?
NO, NOT ME.

. . . got a misleading answer because of the person's fear.

A leading question . . .

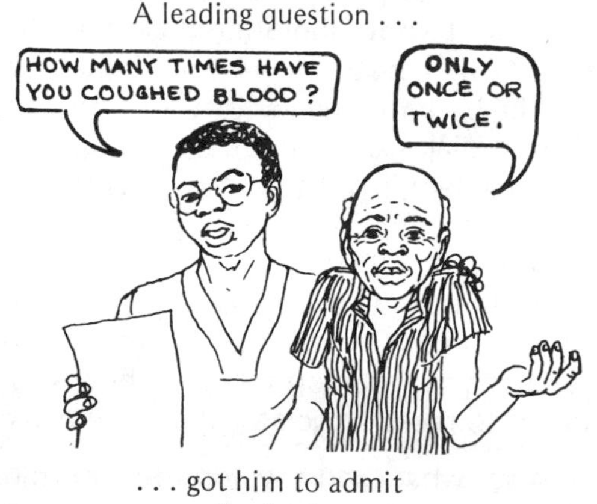
HOW MANY TIMES HAVE YOU COUGHED BLOOD ?
ONLY ONCE OR TWICE.

. . . got him to admit the truth.

Classroom role plays can help students practice asking appropriate questions—in a way that does not offend.

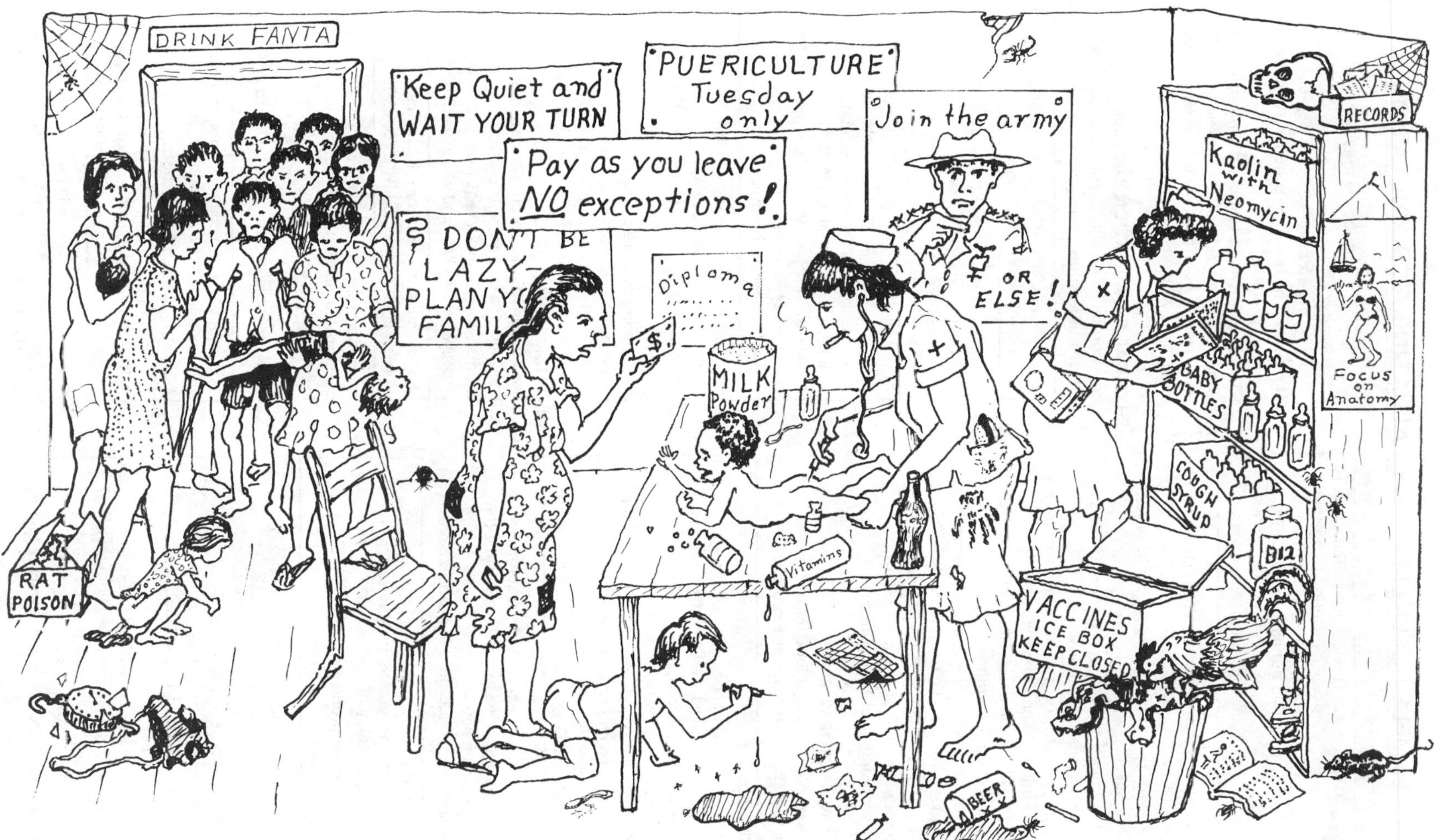
DRINK FANTA
Keep Quiet and
WAIT YOUR TURN
PUERICULTURE
Tuesday
only
Pay as you leave
NO exceptions!
Join the army
OR
ELSE!
DON'T BE
LAZY—
PLAN YO
FAMIL
Diploma
MILK
Powder
Vitamins
Kaolin
with
Neomycin
RECORDS
BABY
BOTTLES
COUGH
SYRUP
B12
Focus
on
Anatomy
VACCINES
ICE BOX
KEEP CLOSED
BEER
RAT
POISON

Ask your health workers how many faults they can find in the clinic shown here. (We find more than 50.) What improvements do they suggest?

SAMPLE CHECKLIST FOR EVALUATING A CONSULTATION

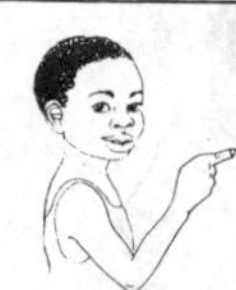

Note: This self-evaluation checklist is a sample, intended for raising questions as well as for evaluation. You do not have to read it in detail as you read through this chapter. Refer to it later if you need to.

PERSONAL APPROACH AND ATTITUDE—
Did you . . .

__attend the person promptly? Or did he have to wait long?
__spot at once if the person was very sick, and if so, see him ahead of others?
__invite the mother or relative to take part in the consultation (if appropriate)?
__ask the sick person and family members to sit down, and make them feel at ease?
__sit close to them, not behind a desk or table?
__ask questions and take the time to listen to personal and family concerns? Were you really interested in the 'patient' as a person?
__touch children and show warmth?

MEDICAL HISTORY

__**Observation:** Did you look for and see obvious signs of illness early in the consultation?

For example:
- general appearance and health (weight, posture, relaxed, nervous, depressed, etc.)
- skin color (normal, pale, yellow, blue)
- eyes (color of whites, pupil size, etc.)
- breathing (sounds, rate, effort, sucking in of skin behind collar bone)
- bulging veins, scars, sores
- specific signs of illness

History (questioning the sick person): Did you . . .

__take an adequate history **before** starting the physical examination?
__ask appropriate questions in a sensible order?

For example:
- What bothers you most **right now?**
- **When** and **how** did this begin?
- What **other problems** do you have?
- When were you last completely well?

__follow up with other searching questions?

For example, if a child has diarrhea:
- When did the problem begin?
- How many stools a day?
- What does the stool look like? (blood? mucus? etc.)
- Has the child vomited? Urinated?
- Has the child been drinking liquids? What? How much? How often?
- Does he eat? What? How often?
- Possible related illnesses? (earache, tonsils, polio, malaria, etc.)

Did you find out about the following, if necessary?

__Details of the problem—signs, dates, etc.?
__If others in the family or community suffer from the same problem?
__The person's living situation, if it might help with diagnosis, treatment, or prevention?
__What medicines or treatments have already been tried? And with what results?

PHYSICAL EXAMINATION Did you . . .

__conduct the physical exam in a sensible order?
__do what is least disturbing first?

For example, listening to a child's lungs before looking in his ears or throat.

__take precautions to make the exam as little disturbing as possible?

For example:
- Explain tests and procedures ahead of time (what you are going to do and why).
- Warm a cold stethoscope by rubbing the bell before examining a child.
- Have the mother remove the child's clothes and hold him on her lap.
- Avoid unnecessary tests.

__make sure enough clothing was removed to allow adequate examination?
__repeat doubtful or difficult examinations 2 or 3 times?
__do all necessary steps of the physical examination, and leave out those not needed for the particular problem?

DIAGNOSIS Did you . . .

__use a systematic approach to problem solving?
__consider different possible causes?
__ask questions or make tests to decide which cause was most likely and which were not?

For example, the test for rebound pain when appendicitis is suspected (***WTND,*** p. 95).

__if you made a diagnosis, did you consider it to be the probable cause of the problem? (Or did you feel absolutely certain—a very risky position to take?)
__make a sensible decision about what to do?

For example if you could not obtain enough information to make a diagnosis, did you:
- Send the person for lab tests.
- Send him to a doctor you trust.
- If it could be done safely, treat the problem according to the most likely diagnosis.

__make good use of available resources for helping make the diagnosis? (books, instruments, people)
__As nearly as can be told, did you make the right diagnosis?

TREATMENT AND MANAGEMENT

Sensible use of medicines or alternatives:

Did you . . .

__use no medicines if they were not needed?

> At least 50% of health problems are best managed without medicines.

__if medicines were not needed, help the person understand why the problem is best managed without them?

__use appropriate non-medicinal treatments?

__use only medicines that were needed?

> Use only 1, or at most 2, medicines. If 3 or more medicines are given at one time, people often cannot remember how to use all of them properly.

__ask if the person is allergic to any medicines?

__before giving a woman medicine, ask if she was pregnant? Give only medicines that are safe for the child in the womb.

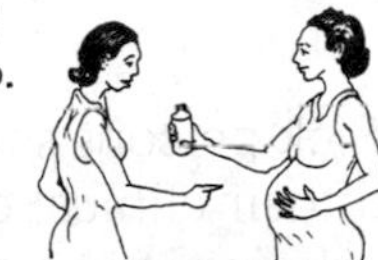

__use the correct dosage of medicines?

__measure or count the medication (pills)?

__write for the person the name of the medicine, its use, the dosage and the person's name, in clear simple form (or in picture code if illiterate)?

__explain the medicine and dosage clearly and simply, and have the person repeat it?

__do your best to make sure the person will take the medicine correctly?

> For example, have him take the first dose at once, especially if it is a single-dose medication (like some worm medicines).

__avoid injections, except when absolutely necessary?

__consider the cost of different possible medications, and choose the cheapest one likely to do the job adequately?

__emphasize the importance of taking the medicine as directed and for the time necessary?

__give advice about risks and precautions?

Traditional medicines and beliefs: Did you . . .

__use traditional medicines or healing methods, if appropriate?

__explain about diet and other traditional concerns people have when taking medicines?

__explain things in such a way as to respect and build upon people's traditions and beliefs, rather than reject them?

__**Follow-up:** Did you make arrangements for follow-up, if necessary?

Referral: Did you . . .

__recognize your limitations, if the problem was beyond your ability to diagnose and treat?

__openly explain your limits and help arrange for the person to receive care elsewhere (hospital or clinic)?

HEALTH EDUCATION AND PREVENTION

Communication about the health problem:

Did you . . .

__discuss with the sick person and his family: the illness, its causes, and its prevention?

__use simple, clear language, and local words?

__include the child, as well as the mother when discussing the health problem and its prevention?

__use books, teaching aids, examples, or stories to make points clearer?

Prevention:

__Did you place enough emphasis on prevention?

__Were the preventive measures you suggested clearly related to the problem in question?

__Did you consider the feelings and concerns of the sick person and his family?

> For example, did you talk about prevention only after providing for treatment?

__Did you try to make sure that the preventive measures you suggested would be followed?

> For example, in case of typhoid, did you:
> - Offer to visit the home and plan with neighbors to help construct a latrine?
> - Help the family make a water filter or a rain water collecting system.

__Did you do your best to share your knowledge and show there is nothing magic or secret about your medical abilities? Or did you look things up secretly (or not at all) in order to give the impression that you 'know it all'?

USE OF BOOKS Did you . . .

__make good use of your reference book(s) during the consultation?

__openly look things up in the book while with the sick person and his family?

__show the sick person or a parent the sections or pictures in the book that explain the problem?

__double check dosage or other information by looking it up, even if you were fairly sure?

RECORDS Did you . . .

__write a record of the consultation?

> - Name, age, date, etc.
> - Health history and what you found in physical exam—in enough detail for another health worker to understand.
> - Possible alternatives for diagnosis.
> - Tests and information in order to rule out or confirm possible causes.
> - Conclusion (most probable diagnosis).
> - Care and treatment (or decision to refer).
> - Preventive advice given.

__record the information so that it is **clear** and **well organized?**

__record the information in a way that did not disturb your conversation with the sick person?

__fill out any other necessary forms?

ROLE OF THE INSTRUCTOR IN THE CLINICAL SITUATION

The role of the clinical instructor—whether an experienced health worker, a doctor, or someone else—is of key importance. The instructor needs to do far more than question, examine, and treat the patient while the students watch. It is up to her to balance consultation with education. She needs to look for every opportunity to help the students learn, yet be sensitive to the needs and feelings of the sick person and her family.

Teaching assistants: In the early stages of clinical learning, it is especially helpful if, apart from the instructor who conducts the consultation, a second instructor or experienced health worker is present. This teaching assistant quietly guides the observing students in where to look in their books and how to record information in the 'patient report' forms. This way, the consultation proceeds with little interruption, yet the students receive individual help and answers to their questions. The teaching assistant can also quietly ask the students questions that lead them to asking the right questions themselves.

Involving the sick person and her family as helpers: Sick persons sometimes feel angry about having students observe or take part in their clinical consultation. They may feel they are being used, without having any choice in the matter. Unfortunately, this is often true.

You can often transform this situation by looking at the sick person as a *person,* not as a patient. To do this:

- Explain to the sick person and her family about the training course, and the need for health workers to gain experience in order to serve their communities better. Then ask if they are willing to help teach the student health workers about the problem.
- Respect the decision of those who say no. Do not try to pressure or shame them into saying yes.
- Keep the student group small—usually not more than 3 or 4.
- Include the sick person and any family members in the discussion of the problem. Make sure that details of the physical examination, diagnosis, treatment, and prevention are discussed clearly and simply.

If the sick person is involved in this way, you will be surprised how often she will end up feeling good about the consultation and the presence of the students. Several times we have seen persons thank the group warmly and say:

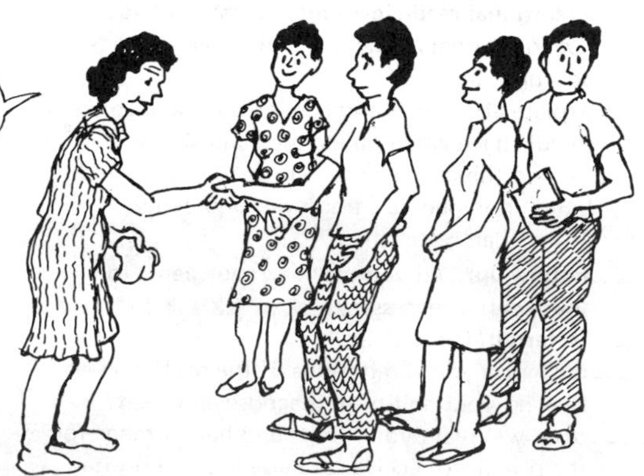

THANK YOU ALL SO MUCH! THIS IS THE FIRST TIME I'VE GONE TO A CLINIC AND HAD PEOPLE EXPLAIN THINGS SO I COULD UNDERSTAND!

If the person's illness is an especially common one, and not embarrassing to her, she may not mind if other people waiting for consultation also hear about its signs, causes, prevention, and treatment. They may even have helpful ideas or experiences to contribute.

STAGES OF CLINICAL LEARNING

The role students take in clinical consultations depends on a number of factors. But generally they are given more responsibility as their training progresses.

At first students may be mainly observers, staying in the background and saying little. As they gain more knowledge and experience, they usually take an increasingly active role (and the instructor a less active one). By the end of the training program, students should be able to take charge of the consultations. The instructor stays very much in the background, participating only when her advice is asked or when students forget an important step or make an error.

STAGE 1:

Instructor takes the lead; students observe.

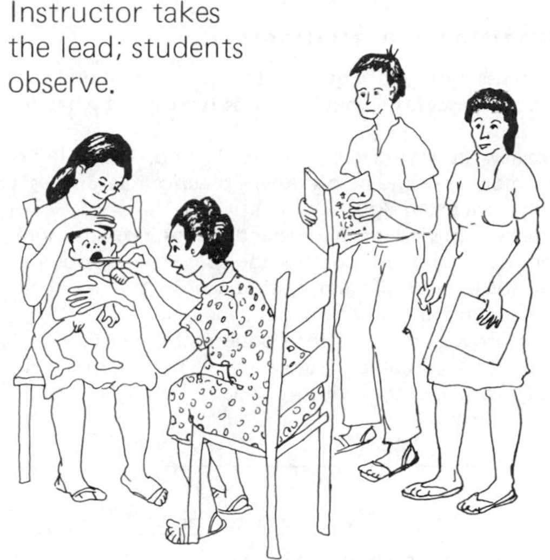

STAGE 2:

Instructor still leads, but students take increasing responsibility.

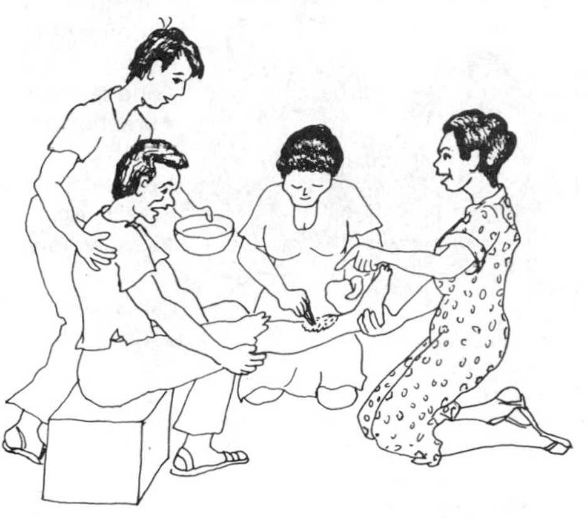

STAGE 3:

Students conduct the consultation; instructor observes.

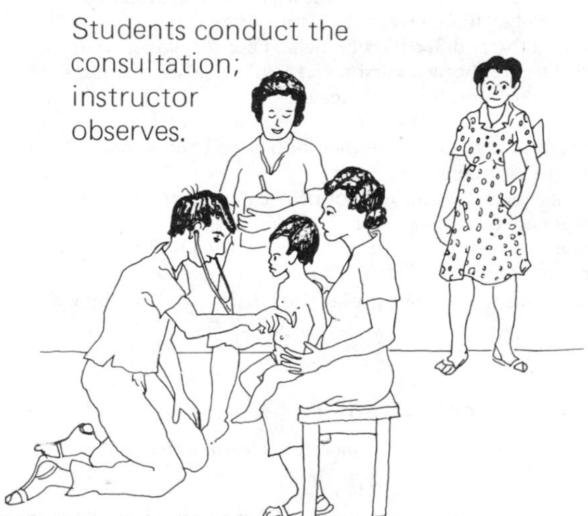

STAGE 4:

Students in charge: instructor absent but on call if needed.

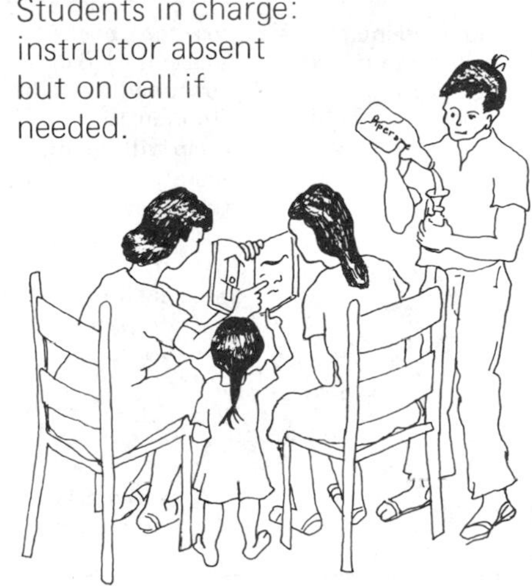

POSSIBLE STAGES IN CLINICAL PRACTICE

STAGE 1:

(about 1-2 weeks)

Instructors take the lead;

students observe.

What health workers can do

- mostly observe
- look up the problem in their books and try to figure it out
- ask instructor some questions (but with care not to disturb the sick person)
- practice filling out record sheets about the sick person

What instructor can do

During the consultations:

- ask the sick person or family if students may observe
- conduct the consultation
- explain steps of history taking, physical exam, diagnosis, and treatment to both the sick person and the students (with care not to disturb the sick person)
- ask occasional questions of the students to help them think things through
- be sure information gathered is clear enough for students to fill out record sheets properly
- discuss appropriate preventive measures with the sick person (or family)

After the consultations:

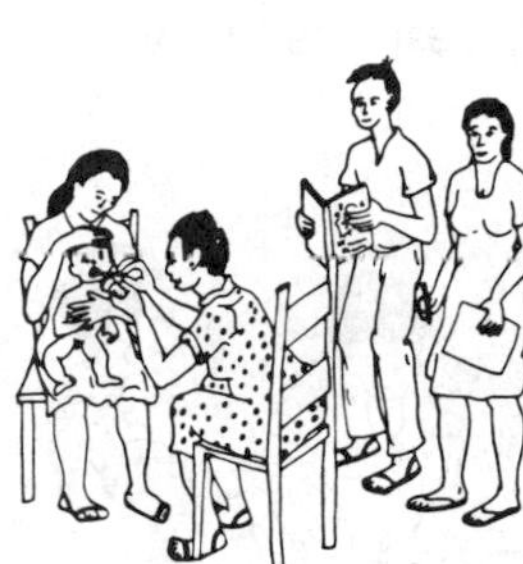

What health workers can do:

- ask instructor questions and comment on what they saw and learned
- practice on each other any physical exam skills used
- review how consultation was carried out

What instructor can do:

- discuss important points of the consultation and the health problem, pointing out what was typical and what was not typical
- review student record sheets and compare with her own
- demonstrate and help students practice relevant tests and physical exam skills
- make sure students understand the inter-relationship and importance of each part of the consultation (observation, history, physical exam, tests, diagnosis, management and/or treatment, prevention, education)
- discuss with students their doubts, abilities, limits, and how they could best handle a similar problem when they confront it in their villages (what to do or not do; if and when to refer)

STAGE 2:

(2-3 weeks)

Instructor still leads;

but students take a more responsible role.

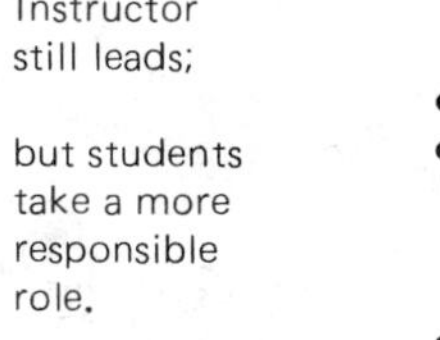

What health workers can do

- help take history
- perform parts of the physical exam that they have already studied and practiced
- fill out record sheets
- use their books to diagnose and determine treatment (with help from instructor)
- help with simple curative measures
- give preventive advice or read preventive measures from their books for the sick person (or family)

What instructor can do

During the consultations:

- let students take the lead in history taking and examination when problems appear to be those with which they have experience, but be quick to step in when they need help
- make suggestions and ask questions to help students remember to make the right tests, interpret results correctly, and ask the sick person appropriate questions
- make sure the sick person and family feel comfortable with the consultation process
- take over when necessary
- make sure students use their books well and explain things to the sick person
- if necessary, repeat tests or physical exam to check if students did things right
- review treatment (medicine, dosage, etc.) and advice given by students
- be sure students give preventive advice, in a friendly way

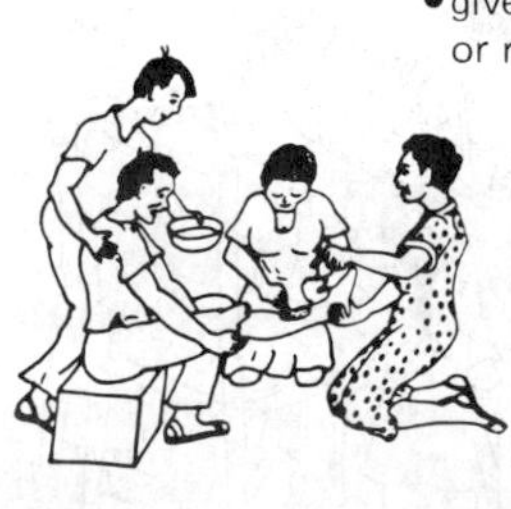

After the consultations:

- as in STAGE 1, but by now students can also take turns leading the review discussions and asking each other questions

FOR HEALTH WORKERS-IN-TRAINING*

STAGE 3:

(about
2-3 weeks)

Students conduct the consultation;

instructor observes.

During the consultations:

What health workers can do

- conduct the entire consultation
- use books as much as possible, and ask for suggestions or help from instructor only (but always) when unsure of what to ask or do
- together with the sick person (or family) make the decision about how to handle the sick person's problem; whether to instruct the person on treatment or refer him to a clinic or hospital

What instructor can do

- be present as an observer. If possible, remain silent throughout the entire consultation, taking notes on points to discuss after the consultation.
- take an active part only when the health workers make an error that might result in harm or inadequate treatment
- when necessary, help health workers gain the person's confidence by agreeing with their conclusions or approving of their methods

After the consultations:

As much as possible, the situation should be like that in which health workers will later work—except that the instructor is nearby.

What health workers can do

- similar to STAGE 1, except that the health workers take more responsibility for the review, evaluation, and questioning of each other.

What instructor can do

- review the handling of the consultation: comment specifically on the strong and weak points, and what might have been done better
- encourage health workers to evaluate each other's handling of the consultation and to review each other's records for clarity, accuracy, and completeness

STAGE 4:

(about
1-2 weeks)

Students completely in charge;

instructor absent, but on call.

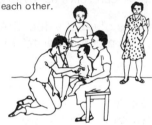

What health workers and instructor can do

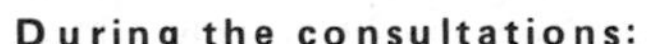

During the consultations:

Similar to STAGE 3. This time, however, the instructor is not only silent, but absent, although on call when needed. In this way, by the end of the training period the clinical consultation is quite similar to the actual situation of a health worker at work in his village or community. He assumes much of the same responsibility. Although the instructor is on call if needed, by the end of the course the decision making is completely up to the health worker trainee.

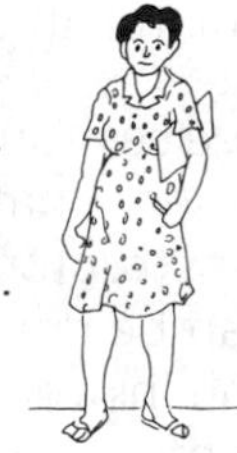

After the consultations:

After the consultation is completed, the instructor can review the record sheets and discuss them with the health workers. This, too, is similar to what will happen when the instructor (or 'supervisor') visits the health workers' villages to help them review their records and 'trouble shoot' problems.

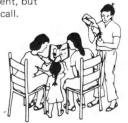

*Timing suggestions are for a two-month course.

ADAPTING CLASSWORK TO PROBLEMS SEEN IN THE CLINIC OR HOME

If the course plan is flexible, instructors can schedule classes about specific illnesses or problems that students have just seen in the clinic or community.

Suppose that one day a badly burned child is seen by the students in the clinic. If class discussion that same day covers burns (their causes, prevention, and treatment), the students are likely to take great interest. Then follow this with more classes on burns, as well as follow-up care and home visits to the burned child, until he is completely well.

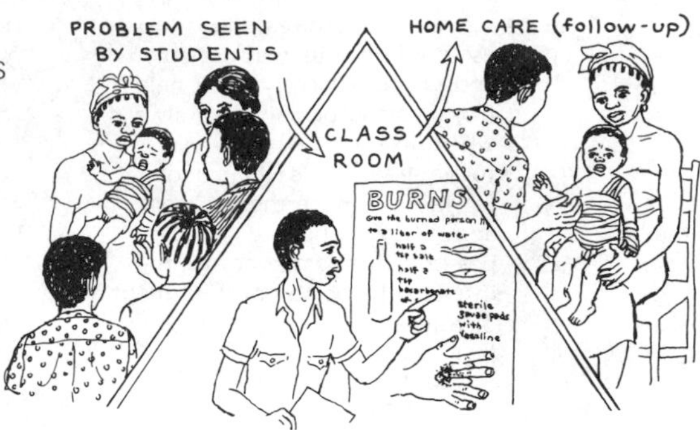

Students learn better when classes relate to problems they have just faced in real life. Such unplanned classes can cover the subject matter for the first time. Or if the subject has already been covered, they can serve as review.

This kind of flexibility in scheduling classes is of great value. But it can create difficulties with planning and coordination. It is much easier to do with a small learning group at the village level.

FOLLOWING THE CLINICAL CONSULTATION

In order to take full advantage of the consultation as a learning experience and still keep classes more or less on schedule, a special period can be planned for discussing problems seen in clinical practice. Some programs allow a half hour or an hour for this each day, immediately after the consultations.

In these sessions, students describe to the rest of the group a problem they have just seen that day in clinical practice. They review the consultation process and the instructor helps emphasize the most important points to be learned. This review can be done mostly in the form of questions and answers. In the early stages, the instructors may take the lead. Later in the course they can encourage the students to summarize what they have learned and to question and evaluate each other.

Remember the importance of clinical skills:

The confidence that villagers have in their health worker depends greatly on his ability to treat their most common and serious illnesses. For this reason it is essential that the training course provide a solid base for curative skills and clinical experience. With this training, and good support from the program and the community, the health worker can help his people meet their felt needs for curative care. Then he will be more able to help people recognize the underlying causes of ill health and work toward effective prevention.

CHAPTER 9

Examinations and Evaluation as a Learning Process

TESTS AND EXAMS

The purpose of tests and exams needs to be carefully reconsidered.

In the typical school, exams provide a way for the teacher to judge (to 'pass' or 'fail') the students. Yet students are given little opportunity to criticize the teacher. The teacher is on top, the students on the bottom—especially at exam time!

Also, the use of number or letter grades for exams encourages competition rather than cooperation. Students who get high marks are usually praised and moved ahead. Those who fail are punished or left behind.

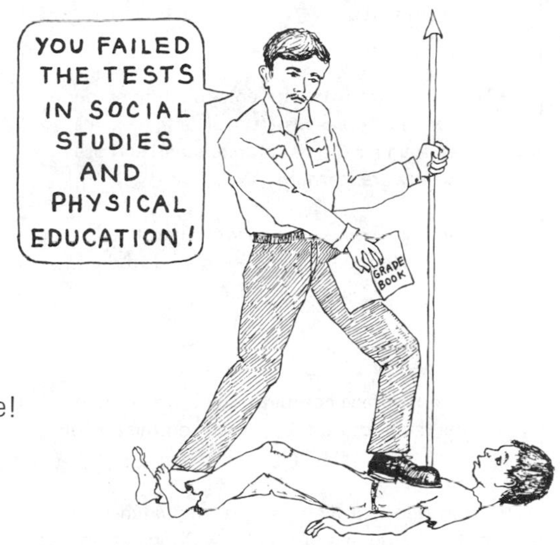
YOU FAILED THE TESTS IN SOCIAL STUDIES AND PHYSICAL EDUCATION!
GRADE BOOK

In education that resists change, tests and exams make it clearer than ever that the teacher has power over the student.

In 'education for change', tests and exams serve a different purpose: to find out how effectively the instructors are teaching. The exams let everyone know what subjects have been covered well and which need more review, or a different approach.

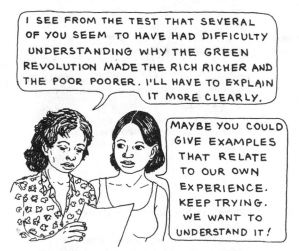

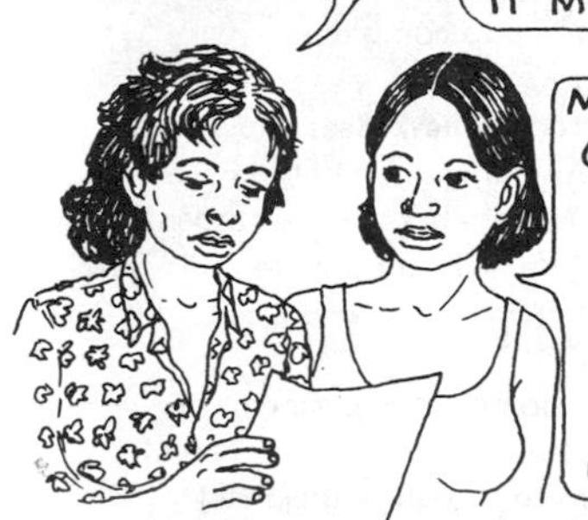
I SEE FROM THE TEST THAT SEVERAL OF YOU SEEM TO HAVE HAD DIFFICULTY UNDERSTANDING WHY THE GREEN REVOLUTION MADE THE RICH RICHER AND THE POOR POORER. I'LL HAVE TO EXPLAIN IT MORE CLEARLY.
MAYBE YOU COULD GIVE EXAMPLES THAT RELATE TO OUR OWN EXPERIENCE. KEEP TRYING. WE WANT TO UNDERSTAND IT!

In education for change, tests are a way of finding out how well both teachers and students are doing. They help teacher and student feel more equal.

Also, in education for change it is the responsibility of the entire group—instructors and students—to make sure that those who learn slowly get the help they need. The quicker students become teaching assistants, helping to explain things to those who are slower. Then, if a slow learner does not do well on a test, the quick learner and the teacher share in the 'failure'. Praise is given when everybody does well.

This approach helps keep quick learners from getting bored, and slow learners from falling behind. The quick students learn not only the material studied, but how to teach it.

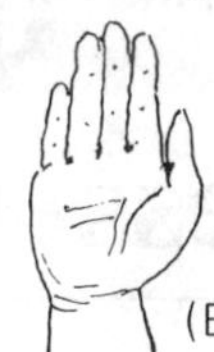

The Function of Tests and Exams in Two Different Approaches to Teaching Health Workers

Conventional Schooling (Education that resists change)	**People-centered Learning** (Education for change)
• Tests and exams serve mainly to help teachers judge students.	• Tests and exams serve to let both instructor and students know how well the instructor is teaching.
• Tests may motivate students to study harder, but for faulty reasons—fear of failing exams rather than eagerness to understand and use what they are learning.	• Tests motivate students by helping them find out what they need to learn in order to serve their people better.
• A grading or pass-fail system is used that compares 'good students' with 'bad students'.	• No grades. No pass or fail. If any student who wants to learn falls behind, this reflects the failure of the group, not the individual, because quick learners are expected to help teach slow learners.
• Tests encourage **competition** between students (some come out on top, others on the bottom).	• Tests encourage **cooperation and sharing** (everyone helps each other come through together).
• Atmosphere of distrust. Teacher watches or 'polices' students during tests. Cooperation between students during tests is called 'cheating'.	• Atmosphere of trust. Teacher may leave room during tests. 'Cheating' makes little sense because the main purpose of tests is to help the instructor teach better and be sure that everyone understands the material. The teacher or other students may assist those who have trouble understanding the questions.
• Strong emphasis on **memorizing.** Students usually are forbidden to use notes or open books during exams.	• Strong emphasis on **understanding.** Notes or books may be used during most exams. Since exams test how well students can apply their learning in real-life situations, the use of books and other available resources is encouraged.
• Tests reward those students who learn to **repeat** like parrots.	• Test questions are designed to help the students **think**—not simply repeat.
• Strict time limit for tests. Slower students fail questions they do not have time to answer.	• No strict time limit. Extra time is allowed after the test so slower readers can finish. Or they can take tests home to complete.
• Tests review only material and ideas already covered in class. **Nothing new.** So tests are usually boring.	• Tests try to introduce **new ideas** and understanding, building on material covered in class and the experiences of the students. Focus is on lifelike problem solving. This can make tests fun!
• All test questions have a right or wrong answer, not open to question by the students.	• Some questions do not have clear right or wrong answers, but ask for students' opinions. These help them to recognize unsolved problems, or to examine their own attitudes.
• Teacher usually corrects the tests.	• Students often correct each others' tests during a group discussion.

THE IMPORTANCE OF OPEN-BOOK EXAMS

There are good reasons to **encourage students to use their books and notes during exams:**

Open-book tests place value on looking things up when in doubt, rather than trying to rely purely on memory. In this way, classroom tests can help health workers develop a careful approach to looking for answers to problems in their communities.

When a health worker is attending a sick person, he may think he remembers all the signs and symptoms and the correct medication. But if he has the slightest doubt, it is safer to look things up. During training programs, we have often seen slower students answer test questions more correctly than quicker students. Why? Because they did not try to rely on their memories. They looked things up!

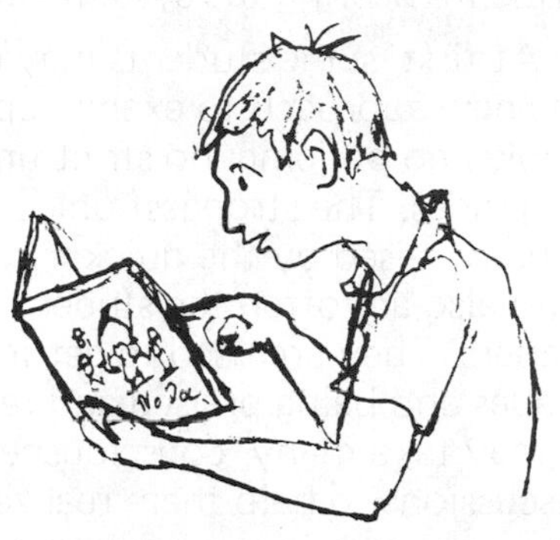

The best student and health worker is not the one who has the best memory. He is the one who takes the time to look things up.

Encouraging students to use their books during exams will help them to use their books openly with sick persons and their families. They will be less tempted to pretend they know it all. This results in fewer mistakes and better health education, and helps take some of the magic out of modern medicine.

TEST QUESTIONS THAT PREPARE STUDENTS FOR PROBLEM SOLVING IN THE COMMUNITY:

Yet another advantage to open-book exams is that they encourage teachers to think of more creative, problem-oriented questions. Questions that call for a good memory, but no thinking, become pointless if students can simply copy the answers from their books. So instructors have to think of questions that **test the students' ability to use what they have learned.**

TWO SORTS OF EXAM QUESTIONS

LESS APPROPRIATE:

What are the common signs of anemia?

MORE APPROPRIATE:

A pregnant woman complains of weakness.
She breathes very hard when she walks uphill.
What might be her problem?
What other signs would you look for?
What questions would you ask?

The second question tests the students' abilities both to apply their knowledge and to use their books. It takes them one step closer to being able to solve real problems they will meet as health workers.

HELPING STUDENTS UNDERSTAND THE NEW APPROACH TO TESTS AND EXAMS

From their previous school experience, most student health workers have very fixed ideas about tests and exams. Those who are most clever often insist on being given tests and grades. Those who are slower may be ashamed to admit their fear of exams. Those who are most honest or independent may even learn to take pride in 'beating the system'—by cheating!

At first, some students may object to the new approach to exams: open books, no policing, no strict time limit, no grades. The strongest objections are usually raised by the quicker students, who also are often the student opinion leaders. They are used to getting top grades and being praised and rewarded. It may take many 'consciousness-raising' discussions to help them realize that a new approach is needed—one that does not always favor the strong.

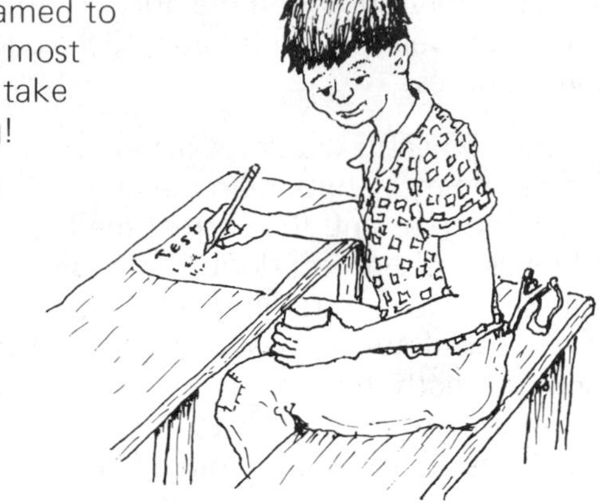

In an attempt to 'beat the system', those who are most honest often learn to cheat!

Some students, out of habit, may still try to cheat, even though cheating no longer serves an obvious purpose. Help them discover that, **instead of trying to 'beat the system' by cheating within it, it makes more sense to work together to change it!**

WHO PREPARES THE EXAMS—AND WHEN?

In some training programs, each instructor gives exams on the material he or she has covered. In others, joint or coordinated exams are given.

Project Piaxtla in Mexico gives a test each week, usually on Friday morning. The test combines and tries to interrelate the different subjects taught during the week. The test is designed to take about one hour, but a second hour of free time is allowed for those who need it.

Each week an instructor is chosen to organize and mimeograph the test. The other instructors prepare questions and give them to him by Thursday afternoon.

The instructors are asked not to wait until the last minute (or day) to prepare their test questions. They are encouraged to write them down **right after class,** when details and points needing reinforcing are fresh in their minds. To help ensure that this gets done, the students are involved in helping prepare their own tests. At the end of each class, **each student is asked to write one question to possibly appear on the Friday test.**

By helping to prepare their own test questions, the students feel more on an equal level with their instructors. They also get a good exercise in thinking about the importance and usefulness of what they study.

From the test questions written by the students, the instructors pick the best ones for the Friday test. They may improve the wording, or add questions of their own.

The instructor coordinating the exam tries to include some problem-solving questions that combine ideas from different classes. For example, if during the week the group has studied eye problems, skin problems, and child nutrition, a test question might be:

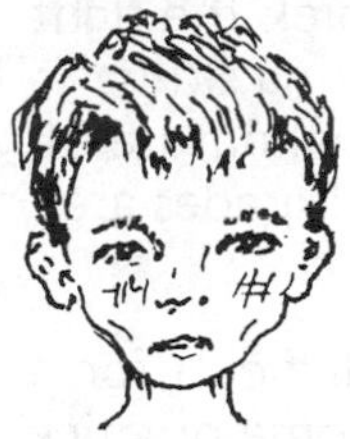

A mother brings a 3-year-old boy whose eyes look dull and dry, with little wrinkles. He also has dry, cracking skin on his cheeks, arms, and legs. What problems would you suspect? What advice would you give?

GUIDELINES FOR PREPARING APPROPRIATE TEST QUESTIONS

Try to ask questions that . . .

- **make people think**
- **present a problem-solving situation** similar to ones health workers may encounter in their villages
- **deal with priority needs**
- **are stated clearly and simply** (not confusingly)
- can be answered in relatively few words (especially important when some students are slow writers)
- **test and strengthen skills** rather than just testing memory
- cannot be answered by simply copying from the book
- do not simply review information already covered, but help health workers form new ideas or gain practical experience

WHAT STYLE OF TEST QUESTIONS TO USE

Test questions can be asked and answered in a number of ways:

Type of question	Type of answer	Examples
1 **Open-ended** Student writes the answer in his or her own words.	A **Long written answer,** or essay—in which the student may analyze or describe a problem, situation, or method.	*Describe in detail what you would do if a mother brought you her 2-year-old child, hot with fever, all wrapped up in a blanket?*
	B **Brief written answer**—one or more words, a sentence, or a short list.	*Mention 3 things you would do right away if a mother brought you a feverish child wrapped in a blanket.*
2 **Closed** Student picks the right answer from choices listed on the answer sheet.	A **True or false**—a statement is given, and the student identifies it as either right or wrong.	*A baby with high fever should be wrapped in a blanket so she will sweat.* *True or False*
	B **Multiple choice**—4 or 5 possible answers are given, and the student is asked to mark one of them.	*A child with high fever should . . .* *a) be cooled so fast that she shivers.* *b) be wrapped up so she does not get cold.* *c) eat nothing until the fever drops.* *d) be cooled by removing her clothing and placing wet cloths on her body.*

Each of these types of question has advantages and disadvantages. Which is most appropriate for your student group?

Open-ended questions (1A and 1B) usually require more thinking and organizing ability than questions that simply have the student pick the right answer. But they may be difficult for students with limited writing skills, especially if they call for longer, essay-type answers. The personal nature of the essay question also makes it more difficult to grade fairly (if grades are given).

Open-ended questions that require short answers (1B) are less difficult for slow or inexperienced writers. Yet they provide students with some practice in writing and expressing themselves. Also, because they take less time to answer, more questions can be asked and the test can cover more subject matter. This kind of question is often easier for students to understand than multiple choice questions, which take time to get used to and may prove confusing.

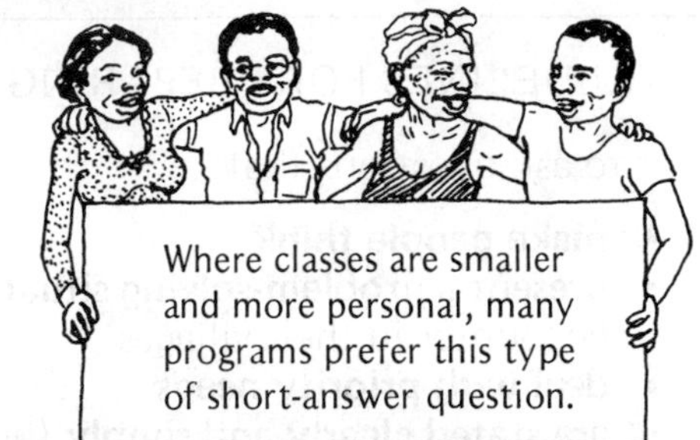

Where classes are smaller and more personal, many programs prefer this type of short-answer question.

True or False questions (2A) are usually easy for students to understand. But they invite guessing at answers—which is not the best approach to solving health problems! True or False questions must be very carefully designed if they are to test students' problem-solving abilities, and not just their memories or guessing skills.

Multiple choice questions (2B), if well designed, are better for testing people's problem-solving and thinking skills. They do not allow as much guessing as True or False questions. But because each question lists 4 or 5 choices, they put slow readers at a disadvantage.

For instructors, also, there are both advantages and disadvantages. Multiple choice tests can be corrected easily and quickly by anyone with a 'master sheet', so they are especially useful when you have a large group of students. However, good multiple choice questions take considerable skill and time to prepare. Also, the longer questions require more paper and stencils. (For sample questions and more ideas about preparing multiple choice tests, see ***Primary Child Care, Book Two,*** by Maurice King, available from TALC.)

The style of question you choose will depend on several considerations, including the size of the group, who will be correcting the papers, and how much formal education the students have had.

Many small, community-based programs prefer questions requiring brief written answers. Large programs often prefer the closed-type questions that permit easy, objective grading and give a sense of statistical control.

In truth, some types of questions lend themselves to certain subjects more than others. For the sake of variety, you might try using a combination of the different styles. This can make a test more interesting. But take care that switching from one form of question to another does not confuse the students.

Trick questions. Life is full of surprises that make us stop and think. Tests can have surprises, too. Trick questions on tests (or in class) sometimes make students angry—but they are also fun! They trap students into looking at important things in new ways. For example:

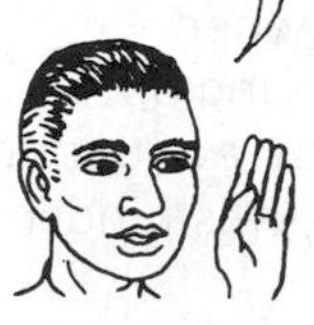
YOU SHOULD NEVER GIVE A PERSON MEDICINE UNLESS YOU ARE ABSOLUTELY SURE WHAT HIS ILLNESS IS. TRUE OR FALSE?
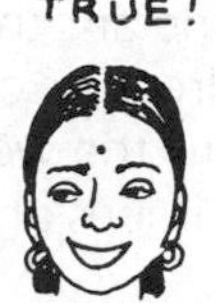
TRUE!
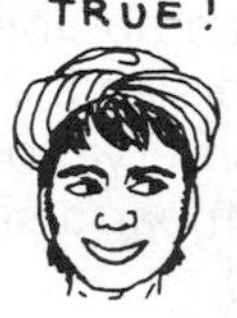
TRUE!
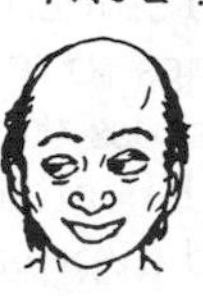
TRUE!
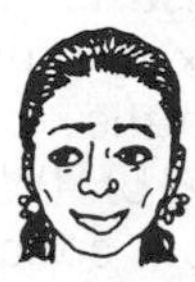
TRUE!
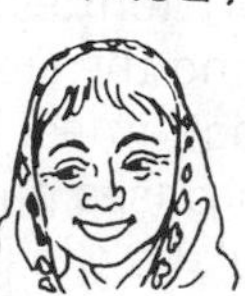
TRUE!

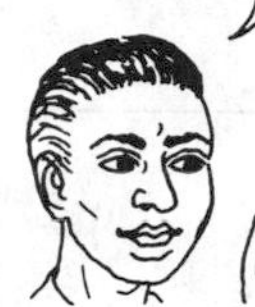
NO! THE STATEMENT IS FALSE! TO BE ABSOLUTELY SURE IS TO CLOSE OUR MINDS TO POSSIBLE ERROR. A HEALTH WORKER SHOULD NEVER BE ABSOLUTELY SURE OF HER DIAGNOSIS. SHE SHOULD ALWAYS KEEP A CERTAIN AMOUNT OF DOUBT, AND BE OPEN TO ANY SIGN THAT SHE MIGHT BE MISTAKEN... REMEMBER OUR CLASS ON SCIENTIFIC METHOD?
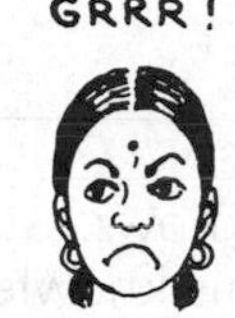
GRRR!
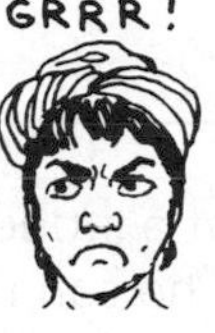
GRRR!
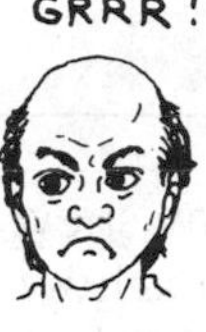
GRRR!
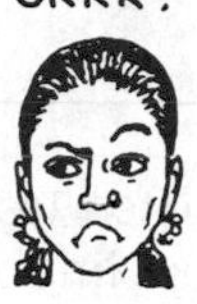
GRRR!
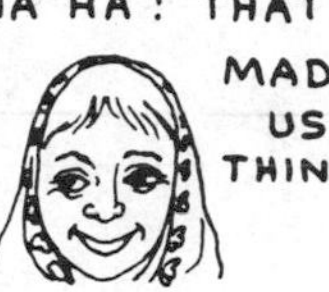
HA HA! THAT MADE US THINK!

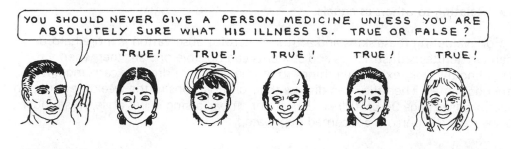

THINGS THAT CANNOT BE MEASURED IN WRITTEN TESTS

Both instructors and students need to find out how well they are helping prepare each other to do their jobs better. Written tests provide some idea about what knowledge students have mastered.

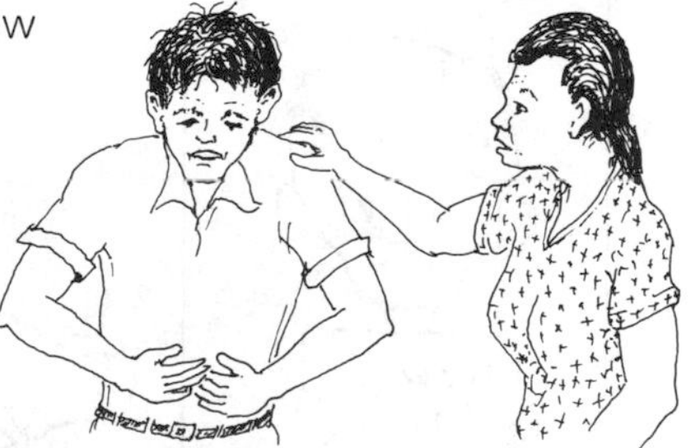

However, many of the skills and attitudes needed for community work cannot be easily evaluated through written tests. These include:

- **Manual skills (skills using the hands)** such as giving an injection, cleaning a wound, or casting a cement platform for a latrine.
- **Communication skills** such as giving preventive advice in a consultation, leading nutrition classes for mothers, or working with children on CHILD-to-child activities.
- **Leadership and organizational skills** such as planning and getting people to work on a community garden or water system.
- **Thinking and problem-solving skills** needed to deal with unexpected difficulties. (For example, what do you do when a mother refuses to take her gravely ill child to the hospital? What do you do when a person asks you to inject a medicine prescribed by a doctor, and you know the medicine is not needed and may cause harm?)

- **Attitudes toward people in need.** (Does the student feel respect, kindness, and concern for sick persons, old persons, women, children, and very poor persons? Is he eager to share his knowledge, or does he like to make people think he has mysterious healing powers?)

- **Relating to others as equals.**

For evaluating these skills and attitudes, careful observation is more helpful than written tests. Instructors and students can observe one another when attending the sick, explaining things to mothers and children, or carrying out other activities. Then they can discuss their observations in the weekly evaluation meetings (see page **9**-15). (When delicate or embarrassing issues arise, it is kinder to speak to the persons concerned in private.)

It is important that each health worker develop an attitude of self-criticism, as well as an ability to accept friendly criticism from others. These can be developed through evaluation sessions, private discussions, and awareness-raising dialogues (see Ch. 26). In the long run, the development of an open, questioning attitude can contribute more to a health worker's success than all his preventive and curative abilities put together.

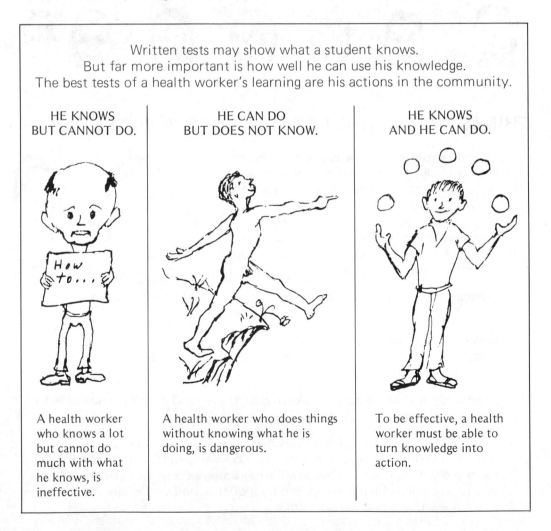

Written tests may show what a student knows.
But far more important is how well he can use his knowledge.
The best tests of a health worker's learning are his actions in the community.

HE KNOWS BUT CANNOT DO.

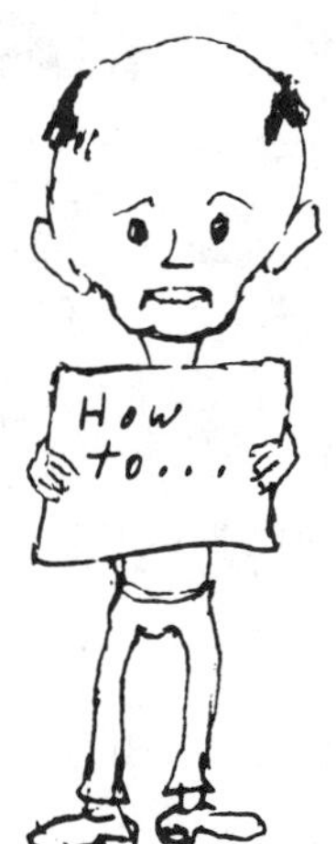

A health worker who knows a lot but cannot do much with what he knows, is ineffective.

HE CAN DO BUT DOES NOT KNOW.

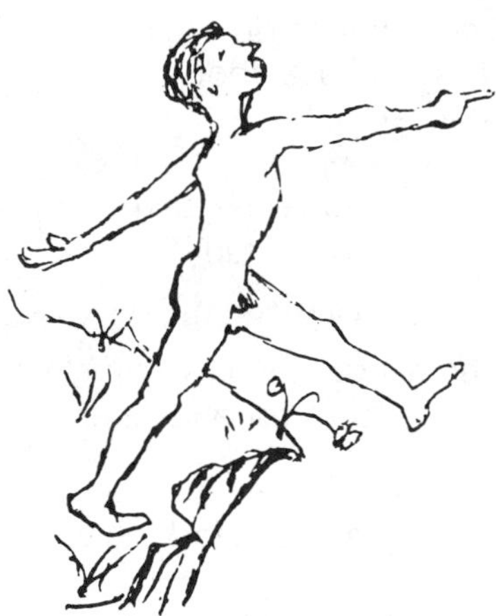

A health worker who does things without knowing what he is doing, is dangerous.

HE KNOWS AND HE CAN DO.

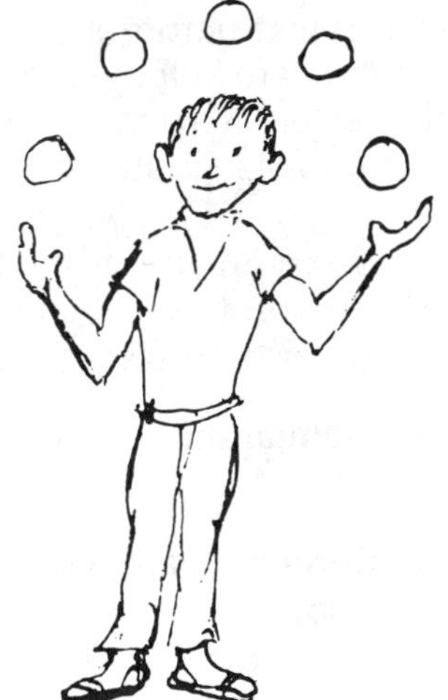

To be effective, a health worker must be able to turn knowledge into action.

SELF-TESTING BY STUDENTS AND HEALTH WORKERS

Learning is, or should be, a continual process—not just something that begins and ends in a training course. To work effectively, health workers need to keep studying and learning on their own once the course is over. So it helps if they gain experience in **independent study** and **self-testing** during their training. They also need to know **how and where to get the books and tools** for continued independent study.

Programmed learning

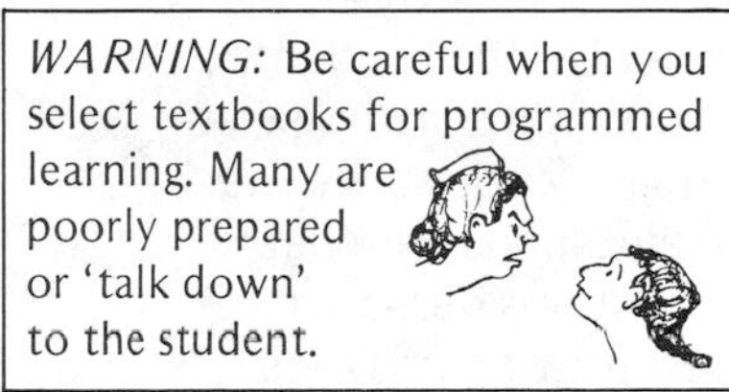

WARNING: Be careful when you select textbooks for programmed learning. Many are poorly prepared or 'talk down' to the student.

One approach to independent study is called programmed learning. Special books take the student step by step through the subject matter. They ask questions to let the student know how well he or she has learned or understood the material. The books are designed so that students can test themselves before looking at the answers.

Answers may be located at the edge of the page. The student can cover them with a strip of cardboard or paper until he has answered the questions (in his mind or in writing). Then he lowers the strip to check the answers. If he has answered right, he goes ahead to a new section. If he answered wrong, he is guided through a review until he can answer correctly. In this way, each person moves ahead at his own pace.

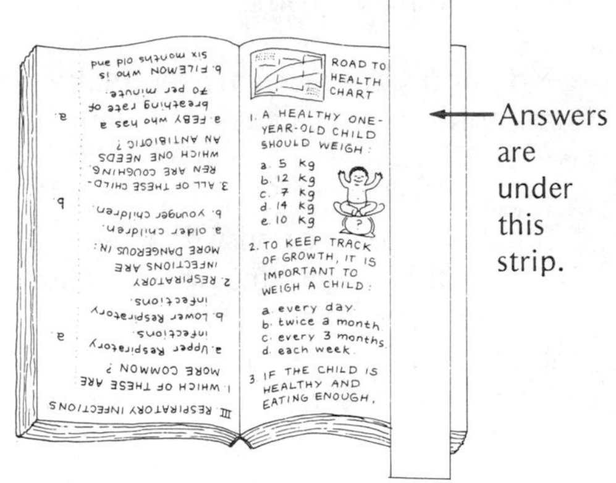

Separate learning guides

Some books on health care, although not written for programmed learning, have accompanying 'learning guides' to help students with independent study and self-testing.

An outstanding example is the learning guide to be used with Maurice King's handbook, ***Primary Child Care.**** Carefully designed test questions have been prepared for use with each part of the book. Most of these multiple choice questions present the subject matter in lifelike, problem-solving situations.

Magic answer sheets: To help health workers with self-testing, Maurice has designed an answer sheet that corrects itself! A simple kit contains the equipment needed for preparing these sheets. It includes a stencil for mimeographing answer sheets, a plastic overlay with holes that line up with the right answers, and 2 packets of chemicals.

---

*The ***Handbook (Book One),*** the ***Teaching Guide (Book Two),*** and an answer sheet kit are available through TALC (see p. **Back**-3).

One chemical (phenolphthalein) is dissolved in alcohol and applied to the answer sheet through the holes in the plastic overlay. The other chemical is baking soda (sodium bicarbonate) with brown dye. It is used by the student, who dips a damp swab into it and marks the treated answer sheet. Right answers turn red. Wrong answers stay brown.

MATERIALS FOR MAKING SELF-CORRECTING MULTIPLE CHOICE QUESTIONS

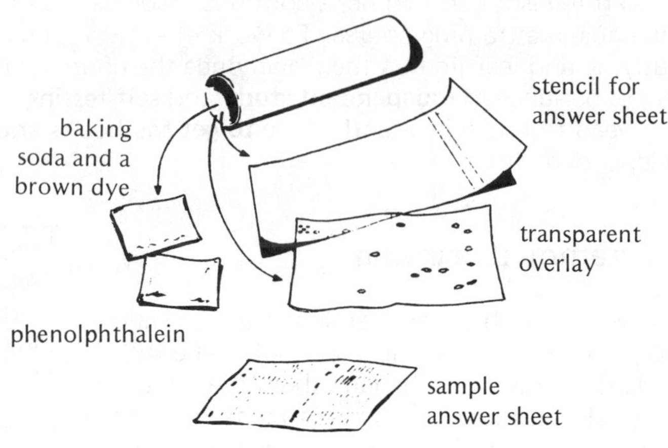

This way, the student knows at once if he has answered correctly. It turns self-testing into a game!

You and your students can make your own self-correcting answer sheets. Phenolphthalein is usually available at laboratory supply centers, and is low in cost.

Small numbers of answer sheets can be individually treated in advance, although this takes time. If you want to prepare a large number of multiple choice answer sheets in a short time, prepare a plastic master sheet. It can be made from an old X-ray film. First soak the film for a day in water with lye, caustic soda, or wood ashes. Then wipe off the dark coating. Next . . .

Place the plastic master sheet over an answer sheet that has the right answers marked. Put a dot of ink over each right answer.

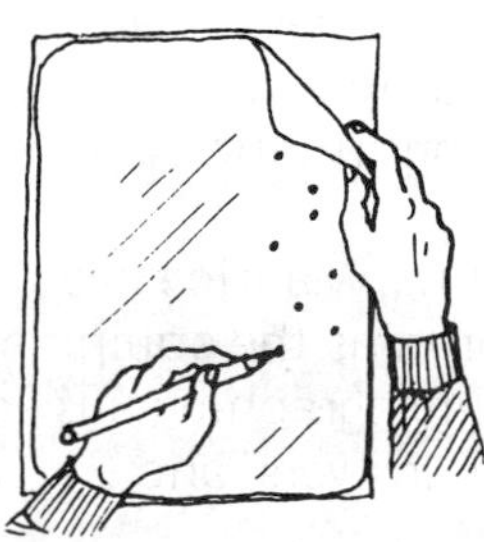

Punch out the ink dots with a leather or paper punch. Now you are ready to mark the right answers with the 'magic' ink.

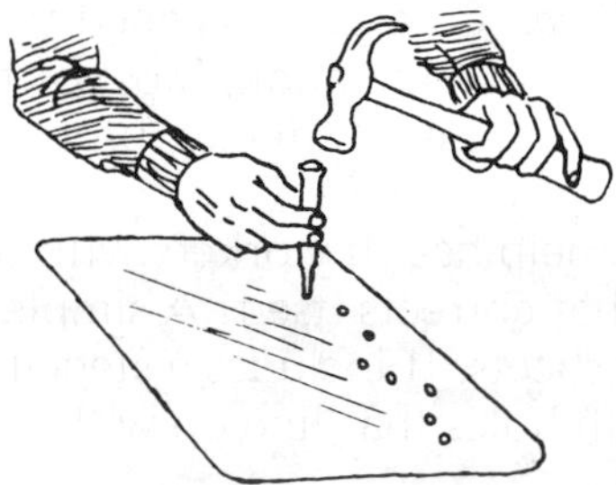

Put the plastic master sheet over each answer sheet. Moisten a cloth with phenolphthalein dissolved in alcohol, and dab it over the punched holes to mark the sheet underneath.

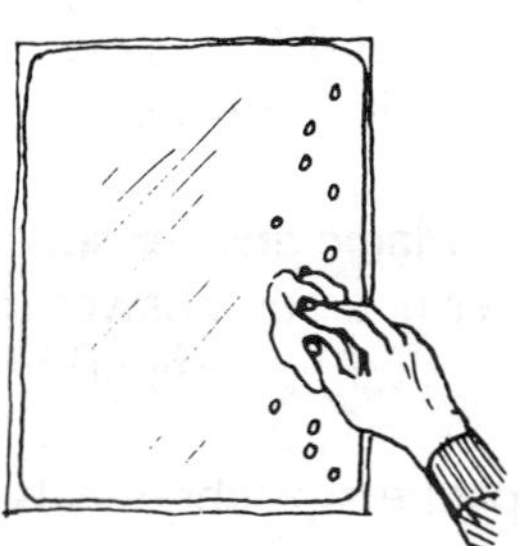

Your 'magic answer sheets' are now ready for students to use. They will help make self-testing fun!

EVALUATION:

Finding out how effective your program is

Evaluation is the process of finding out how well things are being done. It tries to answer the questions:

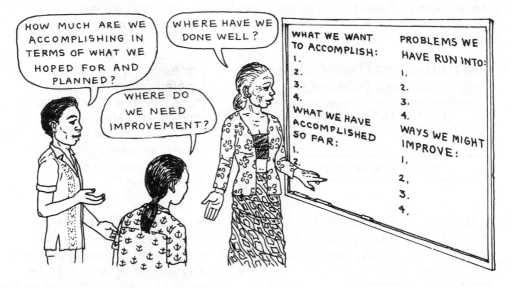

Evaluation of training programs has been approached in many ways, and for many purposes. Some approaches help to increase the understanding, sense of equality, and shared respect of all concerned. Other approaches tend to reduce groups of persons to being the 'objects' of studies largely outside their control—studies through which they are judged, but may not openly judge in return.

EVALUATION—FOR WHOM AND BY WHOM?

Evaluations run by outsiders: Sometimes an evaluation of a training program is requested by a funding agency or by program administrators in a distant city. The design for such an evaluation usually comes from the outside. Or an 'expert' is sent in to conduct it. Too often, both the process and results serve the needs of those requesting the evaluation more than the needs of those actually involved in the program. This kind of top-down evaluation is not our concern in this book.

Note: Sometimes help with evaluations from persons outside the program is beneficial—as long as they understand the local situation, assist only where asked, and do not take charge.

Evaluations run by participants: Some community-based programs are recognizing the importance of having **all** those involved with the program take part in a continual evaluation process. In this way, evaluation becomes a cooperative effort of self-criticism and reflection. It not only considers the results of community-based education and action, it is a part of the process.

The rest of this chapter is about this second kind of evaluation.

EVALUATION AS AN INFORMAL, ONGOING GROUP PROCESS

Many people think of evaluation as a complicated study conducted during a limited time. But the most important evaluation is simple, friendly, and continuous. It happens whenever persons involved in an activity discuss how things are going. However, periodic and more structured evaluation also has a place. In terms of timing, we can consider 4 types of evaluation, all of which are parts of an ongoing process:

1. **CONTINUAL EVALUATION** takes place throughout a project or activity.

CONTINUAL EVALUATION

PROJECT OR ACTIVITY

For example, throughout a training course, instructors and students can ask themselves or each other: "How effective is this class?" "How well does this activity prepare us to solve an urgent problem in our communities?"

2. **PERIODIC EVALUATION** takes place at certain times during a project or activity (once a week, once a month, once a year).

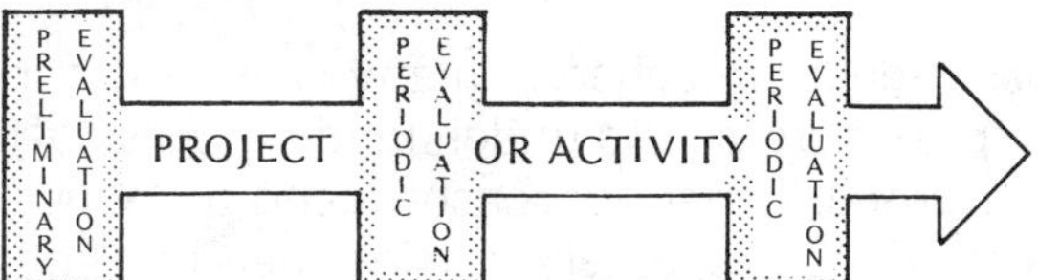

Instructors, students, and concerned members of the community can get together every so often to look at the overall progress of the course and of particular activities. In a one-month course this could be done once a week.

3. **FINAL EVALUATION** takes place at the end of a project or activity, before the next one begins.

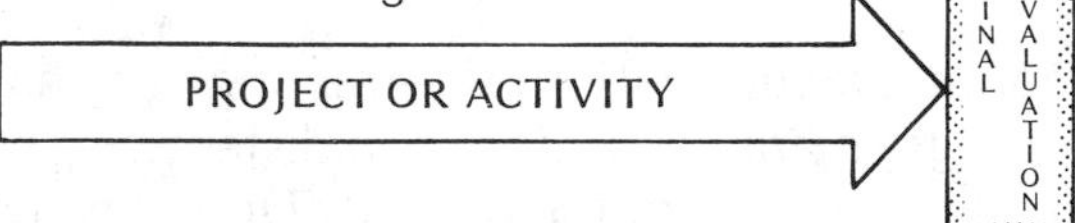

At the end of a course, everyone involved can join together to evaluate the course as a whole. They can discuss strengths and weaknesses, and how it might be improved the next time.

4. **FOLLOW-UP EVALUATION** is based on the results or effect of an activity after it has been completed.

The true effectiveness of a training course is determined by how successful the health workers are at helping people meet their needs in the community. The effect or 'impact' on the community is not easy to evaluate.

You can base it on:

- response of the community
- follow-up visits by the instructors
- health indicators (see p. **6**-10)
- reports or 'feedback' from the health workers about their accomplishments and difficulties

EVALUATION DURING TRAINING AS A TWO-WAY PROCESS

As we mentioned in the section on tests and exams, in the typical school evaluation is usually a one-way process. The teacher judges; the students are judged—the weakest most severely. This top-down approach is based on the convention that the strong may pass judgement on the weak, but that the weak have no right to criticize the strong.

Top-down evaluation favors the strong and resists change.

Another kind of evaluation is one that goes both ways. Instructors and students all take part in evaluating each other and the program. This helps prepare health workers to work with people, not as bosses or authorities, but as equals.

If health workers are to help people work toward social change, evaluation during training needs to be encouraged in all directions, not just one.

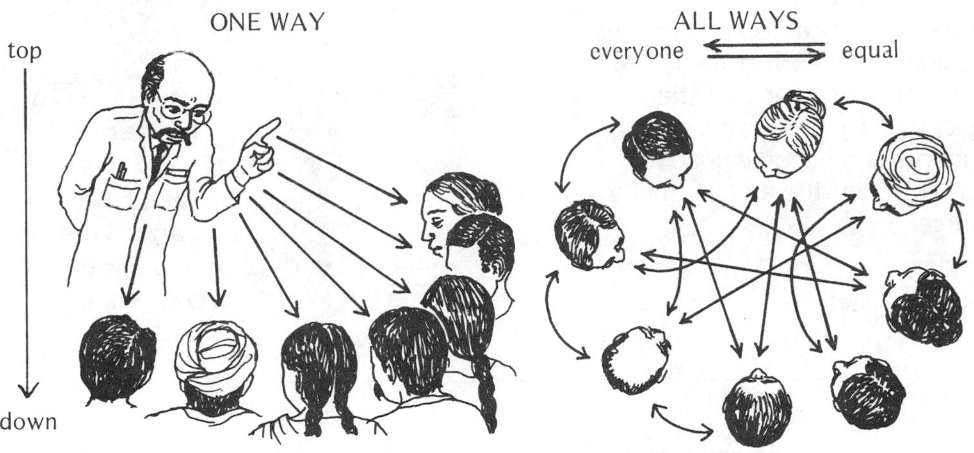

Teacher tests and evaluates students (but not the other way around).

Teacher and students evaluate each other, and the course.

Which of these approaches does your training program take? Which one better prepares health workers to help the poor meet their needs? Why is it important to discuss these questions with health workers during training?

ADVANTAGES TO INVOLVING STUDENTS IN THE EVALUATION PROCESS:

- Evaluation by students helps instructors learn how effective and appropriate their teaching is.
- Two-way evaluation helps instructors relate to student health workers as equals. Then the health workers will be likely to show the same respect for others when they teach people in their communities.
- Two-way evaluation helps everyone to question the accepted social norms or 'rules of the game' that keep the poor on the bottom. It helps people gain the confidence and courage to criticize authority and defend the interests of the weak.
- Taking part in evaluation during the course gives student health workers the practice and skill they will need for evaluating their work in their communities.

WAYS TO INCLUDE STUDENTS IN EVALUATION DURING TRAINING

(based on evaluation and self-testing methods used in Project Piaxtla, Mexico and in the Women's Health Promoter program in Olancho, Honduras)

1. **Short evaluation discussions at the end of each class.** These can happen in both of the following ways:

Instructor asks students to comment on how they liked the class, what they learned, and how it might have been better.

At first it may be hard for students to speak up and criticize the instructor. But if the instructor makes it very clear that she welcomes friendly criticism, students can become good evaluators by the end of the course.

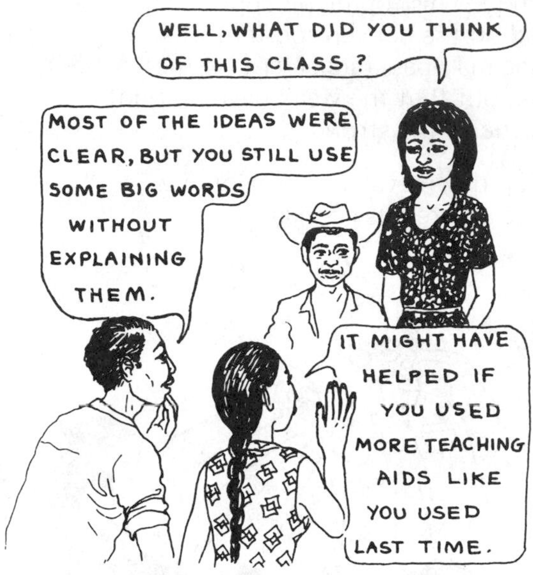
WELL, WHAT DID YOU THINK OF THIS CLASS ?
MOST OF THE IDEAS WERE CLEAR, BUT YOU STILL USE SOME BIG WORDS WITHOUT EXPLAINING THEM.
IT MIGHT HAVE HELPED IF YOU USED MORE TEACHING AIDS LIKE YOU USED LAST TIME.

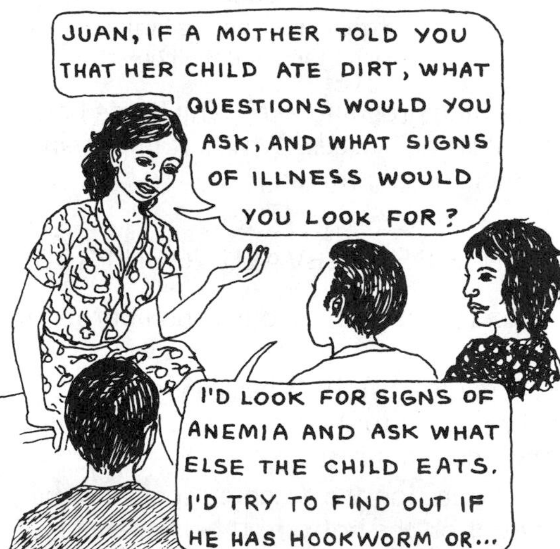
JUAN, IF A MOTHER TOLD YOU THAT HER CHILD ATE DIRT, WHAT QUESTIONS WOULD YOU ASK, AND WHAT SIGNS OF ILLNESS WOULD YOU LOOK FOR ?
I'D LOOK FOR SIGNS OF ANEMIA AND ASK WHAT ELSE THE CHILD EATS. I'D TRY TO FIND OUT IF HE HAS HOOKWORM OR...

Students test themselves by asking each other about what they have learned. They try to ask questions that relate their learning to real situations, questions that make each other think.

The main purpose of this kind of questioning is to see how well everyone can understand and apply what was covered in class. In this way the students help the instructor learn how effective her teaching was. She finds out where she needs to make things clearer, or to teach the material differently.

At first students may find it difficult to think of good questions, but with helpful suggestions, many will become quite skillful at this by the end of the course.

2. **A rotating evaluation committee.** Students can take turns forming an evaluation committee to help make known the ideas and reactions of both students and instructors. A new committee can be formed every week or two, so that everyone gets some experience in evaluating.

The responsibilities of the committee can be decided by the group. They might include:

- Observe classes and comment on their strengths, weaknesses, and ways they might be improved. (See list of questions, page **9**-17.)
- Consider how well course content prepares students for their future work.
- Observe attitudes and actions, both helpful and harmful, of the students and teachers; recommend possible ways to improve.
- Plan and lead weekly all-group evaluation sessions.

3. **Weekly evaluation sessions.** These are attended by all students and staff, and, if possible, by members of the local community or health committee. The sessions can be coordinated by the student evaluation committee. This gives students a chance to learn organizing and leadership skills.

The sessions can cover evaluation of classes and activities, plus any concerns, complaints, problems, and outstanding events that come to mind.

DEVELOPING THE SKILL OF CONSTRUCTIVE CRITICISM:

In the evaluation sessions just described, both students and instructors will quickly discover how difficult it is for most people to accept criticism. But with a few suggestions, everyone can begin to learn ways of criticizing that are less likely to offend.

When offering criticism, be sure to comment on the good as well as the bad. And mention the good things first.

Try to praise 3 things a person does well each time you point out 1 thing he does wrong.

NEGATIVE CRITICISM

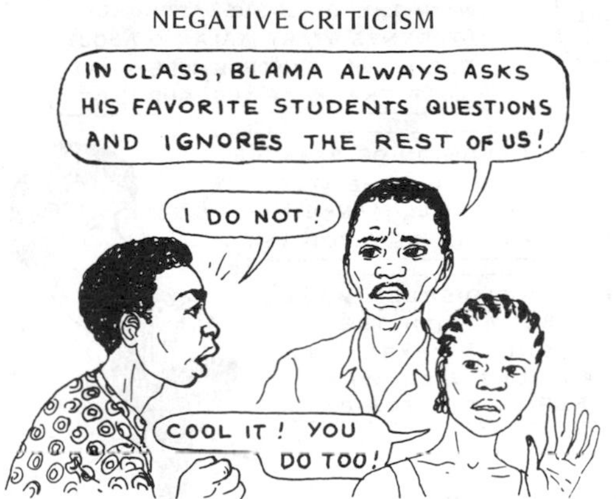
IN CLASS, BLAMA ALWAYS ASKS HIS FAVORITE STUDENTS QUESTIONS AND IGNORES THE REST OF US!
I DO NOT!
COOL IT! YOU DO TOO!

POSITIVE CRITICISM

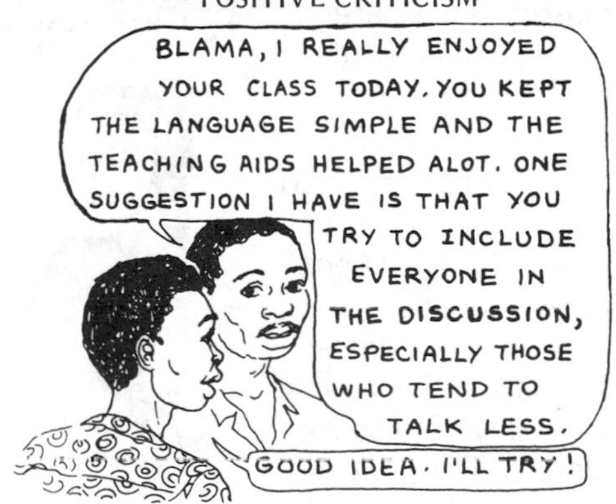
BLAMA, I REALLY ENJOYED YOUR CLASS TODAY. YOU KEPT THE LANGUAGE SIMPLE AND THE TEACHING AIDS HELPED ALOT. ONE SUGGESTION I HAVE IS THAT YOU TRY TO INCLUDE EVERYONE IN THE DISCUSSION, ESPECIALLY THOSE WHO TEND TO TALK LESS.
GOOD IDEA. I'LL TRY!

What 4 important differences can you find in these 2 examples?

INSTRUCTORS' SELF-EVALUATION AND GROUP EVALUATION

In addition to evaluation sessions with students, it is wise for instructors to do their own evaluation of classes and activities. Here are some possibilities:

Self-evaluation of classes. This is easier if you make a fairly complete class plan in advance, listing points to emphasize and the teaching methods you intend to use (see p. **5**-3). When the class is over, you can then see how well you covered each of these.

It helps to make a **checklist** (like the one on the next page) to be sure your evaluation covers each important aspect of teaching, such as:

- coverage of what was planned
- participation by all students
- use of teaching aids and appropriate methods
- relating material covered to students' experiences
- fairness and friendliness
- communicating clearly and simply
- review of important points
- final evaluation to find out what students learned and how they feel about the class

To make the evaluations more useful for you or anyone who may teach a similar class, **write down your suggestions for improving the class.** File them with the class plan. This takes extra time, but it helps the class to become better each time it is taught.

The silent observer. A 'training adviser' or another instructor sits at the back of the class, observes, and takes notes. If possible, the observer should have a copy of the class plan to see how much of the planned material is covered. She also may want to use a checklist such as the one on the next page. After the class, she and the instructor discuss the strengths and weaknesses of the class, and how it might be improved.

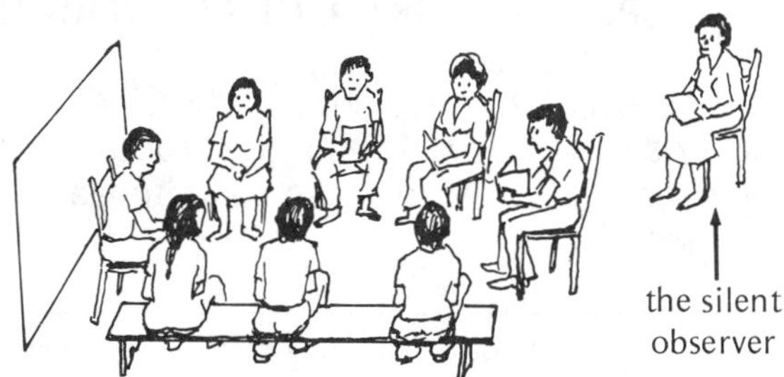
the silent observer

Daily evaluation sessions to discuss classes. These are especially helpful when the teaching team is not very experienced. Instead of discussing each class privately, the silent observers and instructors all meet for half an hour or so each day to discuss the classes. This way everyone benefits from the suggestions and criticisms.

I STILL HAVE TROUBLE COVERING THE MATERIAL I HAD PLANNED.
ME TOO! IT'S A PROBLEM WITH THE DIALOGUE APPROACH. STUDENTS START TALKING ABOUT THEIR OWN EXPERIENCES-- AND LOSE TRACK OF THE SUBJECT.
IT'S A QUESTION OF BALANCE BETWEEN LETTING THE STUDENTS TALK, AND STILL MANAGING TO COVER THE KEY POINTS.
WHY NOT DISCUSS YOUR PROBLEM WITH THE STUDENTS? MAYBE THEY CAN HELP EACH OTHER KEEP TO THE TOPIC.

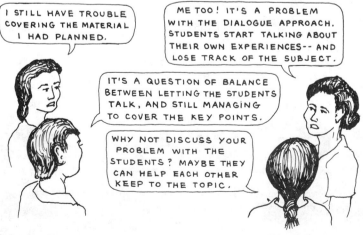

CHECKLIST FOR EVALUATING TEACHING*

Does the teacher:

1. Show enthusiasm?
2. Relate the subject to everyday life and the students' experience?
3. Encourage participation by asking questions and presenting problems?

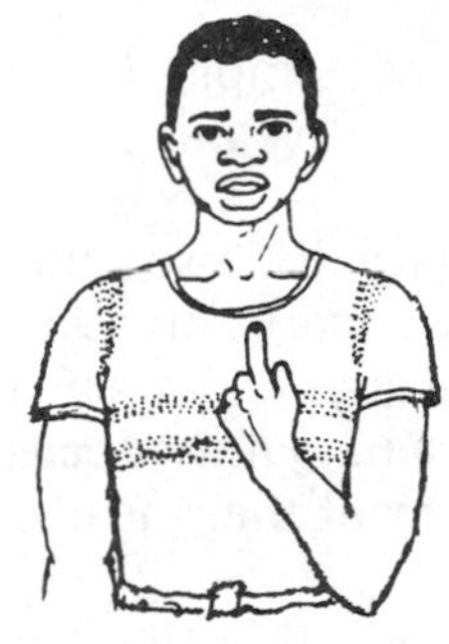

HOW WELL DOES THE WAY I TRAIN HEALTH WORKERS PREPARE THEM TO WORK WITH PERSONS IN A COMMUNITY-STRENGTHENING PEOPLE-CENTERED WAY?

4. Use imaginative teaching aids?
5. Speak and write clearly?
6. Use the vocabulary of the local people and avoid big words?
7. Match the teaching methods to the learning traditions of the local people?
8. Give examples or tell stories to illustrate ideas and new ways?
9. Encourage active learning?
10. Treat the students as friends and as equals?
11. Make sure the shyer students are given a chance to speak?
12. Make himself or herself available to students for discussion after class?
13. Provide enough time for study and review?
14. Avoid embarrassing the students?
15. Encourage quicker students to help those who have more difficulty?
16. Prepare teaching plans and materials in advance?
17. Know the subject adequately?
18. Encourage and respond positively to ideas and criticism from students?
19. Show honesty and openness?
20. Openly admit mistakes or lack of knowledge?
21. Respond to student errors with positive criticism and patience?
22. Provide plenty of opportunities for practical experience?
23. Emphasize how what they learn can be used in the students' future work?
24. Cover the material that was planned?
25. Emphasize and repeat the most important points?
26. Leave out what is not important or too detailed?
27. Evaluate whether students will be able to use their learning in real-life situations?
28. Show loyalty to students?
29. Show loyalty and respect for those whose needs are greatest?

---

*Adapted from a list developed during a training program for students of community health led by Fred Abbatt, author of ***Teaching for Better Learning.*** It is not a complete list. You may add to it or change it to suit the needs of your own situation. The list can be used for you to evaluate yourself, for your students to evaluate your teaching, or for you to evaluate the teaching of others.

OVERALL EVALUATION OF A TRAINING PROGRAM

RELATING EVALUATION TO NEEDS

To be useful, evaluation must be kept simple. It cannot cover every aspect of training in depth. On what, then, should evaluation focus?

In several places in this book we have discussed the problem of faulty training. Students may study hard and get good marks on tests. Yet, on return to their communities, they may find themselves at a loss when faced with real needs. To be meaningful, then, **evaluation of training must focus on how well health workers are prepared to help people meet their needs.**

From before a training course begins until after it is over, the planning and evaluation process should be based on recognizing and meeting people's needs.

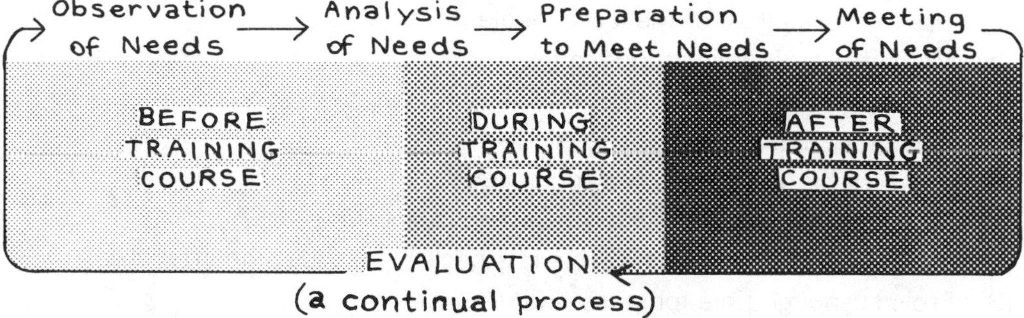

Evaluation of a training program—before, during, and after—is like a key section that completes a wheel.

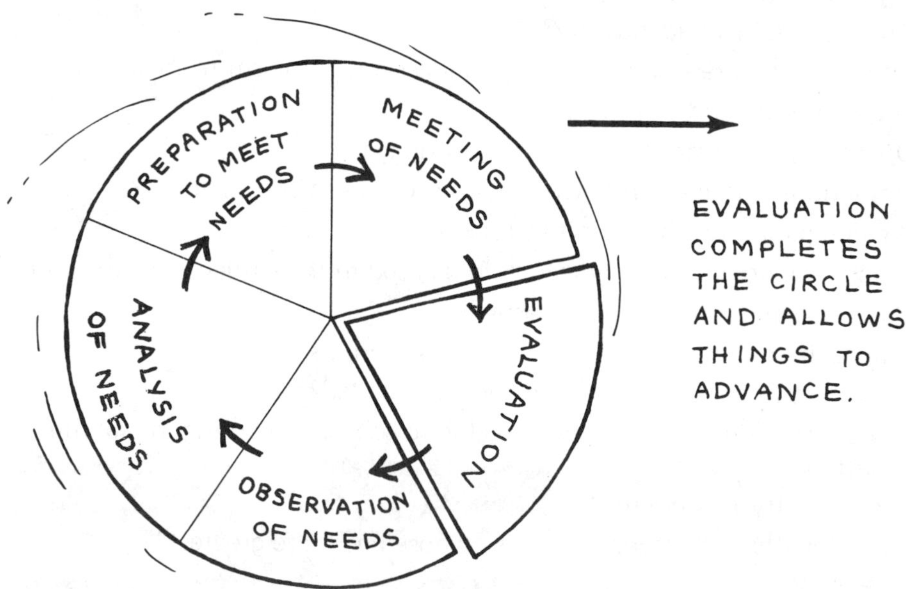

Evaluation is needed if we are to move forward, because it allows us to learn from our successes and mistakes.

SUGGESTED STAGES FOR OVERALL EVALUATION OF A TRAINING PROGRAM

BEFORE TRAINING COURSE

DURING TRAINING COURSE

AFTER TRAINING COURSE

OBSERVATION OF NEEDS & RESOURCES

Gather information about:

Needs and **Problems**
- Environment (physical and biological)
- Social (economic, cultural, political)
- Frequency of diseases, death, injustices
  - At local level
  - At national or regional level

Resources and **Strengths**
Within the community
Outside the community
Including:
- People
- Skills
- Traditions
- Education (formal and practical)
- Materials (animal vegetable, mineral)
- Leaders
- Possible instructors, advisers, health workers, etc.

Conflicts of interest
Between different groups, strong and weak
- Within the community
- Between the community and outside agents or institutions

ANALYSIS OF NEEDS & RESOURCES

Which needs are of greatest importance?
To whom? (local people, ministry, government, international agency)

Whose needs are greatest?
Why? (age, sex, income, race, location)
In what way do the environment and social order affect people's needs and health?

What are the biggest obstacles to resolving people's needs:
- within the community?
- within the country?
- within the government and health ministry?
- around the world?

In what ways might some of the resources (money, MD's, health authorities) be obstacles to the health and well-being of those in greatest need?

How can the resources best be used to increase the self-reliance, health, and well-being of those whose needs are greatest?

PREPARATION TO MEET NEEDS

What is the long-range social or human vision of the program? Does it include fairer distribution of resources, decision making and power? Is community organization considered necessary, or dangerous? Are there differences of opinion or hidden motives among the planners? (These issues are of great importance, as they help determine whose needs the training program is designed to meet.)

Goals and specific learning objectives:
- How well do they fit the real and felt needs of people in the health workers' communities?
- How realistic are they in terms of the students' abilities and limitations?

How appropriate are the following:
- Selection of instructors and health workers.
- Extent and nature of community and student participation in planning different aspects of the program.
- Attitudes and actions of instructors.
- Time, length, location, etc.
- Content of the course and teaching methods used.
- Flexibility of content and plans.
- Teaching methods.
- Balance of power and decision making during course.
- Balance between practical and classroom learning.
- Balance between curative, preventive, teaching, and organizing skills.
- Student and community participation during the course.
- Use of alternative and local resources.
- Emphasis on memorization or on problem solving.

How well does the training program prepare health workers to help people meet their needs in terms of:
- Specific health-related knowledge and skills?
- Motivation, organization, and leadership?
- Teaching skills?
- Social awareness, problem solving, and thinking skills (observation ⟶ analysis ⟶ action ⟶ evaluation)?

MEETING OF NEEDS

How well are community needs being met with the health workers' help?
(Where appropriate, compare with information gathered before or when the health workers began work.)

Measurable indicators:
- How many deaths? births?
- How much illness?
- How many latrines, etc.?

Non-measurable indicators:
- People's response to program?
- More self-reliance and sharing?
- Greater awareness of problems and possible solutions?
- Poor people better organized?
- More resistance to abuses by those in power?
- More justice? (often preceded by greater repression or abuse)
- More hope and dignity?

Program function after training:
- Support system (back-up and supplies).
- Formation and role of health committee.
- Involvement of mothers, school children, and others.
- Health-related activities (family gardens, co-ops, water system, health theater, etc.).
- Health workers' suggestions for improving training.
- Follow-up training

For more ideas on evaluating the health worker's role in the community, see the next page.

FOLLOW-UP EVALUATION

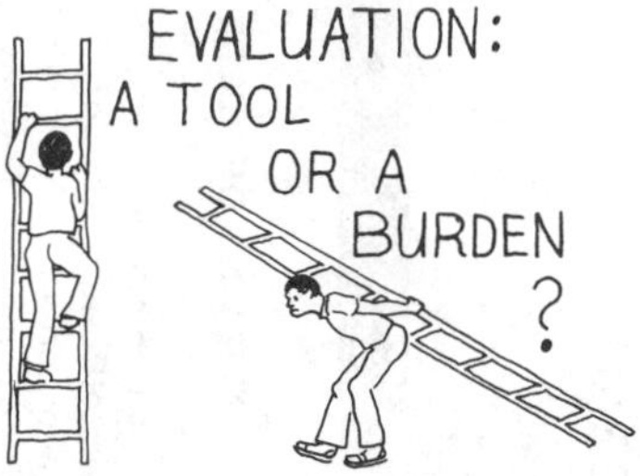

The final measure of a training course is how effectively the health workers serve their communities. In an article called "Evaluation—A Tool or a Burden?"* Mary Annel discusses this issue. Mary works with the Huehuetenango Health Promoter Program, which has trained over 400 village health workers in Guatemala.

EVALUATION: A TOOL OR A BURDEN ?

Mary points out that most of the volunteer workers have limited reading skill, and many find long evaluation questionnaires terrifying. They complain, "We were trained in health care, not statistics." Evaluation is far more practical if it "fits into the daily running of the program and makes sense to people in the village." Instead of trying to gather mountains of facts, Mary suggests that an easier way to evaluate is to observe "the change in the way people act."

> "For example . . . families used to bring undernourished children into the health center when the children had been ill for a month or more. The children were dying, and the center was considered the last resort. In areas covered by health promoters, families now bring children to the promoter much earlier, long before hospitalization is necessary. We use such criteria to measure the success of our program."

To evaluate their program, they try to answer these questions:

THE COMMUNITY

- **Does the community work with the promoter in common projects?** For example, does the community build its own health clinic, or help pay for the promoter's expenses for training courses? All of the promoters may have been elected by their communities; but voluntary labor and/or monetary contributions imply a strong commitment to the health program.
- **Do neighboring villages without promoters ask for their own health workers?** In the last five years, over 225 villages have requested promoters and our program has more than doubled in size.
- **Do the sick follow the health promoter's advice?** Do they complete a prescribed series of injections, or do they stop after the first or second of the series? (The Indians see illness as caused by God's will and they accept illness fatalistically. If members of the community follow the promoter's advice, they are more actively controlling their own health and lives.)
- **Do sick people referred to medical centers actually show up at the centers?**
- **Do the mothers of the village bring their children to be weighed in the under-fives clinic each month?** Preventive medicine is always one of the most difficult concepts to communicate. If the health promoter can convince the mother that a relatively healthy-looking baby is showing early signs of malnutrition when the baby's weight gain falls off, great strides have been made toward eliminating malnutrition in the village.

THE PROMOTERS (village health workers)

- **Do the promoters come up with new ideas and initiate projects?** Or do they simply accept what they learn in training sessions?
- **Do the promoters have more responsibility** for administration, supervision, and continuing education within the program than they did six months or a year ago?
- **Do health promoters want to learn more?** Do they regularly attend continuing education courses? Do they spend free time during the training sessions doing optional reading? Do they stay after class to ask questions? Do they bring patients to the course for advice on difficult cases? Do they bring lists of patients with their symptoms for consultation?

To be used by other programs, the questions asked will need to be different. But the advantages of this approach to evaluation are clear:

- It can be used in a community-based program administered by health workers who have had little schooling.
- It considers changes in ways people act in a community rather than charts and graphics based on often inaccurate statistics.
- It makes evaluation a tool, not a burden. The findings can be understood and used by those involved in the program.
- It is inexpensive. In fact, in many programs the information is already available or can be put together easily from existing records.

*From *Salubritas,* American Public Health Association, July, 1980.

OTHER ORIGINAL IDEAS FOR EVALUATION

The first two ideas come from the Community-Based Health Program newsletter, ***Tambalan,*** from the Philippines (November, 1979).

USING DRAWINGS

"In Bukidnon, instructors once grappled with the task of evaluating their first training session with a group of farmers who had reached only the lower grades in elementary school.

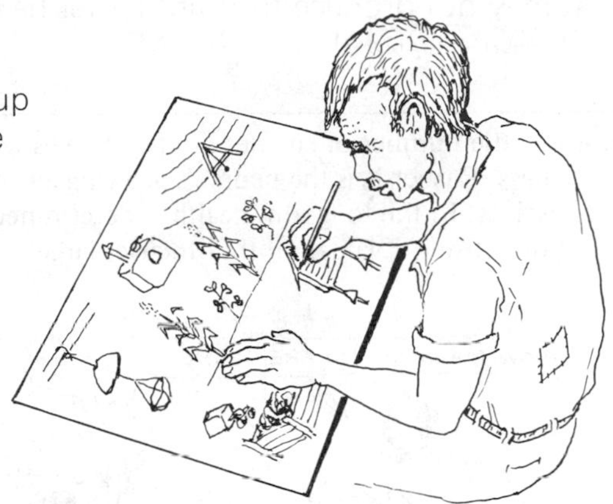

"Solution: they had the farmers put into drawings what they had learned during the session. The drawings weren't any more sophisticated than what most non-artists would produce, but in terms of content, the drawings conveyed a lot more than would have been expected from a written report."

USING DRAMATICS (ROLE PLAYING)

"Instructors had used two different training processes in two ***barrios.*** Curious about the consequences of their use of different approaches, the staff asked the ***barrios*** to present skits centering on how they looked at their situation.

"The differences in training methods, the instructors found out, were very strongly reflected in the plays presented by the ***barrios.*** In the ***barrio*** where health skills were emphasized, the people's perception of their situation was passive, almost fatalistic.

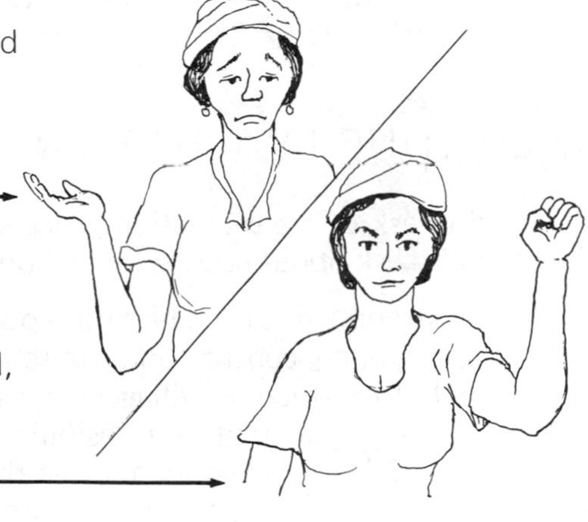

"But in the other ***barrio,*** where organization skills were emphasized, the people depicted their situation the same way as the neighboring ***barrio*** did, with one important difference. Instead of showing passive acceptance, they portrayed themselves as people aware of their own potential to change their situation.

"That experience set the instructors to thinking about the program as a whole and impressed them with the need to change their own orientation and methods."

USING VISITORS

In Ajoya, Mexico, the village health team asks all visitors to write down their observations and opinions of the program. The team uses these outside viewpoints to help evaluate and improve their program.

THE LIMITATIONS OF EVALUATION

The long-range impact of a training course can never be fully measured or known. The human factors in a health worker's training and work may, in the long run, be what influence the people's well-being most. But these human factors may only affect health statistics years later. The seeds the health worker plants deepest may not produce fruit until after he or she is dead and gone. Humanity moves forward slowly!

It is not the number of latrines built or babies weighed that determines a health worker's effectiveness. Rather it is the people's growing awareness of their ability to meet their needs for themselves. In the long run, health is determined more by human qualities than by physical quantities. Evaluation that focuses largely on numbers often tends to forget this.

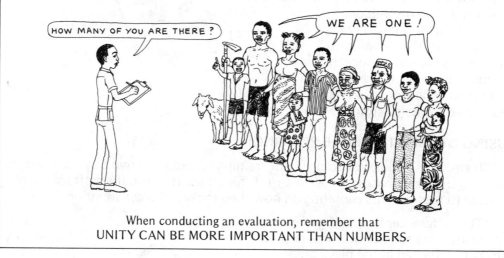

When conducting an evaluation, remember that
UNITY CAN BE MORE IMPORTANT THAN NUMBERS.

EVALUATING EVALUATION

We need to ask of the evaluation process the same searching questions that we continually ask about each aspect of our training or health program:

- Does it strengthen the voice of the powerless? Does it help lead to greater decision making, control, and self-reliance on the part of those who have less? (whether students, villagers, workers, etc.)
- Does it encourage trust, responsibility, and greater equality among all concerned? (teachers, students, health workers, mothers, advisers, etc.)
- Does it help equip people with the knowledge, skills, attitudes, and examples they need to understand and work together to solve their biggest needs?
- Does it consider the group's long-term goals, or vision, as well as short-term objectives?

Evaluation should not only measure whether we have achieved our goals. It should help us judge whether our goals were appropriate in the first place.

CHAPTER 10

Follow-up, Support, and Continued Learning

What and how health workers continue to learn after a training course has ended is just as important as the course itself. The support and advice they receive, and the people who provide it, can make a big difference in the health workers' success or failure once they return to their communities.

'SUPERVISION' OR SUPPORT?

The word ***supervision*** is often used to refer to the process of advising and giving support to health workers. But the word ***supervisor*** brings to mind an overseer or policeman—someone bigger and better than the persons being 'watched over'. Many health programs speak of ***supportive supervision,*** in which the supervisor's role is more to assist and give suggestions than to discipline and make sure orders are followed. Some community-based programs have dropped the terms 'supervision' and 'supervisor' altogether. They prefer friendlier, more equal sounding terms, such as 'follow-up' conducted by 'advisers' or 'fellow members of the health team'. In this book we usually speak of ***support, back-up,*** and ***advisers.***

Clearly, the words used are not as important as the attitudes and relationships behind them. But without a doubt, effective support involves far more than just supervision.

The ideal support system is made up of 4 different sources:

1. The health worker's village or community. This is especially helpful if an honest, active health committee has been formed.

2. Other health workers in nearby villages or communities. Those who have been working longer and have more experience can be especially helpful.

3. Instructors or advisers from the local health program (or the local branch of a larger program).

4. Hospitals, clinics, and agencies to which special problems can be referred. Health officers, agricultural experts, veterinarians, and others may be asked for help and advice when needed.

SUPPORT SYSTEM
FOR THE VILLAGE HEALTH WORKER
(arrows indicate two-way communication and assistance)

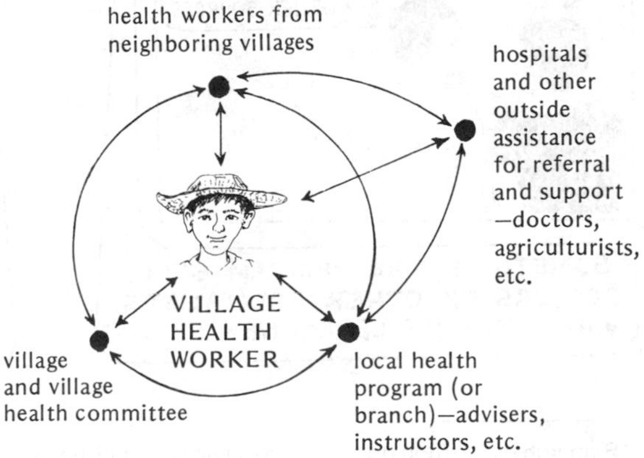

WHERE CAN A VILLAGE HEALTH WORKER LOOK FOR SUPPORT?

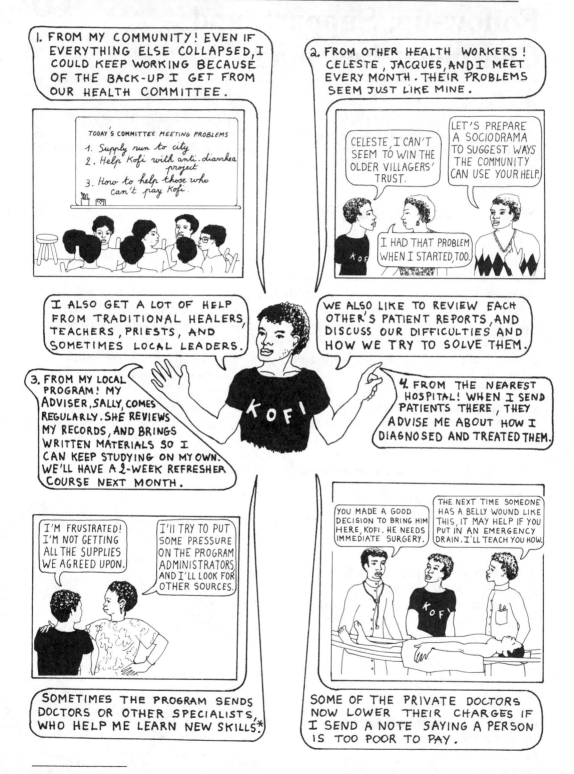

1. FROM MY COMMUNITY! EVEN IF EVERYTHING ELSE COLLAPSED, I COULD KEEP WORKING BECAUSE OF THE BACK-UP I GET FROM OUR HEALTH COMMITTEE.

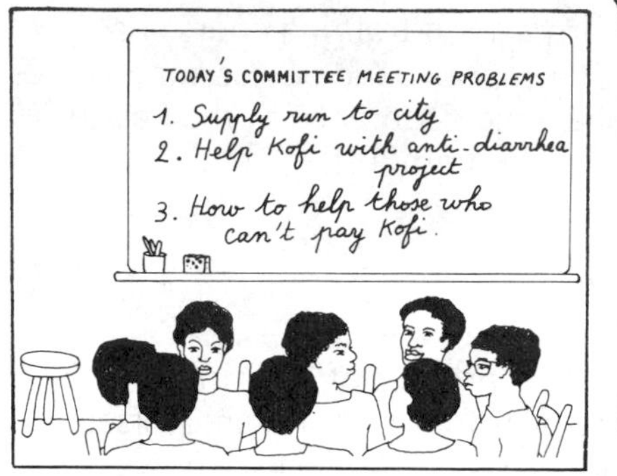

TODAY'S COMMITTEE MEETING PROBLEMS
1. Supply run to city
2. Help Kofi with anti-diarrhea project
3. How to help those who can't pay Kofi.

2. FROM OTHER HEALTH WORKERS! CELESTE, JACQUES, AND I MEET EVERY MONTH. THEIR PROBLEMS SEEM JUST LIKE MINE.

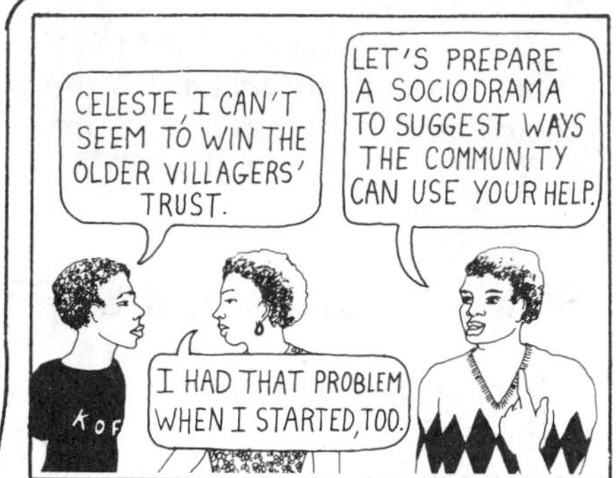

CELESTE, I CAN'T SEEM TO WIN THE OLDER VILLAGERS' TRUST.
I HAD THAT PROBLEM WHEN I STARTED, TOO.
LET'S PREPARE A SOCIODRAMA TO SUGGEST WAYS THE COMMUNITY CAN USE YOUR HELP.
KOFI

I ALSO GET A LOT OF HELP FROM TRADITIONAL HEALERS, TEACHERS, PRIESTS, AND SOMETIMES LOCAL LEADERS.

WE ALSO LIKE TO REVIEW EACH OTHER'S PATIENT REPORTS, AND DISCUSS OUR DIFFICULTIES AND HOW WE TRY TO SOLVE THEM.

KOFI

3. FROM MY LOCAL PROGRAM! MY ADVISER, SALLY, COMES REGULARLY. SHE REVIEWS MY RECORDS, AND BRINGS WRITTEN MATERIALS SO I CAN KEEP STUDYING ON MY OWN. WE'LL HAVE A 2-WEEK REFRESHER COURSE NEXT MONTH.

4. FROM THE NEAREST HOSPITAL! WHEN I SEND PATIENTS THERE, THEY ADVISE ME ABOUT HOW I DIAGNOSED AND TREATED THEM.

I'M FRUSTRATED! I'M NOT GETTING ALL THE SUPPLIES WE AGREED UPON.

I'LL TRY TO PUT SOME PRESSURE ON THE PROGRAM ADMINISTRATORS, AND I'LL LOOK FOR OTHER SOURCES.

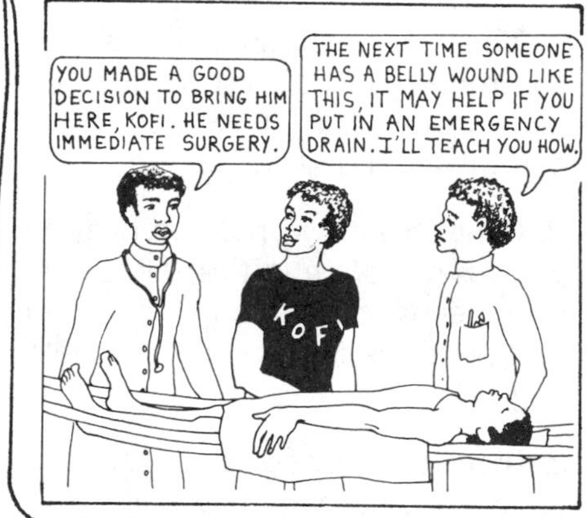

YOU MADE A GOOD DECISION TO BRING HIM HERE, KOFI. HE NEEDS IMMEDIATE SURGERY.
THE NEXT TIME SOMEONE HAS A BELLY WOUND LIKE THIS, IT MAY HELP IF YOU PUT IN AN EMERGENCY DRAIN. I'LL TEACH YOU HOW.
KOFI

SOMETIMES THE PROGRAM SENDS DOCTORS OR OTHER SPECIALISTS, WHO HELP ME LEARN NEW SKILLS.*

SOME OF THE PRIVATE DOCTORS NOW LOWER THEIR CHARGES IF I SEND A NOTE SAYING A PERSON IS TOO POOR TO PAY.

***Remember:** Visiting doctors or specialists should stay in the background and help the village health worker, not the other way around. It must be clear that the village health worker is in charge and the doctor is an auxiliary.

COMMUNITY HEALTH COMMITTEES

Of the four groups that form the support system for the health worker, the most important is the community. Even if the outside health program is discontinued (as often happens), a health worker with strong community support can continue to work effectively.

A well-organized village health committee can be an enormous help in leading activities and encouraging people to take part. Unfortunately, many 'community health committees' do little. They start off full of enthusiasm, but because of problems with selection of members, leadership, or motivation, they gradually become inactive.

The selection of a responsible, hard-working committee can be a first step toward helping the poor gain fairer representation and more control over factors that affect their health and lives. **To be effective, health committees need members who will actively represent the poor.**

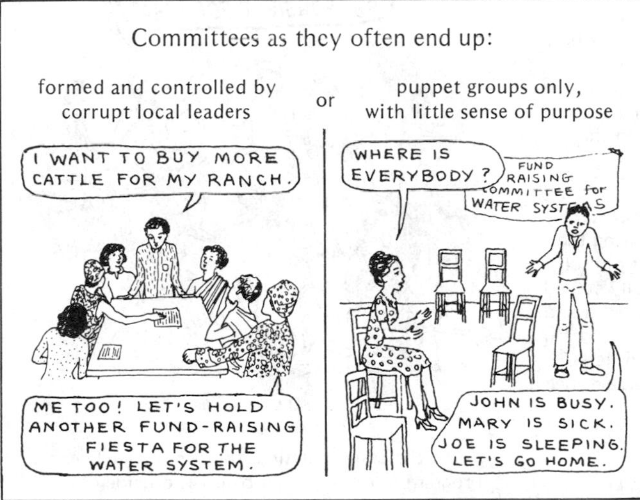
Committees as they often end up:
formed and controlled by corrupt local leaders
or
puppet groups only, with little sense of purpose
I WANT TO BUY MORE CATTLE FOR MY RANCH.
ME TOO! LET'S HOLD ANOTHER FUND-RAISING FIESTA FOR THE WATER SYSTEM.
WHERE IS EVERYBODY?
FUND RAISING COMMITTEE for WATER SYSTEMS
JOHN IS BUSY. MARY IS SICK. JOE IS SLEEPING. LET'S GO HOME.

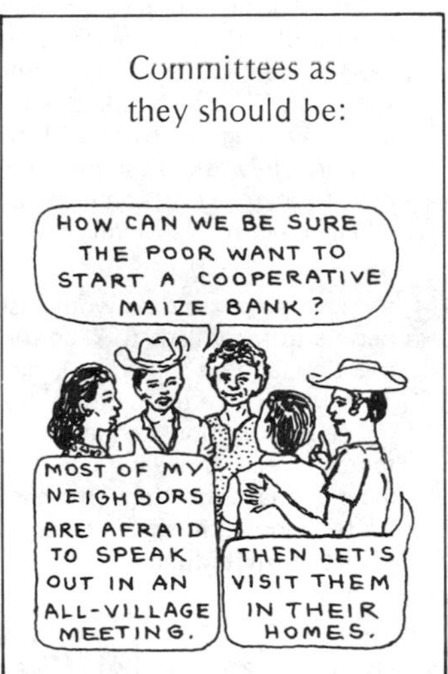
Committees as they should be:
HOW CAN WE BE SURE THE POOR WANT TO START A COOPERATIVE MAIZE BANK?
MOST OF MY NEIGHBORS ARE AFRAID TO SPEAK OUT IN AN ALL-VILLAGE MEETING.
THEN LET'S VISIT THEM IN THEIR HOMES.

TWO STORIES FOR DISCUSSION:

1. Forming a health committee in Ngbokoto

In the village of Ngbokoto lived a health worker named Etienne. He had been instructed by his program leaders to form a community health committee to help organize activities. "Be sure to include the political leaders," he was told. "Then your committee will have the power and leadership it needs."

So Etienne went to the mayor, who welcomed the idea. "I'll do all the work," said the mayor. "Just leave it in my hands. I'll even choose the members." The mayor chose his brother-in-law, some rich friends, a big landholder, and a merchant who had a truck to help carry supplies.

The committee accomplished very little. At meetings, members proposed good ideas for health activities, but nothing ever seemed to get done. It was never made clear who was responsible for anything, so no one did much. There was no special schedule for meetings. Some meetings ended early because nothing had been planned or because so few persons attended.

Soon Etienne had other problems. Committee members expected free care and medicines for their families. Finally they took control of Etienne's village medicine supply, saying they would "help with the distribution." The committee ended up selling some of the drugs secretly for personal profit.

What do you suppose went wrong with this committee? What would your health workers do to form a better one? Before reading the next story, have the group make a list of ideas for choosing and running an effective health committee.

2. Forming a health committee in Bodila

Marcel, a health worker who lived in the village of Bodila, heard about the problems Etienne was having. Still, he needed the support of a village committee. So he asked Etienne and several other health workers in the area for their ideas.

They agreed that the committee should represent and be selected by the poorer families in town. "But how?" asked Marcel. "If we hold an all-village meeting, the mayor, the big landholders, and the merchants will dominate it like always. The poor won't dare open their mouths."

"Maybe we could change that!" said Etienne. And together they made a plan.

A village meeting was to be held. But before it took place, Marcel and the other health workers talked with some of the leaders among the poor. They also talked with the village priest, who agreed to go with them to visit the mayor. They asked the mayor's advice about how to involve everyone who attended the village meeting, especially the poor.

The mayor said he would ask the powerful people in the village to keep silent during the meeting, and he agreed to keep silent himself. This would give the people who usually stayed in the background a chance to sit up front and take the lead. Since women did not customarily attend village meetings, the health workers visited women in their homes and made a special effort to invite them.

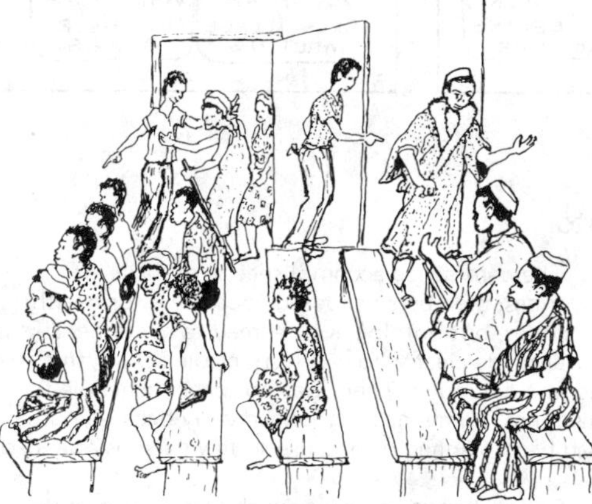

The health workers showed the persons who usually dominated to the back of the room, and asked the poor to sit up front.

The community meeting was a great success. Persons who were normally silent began to speak up. The people elected committee members who would represent the poor. They also made guidelines for their committee. It would meet twice a month, always on a Thursday at sunset at Marcel's house. Any person who missed 3 meetings in a row would be replaced. The members would take turns being responsible for planning and leading the meetings. A monthly financial report would be reviewed by the school teacher and the priest, and read to the group. Meetings would not be closed until necessary decisions had been made.

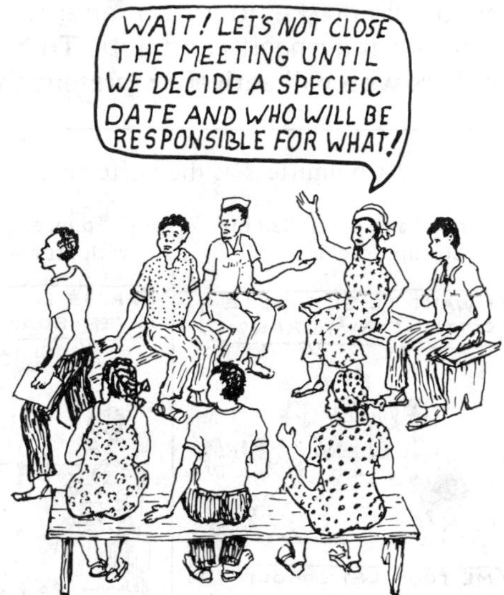
WAIT! LET'S NOT CLOSE THE MEETING UNTIL WE DECIDE A SPECIFIC DATE AND WHO WILL BE RESPONSIBLE FOR WHAT!

At their first meeting, the committee began a program to dig a safe garbage pit outside of town and clean up the village. Sylvie, a committee member, was responsible for this project, and at the second meeting she gave a progress report. Other committee members were impressed by what they had accomplished. But they were also made aware of the problems they still faced in convincing their neighbors to continue to use the new garbage pit and keep the village clean.

The meetings were always interesting, often with Marcel leading flannel-board and filmstrip presentations. Problems and possible solutions were explored with role plays. Attendance was good. The committee remained active and strongly supportive of Marcel's health work.

Why did Marcel's committee succeed? Are there some things you forgot in the list you made before reading this story? Does your list include ideas that Marcel and his friends did not think of?

Marcel was fortunate. He and his fellow health workers succeeded in overcoming obstacles that might have prevented a fair selection process. The people at the village meeting were able to elect a committee that would fairly represent the poor.

In many communities, however, the persons with power will not be willing to remain silent during meetings. And even if they are, the poor may be afraid to speak in public. In places where truly democratic selection was not likely to work, other ways of forming a committee have been tried. Here are two examples.

In Pueblo Viejo, Mexico, the health committee is made up of the village health worker's good friends, relatives, and ***compadres*** (those who are godparents of each other's children). These people have a genuine personal concern in seeing that the health worker keeps doing a good job. (However, several problems have resulted. One is that the health worker's friends and relatives expect free medicines and services, which means there is never enough money to replace supplies.)

In Nigeria, one program has divided the tasks usually done by a health committee among other village organizations. The local women's league is in charge of health activities that affect mothers and children. The older children are responsible for organizing sanitation projects. The religious societies help with supplies, planning, and supervision.

It is not enough simply to hope that a health committee will function effectively. Both the health worker and the program leaders need to give the committee encouragement, advice, and organizational help. But it is important that they **provide support without taking charge!** This requires skill, understanding, and patience.

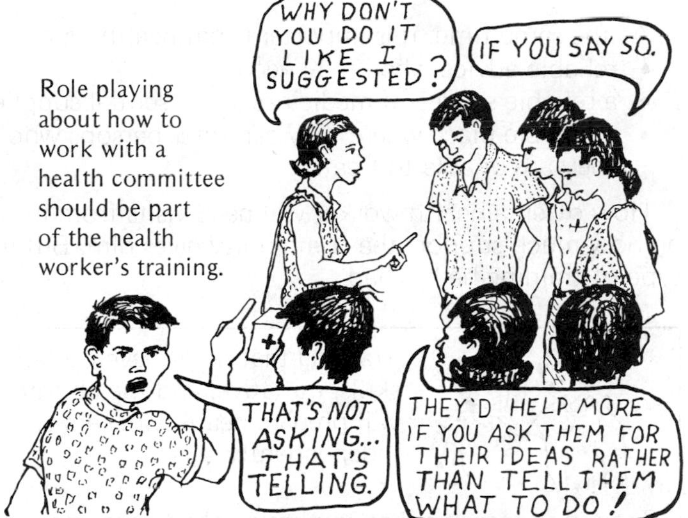
WHY DON'T YOU DO IT LIKE I SUGGESTED?
IF YOU SAY SO.
THAT'S NOT ASKING... THAT'S TELLING.
THEY'D HELP MORE IF YOU ASK THEM FOR THEIR IDEAS RATHER THAN TELL THEM WHAT TO DO!

Role playing about how to work with a health committee should be part of the health worker's training.

SUGGESTIONS FOR AN EFFECTIVE HEALTH COMMITTEE

- Select an active, just committee in a way that is acceptable to the community, yet with strong representation from the poor.
- Meet regularly.
- Talk to each member personally before each meeting to be sure they come.
- Include some kind of fun or excitement in the meetings (perhaps filmstrips or role plays related to an activity the committee is planning).
- Plan activities with specific objectives. Plan enough details so that everyone knows what he or she is expected to do, and when. Post a written plan of action listing the responsibilities, people, and dates the group has agreed upon.
- Have someone check to see that each person completes what is planned or gets the help he needs.
- Plan enough activities to keep everyone interested and active—but not so many that the committee will not have time to carry them out.
- Replace inactive members quickly.

HOW MUCH SUPPORT FROM THE PROGRAM IS NEEDED?

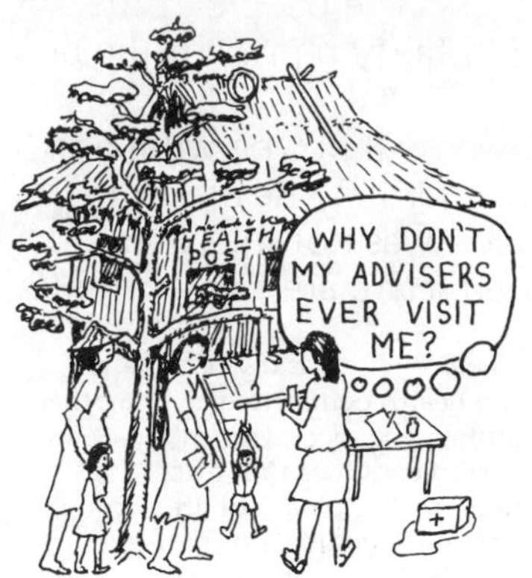
HEALTH POST
WHY DON'T MY ADVISERS EVER VISIT ME?

Some programs provide too little support and assistance for their health workers. Others provide too much regulation and supervised control. And many programs manage to make both mistakes at once.

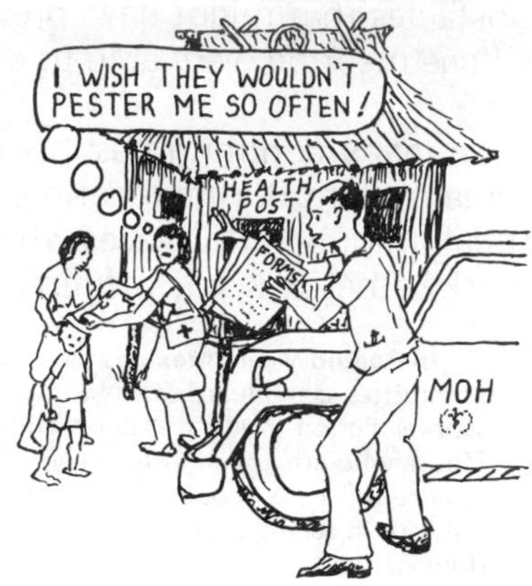
I WISH THEY WOULDN'T PESTER ME SO OFTEN!
HEALTH POST
FORMS
MOH

It is important that health workers be trusted and encouraged to take initiative. They must feel free to help people find their own ways of solving their own problems.

At the same time, it is important that health workers have . . .

- reliable advice when they need it,
- a reliable source of medicines and essential supplies, and
- a reliable place where they can refer persons who have illnesses or injuries they are unable to treat.

How often a health worker will need visits from his adviser will depend, in part, on how much support the community gives him. But mostly it will depend on the type of training he has had.

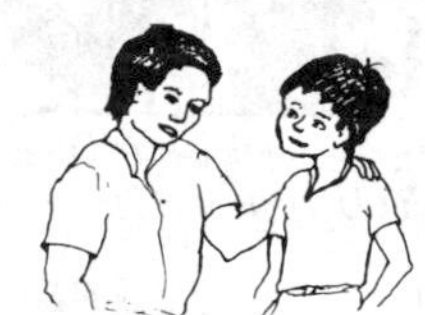

Training that helps develop self-reliance, problem-solving skills, initiative, and the ability to use books effectively will prepare health workers to work more or less independently.

Training programs that emphasize obedience, memorizing facts, and filling out forms create health workers who need a lot of supervision.

Usually, however, the frequency with which support persons visit health workers depends less on need than on the limitations of time and distance. Especially where health workers live in villages reached only by footpath and muleback, visits tend to be very infrequent. Some advisers manage to visit their health workers only once or twice a year. In these cases, support from village health committees and neighboring health workers is particularly important.

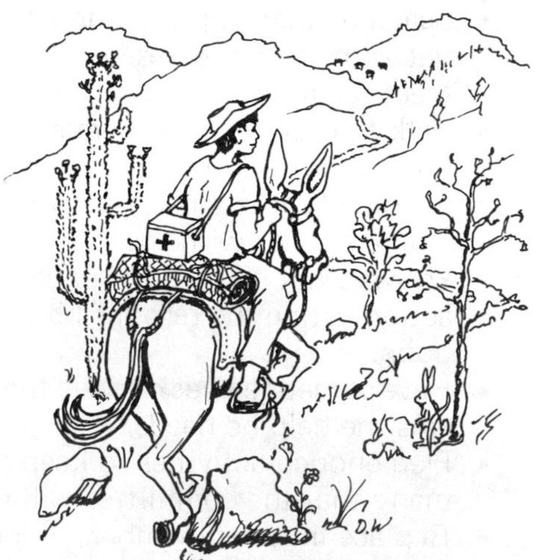

WHO MAKE THE BEST ADVISERS OR SUPERVISORS?

Instructors from the training course are often the best persons to provide health workers with follow-up and support from their program. If instructors and students develop a friendly and trusting relationship during training, this is likely to continue after the course is over.

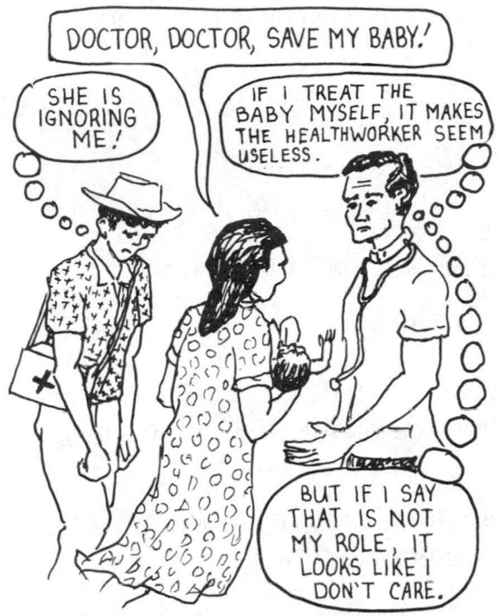
DOCTOR, DOCTOR, SAVE MY BABY!
SHE IS IGNORING ME!
IF I TREAT THE BABY MYSELF, IT MAKES THE HEALTHWORKER SEEM USELESS.
BUT IF I SAY THAT IS NOT MY ROLE, IT LOOKS LIKE I DON'T CARE.

On the other hand, problems often arise when the supervisors are doctors or nurses. They may tend to 'take over' during their visits to village health posts. Even if a doctor tries to remain in the background, the very fact that he is a doctor causes people to seek his advice rather than that of the local health worker. So the doctor finds himself in a 'double bind': If he attends those who beg him for medical care, he weakens the position of the health worker. If he refuses (however politely), he sets an example of someone who denies assistance he could easily give. It takes an unusually sensitive person to handle this situation well.

One way around this problem is to have advisers who have neither the advanced medical knowledge nor the prestige of doctors. In several programs in Guatemala, the more experienced village health workers provide support for the others. In Honduras, young school teachers have been specially prepared to serve as advisers. Their teaching skills, together with special training in sanitation, public health, and community organization, allow them to work effectively with the village health workers in organizing community activities. Yet their relative lack of medical knowledge—and the fact that they are teachers, not doctors—lessens the temptation to provide medical care. They are less likely to take charge and reduce the health worker to the role of a servant.

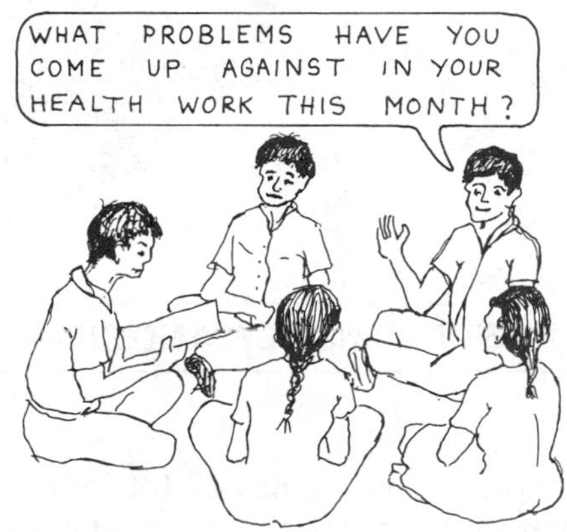
WHAT PROBLEMS HAVE YOU COME UP AGAINST IN YOUR HEALTH WORK THIS MONTH?

A more experienced health worker meets with newer health workers from neighboring villages.

WHAT SORT OF RECORD KEEPING IS NEEDED?

Records can be helpful in several ways. Health workers can use them to evaluate their own work and to get suggestions from their advisers. A training program can use health workers' records to plan appropriate follow-up training. Also, most health authorities require certain records if they are to provide free vaccines, family planning methods, or medicines for tuberculosis, malaria, or leprosy.

Forms for keeping records

Some programs use mimeographed forms for keeping patient records and for making daily, weekly, or monthly reports on health activities and health-related events (births, deaths, and epidemics). **A few simple forms may be useful.** But many programs require health workers to fill out a ridiculous number of forms. Remember, for health workers with little formal education, filling out a lot of forms can be even more painful than it is for those of us who have had more schooling.

When considering what forms to use in your program, it helps to ask yourselves:

- For whom is the information being collected?
- How will the records be used?
- Could the health workers' time be better spent?
- Will the health workers see any value to filling out the form, and be concerned with accuracy?
- Is the form short and easy to use?

If the information being collected is of obvious importance to the health workers and their communities, then it is probably reasonable to use the form. Otherwise, seriously consider whether that form is really needed.

Be sure that during training the health workers practice filling out the forms they will later be using. But do not spend too much time on this. Remember . . .

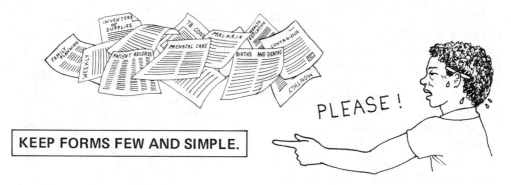

KEEP FORMS FEW AND SIMPLE.

Simple forms can be helpful for keeping ***patient records,*** or records of a sick person from one visit to the next. Examples of forms that can be used for patient records are shown in ***Where There Is No Doctor.*** In Chapter 21 of this book we give ideas for role plays and other ways of teaching about the use of these forms.

PATIENT REPORT, for sending for medical help . . . . ***WTND,*** p. 44
RECORD OF PRENATAL CARE, for pregnant women . . . . . . ***WTND,*** p. 253
CHILD HEALTH CHART, for children under 5 . . . . ***WTND,*** p. 298

Monthly report forms are useful for self-evaluation, and provide an ongoing record of activities in a community. They can be reviewed by both the village health committee and the adviser. The form should emphasize preventive and educational activities, to encourage the health worker to organize and carry out such activities each month. Compare the 2 sample forms on the following pages.

The first sample monthly report, shown below, is a short, problem-related form. It is designed to help health workers, the community, and the health program to work together more effectively. The second sample monthly report, on the next 2 pages, is a longer form intended to gather more information.

Which do you prefer? We would appreciate your ideas. Please send us examples of helpful forms used by your program. Write to the Hesperian Foundation, P.O. Box 1692, Palo Alto, CA 94302, U.S.A.

MONTHLY REPORT 1

Month: ________________

Village: ______________________________ Health worker: ______________________

How many sick people did you see this month? Men___ Women___ Children___

What health problems did you see most often this month? ________________

What was the most serious problem you saw this month? ________________

What were the causes? ________________________________

What are you doing to help prevent these problems from happening again?

Include activities of health workers, health committee, parents' groups, and school children.

What was done in the following areas?

Latrines ________________

Safe water supply ________________

Village cleanliness ________________

Vaccination ________________

Nutrition ________________

Other ________________

Did someone from the program visit this month? ________________

What did you do together? ________________

How is your supply of medicines? ________________

What help or information do you and the health committee need in order to do a better job? ________________

MONTHLY REPORT 2 (front side)

Month: ____________

Village: ____________ Health worker: ____________

BIRTHS:

Name	Weight	Number of brothers & sisters	Age of mother	Name of midwife	Did you attend?	Any problems?

Did you give a ROAD TO HEALTH CHART to the mother of each newborn baby? YES___ NO___

DEATHS:

Name	Age	Cause of death

PREVENTIVE MEDICINE:

Public sanitation

Number of latrines built this month___ Homes with latrines___ Homes without latrines___

Other activities____________ Planned___ In progress___ Completed___

____________ Planned___ In progress___ Completed___

Health education and activities

	Times	What you did	Attendance
With mothers and under-fives			
School-aged children			
Other			

Family planning and prenatal care

		Pill	Injections	IUD	Other	Total
Number of women who started this month						
Total number using birth control						
Number who stopped using birth control						
Number planning who got pregnant . . .						

Total number of pregnant women___ Number receiving prenatal care this month___

Under-fives clinic

AGE:	0-1	1-2	2-3	3-4	4-5
Total number of children in the village					
Number who have Road to Health charts . .					
Number weighed this month					
Number who were healthy					
Number who were ill					
Number with signs of malnutrition: mild . .					
moderate					
severe .					

Did you meet with the health committee this month?___ With what results? ____________

MONTHLY REPORT 2 (back side)

HEALTH PROBLEMS SEEN THIS MONTH

AGE:	0-1	2-5	6-15	16-40	41-65	over 65	new case	repeat visit	gave no medicine*	referred to hospital
Colds and flu										
Pneumonia										
Other respiratory problem										
______										
Diarrhea and dysentery										
Dehydration										
Vomiting										
Urinary problems ______										
______										
Roundworm										
Other parasites ______										
______										
Gastritis or ulcer										
Other belly problem										
______										
Malnutrition										
Anemia										
Skin problems ______										
______										
______										
Accidents: wounds										
fractures										
Other ______										
Measles										
Mumps										
Whooping cough										
Malaria										
Tuberculosis										
Leprosy										
Rabies										
Other problems ______										
______										
______										
Could not figure out										
______										
TOTAL PROBLEMS SEEN										

*The heading "gave no medicine" is included to encourage health workers **not** to give medicine for every problem.

DEALING WITH PROBLEMS

Health workers are as human as any of us. All make honest mistakes, and some make dishonest mistakes. Although we have emphasized the supportive role of advisers (or supervisors), they do need to make sure that health workers are working responsibly and effectively. (Health workers, for their part, need to make sure that the advisers also meet their responsibilities.)

Many common problems in health work can be solved or avoided if the health worker, his adviser, and the community plan and work together. When difficulties arise, it is important to get criticism, suggestions, and cooperation from all parts of the 'support system', including the villagers. Remember that the various parts of the support system may have conflicting interests.

COMMON DIFFICULTIES AND WAYS TO AVOID THEM:

1. Charging too much for medicines or services. In many programs, at least a few health workers will try to turn curative care into a profitable business by charging high prices.

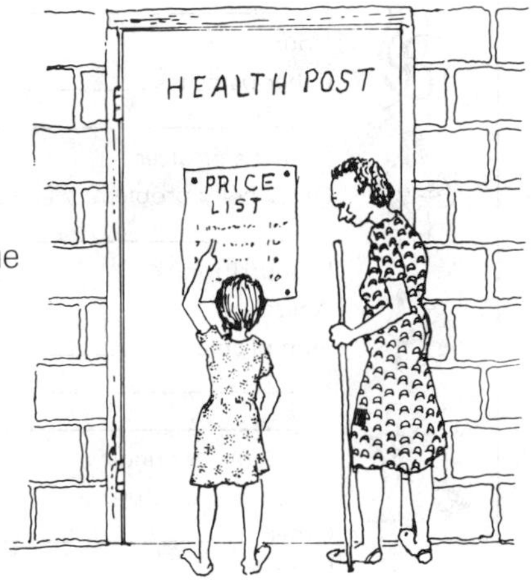

Some health workers are rightfully angry about criticism on this subject from experts or professionals. At a conference in Guatemala, one health worker protested, "So we cheat 25 cents here or there on a few medicines. Remember, we are poor! What is 25 cents compared with the value of the cars, homes, educations, and paid travel enjoyed 'honestly' by those who criticize us?"

In this kind of situation, solutions must be suggested, chosen, and upheld by all parts of the support system, including the health workers themselves. One helpful step is to **nail an agreed-upon price list to the door of the health post.**

HEALTH POST

PRICE LIST

2. Failure of people to pay the health worker for medicines and services. Sometimes people do not have money to pay for health care and medicines when they are sick. In fact, it is the poorest and the hungriest who get sick most often. A health worker will usually give these persons free medicine rather than see them suffer, especially if they are relatives or friends. A village clinic among the Paya Indians in Honduras had to close down because the health workers gave away all the medicines and had no money to replace them.

Getting people to pay is a common problem in programs that try to be self-sufficient. However, most persons can afford to pay something, or may be able to later. The health committee and the program can help determine which people are unable to pay, and perhaps make special arrangements for them. They can also remind those who can afford to pay, but have forgotten. Perhaps persons who are better off can be asked to pay higher rates. One program in Bangladesh uses a simple insurance plan; each family pays a small amount each month. In Ajoya, Mexico, the village health team raises vegetables, chickens, and bees to help cover their expenses. Persons who cannot pay for services are asked to send a family member to help with the work on these self-sufficiency projects.

3. Using too many medicines. Unfortunately, some programs tempt health workers to overuse medicines by permitting them to make a small profit on the medicines they sell. This is often the only money the health workers earn for their services. The temptation to overprescribe can be reduced by allowing health workers to charge a small fee for services. Medicines can then be sold at cost—with prices posted. For more discussion on the overuse of medicines, see Chapter 18.

4. Spending too much time on curative medicine. Many training programs seek a balance between prevention and treatment. But it often happens that community health workers spend much more of their time on curative services than on prevention.

Before protesting this too loudly, we should remember that to be accepted by the community, health workers must respond to people's felt needs. And most people feel a greater need for curative than preventive measures. Only through a gradual process of education and growing awareness will a community choose to place as much emphasis on prevention as on cure. The adviser should respect the community's wish for curative care. But at the same time he must be ready to encourage and support increasing emphasis on preventive activities, as people become aware of the need.

The temptation to put most of their energy into curative medicine will be stronger if health workers earn money only for their curative work. Ideally, of course, health should be more rewarding than sickness. Look for ways to have the health worker's pay reflect this. For example, in ancient Japan each family would pay the doctor every month as long as everyone was healthy. But when someone became ill, his family would stop paying until the doctor healed him. This kind of arrangement would encourage health workers to work hard on prevention.

The adviser can help the health worker and health committee to make specific plans for carrying out various preventive projects. Agreeing on goals and careful planning will help make things happen.

5. Feelings of frustration and need of support. Feelings of discouragement are sometimes overwhelming for community health workers. It is easy for one person to dream of what is needed to make a community healthier. But real changes are part of a slow process that involves all of us.

In addition, village health workers are usually closer to the people they work with than are most medical professionals. They tend to get more personally involved. When something goes wrong or persons get angry with them, they are less protected. So they need plenty of support from their friends and family, the health committee, and the program leaders.

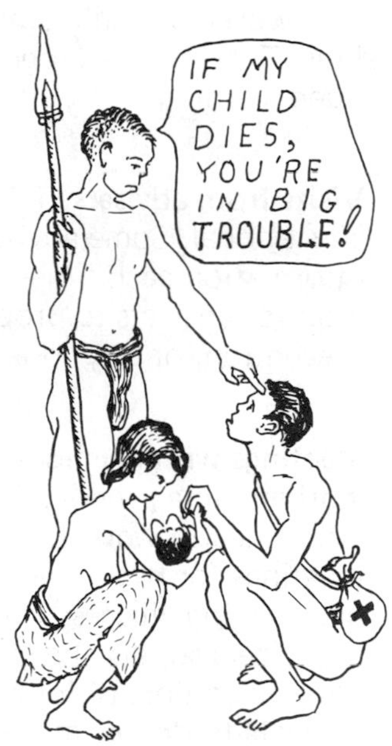

The community health worker is less protected than most doctors, and therefore needs more support.

6. Abuse of knowledge and power. Throughout history, medicine has been a sacred and magic art. Its practitioners—whether folk healers or modern doctors—have often used their special skills to gain power and privilege. Instead of sharing their knowledge, they have kept it secret, leading others to think they are miracle workers. In doing this, the healers have made people as dependent as possible on their services.

TRICKS OF THE TRADE

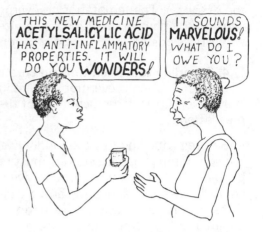

If ordinary aspirin is labeled *'acetylsalicylic acid'*, people think they are getting something new and different. By keeping the truth a secret, the health worker gains power and glory—until people discover they have been tricked!

Some community health workers are tempted to do this also. One way for an adviser to help prevent this problem is to set a good example. If he himself relates to others as an equal, shares freely what he knows, and admits his mistakes, the health workers will be likely to treat people in a similar way. It helps to discuss this problem openly during training.

CONTINUING OPPORTUNITIES TO LEARN

Health workers should always be looking for ways to increase their knowledge and skills. Their health programs can do much to provide opportunities for continued learning:

- **Visits from advisers.** The main purpose of an adviser's visit should be educational. Some advisers make a point of giving health workers new information each time they see them. Also, advisers can help health workers look for answers to problems in community organization, health education, prevention, or diagnosis and treatment.

- **Meetings with neighboring health workers.** In a program in Guatemala, senior health workers lead monthly meetings for health workers from neighboring villages. The program organizers supply the group leaders with 'lesson plans' for suggested subjects to discuss at the meetings. They also send mimeographed sheets answering health workers' requests for information about specific projects or problems.

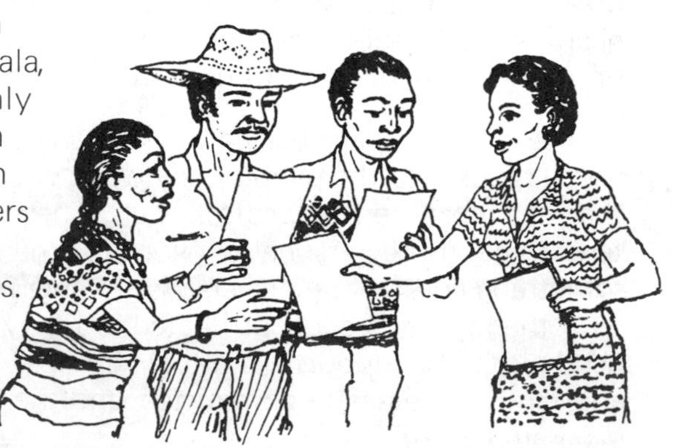

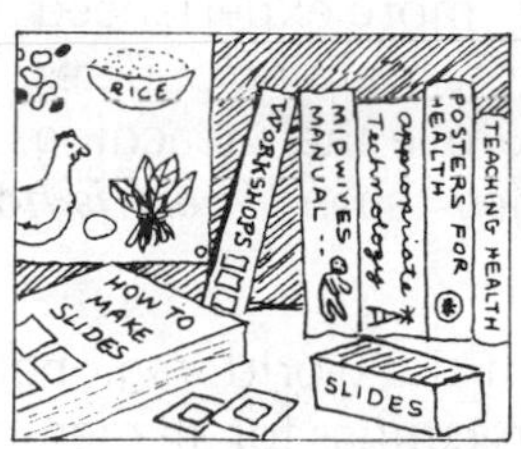

- **Books and other educational materials.** Easy-to-use reference books or pamphlets can be important tools for self-education. Health workers can use them to continue learning about health care, farming techniques, animal breeding, veterinary care, community organization, theater and puppet shows, teaching methods, and other subjects. Health programs often help health workers obtain these materials at low cost.

Many countries now have resource centers that distribute books and educational materials. Examples are TALC in England, ASECSA in Guatemala, and VHAI in India. (See p. **Back**-3.)

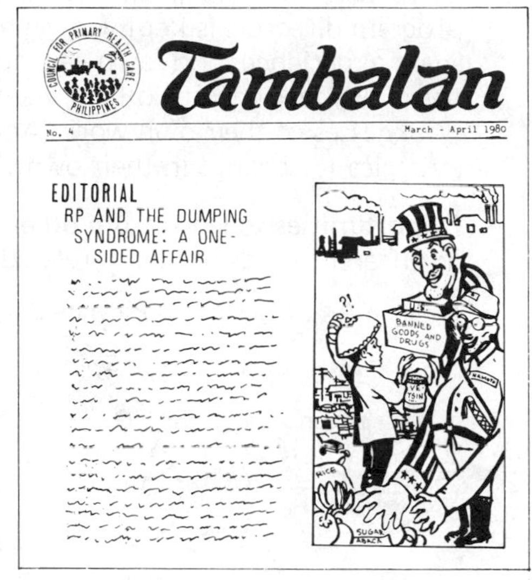

COUNCIL FOR PRIMARY HEALTH CARE · PHILIPPINES

Tambalan

No. 4 — March - April 1980

EDITORIAL

RP AND THE DUMPING SYNDROME: A ONE-SIDED AFFAIR

a community-based newsletter from the Philippines

- **Local newsletters.** A number of health programs and community groups produce newsletters for village health workers. These are usually simply written and well illustrated. They include health information as well as new ideas and approaches that health workers in the area have tried. Good examples of such newsletters are *El Informador,* produced by the Regional Committee for Community Health Promotion in Central America, *AKAP Diary,* published by a network of community-based programs in the Philippines, and *Medico Friends Bulletin,* produced by VHAI in India. For more ideas on village news sheets and how to prepare them, see pages **16**-12 to **16**-17.

- **Refresher courses and continued training.** These can be even more important than the initial training course. Some programs ask health workers to return for group learning sessions one day each week. (In one program, workers must attend weekly sessions in order to continue receiving medicines from the program.) Other programs conduct a 2 to 3 week refresher course, once or twice a year. The approach you decide to use will depend on the distance health workers must travel to the training center, whether they work full time or part time, the seasons for planting and harvesting, and other factors.

- **Apprenticeship opportunities.** The villager-run program in Ajoya, Mexico invites health workers to visit the training and referral center whenever they can. During these visits the health workers help the central team with consultations, care of the sick, training courses, work in the vegetable garden, and community activities. This is a more intimate way of learning than is possible during a large training course. It is especially helpful for persons who have difficulty with classroom learning. One program in Honduras requires a special follow-up apprenticeship for each student who did not learn well during the training course.

- **Teaching assistants.** Some programs invite some of their more experienced village health workers to serve as teaching assistants in the training courses for new health workers. This helps the assistants to improve their teaching skills and gain a better understanding of the subjects they teach. ***There is no better way to learn something than to teach it.***
- **Meetings between different programs.** In several parts of the world, regional associations of community-based health programs hold meetings for all member groups every year or so. These are especially worthwhile when most of the participants are village-level workers and the number of outside experts and program directors is kept very small. At the meetings, health workers can share experiences and learn new approaches to meeting their communities' needs. By talking with others, they come to appreciate the strengths and weaknesses of their own work. Above all, they do not feel so alone in their struggles for change in their own villages.
- **Opportunities to learn from other programs.** Different programs are strong in different kinds of health-related activities. For example:

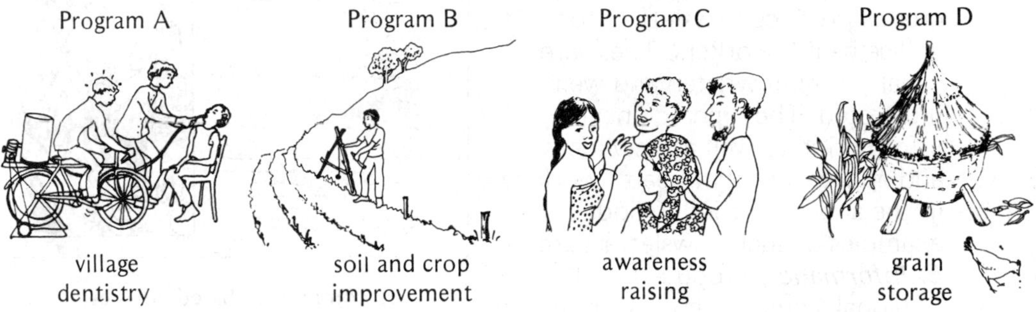

Suppose a program near to yours has developed special skill in dental care or midwives' training. And your own program has particular ability in food production, or land rights organizing. It may be possible for health workers from different programs to visit and learn from each other. Perhaps programs with special skills can give short courses, inviting health workers from other programs. This sort of educational exchange has already begun among programs in Mexico and Central America.

INSTRUCTORS ALSO NEED SUPPORT AND LEARNING OPPORTUNITIES:

Village health workers are not the only ones who need a support system and a chance to learn new ideas. We all would grow stale if we did not meet new people, start new projects, and constantly try out new ways to work.

Most of the suggestions we have given for helping health workers to continue learning also will work for instructors. In addition, some groups sponsor short courses on teaching methods and materials for training health workers.

Perhaps the most effective way for outside instructors to renew their interest and dedication to training village health workers is to spend more time with people in a village. Living with villagers, sharing their daily needs and problems, fun and frustrations, helps reawaken the spirit to work with people toward a healthier village—and world.

VILLAGE HEALTH WORKERS WHO FORM THEIR OWN SUPPORT SYSTEM

In most large health programs, the direction of control is from the city or government center to the communities. But in a people-centered approach, the direction of control is ideally just the reverse: control and decision making are based mainly in the community.

In many programs today, communities select their own health workers and health committees. But seldom do community health workers have the opportunity to select their own support systems for follow-up training and referral.

In Ajoya, Mexico, however, the village health team has succeeded in building its own support system. The village workers invite outside professionals, and have worked out an effective referral system on their own terms. These are the team's guidelines for visiting professionals:

1. Outside professionals come only by invitation, and only for short visits. This way it remains clear that the health team is self-run and not dependent on the continued presence of outsiders.
2. Visiting professionals must speak the local language and are asked not to dress in white.
3. Doctors are asked to teach, not to practice their skills. They serve as the auxiliaries to the primary health workers.
4. Outside instructors and advisers come to learn as well as to teach. They are expected to relate to the health workers as friends and equals.
5. To strengthen the sense of equality, visiting professionals and advisers are expected to help with the daily agricultural work, and to clean up after themselves.

The health team is very careful in deciding which professionals and advisers to invite to their village. They recognize the tendency of doctors, especially, to think of themselves as superior to others, and to set themselves up as authorities, even in areas of health care they know little about.

The village workers have found that getting visiting doctors to clean up after themselves is especially difficult. But they gently insist on it. One time a visiting doctor demonstrated how to do a pelvic exam of a woman, but afterward neglected to wash the instrument, a ***speculum.*** The health workers kept reminding the doctor to clean it, but he kept putting it off. One night when he went to bed, the doctor felt a lump under his pillow cover. It was the unwashed speculum! Fortunately, the doctor was good natured and took the lesson well. From then on he was careful to clean up after himself.

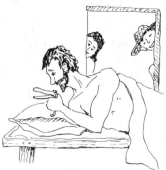

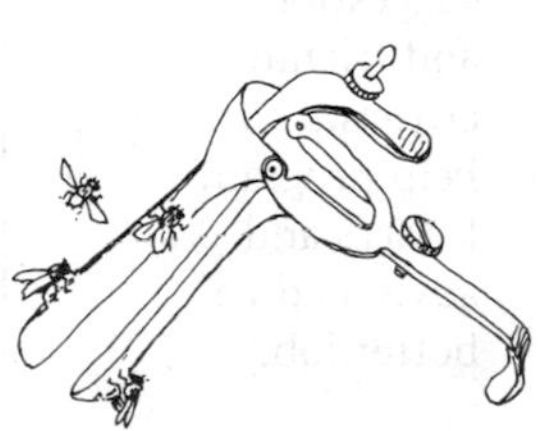

The team of health workers has also managed, over the years, to build an effective referral system in the nearest city, about 4 hours away by bus. The health workers used to have difficulty getting adequate treatment for persons they referred to the city. Private hospitals were too expensive and public hospitals often provided such poor, disrespectful care that no one wanted to go to them.

In time, however, the village team found a few doctors who agreed to provide surgery and care for the poor at low cost. A small private hospital also began to cooperate by lowering its charges, and by asking women's groups in the city to help cover expenses for very poor families. Today, when the health workers refer a person to one of 'their' doctors in the city, they send along a note explaining the family's economic situation. If the family is very poor, the doctor charges little or nothing. If the family is rich, the doctor collects his usual fee.

Some of the doctors have gained so much confidence and respect for the village workers that they sometimes invite them into the surgery room or teach them emergency procedures that can help save lives in a remote village.

The most remarkable aspect of this referral system is that it was developed by the Project Piaxtla health team—from the bottom up. This example gives an idea of how community-based health workers can begin to work with—and help to educate and change—the established medical system.

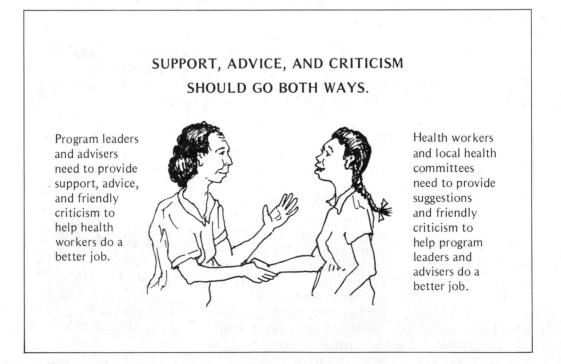

SUPPORT, ADVICE, AND CRITICISM SHOULD GO BOTH WAYS.

Program leaders and advisers need to provide support, advice, and friendly criticism to help health workers do a better job.

Health workers and local health committees need to provide suggestions and friendly criticism to help program leaders and advisers do a better job.

PART TWO

LEARNING THROUGH SEEING, DOING, AND THINKING

IF I **HEAR** IT
I FORGET IT.

IF I **SEE** IT
I REMEMBER IT.

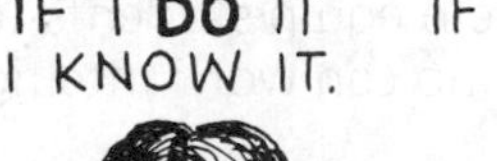

IF I DO IT
I KNOW IT.

IF I DISCOVER IT
I USE IT.

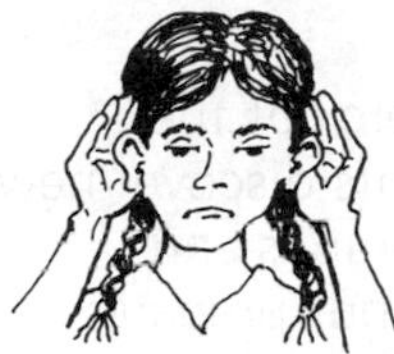

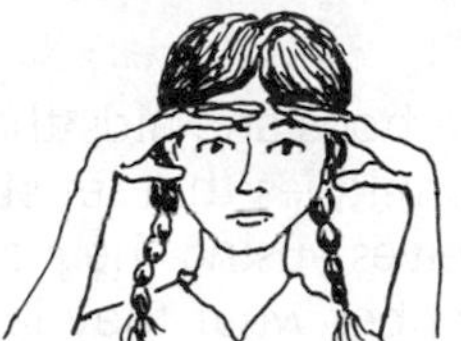

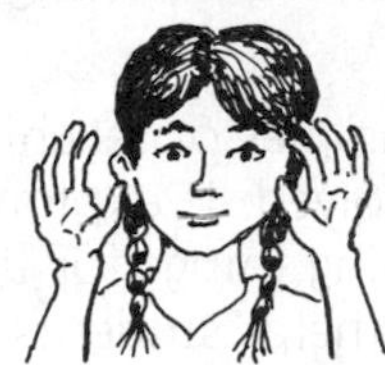

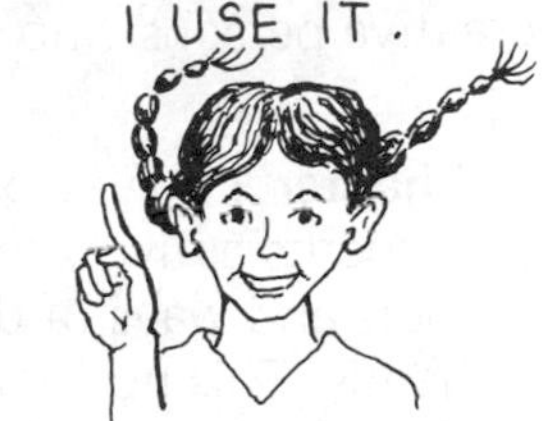

This part of the book gives ideas for bringing learning to life. It suggests ways to make learning more meaningful, useful, and adventurous.

To be effective, health education must be practical. **Health workers need to learn skills that help them observe, understand, and explore ways to improve the life and health of their people.**

An effective training program puts emphasis on these three ways of learning:

1. **Observation:** encouraging students to look at things closely and fearlessly, and to ask searching questions.
2. **Understanding:** helping students learn to analyze problems critically and work together toward finding appropriate solutions.
3. **Action:** students and instructors learn together through experience and practice.

Put simply, observation, understanding, and action mean ***seeing, thinking,*** and ***doing.*** Unfortunately, many training programs do little to encourage students to think. They focus on memorizing facts and carrying out specific instructions. Even standard teaching aids tend to demonstrate information rather than help students discover answers for themselves. Students learn to follow directions (or sometimes flow charts) step by step, without having to think or make decisions. Their training is oriented toward 'performing tasks' rather than 'solving problems'.

Such a mechanical, not-quite-fully-human approach to learning may be a suitable way to train animals—but not people! It can turn students into typical civil servants. They may carry out their duties obediently (or they may become careless or corrupt). But they will probably not become leaders of the poor in their struggle to overcome the biggest causes of ill health.

The human mind is made to think and explore. It grows stronger with exercise. But it grows weak, lazy, or resentful when limited to 'clearly defined tasks'.

If health workers are to become leaders who will defend the interests of the poor, their training must help them learn to use the tools best suited for this purpose.

The best tool a person has for understanding and changing the conditions that affect his world is the human mind. Health workers must be prepared to analyze problems, take initiative, and search for the ways of doing things that will help people meet their needs. Training should encourage people to think!

Part Two includes more than just 'teaching aids'. It is a collection of suggestions and methods to help equip students (and instructors) to be thinking, questioning, creative persons who can work intelligently to deal with their communities' needs.

Chapter 11 gives examples of teaching methods and aids that help get the students actively involved. It explores techniques that let students discover new facts and ways of doing things for themselves—using their own minds and hands. This not only helps students remember what they learn, but prepares them to take initiative in solving still bigger problems they will face in their own villages or communities.

Chapter 12 looks at ways of making and using pictures—valuable skills that help health workers share what they know with others. Both drawings and photos are considered.

Chapter 13 discusses ways that story telling can be used as a tool for teaching. It gives examples of spoken stories and stories told with drawings, filmstrips, and comic strips.

Chapter 14 explores role playing and 'sociodrama' as ways of bringing learning closer to the lives, feelings, and needs of real people. (Examples are also found in Chapter 27.)

Chapters 15 and 16 explore inappropriate and appropriate technologies—both 'soft technology' (methods and ideas) and 'hard technology' (things to make and use). We consider appropriate those ideas, methods, and tools that are controlled and understood by the people who need and use them. Chapter 16 looks at homemade, low-cost equipment, as well as appropriate ways of writing and copying written materials.

Chapter 17 looks at ways to help health workers take a thoughtful, organized approach to solving problems. We call this 'scientific method'.

Chapter 18 examines the problem of overuse and misuse of medicines, both by medical professionals and by people in general. It discusses ideas for helping health workers and other people to use medicines more sensibly.

Chapter 19 follows up on Chapters 11 and 18. It gives examples of imaginative teaching aids for learning how to use antibiotics intelligently, and for understanding the measurement of blood pressure. Blood pressure is discussed in detail, as this is an important skill for health workers in many communities, yet is not covered in ***Where There Is No Doctor.***

CHAPTER 11

Making and Using Teaching Aids

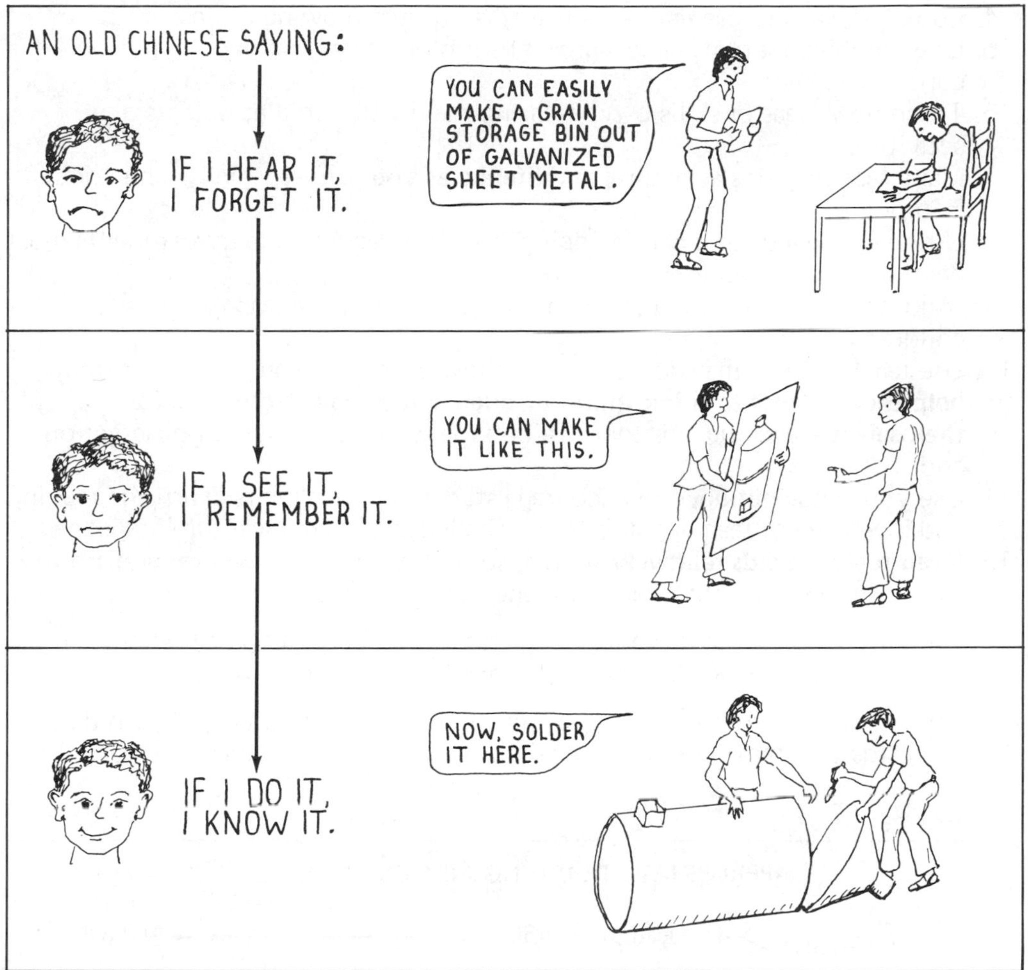
AN OLD CHINESE SAYING:
IF I HEAR IT, I FORGET IT.
YOU CAN EASILY MAKE A GRAIN STORAGE BIN OUT OF GALVANIZED SHEET METAL.
IF I SEE IT, I REMEMBER IT.
YOU CAN MAKE IT LIKE THIS.
IF I DO IT, I KNOW IT.
NOW, SOLDER IT HERE.

We all learn best when we take an active part in finding out things that are new to us!

- A class in which we **take part in discussions** is more interesting than a class in which we just listen to a lecture.
- A class in which we can **see for ourselves** what things look like and how they work, is more interesting than a class in which we only talk about things.
- A class in which we not only talk and see, but actually **do and make and discover things** for ourselves, is exciting! When we learn by finding things out for ourselves, by building on experience we already have, we do not forget. What we learn through active discovery becomes a part of us.

GUIDELINES FOR APPROPRIATE TEACHING AIDS

Whenever possible:

1. **Make your own teaching aids,** using low-cost local materials.
2. When making teaching aids, **use and build on skills students already have.**
3. Try not to make the aids *for* the students, but rather **involve students** or members of the community in making them for themselves.
4. Look for ways to **use real objects** instead of just drawing things.
5. Draw human anatomy (and signs of health problems) on people, not on paper.
6. Teach new ideas or skills by comparing them with familiar objects or activities.
7. **Make teaching aids as natural and lifelike as you can,** especially when detail is important.
8. Use teaching aids that call for doing as well as seeing—aids that students must handle or put together.
9. Make them as fascinating or fun as possible, especially teaching aids for children.
10. Use teaching aids that do not simply show or explain something, but that **help the students to think things through and discover solutions for themselves**—teaching aids that exercise the learners' powers of observation and reason.
11. **Use your imagination,** and encourage students to use theirs. Turn the making and inventing of teaching aids into a challenge and an adventure.
12. **Keep teaching aids relatively simple,** so that when health workers return to their communities, they can make their own and teach others.

In summary: Create and use teaching aids that help develop self-reliance in both acting and thinking—in helping persons find things out for themselves.

In this chapter, we give detailed examples of these 12 points, and then discuss teaching aids that make use of flannel-boards, flip charts, puzzles, and games.

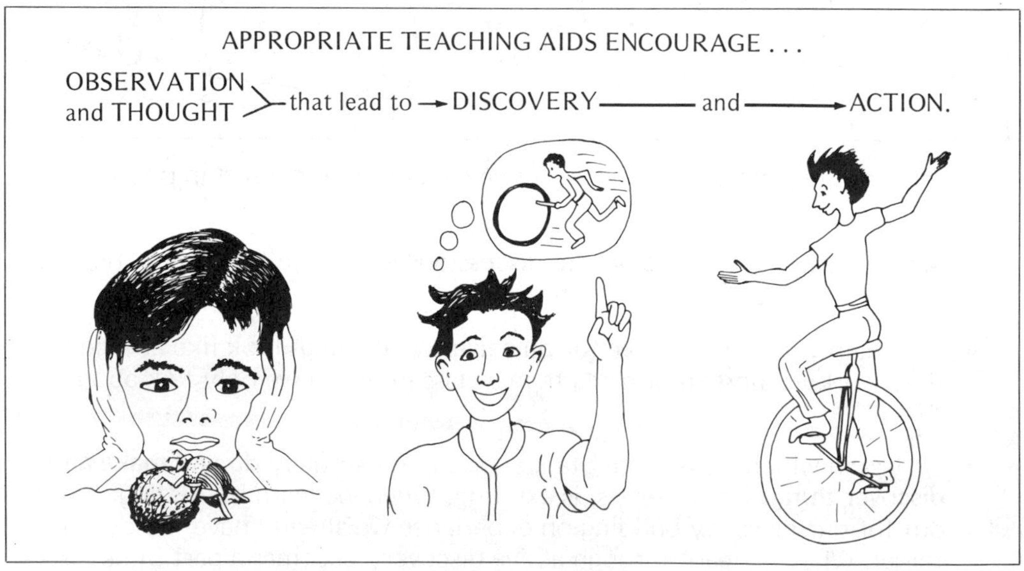

APPROPRIATE TEACHING AIDS ENCOURAGE . . .
OBSERVATION
and THOUGHT
that lead to
DISCOVERY
and
ACTION.

1. MAKING YOUR OWN TEACHING AIDS FROM LOW-COST MATERIALS

Example: **Learning about childbirth**

LESS APPROPRIATE

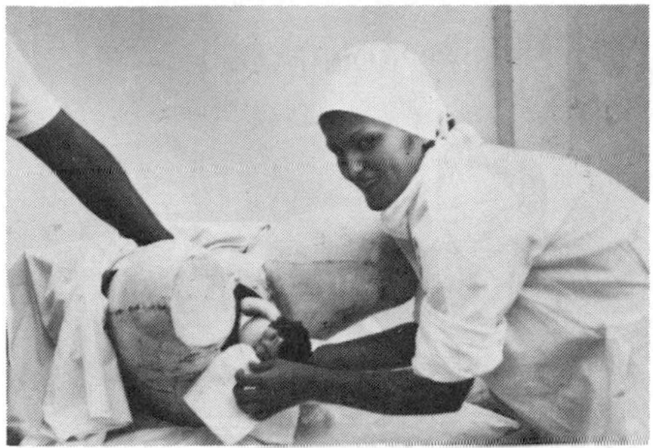

Some programs use an expensive plastic model of a woman's hips to teach health workers or midwives about childbirth. Although such models look natural and are easy to practice with, they are not something health workers can make in their villages to teach local people. (photo from Venezuela)

MORE APPROPRIATE

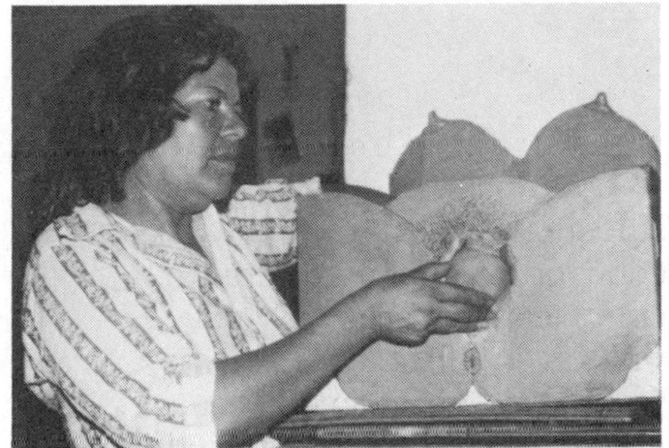

A surprisingly lifelike model for teaching about childbirth can be made by cutting and painting a cardboard box. Health workers or midwives can make this 'birth box' at almost no cost. The back flap, cut to look like breasts, is used to teach the importance of putting the baby to the breast right after birth. This helps to deliver the placenta and reduce bleeding.

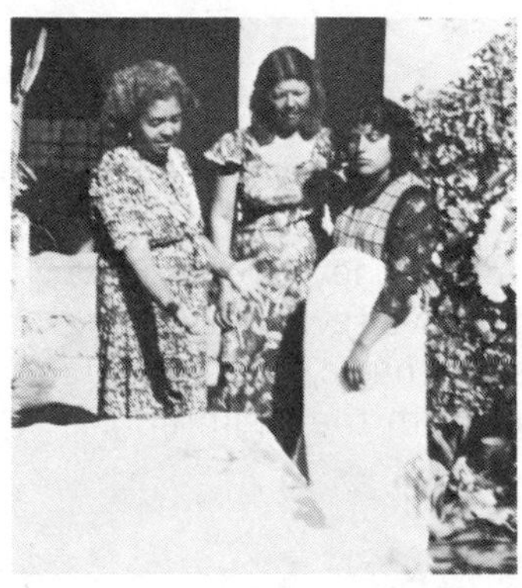

STILL MORE APPROPRIATE

In these photos, student health workers and a midwife act out a birth. (Mexico)

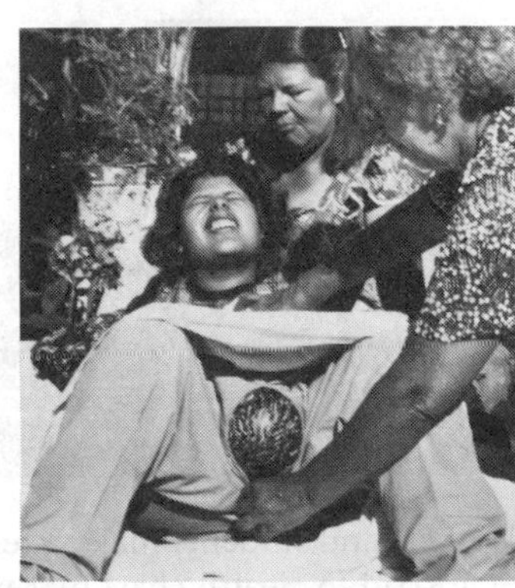

Teaching about birth can become even more lifelike with the use of two local resources: a student and a pair of old pants. The student dresses like a woman about to give birth, and has a doll 'baby' hidden in her clothing. The pants are cut to form a 'birth opening'. The student wears other pants underneath to avoid embarrassment. If possible, sew elastic around the opening so it will stretch.

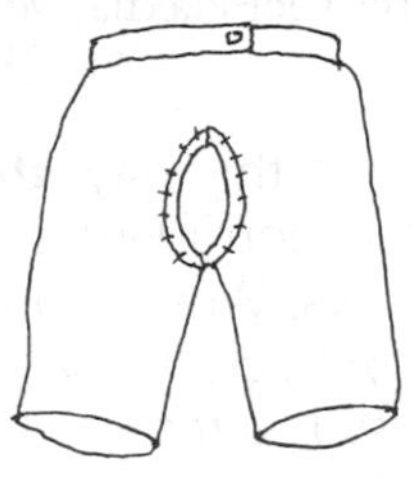

In this way, the students can explore the hope, fear, pain, and joy of childbirth. They learn about the mother's feelings, as well as the mechanics of delivery. By using real people, students learn to feel more relaxed about this natural process. (For more ideas for learning about childbirth, see p. **22**-8 and **22**-9.)

2. MAKING TEACHING AIDS BY BUILDING ON SKILLS PEOPLE ALREADY HAVE

Example: **Making a large Road to Health chart for a flannel-board**

LESS APPROPRIATE

If mothers, midwives, or students with little formal education are asked to draw a complicated chart, they may find it very difficult. They may feel foolish or ashamed because drawing charts is something they have never done before.

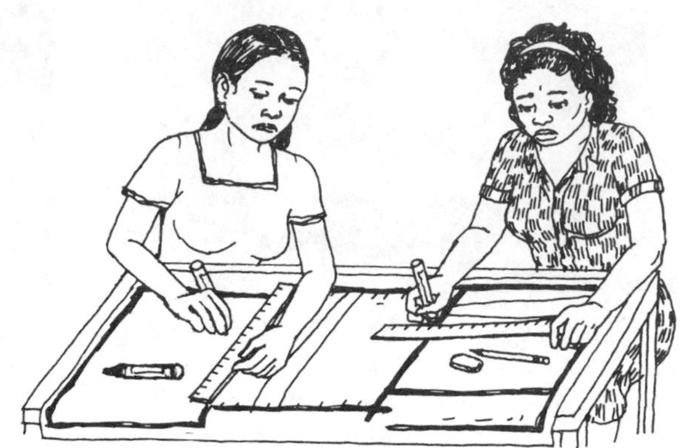

Mothers who have had little schooling try to draw a large teaching model of a Road to Health chart (see *WTND*, p. 299).

MORE APPROPRIATE

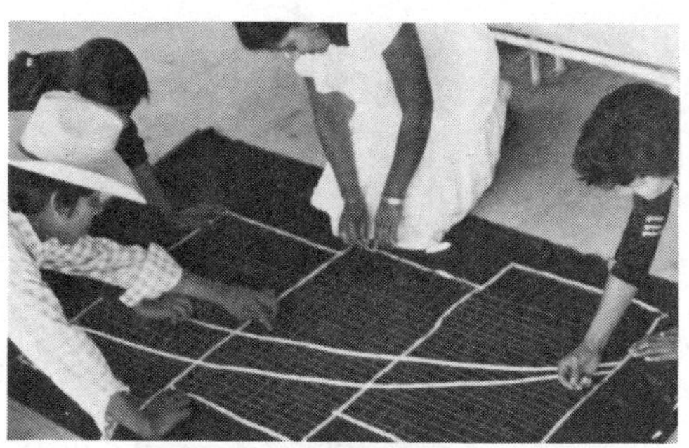

Mothers and students make a teaching model of a Road to Health chart by sewing ribbons and threads onto a big piece of flannel. (Project Piaxtla, Mexico)

Here, however, some mothers and students are making a chart by sewing rather than drawing the lines. Because they are using a skill they already have and enjoy (decorative sewing), some of the strangeness, or magic, is taken out of chart making from the beginning.

In this way, **the students develop a new skill by building on an old one.** They feel confident and proud to put their traditions and knowledge to use in new ways. Where you live, people may be skilled in weaving straw mats or cloth, dying cloth (batik), or carving wood. Any of these traditional skills could be used to make a large teaching model of a Road to Health chart. (In some regions, of course, people may have more experience in drawing. In that case, it would make more sense to draw the chart.)

For ideas about using the flannel-board Road to Health chart, see p. **22**-15.

3. INVOLVING STUDENTS IN MAKING THEIR OWN TEACHING AIDS

Example: **Health posters**

LESS APPROPRIATE–
poster made by outside artist

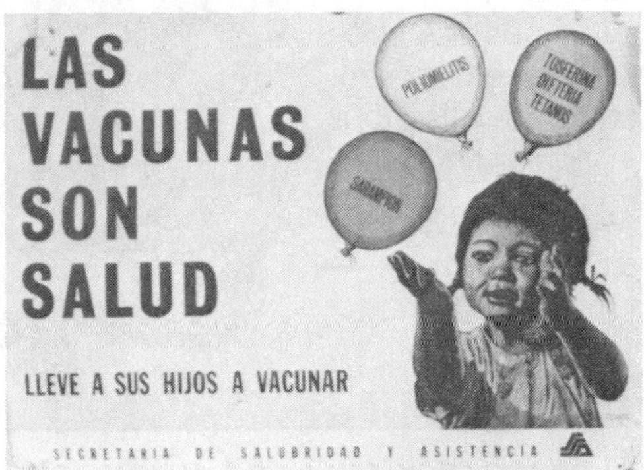

Many programs use posters made by professional artists when drawings by health workers and other local persons might work as well and involve people more.

MORE APPROPRIATE–
poster made by outside artist

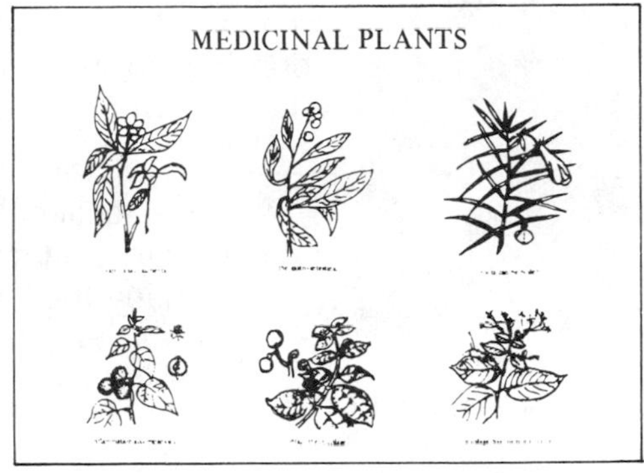

However, it may make sense to use some professionally made posters and displays, especially when details are important.

Instructors or a local artist can help students learn to draw or copy pictures (see p. **12**-9). The health workers can then help school children to make posters about health subjects. The best posters can be displayed in public. This way, the health workers and the children learn the messages of the posters extra well. They also learn a valuable skill—drawing—and have fun at the same time.

MORE APPROPRIATE

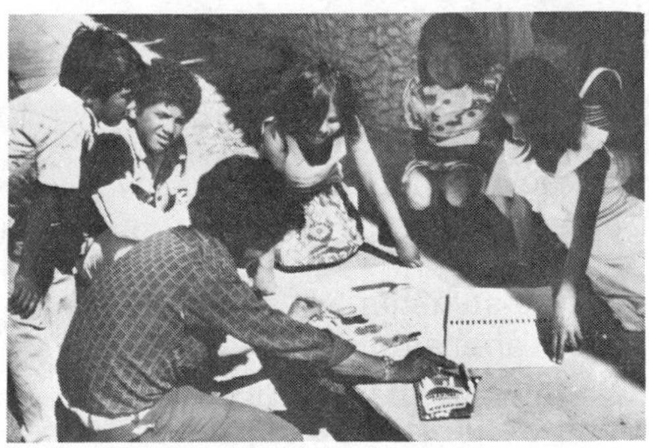

Health worker showing children how to make health posters.

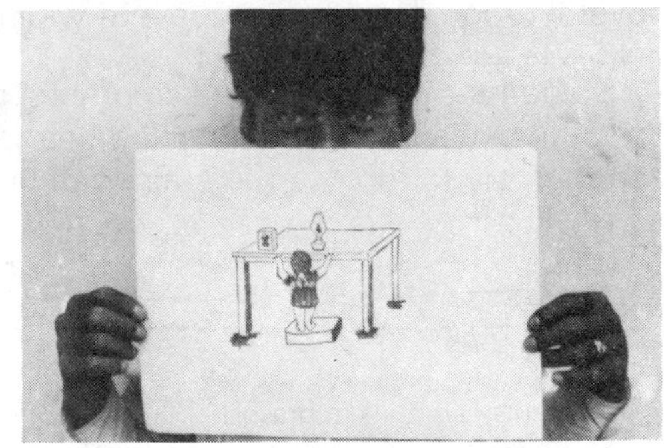

Poster made by school child.

For more ideas on making drawings and posters, see Chapter 12.

4. USING REAL PEOPLE OR OBJECTS INSTEAD OF JUST DRAWINGS

Example 1: **Snakebite**

LESS APPROPRIATE

MORE APPROPRIATE

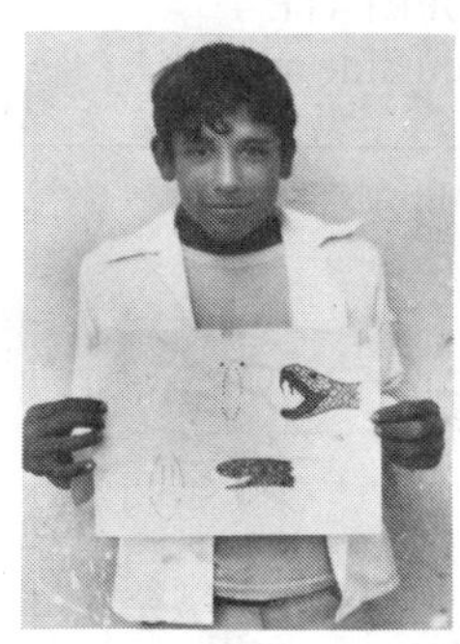

For the CHILD-to-child activity on preventing accidents (see p. **24**-7), a school teacher in Ajoya, Mexico used drawings to show the difference between the bites of poisonous and non-poisonous snakes.

But a local health worker drew red fang marks right on a child's arm. This made the lesson much clearer.

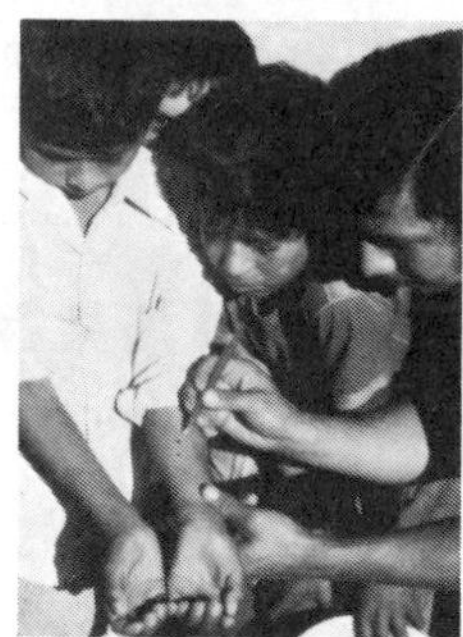

STILL MORE APPROPRIATE

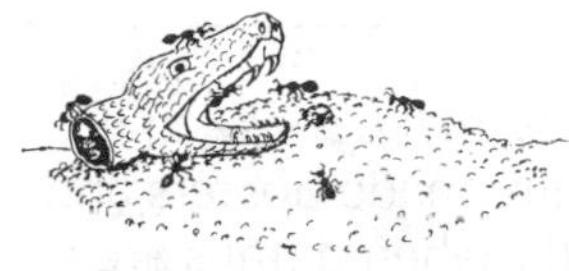

It is even better if you can show students the teeth of live snakes (be careful!) or the skulls. A skull can be cleaned of flesh by putting it on an ant hill for a day or so, and then soaking it in potash (water with ashes) or lye.

Example 2: **Learning about cleaning teeth**

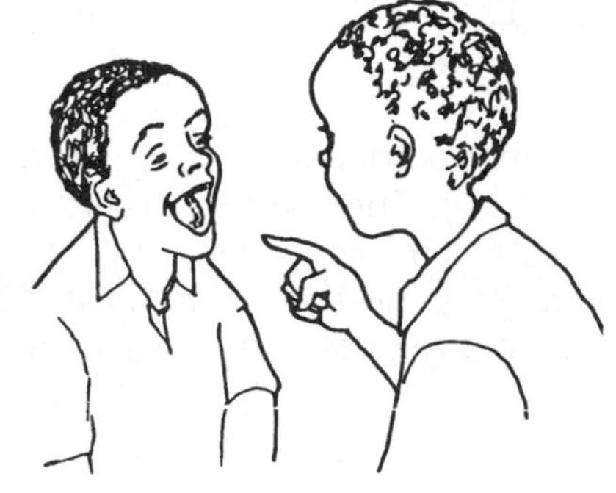

Instead of simply learning that germ colonies, called plaque, form on teeth and gums, students can actually see where the plaque is and learn the best way to remove it with a simple experiment.

Students can gather in pairs or groups and color their teeth with an ordinary household food dye (or try betel nut or berry juice). It can be applied with a clean cloth, or simply by putting several drops onto the tongue and wiping the tongue around the teeth.

Students then look into each others' mouths or into a mirror to see where the staining is heaviest. It will be heaviest where the plaque is heaviest. They can then try to remove the stain with brushes, chewing sticks, or using any other local method.

Students can make a brushstick like this one, using the twig of a tree in their area. The teeth can be sharpened with one end and brushed with the other (***WTND,*** p.230).

The students will also see what teeth are hard to clean and what teeth need the most cleaning to remove the stains and plaque. They can also learn which ways of cleaning work best by checking others' teeth and comparing the different cleaning methods.

For some students one method will work best, for others a different one will work best to clean teeth and remove plaque.

5. DRAWING PARTS OF THE BODY (AND SIGNS OF HEALTH PROBLEMS) ON PEOPLE, NOT PAPER

Example: **Anatomy of the belly or chest**

LESS APPROPRIATE

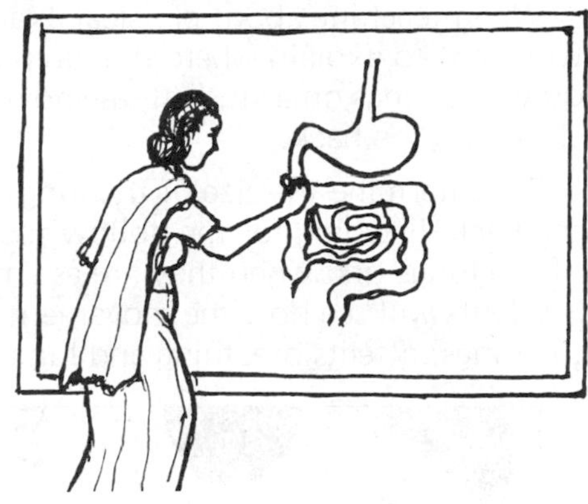

Drawing anatomy on paper or on the blackboard makes things not only flat, but dull.

MORE APPROPRIATE

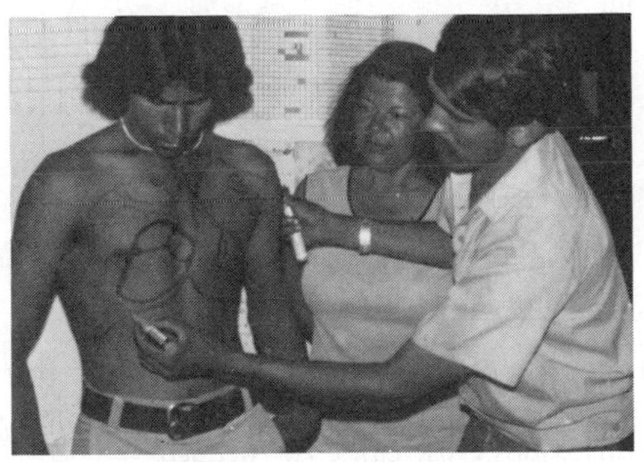

Whenever possible draw on people, not paper.

Drawing the inner parts or organs of the body directly on a person has 3 advantages:

- It is more interesting, and therefore easier to remember.
- The organs are seen in relation to the rest of the body and appear more lifelike.
- It is a good way to get students to feel more comfortable about touching and examining each other—and eventually a sick person.

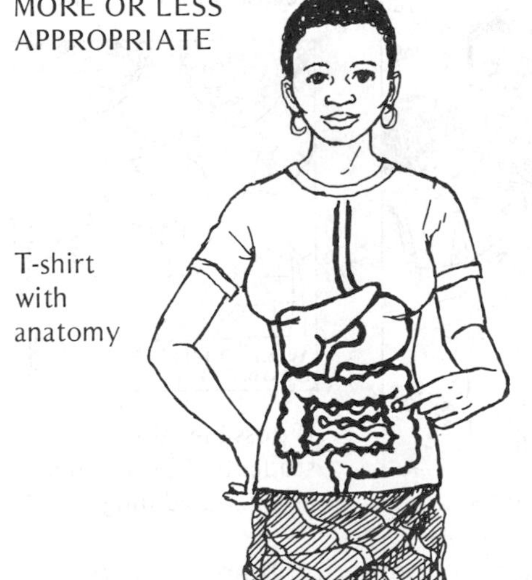

One disadvantage of drawing on people in class is that it takes time.

A quicker way is to use T-shirts with drawings of different body systems already on them: one for the digestive system, one for the bones, one for the heart and blood system, and so on.

T-shirts with anatomy printed on them can be purchased in some countries. But these may be expensive and more detailed than you need. It is better to draw or paint the anatomy on T-shirts with your student group. You can even try 'silk screening' them using the method described on page **16**-12.

6. TEACHING NEW SKILLS OR IDEAS BY COMPARING THEM WITH THINGS THAT ARE FAMILIAR

Example: **Thumping (percussing) the lungs**

When teaching about physical exam or respiratory problems, you probably will want to explain where the lungs are and how they work. For this, it helps to draw the lungs on a student, as shown on page **11**-7. Draw them on both the chest and the back.

To determine the size of the lungs, show students how to thump or *percuss* the back, listening for the hollow sound of air in the lungs. Draw the bottom line of the lungs first when they are as empty as possible, and then when they are full. Students will see how the movement of the *diaphragm* (a muscular sheet below the lungs) affects breathing and lung size (also see p. **11**-13).

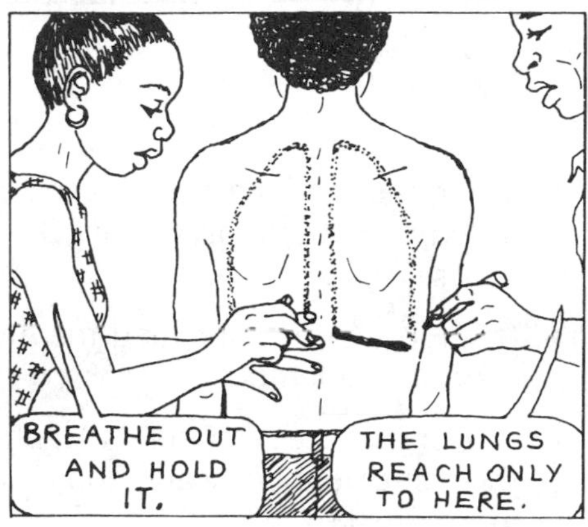

BREATHE OUT AND HOLD IT.
THE LUNGS REACH ONLY TO HERE.

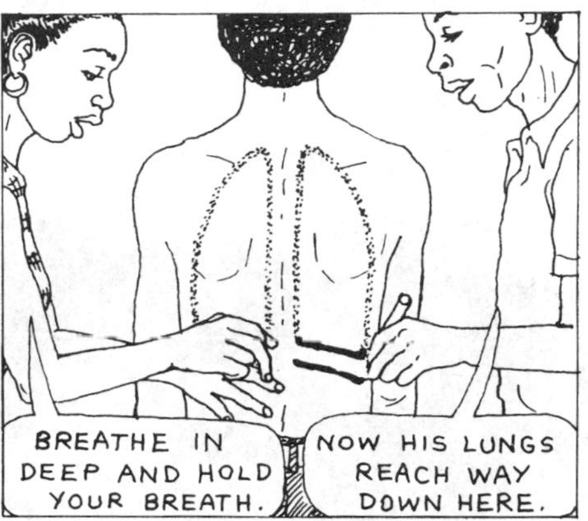

BREATHE IN DEEP AND HOLD YOUR BREATH.
NOW HIS LUNGS REACH WAY DOWN HERE.

By doing this, students not only learn about the position, size, and work of the lungs, they also learn a useful skill for physical examination—thumping the lungs to listen for relative hollowness. This can help them spot signs of disease.

To help students understand the different sounds they hear when thumping, have them determine the level of water (or gasoline) in a large drum or barrel.

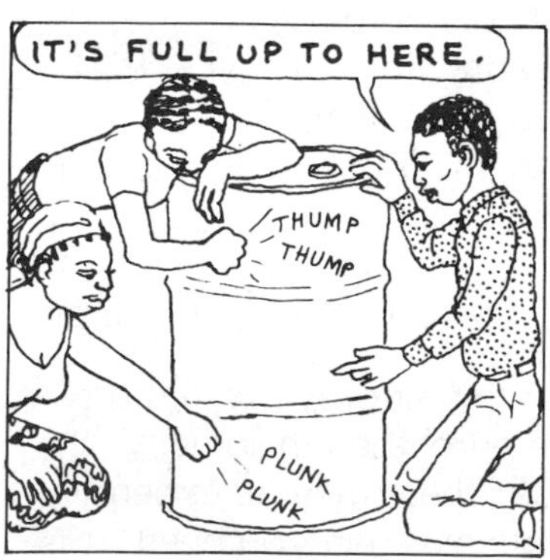

Then thump the chest of a student.

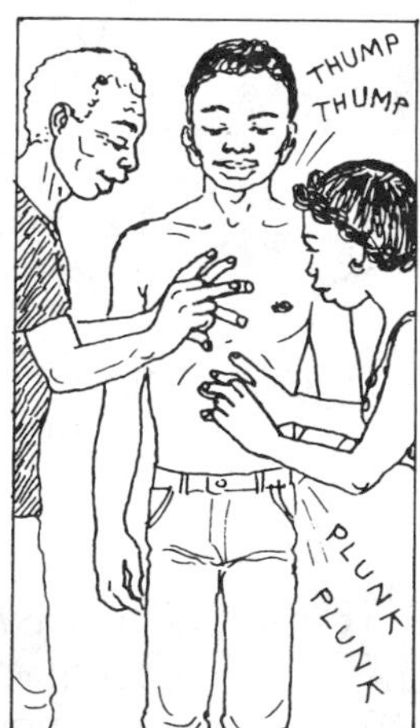

Next, compare with a person who has a solid (diseased) area or liquid in a lung.

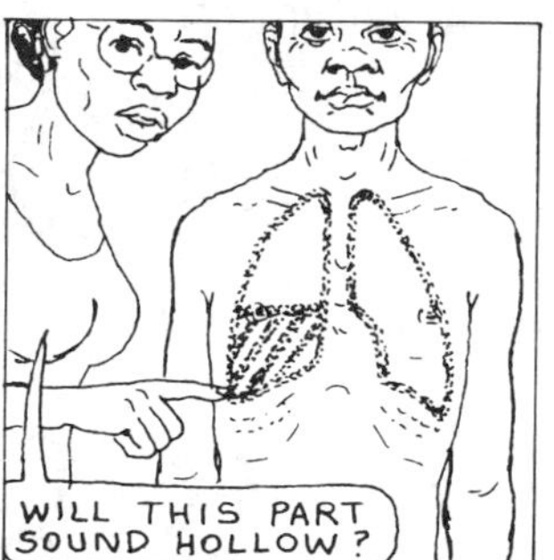

WILL THIS PART SOUND HOLLOW?

If possible, also show the students X-rays of normal and diseased lungs.

For other examples of teaching new things by comparing them with something familiar, see 'how flies spread germs', p. **7**-11; the story from India, p. **13**-1; and the use of plants and fruit to teach about dehydration, p. **24**-19.

7. MAKING TEACHING AIDS AS LIFELIKE AS POSSIBLE

Example: **The belly wrinkle test**

APPROPRIATE (A DRAWING)

When teaching mothers and children about the signs of dehydration, health workers can tell them about the 'belly wrinkle test', or even show drawings like this:

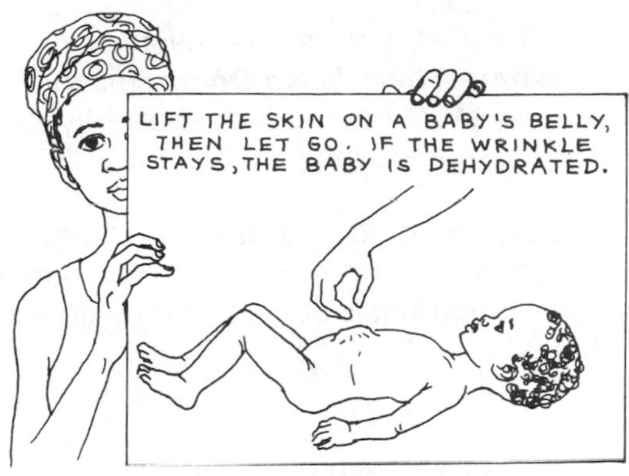

It is much better, however, if students actually **do** the test and find out how it works.

Students can practice doing the test on the back of someone's hand. (The hand of an older person works better than the hand of a child.)

MORE APPROPRIATE (ACTUALLY DOING IT)

In this position, wrinkles will not stay after the skin is pinched.

Pinch here. Wrinkles disappear.

This is like the skin on the belly of a healthy baby.

But in this position, the pinched skin stays wrinkled for a moment—just as on the belly of a dehydrated child.

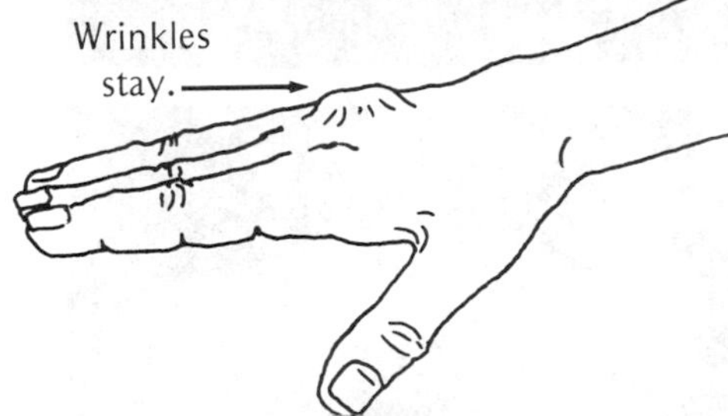

This is like the skin on the belly of a dehydrated baby.

When you show the belly wrinkle test to children, make sure they realize that the test should be done on the belly of a baby, not on the hand. You can have the children make a doll like this, out of an old glove or stocking and an egg.

STILL MORE APPROPRIATE

When the 'belly' is pinched, the wrinkle stays.

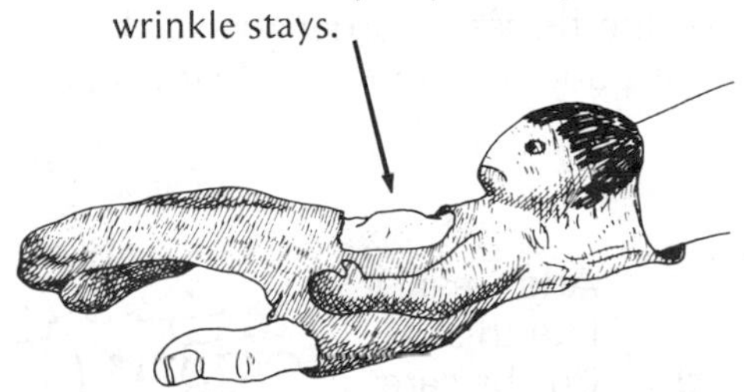

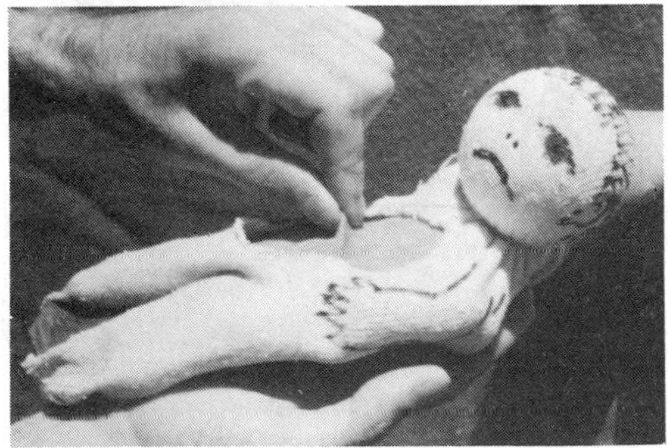

Using a doll like this makes the test more realistic. It also turns learning into a game.

8. TEACHING AIDS THAT REQUIRE DOING AS WELL AS SEEING

Example: **Closing a cut or wound**

The poster at right is adapted from a drawing in ***Where There Is No Doctor*** (p. 85). It shows, step by step, how to make butterfly bandages and close a wound.

But it does not, by itself, give students a chance to learn through practice. Students see how something is done, but they do not actually do it.

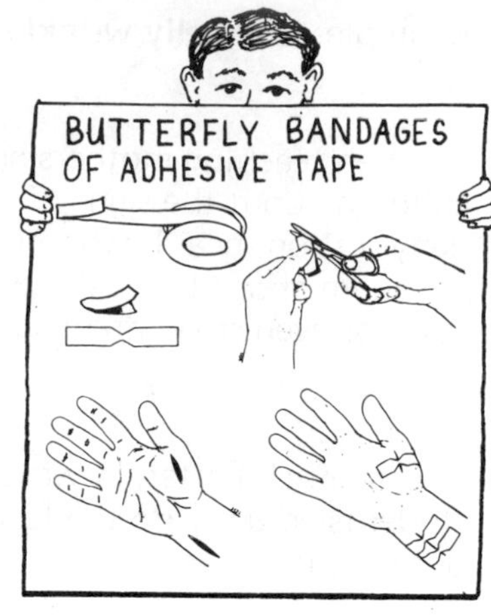

LESS APPROPRIATE

MORE APPROPRIATE

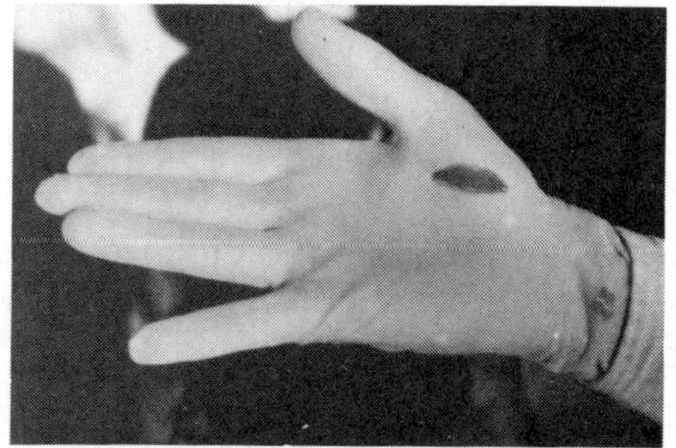

A lifelike way to practice closing wounds is to have someone wear a tight-fitting rubber (surgical) glove. Make a cut in the glove, and color the skin under the cut red to make it look like blood.

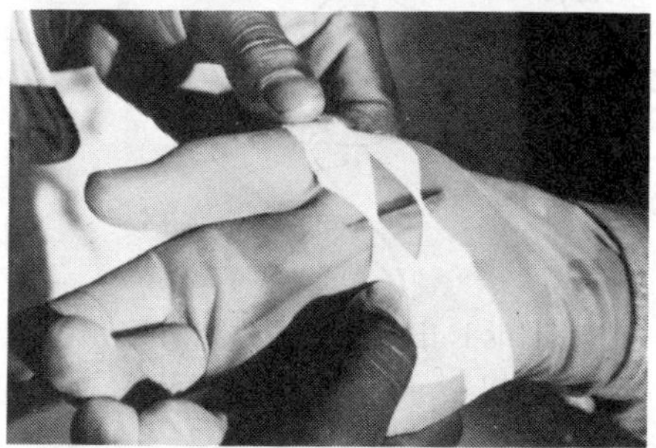

The rubber glove tends to stretch and pull apart like real skin. The students can prepare butterfly bandages and close the 'wound' by pulling the sides of the cut together.

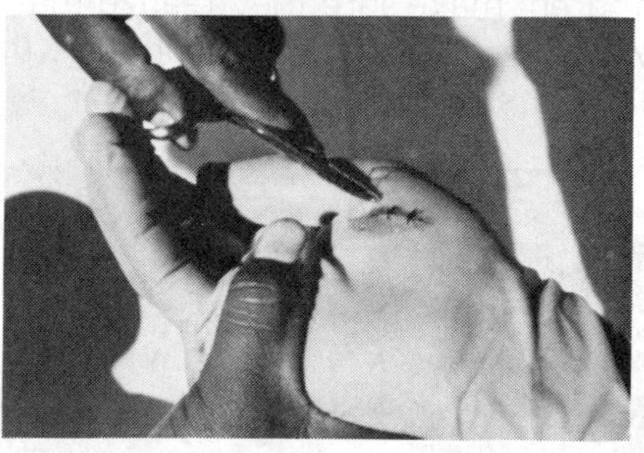

The students can also practice sewing or suturing a wound using the same rubber glove. As with a real wound, care must be taken with the placement and tension (pull) of the thread in order to avoid tearing or bunching up the delicate 'skin'.

If you do not have surgical gloves, try using a large balloon. Cut holes for the fingers, like this.

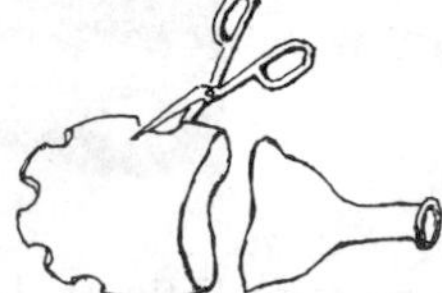

And wear it like this. But be careful. It tears easily.

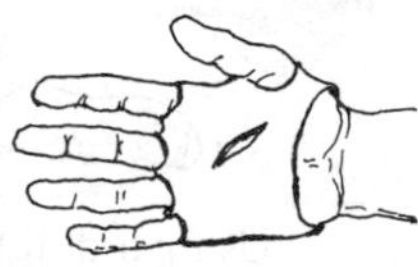

A common mistake when suturing wounds is to make the stitches too shallow. If the wound is not completely closed inside, it heals more slowly and is more likely to become infected.

WRONG

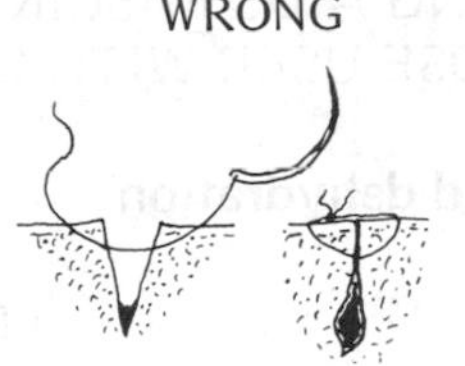

RIGHT

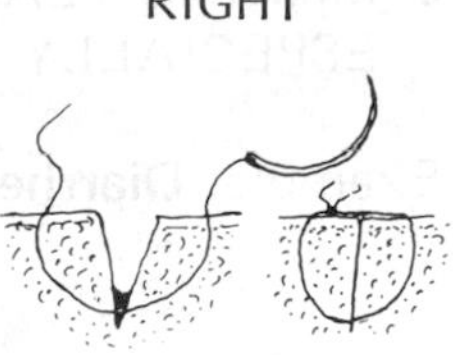

EVEN MORE APPROPRIATE

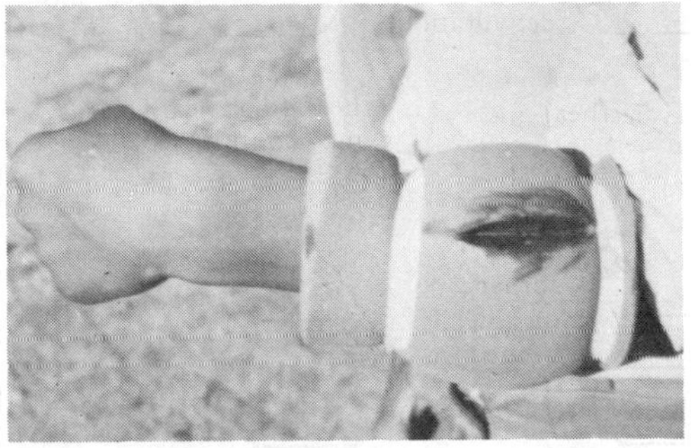

Foam rubber helps students learn how deep to sew stitches.

Unfortunately, the rubber glove teaching aid does not let students practice deep suturing. A better teaching aid for this can be made by wrapping a piece of foam rubber or thick felt around someone's arm. Make a deep cut in the foam and color it red.

STILL MORE APPROPRIATE

Students will learn even better if they can practice on real wounds. It is, of course, best if they do not practice on people until they have gained some skill. Try to use freshly killed animals—especially pigs.

(In the Philippines, health workers make cuts and practice suturing on live dogs. But this also teaches them that cruelty can sometimes be justified. Do you think this is right?)

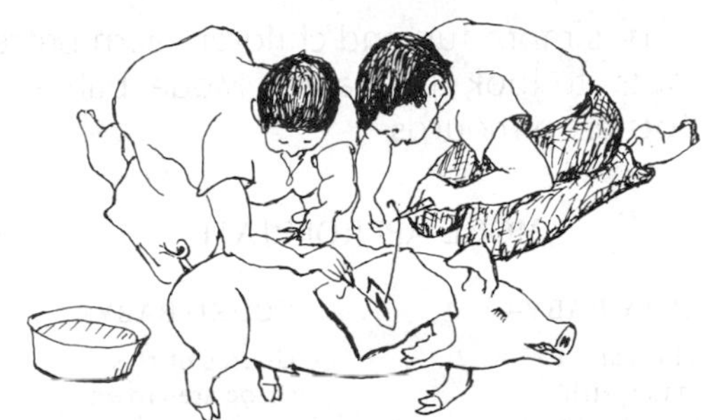

Students practice closing a wound on a dead pig.

MOST APPROPRIATE (after learning the skill through other practice)

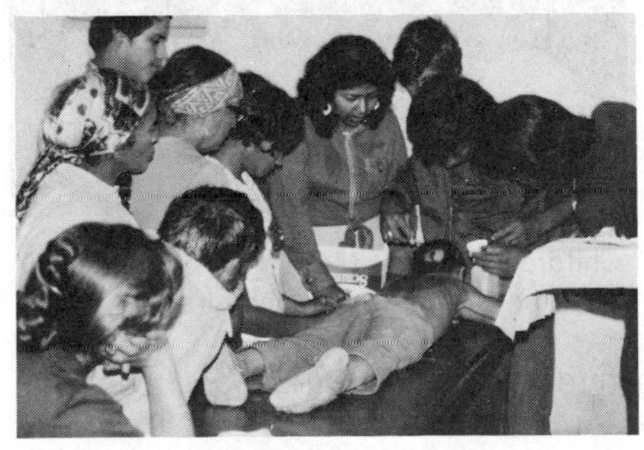

After students have had plenty of practice, they should be given every opportunity to close real human wounds—even if this sometimes means interrupting a class.

In this photo, student health workers are helping to close the head wound of a boy hit by a rock.

(Ajoya, Mexico)

9. MAKING TEACHING AIDS FASCINATING AND FUN—ESPECIALLY THOSE USED WITH CHILDREN

Example: **Diarrhea and dehydration**

LESS APPROPRIATE

Drawings like these contain important ideas. But children, especially, may have trouble understanding them. Also, they are not much fun—even when actual pots are used along with the drawings.

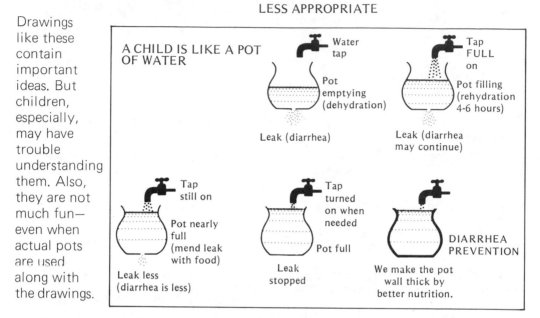

A CHILD IS LIKE A POT OF WATER

Water tap

Pot emptying (dehydration)

Leak (diarrhea)

Tap FULL on

Pot filling (rehydration 4-6 hours)

Leak (diarrhea may continue)

Tap still on

Pot nearly full (mend leak with food)

Leak less (diarrhea is less)

Tap turned on when needed

Pot full

Leak stopped

DIARRHEA PREVENTION

We make the pot wall thick by better nutrition.

It is more fun and children learn better if they can make or paint their own 'pots' to look like babies. Model babies can be made out of clay, tin cans, plastic bottles, or gourds.

MORE APPROPRIATE

CLAY BABY—

This can be made with the help of mothers who make their own pottery.

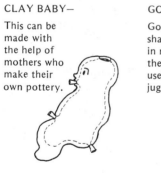

GOURD BABY—

Gourds of this shape are grown in many parts of the world for use as water jugs.

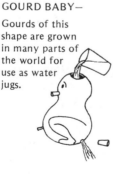

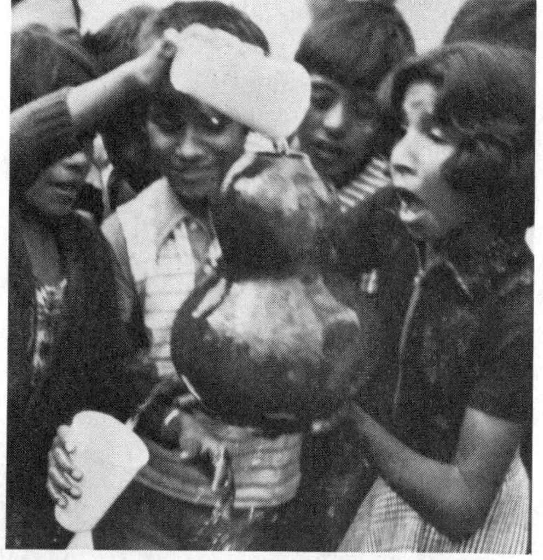

Children in Ajoya, Mexico use a gourd baby to demonstrate signs of dehydration.

The children then experiment with the model baby to find out about dehydration. Because they make their own teaching aid and discover answers for themselves, learning becomes an adventure. It is fun and they never forget what they learn.

For more ideas on how to teach about dehydration using these model babies, see page **24**-18.

10. USING TEACHING AIDS THAT GET STUDENTS TO FIGURE THINGS OUT FOR THEMSELVES

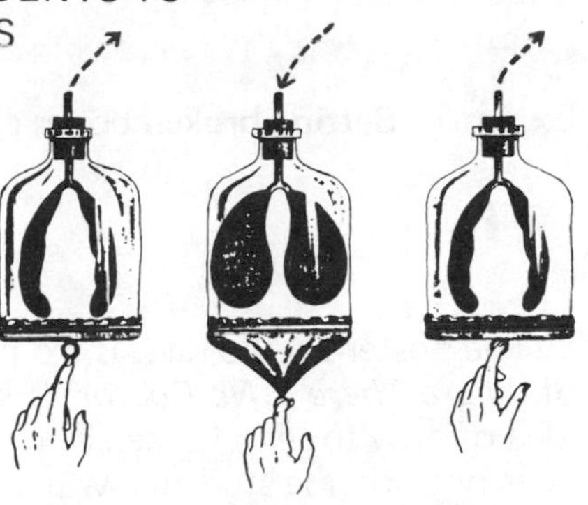

Example 1: **Learning about injuries to the chest and lungs**

The pictures to the right are taken from a popular Venezuelan health magazine called *Ser.* They show how the movement of the *diaphragm* (the muscular sheet below the lungs) helps the lungs fill with air.

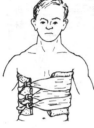

In the mountains of Mexico, gunshot and knife wounds to the chest are common. If air is being sucked through the wound when the person breathes, the hole should be covered at once with an air-tight bandage. (See ***WTND,*** p. 91). To help students discover why this is important, the instructors in Ajoya designed a teaching aid based on the idea shown above.

1. They drilled a small hole in a glass bottle (using a dental drill).
2. They put a balloon in the bottle and blew it up. Then they plugged the hole with wax.
3. They asked the students to pretend the bottle was a man's chest and the balloon his lung. The students were amazed that the balloon stayed full of air although it was open at the top. (They discovered the principle of the vacuum.)
4. To show why it is important to cover a chest wound at once, a student slowly sucked the air out of the bottle until the 'lung' filled up again. (In the body, the air is slowly absorbed.)

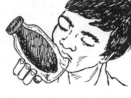

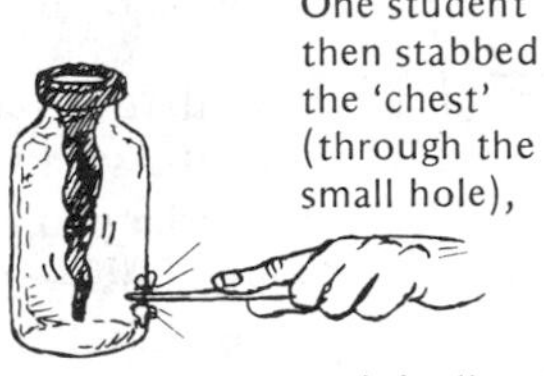

One student then stabbed the 'chest' (through the small hole),

and the 'lung' inside collapsed.

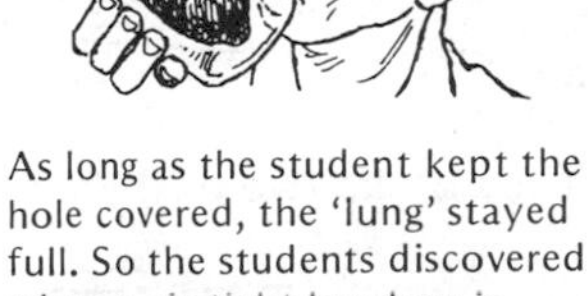

As long as the student kept the hole covered, the 'lung' stayed full. So the students discovered why an air-tight bandage is important.

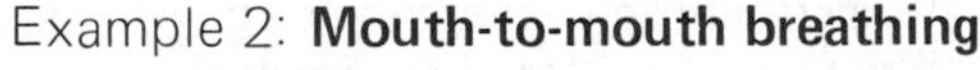

Example 2: **Mouth-to-mouth breathing**

Students can use the following model to find out how mouth-to-mouth breathing works and practice doing it.

Cut holes in a plastic bottle, like this or like this.

Paint it to look like a head.

Use a piece of old bicycle inner tube to attach it to a cow's bladder or a plastic bag.

One person gives mouth-to-mouth breathing while another presses on the 'chest' as it rises and falls.

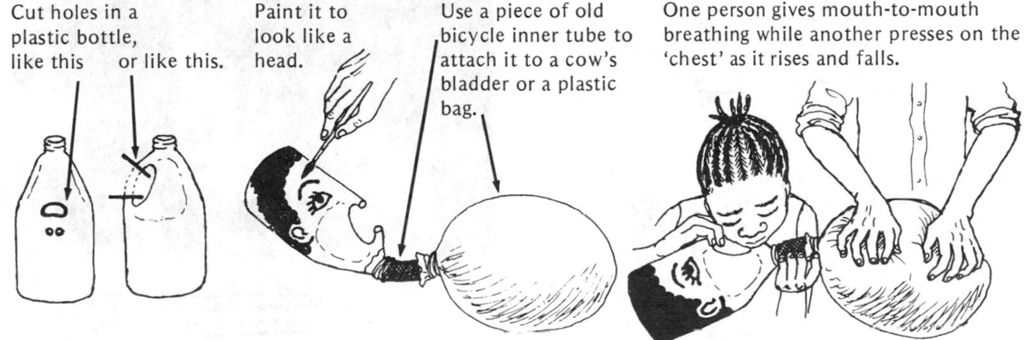

A still better way to learn about mouth-to-mouth breathing, of course, is for students to practice on each other.

11. USING IMAGINATION TO DEVELOP NEW TEACHING AIDS

Example: **Setting broken bones**

LESS APPROPRIATE

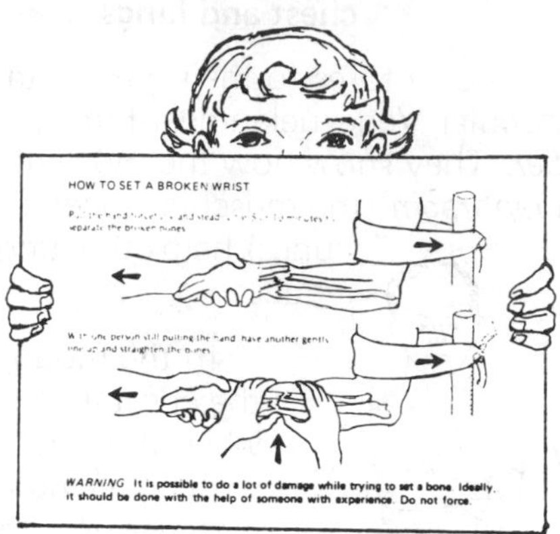

The poster on the right is from page 98 of ***Where There is No Doctor.*** It gives an idea of how to set a broken arm, but does not provide students with a chance to practice it—to learn by doing.

MORE APPROPRIATE

An experienced village health worker, Pablo Chavez, and his students invented the following teaching aid:

(1) They found an old glove, and three sticks about the size of arm bones.

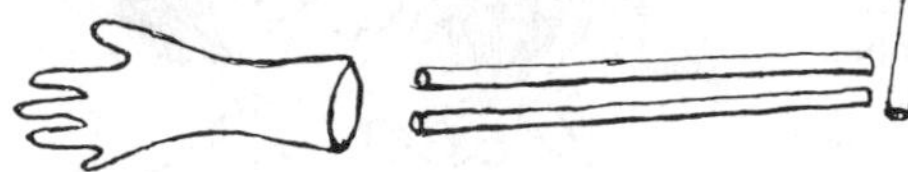

(2) They broke two of the sticks.

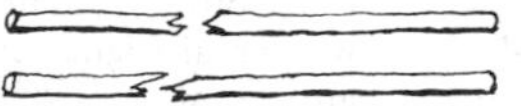

(3) Then they fastened them back together with tightly stretched pieces of an old inner tube (rubber).

(4) They put the sticks inside a stocking, and packed it with wild kapok to make an 'arm'.

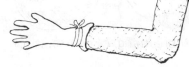

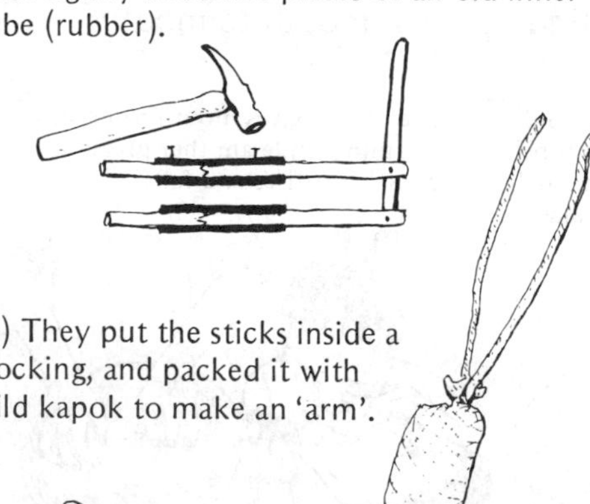

(5) The 'arm' was tied to a person's neck in such a way that it looked natural.

The 'arm' was then 'broken', like this

so that the ends of the sticks overlapped, like this

inside view

(6) Students then practiced setting the broken 'bones'. Just as with a real break, two persons had to stretch the arm while a third person positioned the bones.

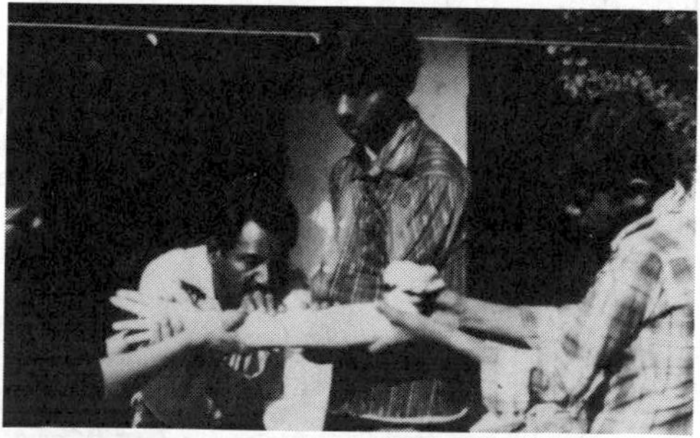

Pull apart,

then set 'bones'.

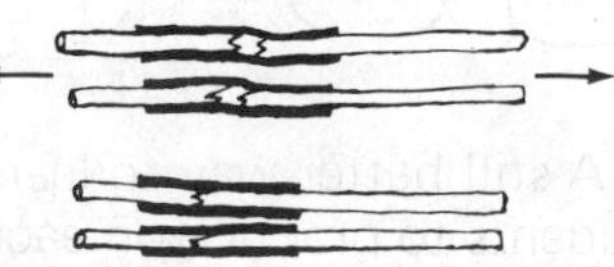

12. KEEPING TEACHING AIDS SIMPLE, SO THAT STUDENTS CAN MAKE THEIR OWN FOR TEACHING IN THEIR COMMUNITIES

Example: **Cardboard babies**

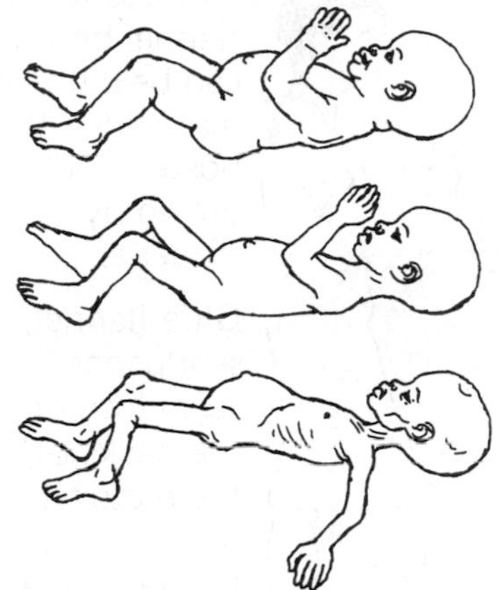

A set of life-size 'babies' cut out of cardboard can be used for teaching many things in many ways.

The 'babies' should be drawn and colored to look as lifelike as possible. If students find it hard to draw realistically, they can copy or trace the program's teaching models.

Ways of using the cardboard babies:

(1) **On flannel-boards.** You can paste flannel on the backs of the cardboard babies, and use them for many different flannel-board presentations. Here the babies are shown with different kinds of worms. The worms and the labels are also cut out of cardboard. (For other flannel-board ideas, see the Index.)

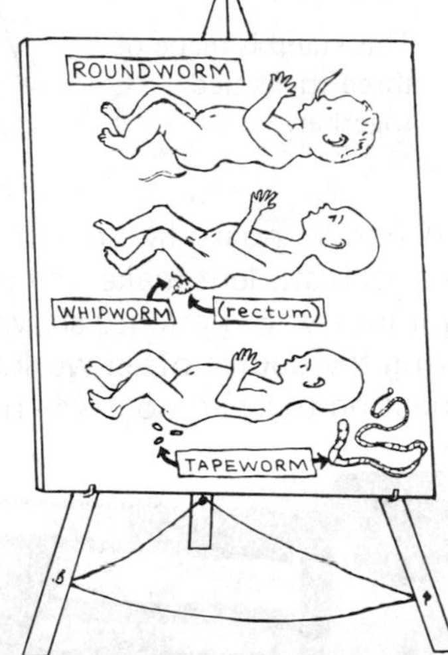

(2) **In role playing.** For classroom learning, health workers can act out the diagnosis, treatment, and prevention of different health problems. The use of cardboard babies makes the role plays more fun and more realistic. (See Chapter 14.)

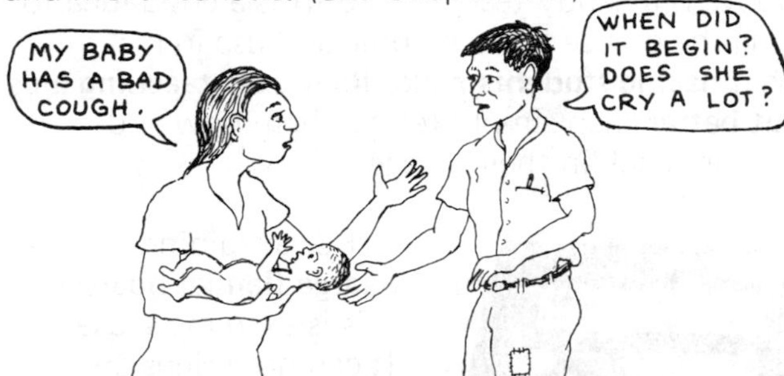

(3) **For public plays and farmers' theater.** The cardboard babies can be used on stage instead of real babies. See the play on "The Importance of Breast Feeding," page **27**-31.

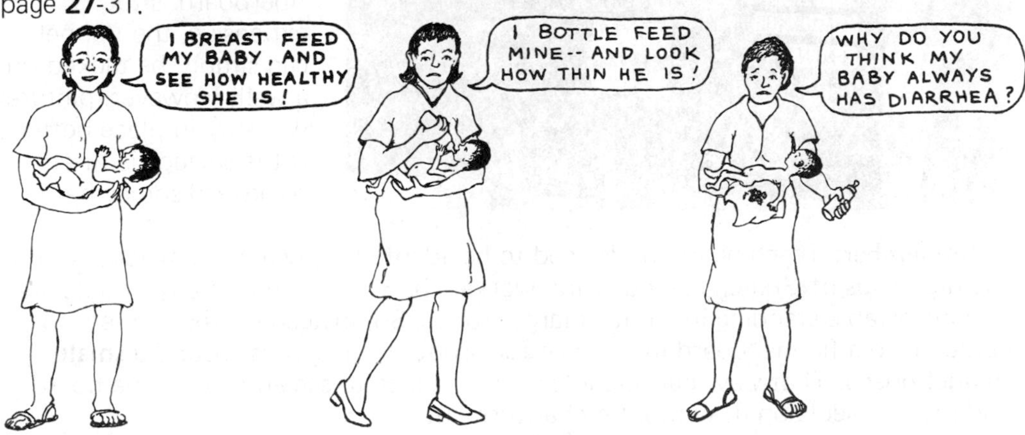
I BREAST FEED MY BABY, AND SEE HOW HEALTHY SHE IS!
I BOTTLE FEED MINE-- AND LOOK HOW THIN HE IS!
WHY DO YOU THINK MY BABY ALWAYS HAS DIARRHEA?

IDEAS FOR PRESENTING TEACHING AIDS

FLANNEL-BOARDS

A flannel-board is a display board on which you can easily place and remove pictures. It consists of:

- A frame with a firm surface made of boards, plywood, fiberboard, masonite, or strong cardboard.
- A large sheet of flannel or soft cloth stretched over the frame.
- Some sort of stand to hold it up (even a chair will do).

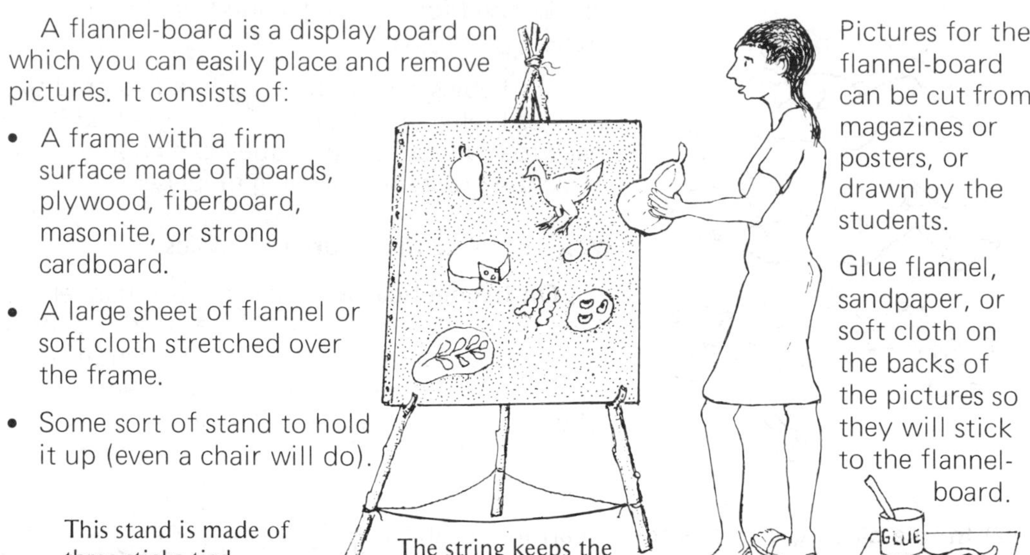

This stand is made of three sticks tied together.

The string keeps the legs from spreading too far apart.

Pictures for the flannel-board can be cut from magazines or posters, or drawn by the students.

Glue flannel, sandpaper, or soft cloth on the backs of the pictures so they will stick to the flannel-board.

A flannel-board like the one above is a handy teaching aid. It is a good idea to have each student make one during the course to take home and use in his community. Experience shows that **having students make their own teaching aids during the course often works out better** than simply telling them how and expecting them to do it when they are back in their villages.

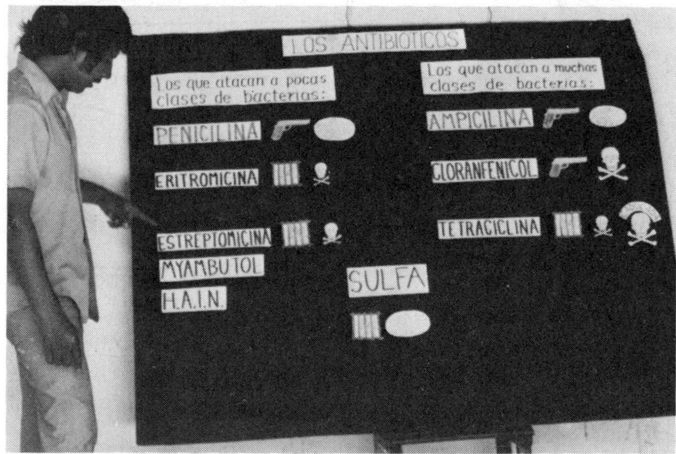

For a training program, a **large flannel-board** like this is extremely useful. It can hold signs and objects large enough for everyone to see clearly. If plywood, masonite, or fiberboard is too expensive, the flannel can simply be tacked on a wall. However, pictures will stay in place better if the surface is tilted backward somewhat.

Remember: Teaching methods need to be adapted to local circumstances. In the highlands of Guatemala, nutrition workers have found that many people are uncomfortable standing in front of large groups. So, instead of asking them to come up to a flannel-board in front of the group, leaders pass around a **small flannel-board.** That way, participants have a chance to see and touch the board, and place objects on it, without embarrassment.

If classes are often held in a particular spot outdoors, a low-cost 'billboard' of ***bajareque*** (mud on bamboo or sticks) can be made to hold up a flannel sheet and posters. Be sure the surface tilts backward a little so that flannel-board pieces will not fall off easily. Try to build it in a place that is protected from the wind.

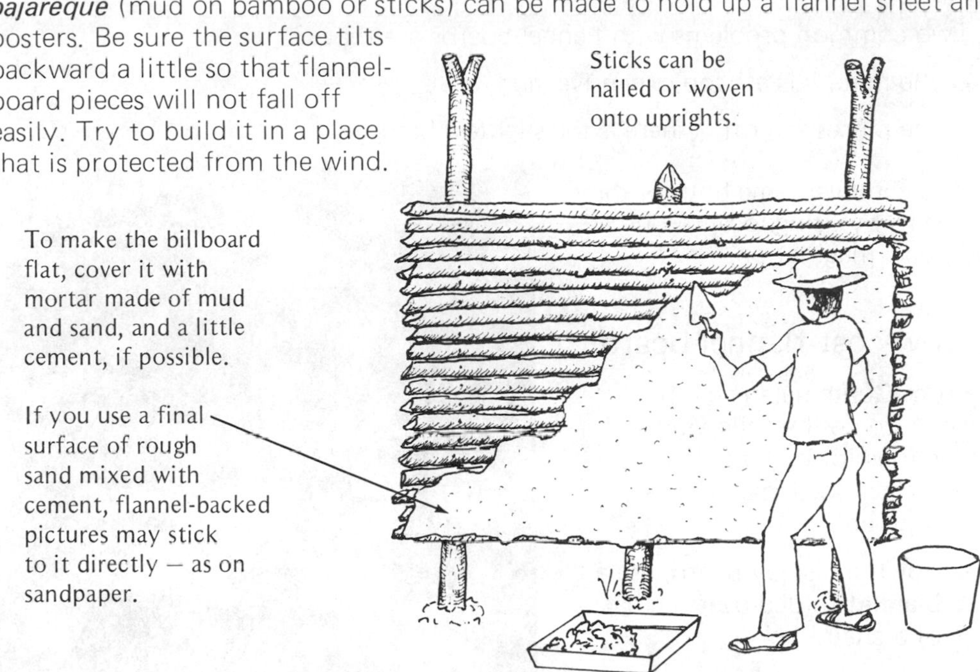

Sticks can be nailed or woven onto uprights.
To make the billboard flat, cover it with mortar made of mud and sand, and a little cement, if possible.
If you use a final surface of rough sand mixed with cement, flannel-backed pictures may stick to it directly — as on sandpaper.

You can build a small roof over the billboard to protect it from the weather.

The flannel sheet or blanket can be hung on the billboard for class, and then taken down and stored in a safe place.

Between classes the billboard can be used for posters and announcements. If children make health posters, try displaying the best ones on the billboard every week.

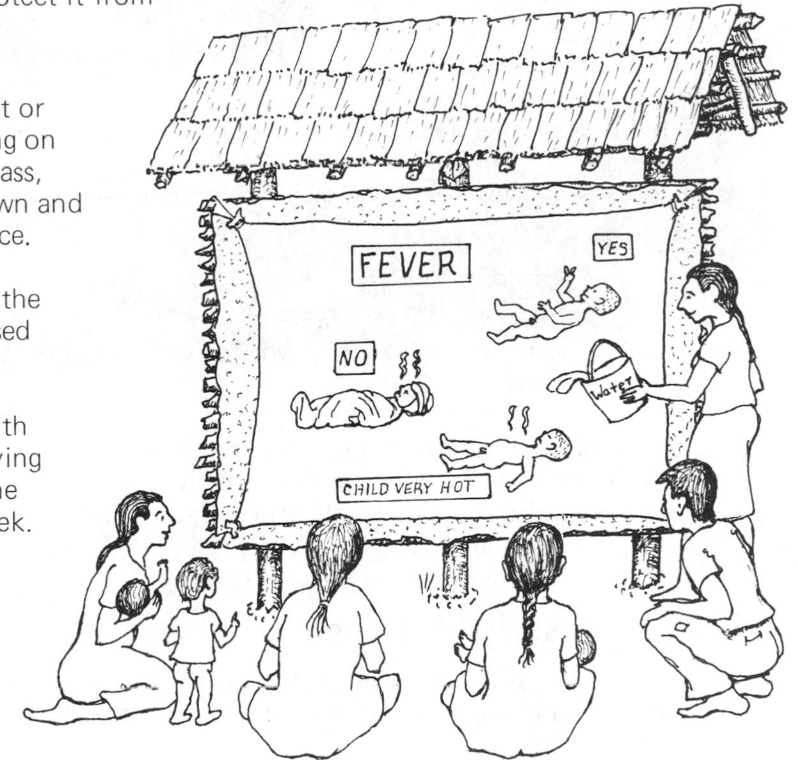

FLANNEL-BOARD ALTERNATIVES

Two common problems with flannel-boards are that . . .

- the materials are too expensive, and
- the pieces fall off if there is the slightest breeze.

You can overcome both of these problems by using local resources and your imagination.

1. Low-cost flannel-board

From Guatemalan health workers come the following suggestions for making flannel-boards from local materials at almost no cost:

- For the display board, use a **blanket** folded over the back of a chair.
- To make the pictures stay in place, make a paste of flour and water and smear it on the backs of the pictures. Then sprinkle **wheat chaff** (the waste husks of the grain) over the wet paste. The tiny barbs of the chaff work better than sandpaper or flannel to hold the pictures on the blanket.

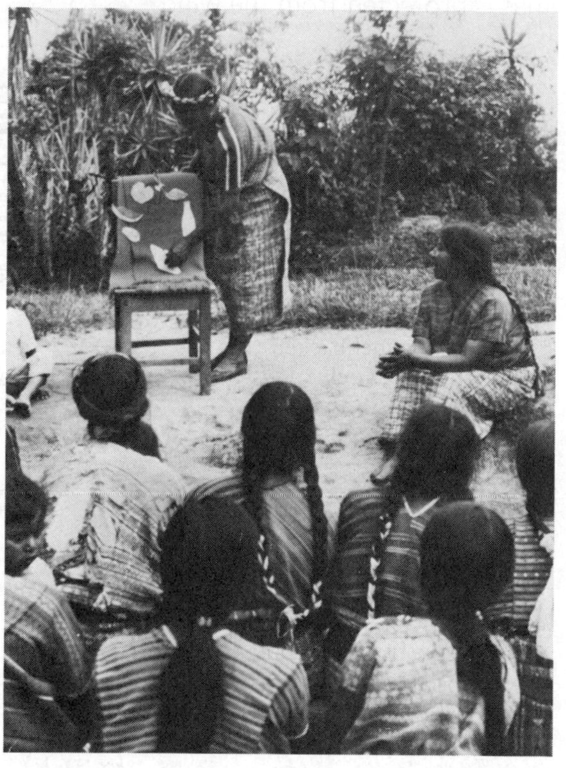

A Guatemalan health worker uses a blanket over a chair as a flannel-board.

Mix white flour → in water. → Spread on back of picture → and sprinkle with wheat chaff.

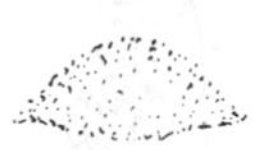
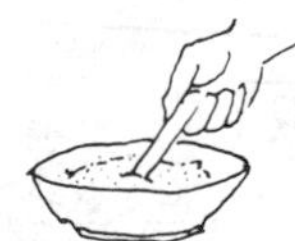
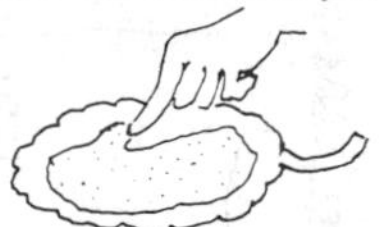
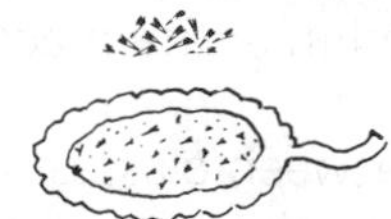

Rice chaff or other grain husks may work as well. (Please let us know the results if you try them.)

Homemade glue can also be made from certain local plants. In Mexico, villagers make a strong glue by squeezing the juice from the bulbs of certain wild orchids, and boiling it into a thick syrup.

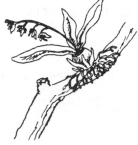

2. Masonite instead of flannel

In Mexico, health workers found that the rough back side of a sheet of masonite (fiberboard) works just as well as a flannel-board. It does not need to be covered with cloth.

3. String-board

To prevent pictures from falling off or blowing away, you can use a string-board instead of (or combined with) a flannel-board.

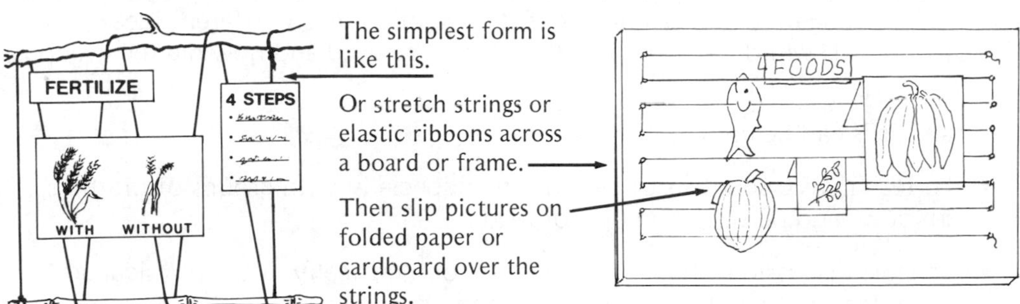

The simplest form is like this.

Or stretch strings or elastic ribbons across a board or frame.

Then slip pictures on folded paper or cardboard over the strings.

Imaginative string-board teaching aids were developed in the Gambia, Africa by a Peace Corps volunteer. This one is used to teach mothers and children about malaria. The learners can place the mosquito so it actually 'bites' the arm.

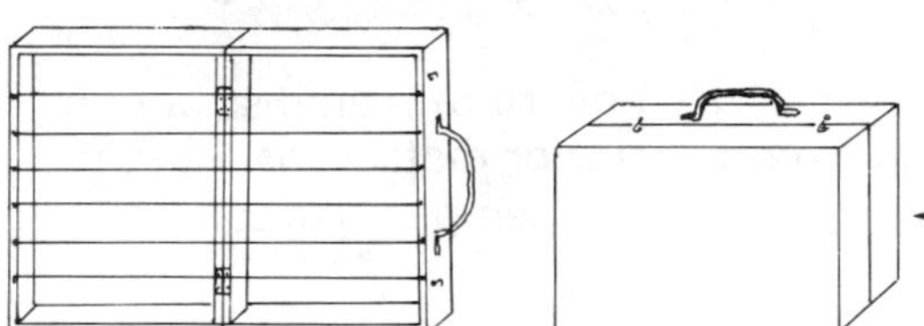

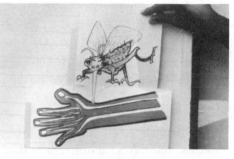

This is a combination string-board and flannel-board. It folds into a simple case for carrying and storing the pictures.

4. Magnet-board

This is another wind-resistant alternative to the flannel-board.

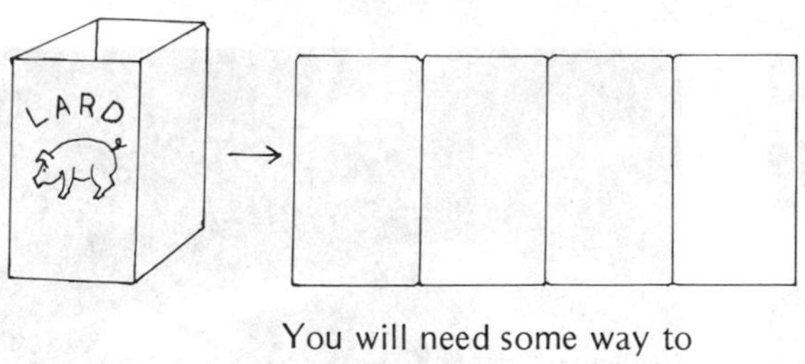

Use a thin piece of tin-plated steel. Perhaps you can find an old metal sign board or open up and flatten an old lard tin.

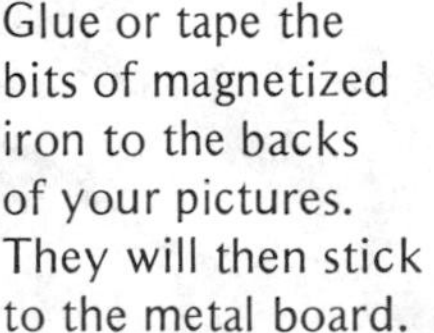

You will need some way to magnetize small pieces of iron. One way is to use an old induction coil from an automobile. Ask a school teacher or mechanic to help you.

Glue or tape the bits of magnetized iron to the backs of your pictures. They will then stick to the metal board.

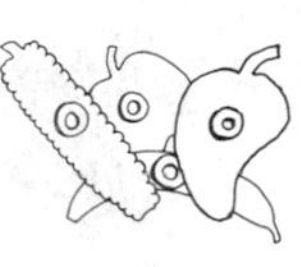

If you paint the magnet-board with black non-glare paint, it can be used as a chalkboard as well.

FLASH CARDS

Flash cards are cards showing a series of pictures or messages. Like flip charts (see p. **11**-23), they can be used to tell stories or to teach skills step by step. But they allow more flexibility because they are not attached together in a given order. You can rearrange them to tell different stories, or to teach different ideas. The size of the cards will depend on how they are to be used and how big the group is.

Flash cards can be used . . .

- To teach basic concepts of health care—especially with groups of mothers, children, and persons who cannot read.
- To start discussions that help people to look critically at the physical and social factors that affect their health and well-being.
- For playing educational games. In this case the cards are often smaller. Each person is given several to 'play' or match with other cards, according to the rules of the game (see p. **11**-22).

Flash cards are usually drawn on cardboard. But they can also be made of heavy cloth that can be rolled up for carrying.

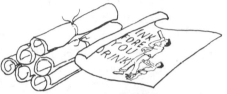

The Voluntary Health Association of India (VHAI) distributes an instruction sheet explaining how to prepare **flash cards from old tins or metal cans.** First the tin is hammered flat, cut into cards, and painted white. Then pictures can be drawn or painted on the cards.

On these 2 facing pages, we showthe 8 photographs from the VHAI's instruction sheet. This printed sheet communicates completely through pictures, without any need for words. It is a good example of an effective teaching material that can be used by persons who cannot read (as well as by those who can).

1.

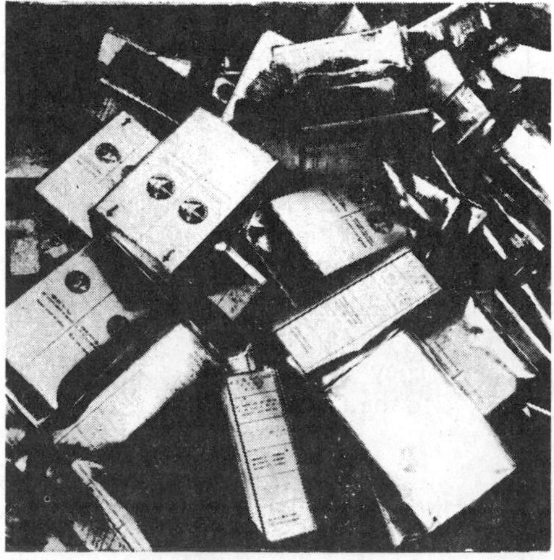

2.

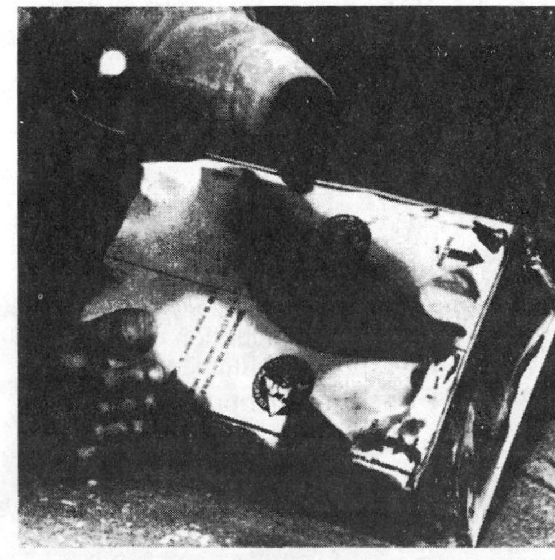

3.

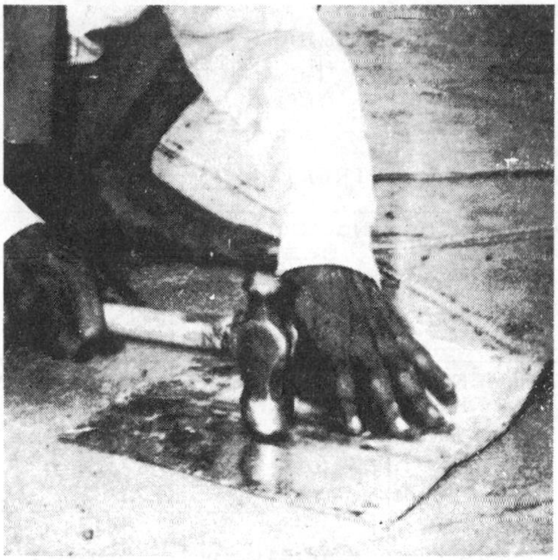

4.

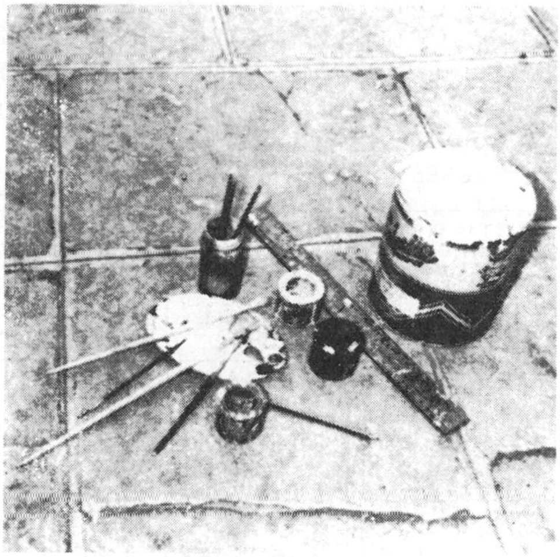

5.

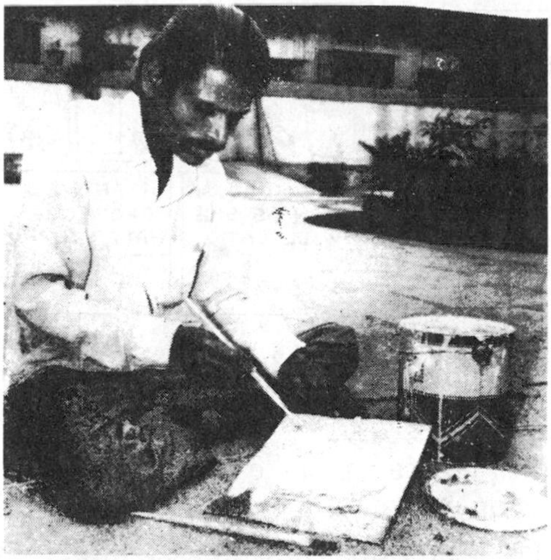

6.

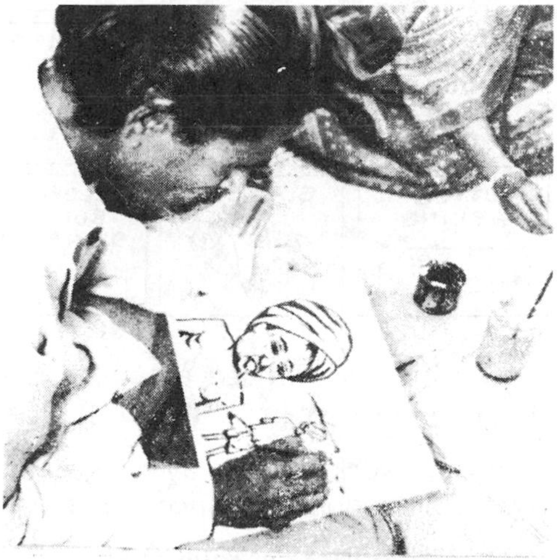

7.

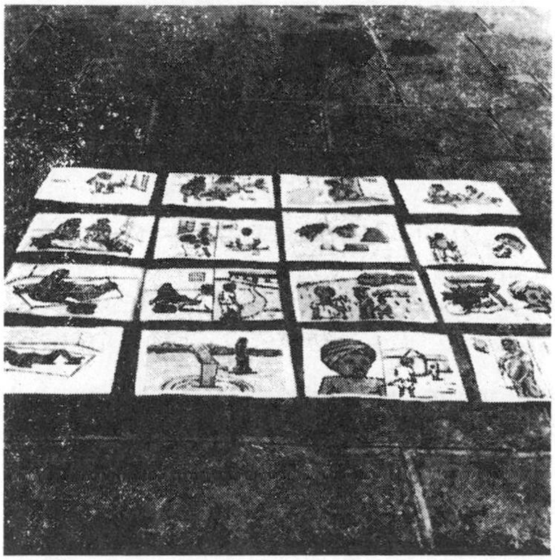

8.

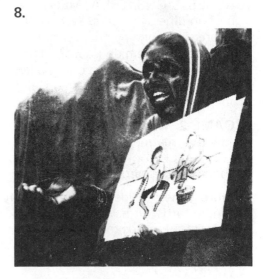

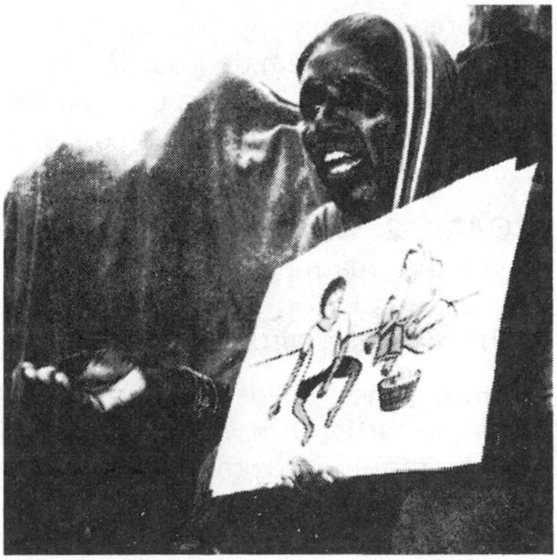

Flash card games

Sets of flash cards can be used to play games that help students learn about particular health problems. For example, for games about the different problems that cause diarrhea, students can make a set of flash cards like these:

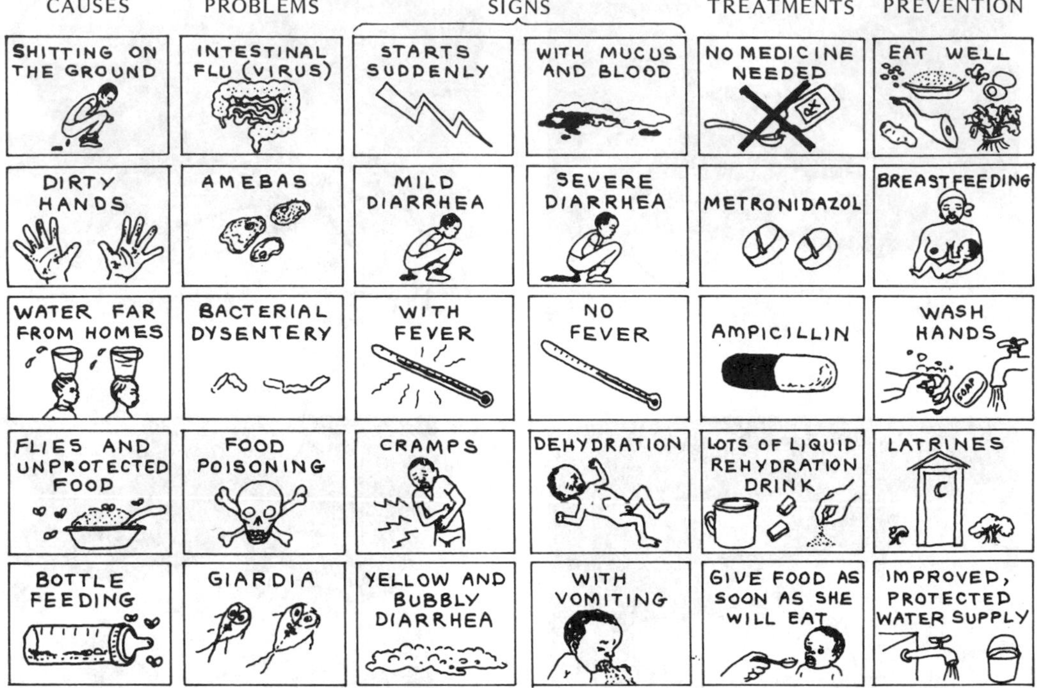

CAUSES
PROBLEMS
SIGNS
TREATMENTS
PREVENTION
SHITTING ON THE GROUND
INTESTINAL FLU (VIRUS)
STARTS SUDDENLY
WITH MUCUS AND BLOOD
NO MEDICINE NEEDED
EAT WELL
DIRTY HANDS
AMEBAS
MILD DIARRHEA
SEVERE DIARRHEA
METRONIDAZOL
BREASTFEEDING
WATER FAR FROM HOMES
BACTERIAL DYSENTERY
WITH FEVER
NO FEVER
AMPICILLIN
WASH HANDS
SOAP
FLIES AND UNPROTECTED FOOD
FOOD POISONING
CRAMPS
DEHYDRATION
LOTS OF LIQUID REHYDRATION DRINK
LATRINES
BOTTLE FEEDING
GIARDIA
YELLOW AND BUBBLY DIARRHEA
WITH VOMITING
GIVE FOOD AS SOON AS SHE WILL EAT
IMPROVED, PROTECTED WATER SUPPLY

The cards shown here are only a beginning. Add more according to the common diarrheal diseases in your area.

Health workers can play several games with these cards. Make the games lively by having people announce or act out what is on each card they play.

GAME 1: What and why? First, hand each person some cards of each kind (CAUSES, SIGNS, TREATMENTS, etc.). One student holds up a card with a sign of an illness and asks, "What other signs might I have?" Other students hold up more signs, one by one, forming a description of a particular problem. They ask, "What problem do I have?" Then the student who has the card naming that problem holds it up. If no one challenges the diagnosis, that student asks, "Why did I get sick?" Now each person who has a card with a possible cause of the problem holds it up. The group discusses how the illness is spread.

GAME 2: What to do? Following GAME 1, a similar game can be played to review the treatment and prevention of different kinds of diarrhea. Encourage the students to look in their books and to add information and suggestions not included on the cards.

More games: Students can divide into small groups to think of new games using the cards. Or have them design new cards about other health problems, or cards without words to use with children or people who do not read. This way students use their imaginations to create learning games for people in their communities.

FLIP CHARTS AND OTHER WAYS TO TELL STORIES WITH PICTURES

Pictures—hand drawn, silkscreened, or mimeographed—can be used as aids for telling stories or teaching skills step by step.

It is easier to keep pictures in order if they are joined together in some way. They can be rolled on a stick, linked together, or made into flip charts. Attach them together any way you like—by stapling, sewing, gluing, attaching them to rings, or bolting them between 2 thin boards.

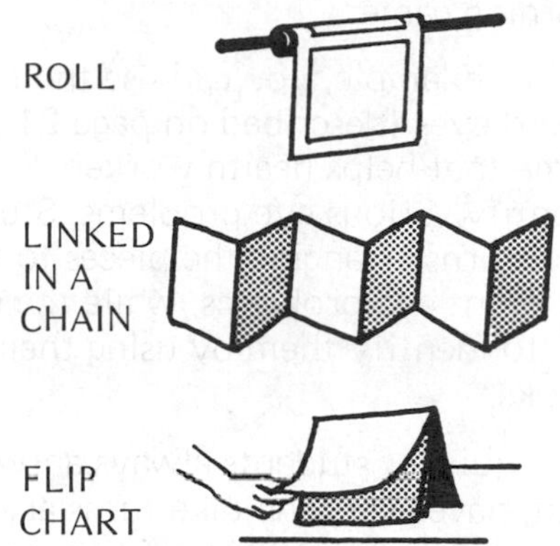

Pictures are doubly effective if the learning group—health workers or mothers or children—helps to make them. The group may want to use a flip chart or story from some other source as a model, and adapt the pictures and events to the local situation.

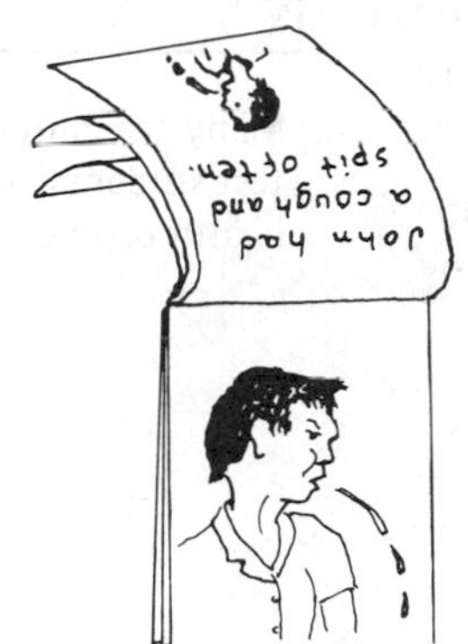

To make it easier to read a flip chart story to a group, write the part of the story that goes with each picture on the back of the page before. With the writing, include a small copy of the picture being shown. This lets you know what the group is looking at.

But even better than telling people the story is to let them tell you what they see happening in the pictures.

FOLDABLE POSTERS ON THIN PLASTIC SHEETS:

You can make large posters from thin sheets of white plastic or old plastic mattress covers. Draw on them with 'waterproof' marking pens. These posters can easily be folded, carried about, and even washed.

FOLDED UP

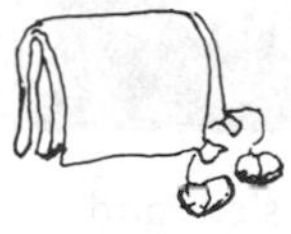

UNFOLDED

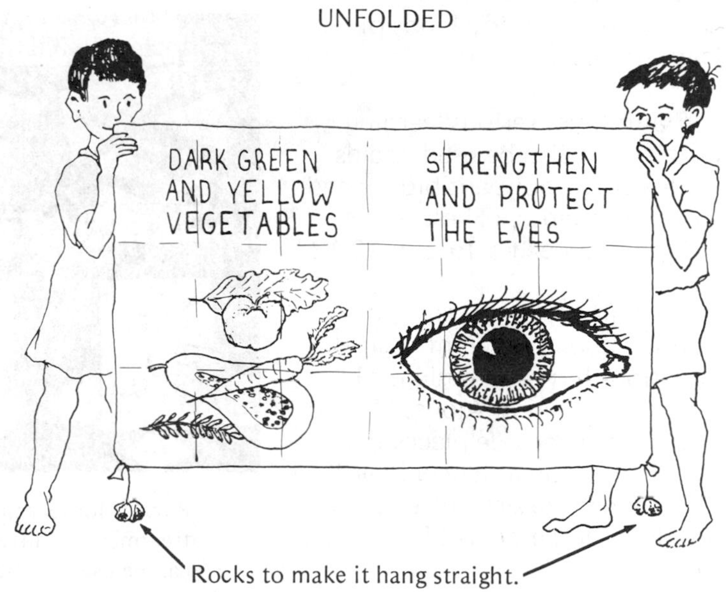

Rocks to make it hang straight.

GAMES THAT HELP PEOPLE LEARN

Many of the teaching aids described in this book can be used for group learning games.

For example, you can use the flannel-board eyes (described on page **21**-8) in a game that helps health workers learn to identify various eye problems. Students take turns arranging the pieces to form different eye problems, while the others try to identify them by using their books.

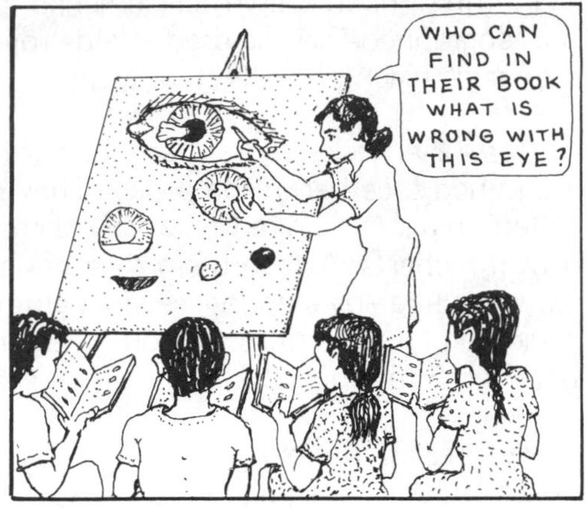
WHO CAN FIND IN THEIR BOOK WHAT IS WRONG WITH THIS EYE?

Many teaching aids can be used as games to test students' abilities to identify different health problems.

If quicker students always answer first, have everyone take turns answering. Or you can decide who will answer next by spinning a bottle (p. **4**-8), throwing dice, or picking numbers out of a hat.

You and your students can invent similar games for learning about skin problems or other illnesses.

Puzzles

Students can make their own puzzles by cutting pieces of cardboard, wood, or cloth to fit together in certain ways. They can design 'jigsaw' puzzles that fit together to form one picture or shape (like the puzzle about diarrhea on the next page). Or they can make puzzles that have separate pieces representing signs of illnesses that fit onto a human figure (see the teaching aid about swollen lymph nodes, p. **21**-6). Either of these can be used in many kinds of learning games.

Playful, yet serious learning puzzles can also be used as aids for learning about antibiotics and worm medicines. (These are described on pages **19**-2 to **19**-12.)

A similar set of puzzles for learning about different vaginal infections has been designed by the health team in Ajoya, Mexico. The puzzles include pieces that fit together (on a flannel-board) to demonstrate signs of the problems and aspects of treatment.

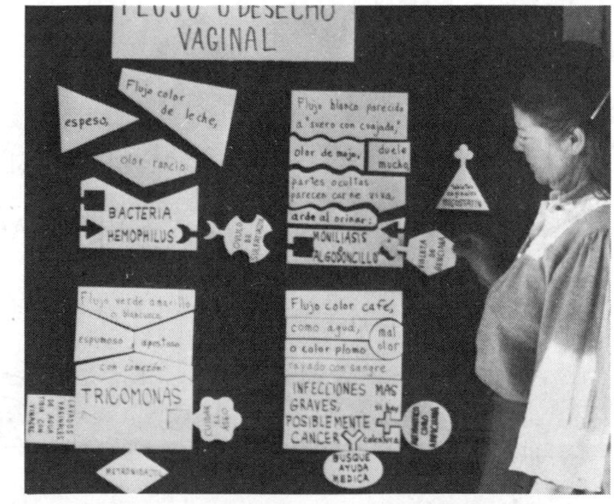

Puzzles for learning about signs and treatment of different vaginal infections can be used for 'self-testing' games.

'JIGSAW' PUZZLE SHOWING THE CAUSES OF DIARRHEA:

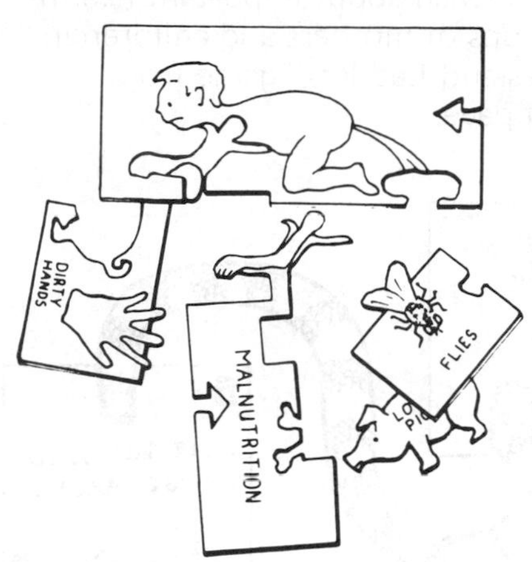

Life itself is full of puzzles. A responsible health worker helps people look at their many problems to see how they fit together to form a whole picture. It is like putting together the pieces of a puzzle.

Teaching aids in the form of puzzles can help students see for themselves how many different conditions and problems in their lives are related.

Putting together the puzzle shown here helps students to recognize how various factors combine to cause death by diarrhea. Poor personal hygiene and poor public sanitation lead to the spread of infection. Several factors cause malnutrition, and poorly nourished children get sick more often and are more likely to die because they cannot fight off disease. The students also see how the whole unhealthy situation is locked in place by unjust social factors.

To encourage students to think and choose, include alternative pieces for different diseases, signs, and causes. Or have some blank pieces that students can fill in based on their own ideas and experience.

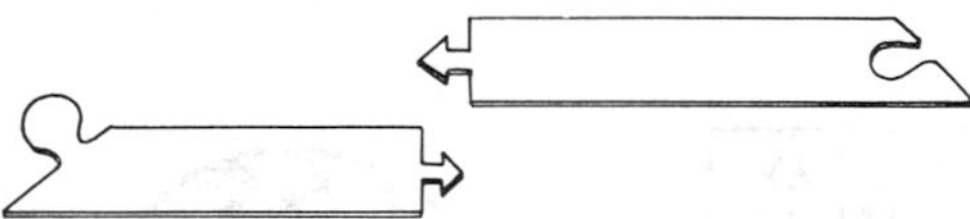

Many exciting discussions can result from putting together this kind of puzzle.

After the group explores how the different causes relate to each other, a whole new area of discussion can be opened by asking questions such as these:

- What should be done about this situation?
- What can be done about each of the contributing causes?
- Will treating the diarrhea solve the problem? What will?
- Where should we begin?

Encourage students to make their own puzzles based on problems and causes in their communities.

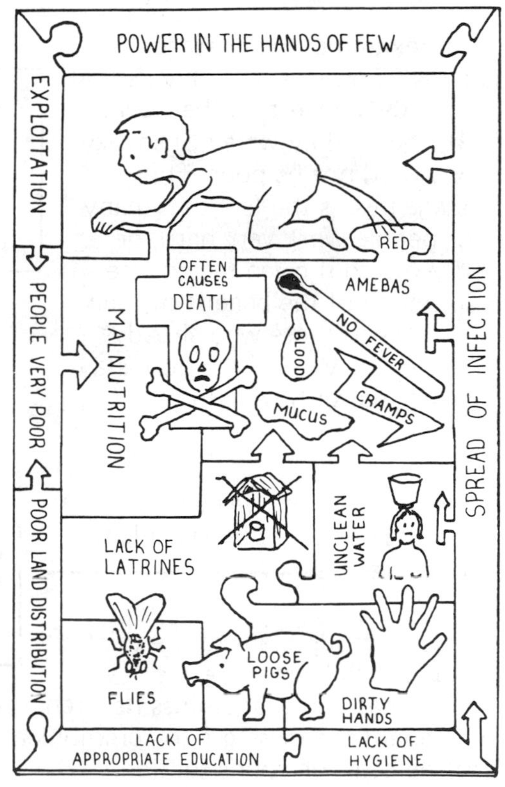

Games health workers can introduce in their villages

Games can be fun to play and at the same time teach about important health practices. Some learning games are used with groups of mothers and children in community programs. An example is the "Snakes and Ladders" game from Liberia, Africa shown and explained on the next page.

One of the strengths of this version of "Snakes and Ladders" is that the pictures, messages, and language have been adapted to the local situation. For instance, in squares 74 and 8 it says that a bottle-fed baby is "quick to go back"—which to the Liberian people means to go back to God, to die. Also, "running stomach" in square 24 is the local term for diarrhea.

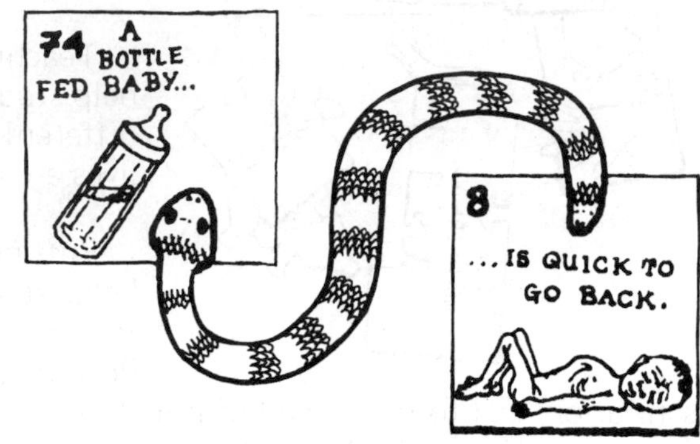

One of the weaknesses of this version of the game is that it focuses mainly on the physical causes of poor health. Where social causes are mentioned, the messages tend to put the blame on the poor themselves rather than on problems in the social system. This reinforces poor people's sense of powerlessness and worthlessness, rather than strengthening their self-confidence and their will to act to change their situation.

For example, the message in squares 73 and 31 tells players that **the family's poverty is their own fault,** that if they were not so lazy they would not be poor. This message misses the fact that many poor people work very hard, or gladly would if given the chance. Also, much of the benefit of their work goes to those who already have plenty. Most of the poor stay poor no matter how hard they work.

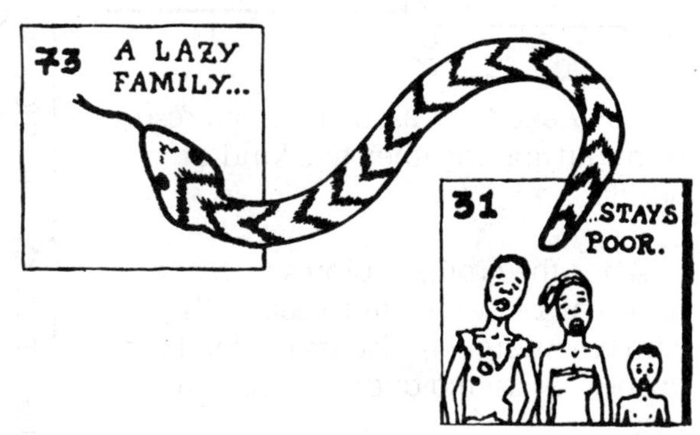

A much more positive message about the cause of poverty might be one like this ⟶

If your group plans to use this snakes and ladders game, we suggest that you first discuss its strengths and weaknesses. Then adapt the messages to communicate what you decide is most helpful for your situation.

HEALTH EDUCATION SNAKES AND LADDERS*

RULES:

2, 3, or 4 people can play this game. Each player uses a seed to show what place he or she has on the board.

Each player throws the die. The player with the highest number starts the game.

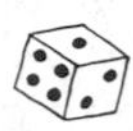

The first player throws the die and moves his or her seed according to the number shown on the die, beginning from square 1, marked **START.**

If a player rolls a 6, the die can be thrown again for another turn.

If a marker stops on the head of a SNAKE, the snake swallows it. The player then moves the seed down to the tail of the snake, and reads the message to all the players. That player's turn is over, and his next turn begins from the square at the tail of the snake.

If a seed lands on a square that has the foot of a LADDER, the player moves it to the top of the ladder, and reads the message to all the players. That player's turn ends at the top of the ladder, and his or her next turn begins from there.

The first player to reach square 100 wins the game, but **the player must throw the exact number needed to land on that final square.**

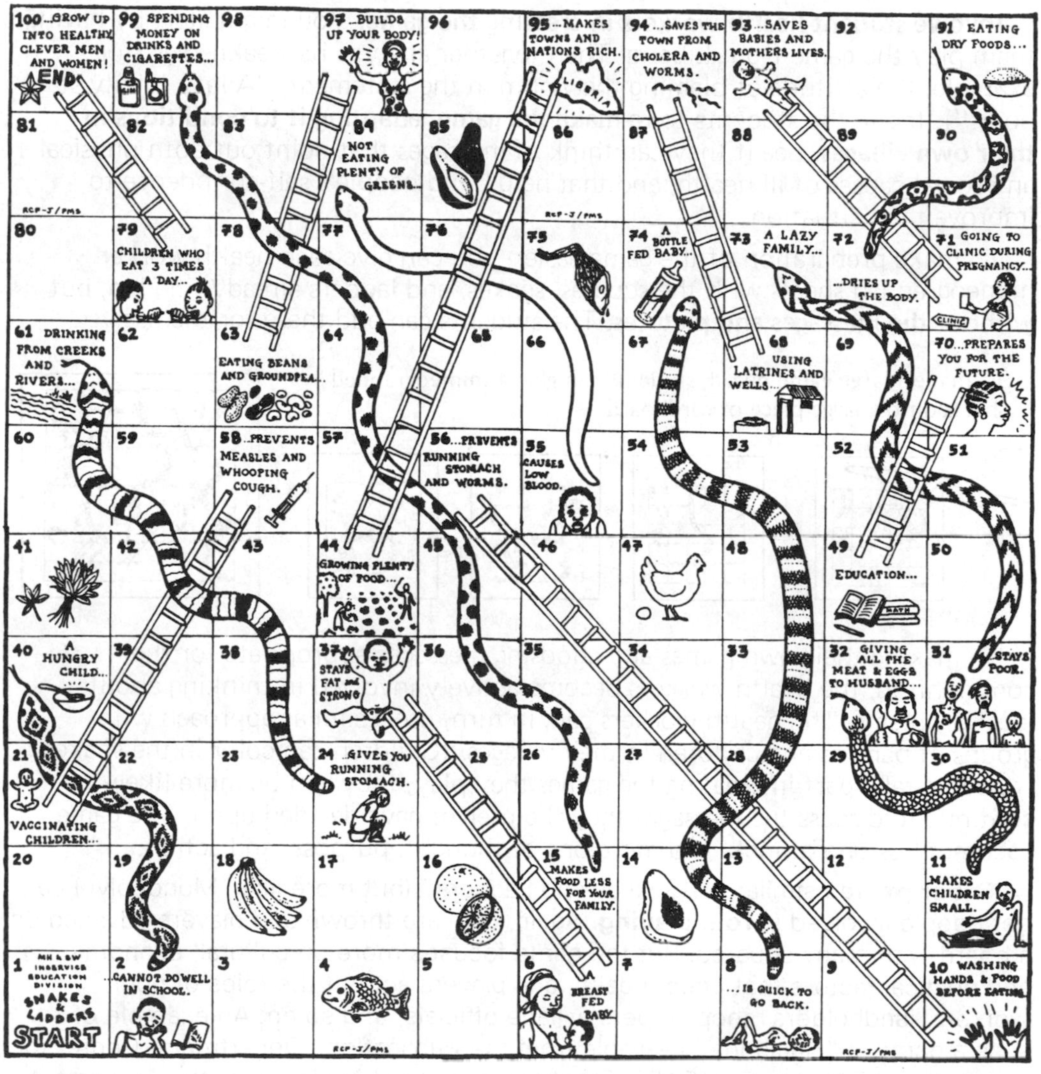

100 ...GROW UP INTO HEALTHY CLEVER MEN AND WOMEN! END	99 SPENDING MONEY ON DRINKS AND CIGARETTES...	98	97 ...BUILDS UP YOUR BODY!	96	95 ...MAKES TOWNS AND NATIONS RICH. LIBERIA	94 ...SAVES THE TOWN FROM CHOLERA AND WORMS.	93 ...SAVES BABIES AND MOTHERS LIVES.	92	91 EATING DRY FOODS...
81	82	83	84 NOT EATING PLENTY OF GREENS...	85	86	87	88	89	90
80	79 CHILDREN WHO EAT 3 TIMES A DAY...	78	77	76	75	74 A BOTTLE FED BABY...	73 A LAZY FAMILY...	72 ...DRIES UP THE BODY.	71 GOING TO CLINIC DURING PREGNANCY... CLINIC
61 DRINKING FROM CREEKS AND RIVERS...	62	63 EATING BEANS AND GROUNDPEA...	64	65	66	67	68 USING LATRINES AND WELLS...	69	70 ...PREPARES YOU FOR THE FUTURE.
60	59	58 ...PREVENTS MEASLES AND WHOOPING COUGH.	57	56 ...PREVENTS RUNNING STOMACH AND WORMS.	55 CAUSES LOW BLOOD.	54	53	52	51
41	42	43	44 GROWING PLENTY OF FOOD...	45	46	47	48	49 EDUCATION... MATH	50
40 A HUNGRY CHILD...	39	38	37 STAYS FAT and STRONG	36	35	34	33	32 GIVING ALL THE MEAT & EGGS TO HUSBAND...	31 STAYS POOR.
21 VACCINATING CHILDREN...	22	23	24 ...GIVES YOU RUNNING STOMACH.	25	26	27	28	29	30
20	19	18	17	16	15 MAKES FOOD LESS FOR YOUR FAMILY.	14	13	12	11 MAKES CHILDREN SMALL.
1 MH & SW INSERVICE EDUCATION DIVISION SNAKES & LADDERS START	2 ...CANNOT DO WELL IN SCHOOL.	3	4	5	6 BREAST FED BABY.	7	8 ...IS QUICK TO GO BACK.	9	10 WASHING HANDS & FOOD BEFORE EATING.

*This game was adapted for Liberia from one prepared by the National Food and Nutrition Commission of Zambia, in *PSC Newsletter,* UNICEF.

"Snakes and Ladders" and similar games generally have two big weaknesses as teaching aids:

1. **The messages are given to the players.** The players land on the squares and read the messages, but they do not need to think or solve anything for themselves. It is doubtful whether such pre-packaged messages will be effective unless people discuss them and relate them to their own lives during and after the game.

2. **The game is primarily one of luck or chance.** Apart from the written messages, the game carries the unwritten message that the health of a child is determined by lucky or unlucky rolls of the die. Although the game is intended to help people learn what they themselves can do to protect their children's health, there is a danger that it may reinforce people's sense of 'fatalism'. It may make them feel that their children's health is also a matter of luck or fortune, outside their control.

There is one way to get around these weaknesses of the game, at least in part.

Involve student health workers in creating the game. You might start by having them play the game from Liberia. Then together analyze its weaknesses (for example, the attitude of blaming the victim in the statement, "A lazy family stays poor."). Invite the students to **re-make the game, adapting it to conditions in their own villages.** See if they can think of messages that point out both physical and social causes of ill health, and that help build people's self-confidence to improve their situation.

To make preparation of the game easier, you can give each health worker mimeographed sheets with the squares, snakes, and ladders already filled in, but **without the messages and pictures.** The students can add these for themselves.

To make a large game board, students can glue 4 mimeographed sheets onto a large piece of cardboard.

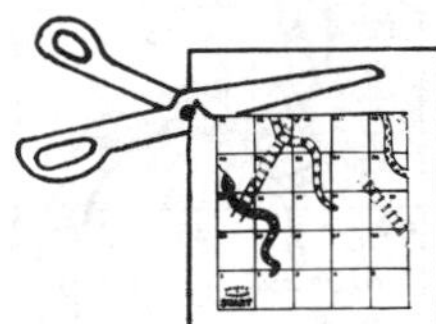

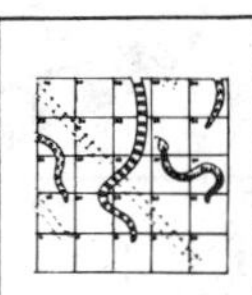

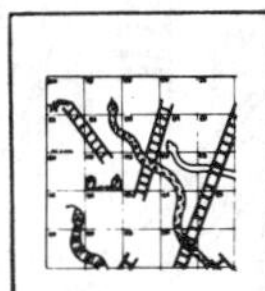

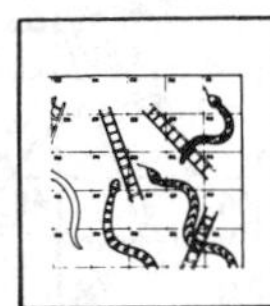

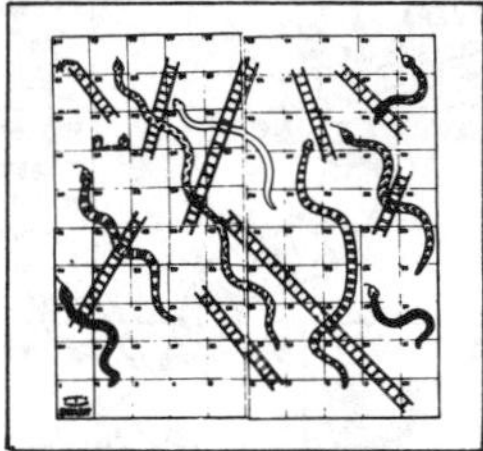

By making their own games and choosing messages appropriate for their communities, the health workers become actively involved in thinking about local problems. The health workers can, in turn, use a similar approach with groups of parents and children in their villages. (Children can color in the snakes.) If people take part in creating the games they play, they will be more likely to continue to discuss the messages they themselves have decided upon. The game becomes less one of luck, and more one of thought, purpose, and action.

Other games similar to "Snakes and Ladders" (but more like "Monopoly") can get people involved in **role playing.** Again, dice are thrown and players advance on a board with many squares. But the game focuses more on cultural, economic, and political factors that affect health, and players act out the roles of poor workers, landholders, shopkeepers, village officials, and so on. An example of such a game is "Hacienda," available from the Publications Department, Center for International Education, 285 Hills South, University of Massachusetts, Amherst, Massachusetts 01003, USA.

HOW TO 'SHOW' PEOPLE THINGS THAT ARE TOO SMALL TO SEE

One especially difficult idea to teach is the extreme smallness of things like bacteria and amebas, which can only be seen with a microscope. If a microscope is available, it helps to have students use it to look at bacteria, worm eggs, and amebas, even if they will not have microscopes in their villages.

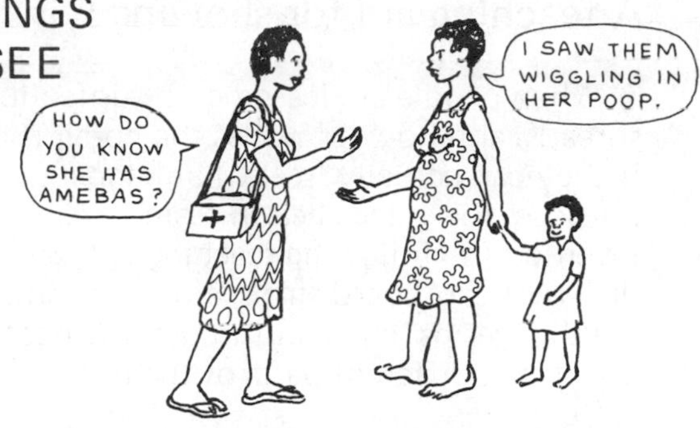
HOW DO YOU KNOW SHE HAS AMEBAS?
I SAW THEM WIGGLING IN HER POOP.

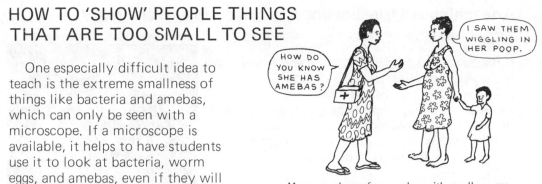

Many people confuse amebas with small worms because they cannot imagine that amebas are too small to see.

Here is one way to help students understand how small bacteria, amebas, and worm eggs are:

1.

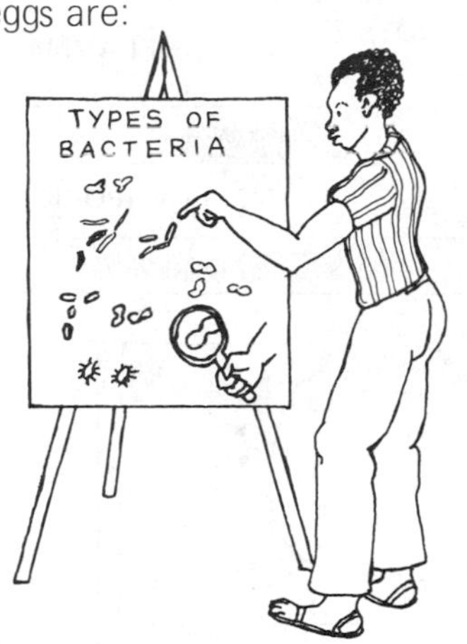

TYPES OF BACTERIA

2.

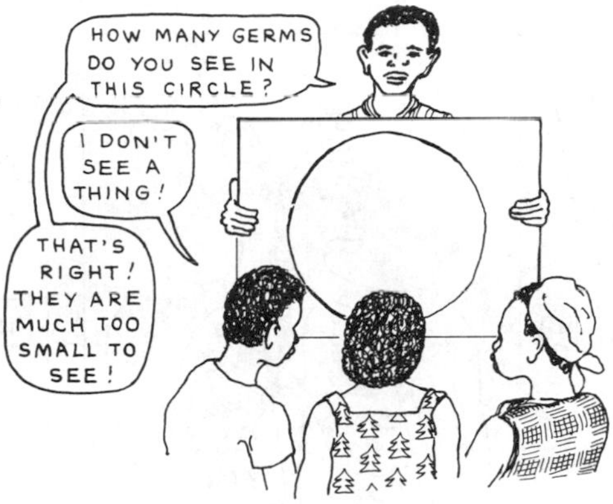

HOW MANY GERMS DO YOU SEE IN THIS CIRCLE?

I DON'T SEE A THING!

THAT'S RIGHT! THEY ARE MUCH TOO SMALL TO SEE!

3.

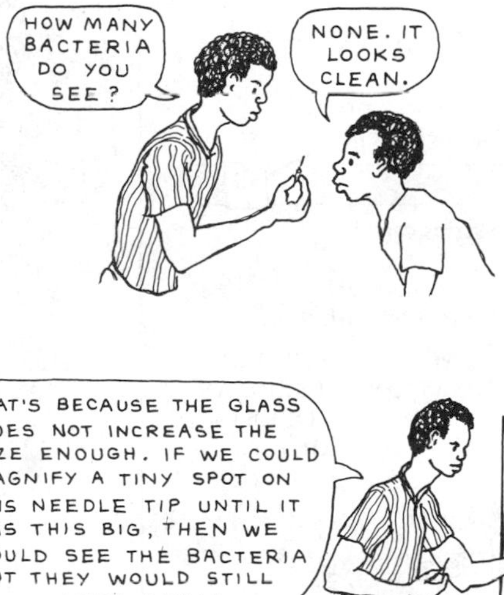

HOW MANY BACTERIA DO YOU SEE?

NONE. IT LOOKS CLEAN.

4.

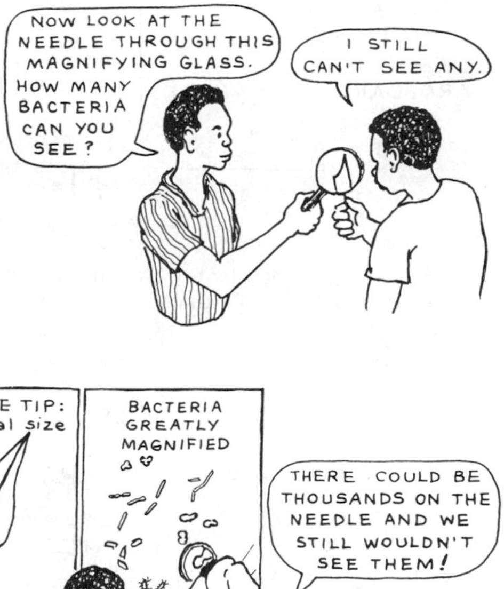

NOW LOOK AT THE NEEDLE THROUGH THIS MAGNIFYING GLASS. HOW MANY BACTERIA CAN YOU SEE?

I STILL CAN'T SEE ANY.

5.

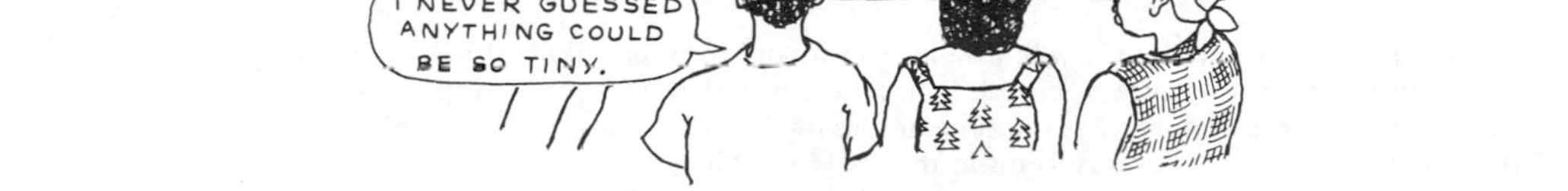

THAT'S BECAUSE THE GLASS DOES NOT INCREASE THE SIZE ENOUGH. IF WE COULD MAGNIFY A TINY SPOT ON THIS NEEDLE TIP UNTIL IT WAS THIS BIG, THEN WE WOULD SEE THE BACTERIA BUT THEY WOULD STILL LOOK SMALL.

NEEDLE TIP: ← actual size

greatly magnified

BACTERIA GREATLY MAGNIFIED

THERE COULD BE THOUSANDS ON THE NEEDLE AND WE STILL WOULDN'T SEE THEM!

I NEVER GUESSED ANYTHING COULD BE SO TINY.

A teaching aid for showing how germs invade the body

When people are learning how infection spreads, and how it invades the body, it helps if they can actually 'see' what happens. For this purpose, the village health team in Ajoya invented the following teaching aid. By pulling different cardboard strips, students can actually see the 'germs' move in through the nose and attack the different parts of the respiratory system.

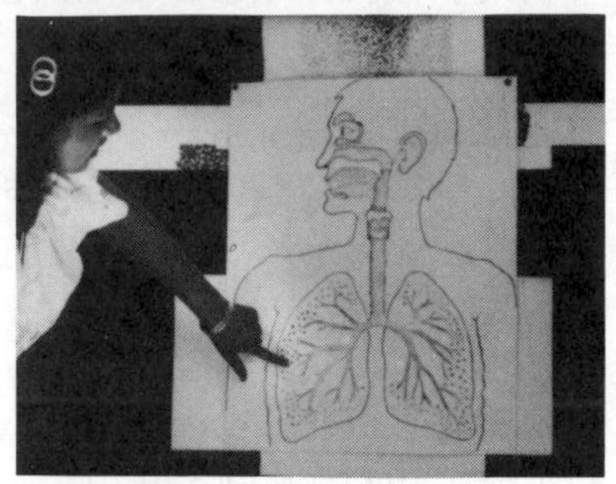

WHOLE TEACHING AID ASSEMBLED

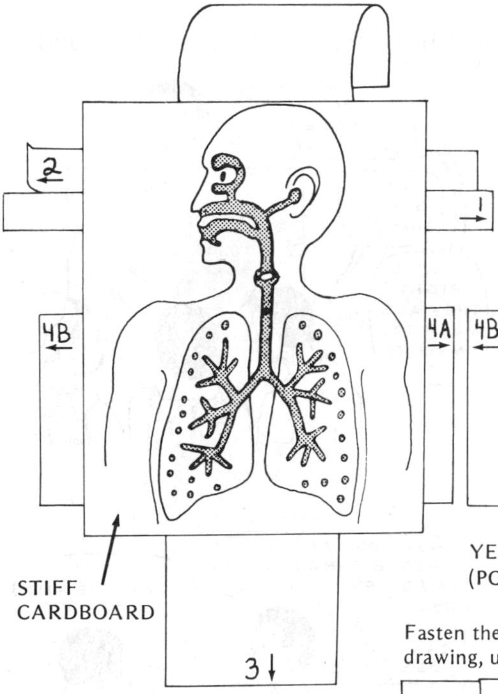

FOUR MOVABLE STRIPS

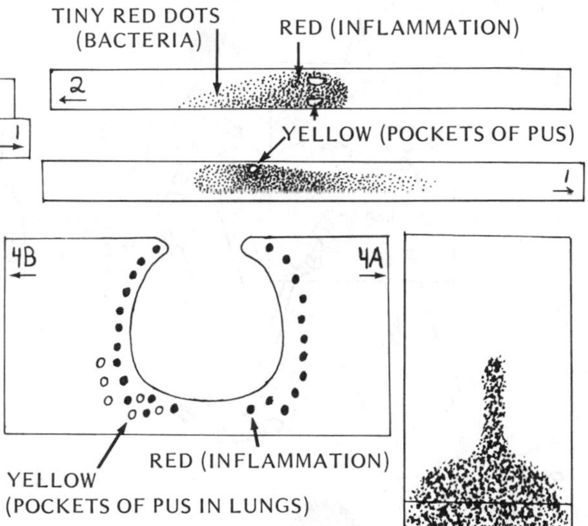

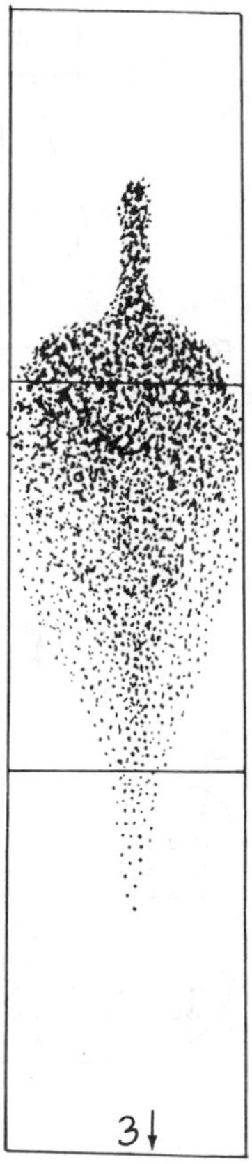

Fasten the strips to the back of the drawing, using paper 'belt loops' through which the strips can slide.

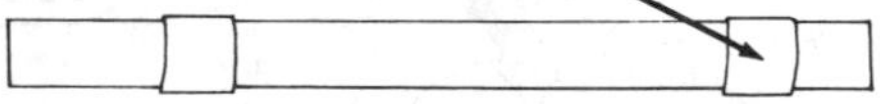

By pulling the different strips in the direction of the arrows, you can see the bacteria invade, followed by inflammation, and then infection with pus.

PULL STRIP 1, AND SEE THE GERMS BEGIN TO ENTER THE NOSE.

PULL STRIP 2, AND THEY INVADE THE SINUSES . . .

AND CAUSE INFLAMMATION.

FINALLY THERE ARE POCKETS OF PUS.

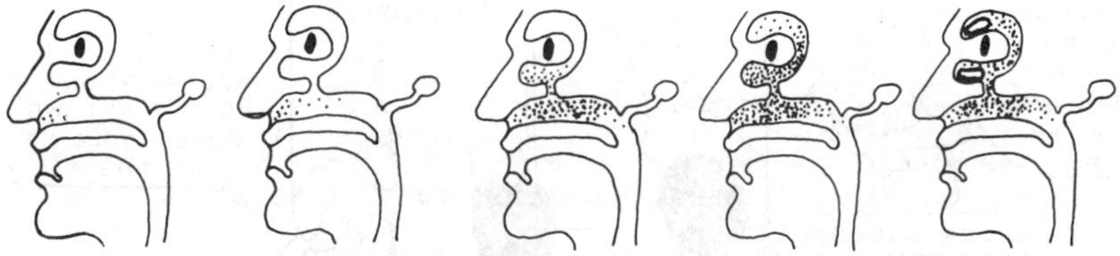

Pull strip 1 farther and the germs will invade the ear, and form pus. Pull strip 3 to show an infection of the voice box, and then the tubes in the lungs (bronchitis). Pull strip 4A and the infection reaches the tiny air sacs of the lungs, causing pneumonia. Pull strip 4B and a pocket of pus forms in the lower right lung.

PHOTOS OF THE 'INVADING GERMS' TEACHING AID

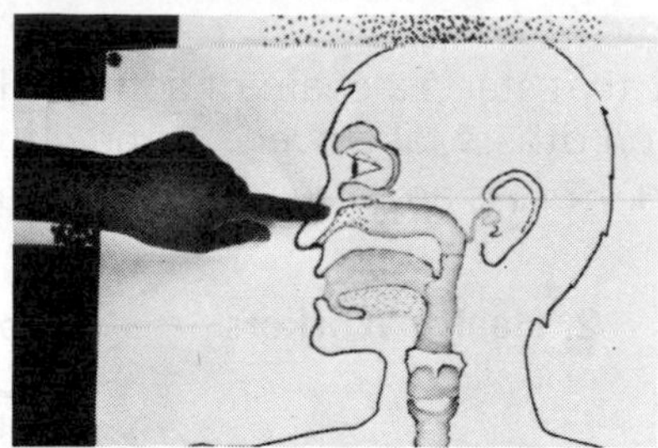

GERMS BEGIN TO INVADE.

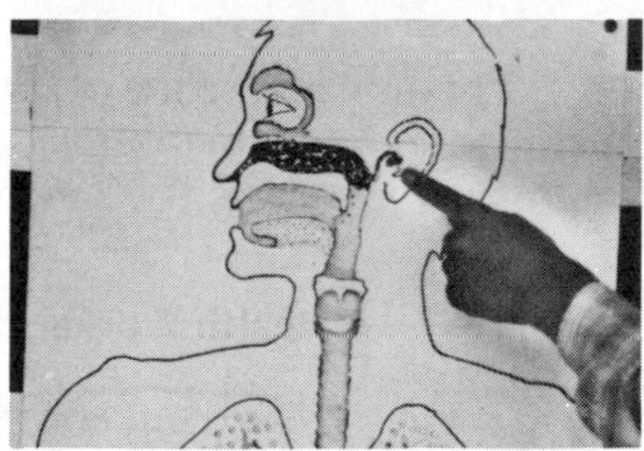

PUS IN EAR.

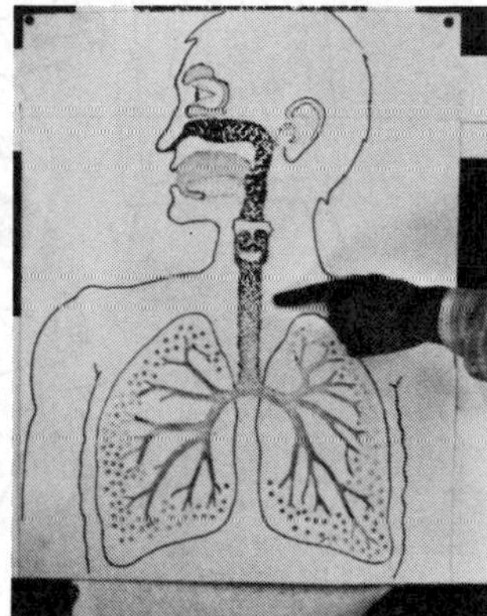

GERMS AND INFECTION SPREAD TO LOWER RESPIRATORY TRACT.

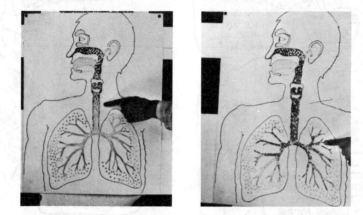

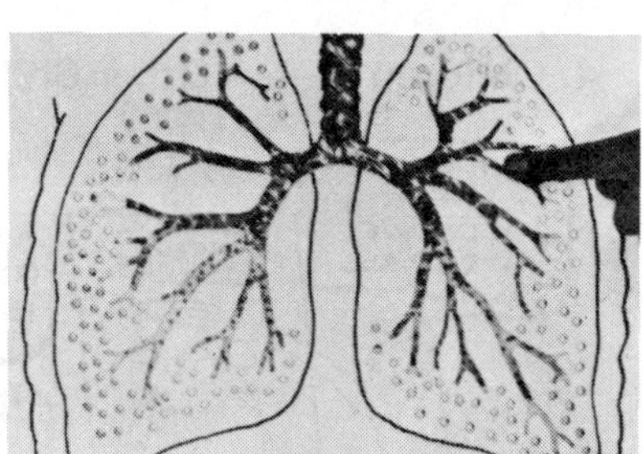

BRONCHITIS
Bronchi (tubes) are infected, but *alveoli* (little sacs) are clear.

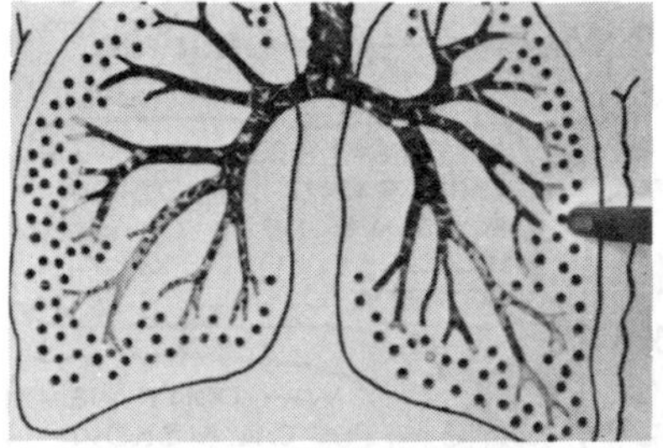

PNEUMONIA
Infection has spread to even the tiny air sacs.

ENCOURAGING HEALTH WORKERS TO BE CREATIVE:

The 'invading germs' teaching aid was designed and put together by instructors and students during a health worker training course in Ajoya, Mexico. The invention of new and better teaching aids has become one of the most challenging and exciting parts of the training program. Teaching aids designed during the course are doubly valuable. They not only help health workers to learn and teach basic health principles, they also help the health workers and their instructors become more creative. Together they begin to think in terms of hunting for new and better answers. **Learning—and life itself—becomes an adventure!**

EACH ONE TEACH ONE

A good teacher is like a spark or *catalyst* that starts a chain of action. He or she sets a process or a project in motion . . . soon others take over . . . they, in turn, get still more people involved . . . and so on. Here is an imaginary example:

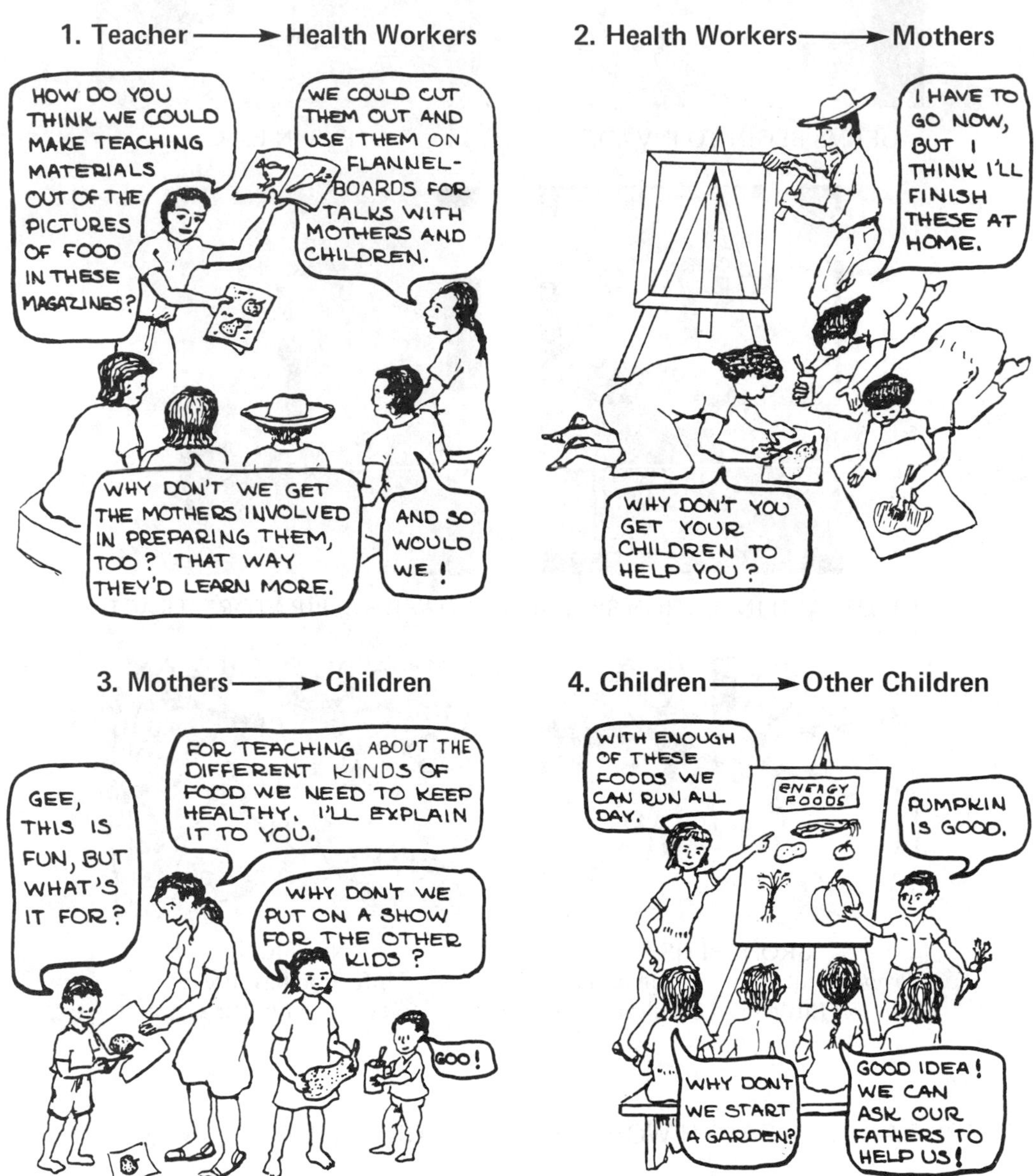
1. Teacher → Health Workers
HOW DO YOU THINK WE COULD MAKE TEACHING MATERIALS OUT OF THE PICTURES OF FOOD IN THESE MAGAZINES?
WE COULD CUT THEM OUT AND USE THEM ON FLANNEL-BOARDS FOR TALKS WITH MOTHERS AND CHILDREN.
WHY DON'T WE GET THE MOTHERS INVOLVED IN PREPARING THEM, TOO? THAT WAY THEY'D LEARN MORE.
AND SO WOULD WE!
2. Health Workers → Mothers
I HAVE TO GO NOW, BUT I THINK I'LL FINISH THESE AT HOME.
WHY DON'T YOU GET YOUR CHILDREN TO HELP YOU?
3. Mothers → Children
GEE, THIS IS FUN, BUT WHAT'S IT FOR?
FOR TEACHING ABOUT THE DIFFERENT KINDS OF FOOD WE NEED TO KEEP HEALTHY. I'LL EXPLAIN IT TO YOU.
WHY DON'T WE PUT ON A SHOW FOR THE OTHER KIDS?
GOO!
4. Children → Other Children
WITH ENOUGH OF THESE FOODS WE CAN RUN ALL DAY.
ENERGY FOODS
PUMPKIN IS GOOD.
WHY DON'T WE START A GARDEN?
GOOD IDEA! WE CAN ASK OUR FATHERS TO HELP US!

Here you see how the instructor sparks an idea, and how it grows. In this example, it goes from:

TEACHER → HEALTH WORKERS → MOTHERS → CHILDREN → OTHER CHILDREN → FATHERS

(Of course, in real life the spread of ideas usually happens more slowly and is not as obvious as shown here.)

CHAPTER 12

Learning to Make, Take, and Use Pictures

Being able to make and use pictures effectively is one of the most valuable skills a health worker or teacher of health workers can learn. In this chapter we look at:

- different ways of presenting ideas through pictures
- making sure your drawings communicate what you want
- when to use cartoons and when to draw people as realistically as possible
- learning to draw
- how to draw the human body
- techniques for copying
- suggestions for taking and using photos (for ideas on use of filmstrips and color slides, see Ch. 13)
- use of symbols
- the importance of a sense of humor

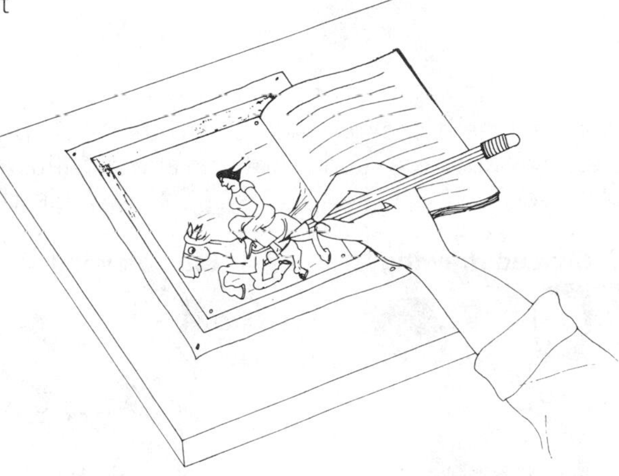

This drawing and many others in this book were done by Pablo Chavez, a village health worker from Mexico who taught himself to draw.

DIFFERENT WAYS TO ILLUSTRATE THE SAME IDEA

On the next page are 5 different kinds of illustrations: 2 photos and 3 drawings. Each kind is useful in certain circumstances.

Photos are often more exact (if well done), and they can give a sense of reality to a message. But they are more expensive to reproduce in manuals, information sheets, and posters than are line drawings. Photos cannot be mimeographed or easily copied by health workers.

Drawings have the advantage of being less costly to make and reproduce. Health workers can learn to copy drawings to use for their own teaching materials. Also, a careful drawing often can illustrate a specific health problem more clearly than a photo.

FIVE KINDS OF ILLUSTRATIONS*

1. **Photo with background complete**

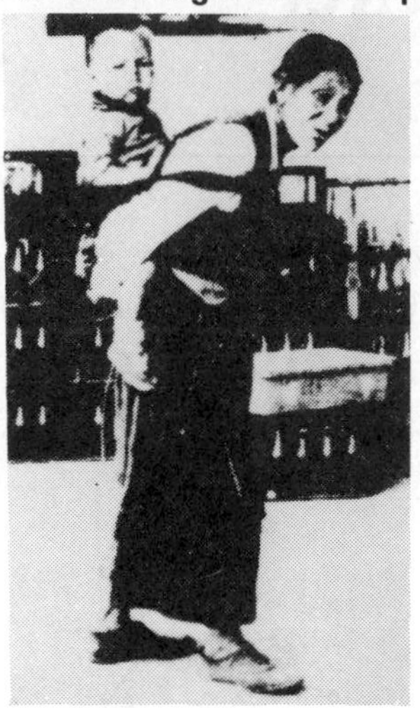

Appropriate if background adds to the message (but here it adds nothing and confuses).

2. **Photo with background cut away or 'whited out'**

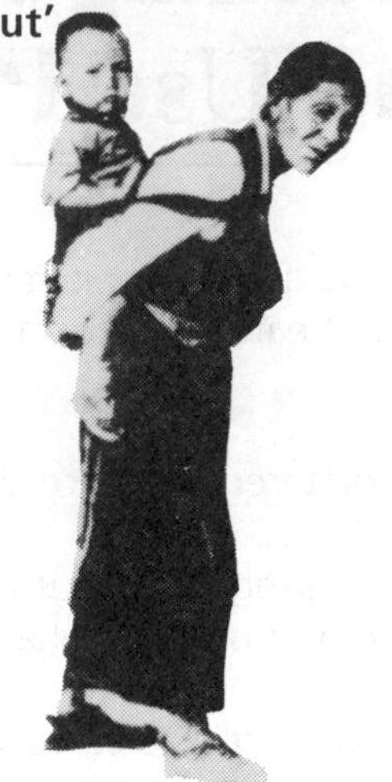

Appropriate for many health illustrations. Subject stands out more clearly. Less confusing.

3. **Shaded drawing**

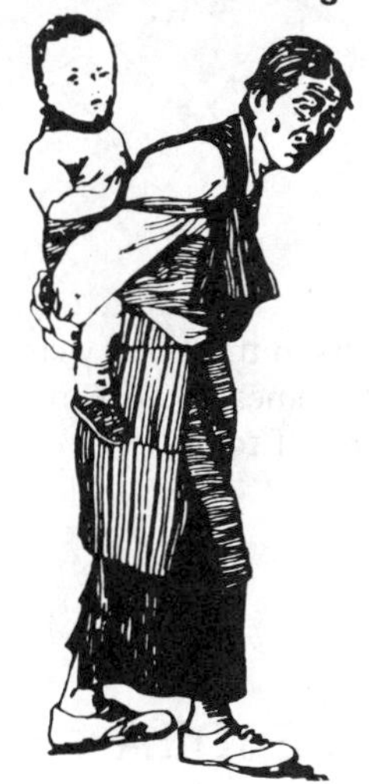

Usually less appropriate because it is difficult for people to copy and because heavy shadows can be confusing. (People might wonder, "Why is the baby's neck black?")

4. **Line drawing**

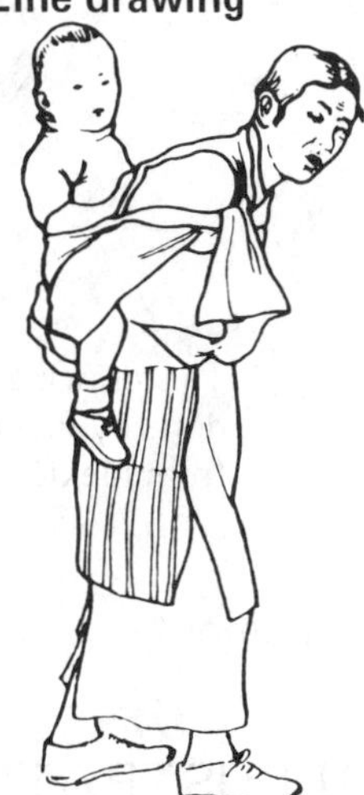

Often most appropriate because it is relatively simple, yet adequately detailed. Relatively easy for people to copy for flip charts or posters.

5. **Stylized drawing**

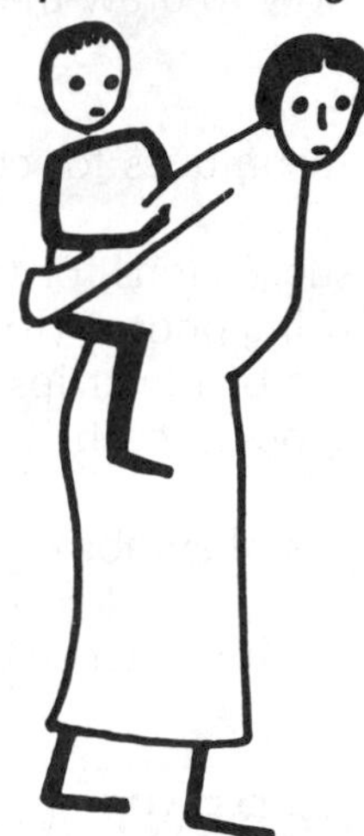

Usually less appropriate. Simplified so much that personal quality is lost. People will not identify as much with these characters.

Notice that in this book and in *Where There Is No Doctor* we mostly use simple line drawings. As a result, many health workers have copied them for posters and other health education materials.

---

*These drawings and photos are from ***Teaching For Better Learning,*** by Fred R. Abbatt, World Health Organization, 1980.

MAKE SURE DRAWINGS COMMUNICATE WHAT YOU WANT

A picture is worth a thousand words. But this is true only if the picture says what you want it to say—to the people you are trying to reach.

Confusion about size

Pictures can mean different things to different people.

For example: The instructor here believes that this huge picture of a malaria mosquito will help students tell it apart from other mosquitoes. But the students do not recognize it as anything they have ever seen. The mosquitoes that bite them are not nearly so big or frightening.

LESS APPROPRIATE

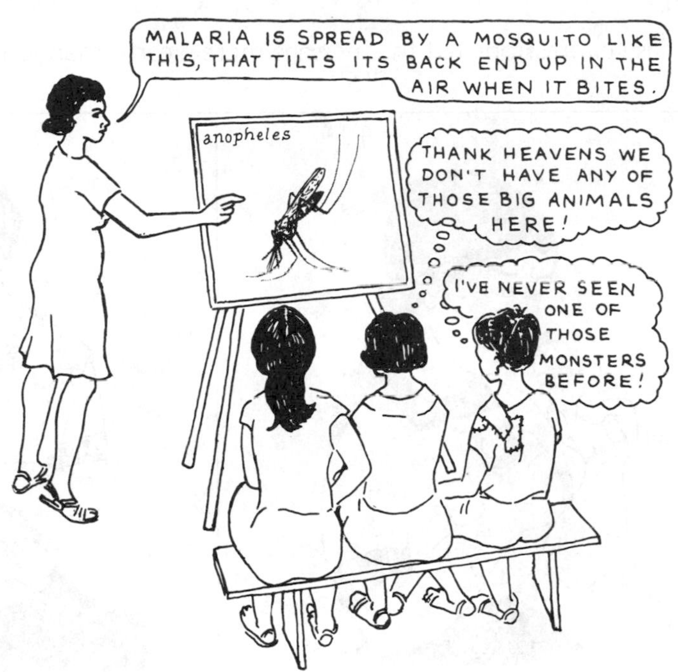

MALARIA IS SPREAD BY A MOSQUITO LIKE THIS, THAT TILTS ITS BACK END UP IN THE AIR WHEN IT BITES.
anopheles
THANK HEAVENS WE DON'T HAVE ANY OF THOSE BIG ANIMALS HERE!
I'VE NEVER SEEN ONE OF THOSE MONSTERS BEFORE!

THE BLACK FLY THAT SPREADS RIVER BLINDNESS LOOKS LIKE THIS:

BUT IT IS REALLY ONLY THIS BIG:

MORE APPROPRIATE

Whenever oversized, bigger-than-life drawings are used, it is a good idea to include a small drawing of the thing showing its actual size.

STILL MORE APPROPRIATE

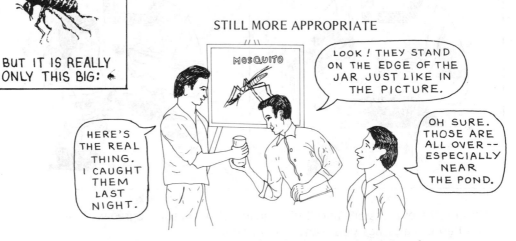

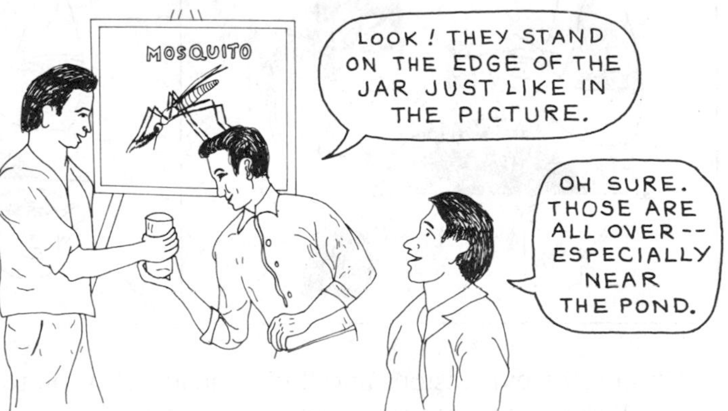

MOSQUITO
LOOK! THEY STAND ON THE EDGE OF THE JAR JUST LIKE IN THE PICTURE.
HERE'S THE REAL THING. I CAUGHT THEM LAST NIGHT.
OH SURE. THOSE ARE ALL OVER -- ESPECIALLY NEAR THE POND.

Even better than a drawing at actual size is, of course, to show the real thing—better alive than dead.

The importance of drawing people's expressions

The drawings below are part of a series produced in Guatemala for teaching mothers about child nutrition.* The health worker holds up a picture and asks, "What do you see?" or "What is happening here?" The women look at the pictures and at once they notice the expressions on the faces of the mother and child.

These expressions tell the message more clearly than words.

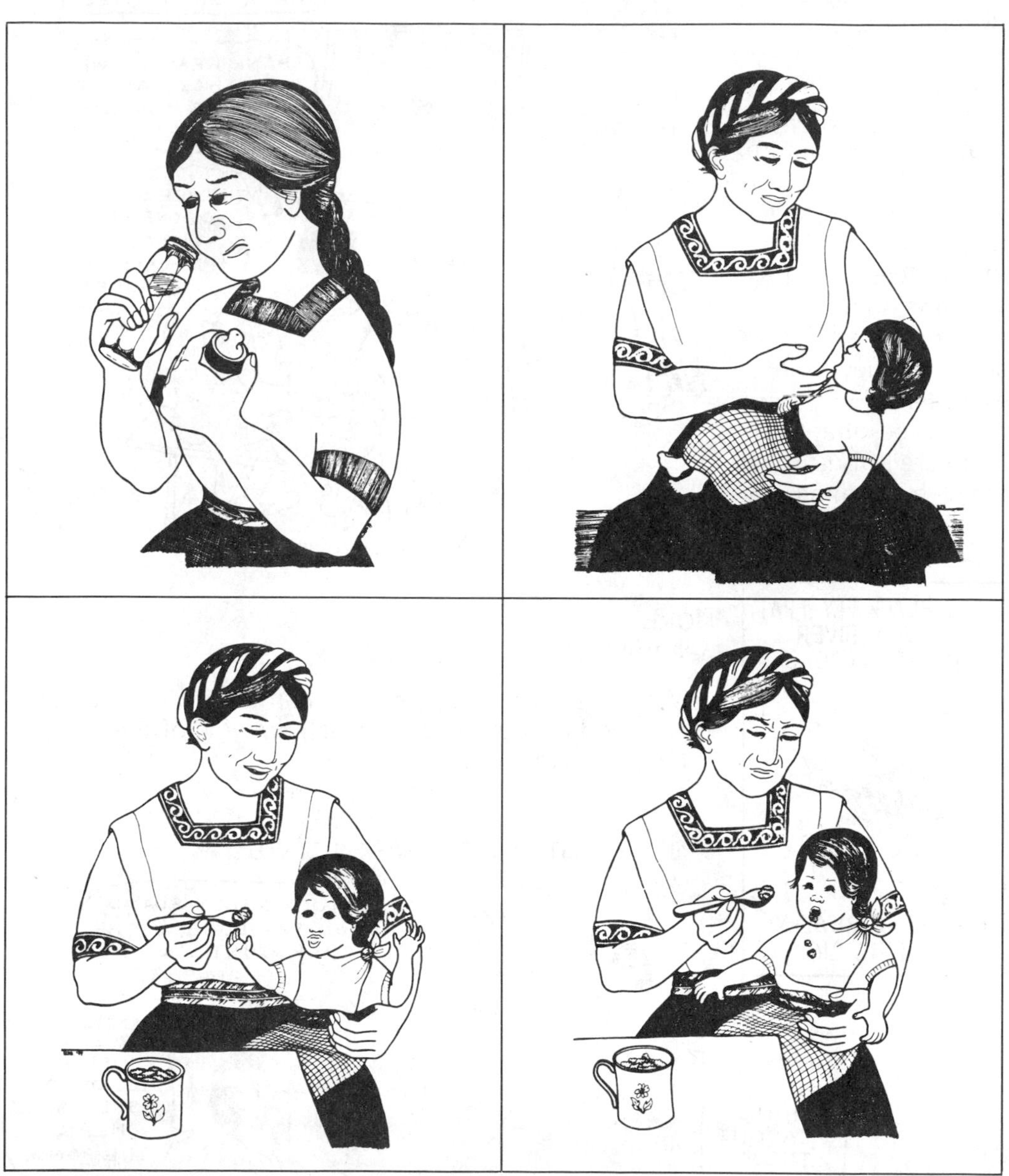

Be sure the expressions and 'body language' of pictures agree with and strengthen the message you want to communicate.

*Materiales Maria Maya, Apdo. 205, Quetzaltenango, Guatemala, Central America.

Be sure your drawings communicate care and respect

This picture, from a World Health Organization manual for the primary health worker, fails to communicate what it is supposed to.* Readers will first notice the baby's ugly, over-sized head, his twisted ear, or the ink on the mother's elbow. Even the baby's eye problem is not recognizable. It must be spelled out.

LESS APPROPRIATE

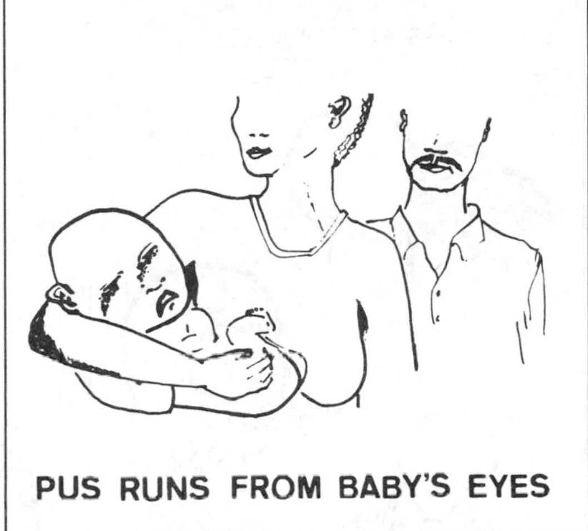

PUS RUNS FROM BABY'S EYES

Notice also that the parents have mouths, but lack eyes and brains. What does this tell you about how the authors of the manual view villagers or poor persons?

Artwork like this is typical of manuals prepared for the poor by highly paid experts. It communicates the authors' carelessness and unspoken disrespect for the 'primary health worker' and others at the village level.

This picture, from a flipchart called *"Las Moscas"* ("The Flies"), was produced in Peru by the Summer Institute of Linguistics and the Ministry of Education. It, too, shows a child with pus running from her eyes. But here the child looks real. Anyone looking at the drawing notices the eye problem at once—because when people are real, we look first into their eyes.

MORE APPROPRIATE

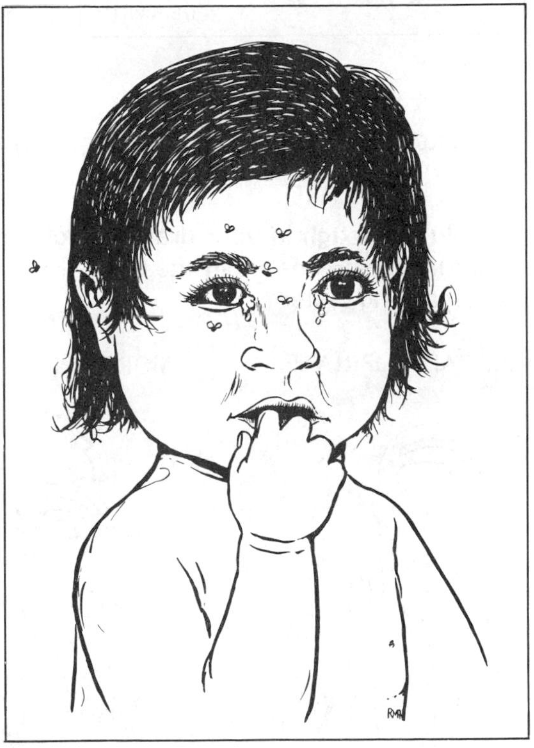

The picture also tells us something about whoever was responsible for this flipchart. He or she cared. The drawing is warm and human. It communicates deep respect for the health workers and other persons who may use or see the flipchart.

Clearly, not everyone can draw this well. But if we all try to do the best we can, people will at least see that we care. And that is one of the most important health messages of all.

*In a newer edition of the WHO manual, the pictures are much better.

Techniques for illustrating parts of the body

1. **Avoid making people look inhuman.** Make drawings as human and friendly as you can.

LESS APPROPRIATE

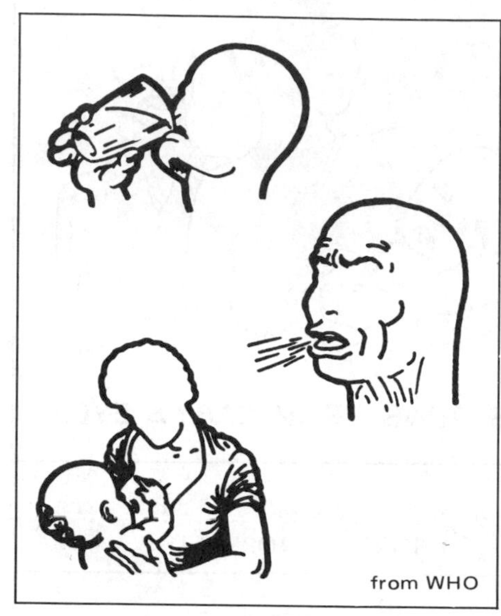
from WHO

MORE APPROPRIATE

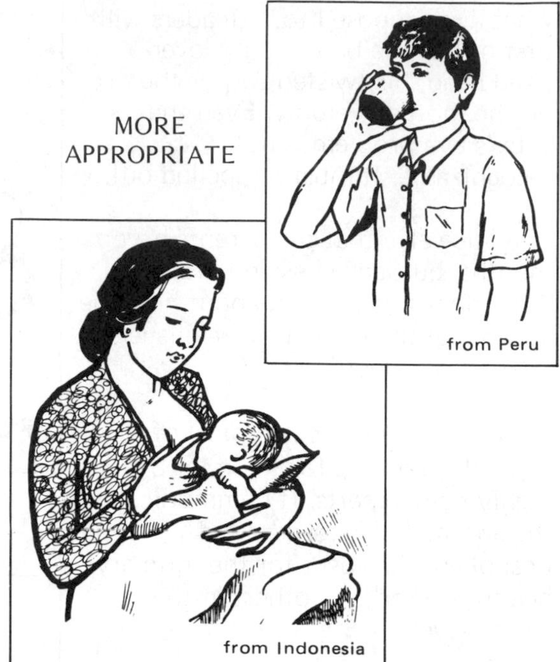
from Peru

from Indonesia

Whatever you do, **give people faces—eyes, mouths, noses, ears:**

2. **Include enough in your drawings to be sure people can tell where different structures or organs are in the body.** For example, look at these ways of showing the breathing system:

LESS APPROPRIATE

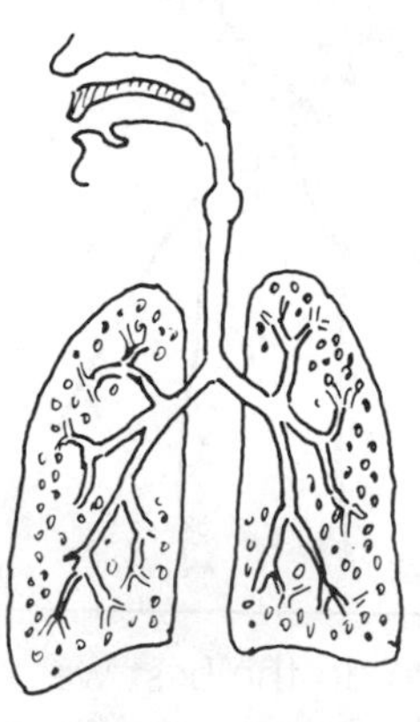

Instead of drawing only the insides, like this . . .

MORE APPROPRIATE

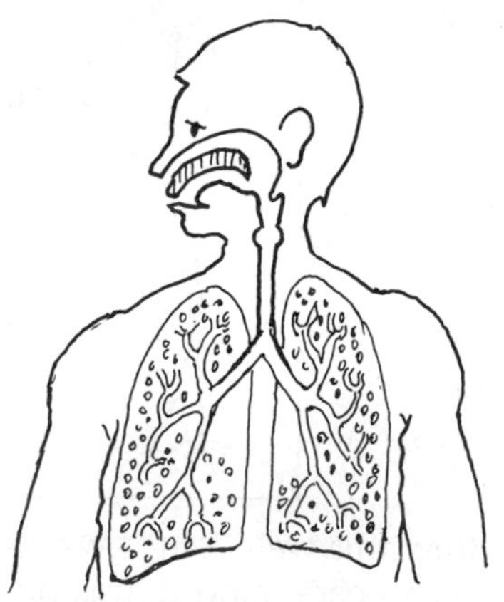

draw also the outline of the body, like this.

STILL MORE APPROPRIATE

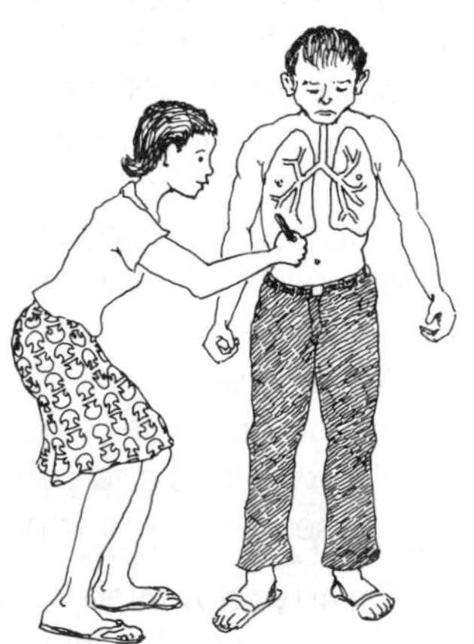

Or better still, draw directly on a person, like this.

Avoid cutting off arms and legs. Try to draw enough of the body to be sure people can recognize what is shown.

LESS APPROPRIATE

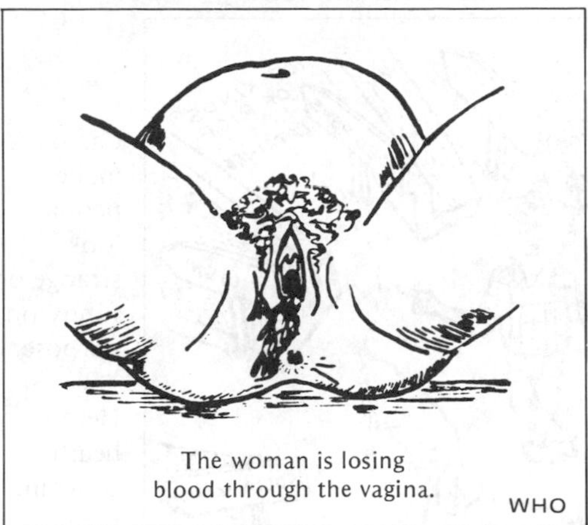

The woman is losing
blood through the vagina.
WHO

Here we must read the caption to find out what is happening. We cannot tell from the picture.

MORE APPROPRIATE

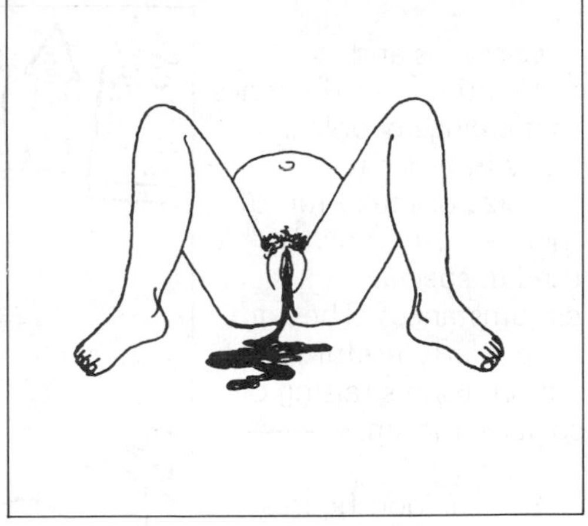

Here we do not need to be told. We see what is happening.

3. **When using pictures to teach skills, include landmarks people will recognize.** Compare these illustrations of breech birth:

When possible, show **outside anatomy** (what people actually see and are familiar with) . . .

MORE APPROPRIATE

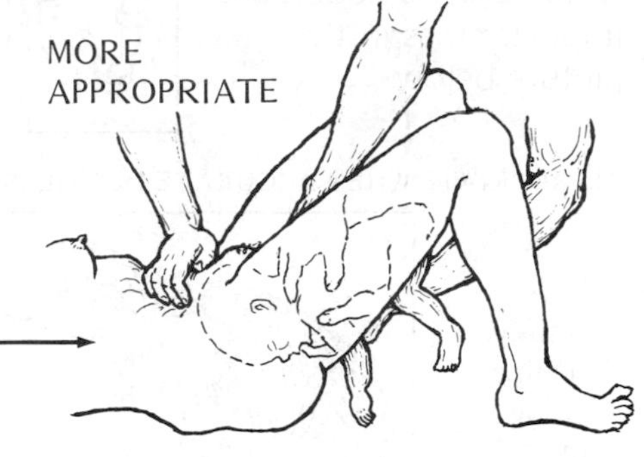

rather than **inside anatomy** (what people do not usually see and may not recognize).

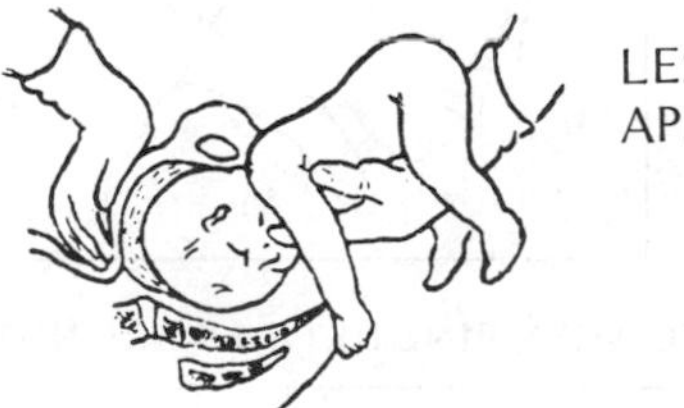

LESS APPROPRIATE

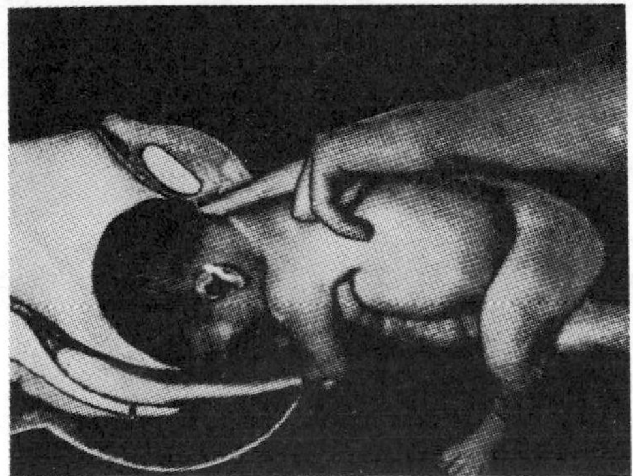

From ***Manual Practico Para Parteras,*** by Esther Gally, Editorial Pax, Mexico, 1977.

Combining real people (or photos) with drawings:

Another effective method is to combine drawings with real persons or things in the same presentation. The picture you see here was made by holding a real baby in front of a drawing showing the inside of a mother's body. The same method, using a drawing of the mother's whole body, is shown on p. **22**-9.

When to use cartoons and when to make people look real

APPROPRIATE FOR SOCIAL CRITICISM

Cartoons and 'caricatures'—or drawings that change people's looks in order to criticize or make fun of them—should only be used in special circumstances. They are particularly useful for consciousness raising or social criticism.

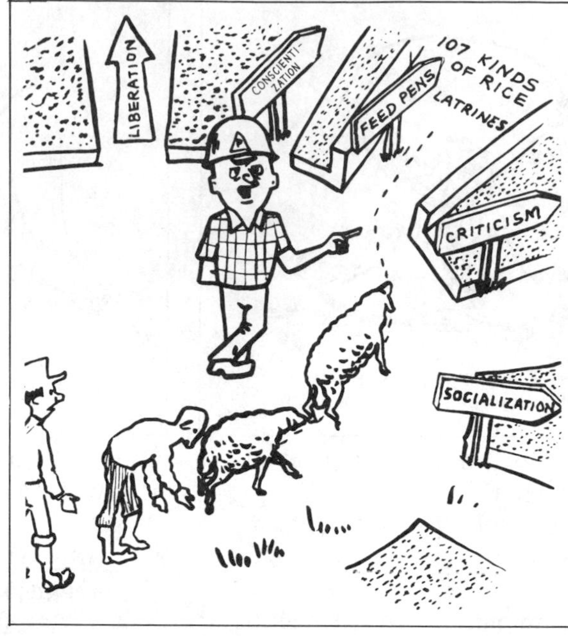

Cartoons make people look strange or funny on purpose.

Here a health program turns people into sheep.

But cartoon figures usually should **not** be used for illustrations in which precise details are important, as in the picture below.

APPROPRIATE WHEN ACCURATE DETAIL IS NEEDED

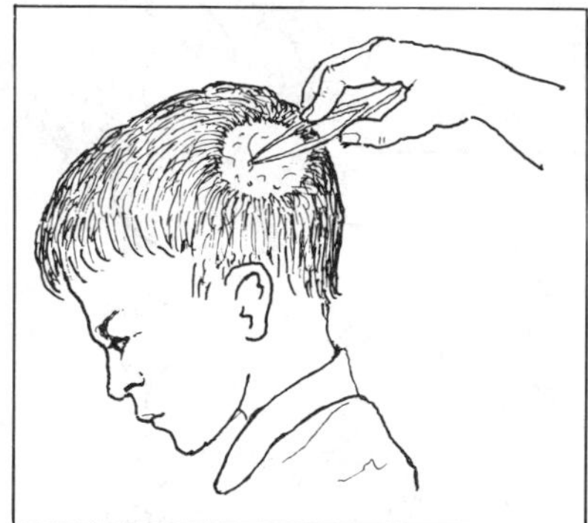

Carefully done line drawing with correct physical proportions

When showing how to do something or how to tell different health problems apart, try to make the drawings as lifelike as possible. The details should be clear and accurate.

APPROPRIATE WHEN FINE DETAILS ARE NOT IMPORTANT

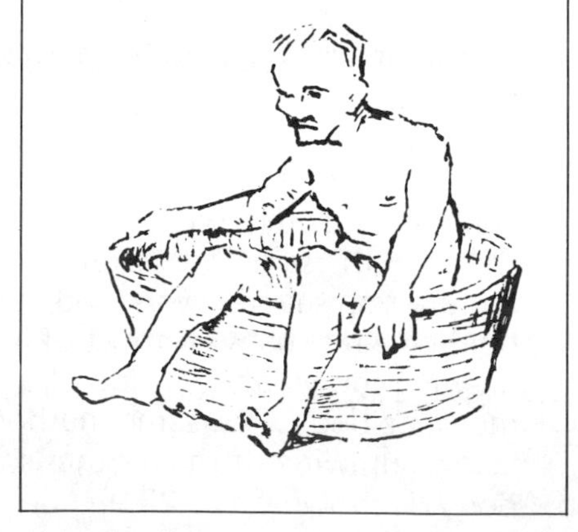

Free artistic sketch

Freer, less precise, or more artistic drawing can be used when fine detail is not so important.

But notice that, although the drawing shown here is less detailed and some lines are not complete, the physical proportions are quite accurate. This is what gives the drawing life.

LEARNING TO DRAW

Learning to draw is mainly a process of learning to see! To be able to observe things accurately and draw them well is a skill of great value to a health worker or instructor.

Almost anyone can learn to draw. What it takes is care and practice.

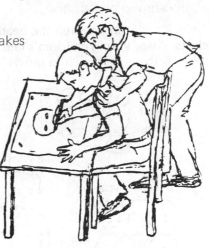

To draw fairly well you do not need to be an artist, or to study art. You do need to look at things carefully. And you need lots of practice.

Tracing and copying from others

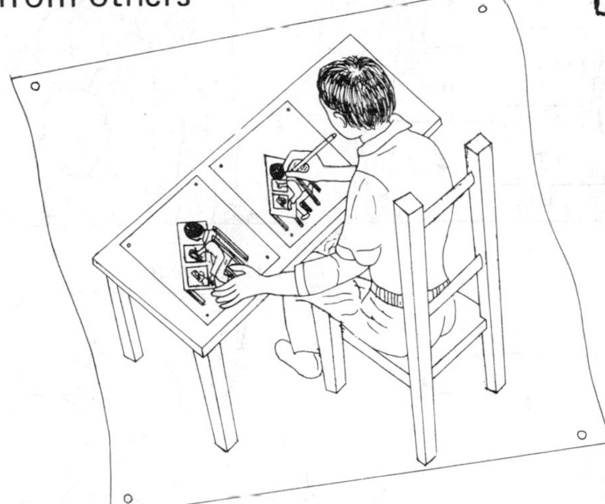

One of the best ways to learn how to draw is to practice copying other drawings or photographs. At first this often is easier than drawing people or things from real life.

In making posters, leaflets, working guides, and other teaching materials, do not be afraid to 'borrow' from other people's work. Lots of people do it.

Drawing people

When drawing people, do not start with details. First sketch the general shapes in light pencil, and check if the proportions are right.

If you want your drawings of children and adults to look convincing, watch for these 3 important things:

- relative **size of the head**
- relative **position of the eyes** on the face
- relative **length of arms and legs**

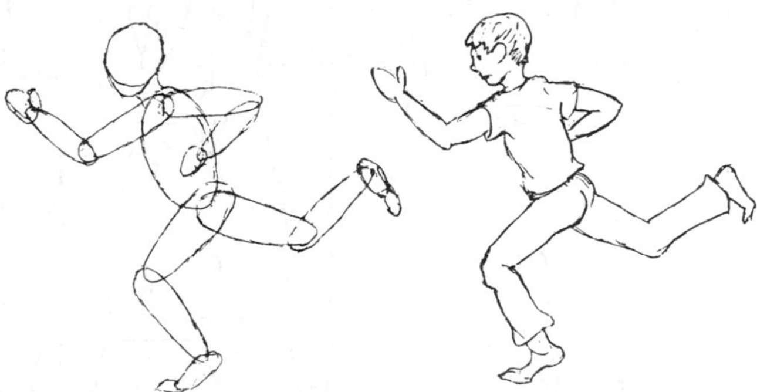

When drawing people, remember their muscles and bones! It helps to draw bodies naked first and then add the clothes.

Proportions

In order to draw people so they look human, try to get the proportions right. This means making sure the different parts of the body are the right size in relationship to one another.

Notice that **in children the head is much bigger, relative to the body, than in adults.** Also, **young children's legs are relatively shorter.** Notice how the halfway line gets lower as the child grows.

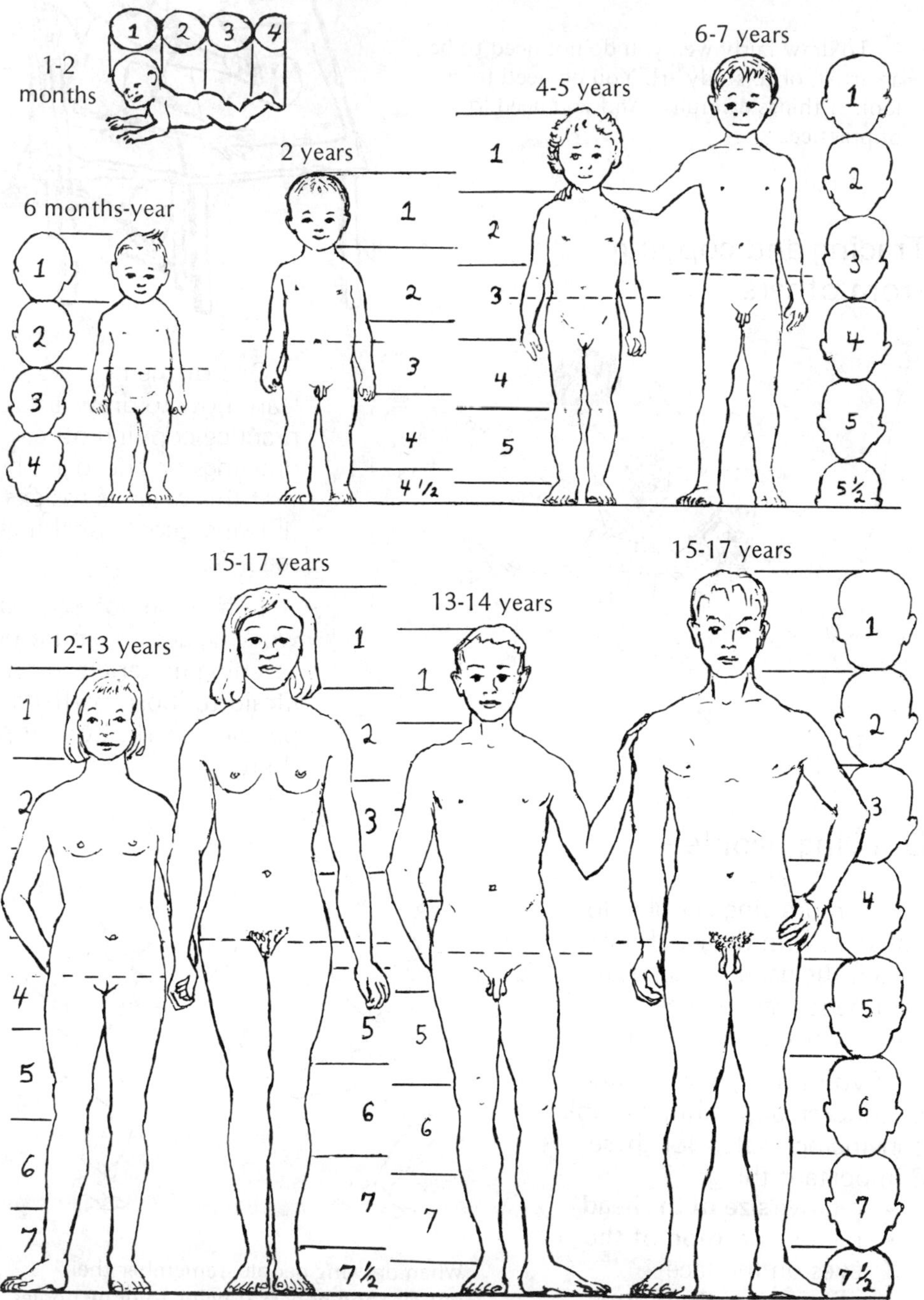

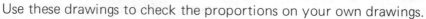

Use these drawings to check the proportions on your own drawings.

Drawing faces

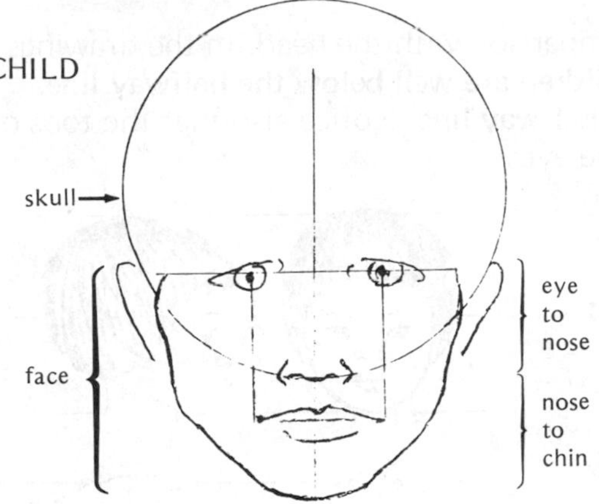

The child has a smaller face and jaw.

You can practice drawing heads by first putting a circle for the skull. Then add the line of the jaw.

Notice that in both drawings shown here, the nose lies on the circle. And the distance from eyes to nose is about equal to that from the nose to the chin. So the lower you put the line of the eyes, the smaller the jaw should be—and the younger the child you draw will look.

In the adult, the face is relatively big.

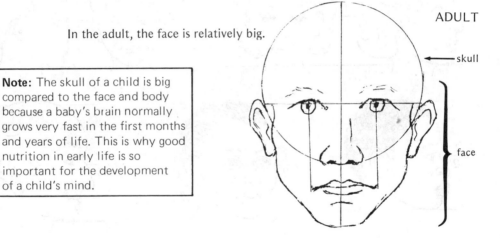

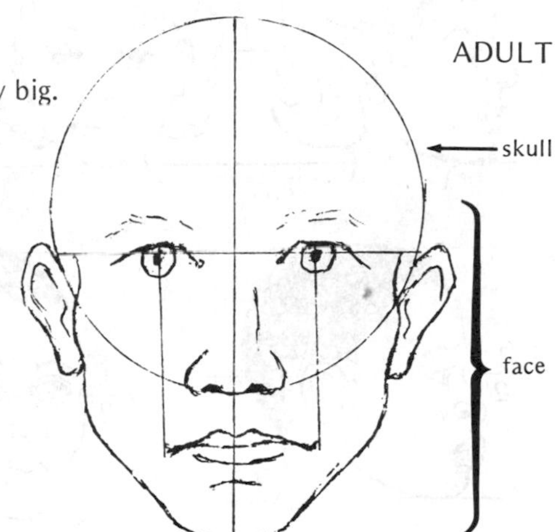

Note: The skull of a child is big compared to the face and body because a baby's brain normally grows very fast in the first months and years of life. This is why good nutrition in early life is so important for the development of a child's mind.

Face features: Try to make them like those of people in your area. Pay special attention to the shapes of the forehead, nose, and lips.

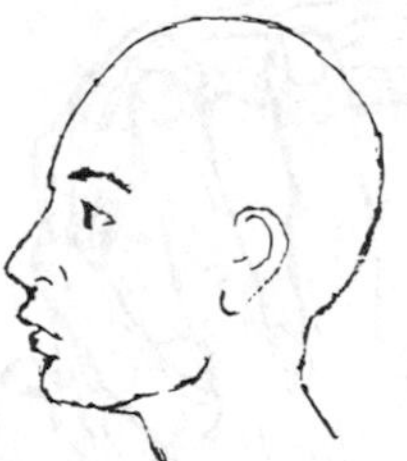
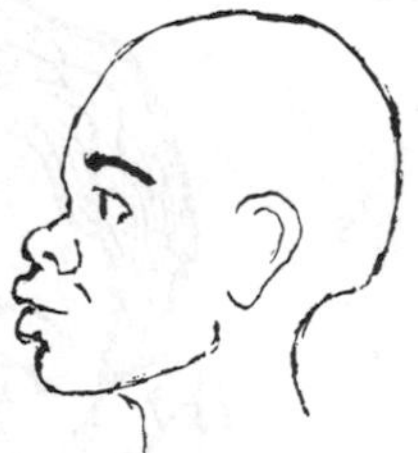
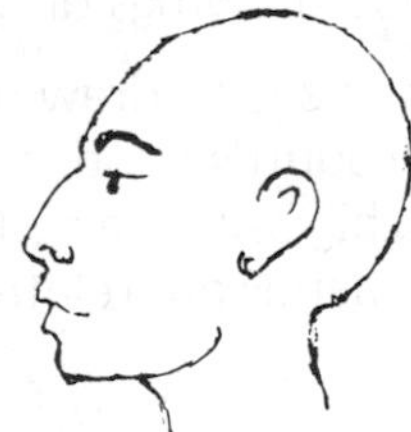
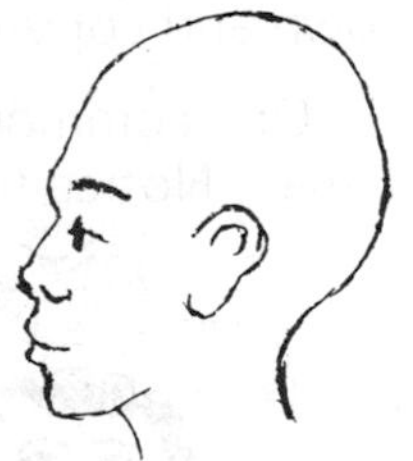

Face expressions: To change expressions, change the shapes of the eyebrows and mouth.

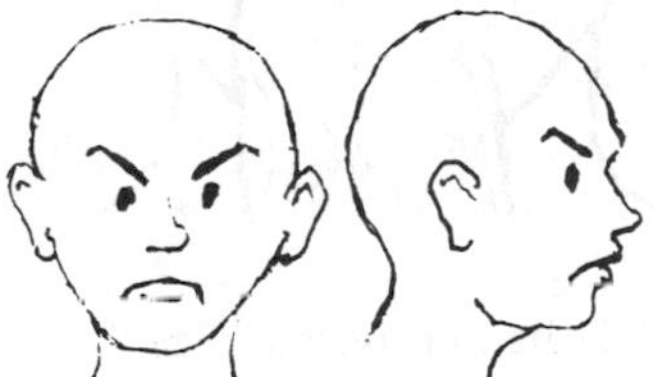
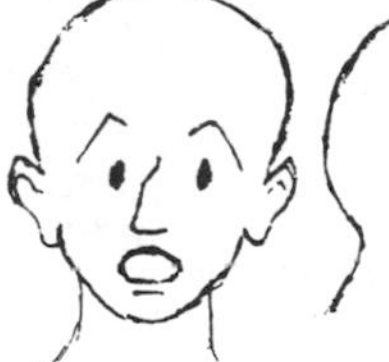
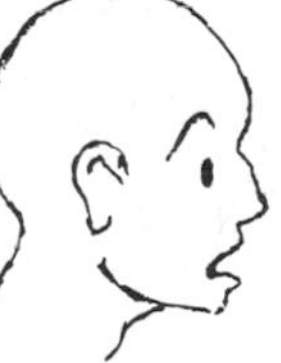
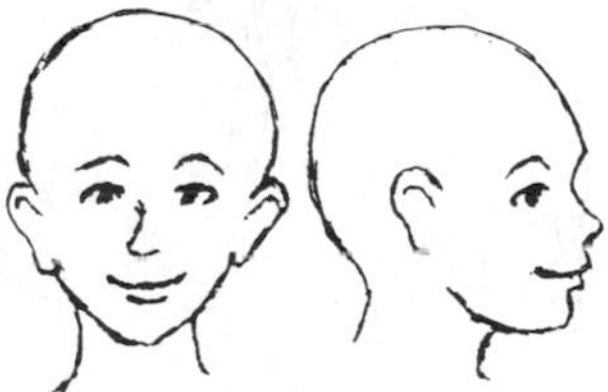

Face proportions

A child's face is relatively small in comparison with the head. In the drawings below, notice that **the eyes of young children are well below the halfway line. In adults the eyes are slightly above the halfway line.** Notice also that the tops of the ears are at about the same level as the eyes.

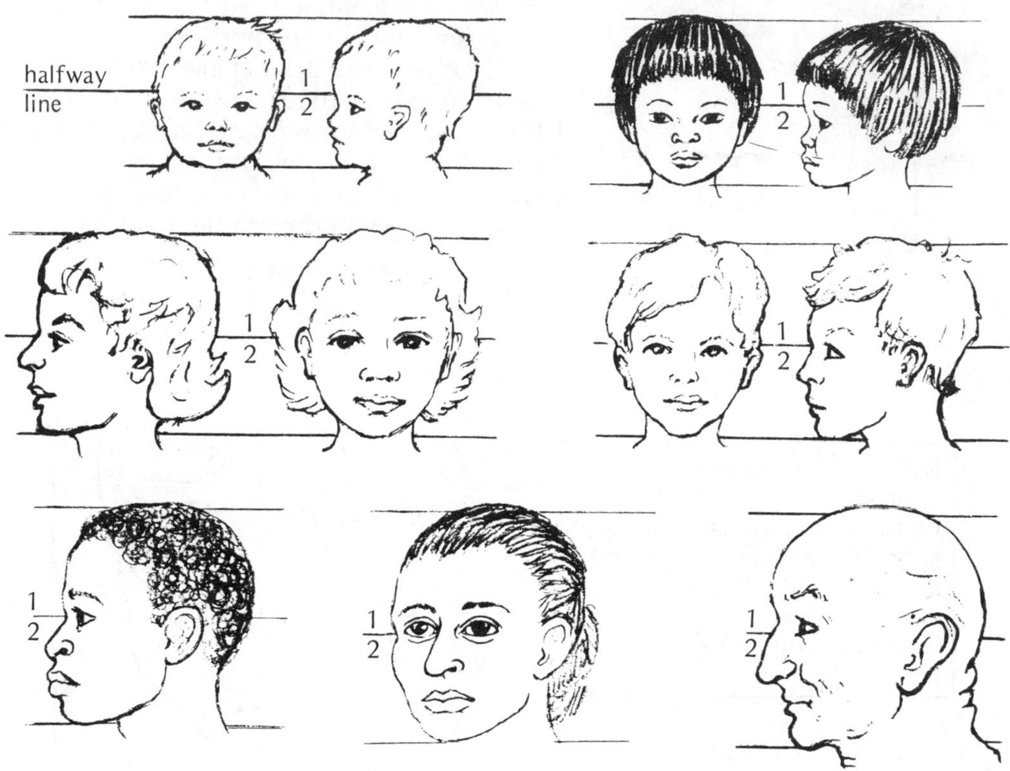
halfway line
1
2

Drawing hands

Hands are hard to draw. Practice drawing your own and copying good drawings or photos.

One common mistake is to draw hands too small. Notice that an adult's hand is almost as big as his face. (Children's hands are relatively smaller.)

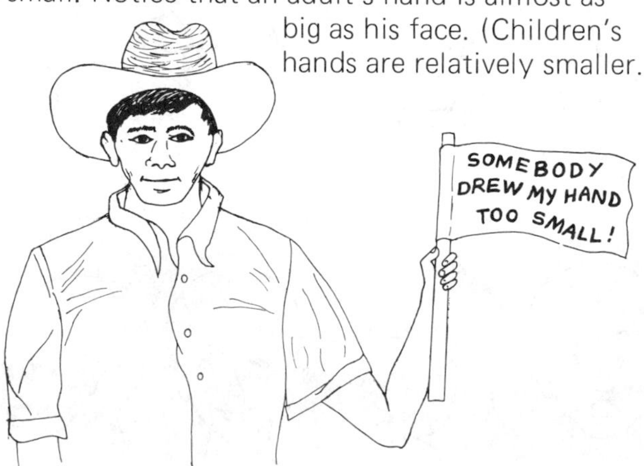
SOMEBODY
DREW MY HAND
TOO SMALL!

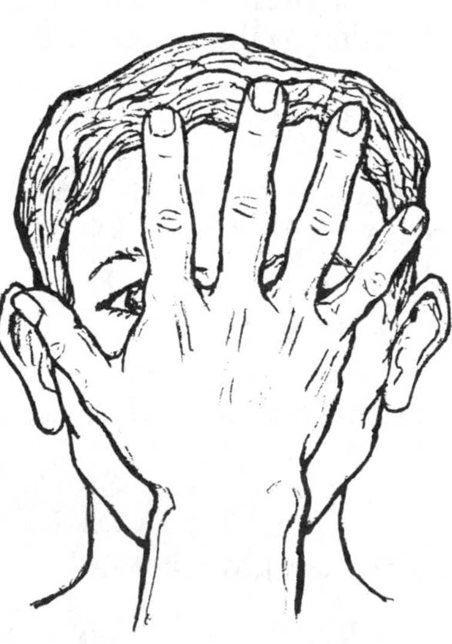

"My hand is normal size."

Learning to draw human proportions correctly

This method was developed at an 'educational exchange' for instructors of village health workers, held in Ajoya, Mexico in 1979.

Have students cut out figures like those below, but much larger. They can be made of flannel, or cardboard fixed for flannel-board use.

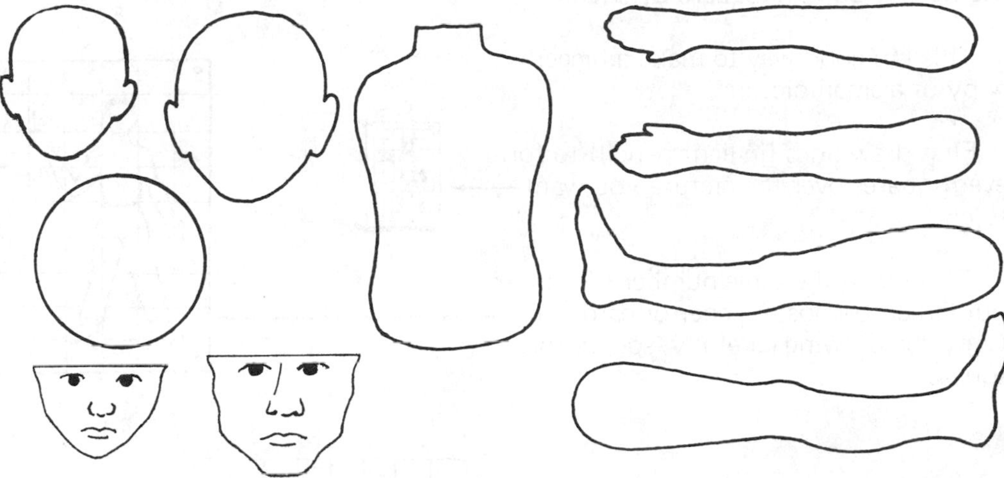

By putting the pieces together in different ways, the students can form persons of different ages.

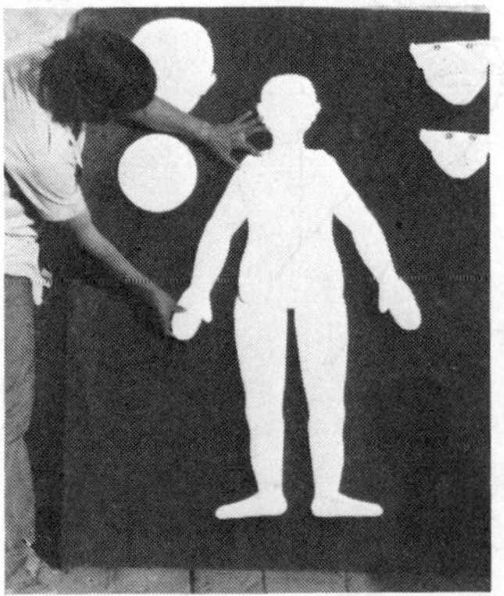

The small head on the body forms an adult.

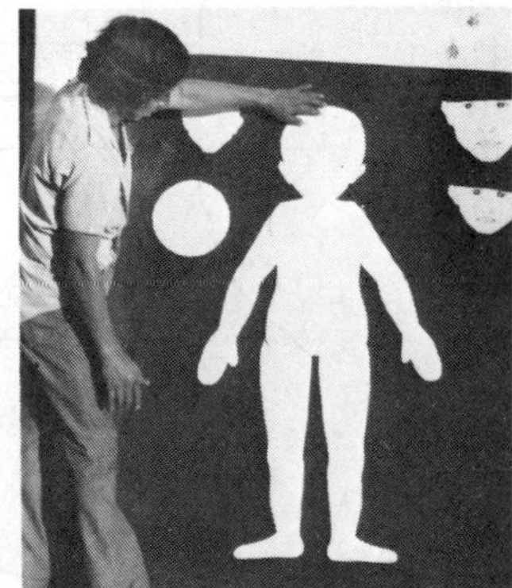

The big head on the body forms a child.

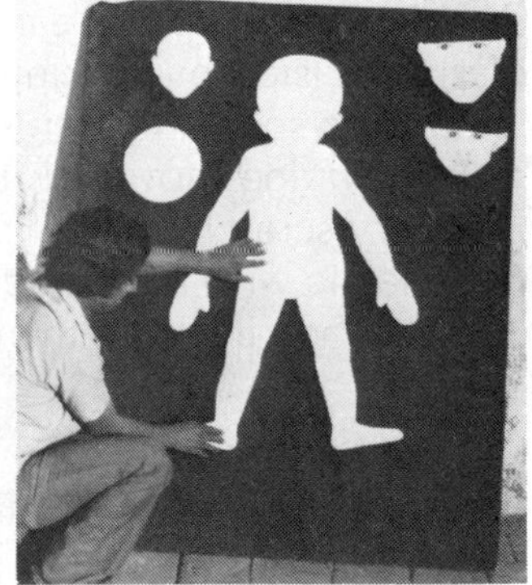

The child can be made younger by pushing up the arms and legs to make them shorter.

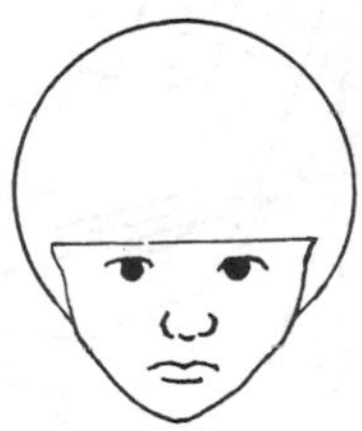

The small face on the skull forms a child.

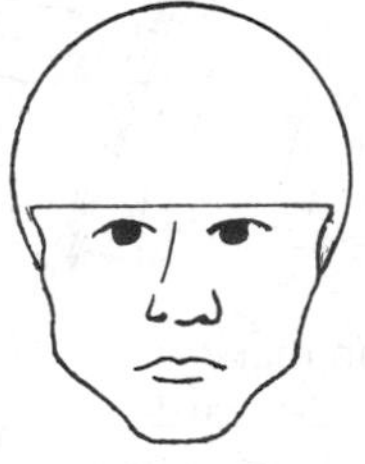

The large face on the same skull forms an adult.

Health workers can make their own sets of figures during training. Then they can use them in their villages to help others learn to draw.

TECHNIQUES FOR COPYING

When copying, again it is important to get the proportions right: the head the right size in relation to the body, and so on. There are several ways this can be done.

Method 1: Copying square by square

This is a good way to make a bigger copy of a small picture.

First draw lines (in light pencil) to form even squares over the picture you want to copy.

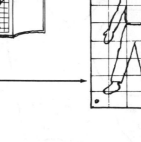

Then draw the same number of squares, but larger, on poster paper or cardboard. Copy the drawing carefully, square for square.

To make copies without marking up the original, and to save time, you can prepare a sheet of plastic by carefully drawing squares on it. (Use heavy, clear plastic. An old X-ray plate is ideal. Clean off the dark emulsion by soaking it in lye or caustic soda and then scrubbing it.) If ink does not mark the plastic well, try scratching the lines into the plastic with a pointed piece of metal. Then ink over them.

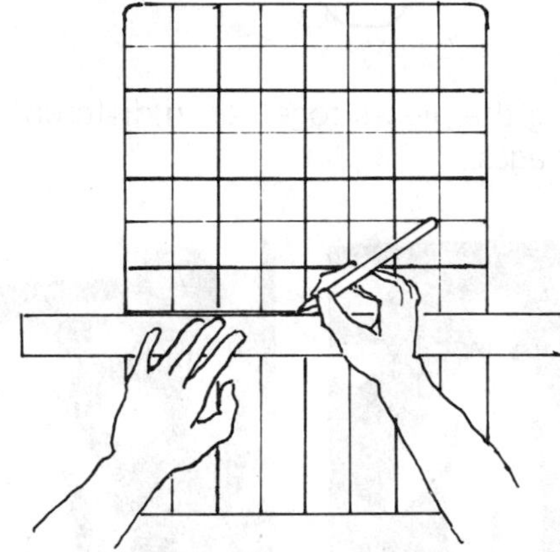

It helps to make every second or third line darker.

To copy, simply place (or pin) the marked sheet of plastic over the picture you want to copy. Draw the same number of squares on poster paper, and copy.

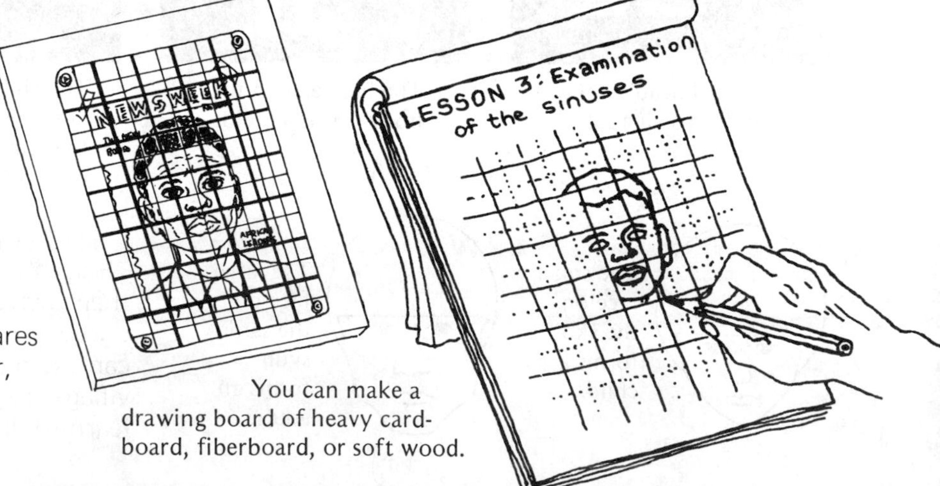

You can make a drawing board of heavy cardboard, fiberboard, or soft wood.

Method 2: The elastic string method*

This can be used for making bigger copies of small pictures, especially on the blackboard but also on posters and flip charts.

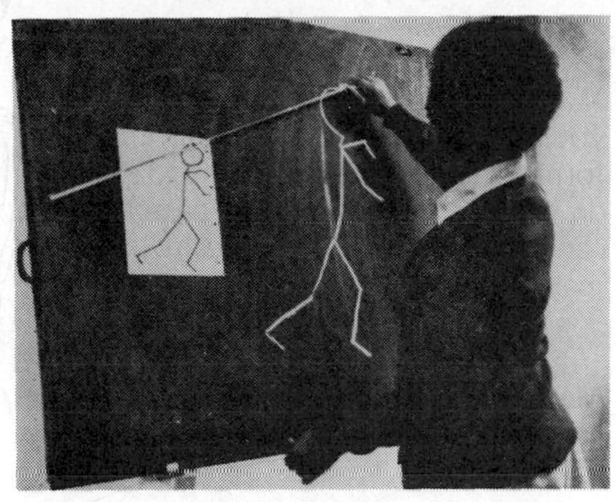

After attaching the original drawing to the blackboard, pin one end of an elastic string to the left of the drawing. A knot should be tied in the middle of the string so that, when the string is stretched across the drawing, the knot may cover any point on the drawing. At the other end of the string, tie a piece of chalk (or a pencil, if you are drawing on paper or cloth).

Now begin to copy, taking care that the knot in the string follows the outline of the original drawing.

The larger the distance between the chalk and the knot, the greater the enlargement will be.

Method 3: The punched pattern or template method

Use this method for pictures of the human body, maps, or other things that you want to put frequently on the blackboard or on posters, but have trouble drawing freehand. Patterns or 'templates' can be prepared for repeated use.

First prepare a full-size drawing on heavy paper or cardboard. Then use a leather punch to make small holes, 2 to 4 mm. across, over the lines of the drawing. Now place the cardboard pattern against the blackboard and rub a dusty eraser (or a cloth with chalk dust) over the surface. An outline of the picture will be formed by chalk dots on the blackboard. Remove the pattern and connect the dots with chalk.

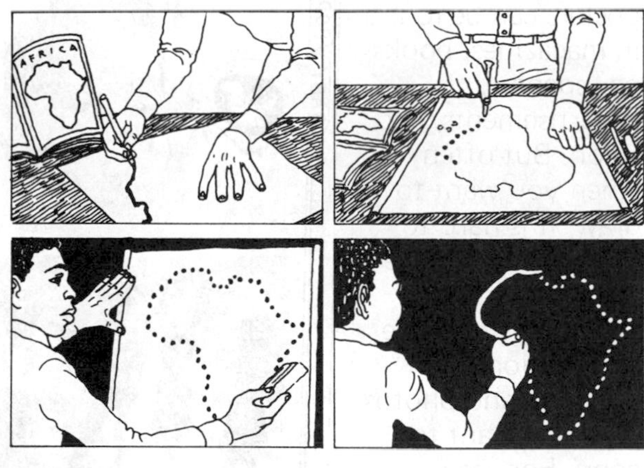

*These ideas and photographs come from a booklet entitled "Blackboard Tips." It was developed in a workshop in Botswana and published by the Werkgroep Ontwikkelings Technieken, Technische Hogeschool Twente, Postbus 217, Enschede, Holland.

Method 4: Cut-outs

Another way to make a pattern, instead of using punched holes, is to carefully cut out the drawing. Cut along its outer edges so that you have a cardboard image in the form of the object you want to draw. This type of cut-out pattern can also have punched holes to mark lines inside the drawing.

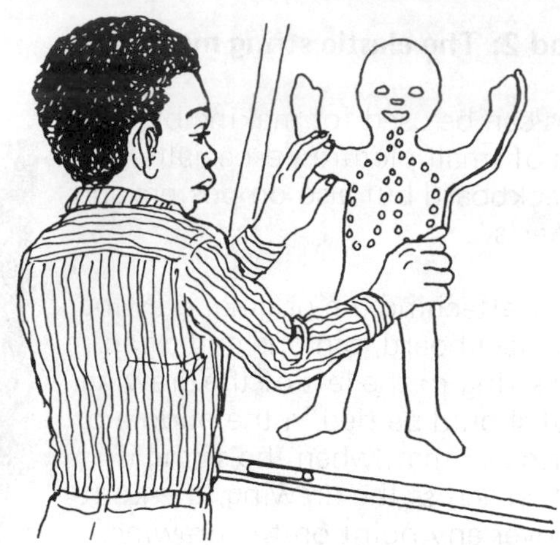

Method 5: Tracing a color slide projection

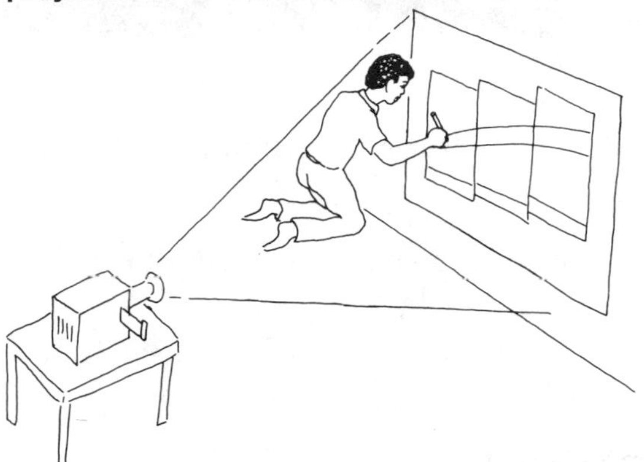

This is a good way to make accurate enlargements of pictures from color slides or transparencies. Project the slide against a large paper or a wall. Then trace the picture exactly.

This method is especially useful for Road to Health charts, thinness charts (see page **25**-10), etc. Slides of both these charts are available from TALC (see page **Back**-3).

KEEPING A 'SCRAPBOOK' OF GOOD PICTURES FOR COPYING

Good pictures for making drawings or posters can be found in magazines, books, newspapers, advertisements, and so on. But often when you want to draw, it is hard to find a good picture to use as a model. So it helps to make a collection of drawings and photos you may want to copy. For easy reference, you can organize them by subjects in a scrapbook (notebook or album). It is also helpful to keep a list of books and the pages with pictures you may want to copy.

BODY
BABY
LIST OF EXTRA GOOD BABY PICTURES IN BOOKS WE HAVE
(continued)
7. KING -"Primary Child Care" pages: 152, 285, 340, 413, 444
8. ARMS -"A Season To Be Born" pages: 90, 92, 93
9. GALLY -"Manual Practico Para Parteras" pages: 406, 452, 487, 488, 526, 529
10. WERNER -"Where There Is No Doctor" pages: 271, 273, 274, 302, 316, 317, 319
11. REICH - "Children of Many Lands" pages: 2-5, 8, 4, 9, 104
FACE
HANDS
MOTHER
HOME
FOOD

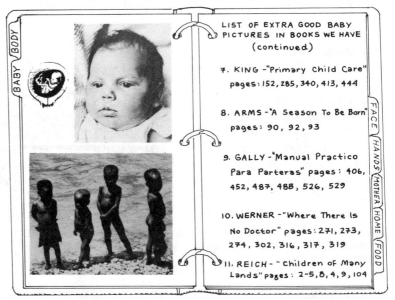

USING PHOTOGRAPHS AS TEACHING AIDS

Photographs can be used for teaching in many ways:

- in pamphlets and books
- on posters or flannel-boards
- in the form of filmstrips or slides for projection (see p. **13**-11)

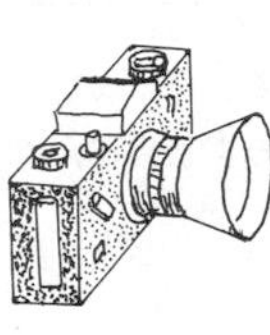

If your program can buy or borrow a camera and afford the film, you can take many photos to use for health education. A 35 millimeter camera is usually a good choice—especially for taking color slides.

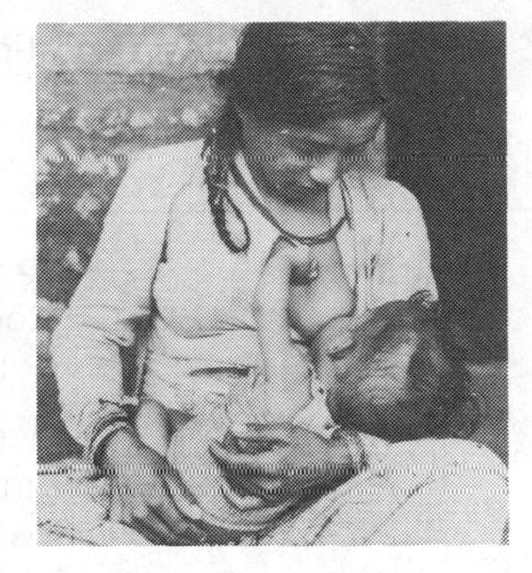

Good photos can help bring ideas to life and make them convincing.

Whether you have a camera or not, good photos can be cut from magazines or newspapers to make posters, flannel-board figures, and other teaching aids.

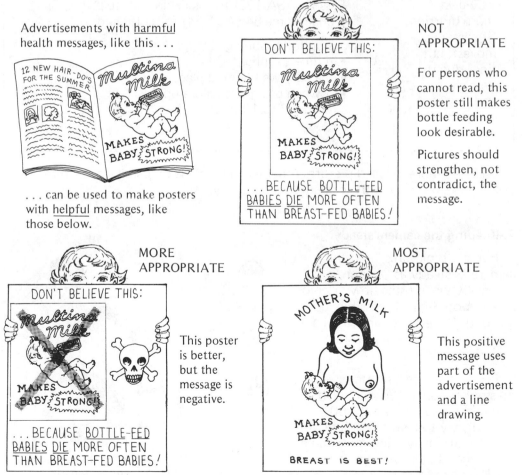

Advertisements with harmful health messages, like this . . .

. . . can be used to make posters with helpful messages, like those below.

NOT APPROPRIATE

For persons who cannot read, this poster still makes bottle feeding look desirable.

Pictures should strengthen, not contradict, the message.

MORE APPROPRIATE

This poster is better, but the message is negative.

MOST APPROPRIATE

MOTHER'S MILK
MAKES BABY STRONG!
BREAST IS BEST!

This positive message uses part of the advertisement and a line drawing.

Be sure the picture carries a helpful message—with or without the words.

How to get better photos with your camera

In this book we cannot explain how to use different cameras. You will want to read an instruction book or, better still, to learn from someone who has experience.

Here are just a few suggestions for getting good quality pictures.

1. **Film speed**

Fast film gives less blurring but coarser quality (grain).	Use faster film (ASA rating above 200) such as Kodak Tri-X (ASA 400) for black and white prints, or Ektachrome (ASA 400) for color slides when photographing . . . • indoors • where the light is poor • or when the subject is moving fast } except when using flash **close up**
Slow film may give more blurring (if camera moves), but finer quality (less grain) and better color. Better for enlargements.	Use slower film (ASA rating below 200) such as Plus X (ASA 125) for black and white prints, or Kodachrome 64 (ASA 64) for color slides when photographing . . . • in direct sunlight • in a very well lighted place • or when using flash close up (within 7 to 10 feet) } when subject is still or moves slowly

Sharper, more detailed pictures usually can be made by using slower film in good light—but only if the camera is kept steady.

2. **Keeping the camera steady**

For sharp pictures, hold the camera as steady as you can, especially when using slow or color film in poor light. If possible, use a tripod. Or rest the camera on a wall or chair, to keep it from moving.

If possible, use a shutter speed no slower than 1/125 second. If you must take it slower (1/60 second), try to rest the camera on something steady. Pictures taken at 1/30 second or slower are very hard to keep from blurring unless you use a tripod.

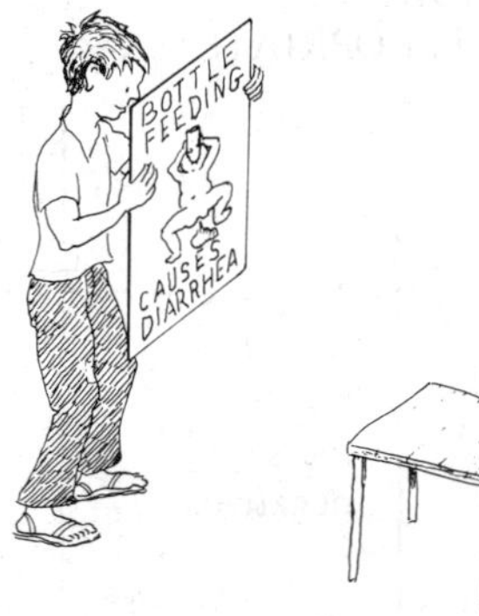
BOTTLE FEEDING
CAUSES DIARRHEA

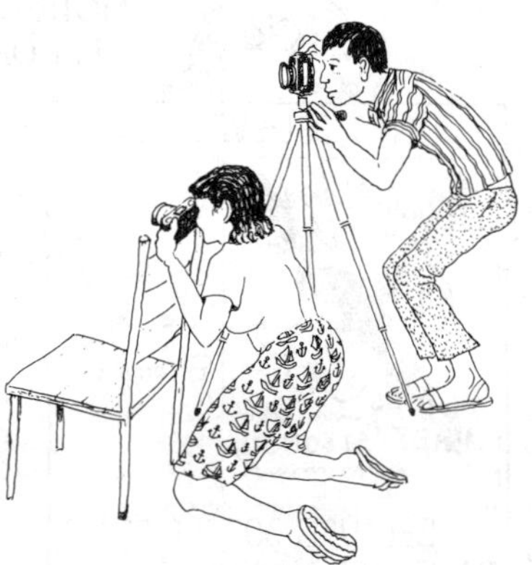

Keep the camera as still as you can.

3. **Lighting**

Good lighting is important. Before clicking the shutter of your camera, always check to be sure the light falls well on the faces of people and on the details of whatever you are trying to photograph.

Sometimes good pictures can be taken in direct sunlight, but usually the shadows come out very dark.

If you take pictures outdoors, they will often be better if you **take them when the sun is not too high overhead**—an hour or two after sunrise or an hour or two before sunset.

Also, to avoid shadows that are too dark, try to take pictures on a cloudy or hazy day.

For taking pictures of charts, skin problems, and other subjects to be used for teaching, indirect lighting is often best. Light can be shined against a white wall so that it reflects onto the subject. Or hold a white sheet so that the sunlight reflects onto the object to be photographed.

USUALLY NOT SO GOOD—SHADOWS TOO DARK

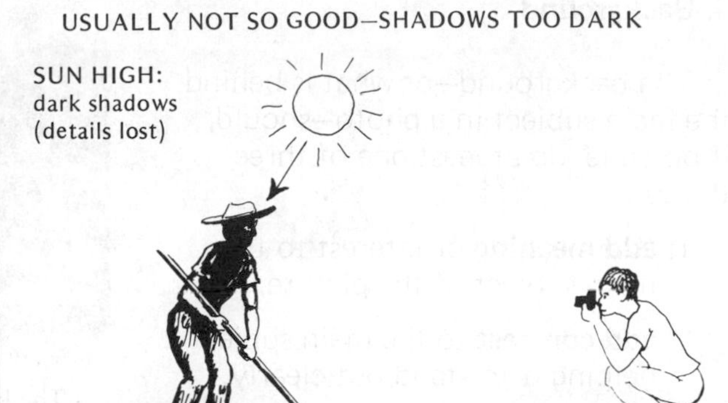
SUN HIGH:
dark shadows
(details lost)

GOOD FOR PHOTOGRAPHING PEOPLE OR ACTIVITIES

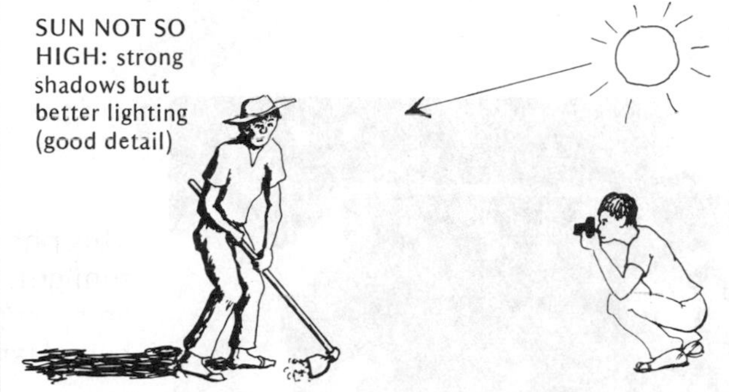

SUN NOT SO HIGH: strong shadows but better lighting (good detail)

GOOD FOR PHOTOGRAPHING PICTURES, FLANNEL-BOARDS, CHARTS, SKIN PROBLEMS

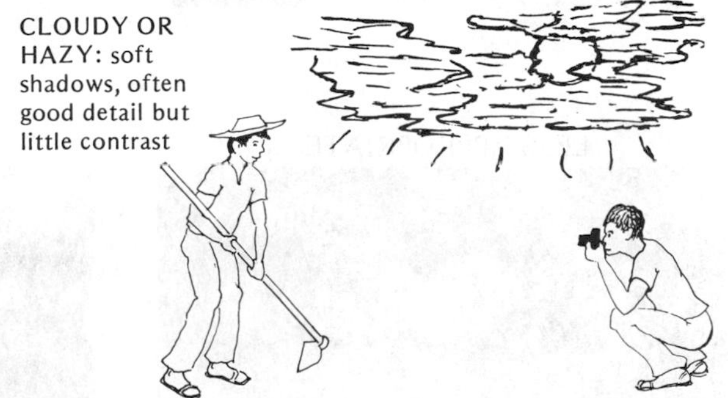
CLOUDY OR HAZY: soft shadows, often good detail but little contrast

GOOD FOR PHOTOGRAPHING DISPLAYS, PICTURES, CHARTS, FLANNEL-BOARDS, ETC.

INDIRECT LIGHTING: shadows soft, but good contrast (details good)

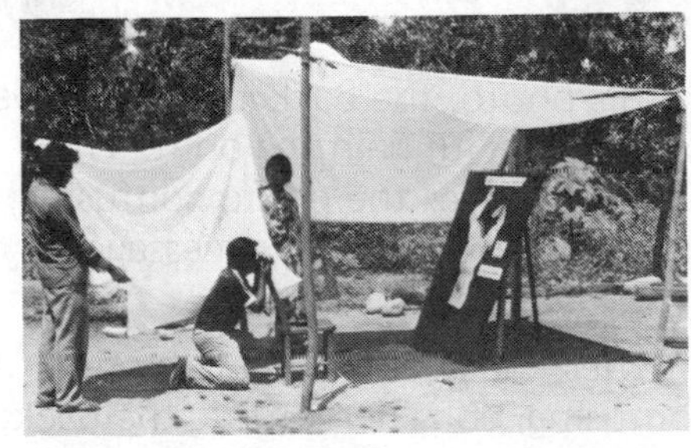

4. **Background**

The background—or what is behind the main subject in a photo—should, if possible, do at least one of three things:

1. **add meaning** or interest to the main subject of the picture,
2. **add contrast** to the main subject, helping it to stand out clearly,
3. **not detract** or take attention away from the main subject.

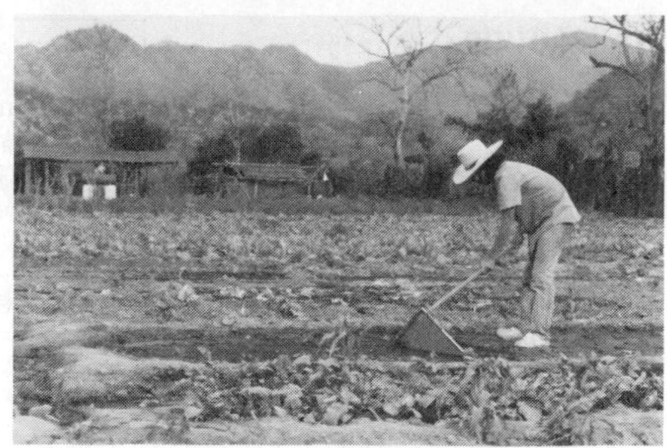

The background in this picture of a community garden adds to the message.

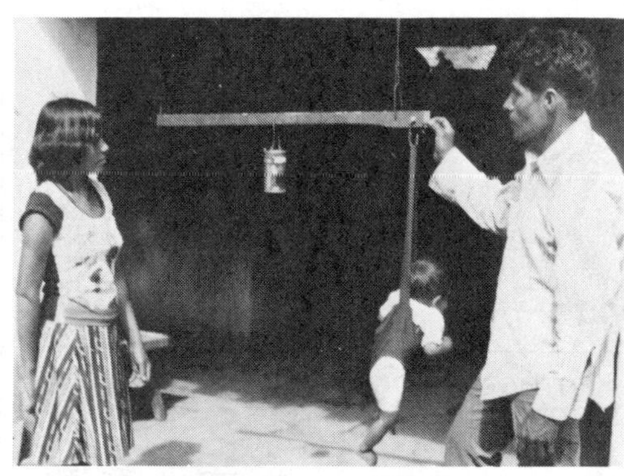

This photograph was taken in the sunlight, against the dark background of an open doorway. The scales and the baby stand out clearly.

LESS APPROPRIATE

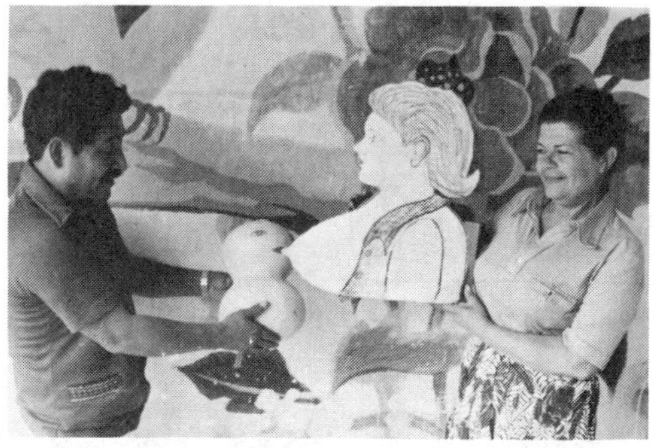

In this photo, the background is a wall with a colorful painting on it. The painting makes the photo confusing, and adds nothing to the message.

MORE APPROPRIATE

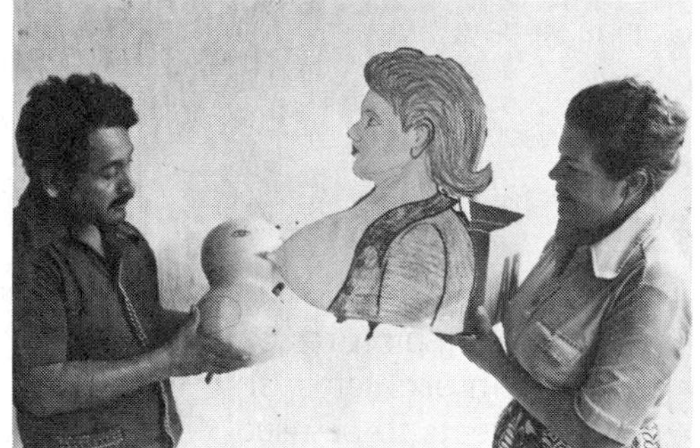

This photo was taken against a plain white wall. The subject of the picture stands out clearly, and the background does not disturb.

When the background in a photo does not add anything and makes the subject confusing, consider cutting the background away with scissors and mounting the subject on plain paper. (Compare the first two photos on page **12**-2.)

USE OF SYMBOLS IN PICTURES

By combining things in unexpected ways, drawings can make people stop and think.

For example, a gun is a well-known symbol for killing. When tablets are compared with bullets, people can at once see how dangerous medicines can be.

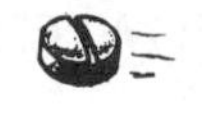
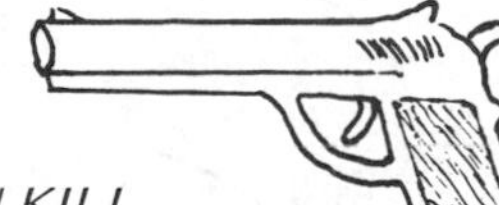
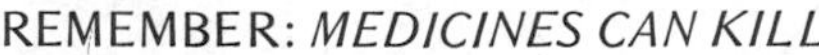

REMEMBER: *MEDICINES CAN KILL*

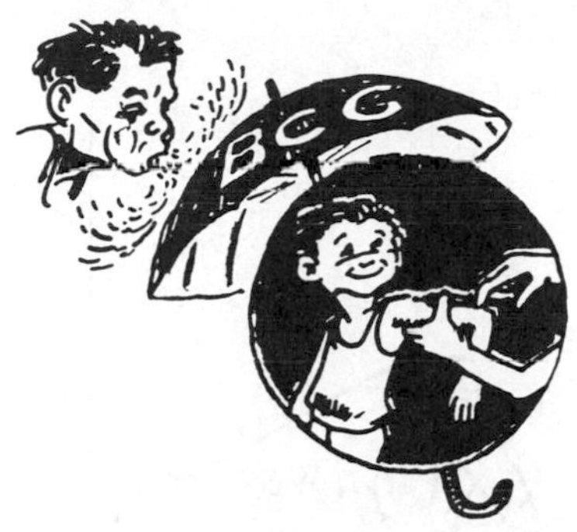
BCG

Here, an umbrella is used as a symbol of protection. However, the symbol will only work where people use umbrellas. (From ***The Control of Tuberculosis, Course of Instruction for Community,*** AKAP, Philippines.)

> *CAUTION:* When using pictures—especially those with unexpected symbols or comparisons—try showing them to a few people first to see what they actually understand and remember. (This is called 'field testing'.)

The importance of a sense of humor

In health work as well as in other human activities, it is important to keep a sense of humor. Humor takes us by surprise and makes us laugh. But it also makes us think.

The idea for these drawings appeared in a health care manual printed in a city slum in Mexico. Pictures like these (drawn by a village health worker) catch the imagination, especially of children. There is no harm if they laugh!

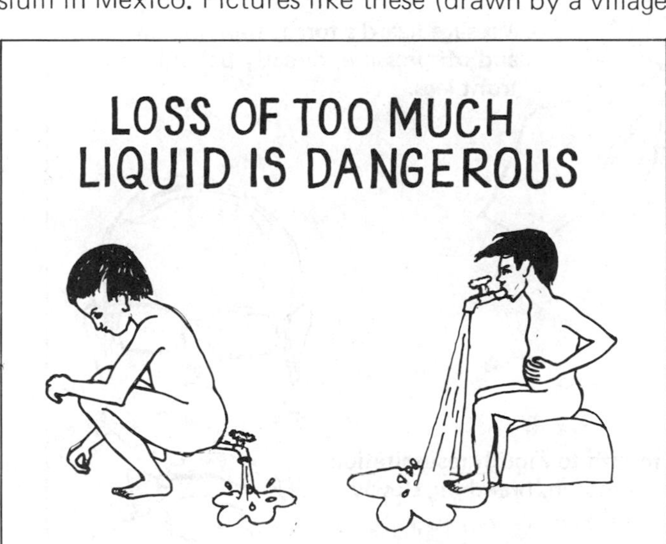
LOSS OF TOO MUCH
LIQUID IS DANGEROUS

After seeing these, they will not forget the danger of losing too much liquid with diarrhea or vomiting.

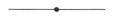

Surprising, ridiculous pictures or remarks by the instructor help people realize the need to question and doubt everything educators and experts say. Help your students to keep asking, "How many of these ideas are appropriate for my work?" "How much of all this is nonsense?" Here is a good example to use with your students. Is this appropriate or nonsense?

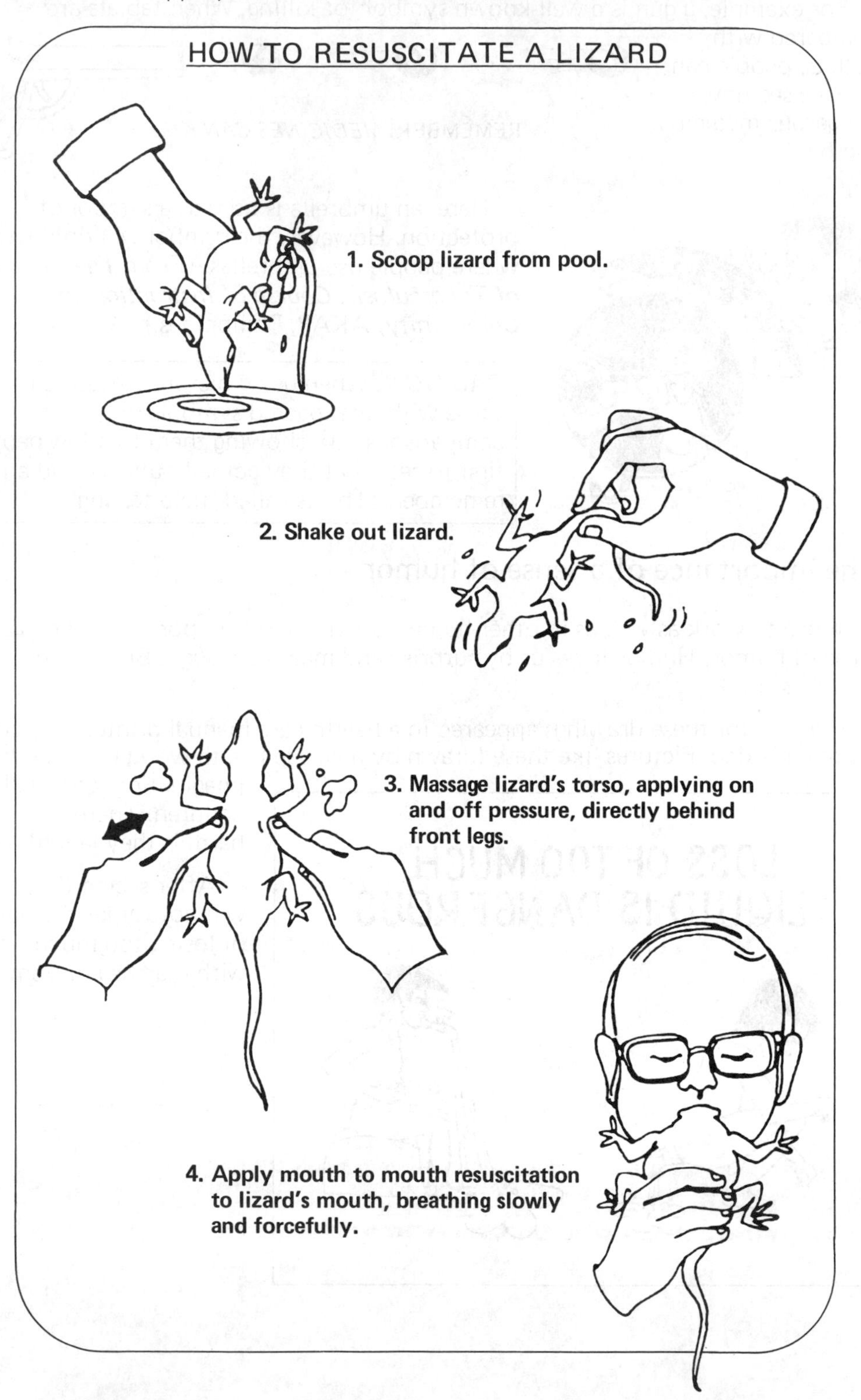

HOW TO RESUSCITATE A LIZARD
1. Scoop lizard from pool.
2. Shake out lizard.
3. Massage lizard's torso, applying on and off pressure, directly behind front legs.
4. Apply mouth to mouth resuscitation to lizard's mouth, breathing slowly and forcefully.

CHAPTER 13

Story Telling

Janaki and Saraswati: a story from India*

Once upon a time, not long ago, there was a young health worker named Janaki, who lived in a small village called Mumabundo in northern India. After making a list of the health problems in her village, Janaki realized that one of the biggest problems was that women did not eat well during pregnancy. They ate too little, and were very thin and anemic. As a result, many babies were born small, thin, and weak. Many of them died. Some of the mothers died too, from bleeding or infection following childbirth.

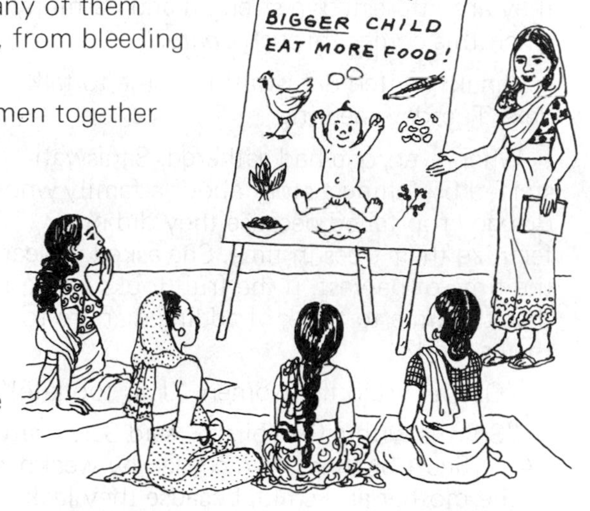

Janaki began to call pregnant women together on Tuesday afternoons to teach them about nutrition. She explained the different food groups and the importance of getting enough to eat. She told the women about vitamins and minerals, and which foods contained iron that would keep them from becoming anemic. To make the meetings more interesting, Janaki used flash cards and a flannel-board, and even had the mothers bring different foods from their gardens and the market.

But as the months went by, nothing changed. Pregnant women continued to come to the Tuesday meetings. And they continued to eat poorly.

One night, one of the mothers who had regularly attended the Tuesday meetings gave birth. She had become more and more anemic during pregnancy, and from the loss of blood following childbirth, she died. Her baby died, too.

Janaki felt partly to blame. She decided to go talk to Saraswati, a wise old woman whom everyone went to for advice. Saraswati also practiced *ayervedic* medicine—the traditional form of healing.

Janaki explained her problem to the old woman.

Saraswati put her wrinkled hand on Janaki's shoulder. "I think your problem is this," she said. "You started with what you were taught in your health training, instead of with what the women in the village already know. You must learn to see things through their eyes."

"How do you mean?" asked Janaki.

*Many of the ideas in this story have been taken from "Education by Appropriate Analogy," a paper by Mark and Mimi Nichter, 2952 Park Street, Honolulu, Hawaii, U.S.A.

"You have been telling the women that eating more during pregnancy will make their babies weigh more at birth. But mothers here are afraid to have big babies. Sometimes, if a baby is too big for her hips, the mother cannot give birth. So women have learned to eat little during pregnancy, in order to have smaller babies."

"No wonder my teaching failed!" said Janaki. "Why didn't they tell me? I tried to encourage them to express their ideas."

"Maybe you spoke your own new ideas too quickly and too strongly," said Saraswati. "The women do not like to contradict you."

"Then how can I teach them?" asked Janaki.

"Begin with what they know and believe. Build on that," answered Saraswati. "For example, talk to them about ***dhatu.*** According to our tradition, ***dhatu*** is a substance that brings strength and harmony. It is related to eating certain foods. Pregnant women are not interested in gaining weight or having larger babies. But they are interested in strength and harmony for themselves and their babies, when this comes through ***dhatu."***

Janaki invited Saraswati to come to talk with the women about ***dhatu*** at the next Tuesday meeting.

When everyone had gathered, Saraswati started by telling a story about a family whose mango crop failed because they did not fertilize their trees in time. She asked, "Near the time of harvest, if the fruit looks weak, is that the time to think of adding manure to the ground?"

"Oh no," said the women. "It is too late!"

"So it is with giving birth," said Saraswati. "A difficult birth is often caused by weakness of the mother and child, because they lack ***dhatu.*** Since a mother must share her ***dhatu*** with her child, she needs to eat plenty of ***dhatu***-producing foods. But ***dhatu*** takes time to be made. Foods that make blood and ***dhatu*** need to be eaten all through pregnancy."

The women were excited and began to discuss what they knew about ***dhatu***-producing foods. They begged Saraswati to come back and talk to them again.

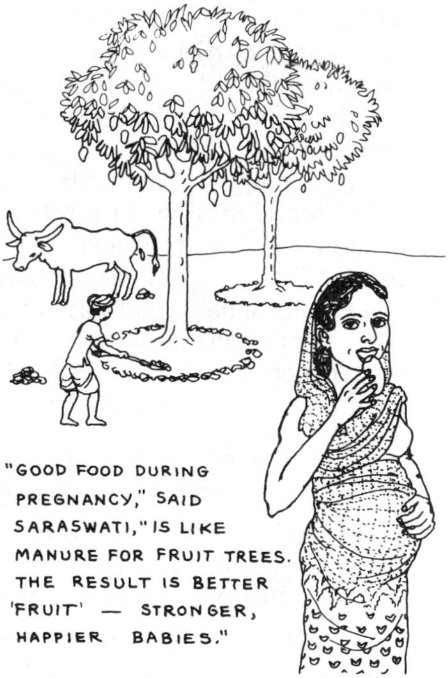

"GOOD FOOD DURING PREGNANCY," SAID SARASWATI, "IS LIKE MANURE FOR FRUIT TREES. THE RESULT IS BETTER 'FRUIT' — STRONGER, HAPPIER BABIES."

The following Tuesday Saraswati did not go to the meeting. But before it began, she talked to Janaki about ways that Janaki might interest the mothers in eating foods with iron. Saraswati reminded her that redness of the body and blood is considered a sign of health. In Mumabundo, pregnant women are said to be in danger of 'impurities of the blood', and iron is traditionally used to protect and purify the blood in times of danger. Also, teas made from iron-rich plants like fenugreek and sesame are given to girls when they begin to menstruate and before they marry, to strengthen blood and increase beauty. Saraswati suggested that Janaki build on these traditions, to help the women realize the need for iron-rich foods during pregnancy.

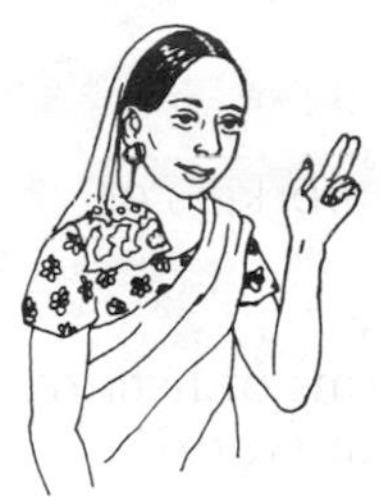

So Janaki discussed these customs during the Tuesday meeting:

"When one of us is 'impure' during menstruation or after childbirth, or when lightning flashes, or someone has fits, we hold a piece of iron in our hand or throw it in front of the house. Why is that?"

"It is to protect us from ***sandhi***—the evil spirits."

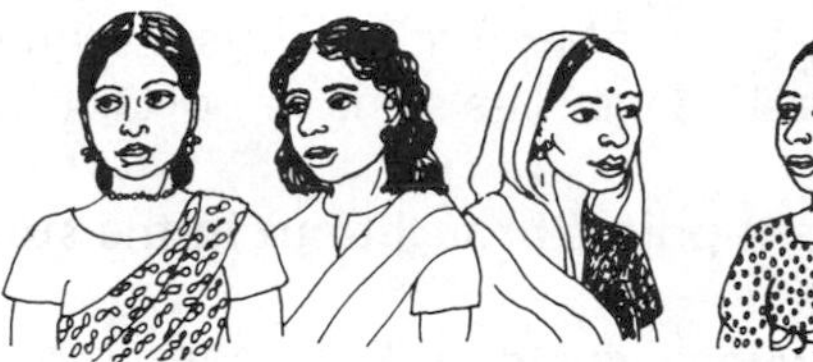

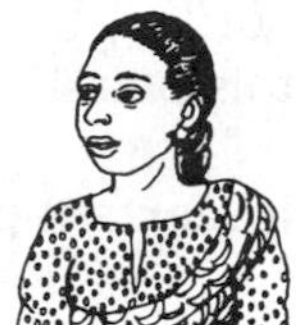

"When a chicken dies suddenly, we cook it with a piece of iron in the pot. Why?"

"To purify it from ***visha***—poison."

"Yes," said Janaki. "We all know iron has ***guna***—the power to protect and purify. This is also true inside the body. Iron makes the blood red and strong. We can see by the red color of our tongues and fingernails that our blood is strong. If the blood is weak, these are pale, not red."

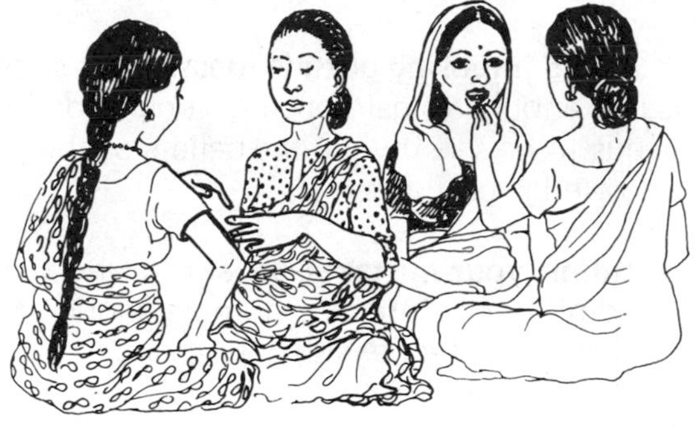

The women began to examine each others' tongues and fingernails. Soon they became concerned. "Some of us have very weak blood," they said. "We need ***guna*** to purify and protect us. Should we hold a piece of iron?"

"Iron will help," explained Janaki, "but only when it is inside us. There are plants that are rich in iron. What plants do we give in tea to girls when they begin to have monthly bleeding, or before marriage, to increase their blood and beauty?"

"Fenugreek and sesame seed!" said the women.

"Yes," said Janaki. "These plants are rich in iron. So we should eat them during pregnancy, to strengthen our blood."

"What other foods are rich in iron?" the mothers asked eagerly. Janaki had already told them many times. But this was the first time they had shown real interest and asked for the information themselves.

As the weeks and months went by, more and more women came to the Tuesday discussions. Each week they examined each others' tongues and fingernails. And changes began to take place. They had discovered that the ***guna*** in the iron-rich foods strengthened their blood. They also had begun to eat more so that they and their babies, through ***dhatu,*** would gain more strength and harmony.

Today, eating well during pregnancy has become part of the tradition in Mumabundo. Babies are born healthier. And fewer women die in childbirth.

DISCUSSION FOLLOWING STORIES

A story like this one from India can be useful for helping health workers or instructors think about appropriate ways of teaching.

After telling or reading the story to a group, you can ask, "In terms of health education, what important points or methods are brought out in this story?"

The group might make a list of ideas similar to the one below. (Before you read our list, think of as many points as you can. Then compare your own list with this one. Did we miss some important ideas?)

Important points brought out in the story:

Know local customs. Before teaching about health, it helps to be familiar with local customs and beliefs. Make sure that your teaching does not conflict with them.

Build on traditions. Teaching is more effective if you respect people's traditions and use them as a basis for introducing new ideas.

Avoid imposing outside ideas. The use of teaching aids and a 'dialogue' approach is not enough to gain open participation in group discussions. The health worker needs to be sensitive to the beliefs of the group, and not try to impose her new knowledge on them.

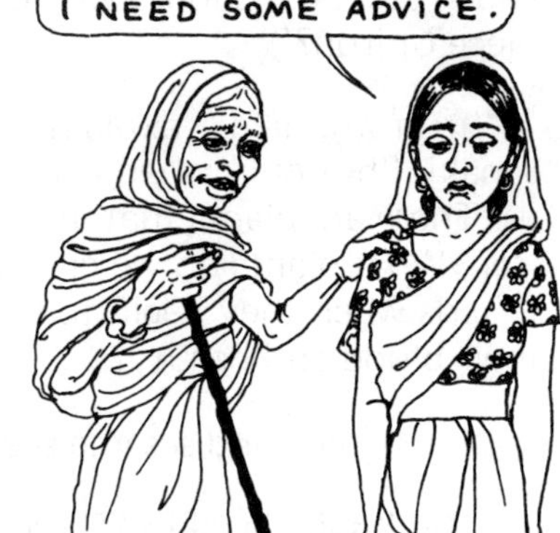

Admit your mistakes. Janaki was honest enough to admit her failure, and humble enough to seek help from someone with little training but much practical experience.

Old people are a valuable resource. Health workers can benefit from the knowledge and wisdom of old people and folk healers.

Set a good example. Saraswati taught Janaki by giving an example of a better way to teach.

A wise adviser stays in the background. Saraswati did not go to the second meeting. She helped strengthen Janaki's leadership rather than taking over.

Use comparisons. Saraswati and Janaki helped the women understand new ideas by comparing these with things that were already familiar to them. (For example, they compared nutritious food for pregnant women with fertilizer for fruit trees.)

Encourage a questioning attitude. The women did not remember Janaki's lessons until they themselves asked for the information. Only when people begin to question, will important changes begin to take place.

Stories can be tools for teaching. The whole story is an example of how stories can be used as teaching tools. They help bring ideas to life.

STORY TELLING AS A TOOL FOR TEACHING

An example from Nigeria

An excellent example of how traditional forms of learning can become the basis for health worker training comes from Lardin Gabas, Nigeria. The Lardin Gabas Rural Health Programme has been described as follows:*

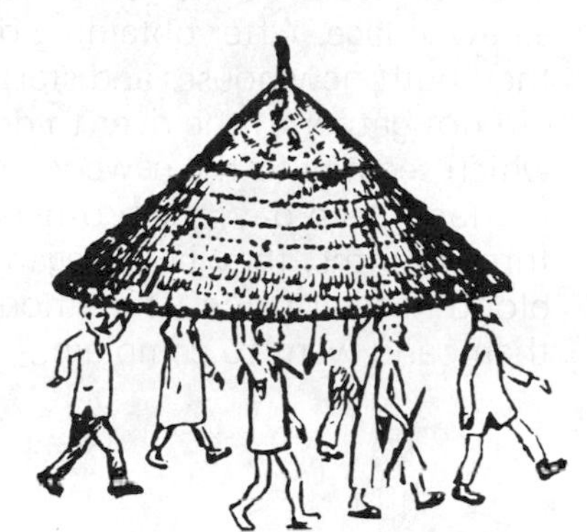

There is a saying in Lardin Gabas, *One head can't carry a roof.* It refers to the need to lift heavy thatched roofs onto the walls of the huts. This requires the effort of many villagers lifting together. Local health workers build a story around this saying to help people realize the need for cooperative action in solving health problems.

"The unique feature of the training programme is its **extensive use of** *parables,*** **drama, songs, and riddles,** the traditional methods of learning among people who still depend heavily on the oral traditions. **These techniques are used both in teaching the course and in teaching in the villages.**

"Teaching in the village is often laughed at or simply ignored if it conflicts openly with current beliefs. For this reason, **stories are constructed to include the traditional knowledge or belief and to move, through the means of the story, to an action which will help solve the problem.** Customary ways of telling stories in the village are imitated as much as possible. The instructors must be sensitive to the differences in patterns and customs among the various villages, as those differences are reflected in the form and content of the traditional stories."

In Lardin Gabas, even clinical teaching, which has a heavy emphasis on prevention through changing health practices, is based on story telling:

"The diagnostic method taught is based on symptoms. Each set of symptoms suggests a disease about which health workers will teach their fellow villagers through story telling, taking into account the traditional beliefs and taboos.

"Use of simple medicines is taught in practice clinics with real patients. Brief history taking and a physical examination are followed by a story conveying the knowledge of what factors contributed to these symptoms and what actions could be taken to alter the development of this health problem. **Teaching through stories avoids confronting the patient directly with his inadequate knowledge, and allows him to identify with the story character who finds the solution to the same problem.** Finally, the appropriate medication is given."

---

*The complete article—which is excellent—appears in ***CONTACT*** 41, Oct., 1977. It is available from the Christian Medical Commission, 150 Route de Ferney, 1211 Geneva 20, Switzerland. Also see p. **13**-9.

***Parable:** A story that teaches a lesson.

TWO STORIES FROM LARDIN GABAS, NIGERIA

Blood worms (schistosomiasis)

Once two brothers' farmland was wearing out, so they decided to move to a new village. After obtaining permission from the chief of a nearby town, they built new houses and started their farming. They found that families did not gather at the river to draw water but rather, each had its own well, which seemed to the newcomers rather unsociable. After finishing work on the farm each day, the brothers bathed in the river before going home. After three months, they both began having belly pains and soon started noticing blood in their urine. They thought that the townspeople were poisoning them, and went to complain.

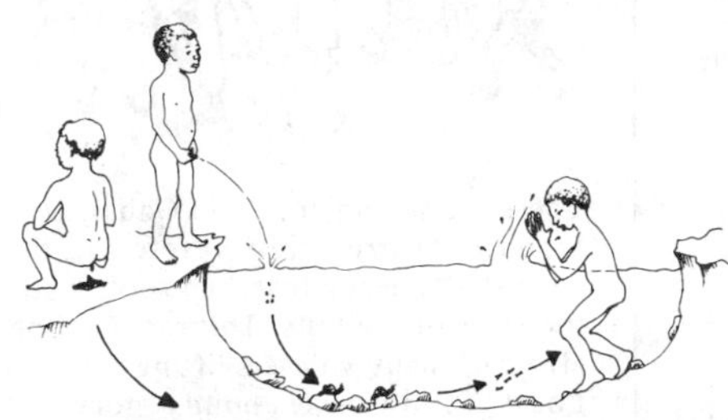

Upon explaining their troubles, the brothers were told that years before this had been a problem for the rest of the villagers, too. The people had been about to move their village to another site when a health worker had advised them that the disease came from tiny organisms living in pools and streams where people bathed. These baby worms went through the skins of the bathers and traveled through the blood to their bellies. The villagers also learned that the eggs of the worms were passed in people's urine or shit, and would be washed by rain into the pools.

The people said that upon the advice of the health worker, they had built and begun to use latrines to bury their shit. They also had dug wells to draw water for drinking and washing. Once those who were ill had completed treatment at the hospital, this kind of belly pain and bloody urine were no longer a problem in their village.

The two brothers followed the example of the rest of the villagers, and soon became healthy again.

Child spacing

A father and his son were planting corn. The son asked his father why the corn wasn't planted closer together in order to obtain more per hectare. The father explained that if there is space between the plants, they grow stronger and healthier and produce more grain. Can you see the relationship between little corn plants and children?

TOO CROWDED

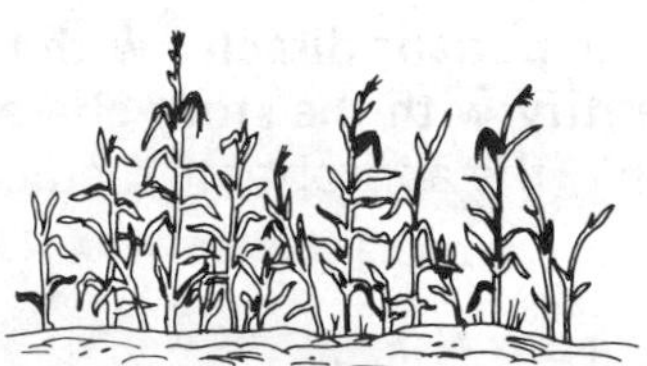

They do not grow well.

WELL SPACED

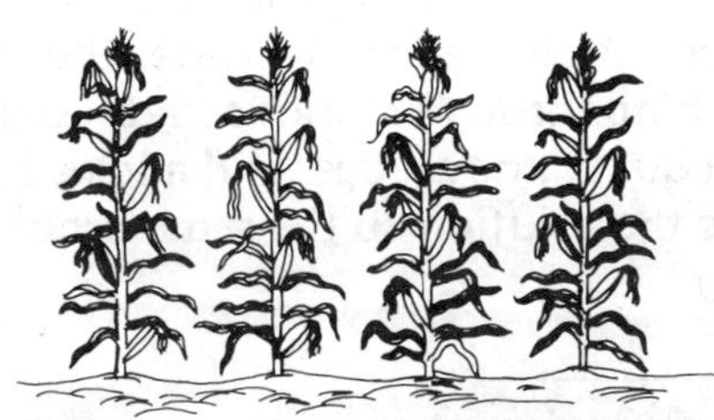

They grow healthy and strong.

In this book we use a lot of stories. (See the list on page **13**-14.) Story telling is useful because it lets us put new ideas in a familiar yet adventurous setting. It allows people to see how new and old ideas fit together—or conflict—in a real-life situation. Also, stories are a traditional form of learning that most people have experienced since childhood.

DIFFERENT WAYS TO TEACH WITH STORIES

1. Parables—or stories with a moral

Some stories teach a lesson, or *moral,* which is stated at the end. These can be make-believe stories with animals (fables), imaginary stories about people (tales), or true stories. Examples of parables are on pages **1**-26 and **5**-7 of this book.

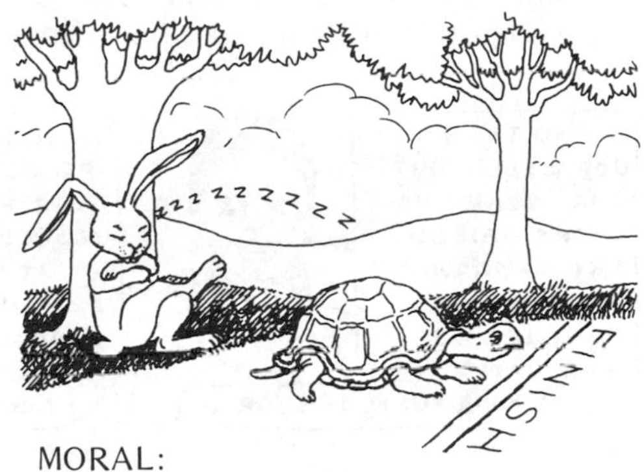

MORAL:
SLOW BUT STEADY WINS THE RACE.

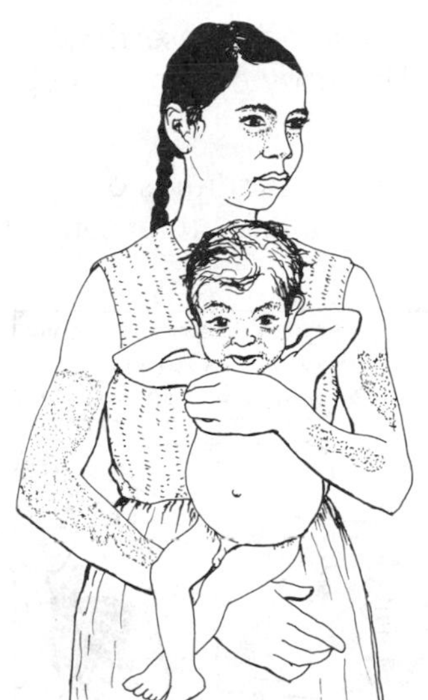

2. Stories that help people think about local problems

Some stories do not give any simple answers or morals, but instead point to existing problems. An example is "The Story of Luis" on page **26**-3. This kind of story can help get people thinking about and discussing social issues.

At first, it is often easier for a group to discuss the problems of imaginary people in a story than to talk about the real problems in their own lives and community. But if they begin by looking at the problems faced by the people in a story, this may help them to reflect on their own difficulties.

3. Stories that students help to write

A community literacy program in Mexico has the students learn to read stories about social problems that are related to their own lives. Parts of the stories are left blank, for the students to fill in themselves. This way the students take part in creating the stories and will relate them more to their own situation.

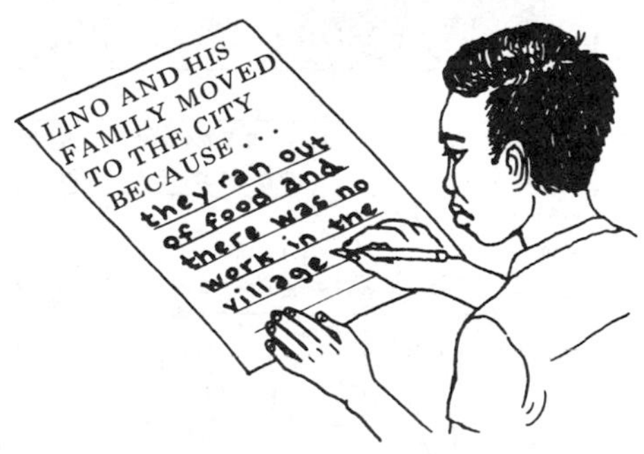

LINO AND HIS FAMILY MOVED TO THE CITY BECAUSE . . .
they ran out of food and there was no work in the village

The best teaching stories often are those the students tell or complete themselves—based on their own experience.

4. Stories told by a group

These are stories that everyone tells together. One person begins telling about a family or community. She gets the characters into a difficult situation and then passes the story on to the next student. He has to tell how the characters resolve their problem, and then creates a new one. The story is then continued by still another student. These group stories are especially useful because they get everyone to think and take part. They are great fun with children.

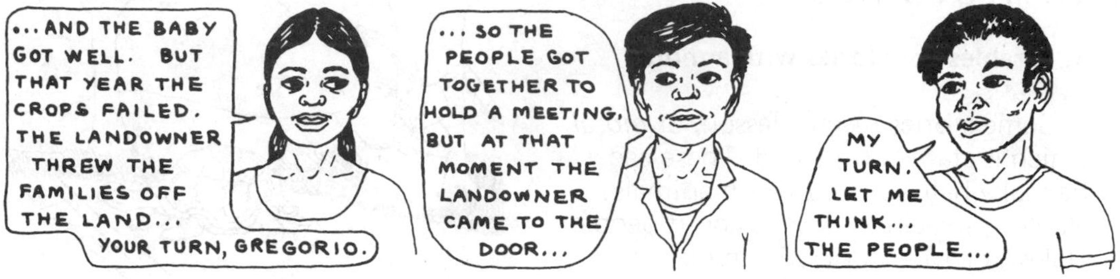

5. Analogies—or comparisons that help people discover healthy answers

The use of comparisons or ***analogies*** to place new ideas in a familiar setting has been discussed, with examples, on pages **7**-11 and **11**-8. The story of Janaki and Saraswati in this chapter also shows how this works.

Some health workers in Liberia, Africa use stories and cut-out pictures of animals to help people realize that breast milk is healthier for a baby than canned or powdered cow's milk:

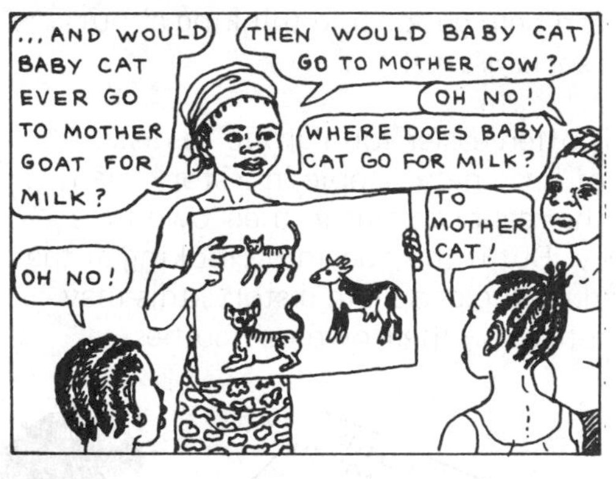

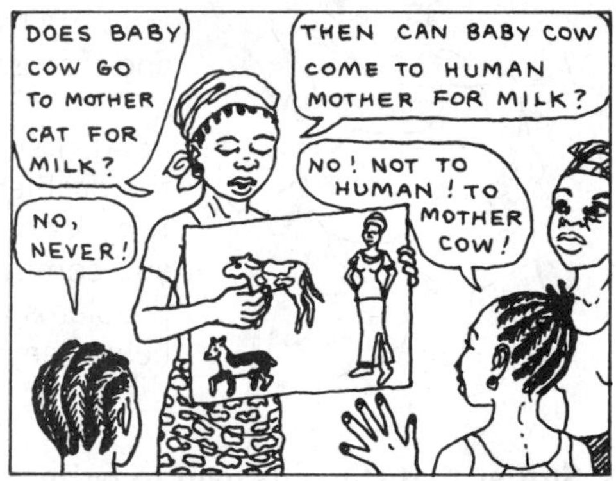

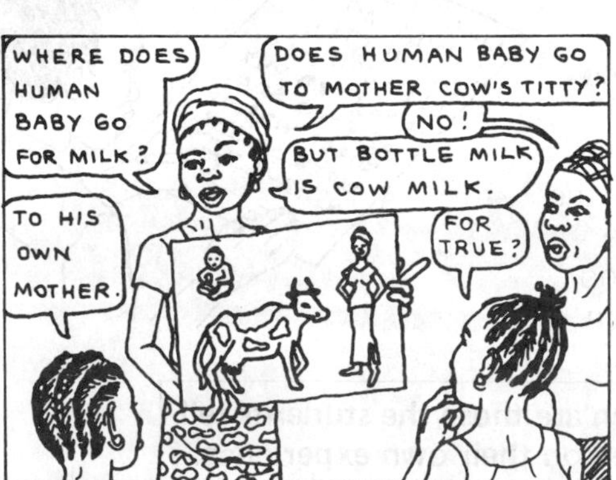

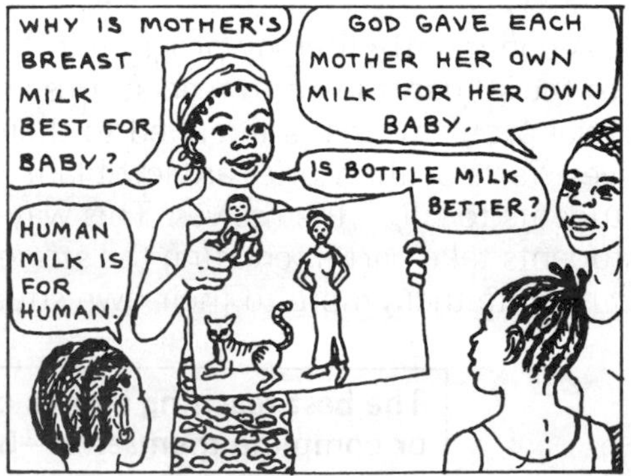

6. Acting out stories

In Lardin Gabas, Nigeria, stories with health messages are often acted out by those who hear them. First a story is told by the group leader. Then one person repeats it and everyone comments on how well it was retold, what details were forgotten, and how it was changed. (Stories are often added to or improved as learners retell them.) Finally, the whole group acts out the story. Here is an example.*

There was a woman called Pokta who sold cans and bottles. All around her yard were cans and bottles with water in them.

Madam Pokta's young son was always getting fever. One day the boy had a terrible headache and a high fever with chills. Madam Pokta went to the store and bought ***Caffenol*** (aspirin with caffeine) for the boy, but it did not bring the fever down. So she took him to the native healer, who took a knife and cut the boy's chest and sucked out some blood.

Soon after, the boy died. Madam Pokta was unhappy for a long time. She could not understand why the boy had had so much malaria. She thought perhaps the boy was not meant to live.

One day she heard about a health worker close to her village. She went and told him about her son's death. So the health worker went with Madam Pokta to her house. When they arrived, mosquitoes were buzzing everywhere because it was late afternoon. The health worker saw the cans and bottles lying around with water in them. And he found little 'summersaulters' (baby mosquitoes) in the water.

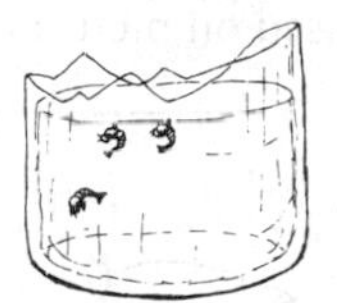

He showed these to Madam Pokta and told her that mosquitoes biting her son had caused him to get malaria and die. Together they cleaned up her yard. Then he told her she should bring her other children to the clinic every month so they could receive ***Daraprim*** pills to prevent malaria. They became healthier and all were happier.

After the story has been acted out, people in the group ask each other questions about it and make up songs about the main health messages. With all this repetition through stories, acting, discussion, and songs, people remember well.

7. Analyzing stories for hidden or harmful messages

Sometimes stories used for health teaching carry hidden messages that were not intended. **If story telling is to help people gain confidence in themselves and pride in their own culture, care must be taken not to make local ways or persons look all bad, and outside ways or persons look all good.** If the weakness of a local custom is pointed out, a beneficial custom should also be mentioned. If a story tells of a traditional healer who does something harmful, it is best if another traditional healer (rather than an outsider) finds out and shows people a better way.

In the story about malaria, notice that Madam Pokta first tries ***self-care*** (she buys *Caffenol*). This fails. Next she goes to a ***traditional healer.*** His treatment also fails, and may even have made the child worse. At last she goes to an ***outside health worker,*** whose advice is successful.

The hidden messages in the story are "Self-care is wrong," "Traditional medicine is wrong," and "Outside advice is right." Although the story of Madam Pokta is in many ways excellent, such messages can actually weaken people's confidence in their own experience and ability to find answers for themselves.

Health workers need to analyze the stories they use to make sure that hidden messages are community strengthening. (Compare this story from Lardin Gabas with the story from India at the beginning of this chapter.)

---

*Adapted from a booklet called ***Health Teaching for West Africa: Stories, Drama, and Song,*** edited by David Hilton. Available from MAP International, Box 50, Wheaton, Illinois 60187, U.S.A.

STORIES TOLD WITH PICTURES

Using pictures with story telling helps in several ways:

- Pictures let people 'see' what is happening in the story.
- A series of pictures can serve as a guide for the story teller.
- Pictures can be used to help a group tell a story from their own experience.
- Health workers can use flash cards or flip charts in discussing health problems with groups of villagers, letting the group try to explain what is happening in the pictures. This way **students discover the health message themselves and tell it to the teacher** (rather than the teacher telling them).

This set of flash cards is based on pictures from page 132 of *Where There Is No Doctor.*

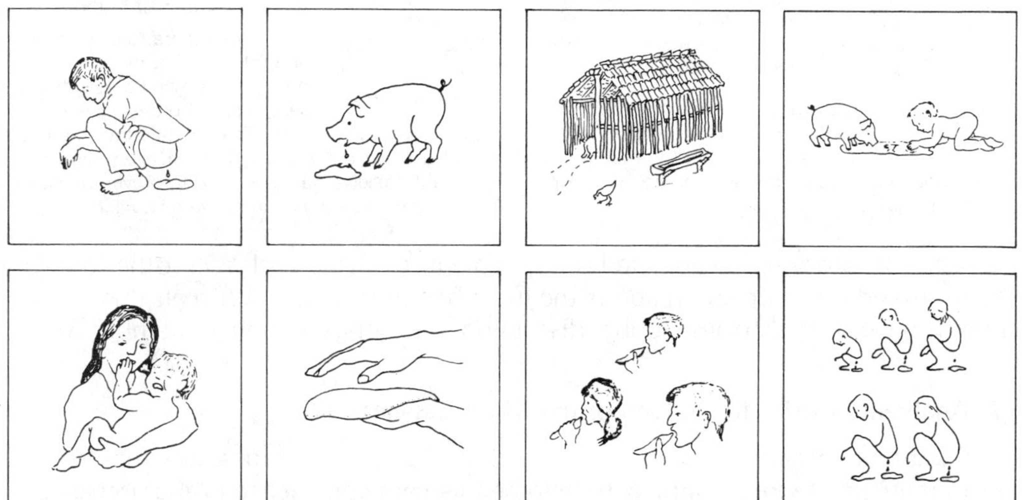

In Chapter 11 we discussed the use of pictures on **flash cards and flip charts.** But pictures can also be used to tell stories in **comic strips, photonovels, color slides** (transparencies), **filmstrips,** or **moving pictures** (movies).

Comics and photonovels

In many countries, especially in Latin America, people read comic books more than any other written materials. As a result, many comic books and ***photonovels**** have been produced on a variety of health topics. A few of them are excellent, but many are a boring mixture of preaching and brainwashing, masked by a silly story.

Instead of using prepared materials, health workers can make their own comic strips on health themes, or organize school children to make them. They can make up stories and draw pictures to go with them, or copy pictures from other comic books. If someone has a camera, the group may even be able to make photonovels using local people as 'stars'.

---

*Photonovels or ***fotonovelas*** are comic books that use photographs instead of drawings.

This comic strip, or 'picture story', is from the Voluntary Health Association of India edition of *Where There Is No Doctor.*

Teaching idea:

Try showing this comic strip to a group of health workers, mothers, or children. Discuss with them what the family in the story could do to stop the problem from spreading. Then have the group make their own picture story about a common problem in their area.

Note: People will find stories more real and more interesting if the characters have names (instead of just being called 'this boy' and 'the mother'). Try to make the people in the story seem as lifelike as possible.

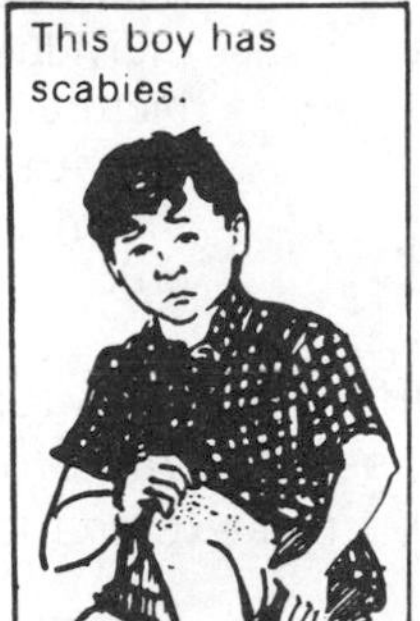

This boy has scabies.

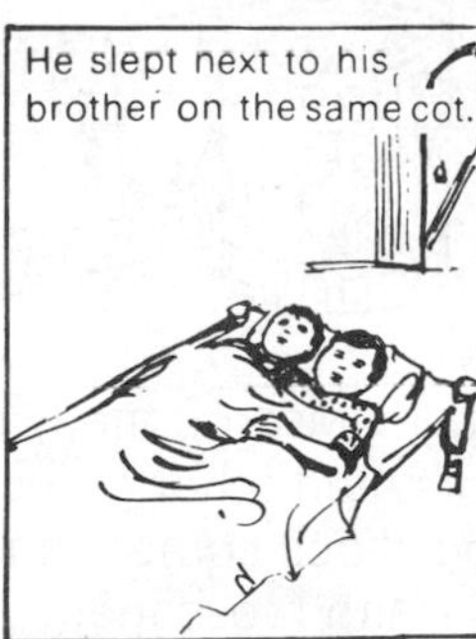

He slept next to his brother on the same cot.

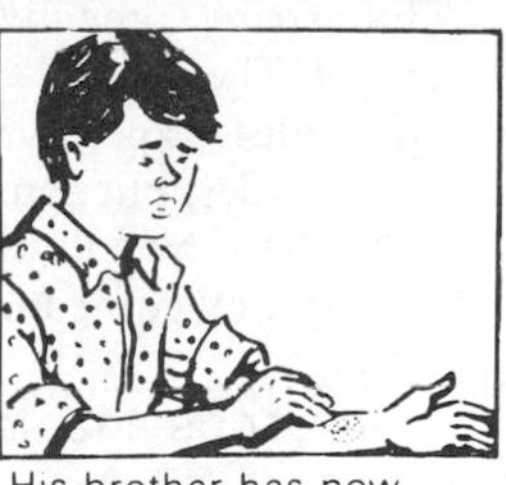

His brother has now got scabies.

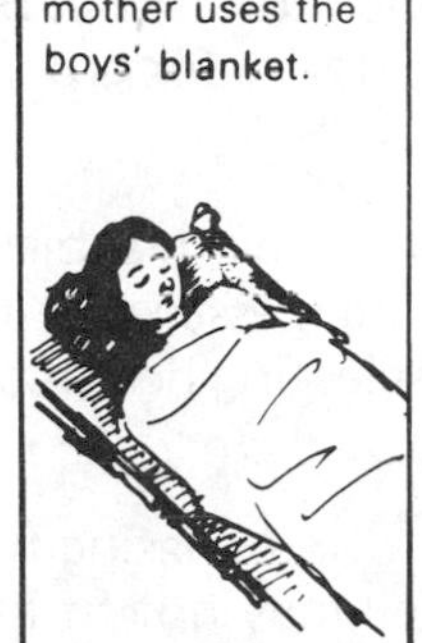

The next day, the mother uses the boys' blanket.

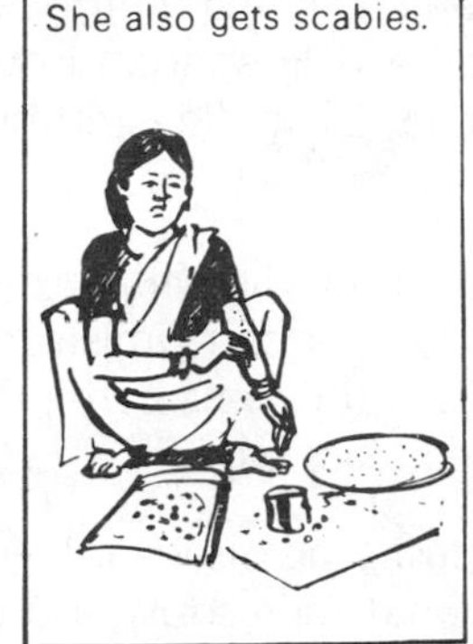

She also gets scabies.

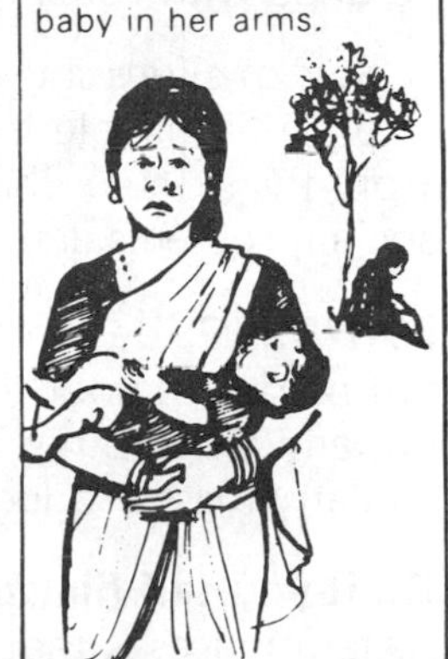

She holds her crying baby in her arms.

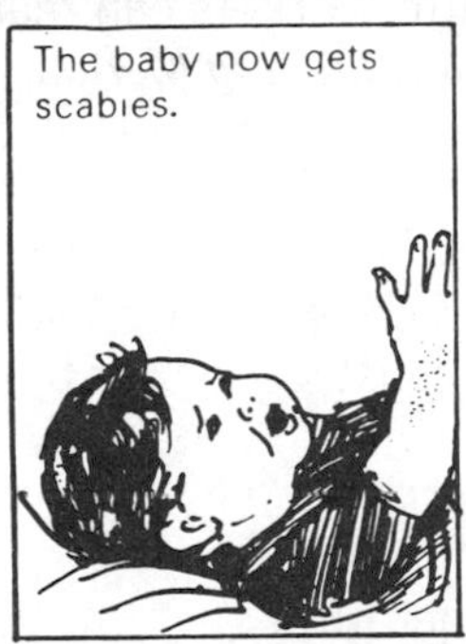

The baby now gets scabies.

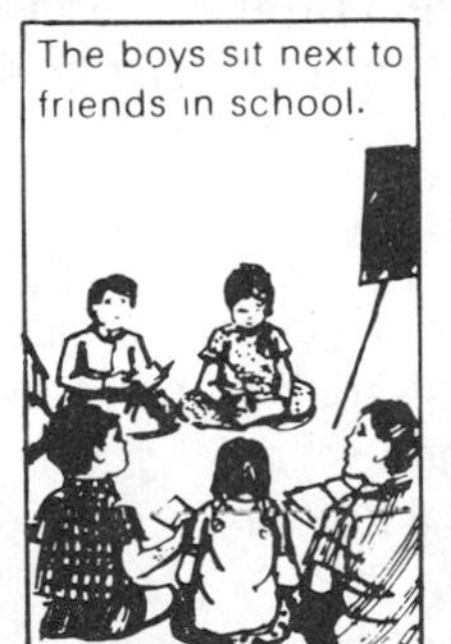

The boys sit next to friends in school.

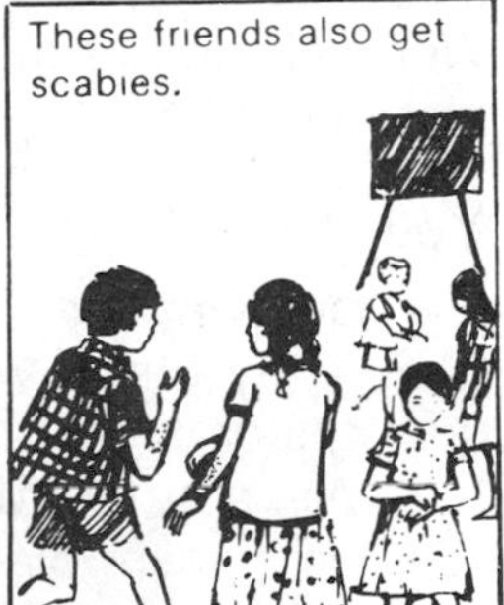

These friends also get scabies.

Filmstrips and slides

Filmstrips and slides are both forms of pictures (either photos or drawings) that can be projected against a wall, sheet, or screen. Usually, they must be shown at night or in a dark room, although a special (very expensive) screen for daylight showings has been developed. Battery-operated projectors can be obtained in some countries, for use in areas that do not have electricity.*

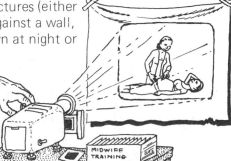

*For information on projectors and 'daylight screens', write to World Neighbors (see page **Back**-3).

Filmstrips and color slides are similar, except that . . .

Filmstrips come in a roll. They are much less expensive than slides, but can only be shown in the order they come in.

Slides are individual pictures. They can be shown in any order.

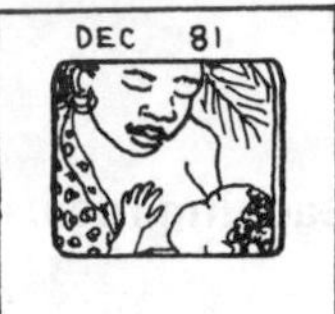

Filmstrips and sets of slides on many different health topics are available from TALC, World Neighbors, and other groups (see p. **Back**-3 or ***WTND,*** p. 429). Many of these filmstrips and slides come with written explanations to help in telling stories with specific health messages.

Sets of slides showing teaching methods and village theater discussed in this book are available from the Hesperian Foundation (see p. **Back**-3). The slides from the skits in Chapter 27 make exciting stories for group discussion about social problems and health.

WARNING: Be careful in buying filmstrips on health subjects. Some are excellent, but many are poorly done or carry misleading messages—especially some of those on family planning. Take the same care in selecting health comics, photonovels, and any mass-produced teaching aids.

Do-it-yourself filmstrips: One disadvantage of purchasing filmstrips or slides from distant places is that what they show and tell may not fit the situation in your area. However, you and other local health workers can make your own filmstrips. World Neighbors distributes a ***Visual Aids Tracing Manual*** that gives complete instructions for this.

You will need:

- polyvinyl or acetate plastic strips 5 cm. (2 inches) wide. (You can use old X-ray film if you soak it in lye or caustic soda for a day, and then scrub off the dark coating.)
- pen points and a holder
- permanent black ink
- colored marking pens with permanent ink
- a projector that can be used to project 5-cm. slides

You can draw your own pictures on the plastic strips, and color them in. If you prefer to copy or trace the pictures, the World Neighbors manual contains many drawings that can easily be traced. Here are samples from two sets of drawings.

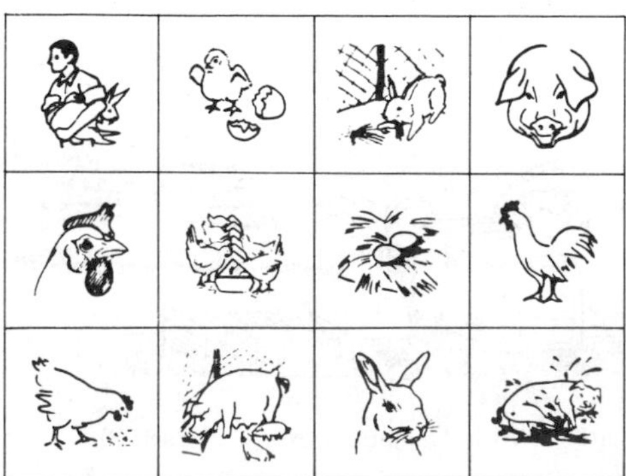

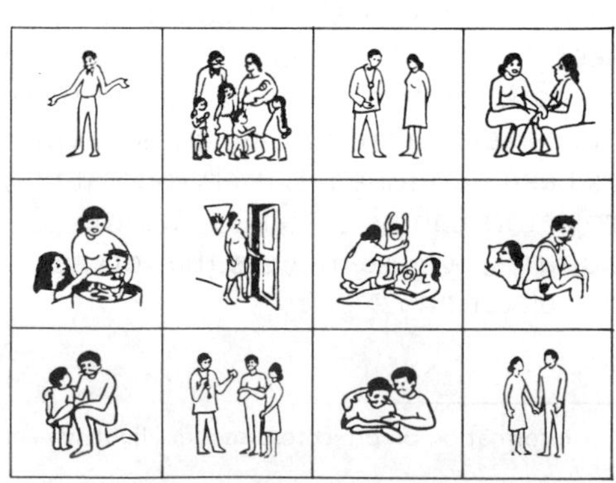

SUGGESTIONS FOR TEACHING WITH PICTURE STORIES

(flash cards, flip charts, filmstrips, comic strips, or photonovels)

- Keep the story simple and clear. Make one or two main points.
- Be sure that both pictures and words relate to the lives of the local people.
- Make every effort to respect and build on local traditions.
- Make the first picture one the audience will understand. If most of the viewers cannot read, start with pictures, not written words.

LESS APPROPRIATE | MORE APPROPRIATE

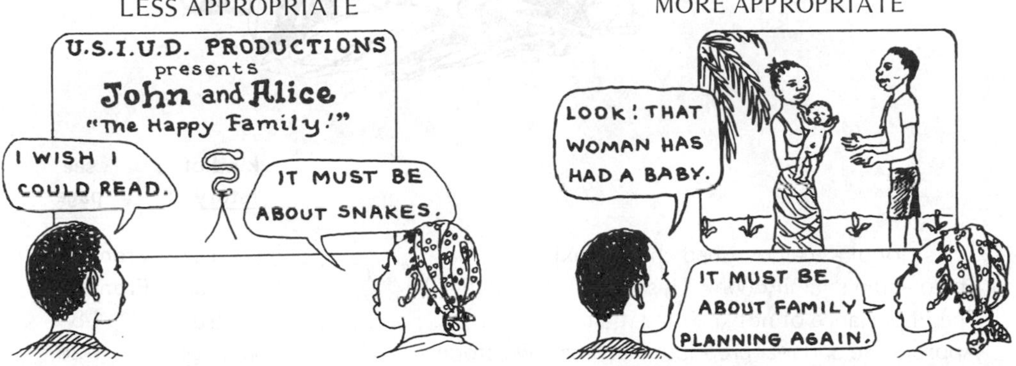
U.S.I.U.D. PRODUCTIONS
presents
John and Alice
"The Happy Family!"
I WISH I COULD READ.
IT MUST BE ABOUT SNAKES.
LOOK! THAT WOMAN HAS HAD A BABY.
IT MUST BE ABOUT FAMILY PLANNING AGAIN.

- Each picture should tell a story, or carry the story forward.
- Keep the pictures simple, so that the main message comes through clearly. Avoid complicated details. But make things look as real as possible—especially the people.
- 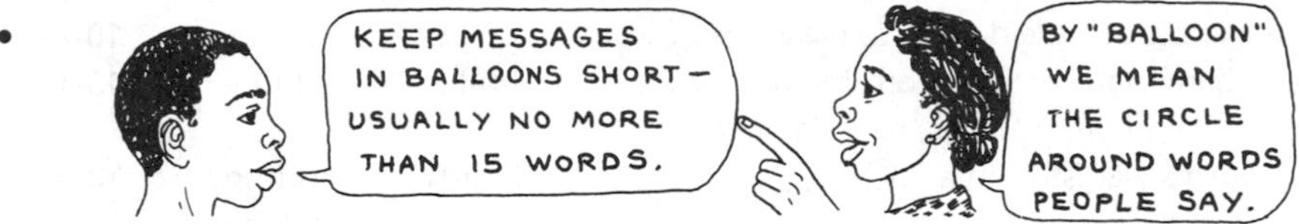
KEEP MESSAGES IN BALLOONS SHORT—USUALLY NO MORE THAN 15 WORDS.
BY "BALLOON" WE MEAN THE CIRCLE AROUND WORDS PEOPLE SAY.

- Use some pictures that show the whole scene, but also include plenty of close-up scenes. Close-ups are good for emphasizing important ideas because they usually move people emotionally.

WHOLE SCENE | CLOSE-UP SCENE

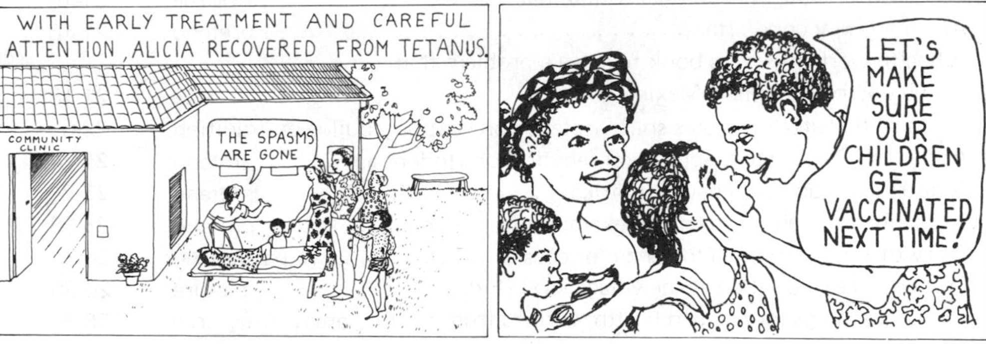
WITH EARLY TREATMENT AND CAREFUL ATTENTION, ALICIA RECOVERED FROM TETANUS.
COMMUNITY CLINIC
THE SPASMS ARE GONE
LET'S MAKE SURE OUR CHILDREN GET VACCINATED NEXT TIME!

- Use color if possible—but make colors as natural as you can.
- Make the story interesting. Try to include situations of happiness, sadness, excitement, courage, serious thought, decisions, and action to solve problems.
- For filmstrips, slides, or flip charts, it is usually a good idea to provide a written guide for the user. (For an example, see page **11**-23.)

EXAMPLES OF STORY TELLING IN THIS BOOK

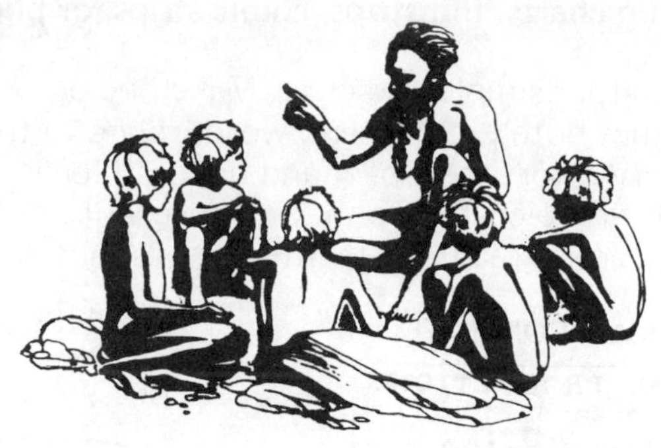

The stories listed here can be spoken or read, or told through pictures. But stories can also be 'acted out' in the form of role plays, theater, and puppet shows. These dramatic forms of story telling are discussed in Chapters 14 and 27.

CHAPTER 14

Role Playing

One of the best ways to learn how to do something is through **guided practice.** To gain skill in doing physical exams, students need to practice examining persons with different sicknesses. To learn how to carry out a home health visit, they need to actually visit different families. To become effective in helping people solve problems, they need to practice solving real problems in a community. There is no substitute for experience.

Yet some sort of preparation is essential. It would not be fair to have students examine a sick person without first learning how. Classroom study about 'what to do' may help. But what is most important is practice.

Role playing provides a lively, realistic way of practicing skills that involve working with people. **It is especially useful for training persons who are more used to learning from life than from books.**

By "role playing" we mean that members of a learning group act out real-life situations. Some may pretend to be persons with particular problems or illnesses. Others may play the roles of relatives, health workers, and so on. **Students act out problem-solving situations similar to those they will encounter as health workers in their own villages.**

Role playing gives students a chance to learn about and practice the human aspects of health care.

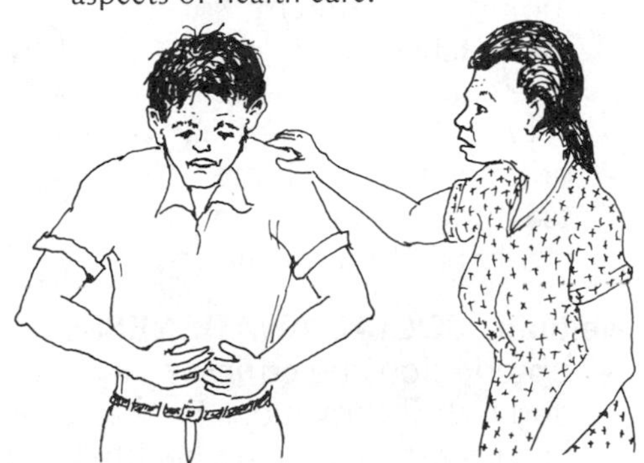

Touching is an especially important way of showing you care.

For role playing, no written script is needed. There is no memorization of parts. Each participant pretends he or she is someone else, and tries to act and speak the way that person would (or should).

Also, few 'props' or special objects are needed. Instead, people can represent many objects by *pantomime.* This means they pretend to do things such as knocking on a door, grinding maize, or picking lice out of the hair, without actually using any doors, maize grinders, or lice. This use of imagination adds to the fun. However, a few simple props, objects, and visual aids can be helpful. Some of these will be discussed here, others in Chapter 27.

Role playing in the classroom is one of the best ways to bring learning close to real life—and to make it fun.

WAYS ROLE PLAYING CAN BE USED IN THE CLASSROOM

Role playing is especially useful for . . .

developing PRACTICAL SKILLS:

- practice in using the book *Where There Is No Doctor* (finding and using information; using the book to help others learn)
- practice in attending a sick or injured person (diagnosis, treatment, advice about prevention)
- practice in step-by-step solving of problems (use of scientific method)

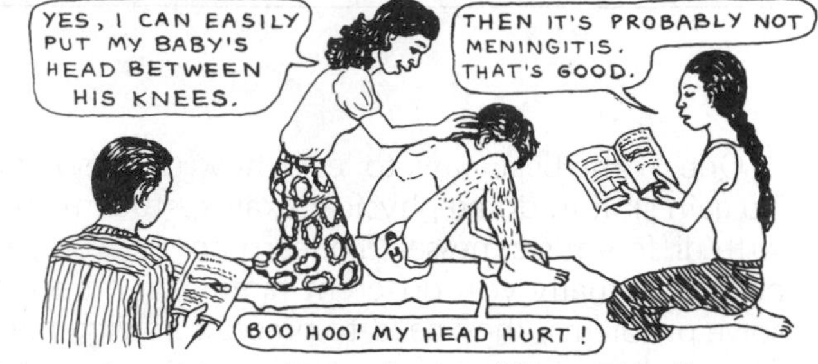

developing SOCIAL SKILLS:

- leadership
- home visits
- community organizing
- relating to people with different needs: the sick, the worried, the proud, the dying, children, doctors, authorities, etc.

developing TEACHING SKILLS:

- looking at different approaches to education (see example on pages **1**-17 to **1**-23)
- practicing appropriate teaching methods (with mothers, children, etc.)

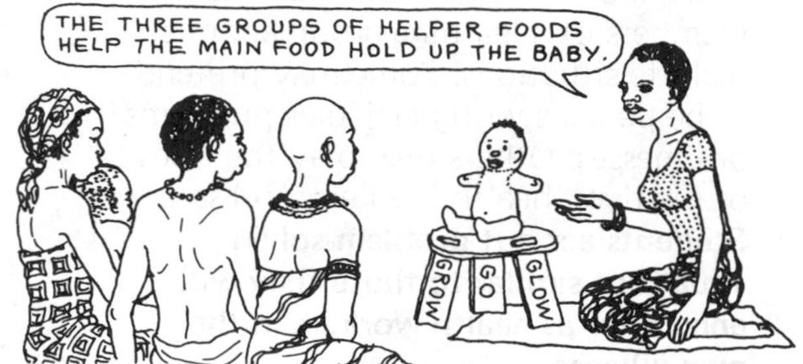

developing SOCIAL AWARENESS:

- observation and critical analysis of how social and political relations between persons and groups affect people's health and well-being
- looking at attitudes, customs, and patterns of behavior—how they affect people's health; how to help people understand them better
- exploring alternative solutions to different problems
- trying out ideas for public skits or farmers' theater. (Many of the plays discussed in Chapter 27 began with simple role playing in health worker training classes.)

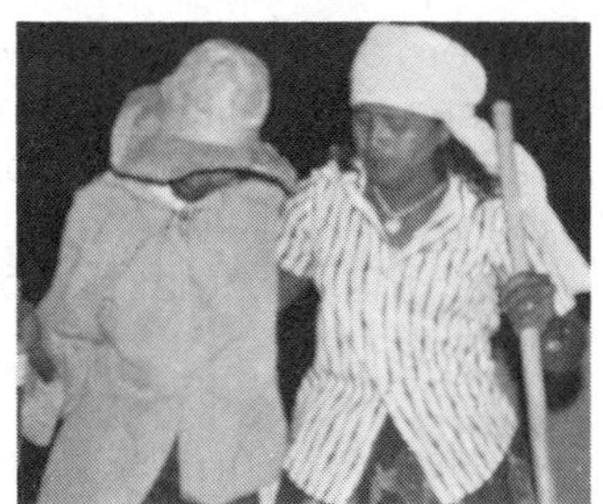

Two women health promoters from Honduras act out problems caused by men's drinking habits. (See p. **27**-19 for another example.)

As you will see from the examples in this chapter, a single role play may explore several of the areas listed above. Because it imitates real-life situations, role playing requires students to combine a range of skills and understanding. They must think things through and use their full powers of observation, analysis, imagination, and human feeling.

SIMPLE VISUAL AND PRACTICAL AIDS FOR USE IN ROLE PLAYING

You will not need many 'props' or special objects for role playing. However, a few simple supplies, visual aids, or pretend instruments sometimes help make role playing more effective. Here are some suggestions:

1. PAINTS, COLORED PENCILS, OR MARKING PENS

Use these for marking various signs of illness on the skin.

For example, mark a row of red dots on someone's back. The person plays the role of a child who is brought to a health worker by his mother. The health worker asks questions, examines the child, and tries to determine the cause of the 'sores'. (Judging from the pattern of these bites, they were probably caused by bed bugs.)

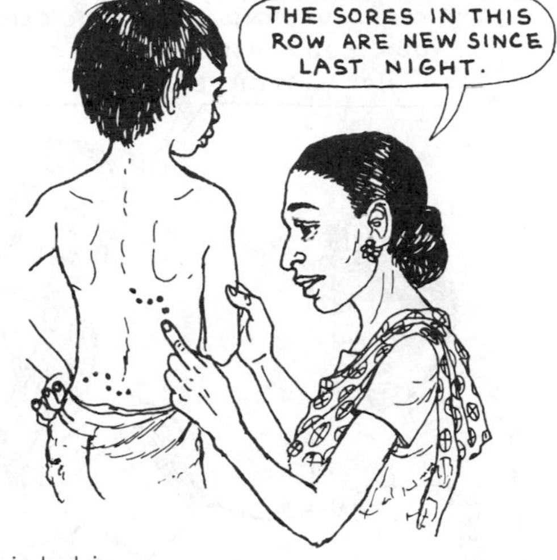

THE SORES IN THIS ROW ARE NEW SINCE LAST NIGHT.

2. CARDBOARD 'BABIES' AND SIMILAR AIDS

Because so much of health care has to do with small children, it is important to do role plays about children's health problems. If your training program has a good relationship with the local community, children may willingly join in role plays with student health workers. Or mothers may agree to take part with their babies.

However, children and babies are not always available or cooperative. It helps if students make a series of cardboard, cloth, or straw dolls or puppets to be used in role playing.

The more lifelike these doll babies look, the better. They can be used along with other visual aids, such as the pretend thermometers on the next page, for many different role plays.

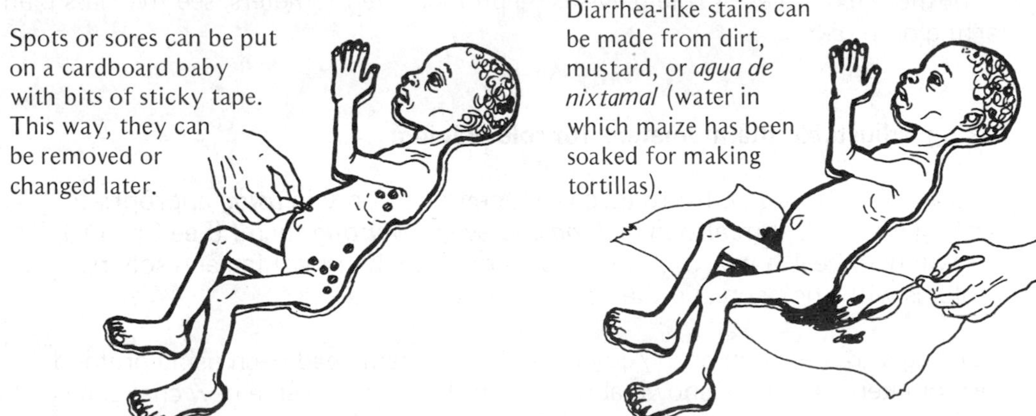

Spots or sores can be put on a cardboard baby with bits of sticky tape. This way, they can be removed or changed later.

Diarrhea-like stains can be made from dirt, mustard, or *agua de nixtamal* (water in which maize has been soaked for making tortillas).

For other ideas of how to use these model babies in role playing and other activities, see pages **11**-15, **14**-4, and **27**-31.

3. PRETEND THERMOMETERS

These can be made of cardboard and covered with cellophane or transparent tape. Students can prepare a series of thermometers showing different temperatures, to use in many different role plays.

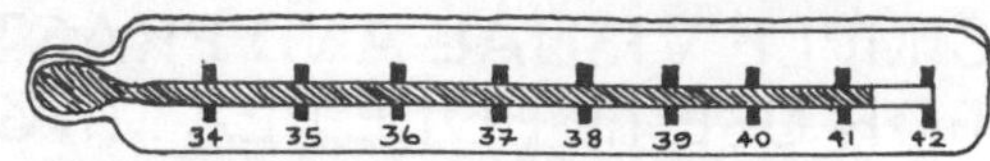

temperature dangerously high (see *WTND*, p.76)

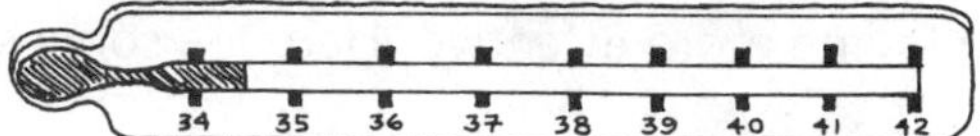

temperature dangerously low (see *WTND*, p.273)

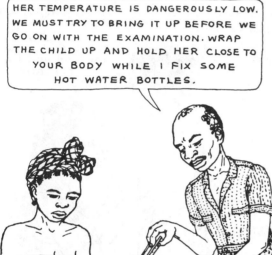

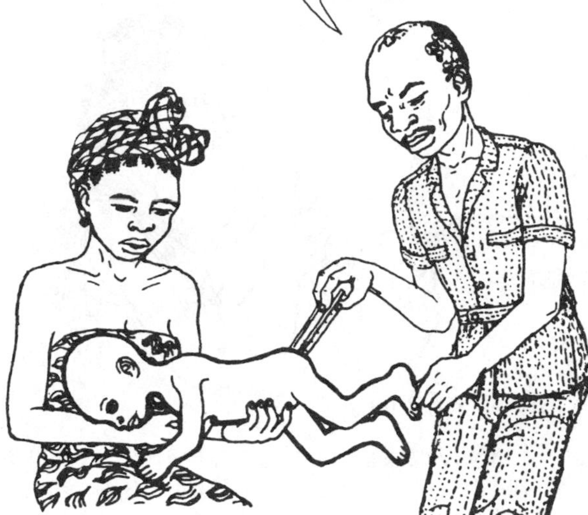

HER TEMPERATURE IS DANGEROUSLY LOW. WE MUST TRY TO BRING IT UP BEFORE WE GO ON WITH THE EXAMINATION. WRAP THE CHILD UP AND HOLD HER CLOSE TO YOUR BODY WHILE I FIX SOME HOT WATER BOTTLES.

In role plays, use a cardboard baby, a doll, or a real baby.

Role plays using pretend thermometers provide practice for what to do in different emergencies. When examining a sick baby, it is important that, as soon as a dangerously high or low temperature is observed, the health worker interrupt his examination and take action to lower or raise the baby's temperature.

For example, if the thermometer shows that a baby has a dangerously low temperature, the health worker needs to correct this problem at once. Only after the child is out of immediate danger from the low temperature should the health worker continue with the rest of the examination and treatment.

For more examples of role plays using pretend thermometers, see the class plan starting on p. **5**-3.

Making 'adjustable thermometers' for role playing:

During their training, try to involve students not only in ***using*** appropriate teaching materials, but also in ***making*** and even ***inventing*** them. (See Ch. 11.) This will help health workers to be more creative when teaching and solving problems with the people in their communities.

During a training course in Ajoya, Mexico, students had been using pretend thermometers like those shown above. Then they were given a new challenge: "Let's see who can make a pretend thermometer with a temperature reading you can change!" Students divided into small groups, and returned an hour later with the inventions on the next page.

EXAMPLES OF ADJUSTABLE THERMOMETERS MADE BY STUDENTS

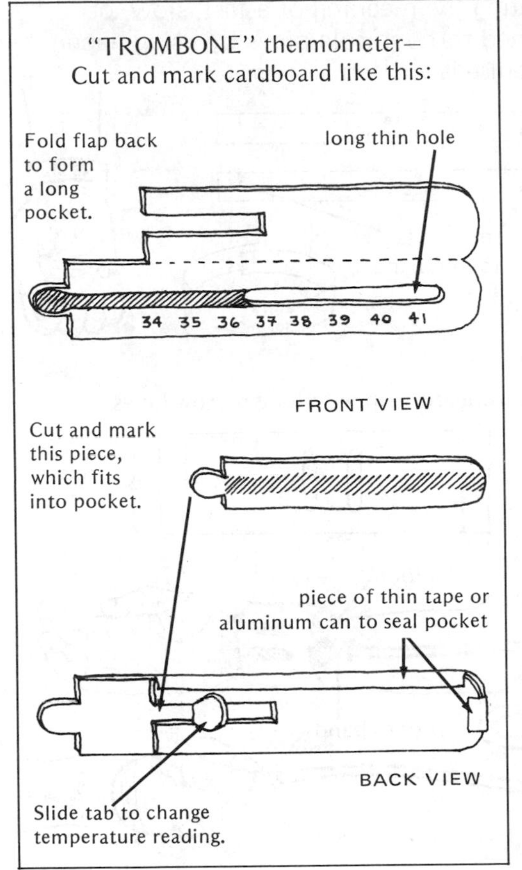

"TROMBONE" thermometer–
Cut and mark cardboard like this:
Fold flap back to form a long pocket.
long thin hole
34 35 36 37 38 39 40 41
FRONT VIEW
Cut and mark this piece, which fits into pocket.
piece of thin tape or aluminum can to seal pocket
BACK VIEW
Slide tab to change temperature reading.

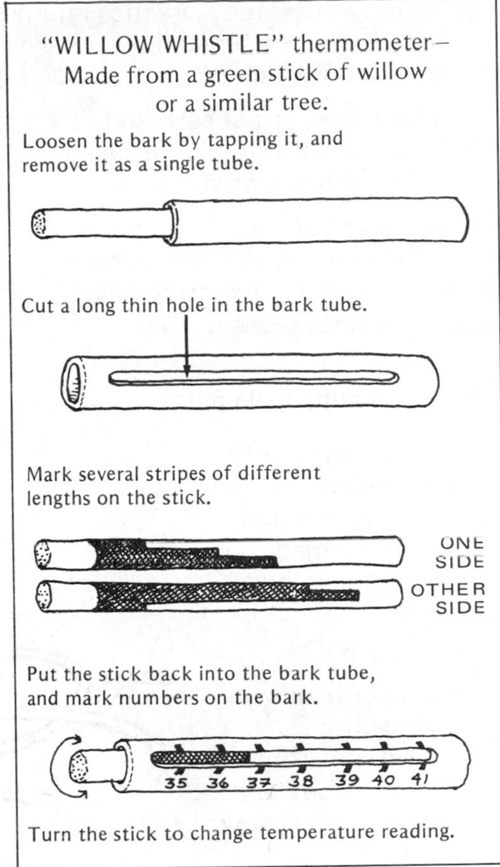

"WILLOW WHISTLE" thermometer–
Made from a green stick of willow or a similar tree.
Loosen the bark by tapping it, and remove it as a single tube.
Cut a long thin hole in the bark tube.
Mark several stripes of different lengths on the stick.
ONE SIDE
OTHER SIDE
Put the stick back into the bark tube, and mark numbers on the bark.
35 36 37 38 39 40 41
Turn the stick to change temperature reading.

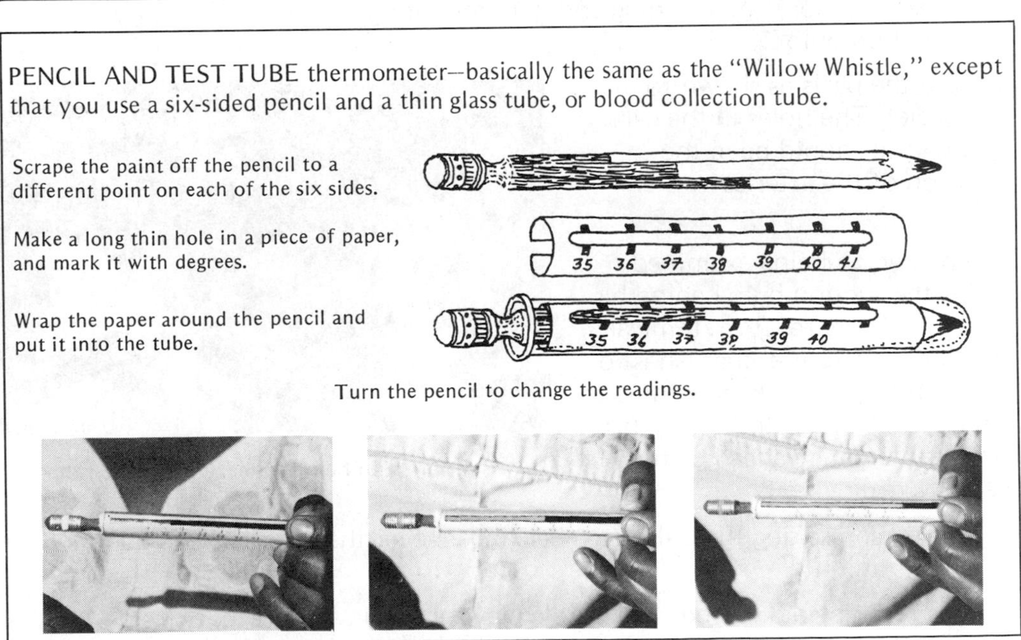

PENCIL AND TEST TUBE thermometer–basically the same as the "Willow Whistle," except that you use a six-sided pencil and a thin glass tube, or blood collection tube.
Scrape the paint off the pencil to a different point on each of the six sides.
Make a long thin hole in a piece of paper, and mark it with degrees.
35 36 37 38 39 40 41
Wrap the paper around the pencil and put it into the tube.
35 36 37 38 39 40
Turn the pencil to change the readings.

You can make one of these adjustable thermometers in a few minutes. Try it. Or see if your students can invent their own.

4. ARTIFICIAL PULSE

Health workers need practice interpreting the meaning of a fast, slow, or changing pulse. Such practice can be gained through role plays by using paper wristbands on which the 'sick person's' pulse is written.

Make a small cut at each end of the band so that it can be fastened around someone's wrist.

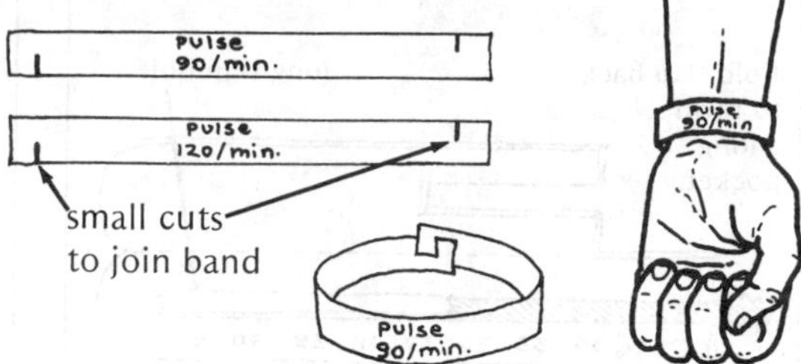

The person checking the 'pulse' reads the number on the wristband and uses this information to help make a diagnosis (see p. **14**-9).

Making an adjustable pulse:

An adjustable pulse that the health worker can actually feel and count can be made from the following materials:

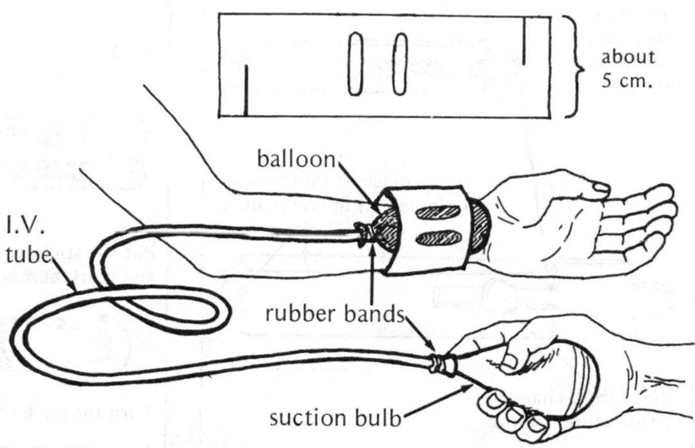

1 balloon
2 rubber bands (or thread)
1 strip of cardboard about 5 cm. wide, with long narrow holes cut in it
1 I.V. tube, or similar tubing about 1 meter long
1 suction bulb

Join the parts as shown to make a bracelet. The holes in the cardboard strip should be in the position of the arteries in the wrist.

The person being examined holds the suction bulb behind his back and squeezes it rhythmically to produce a 'pulse' that is fast or slow, strong or weak, according to the illness being acted out. (This will take practice ahead of time to get it right.)

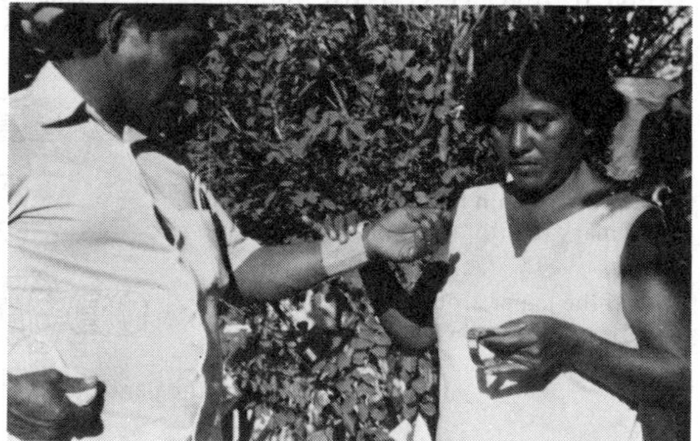

suction bulb being squeezed at pulse rate

The person taking the pulse puts her fingers over the 'arteries' and counts the pulses per minute.

This teaching aid can be used in role plays about fever, shock, extreme fear (hysteria), typhoid (see p. **14**-9), and many other problems. It not only gives students practice in measuring and comparing different pulse rates, but helps them learn where to find the arteries of the wrist.

ROLE PLAYING FILE CARDS OR LOOSE-LEAF NOTEBOOK

It is a good idea to make a collection of notes on different role plays as you develop them during a training program. This collection can be built upon from course to course, as old role plays are improved and new ones are added. Such a collection serves as a memory bank for experienced instructors and as a gold mine of ideas for new instructors. These ideas should, of course, serve only as a starting point. They can be changed and expanded each time a learning group uses them.

The role plays can be grouped by subjects. For each role play, it helps to also list **learning objectives; actors, materials, and preparations needed; manner of presentation; and questions for group discussion.** Here is an example:

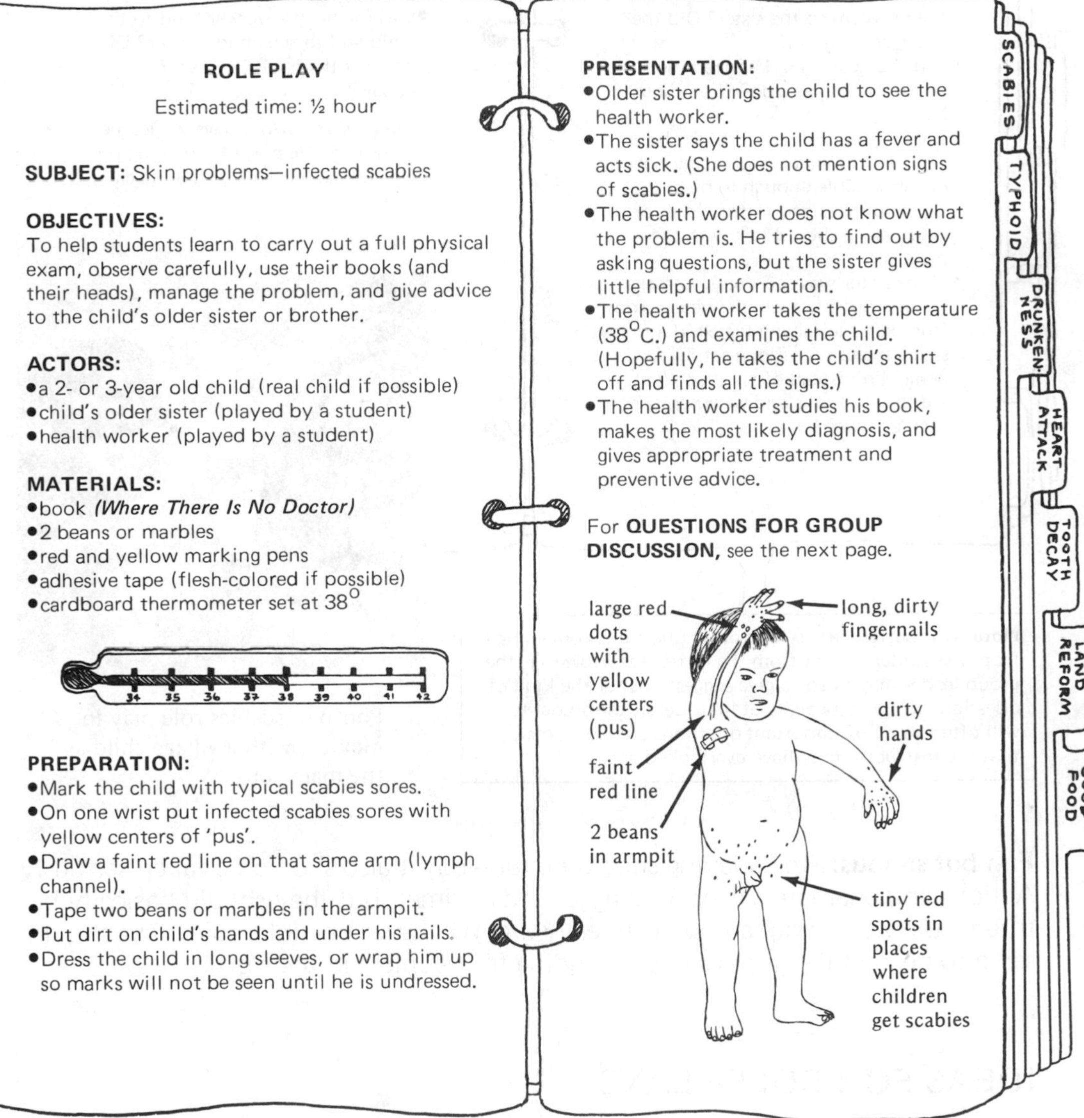

ROLE PLAY
Estimated time: ½ hour
SUBJECT: Skin problems—infected scabies
OBJECTIVES:
To help students learn to carry out a full physical exam, observe carefully, use their books (and their heads), manage the problem, and give advice to the child's older sister or brother.
ACTORS:
•a 2- or 3-year old child (real child if possible)
•child's older sister (played by a student)
•health worker (played by a student)
MATERIALS:
•book (Where There Is No Doctor)
•2 beans or marbles
•red and yellow marking pens
•adhesive tape (flesh-colored if possible)
•cardboard thermometer set at 38°
34 35 36 37 38 39 40 41 42
PREPARATION:
•Mark the child with typical scabies sores.
•On one wrist put infected scabies sores with yellow centers of 'pus'.
•Draw a faint red line on that same arm (lymph channel).
•Tape two beans or marbles in the armpit.
•Put dirt on child's hands and under his nails.
•Dress the child in long sleeves, or wrap him up so marks will not be seen until he is undressed.
PRESENTATION:
•Older sister brings the child to see the health worker.
•The sister says the child has a fever and acts sick. (She does not mention signs of scabies.)
•The health worker does not know what the problem is. He tries to find out by asking questions, but the sister gives little helpful information.
•The health worker takes the temperature (38°C.) and examines the child. (Hopefully, he takes the child's shirt off and finds all the signs.)
•The health worker studies his book, makes the most likely diagnosis, and gives appropriate treatment and preventive advice.
For QUESTIONS FOR GROUP DISCUSSION, see the next page.
large red dots with yellow centers (pus)
long, dirty fingernails
dirty hands
faint red line
2 beans in armpit
tiny red spots in places where children get scabies
SCABIES
TYPHOID
DRUNKENNESS
HEART ATTACK
TOOTH DECAY
LAND REFORM
GOOD FOOD

CAUTION: When putting on this and similar role plays, be sure the group and the person playing the health worker do not know what the problem is beforehand.

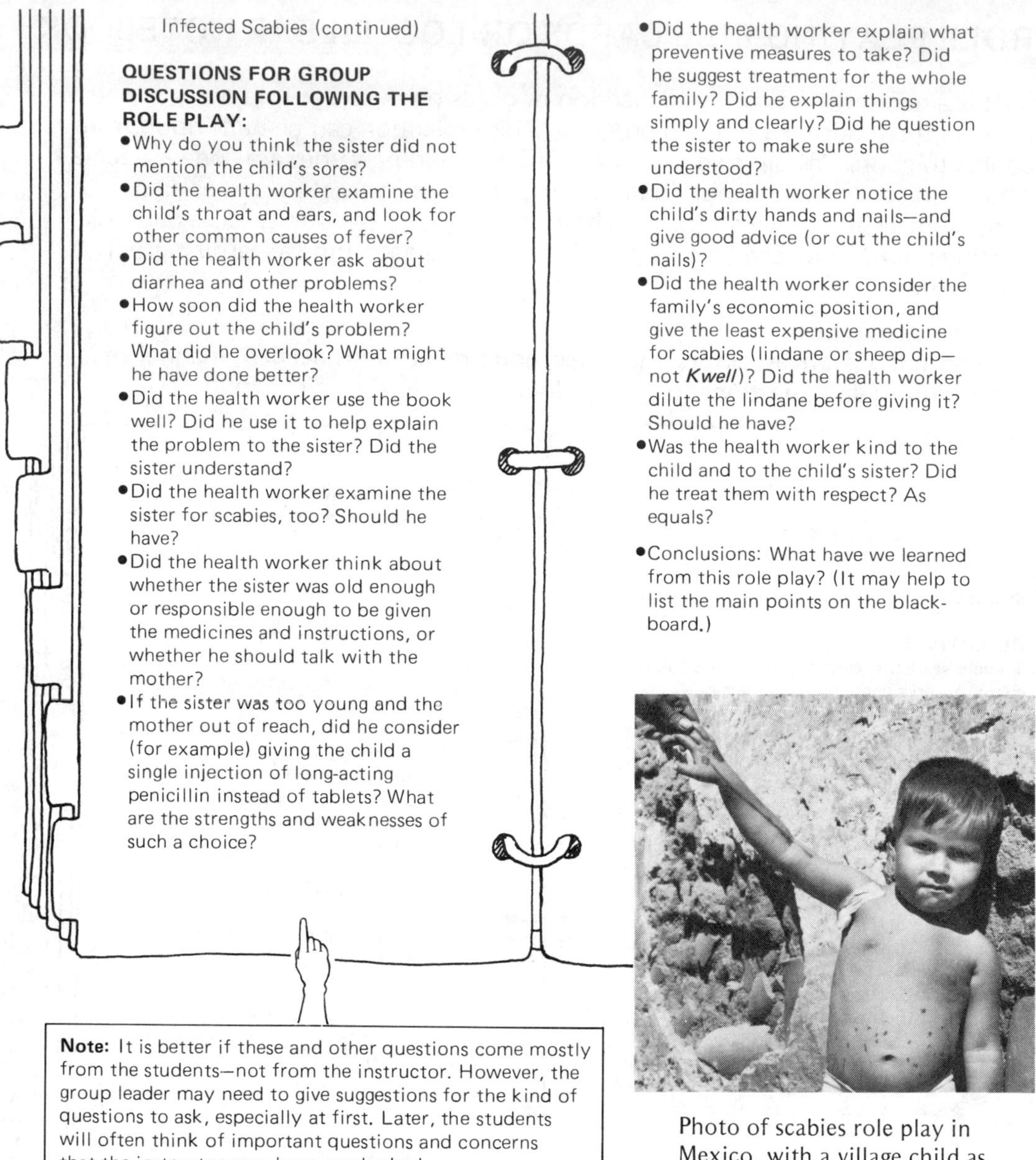

Infected Scabies (continued)

QUESTIONS FOR GROUP DISCUSSION FOLLOWING THE ROLE PLAY:

- Why do you think the sister did not mention the child's sores?
- Did the health worker examine the child's throat and ears, and look for other common causes of fever?
- Did the health worker ask about diarrhea and other problems?
- How soon did the health worker figure out the child's problem? What did he overlook? What might he have done better?
- Did the health worker use the book well? Did he use it to help explain the problem to the sister? Did the sister understand?
- Did the health worker examine the sister for scabies, too? Should he have?
- Did the health worker think about whether the sister was old enough or responsible enough to be given the medicines and instructions, or whether he should talk with the mother?
- If the sister was too young and the mother out of reach, did he consider (for example) giving the child a single injection of long-acting penicillin instead of tablets? What are the strengths and weaknesses of such a choice?
- Did the health worker explain what preventive measures to take? Did he suggest treatment for the whole family? Did he explain things simply and clearly? Did he question the sister to make sure she understood?
- Did the health worker notice the child's dirty hands and nails—and give good advice (or cut the child's nails)?
- Did the health worker consider the family's economic position, and give the least expensive medicine for scabies (lindane or sheep dip—not ***Kwell***)? Did the health worker dilute the lindane before giving it? Should he have?
- Was the health worker kind to the child and to the child's sister? Did he treat them with respect? As equals?
- Conclusions: What have we learned from this role play? (It may help to list the main points on the blackboard.)

Note: It is better if these and other questions come mostly from the students—not from the instructor. However, the group leader may need to give suggestions for the kind of questions to ask, especially at first. Later, the students will often think of important questions and concerns that the instructor may have overlooked.

Photo of scabies role play in Mexico, with a village child as the main actor.

Fun but serious: Role playing should be fun—but it also should be taken seriously. Actions and characters may be exaggerated at times, but they should basically be true to the way things and people really are. Whenever possible, role plays should serve to deepen the group's understanding for people and their problems.

IDEAS FOR ROLE PLAYS

In the rest of this chapter, we give examples of different kinds of role plays. Other examples are found in other parts of this book. Look in the Index under 'Role playing'.

EXAMPLE OF ROLE PLAYING PLAN

SUBJECT: Typhoid Fever

Estimated time for role play and discussion: 1 hour

OBJECTIVES:
1. To help students develop a systematic approach to problem solving.
2. To learn how to record vital signs and use them in diagnosing illnesses.
3. To gain experience in the diagnosis, treatment, and prevention of typhoid fever.

ACTORS:
- the sick person
- parents or relatives of the sick person
- one or two health workers

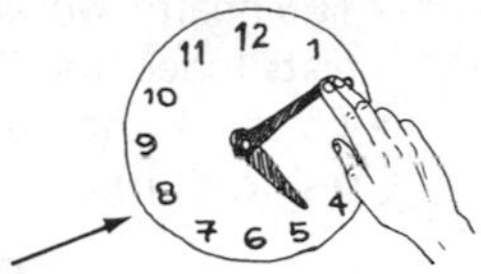

MATERIALS:
- a pretend clock with movable hands to show changes in the hour
- a pretend thermometer with adjustable temperature readings (see p. **14**-4)
- an adjustable artificial pulse (see p. **14**-6)
- a watch with a second hand, or a homemade one-minute timer (see p. **16**-7)
- pink marking pen for painting 'rose spots' on skin
- poster paper for making a vital signs chart everyone can see

PREPARATION:
- Paint 4 or 6 pink spots—each about 3mm. across—on the chest of the 'sick person'.
- Plan with the 'sick person' and 'parents' how to act the role of a person with typhoid (see *WTND,* p. 189) and what history to give (flash flood, no latrines, work on coastal plantation, etc.—whatever fits your area).
- Advise the 'sick person' and the 'parents' not to provide any of this information unless asked by the 'health workers'.
- Have the 'sick person' practice with the artificial pulse until he can do it at the correct rate.

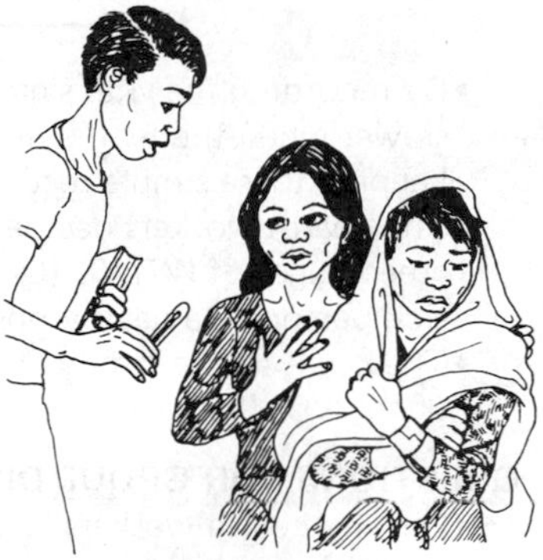

PRESENTATION:
- Parents come in with 'sick person', saying he has a fever and has been getting sicker for several days. Now he is too weak and sick to eat. He is wrapped in a blanket.
- **The students playing health workers have not been told what the illness is.** They try to find out by using their books, asking questions, and examining the 'sick person'.
- The health workers take temperature and pulse, using the pretend thermometer and adjustable artificial pulse. On the first reading they find:

temperature 40°C.	(These readings and those to follow
pulse 82/min.	are set by sick person or parents.)

- Because the fever is high, the health workers should ask the parents to uncover the sick person, and give him aspirin and cool water to drink. Together they can put cool, damp cloths on his chest and forehead.
- The health workers should recognize that the pulse is unusually slow for a 40° fever. They can check in their books under 'Pulse' (*WTND,* p. 32-33) and find that this may be a sign of typhoid fever.

- Half an hour later (according to the pretend clock, which someone sets ahead), the health workers take the temperature and pulse again. This time they find:

  temperature 39°C. pulse 88/min. (Parents have reset the temperature, and the sick person speeds up the fake pulse according to plan.)

- The health workers notice that the pulse is faster now, even though the temperature has dropped.
- Health workers may find various clues that lead them to consider typhoid fever (pinkish skin spots—in skin chapter, ***WTND,*** p. 198; comparison of different 'fevers'—***WTND,*** p. 26; pulse—***WTND,*** p. 32). If the health workers are having difficulty, other students in the class—who are also looking in their books—can give suggestions. On page 189 of ***WTND,*** under 'Typhoid fever', they may read that, **"If the pulse gets slower when the fever goes up, the person probably has typhoid."**
- The health workers make the probable diagnosis based on **history, examination,** and **tests** (checking fever and pulse several times).
- To check their diagnosis, they continue to take 'vital signs' (temperature, pulse, and respiration) every half hour, and they record the results on a simple chart.

Time	Temp.	Pulse	Respiration
9:00 AM	40°	82/min.	30/min.
9:30 AM	39°	88/min.	28/min.
10:00 AM	38.5°	95/min.	28/min.
10:30 AM	39°	82/min.	30/min.

- By recording the vital signs in this way, students can see how the pulse actually gets slower when the temperature rises—a sign of typhoid. (All students should practice keeping these simple records.)
- The health workers decide on treatment, checking medicines and dosages in the green pages of ***WTND.*** (Or, if the family can afford it, they may decide to refer the sick person to a nearby hospital.)
- They talk to the family about care of the sick person, the causes, course, and dangers of the disease. They explain what to do to prevent it from spreading.

QUESTIONS FOR GROUP DISCUSSION FOLLOWING THE ROLE PLAY:

- Did the health workers go about diagnosing the illness in a reasonable way? How could they have done better? (See Chapter 17 of this book.)
- Did they check for signs and history of other possible illnesses?
- When they found the person's temperature so high, did they try to lower the fever at once? Once they decided that it was probably typhoid, did they stop giving him aspirin? (Aspirin reduces normal clotting of blood and may increase the danger of hemorrhage in the gut.)
- Did they weigh the advantages and risks of treating the person themselves, or of sending him to a hospital?
- Did they ask if any neighbors had the same illness? Did they consider public health measures?
- Did they explain to the family what to do to prevent the spread of typhoid?
- Was their advice realistic? For example, did they offer to get some neighbors together to help dig the family a safe latrine (or whatever might be appropriate in the area)?
- Did they show sympathy, concern, and respect for the sick person and his family?
- Did the student group observing the role play make suggestions and criticisms in a kind, supportive way? Did the instructor do likewise?
- What different things were learned through the role play? About health care? About teaching? About human behavior? How could the group have learned better?

DIAGNOSIS GAMES

This is a different sort of role playing. One person acts out a series of similar health problems, one after the other, and the group tries to identify them. Here is an example.

SUBJECT: Noticing how a person breathes

OBJECTIVES:
1. To help health workers recognize various ways of breathing as signs of different illnesses.
2. To improve students' powers of observation.

USE: This game can be played when studying how to examine a sick person or when reviewing different respiratory illnesses.

METHOD: The instructor (or a well-prepared student) asks the group if they can guess his 'illness' by the way he breathes. In some cases he may want to give a few additional clues. For example, if students ask him, he might say whether or not he has a fever. Students can use their books to find the illness. After the instructor has demonstrated the different types of breathing, students can take turns demonstrating and testing each other.

1.

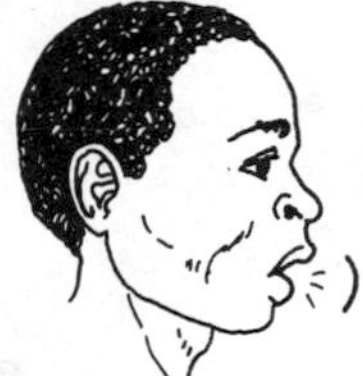
WHAT ILLNESS DO YOU THINK I HAVE ?

Breaths **rapid and shallow;** nostrils spread and person grunts slightly with each breath; fever.

50-80 breaths/minute

"What is it?"

(Pneumonia? ***WTND,*** p. 171)

2. Breaths **rapid and deep;** person very weak.

40-80 breaths/min.

"What is it?"

(Severe dehydration? ***WTND,*** p. 151)

3. Breaths **rapid and deep;** person very frightened.

60-80 breaths/min.

"What is it?"

(Hyperventilation? ***WTND,*** p. 24)

4.

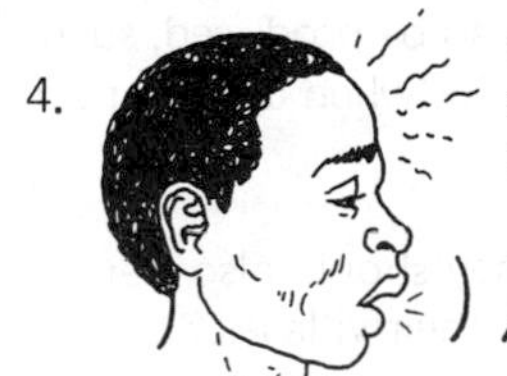

Breaths **rapid** but neither shallow nor deep; high fever.

30-40 breaths/min.

"What is it?"

(Rapid breathing that accompanies high fever? ***WTND,*** p. 32)

5.

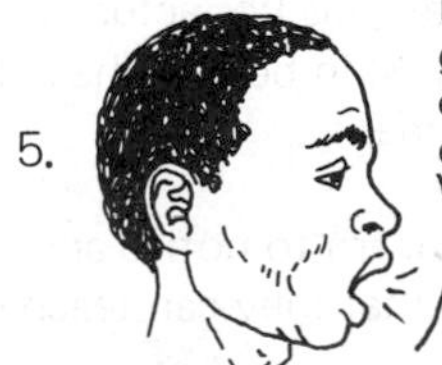

Breaths **very deep,** gasping for air, especially after mild exercise.

"What is it?"

(Severe anemia? ***WTND,*** p. 124, Heart problem? ***WTND,*** p.325)

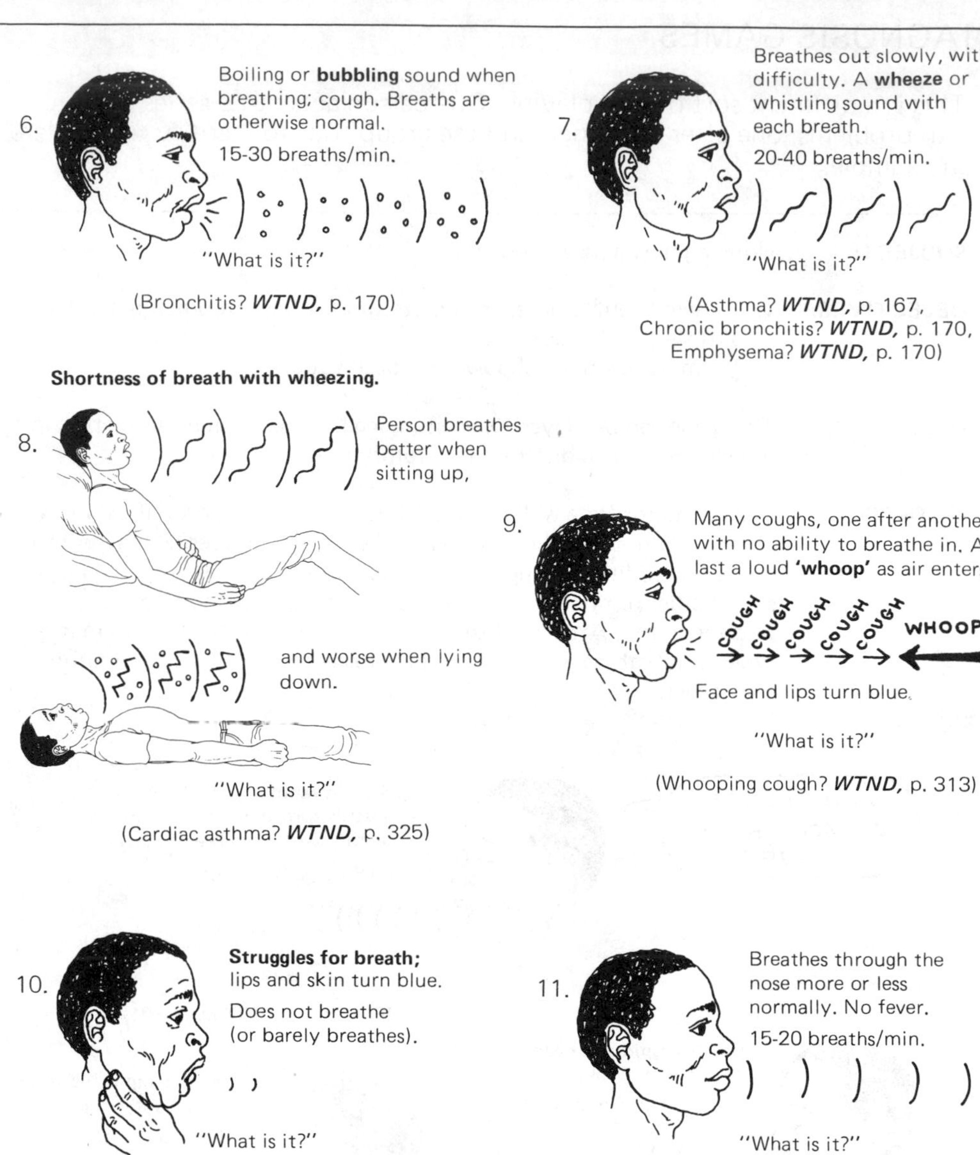

6.
Boiling or **bubbling** sound when breathing; cough. Breaths are otherwise normal.
15-30 breaths/min.
"What is it?"
(Bronchitis? ***WTND,*** p. 170)
7.
Breathes out slowly, with difficulty. A **wheeze** or whistling sound with each breath.
20-40 breaths/min.
"What is it?"
(Asthma? ***WTND,*** p. 167, Chronic bronchitis? ***WTND,*** p. 170, Emphysema? ***WTND,*** p. 170)
Shortness of breath with wheezing.
8.
Person breathes better when sitting up,
and worse when lying down.
"What is it?"
(Cardiac asthma? ***WTND,*** p. 325)
9.
Many coughs, one after another, with no ability to breathe in. At last a loud **'whoop'** as air enters.
COUGH COUGH COUGH COUGH COUGH
WHOOP!
Face and lips turn blue.
"What is it?"
(Whooping cough? ***WTND,*** p. 313)
10.
Struggles for breath; lips and skin turn blue.
Does not breathe (or barely breathes).
"What is it?"
(Choking—something stuck in the throat? ***WTND,*** page 79, Diphtheria? ***WTND,*** p. 313)
11.
Breathes through the nose more or less normally. No fever.
15-20 breaths/min.
"What is it?"
(A normal, healthy person?)

With practice, health workers can learn to imitate the various noises (wheezing, rattling, whooping) and other signs (flaring nostrils, watering eyes, etc.) typical of different respiratory problems. For choking or asthma, the demonstrator can, by not breathing much, make his lips actually turn blue! Other signs can also be produced, such as 'sucking in' of the skin behind the collar bone and between the ribs when demonstrating asthma or emphysema.

Students should learn to notice and recognize all these signs. They should also learn to imitate them, so that they can teach others when they return to their villages.

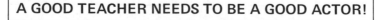

A GOOD TEACHER NEEDS TO BE A GOOD ACTOR!

ROLE PLAYING TO MOTIVATE COMMUNITY ACTION

Role playing has sometimes been used as part of a process to get a whole community of people thinking and taking action to meet their needs.

In Ghana, Africa, role plays were used to involve the people of Okorase in the town's development. To help with the role plays, health program leaders invited a popular cultural group that often performs at local ceremonies. First the group would help lead a 'one-day school' focusing on town problems. Then the group would stage role plays about one or two particular problems and their possible solutions. The following description of these events (somewhat shortened and simplified) is from an article by Larry Frankel in *World Education Reports,* April, 1981.

The cultural group members (with help from the project) purchased food and palm wine to entertain their guests. Then they invited the chief, his elders, and other members of the community to attend the 'one-day school'. After the traditional ceremonies and welcoming speeches, they gave the entire morning to small group discussions of the town's problems and their possible solutions. Each group had a discussion leader whose job was to see that everyone participated freely so that the 'big men' didn't dominate.

Before stopping for lunch, each small group was asked to choose a single problem, one that they considered serious but also solvable by the people's own efforts. The small groups then joined together to choose one or two problems and propose realistic solutions.

After lunch all the people were excused, except the cultural group members. Everyone thanked the chief and elders for their attendance and their help in trying to make the problem's solution a reality.

The cultural group spent the afternoon preparing and practicing two role plays or brief skits. They wanted to show as dramatically and humorously as possible why each problem was important and what could be done about it. In the evening, the chief had the 'gong gong' beater call the entire town to a free show. The role plays were performed, along with drumming, singing, and dancing.

The role plays in Okorase focused on two problems: unhealthy shitting habits and the lack of a health clinic.

In **the first role play,** a big shot from Accra (the capital) returns to visit his birthplace, Okorase. He has come to donate a large sum of money to the town development committee. Feeling nature's call, he seeks a place to relieve himself. When he finds only bushes, he becomes increasingly discomfited. His distress amuses several villagers, who wonder aloud why the bush is no longer good enough for him. The desperation of the actor playing the big shot had the people in the audience laughing until they cried.

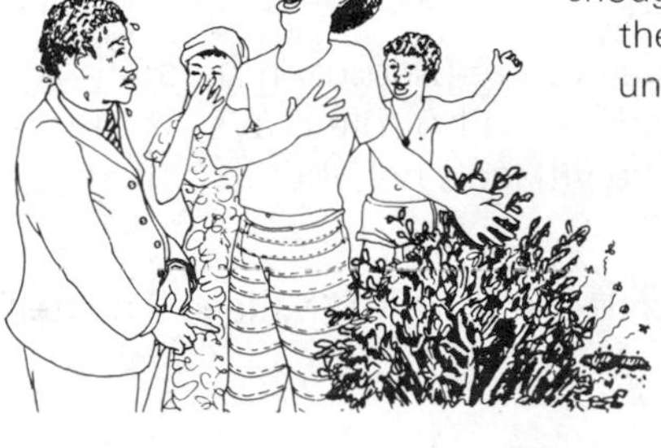

Finally, the big shot flees Okorase without donating any money. Later, each of the people who laughed at him falls ill with some sort of sickness carried in human shit. So now the villagers become interested in trying a suggested solution: using low-cost water-sealed toilets to keep flies off the shit.

As a result of this role play and the discussion that followed, a local mason volunteered to be trained in the construction of toilet bowls. Cement was donated by the People's Educational Association (a private Ghanaian agency). Soon a profitable local industry was started, making water-sealed bowls for Okorase and surrounding villages.

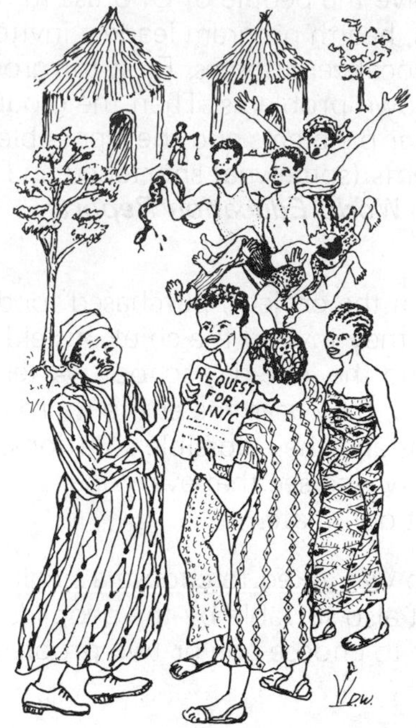

In **the second role play,** a concerned group of villagers approaches the chief for help in starting a clinic. But the chief is not interested. He argues that medical attention is available in Koforidua, only four miles away.

During this discussion, a messenger bursts in and throws himself at the chief's feet. The chief's son has just been bitten by a poisonous snake! Everyone rushes to find a way to get the boy to the hospital in Koforidua, but before a vehicle can be located, the boy dies.

In his grief, the chief sees the error of his ways. He gathers the townspeople together and begs them to contribute money and labor to build a clinic so that no other parent will have to suffer as he has. He also appoints some villagers to negotiate with the regional medical officers for drugs and personnel.

As it happened, the real village chief of Okorase had recently lost a very well-liked relative. This made the role play extra powerful. The people of Okorase determined to build their own clinic and to collect some money for medicines.

The new clinic was soon built. For the ceremony to celebrate its opening, officials from the regional government and a foreign agency, as well as newspaper and television reporters, were invited. On this occasion, the village cultural group put on another, more carefully planned skit telling the story of a young girl who died of snakebite because the clinic had no electricity and so could not refrigerate antitoxin. The skit was presented as a community request to the authorities and development agencies to introduce electricity into their town. As a result, negotiations are presently taking place between the village and the Ministry. There is a possibility that electricity may actually come to Okorase.

This example from Ghana shows how role plays were used to motivate villagers to take action to meet their health needs. Finally, role plays (or skits) were even used to activate the government in the village's behalf.

The use of more organized role plays or skits in the form of 'Village Theater' is explored in Chapter 27.

CHAPTER 15

Appropriate and Inappropriate Technology

'HARD' AND 'SOFT' TECHNOLOGIES

Appropriate technology is a fashionable way to say "doing things in low-cost, effective ways that local people can manage and control."

Development workers often use the term *appropriate technology* to refer to practical, simple THINGS—such as tools, instruments, or machines—that people can make, use, and repair themselves using local resources.

But appropriate technology also refers to METHODS—ways of doing, learning, and problem solving that are adapted to people's needs, customs, and abilities.

The technology of THINGS is called 'hard'; technology of METHODS is called 'soft'. Ideas are more flexible than bricks (if both are appropriate).

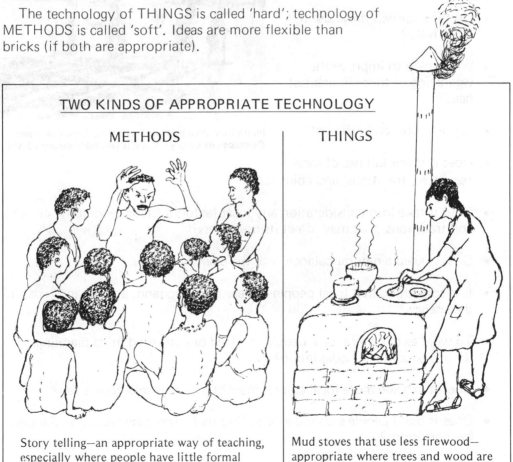

TWO KINDS OF APPROPRIATE TECHNOLOGY

METHODS

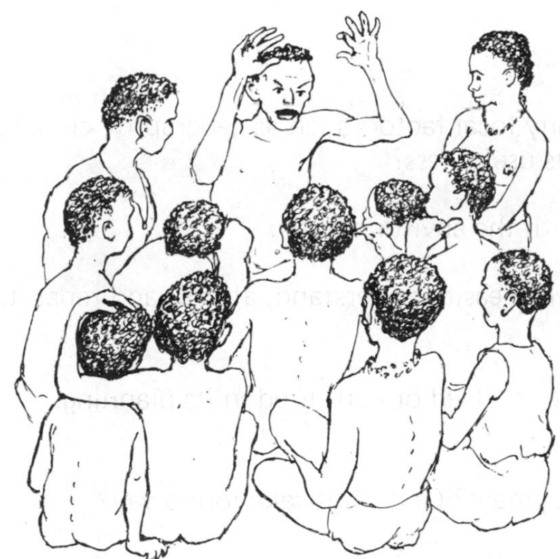

Story telling—an appropriate way of teaching, especially where people have little formal education and story telling is a tradition.

THINGS

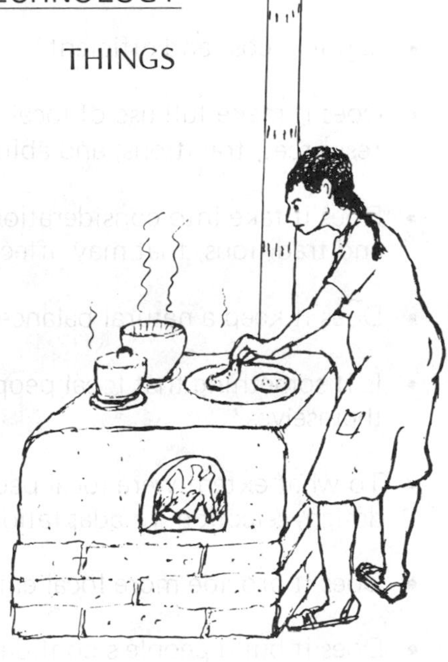

Mud stoves that use less firewood—appropriate where trees and wood are scarce, but only if people will make and use them.

Unfortunately, some of the technologies commonly introduced by health programs turn out to be less appropriate than they seem. In this chapter, we will look at the strengths and weaknesses of some of the advice, methods, and things that are often assumed to be appropriate.

Chapter 16, which follows, also deals with appropriate technology. In it, we will look at some basic tools and pieces of equipment that health workers can make themselves.

HOW APPROPRIATE IS A SPECIFIC TECHNOLOGY?

To determine whether a certain **thing** or **method** is appropriate for your area, you can ask yourself the following questions:

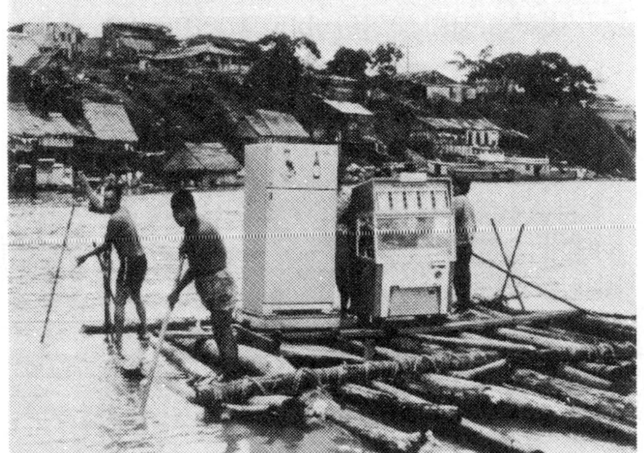

Photo from Peru by Douglas Botting, from *Questioning Development* by Glyn Roberts (available through TALC).

- Is it acceptable to the local people?
- Do they (or will they) use it effectively?
- Will it help to improve the well-being of those in greatest need?
- Is it low-cost and efficient?
- Does it make full use of local resources, traditions, and abilities?
- Does it take into consideration any local factors such as geography, climate, and traditions, that may affect its usefulness?
- Does it keep a natural balance with the environment?
- Is it something that local people can easily understand, afford, and repair by themselves?
- To what extent were local people involved or consulted in its planning, design, selection, or adaptation?
- Does it provide more local employment? Or does it take jobs away?
- Does it build people's confidence to find their own answers and make their own decisions?
- Will it help close the gap between the rich and the poor? Or widen it?
- Does it help the weak to gain greater control and become more self-reliant?

RE-EXAMINING SOME COMMON ASSUMPTIONS

All aspects of a health worker training program—methods, materials, and content—should be continually re-examined. Questions like those on the previous page need to be asked again and again. **It is important that health workers take an active part in this questioning process.**

Much of the standard advice taught to health workers and villagers comes from faraway lands where conditions are very different. Some of it may apply to your own situation. Some may not. And some may even do more harm than good. Often recommendations from outside need to be adapted or completely changed. When planning a course or class, or providing any sort of information to student health workers, it is important to ask yourself:

- How is this information or advice likely to be accepted and used in the particular situation where the health workers will work?
- How is it likely to affect people's well-being—in terms not only of their immediate health needs, but of their long-range environmental, economic, and social needs?

Before giving people standard health advice, consider the reality of their lives.

To follow are 5 examples of standard health recommendations that need to be re-examined: (1) boiling of drinking water, (2) use of hybrid grains, (3) use of 'flow charts', (4) official inspection of food and marketplace, and (5) use of packaged rehydration salts.

Example 1: Drinking water—to boil or not to boil?

Boil all drinking water is standard advice in many health programs. But is it good advice?

Often it is not! In fact, **advising families to boil drinking water may do more harm than good.**

Boiling does kill germs. But there are many other ways that the same germs can reach a child's mouth.

Water piped into homes, even if it is not 'pure', usually proves to be far more helpful in preventing infection. This is because it allows families to keep their homes and their children cleaner. For keeping a family healthy, quantity and availability of water are usually more important than its purity.

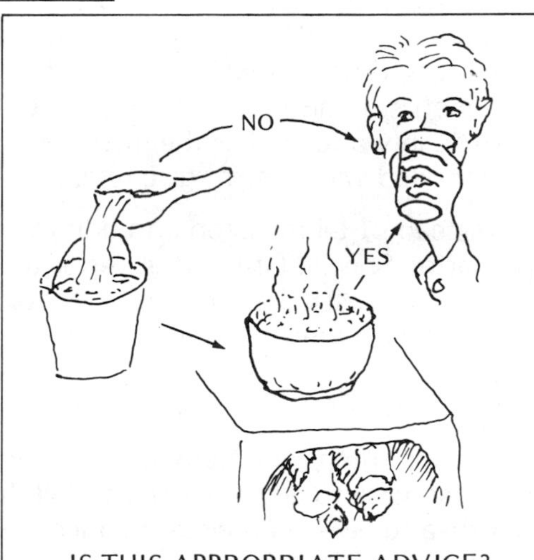

IS THIS APPROPRIATE ADVICE?
Perhaps we should think again about this recommendation in *Where There Is No Doctor.* Health advice needs to be adapted to local conditions.

Before telling people to boil water, be sure to consider the cost to them. Families may be poor and resources limited. To boil water costs firewood (or cow dung), time, energy, and often money. If a poor family has to spend part of its limited food money on firewood, then boiling the water may actually harm their children's health!

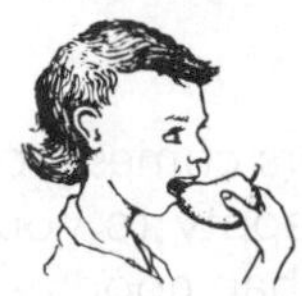

Good nutrition does far more to prevent infection than does boiling of drinking water.

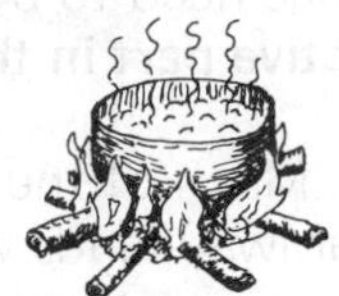

Also consider people's need to live in balance with nature. In many areas, the gathering of firewood is turning forests into deserts. Where forests are destroyed, there is less rainfall, causing drought and crop failure. In these areas, advice on ways to cook with less firewood (such as by using special mud stoves) may be most important to long-term health. Advice to "boil your water" could be a slow death sentence, to both the land and the people.

Fortunately, in such circumstances, villagers tend to be more realistic than health advisers. They simply do not follow the advice. Unfortunately, the villagers are often scolded or made to feel backward for not doing so.

Boiling water for Rehydration Drink: Most dangerous of all is to instruct people to boil water when preparing Rehydration Drink for children with diarrhea (see Special Drink, p. **24**-20). **Telling mothers to boil the water for Rehydration Drink may actually cause more infant deaths.** The reasons are these:

- **Boiling water means extra work and extra cost.** Some mothers will simply not make the Special Drink if told they must boil the water for it.
- **Boiling takes time.** Cooling takes still more time. But a baby with diarrhea needs liquid immediately! The delay caused by boiling increases the danger of dehydration. This increased risk outweighs the germ-killing benefits. In any case, the baby with diarrhea probably already has the infection that the unboiled water might give him.

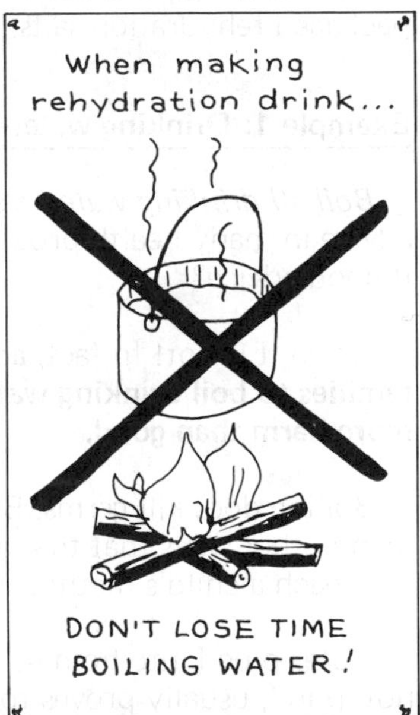
When making
rehydration drink...
DON'T LOSE TIME
BOILING WATER!

Instead of telling people to boil the water when preparing Special Drink, it is better to advise them, "Prepare it fast! Use the cleanest water you have. If you have water that has already been boiled, that is best. But DON'T LOSE TIME BOILING WATER WHEN YOUR BABY HAS DIARRHEA!"

Because preparing Rehydration Drink takes time, it is also wise to advise mothers of children with diarrhea to give plain water at once, and until the drink is prepared.

Note: This advice about boiling, like all advice, needs to be adapted to local conditions. In places where people get their water from open sewers, for example, boiling water may be an essential, even life-saving measure. Where firewood is scarce, you can put water (or Rehydration Drink) in small, tightly sealed plastic bags or clear glass bottles. Leave these in the sun for 2 hours. This will kill all or most of the germs.

Example 2: Native grains or hybrids—which are more appropriate?

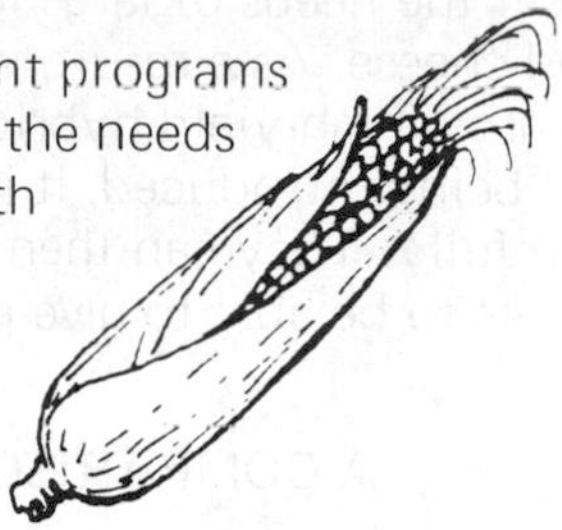

In farming and nutrition, as in other areas, development programs sometimes introduce new technologies that do not meet the needs of the poor as well as the old ways (see Chapter 7). Health workers and their people need to carefully evaluate any new methods that agricultural extension workers or other outsiders try to introduce. As with medicines, **possible benefits must be weighed against possible harm.**

Consider hybrid grains. Hybrids are varieties produced by crossing two closely related types, in order to increase the amount of harvest. Under the best conditions, they often give a higher yield (more harvest per hectare). But they usually require costly fertilizers and insecticides—which may upset the natural balance of plants and animals in the area.

An even bigger problem is that **a new kind of plant disease could suddenly appear and in one season destroy all the hybrid grain planted in the entire region.** The result could be economic ruin and widespread starvation. The crops can be destroyed easily because hybrids lack the natural variation needed to resist disease. Native grains, on the other hand, have enough variation so that only a part of the crop is likely to be ruined by such an epidemic.

Nevertheless, banks, agriculture experts, and governments in some parts of the world have given a great deal of support to the growing and marketing of hybrid grains. As a result, some native grains are in danger of being lost or weakened through crossbreeding with the hybrids. This could lead to disaster in the future because when an epidemic destroys a hybrid crop, the native grain—if it still exists—must provide the reserve from which a more disease-resistant hybrid can be developed.

In the case of maize (corn) grown in Mexico, this danger is near. There the government pays a higher price for hybrid 'white maize', and it is now grown on almost all the large irrigated landholdings. Today, the main reserve of the traditional *criollo* maize lies in the small independent plantings of poor farmers. Although this yellow maize has been the main food in the native people's diet for hundreds of years, many small farmers are now switching to the white hybrids, tempted by the promise of a greater yield and a higher market price.

But **the disadvantages and risks of growing the hybrid are especially great for the poor farmer.** The white maize requires expensive fertilizers and insecticides for good harvests. It is less resistant to disease. And it matures more slowly than the native grain—so if the rainy season is short, the crop fails. All this does not matter much to the large landholder with irrigated fields. But it is of great importance to the small farmer.

The nutritional difference is also a concern. *Criollo* maize is higher in protein and vitamin A than the new white maize. For families that can afford to eat meat and cheese, this difference is not very important. But for poor families, that often lack even beans, the additional protein in *criollo* maize can make the difference between health and malnutrition.

Unfortunately, the training of many agricultural advisers has been designed to meet the needs of large landholders and decision makers who can afford meat and cheese. As a result, village health and development programs are often advised to grow high-yield hybrids instead of native grains. In areas where hybrid crops are being introduced, it is important that program leaders study these questions carefully. They can then help health workers gain enough understanding of the issues to be able to give people sound advice.

A COMPARISON BETWEEN NATIVE AND HYBRID MAIZE

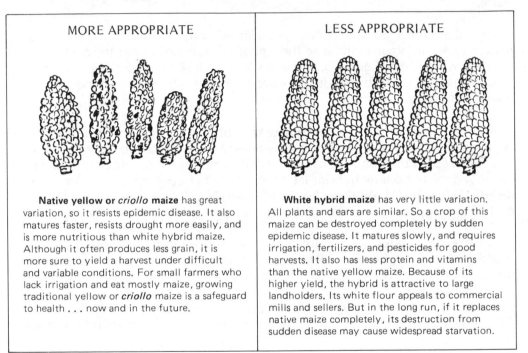

MORE APPROPRIATE	LESS APPROPRIATE
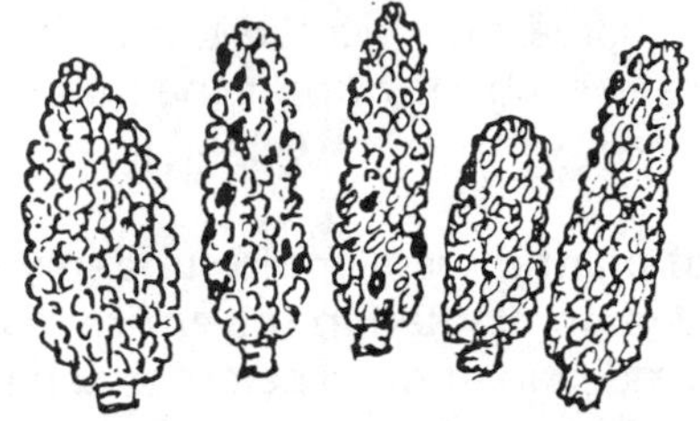	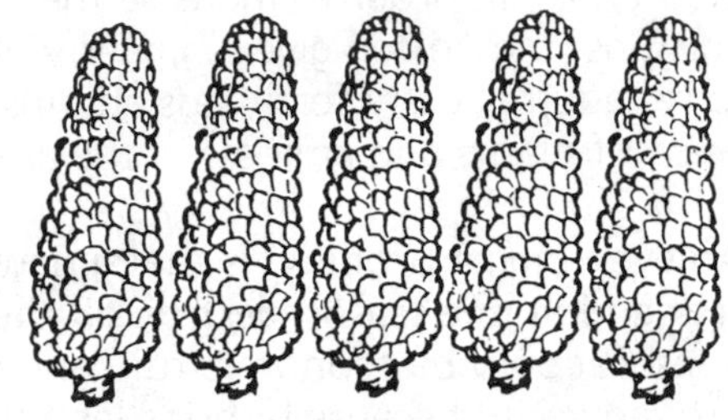
Native yellow or *criollo* maize has great variation, so it resists epidemic disease. It also matures faster, resists drought more easily, and is more nutritious than white hybrid maize. Although it often produces less grain, it is more sure to yield a harvest under difficult and variable conditions. For small farmers who lack irrigation and eat mostly maize, growing traditional yellow or ***criollo*** maize is a safeguard to health . . . now and in the future.	**White hybrid maize** has very little variation. All plants and ears are similar. So a crop of this maize can be destroyed completely by sudden epidemic disease. It matures slowly, and requires irrigation, fertilizers, and pesticides for good harvests. It also has less protein and vitamins than the native yellow maize. Because of its higher yield, the hybrid is attractive to large landholders. Its white flour appeals to commercial mills and sellers. But in the long run, if it replaces native maize completely, its destruction from sudden disease may cause widespread starvation.

Problems similar to those with hybrid maize in Latin America have occurred in many parts of the world. In **Zambia,** a mold called *fusarium* destroyed hybrid maize on big farms, while small farms with traditional maize were not affected. In the **Philippines,** epidemics have destroyed huge crops of hybrid rice. In **Indonesia,** 200,000 hectares of hybrid rice were lost in 1974 and 1975 because of a new virus disease spread by insects. Now the Indonesian government is trying to improve the old local varieties of rice, instead of using hybrids from outside the area.

Note: We are not suggesting that all hybrid grains are bad and should not be used. As long as care is taken to maintain a reserve of native grain, certain hybrids can be of considerable benefit. In a just political climate, they may even help to improve the well-being of the poor. Also, some hybrids—such as ***Opaque 2*** maize—are more nutritious than the native grains, although there have been major problems with rot, fungus, etc. The point we are trying to make is this:

Health workers should not simply accept hybrids—or anything else introduced by outsiders—without first checking to see if they will really meet the needs of the local people.

Raising social awareness using the example of *criollo* and hybrid maize:

When you stop to think about it, the differences between ***criollo*** and hybrid maize have a kind of symbolic meaning.

After health workers have discussed the advantages and disadvantages of each type of maize, have the group imagine that these represent two kinds of people. Hand around samples of each kind of maize and have everyone think quietly for a few moments. Ask them to consider how the two kinds look, whose needs they serve, and their present and possible future effects on people's health. Then ask them to relate their ideas to different approaches to education, health care, and government.

You might start by asking questions like these:

- Who do these two different types of maize remind you of? Why?
- How do the different types (of maize and people) relate to the needs of the poor?
- What type do our schools try to produce? What type does the army try to produce? Why?
- How do these different types of maize compare with the kinds of health workers different programs try to train?

The group can carry on with their own questions and answers. It will be interesting to see where the discussion leads!

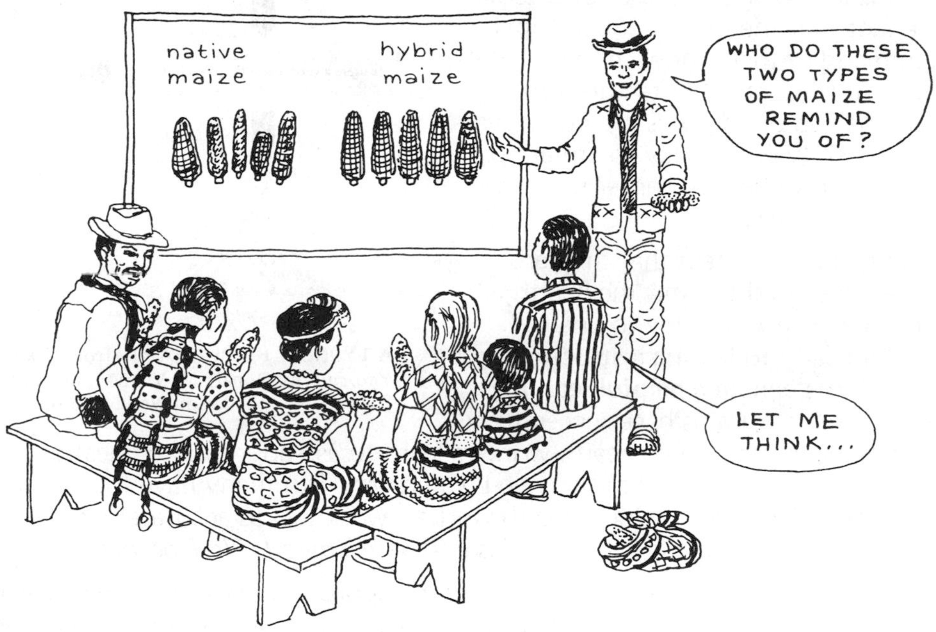

WARNING: In leading a discussion like this one, you will need to be careful that people do not conclude that they, the 'natives'—because they appear darker, more irregular, and 'less perfectly formed'—are less worthy than the more uniform 'white' variety. Help them understand that, in spite of appearances or what they have been told, they have a hardiness, strength, and ability to survive under difficult conditions, that the more demanding, artificially developed, more uniform variety often lacks. If the discussion is led well, people will end up with a new appreciation and respect for both their native crops and themselves.

Example 3: Flow charts

Some health programs make extensive use of flow charts, or ***algorithms.*** These are charts designed to help health workers diagnose illnesses by guiding them through a series of yes-or-no questions.

A few studies done under ideal conditions have shown that health workers make more accurate diagnoses with flow charts than when using more conventional methods. However, some programs have had disappointing results with flow charts. They have found that the charts often make for a less personal relationship between the health worker and the sick person. Also, some health workers with limited formal education find flow charts difficult or confusing.

Our biggest objection to flow charts has to do with the question of who has control. **Flow charts provide a means of keeping control over diagnosis and treatment in the hands of the professionals** who design the charts. Little decision making or clinical judgement is expected of the health worker. The hidden message in most flow charts seems to be, "We don't trust you. Your role is to follow instructions. Not to think. Not to lead!"

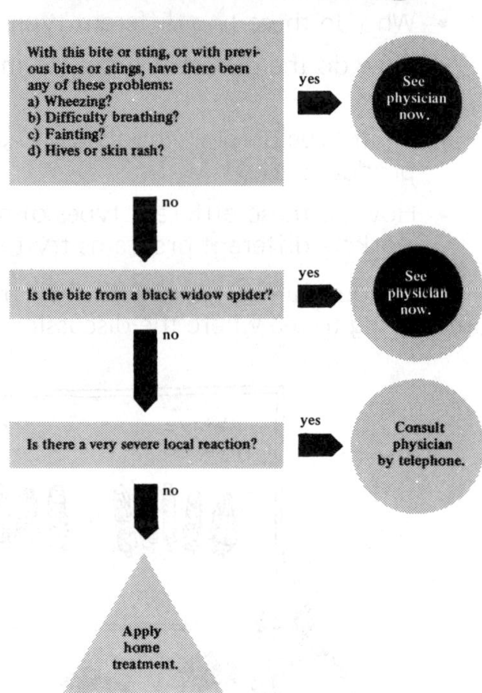
Insect Bites or Stings
With this bite or sting, or with previous bites or stings, have there been any of these problems:
a) Wheezing?
b) Difficulty breathing?
c) Fainting?
d) Hives or skin rash?
yes
See physician now.
no
Is the bite from a black widow spider?
yes
See physician now.
no
Is there a very severe local reaction?
yes
Consult physician by telephone.
no
Apply home treatment.

A TYPICAL FLOW CHART—from *Take Care of Yourself,* by Donald M. Vickery, M.D. and James F. Fries, M.D., Addison-Wesley, 1976.

This lack of trust is also reflected in the fact that the most frequent final command of many flow charts is "Refer to doctor at once." Often no other information or advice is provided, even though early emergency treatment by a community health worker might save the person's life.

In spite of the fact that they are sometimes used to limit the health worker's diagnostic role to one of mechanically following instructions, **flow charts can be a helpful learning tool.** Some programs have successfully used flow charts to help health workers learn to ask appropriate questions and approach diagnosis in a logical, step-by-step way. But many have found that once those skills are learned, their health workers work just as accurately with, and greatly prefer, simple lists of signs (as in ***Where There Is No Doctor).***

As with any other health technology, the appropriateness of flow charts must be judged on social as well as medical grounds. A key question to ask is, **"Does the use of this technology encourage or discourage initiative, critical thinking, and problem-solving skills?"**

As we have seen, flow charts can be used to help health workers develop independent mastery of the problem-solving process. Or they can be used to keep the health worker dependent on the decisions of professionals. Which way they are used will depend largely on the program's trust and respect for health workers and whether they want them to be followers or leaders.

Example 4: Inspection of food and market place—top-down or bottom-up?

A public market where farmers and vendors sell food can be a place where disease is spread through spoilage, dirt, flies, and careless handling.

A variety of approaches have been taken to 'clean up the market place'. In some cases, the authorities take steps that throw small, independent sellers out of the market. Or public health inspectors sometimes fine the vendors or close down stalls that do not meet standards of cleanliness.

Unfortunately, attempts by health authorities and officials to clean up market places have resulted in many abuses and hard feelings. The small farmers selling their produce are often hurt most. This leads to more 'middle men' and higher prices, which means that poor customers also suffer.

Some sort of cleanliness inspection for the market place may be appropriate. But **health workers need to find ways for checks and control to come from the local people rather than from outside authorities.**

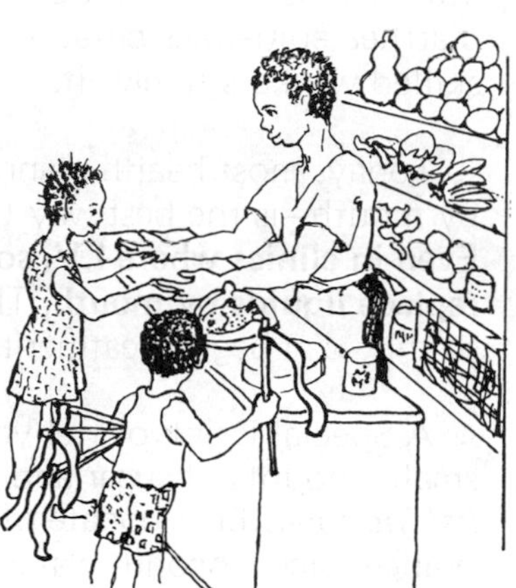

A good example comes from Togo, Africa, where school children have become the local 'health inspectors'. Once a week the children go to the market and observe the cleanliness and condition of all the stalls. They check to see if the vendors' hands are clean, the floors swept, and the food fresh and protected from flies. To each stall that passes their inspection, they award a red ribbon. The people who come to buy have learned to look for these ribbons and prefer to buy where they are displayed. So vendors try to keep their stalls clean in order to pass the children's test.

Teaching suggestions:

Discuss this example from Togo with the learning group and see how many beneficial features they can point out. Here are some:

- It is an example of true community participation. A group that usually has little power (the children) is able to take a leading role in dealing with a problem affecting their health.
- In taking this responsibility, the children not only learn about hygiene and sanitation, but put their knowledge into action.
- The children take part eagerly because they are doing something that matters and because **they are in charge.** It builds their confidence and awareness.
- Rather than focusing attention on those who fail the inspection, the child-inspectors reward those who do best.
- The example shows everyone involved—children, sellers, and buyers—the possibilities of a friendly, community-based approach to solving problems in which the weak gain strength through popular support.

Example 5: Oral rehydration—which method is most appropriate?

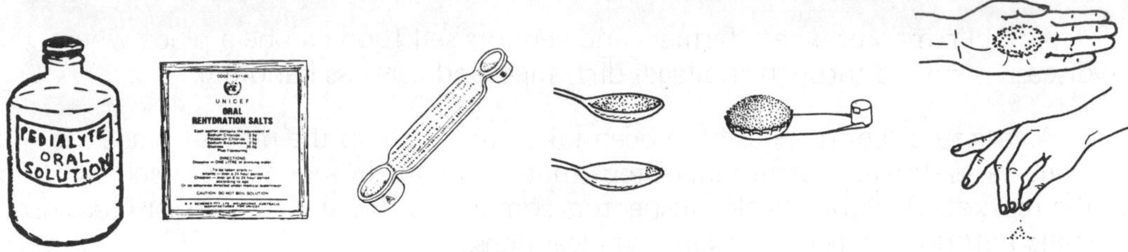

Diarrhea is one of the main causes of death in small children. However, most of these children actually die from *dehydration*—the loss of too much water. It is generally agreed that the most important way to manage diarrhea is to replace the liquid that the child is losing. But there is less agreement about how to do this.

A few years ago, most doctors treated even mild dehydration by giving intravenous (I.V.) solution. But this was expensive, and many children died in diarrhea epidemics because there was not enough I.V. solution, or not enough skilled workers to give it.

Today, most health planners recognize that *oral rehydration*—or giving liquid by mouth—is the best way to manage most cases of diarrhea and dehydration. **Even in clinics where I.V. solution is available, it usually makes more sense to replace liquids by mouth.** This way parents learn how to prepare and give liquids so they can begin treatment early, at home, the next time a child gets diarrhea.

A Special Drink or Rehydration Drink can be made from water mixed with small amounts of sugar and salt. It is even better if the drink contains a little *baking soda* (bicarbonate of soda) and a mineral called *potassium*—found in orange juice, coconut water, banana, and other foods.

- The **salt** in the Special Drink replaces the salt lost through diarrhea, and helps the child's body to keep liquid.
- The **sugar** provides energy and also helps the body absorb liquid more quickly.
- The **baking soda** prevents 'acid blood', a condition that causes fast, heavy breathing and shock.
- The **potassium** helps keep the child alert and willing to drink and eat.

The amounts of sugar and salt in the Special Drink do not have to be very exact. In fact, there is great variation in the amounts recommended by different experts. However, too little sugar or salt does less good, and too much salt can be dangerous.

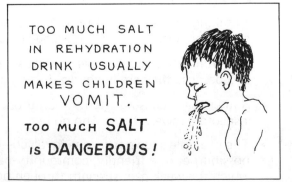

TOO MUCH SALT IN REHYDRATION DRINK USUALLY MAKES CHILDREN VOMIT.

TOO MUCH SALT IS DANGEROUS!

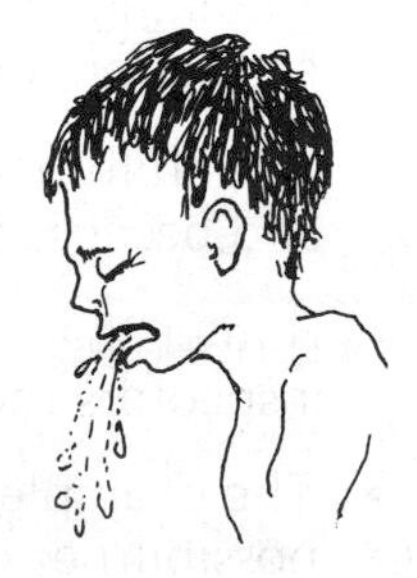

There is much debate among health planners about how a rehydration drink should be prepared. The main disagreements center around 3 issues:

- Whether to use mass-produced 'packets' or homemade rehydration mixes.
- What amount of salt to use.
- Whether methods should be standardized or locally adapted.

Instructors of health workers should be familiar with the different points of view so that they can prepare health workers to make appropriate decisions and advise people well.

1. 'Packets' or homemade mix?

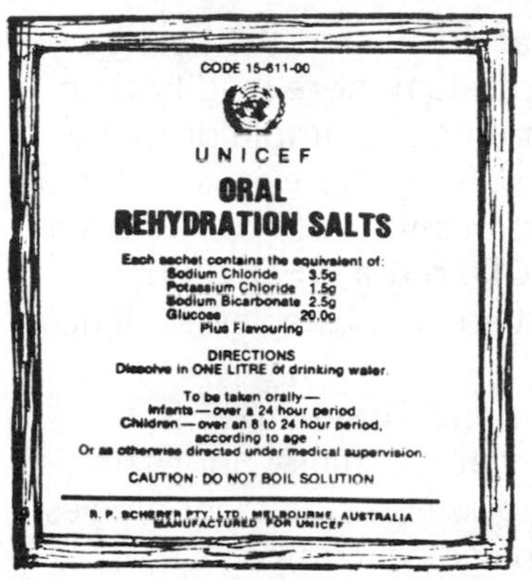

- Which can save more lives?
- Which is more reliable in terms of safety? In terms of being available when needed?
- Which puts more control and responsibility in the hands of the local people?

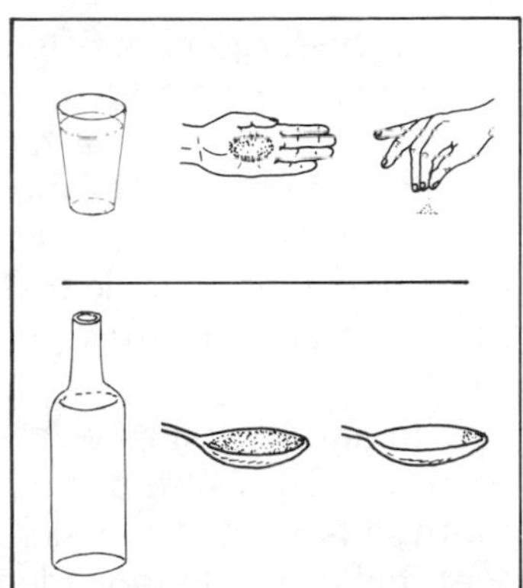

Many large organizations, including the World Health Organization, favor teaching people to use factory-produced 'rehydration salts'. Millions of standard packets have been produced by large drug companies and are now being distributed in many countries by UNICEF and other groups. Each UNICEF packet can be used to make 1 liter of Rehydration Drink.

Smaller, community-based programs often favor teaching families to make their own Special Drink, using water, sugar, and salt that they have in their homes or can buy at the local market.

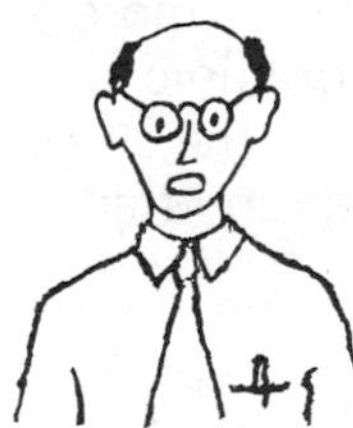

Those in favor of the packets argue that these are safer and work better. "After all," they say, "the contents of each packet are accurately measured. Baking soda and potassium are included. And the special sugar ***(glucose)*** may, in some cases, be more easily absorbed by children with severe diarrhea." (However, studies indicate that ordinary sugar works as well.)

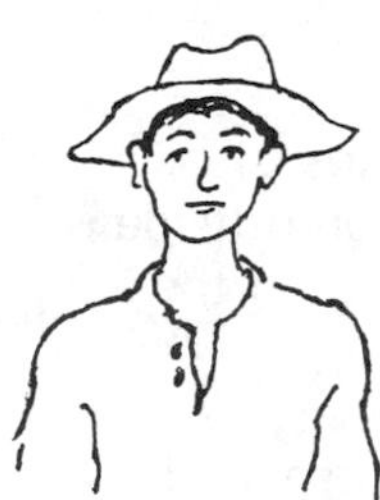

Those in favor of the homemade Special Drink argue that this approach allows more children with diarrhea to be treated, right away, and in their own homes. If packets are used, then for each case of diarrhea families will have to depend on a supply system that involves foreign manufacturers, international organizations, health ministries, transportation networks, and health posts. But in most parts of the world, the sugar and salt needed for home-made mix are common household items. Once they learn how, families can make and use the drink right away whenever it is needed—without having to depend on outsiders.

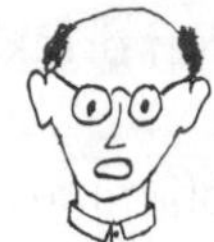

"But you must consider safety!" argue the packeteers. "If people make their own rehydration drink, they may put in too much salt! That can be dangerous!"

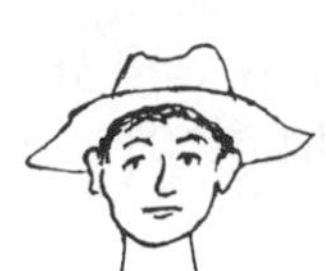

"True," say the home mixers. "But if people mix a standard packet with too little water, the result can be equally dangerous!" And it does happen. John Rohde and others conducted a study with two groups of mothers in Indonesia. One group made Rehydration Drink using packets. Another group mixed salt, sugar, and water, using plastic measuring spoons. **The study showed a slightly higher number of mothers prepared dangerously salty drinks when using the packets.**

Another argument often given by those favoring packets is that the packets seem more like medicines, and therefore people accept them more readily than homemade mixes. This may be true. But, surely, to promote a simple drink by giving it the magic of a medicine is shortsighted. It makes far more sense to help people understand oral rehydration and why it works. Many health workers feel it is important to **look at Rehydration Drink as a FOOD, not a MEDICINE!** Strict medical controls for this basic food supplement are an obstacle, not a help.

The underlying issue in the argument about packets and home mixes is political. Do health planners want to use technology that will make poor families more self-reliant and independent? Or do they want to use outside technologies that make people more dependent on institutions and central control?

We think that, in most circumstances, the arguments in favor of the homemade drink strongly outweigh those in favor of packets. An exception might be in remote areas where sugar or salt is sometimes scarce or unavailable.

What about packets for use in clinics?

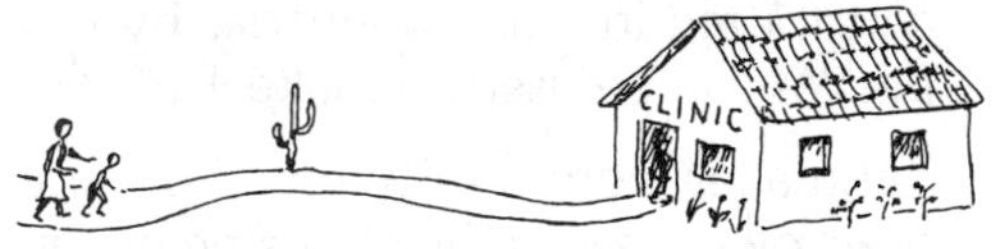

Some health program planners suggest that Special Drink should be prepared by families in their homes, but that packets or more complex mixes might be more appropriate in health posts and clinics. We disagree. The health post or clinic should be a center for parent education. So it is important that, even in the clinic, the parents learn to prepare the Rehydration Drink and give it to their children themselves.

In the health post or clinic, use the same rehydration methods you want families to use in their homes.

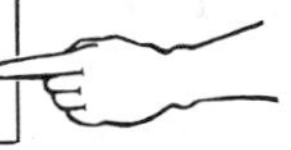

On the following page is a diagram showing many different methods of rehydration. They range from those that are completely dependent on outside resources (I.V. solution) to those that permit the greatest self-reliance on the part of the family.

Discuss these choices with the health workers in your training course, and decide together which approach will best serve the needs of people in your area.

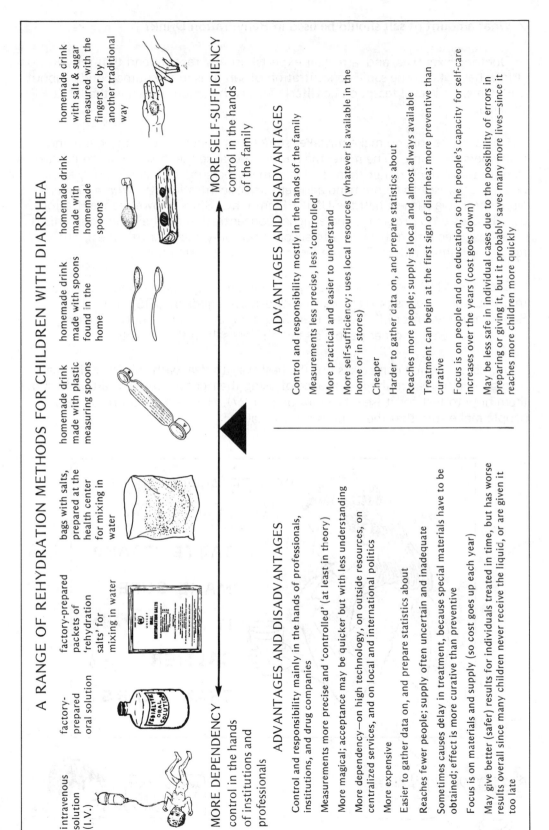

A RANGE OF REHYDRATION METHODS FOR CHILDREN WITH DIARRHEA

- intravenous solution (I.V.)

- factory-prepared oral solution

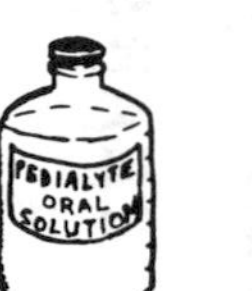

- factory-prepared packets of 'rehydration salts' for mixing in water

- bags with salts, prepared at the health center for mixing in water
- homemade drink made with plastic measuring spoons

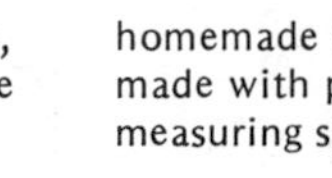

- homemade drink made with spoons found in the home
- homemade drink made with homemade spoons
- homemade drink with salt & sugar measured with the fingers or by another traditional way

MORE DEPENDENCY ⟵ ⟶ MORE SELF-SUFFICIENCY

MORE DEPENDENCY control in the hands of institutions and professionals	MORE SELF-SUFFICIENCY control in the hands of the family
ADVANTAGES AND DISADVANTAGES	**ADVANTAGES AND DISADVANTAGES**
Control and responsibility mainly in the hands of professionals, institutions, and drug companies	Control and responsibility mostly in the hands of the family
Measurements more precise and 'controlled' (at least in theory)	Measurements less precise, less 'controlled'
More magical; acceptance may be quicker but with less understanding	More practical and easier to understand
More dependency—on high technology, on outside resources, on centralized services, and on local and international politics	More self-sufficiency; uses local resources (whatever is available in the home or in stores)
More expensive	Cheaper
Easier to gather data on, and prepare statistics about	Harder to gather data on, and prepare statistics about
Reaches fewer people; supply often uncertain and inadequate	Reaches more people; supply is local and almost always available
Sometimes causes delay in treatment, because special materials have to be obtained; effect is more curative than preventive	Treatment can begin at the first sign of diarrhea; more preventive than curative
Focus is on materials and supply (so cost goes up each year)	Focus is on people and on education, so the people's capacity for self-care increases over the years (cost goes down)
May give better (safer) results for individuals treated in time, but has worse results overall since many children never receive the liquid, or are given it too late	May be less safe in individual cases due to the possibility of errors in preparing or giving it, but it probably saves many more lives—since it reaches more children more quickly

2. What amount of salt should be used in Rehydration Drink?

Doctors, scientists, and 'armchair experts' usually recommend that rehydration drinks have about the same concentration of salt as is in the human body (about 3½ grams, or 1 level teaspoon per liter). This is the amount used in the UNICEF packets.

However, people do make mistakes sometimes. When it comes to medicines, many persons think, "The more, the better." Because the most common mistake is to put in too much rather than too little, many persons with community experience believe it is wiser to recommend a lower salt concentration. (In ***Where There Is No Doctor,*** we suggest half the UNICEF amount.) Since a lower concentration usually causes no problems, and a higher concentration can be dangerous, this is a sensible precaution. It takes into account not only the scientific ideal, but the reality of human nature. This is a factor the experts often forget.

Even the WHO, belatedly realizing this human factor, now often recommends that you "give a glass of plain water between each glass of ORS (Oral Rehydration Solution)." A wiser plan would be to face up to human error—their own as well as other people's—and put less salt in the packets.

Imposing outside controls is not the best way to deal with this issue. Instead, help people to realize the importance of using the right amount of salt. And show them how to test for it (see the story on p. **1**-27). Here is a good test to help people make sure that the drink is not too salty:

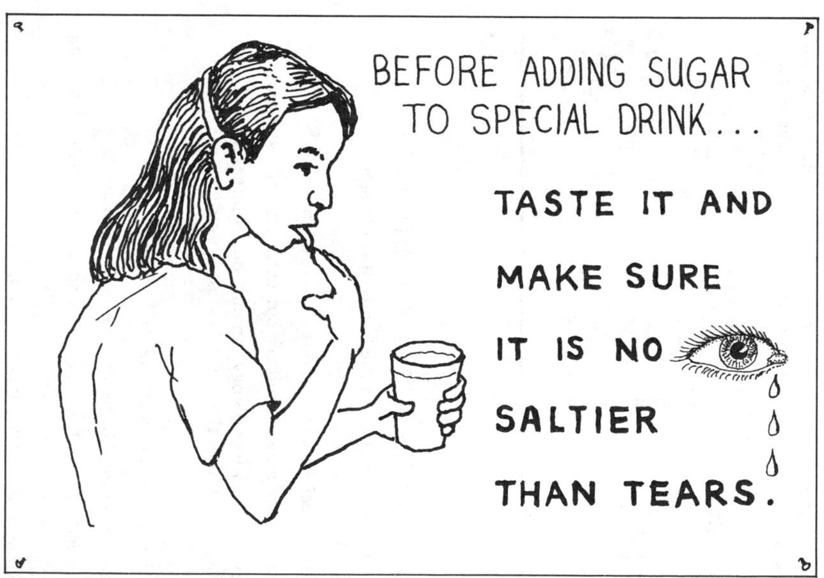
BEFORE ADDING SUGAR TO SPECIAL DRINK...
TASTE IT AND MAKE SURE IT IS NO SALTIER THAN TEARS.

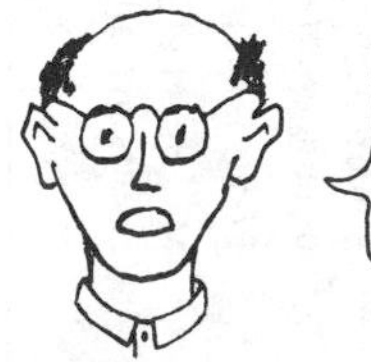
BUT WHO REMEMBERS THE TASTE OF TEARS ?

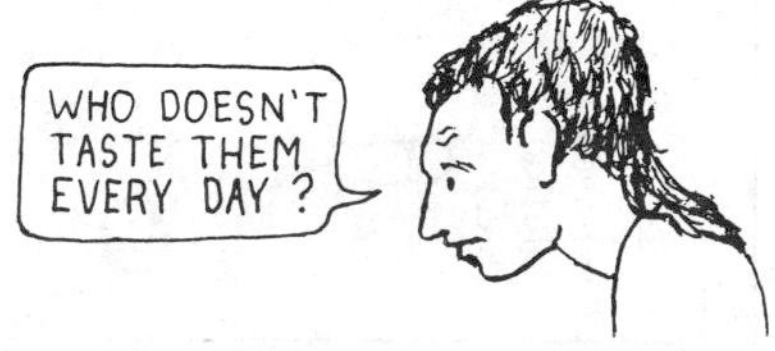
WHO DOESN'T TASTE THEM EVERY DAY ?

3. Worldwide standardization or local adaptation?

Large organizations tend to want to standardize rehydration methods (along with other aspects of life and health). Although, at conferences, WHO and UNICEF experts may speak in favor of "local adaptation," in fact, they are promoting their standardized packets in as many countries as are willing to accept them.

But this standardization has led to the very problem the experts fear. In many places, one-liter containers are not available—so people mix the packets in smaller containers. The resulting drink has too much salt!

It makes more sense to adapt Rehydration Drink to the resources and traditions of each area. In Bangladesh, for example, women learn to make the drink with crude block sugar from home-grown cane. They measure a 'pinch of salt' with their fingers and this works fairly well.

In Nigeria, families use cubes of 'St. Louis sugar' in the universal 600 ml. beer bottle. To help mothers remember how to make the drink, a group of nuns teaches them the following song, sung in Pidgin English. 'Purge' and 'sheet' are local terms for diarrhea. (Compare with the song on p. **1**-27.)

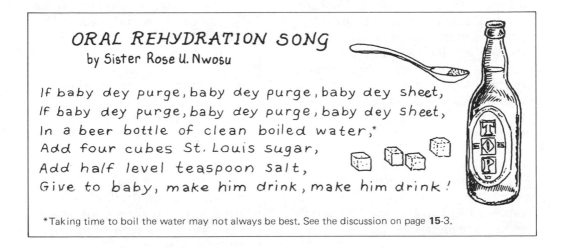

ORAL REHYDRATION SONG
by Sister Rose U. Nwosu

If baby dey purge, baby dey purge, baby dey sheet,
If baby dey purge, baby dey purge, baby dey sheet,
In a beer bottle of clean boiled water,*
Add four cubes St. Louis sugar,
Add half level teaspoon salt,
Give to baby, make him drink, make him drink!

*Taking time to boil the water may not always be best. See the discussion on page **15**-3.

Ways to measure sugar and salt for homemade Rehydration Drink:

One of the biggest problems in making the homemade drink is measuring the right amounts of sugar and salt. Spoons in people's homes are not always the same shape and size.

One method that has been tried is to **'pinch and scoop'** with the hands. Some health experts protest that this method is very inaccurate. And often it is—in areas where people are not used to measuring this way. But in places where people traditionally measure foods and spices with their fingers, the pinch and scoop method appears to be fairly accurate.

Appropriate where people traditionally measure with their fingers:

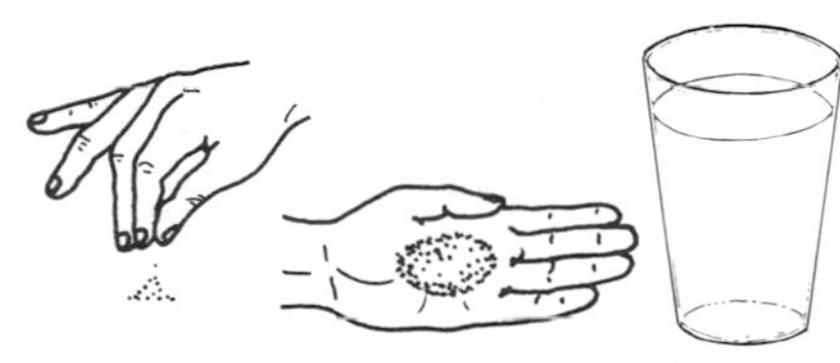

3-finger pinch SALT | 1-hand scoop SUGAR | in 1 glass WATER

Special spoons for measuring the sugar and salt have also been used. Some of these spoons are manufactured in developed countries. Others can be made in villages—even by children. The advantages and disadvantages of several kinds are discussed below.

APPROPRIATE AS A MODEL

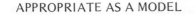

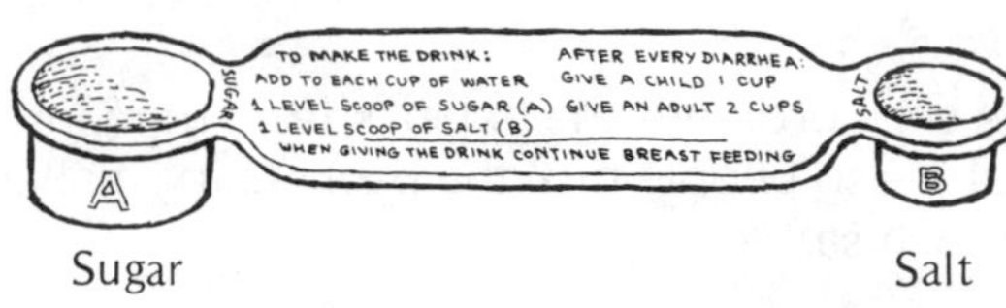
TO MAKE THE DRINK:
ADD TO EACH CUP OF WATER
1 LEVEL SCOOP OF SUGAR (A)
1 LEVEL SCOOP OF SALT (B)
AFTER EVERY DIARRHEA:
GIVE A CHILD 1 CUP
GIVE AN ADULT 2 CUPS
WHEN GIVING THE DRINK CONTINUE BREAST FEEDING
SUGAR
SALT
A
B

Sugar Salt

Plastic measuring spoons for making Special Drink are now being used in several countries. They are distributed by TALC (see p. **Back**-3). For those who can read, a big advantage is that instructions are printed right on the spoon.

Unfortunately, these spoons have some of the same disadvantages as the packets of rehydration salts. They are produced using high technology (plastic), so people must depend on an outside supply. Also, they add a sense of mystery to what is basically a simple process. (A mother may feel unable to make the Special Drink because she has lost her 'magic' plastic spoon.) So TALC now recommends that the plastic spoons be used mainly as models for health groups, school children, and villagers who want to make their own spoons using local resources. For that purpose, TALC will send a free sample spoon on request.

MORE APPROPRIATE

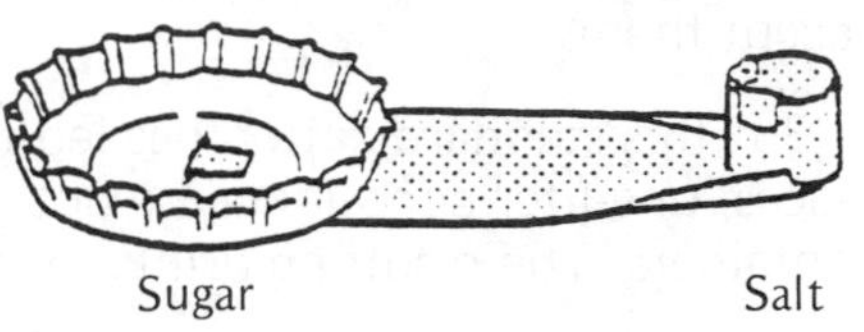

Sugar Salt

A similar spoon can be made from old bottle caps and beer or juice cans—or from other materials commonly found in villages. In Mexico, children have made hundreds of these spoons through the CHILD-to-child program. By making and learning to use the spoons themselves, people realize there is nothing magical about the Special Drink. And if they lose a spoon, they can easily make another one.

In designing an appropriate homemade spoon for your particular area, take care to see that each spoon made will measure about the same amount. For example, the spoon shown above uses a standard sized bottle cap for the sugar scoop. And the salt scoop is made to the diameter of a pencil. For instructions on how to make this spoon, see p. **24**-21.

Another kind of measuring spoon can be made by drilling holes in a small piece of wood.

Drill the holes to be as wide and deep as shown in the drawing at right. Or you can carve the holes, taking care to make them the right size. A model plastic spoon like the one shown above can be used to check the sizes of the holes you have made.

MORE APPROPRIATE

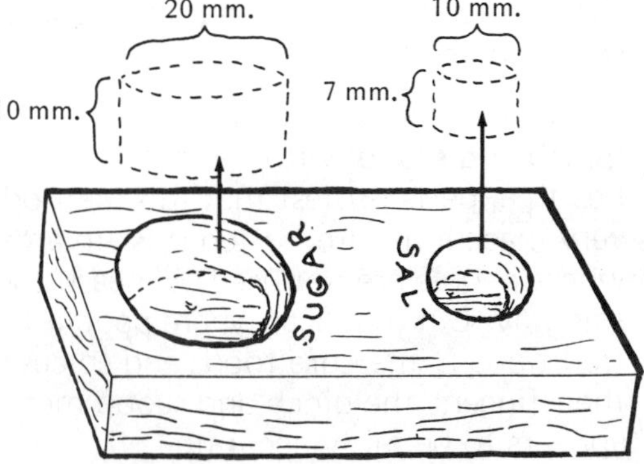

If you do not have a drill for making the wooden measuring spoon, you can try using a red-hot bolt about this size.

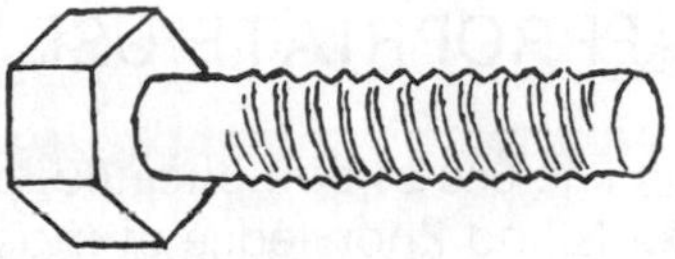

Heat the bolt in a fire, and use it to burn two holes in a piece of wood.

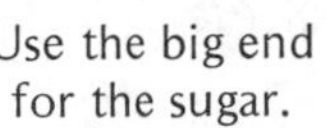
Use the big end
for the sugar.

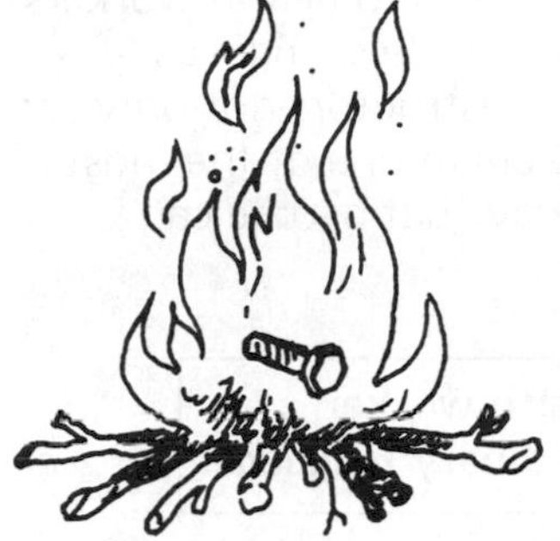

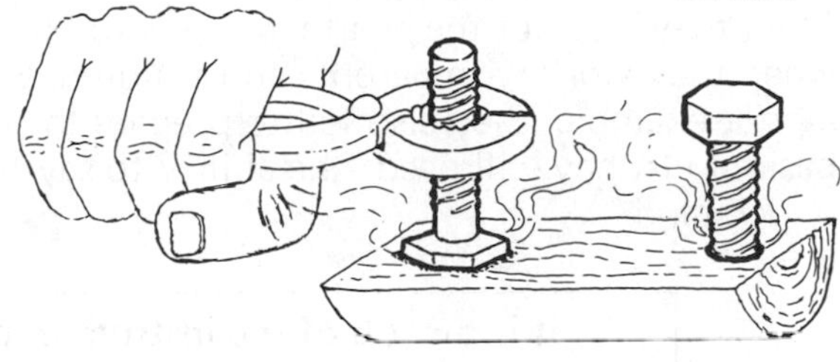
Use the small
end for
the salt.

Use a model plastic spoon (if you have one) to check if each hole is the right size. If the hole is too small, burn it deeper. If it is too big, shave some wood off the top.

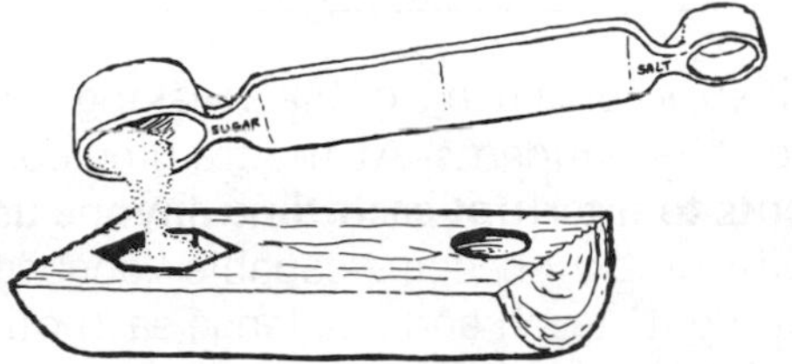
SUGAR
SALT

Yet another kind of measuring spoon can be made out of bamboo. Find 2 pieces of bamboo with hollow centers about as big around as the scoops of the model plastic spoon.

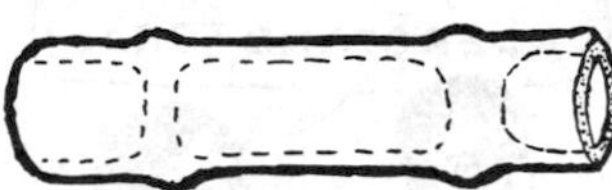

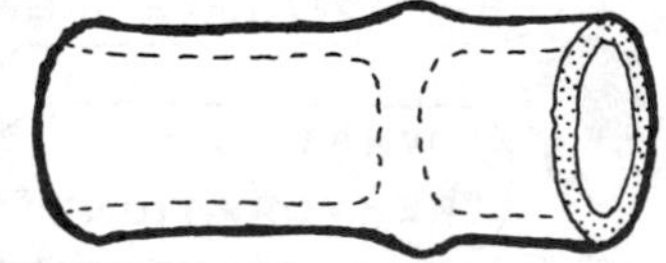

Cut the bamboo so the dividers form cups that can hold just a little more than the scoops of the plastic spoon. File or trim them until they hold the right amounts of sugar and salt. Then slip the two pieces together to form a double-headed measuring spoon.

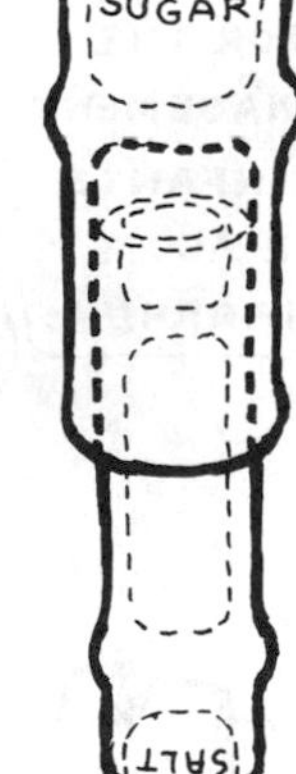
SUGAR
SALT

The important thing in making homemade spoons is to encourage local people to use their imaginations to adapt whatever materials they have on hand. But at the same time, care must be taken to see that the spoons are reasonably accurate.

Helping people use local resources to meet their needs means they will not have to depend as much on outside supplies and assistance. Their increased self-reliance will give them more control over the things that affect their well-being.

APPROPRIATE USE OF LANGUAGE

The use of complicated language is one of the biggest obstacles to making the tools and knowledge of modern health care available to ordinary people. Several times in this book, we have emphasized the need to keep language clear and simple. This point is extremely important.

Many instructors use big, 'scientific' words to explain things to health workers. Then they instruct the health workers to "put it into the people's language" when they work with parents and children. By doing this instructors not only set a poor example, they also fail to prepare the health workers in one of the most basic skills they will need: the ability to say things in a way that people can understand.

It is the job of the instructor, not the health worker, to translate the big words of textbooks into ordinary language.

If instructors have trouble speaking simply, and many do, they can ask the help of their students. At the training course in Ajoya, **the instructors urge students to interrupt each time anyone uses a word they do not understand.** The students quickly become capable 'language watchdogs'. In this way, instructors and students teach and challenge each other. Sometimes visiting instructors, though warned to use simple language, get interrupted several times in their first sentence—a marvelous learning experience for them! (See the story on page 2-16.)

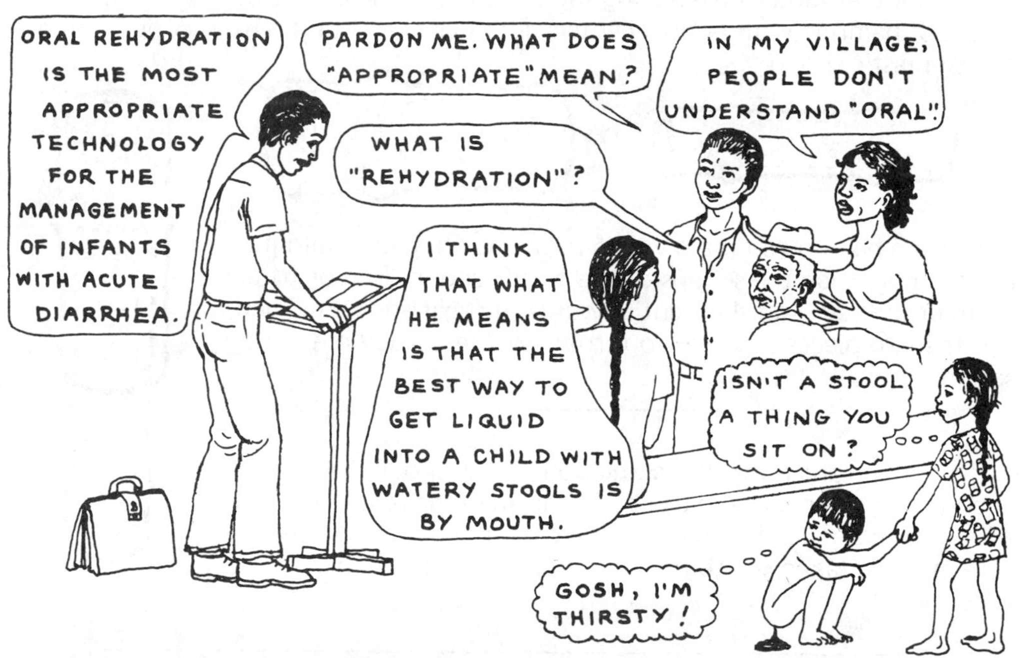
ORAL REHYDRATION IS THE MOST APPROPRIATE TECHNOLOGY FOR THE MANAGEMENT OF INFANTS WITH ACUTE DIARRHEA.
PARDON ME. WHAT DOES "APPROPRIATE" MEAN?
IN MY VILLAGE, PEOPLE DON'T UNDERSTAND "ORAL".
WHAT IS "REHYDRATION"?
I THINK THAT WHAT HE MEANS IS THAT THE BEST WAY TO GET LIQUID INTO A CHILD WITH WATERY STOOLS IS BY MOUTH.
ISN'T A STOOL A THING YOU SIT ON?
GOSH, I'M THIRSTY!

The first rule for any 'appropriate technology' is to explain it in words that people can understand!

CHAPTER 16

Homemade, Low-Cost Equipment and Written Materials

Many of the tools that health workers need are costly to buy. But some can be handmade with local materials by the health workers themselves, blacksmiths, or other local craftsmen.

Homemade equipment can be simple or complex. It can be made from local materials only, or from a combination of local and outside resources. The dental drill shown here combines a high-technology drill with appropriate local power sources—people and bicycle.

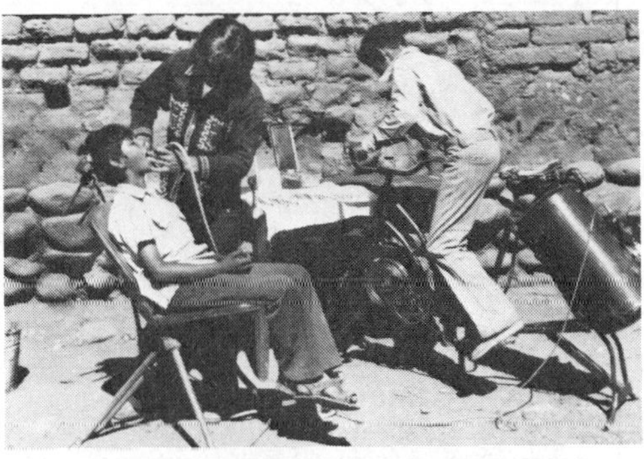

This high-speed dental drill runs on air compressed by bicycle power. It is used by village dental workers in Verano, Mexico.

Most of the homemade equipment we describe in this chapter can be made quickly and easily with materials on hand.

During training, encourage health workers to invent and make some of their own equipment. This develops the imagination and creativity needed to help people solve their problems in their own way.

HOMEMADE SCALES FOR WEIGHING BABIES

During training, health workers can make their own simple scales for weighing babies. Although less accurate and less easy to use than store-bought scales, they have several advantages:

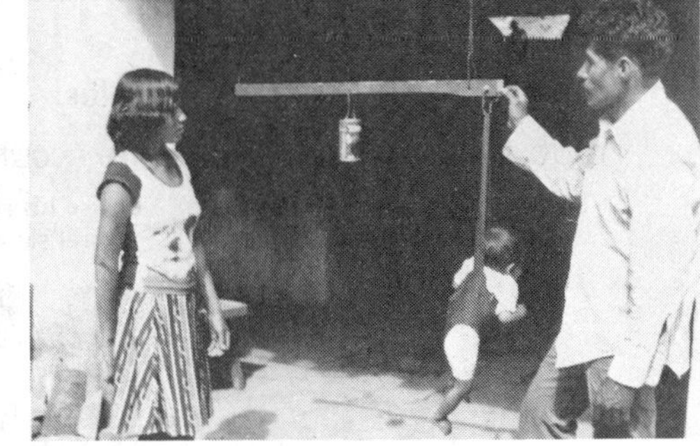

- They are **cheap and easy to make.**
- They can be **made of local materials.**
- By building the scales themselves, the **health workers gain new understanding and skills.**
- By getting the local people to help them, **they extend that knowledge and skill to others.**
- **This gets people, including fathers, to take a more active part.**
- Midwives or parents can make their own scales using the health worker's as a model.
- Homemade scales make the baby-weighing process less mysterious.

Ideas for several types of homemade scales are given on the next page. Be sure to check the accuracy of your scales from time to time, using objects of known weight.

EXAMPLES OF HOMEMADE SCALES

BEAM SCALE: This is the easiest kind to make, and probably the most accurate. The beam can be made of dry wood or bamboo. The movable weight can be a bag, bottle, or tin filled with sand.

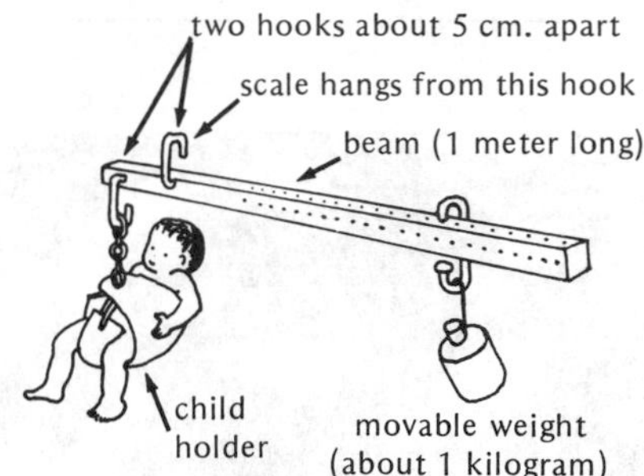

Weight is correct when beam stays horizontal.

FOLDING SCALE: Easy to carry from place to place. Works best if made of metal or plywood strips.

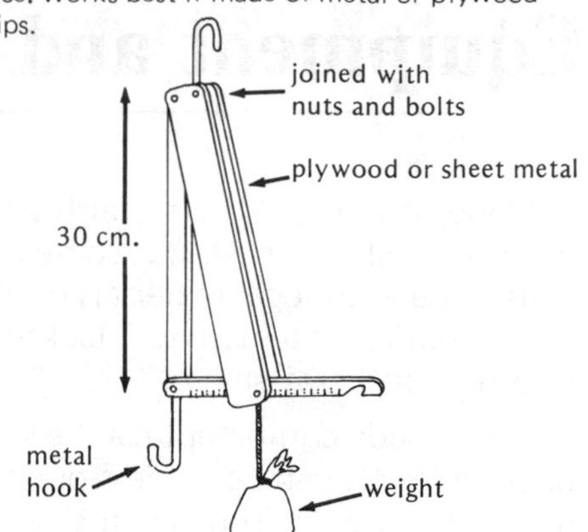

QUARTER-CIRCLE SCALE: If made with plywood, use sheet metal to reinforce upper corner. The weight should be between 1 and 2 kilograms. It can be made from scrap metal or a piece of heavy pipe.

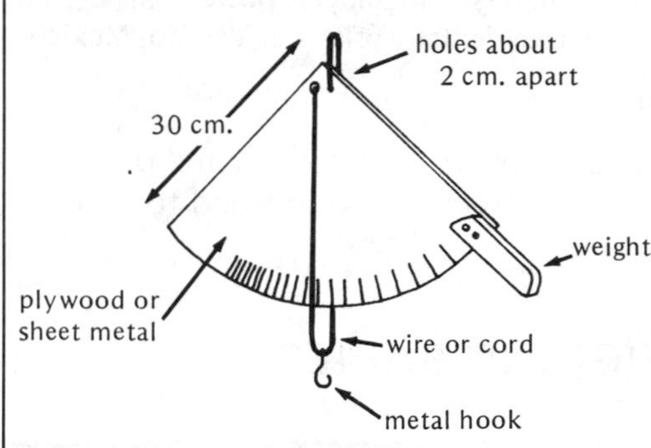

SPRING SCALE: This is made with a coil spring inside a bamboo tube. The spring should be about 30 cm. long and squeeze to half its length with a weight of 15 kilograms.

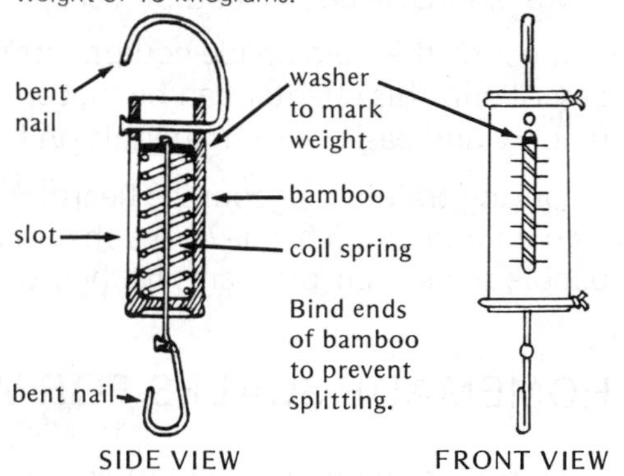

How to mark or *calibrate* the scales:

To do this, you will need some accurate standard weights. Perhaps you can . . .

borrow some weights from a merchant at the market

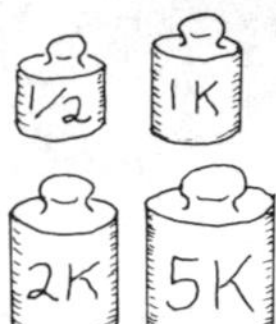

or use his scale to prepare several sand weights

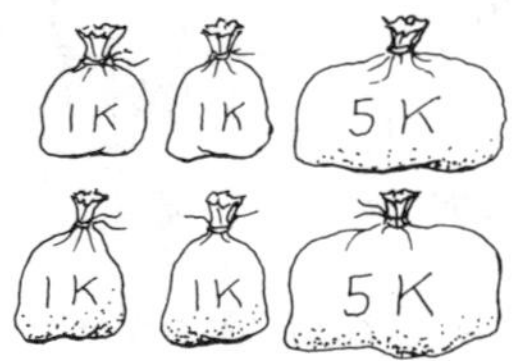

or borrow some 1-kilo packages or cans of food.

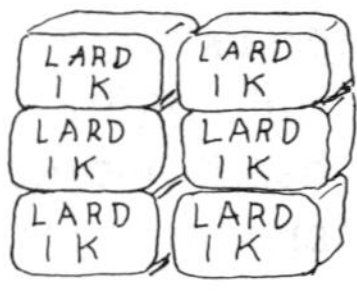

To mark your scale:

1. Hang 2 kilos on it.

2. Balance the movable weight.

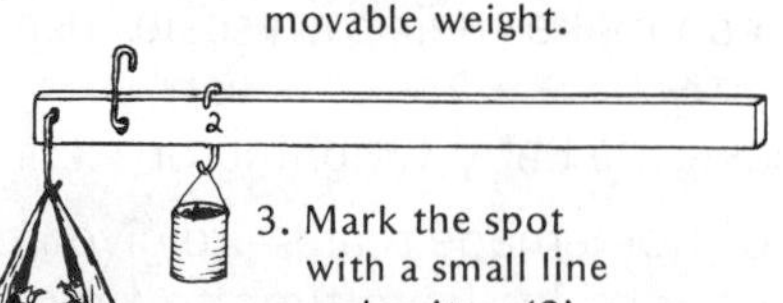

3. Mark the spot with a small line and write a '2'.

4. Now add one more kilo and repeat the process. Keep going until the whole scale is marked. To weigh children up to age 5, mark your scale up to 20 kilos.

AVOIDING THE PROBLEM OF SPOILED VACCINES*

Keeping vaccines cold is important. If they get warm before being used, they spoil and will not protect children against disease.

Vaccines need to be kept cold all the way from the factory where they are made to the village where a health worker vaccinates the local children. The vaccine changes hands many times along the way. If at any time the vaccine gets warm (or in the case of polio vaccine, thaws and is refrozen), it spoils and becomes useless.

Not keeping vaccines cold enough is a very common problem. A great many vaccines get warm and spoil at some point on the way from factory to child. In fact, **in many countries more than one third of the vaccines given do no good—because they were not kept cold enough.**

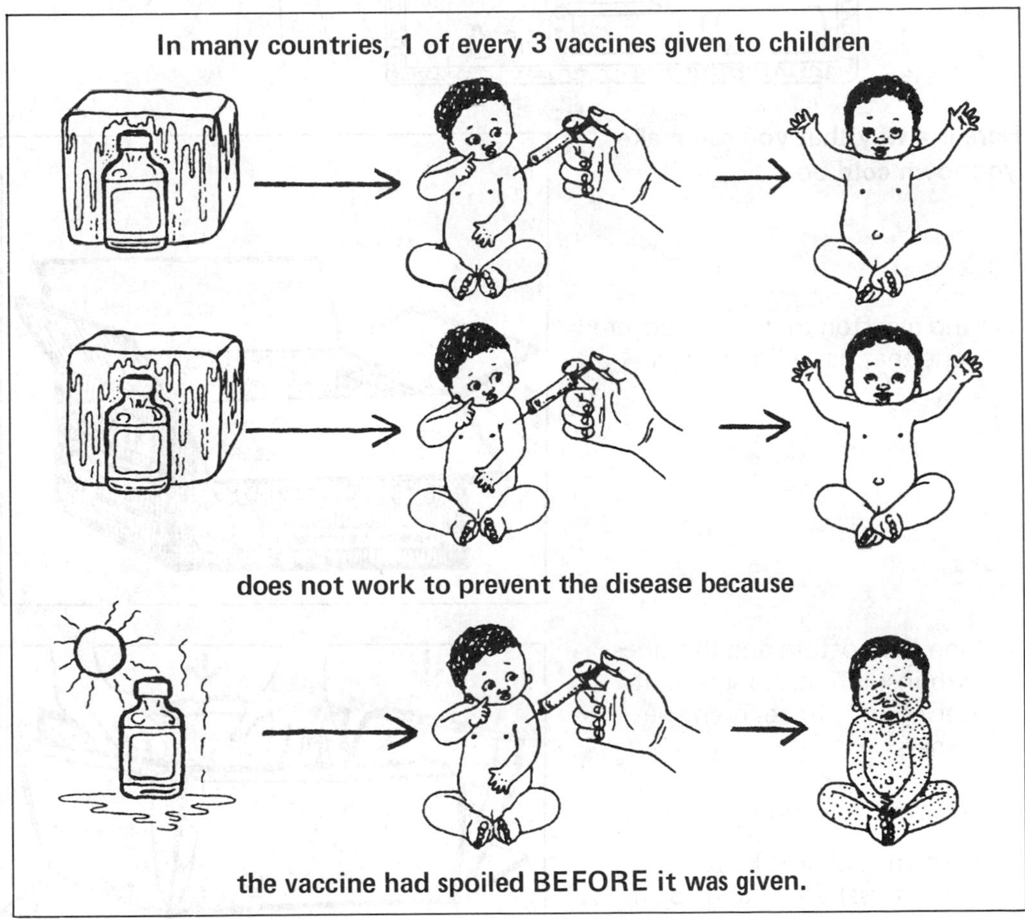

In many countries, 1 of every 3 vaccines given to children
does not work to prevent the disease because
the vaccine had spoiled BEFORE it was given.

*These ideas and drawings are from the Expanded Immunization Project in Liberia, Africa. Their ***Handbook for Health Workers*** is an excellent booklet about vaccination and the 'cold chain'—keeping vaccines cold. It is available from the following:

Christian Health Association of Liberia
P.O. Box 1046
Monrovia, Liberia

Continuing Education Joint Project
Inservice Division
Ministry of Health and Social Welfare
P.O. Box 9009
Monrovia, Liberia

HOMEMADE 'COLD BOX' FOR KEEPING VACCINES COLD:

Sometimes vaccines spoil simply because there are not enough thermoses or 'cold boxes' to allow each health worker to take them quickly to his or her village.

But there is nothing magic or secret about a cold box. It is a box that has been *insulated* or padded so that cold will stay in and heat will stay out. Any box with insulation can be a cold box.

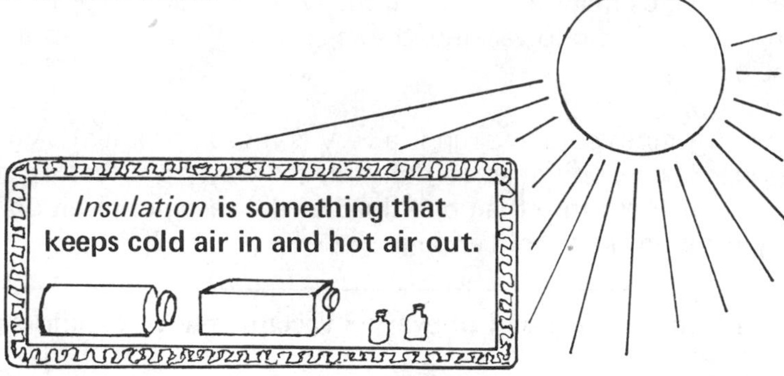
Insulation is something that
keeps cold air in and hot air out.

Here is a way that you can make your own cold box:

1. Find a carton that can be covered —one that has a lid or flaps.

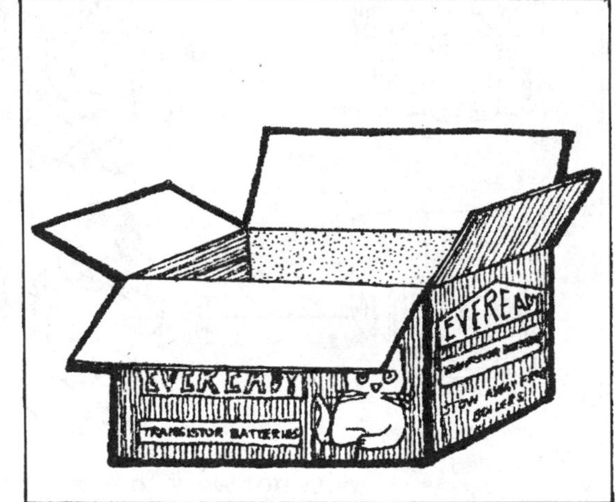

2. Line the bottom and the sides with insulation. Be sure that every part is lined, even the corners.

   For insulation you can use . . .

   - foam rubber (like for a mattress) 2 inches or 5 cm. thick,
   - Styrofoam (what radios are packed in),
   - dry grass, rolled up so it is about 2 inches thick, or
   - many layers of old newspaper.

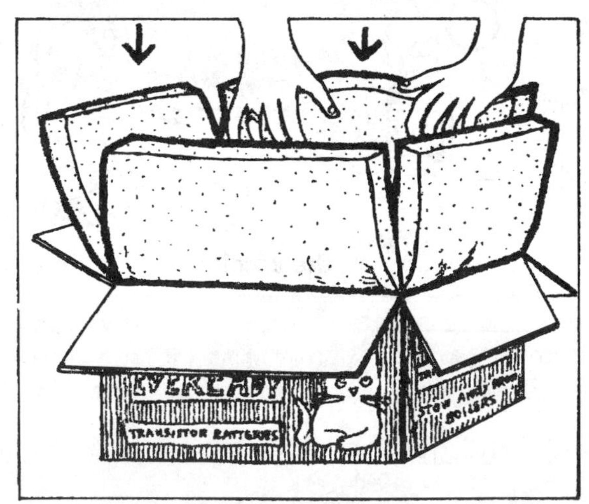

3. Paint the outside of the carton white. The white paint will reflect the sun and keep the box cooler.

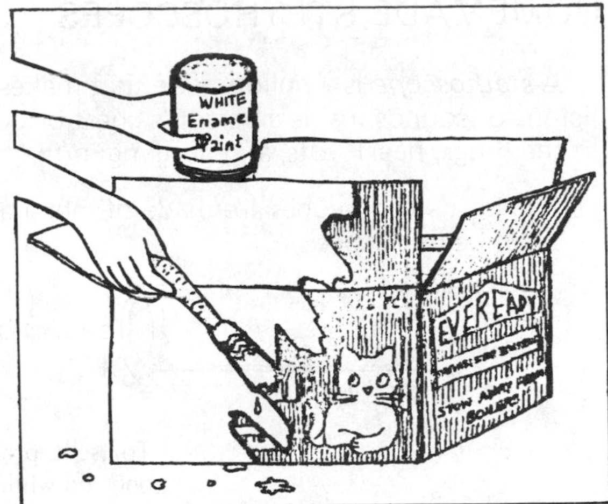

4. Cover the inside with plastic to keep water from getting into the insulation.

   Now you can put 'cold dogs' (ice in tight containers) and vaccines in the box.

   Put more plastic over the cold dogs and vaccines to cover them.

   Put more insulation on the top, and close the box.

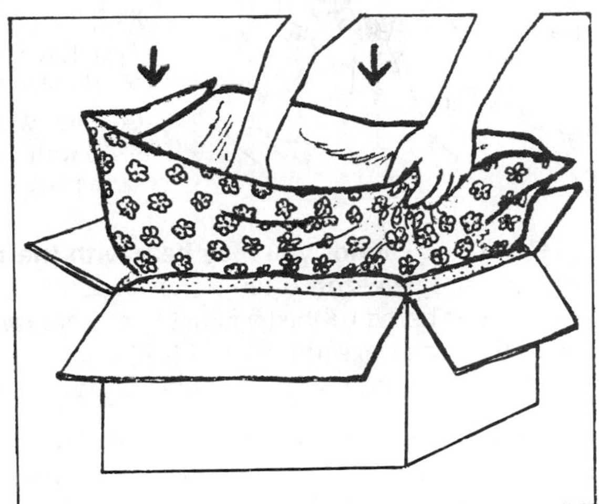

Always keep your cold box in a cool, shady place.

'COLD DOGS' FOR KEEPING THE COLD BOX COLD:

Putting ice directly into the cold box is not a good idea because it makes a mess when it melts. The ice can be put in plastic bags, but these often break or leak. Here is a better idea for making 'cold dogs'.

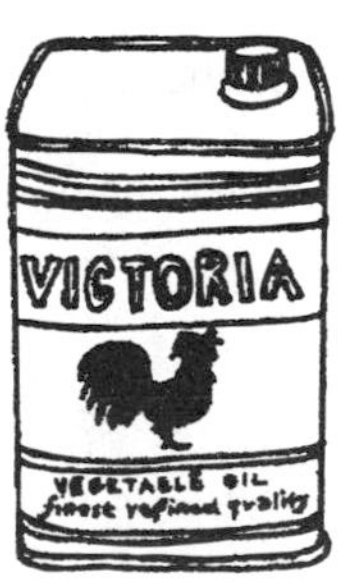

- Find an empty container made of plastic or metal. DO NOT USE A GLASS CONTAINER. (Guess why not.)
- Fill it almost full with water and close it tightly.
- Keep it in the cold part of the refrigerator (not the freezer) until it becomes cold.
- Put it in the freezer part of your refrigerator about 1 day before you want it to be frozen.
- Always have plenty of cold dogs in your refrigerator and freezer **before** you plan to send vaccines to nearby villages. They will be needed to keep the vaccines from spoiling.

HOMEMADE STETHOSCOPES

A ***stethoscope*** is a hollow tube that makes it easier to listen for sounds inside a person's chest or belly: breathing in the lungs, heartbeats, and gurgling in the belly.

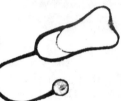

The best stethoscopes are made of metal and plastic, and can be expensive.

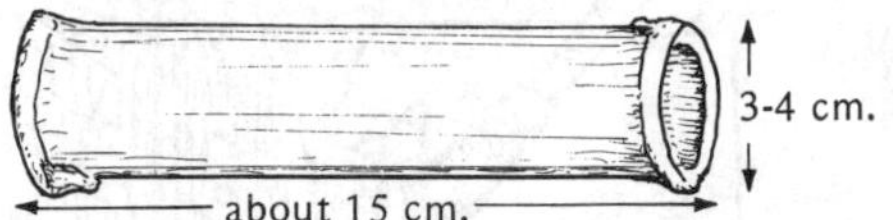

But a simple stethoscope can be made of a hollow tube of bamboo, wood, or clay.

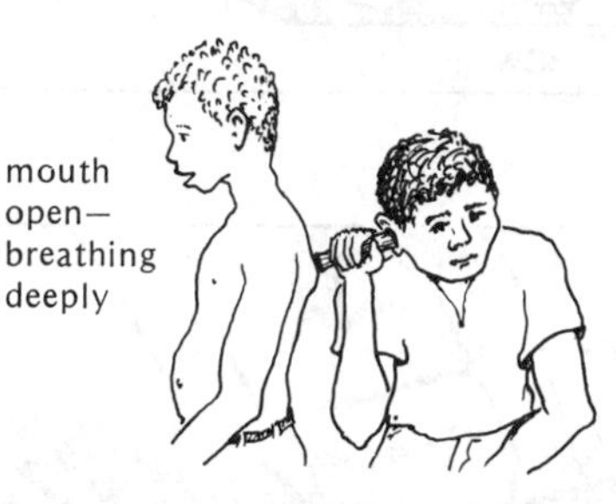

To use it, press your ear firmly to one end while holding the other end flat against the person's back.

Check the lungs by listening on the person's back in 6 places.

Then listen to the front between the shoulders and neck.

Compare what you hear in one place with what you hear in the same place on the other side.

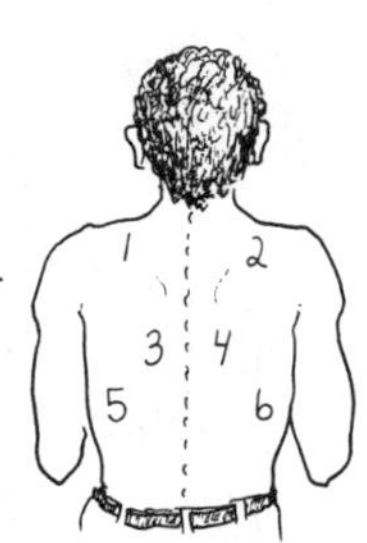

Breathing sounds you may hear with the stethoscope: Long, high-pitched squeaks are ***wheezes,*** often a sign of asthma. Lower-pitched sounds, like silk or thin paper being rubbed against itself, are ***rales,*** often a sign of pneumonia. The lack of normal breathing sounds in one area, but not everywhere, usually means pneumonia in one part of a lung—or advanced tuberculosis.

Heart sounds: Also listen to the person's heart on the front of the chest where it beats hardest. There should be **two sounds for each pulse.** In an older person, a third sound may mean heart disease, especially if he has swollen feet or is short of breath (see ***WTND,*** p. 325). In a child, an extra sound may mean he has had rheumatic fever ***(WTND,*** p. 310). If he is sickly he should see a doctor.

Belly sounds: In a severely ill person, the absence of normal gurgles in the belly is probably a sign of acute abdomen (see ***WTND,*** p. 93).

OTHER KINDS OF HOMEMADE STETHOSCOPES:

Use the top of a narrow-necked plastic bottle and a piece of rubber tube.

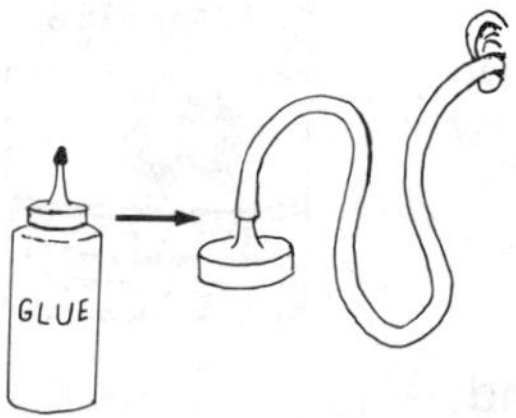

Or cut off the top of a rubber suction bulb.

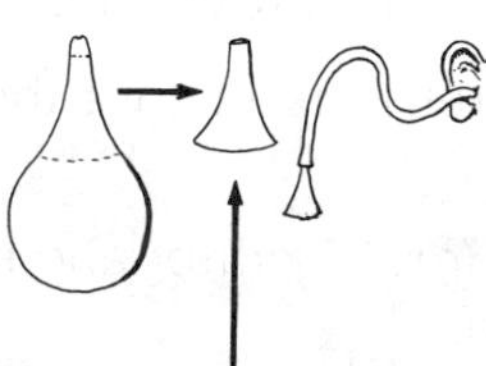

This piece can also be used for looking in people's ears.

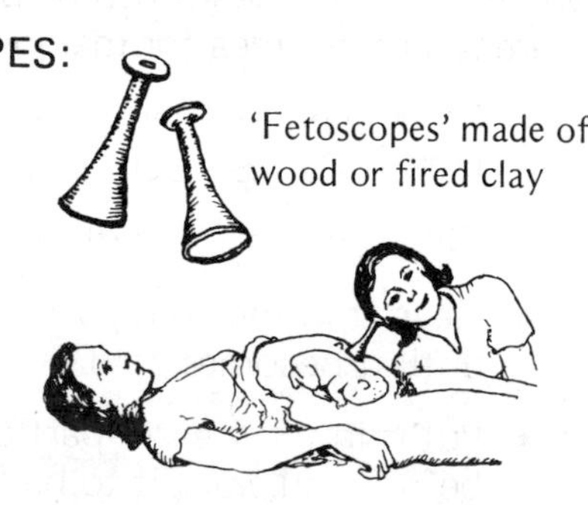

'Fetoscopes' made of wood or fired clay are especially useful for listening to the heartbeats of unborn babies (see *WTND*, p. 252).

HOMEMADE TIMERS

Health workers, midwives, and parents at times need to measure the number of heartbeats (pulse) or breaths (respirations) per minute. But they may not be able to afford a clock or watch with a second hand.

However, simple instruments for measuring time can be made by the health workers themselves. Encourage them to invent and make their own timers. When you first make the timers, be sure you have a watch to 'set' the time. Here are some ideas that have been tried and work fairly well.

WATER TIMERS—easy to make, but less accurate

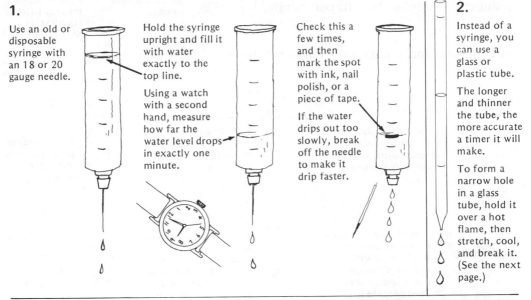

1.

Use an old or disposable syringe with an 18 or 20 gauge needle.

Hold the syringe upright and fill it with water exactly to the top line.

Using a watch with a second hand, measure how far the water level drops in exactly one minute.

Check this a few times, and then mark the spot with ink, nail polish, or a piece of tape.

If the water drips out too slowly, break off the needle to make it drip faster.

2.

Instead of a syringe, you can use a glass or plastic tube.

The longer and thinner the tube, the more accurate a timer it will make.

To form a narrow hole in a glass tube, hold it over a hot flame, then stretch, cool, and break it. (See the next page.)

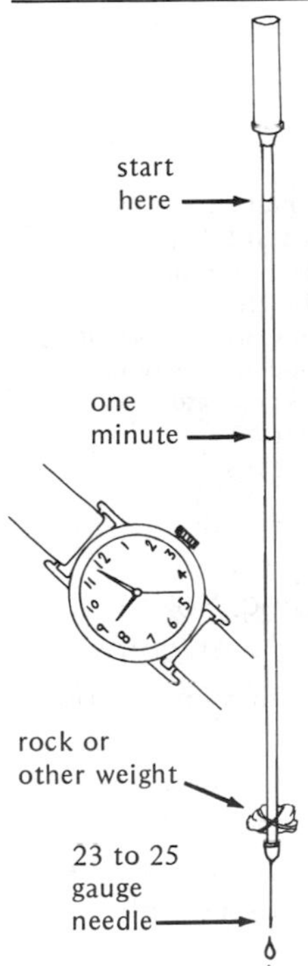

3.

A fairly accurate timer can be made from an old I.V. (intravenous solution) administration kit.

Open the wider tube at the top to serve as a funnel.

Fill the tube with water. (Be sure there is no air in the tube.)

Using a watch with a second hand, mark the distance the water drops in 1 minute. Check it several times to be sure.

To help keep the tube straight, tie a weight at the lower end.

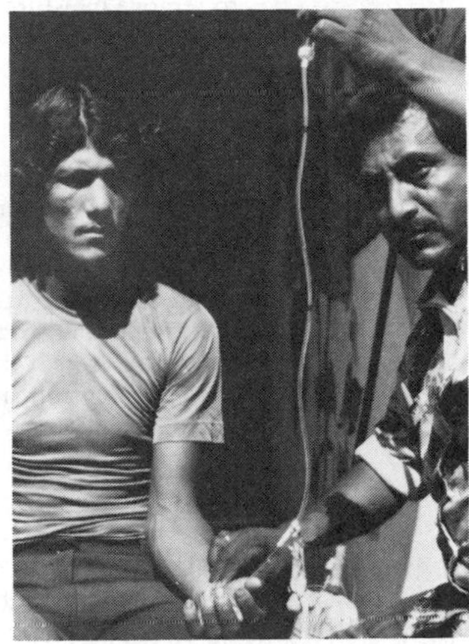

Counting the pulse using an I.V. tube timer.

The I.V. tube timer has the advantage of being fairly accurate and easy to make, and it can be made at no cost from old I.V. sets.

SAND TIMER—harder to make, but more accurate

A sand timer consists of a tube of glass closed at both ends, with a narrow neck in the middle. It is partly filled with fine sand. The sand runs from the upper to the lower half in an exact period of time.

'Egg timers', or 3-minute sand timers, can be purchased at low cost in some areas. To use one, count the number of pulses or breaths for 3 minutes and then divide by 3 to know the number of pulses or breaths per minute.

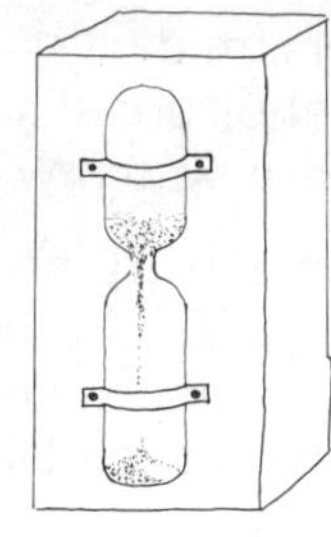

Store-bought 3-minute sand timer.

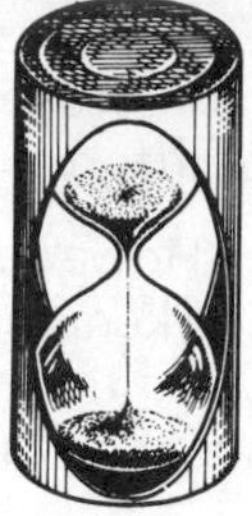

One-minute sand timer available through UNICEF (UNIPAC #0568500).

A **1-minute sand timer** can be made as follows:

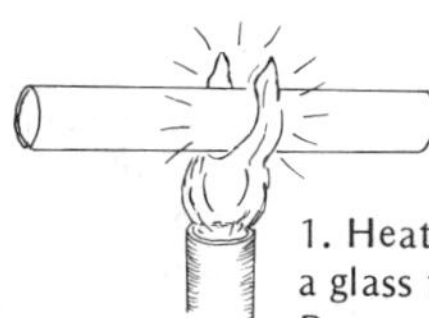

1. Heat the middle of a glass tube over a Bunsen burner or other small, very hot flame.

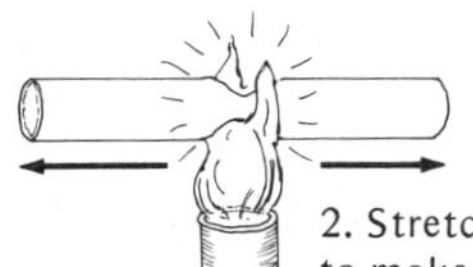

2. Stretch the tube to make a thin neck in the middle.

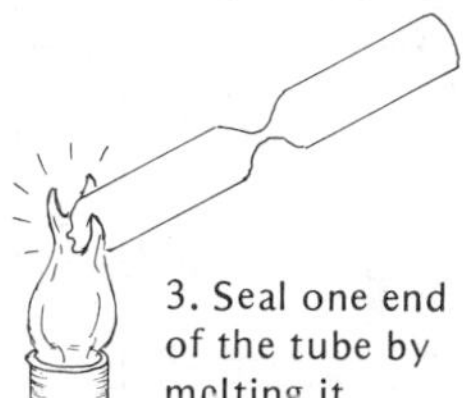

3. Seal one end of the tube by melting it slowly.

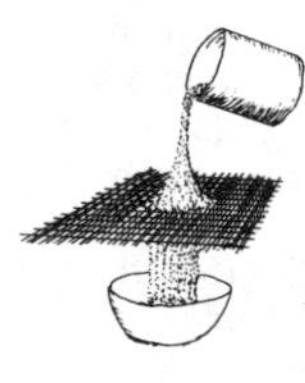

4. Wash some fine sand to remove the dirt. Dry it in the sun, and sift it through a very fine strainer. Then heat the sand to remove moisture.

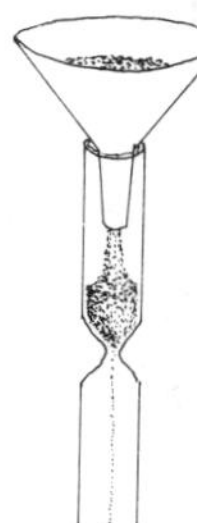

5. Put just enough sand in the tube so that it takes exactly 1 minute for all of it to run from one part to the other. (Use someone's watch with a second hand to check this.)

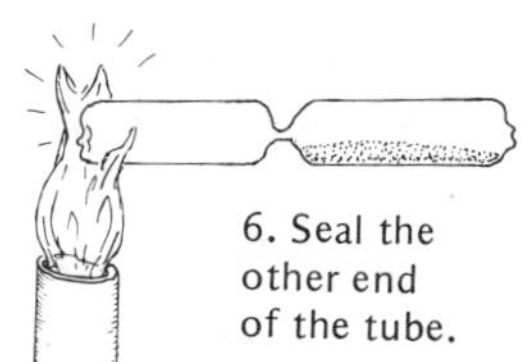

6. Seal the other end of the tube.

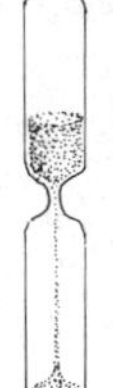

Note: Do not be surprised if you have to make the timer several times before you get it just right. Try to make sure you have the right amount of sand before you seal the tube. If the sand sticks, try to find a smoother, finer sand, and be sure it is absolutely dry. Protect the timer by keeping it in a box with cotton, as it can break very easily at the neck.

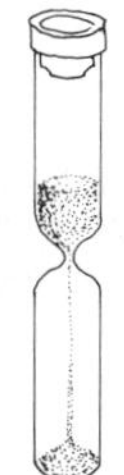

An easier method is to use a 'soft glass' test tube, or a blood collection tube. Instead of melting the end, simply seal it with a cork or rubber stopper. This timer may be less accurate in a moist climate.

Sometimes a timer will get partly clogged and give a false reading. So it is a good idea to check your timer occasionally (especially the water timer) with someone's watch. If this is not possible, you can make 2 timers and check one against the other.

Sand and water timers, if well made, are fairly accurate. They are better than watches in that health workers, midwives, or almost anyone can learn to make and use them. A person using them does not need to know how to read a clock.

MEASURING WITHOUT INSTRUMENTS—A TEST FOR SHOCK

In some cases, rather than using instruments for specific tests, you can make measurements without any instruments at all. Here are some examples from this book:

- In a CHILD-to-child activity, a group of children becomes the 'measuring instrument' for testing hearing. See page **24**-12.
- A simple test for dehydration is described on p. **11**-9.
- A way to check for malnutrition using your fingers is explained on p. **25**-15.
- Ways of checking for anemia are described on p. **25**-18 and **25**-19.

Here is a simple way of **testing for shock without using instruments:**

If you suspect a person is in a state of shock (very weak or unconscious, with rapid weak pulse and cool sweaty skin), quickly do this test:

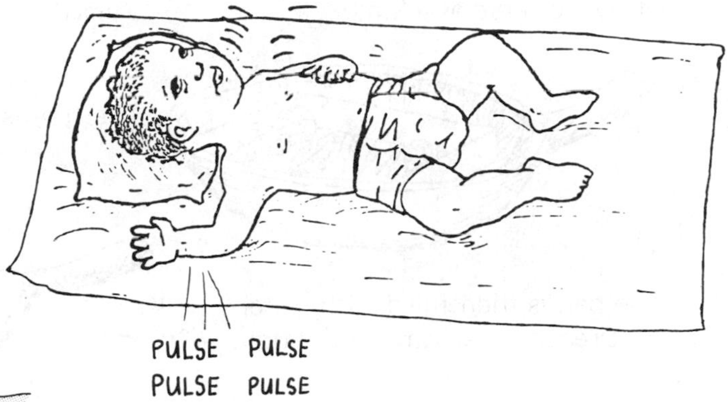

PULSE PULSE
PULSE PULSE

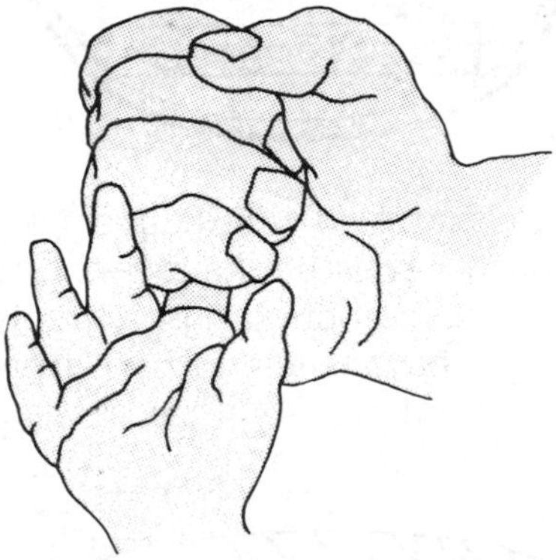

Squeeze one finger hard for a moment, and then let go.

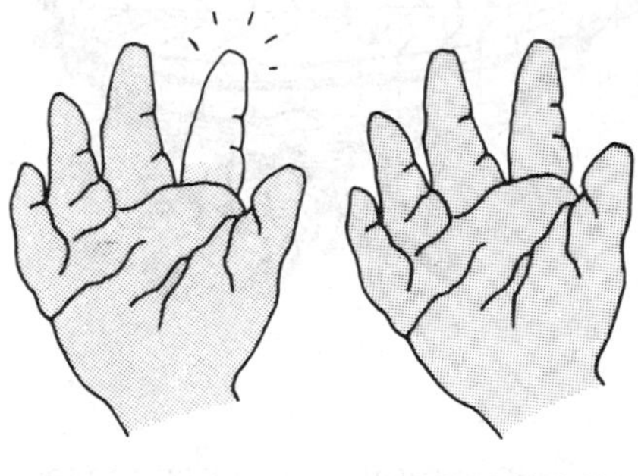

The moment you let go, the palm side of the finger will look white. If it takes more than 3 seconds for the normal pink or reddish color (blood) to return, the person is probably in shock. (You can measure the 3 seconds by quickly saying "Is he in shock?" 3 times.)

IN SHOCK NOT IN SHOCK

This is a good test to do when a child is dehydrated and seems very weak. If the child is in shock, provide emergency care ***(WTND,*** p. 77) and get medical help fast.

MINOR SURGERY IN THE FIELD

Health workers in remote areas sometimes need to do emergency minor surgery, such as closing of wounds, without the basic supplies for sterilizing and suturing. The Medical Mission Sisters in the Philippines have developed these alternative methods, using local resources.

FOR STERILIZING INSTRUMENTS AND BANDAGE MATERIALS:

Instruments and supplies are put into a tray. Bandage materials, thread, and other objects that must be kept dry are wrapped in several layers of **dead, dry banana leaves,** and then a layer of **green banana leaf.** A piece of raw cassava wrapped in banana leaf is also placed in the tray, to serve as a 'timer'.

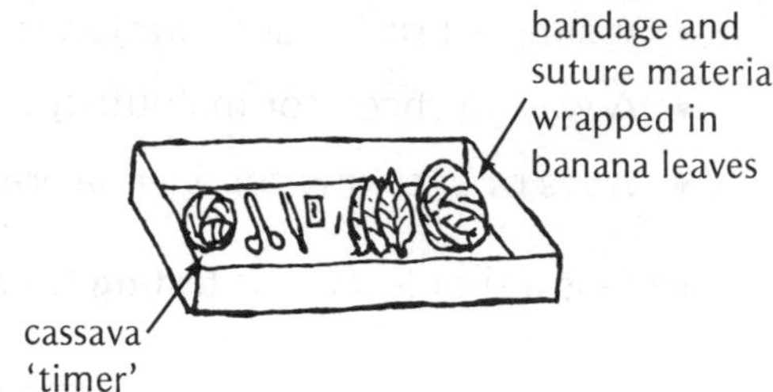

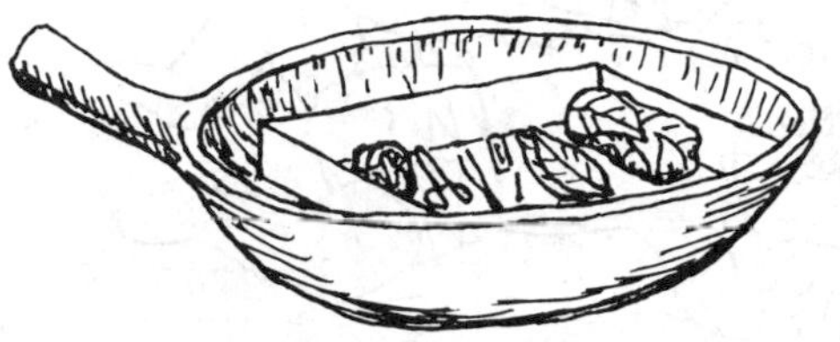

The tray is placed in a cooking pan.

The pan is then filled with water until it reaches halfway up the tray.

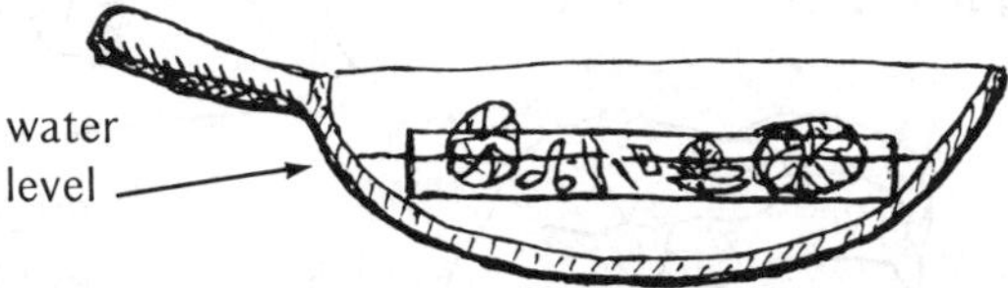

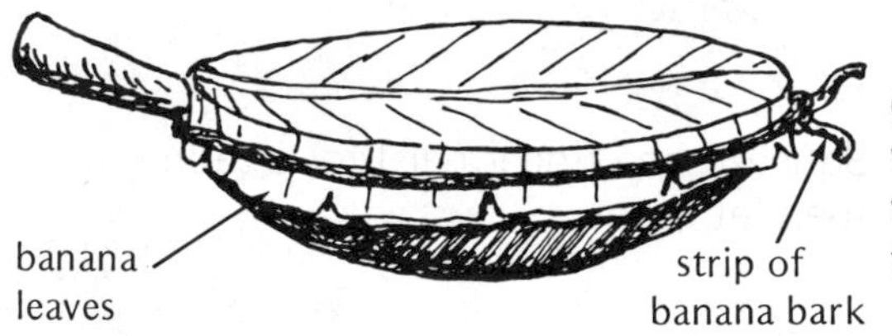

The pan is covered with 8 layers of green banana leaves that have been well washed. These are bound tightly in place with strips of banana leaf or bark from the banana plant.

Then the pan is placed on a low fire.

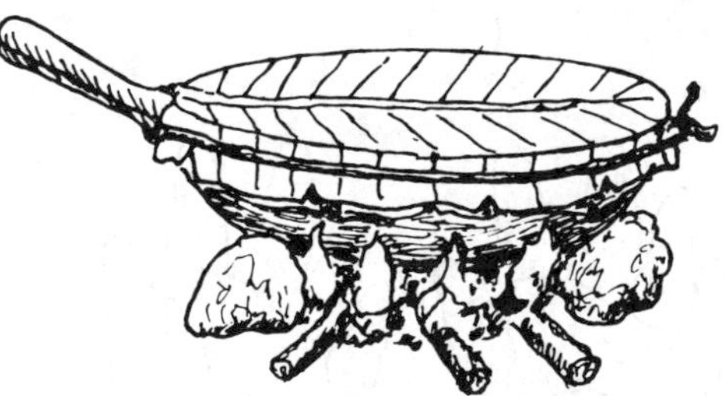

After boiling for about 2 hours, carefully remove the banana leaves and check to see if the cassava is cooked (soft). If it is, your equipment should be sufficiently sterilized.

FOR SURGICAL DRAPES:

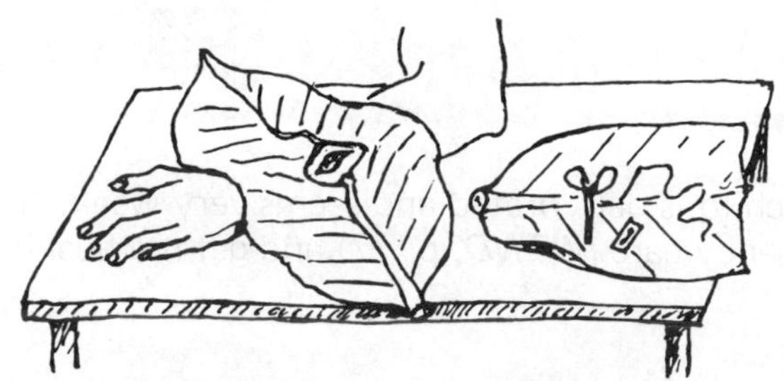

When removing the banana leaves, throw away only the top layer. The inner layers are sterile and can be used as surgical drapes.

FOR SUTURING WOUNDS:

You can use silk or cotton sewing thread, and a sewing needle, also sterilized. (See *WTND,* p. 86.)

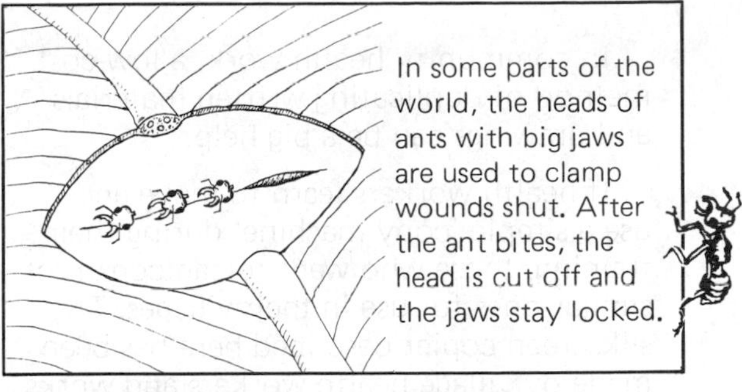

In some parts of the world, the heads of ants with big jaws are used to clamp wounds shut. After the ant bites, the head is cut off and the jaws stay locked.

FOR SURGICAL PADS AND BANDAGES:

Instead of sterile gauze pads, the sisters have used the leaves of a Philippine tree called ***hogonoy.*** These are said to be antiseptic and to help control bleeding. The leaves are first washed and then soaked in soapy water.

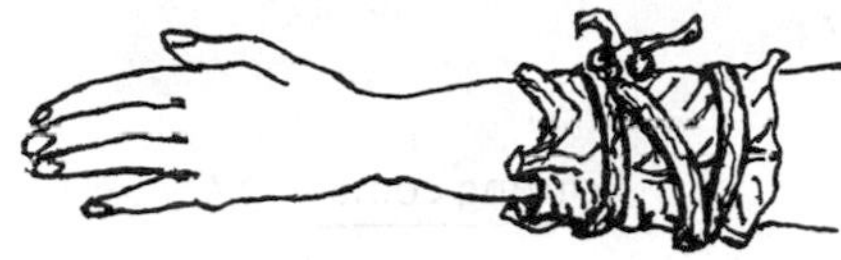

For outer bandages, the sisters use papaya leaves, which they scrub and soak in soapy water, and then bind in place with thin strips of banana bark.

ACUPUNCTURE AND ACUPRESSURE ANESTHESIA:

A number of health programs in the Philippines, including the Medical Mission Sisters, are experimenting with acupuncture and acupressure for anesthetizing parts of the body and for treating a variety of common health problems.

Acupuncture is an ancient Chinese science now being used increasingly in many parts of the world. Thin sterile needles are put into specific parts or points of the body—often distant from those areas being treated or anesthetized. Special 'body maps' showing the many acupuncture points are available.

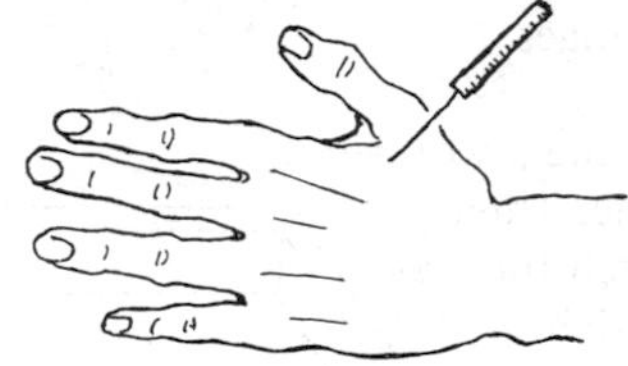

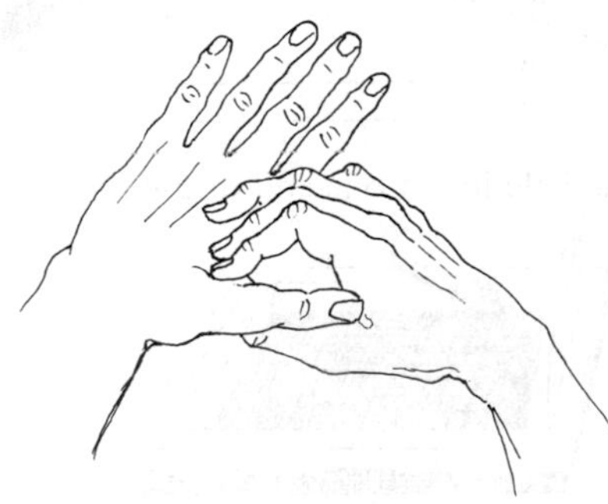

Acupressure, or 'finger pressure', is similar to acupuncture, except that the points are pressed rather than being pierced with a needle. Acupressure is now being taught to health workers in several countries. In the Philippines, some health workers are said to pull teeth painlessly using acupressure as the only anesthesia.

The Medical Mission Sisters recognize that acupuncture and finger pressure usually are most effective for removing pain or other symptoms, not for curing the underlying illness. They do not work for all illnesses or for all persons. Yet for problems like arthritis, headache, backache, sinus trouble, and asthma, they sometimes give great relief—at little cost and with no side effects.

Basic techniques for acupuncture or finger pressure may be appropriate to include in health worker training, especially in places where these methods are already widely accepted. But just as with modern medicine, care must be taken that the learners do not misuse them as magic 'cure-alls'. Books are available on both acupuncture and acupressure. However, the best way to learn is from someone who knows how.

LOW-COST DUPLICATION

In community health work, a low-cost method of duplicating written materials and drawings can be a big help.

If health workers learn to make and use a simple 'copy machine' during their training, those who want to can construct similar ones for use in their villages. The silkscreen copier described here has been made by village health workers and works well.

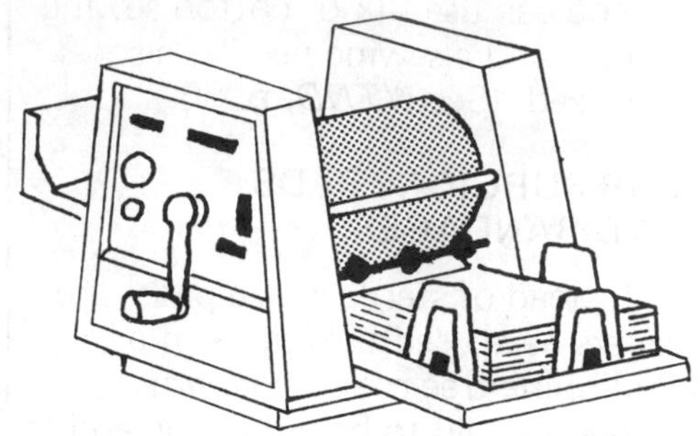

Expensive hand-cranked mimeograph

SILKSCREEN COPIER:

Making the screen

- wood about 5 cm. (2 in.) wide
- screws or nails
- silk or fine nylon cloth (threads must be very fine)
- small nails or tacks
- glue or paint that resists water
- a smooth board for the base
- hinges

1. Make a wooden frame. Then stretch the silk tightly over it and tack it down.

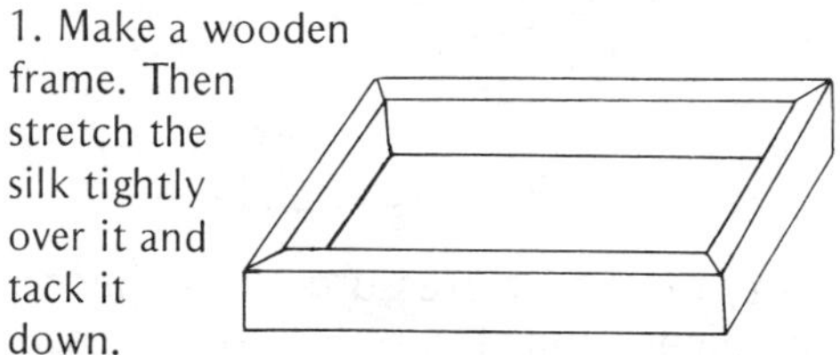

2. Spread glue or paint on the edges of the screen that will not be covered by the stencil. That way ink will not come through.

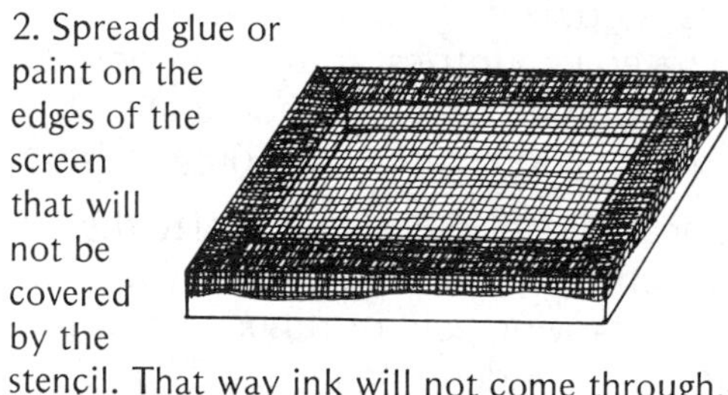

3. When the screen is dry, turn the frame over and attach it to the base with hinges.

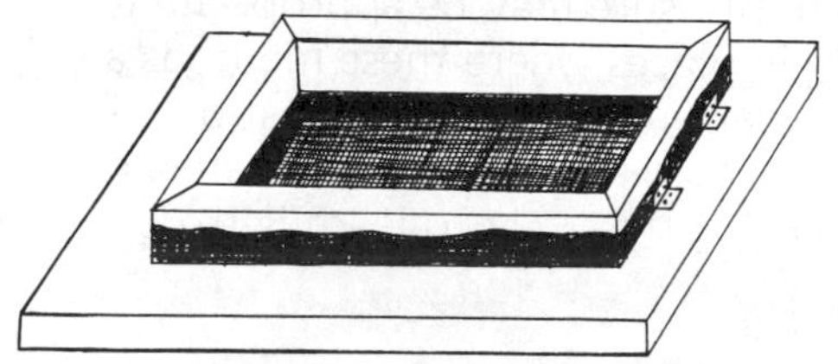

Printing copies

- standard mimeograph stencils
- adhesive tape or sticking plaster
- standard mimeograph ink (or homemade ink)
- squeegee for spreading the ink (see next page)

1. Write, type, or draw on the stencil, and tape it to the bottom of the screen.

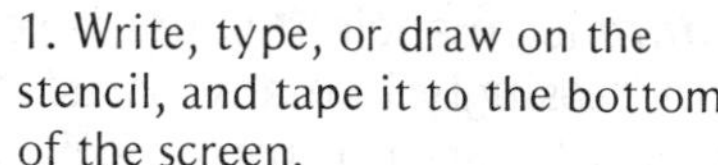

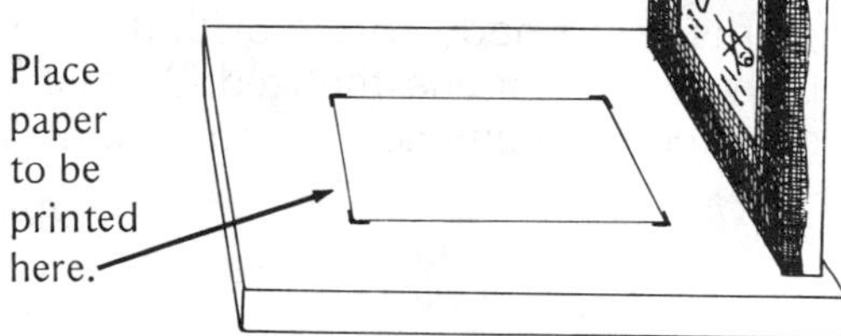

Place paper to be printed here.

2. Pour a little ink at one end of the screen.

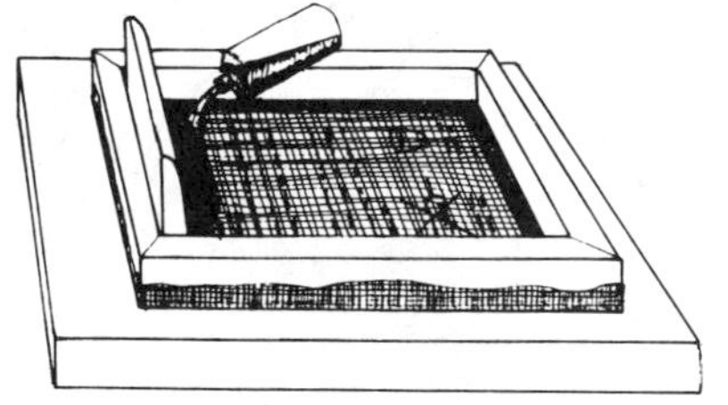

3. In one firm, even motion, spread the ink across the screen with the squeegee.

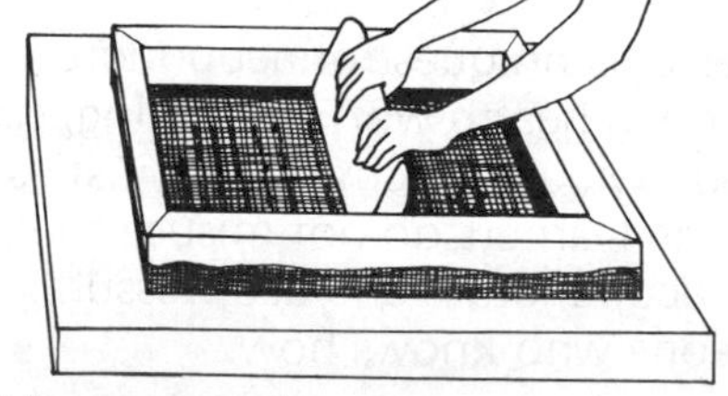

Lift frame and take out copy to dry.

A HOMEMADE SQUEEGEE:

Wrap a piece of inner tube or thin rubber around a stiff strip of metal or thin plywood. Then mount it in a wooden frame.

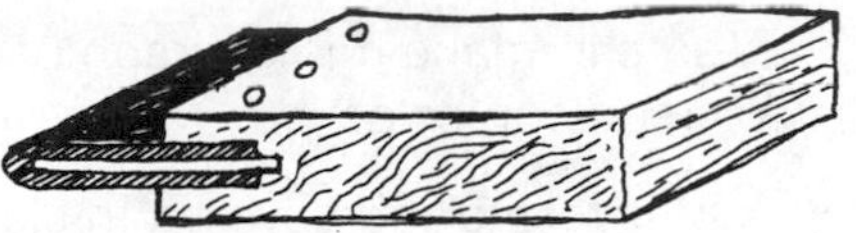

SILKSCREEN PAINTS AND INKS:*

Low-cost inks and paints can be made with materials commonly found in a village store. For coloring you can use ink, food color, tempera (paint) powder, or any kind of dye that will dissolve in water. Tempera powder makes the most brilliant colors.

The following silkscreen paint recipes have been used successfully in a cool climate. If you try them in hot climates, please let us know how well they work.

Recipe 1

- Non-instant starch 120 ml. (½ cup)
- Boiling water 350 ml. (1½ cups)
- Soap flakes 120 ml. (½ cup)
- Coloring

Mix starch with enough cold water to make a smooth paste. Add boiling water, and cool until glossy. Stir in soap flakes while mixture is warm. When the mixture is cool, add coloring.

Recipe 2 (quite lumpy, but this does not affect the printing quality)

- Cornstarch 60 ml. (¼ cup)
- Boiling water 460 ml. (2 cups)
- Soap flakes 30 ml. (1/8 cup)
- Coloring

Mix cornstarch with a small amount of cold water. Stir it into the boiling water. Bring to a boil again, and stir until thickened. Add soap flakes while mixture is warm. Then add coloring.

Recipe 3

- Cornstarch 120 ml. (½ cup)
- Gelatin (unflavored) 1 envelope or 15 ml.
- Soap flakes 120 ml. (½ cup)
- Water 700 ml. (3 cups)
- Coloring

Dissolve cornstarch in 170 ml. (¾ cup) cold water. Dissolve gelatin in 60 ml. (¼ cup) cold water. Heat 460 ml. (2 cups) of water, pour in cornstarch, and add dissolved gelatin. Boil and stir until thickened. Cool and add soap flakes and coloring.

Note: If you add 1 or 2 teaspoons of glycerine to these inks, they will be smoother and easier to use.

These paints should last for several months if stored in jars with tight-fitting lids.

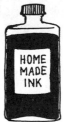

Never let dried particles of paint get mixed into the paint or fall onto the screen, as they may puncture the silk during printing. A small hole in the silk can be repaired with a drop of shellac. (Fine nylon cloth is tougher than silk, and does not puncture as easily.)

Be sure to wash the screen after you have finished making copies. For the homemade inks described above, wash the screen with soap and water. But if you use an oil-based ink or paint, wash it with turpentine, kerosene, or gasoline.

*From ***Village Technology Handbook,*** p. 405. Available from VITA, P.O. Box 12028, Arlington, Virginia 22209, U.S.A.

POSSIBLE USES FOR SILKSCREEN COPIER

You can make mimeograph or silkscreen copies of:

- key information covered in classes (to hand out to students)
- tests, exams, or questionnaires
- lists of health priorities and decisions discussed in group meetings
- notices with health information for the public (see example below)
- a monthly news sheet or 'health bulletin' for health workers or the whole village (see next page)
- information sheets for school children, mothers, midwives, or other groups
- health education posters drawn by school children

Have students help with copying information sheets so they will know how to do this when they return to their villages.

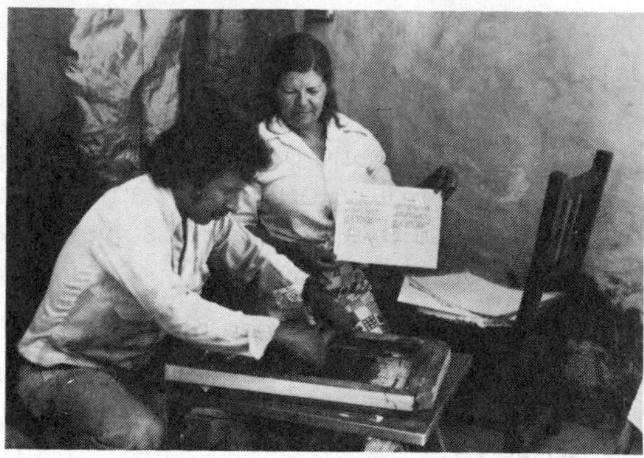

Here Pablo Chavez (a village health worker who drew some of the pictures for this book) teaches students how to use a silkscreen copier.

A HEALTH INFORMATION NOTICE:

The notice shown here was produced with a silkscreen copier by health workers in a Mexican village. They did this example in English so it could be used in this book. The original Spanish notice was distributed to people in their village because many villagers were wrongly using antibiotic injections to treat an epidemic of the 'flu', or common cold.

Notice

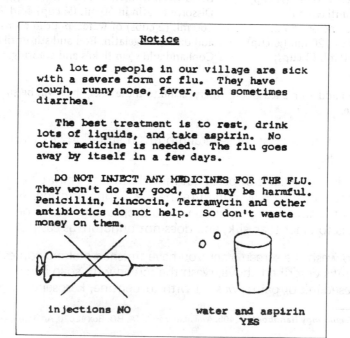

A lot of people in our village are sick with a severe form of flu. They have cough, runny nose, fever, and sometimes diarrhea.

The best treatment is to rest, drink lots of liquids, and take aspirin. No other medicine is needed. The flu goes away by itself in a few days.

DO NOT INJECT ANY MEDICINES FOR THE FLU. They won't do any good, and may be harmful. Penicillin, Lincocin, Terramycin and other antibiotics do not help. So don't waste money on them.

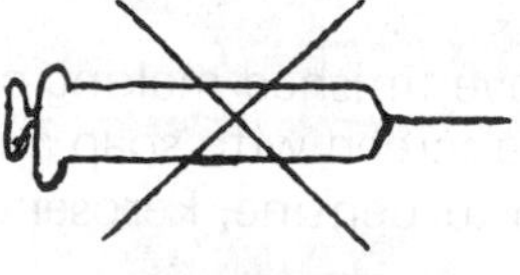

injections NO

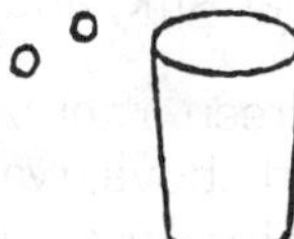

water and aspirin YES

A COMMUNITY NEWS SHEET OR 'HEALTH BULLETIN'

Good communications between a health worker or health team and the community are important. Meetings may be useful, but not everyone attends them.

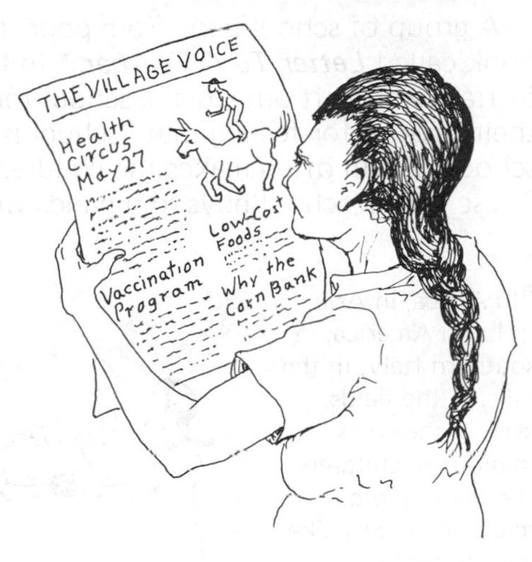

In places where many people can read (even a little), a good way to improve communications is to print news sheets with information and announcements. These news sheets need not be longer than a page or two, and could be produced every month or so.

Invite people in your village to contribute articles and announcements. You might also ask the school teacher to help. He could have the children write about different things they think are important to health in their village. Then the children could choose one or two of their better articles, work together to improve them, and contribute them to the news sheet.

Perhaps some school children, mothers, young men, or other persons in town can help you produce the news sheet. This would not only save time, but give you a chance to work closely with members of the community.

THE SKILL OF CLEAR, SIMPLE WRITING

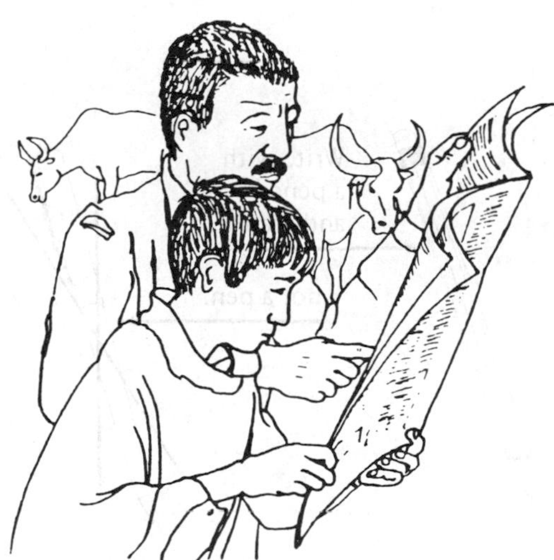

News sheets with simple, clear information can help persons with little formal education learn to read and write better (especially if they help produce them).

The skill of being able to write simply and clearly, to organize ideas, and to say strongly what you feel is one of the most powerful tools a person can have. But it is a skill the poor often lack. Many village schools teach children to read, and to copy letters and words, but do not teach them to express clearly what they want to say.

Clear, simple writing is a skill that can best be learned through practice. Working on a community news sheet is a good way to get such practice. It helps if someone with more writing experience—perhaps the school teacher—can review the articles and make suggestions about clearness, organization, and perhaps spelling. But it is important that whoever gives these suggestions let the writers themselves decide upon and make the corrections.

Suggestions for good writing

A group of school boys from poor farm families in Italy has written a powerful book called ***Letter To A Teacher.**** In this book, they point out that "the peasants of Italy were left out when a school for them was being planned." The boys state their reasons for feeling that "school is a war against the poor." They say the school system often makes the children of the poor feel worthless, lazy, or stupid. These Italian school boys join hands with the children of the world, saying:

"In Africa, in Asia, in Latin America, in southern Italy, in the hills, in the fields, even in the cities, millions of children are waiting to be made equal. Shy like me; stupid like Sandro; lazy like Gianni. The best of humanity."

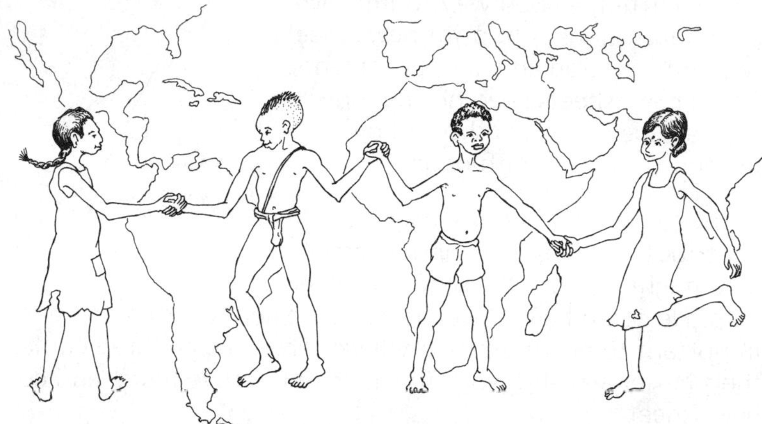

These farm boys have taught themselves to write well, and in doing so have found a strong means of self-defense. Their immediate goal is "to understand others and to make oneself understood." Their ***rules of good writing*** should be a help to any group working on a news sheet or trying to develop writing skills.

RULES OF GOOD WRITING (by the school boys of Barbiana):

- Have something important to say, something useful to everyone, or at least to many.
- Know for whom you are writing.
- Gather all useful materials.
- Find a logical pattern with which to develop the theme.
- Eliminate every useless word.
- Eliminate every word not used in the spoken language.
- Never set time limits.

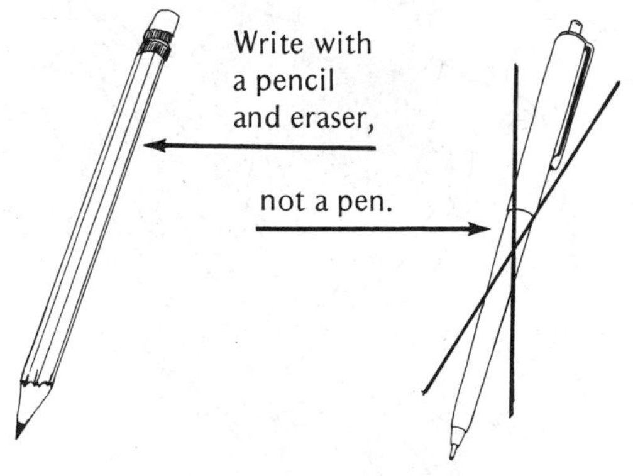
Write with
a pencil
and eraser,
not a pen.

*Published by Vintage Books in the United States and Penguin Books in England.

If you are trying to produce a news sheet, statement, or any other piece of writing **as a group,** the Barbiana school boys' explanation of how they worked together to write ***Letter To A Teacher*** may give you some ideas:

THIS IS THE WAY WE DO IT:

To start with, each of us keeps a notebook in his pocket. Every time an idea comes up, we make a note of it. Each idea on a separate sheet, on one side of the page.

Then one day we gather together all the sheets of paper and spread them on a big table. We look through them, one by one, to get rid of duplications. Next, we make separate piles of the sheets that are related, and these will make up the chapters. Every chapter is subdivided into small piles, and they will become paragraphs.

At this point we try to give a title to each paragraph. If we can't, it means either that the paragraph has no content or that too many things are squeezed into it. Some paragraphs disappear. Some are broken up.

While we name the paragraphs, we discuss their logical order, until an outline is born. With the outline set, we reorganize all the piles to follow its pattern.

We take the first pile, spread the sheets on the table, and we find the sequence for them. And so we begin to put down a first draft of the text.

We mimeograph that part so that we each can have a copy in front of us. Then, scissors, paste, and colored pencils. We shuffle it all again. New sheets are added. We mimeograph again.

A race begins now for all of us to find any word that can be crossed out, any excess adjectives, repetitions, lies, difficult words, overly long sentences, and any two concepts that are forced into one sentence.

We call in one outsider after another. We prefer that they not have had too much school. We ask them to read aloud. And we watch to see if they have understood what we meant to say.

We accept their suggestions if they clarify the text. We reject any suggestions made in the name of caution.

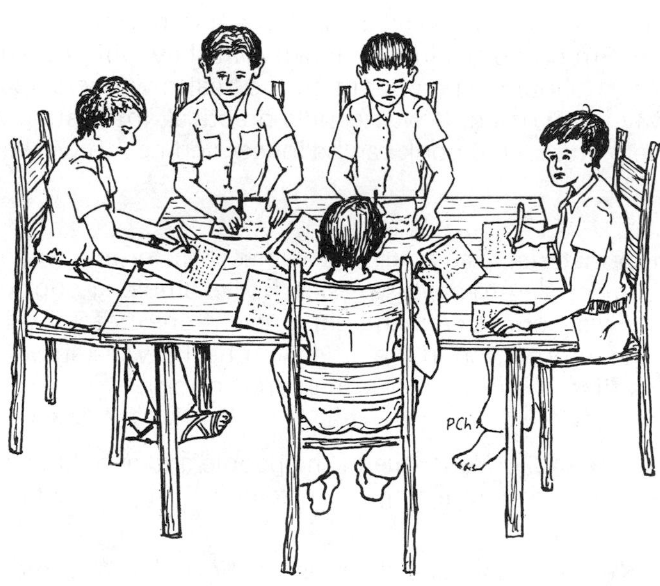

PREPARING TRAINING AND WORK MANUALS FOR HEALTH WORKERS

One of the most valuable tools health workers can have is a clearly written, well-illustrated, easy-to-use manual. Ideally, it should be written for, or adapted to, the local area and its needs. If the health workers' training focuses on learning to use a practical manual effectively, they can accomplish far more than if they are expected to rely on their memories or class notes.

An idea for helping you find things quickly in your manual:

Cut the edges of the pages like this, to mark important sections.

Unfortunately, many manuals written for community health workers are not adequate. Often they are too simple or too complex, or a combination of both. Drawings and photos tend to be carelessly done or hard to understand. The text often provides too little information, or is not arranged for easy problem-solving use.

Here we give a few suggestions that may help in the preparation of interesting, useful manuals:

1. **Content.** Base the content on the most important local needs. Be sure to include concerns of the people—not just of the health authorities. (For example, in ***Where There Is No Doctor,*** we include a discussion of 'Mask of Pregnancy'. Although it is not really a medical problem, it is of concern to village women in Mexico.)

2. **Length.** Include information on all areas that are important for the health workers' work. But do not include so much that they will not read or use the manual. Its length should depend both on the health workers' reading ability and on the way it is written. If written in a practical, interesting way, with lots of informative pictures, the book can be longer and health workers will still use it eagerly.

3. **Organization of material.** Try to arrange subject matter in a way that makes problem solving and day-to-day use easier. For example, group together the information on diagnosis, treatment, and prevention of each health problem. And present the information in the order that health workers will use it (signs and symptoms first, then treatment, then prevention).

4. **Language.** Use the spoken language of the people and avoid big words. For example, say "Press with your finger," instead of "Apply digital pressure."

5. **Writing style.** Keep paragraphs and sentences short. Try to **avoid sentences of more than 20 words.** Use many headings and subheadings to divide up the material and to make specific references easy to find.

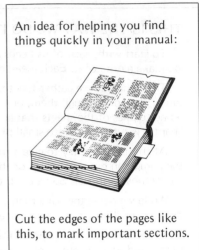

6. Emphasis. Emphasize what is most important by underlining or using **bold** or **dark print.** Also use pictures and 'boxes' to set off important points. For example:

THIS BABY'S CORD WAS CUT SHORT, KEPT DRY, AND LEFT OPEN TO THE AIR.

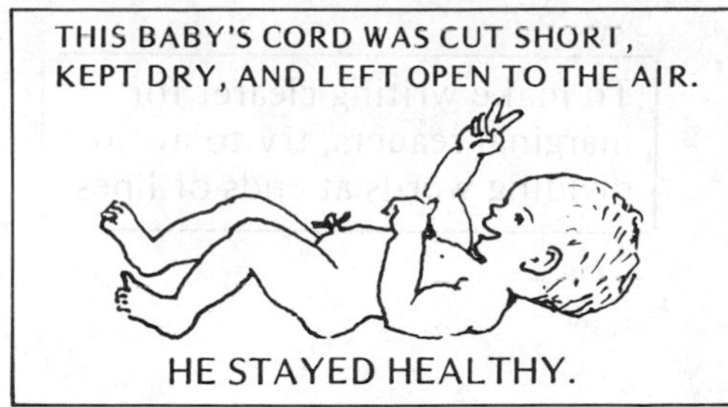

HE STAYED HEALTHY.

THIS BABY'S CORD WAS LEFT LONG, KEPT TIGHTLY COVERED, AND NOT KEPT DRY.

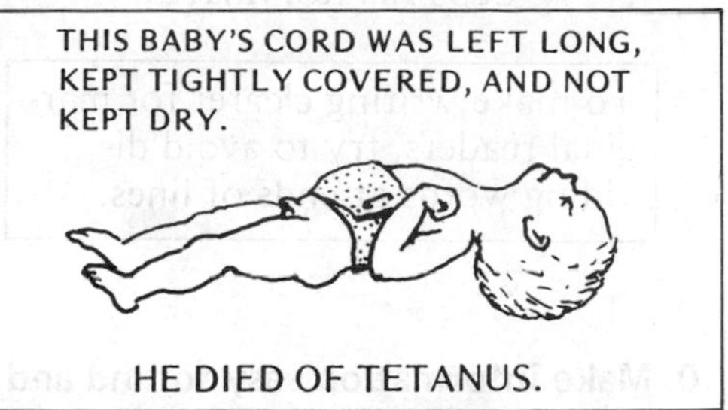

HE DIED OF TETANUS.

7. Pictures. Include plenty of clear, informative line drawings. Integrate the drawings with the text in a way that saves extra words. For example:

SINUS TROUBLE (SINUSITIS)

Signs:

- Pain in the face above and below the eyes, here (It hurts more when you tap lightly just over the bones, or when the person bends over.)
- Thick mucus or pus in the nose, perhaps with a bad smell. The nose is often stuffy.
- Fever (sometimes).

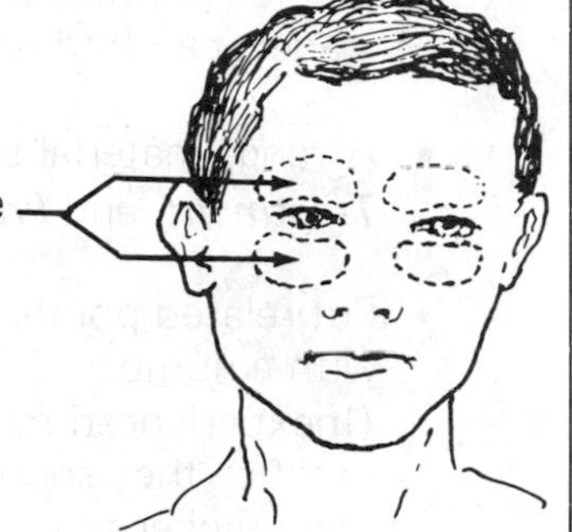

8. Type and layout. Use large, clear type. Keep lines of words relatively short (not more than about 60 letters). Compare these actual-size examples from two different health manuals.

For one who knows about a task and can answer questions and teach others well but is not able to do correctly important tasks like a dressing or giving an injection, we must help him to correct what is wrong and to spend more time doing practical work. So we see why it is important to write what you want the student to be able to do at the end of his training (learning objectives) so that you can see if he has learned these tasks (evaluation) and when and why to go back to correct what is wrong and continue to develop what is good.

from p. 320, *The Primary Health Worker,* WHO

LESS APPROPRIATE—Print is unclear and too small; lines too long, sentences much too long, and the message confusing.

22.2 POISONING

a) Kerosene poisoning

this is a common poison drunk by young children. It is kept in houses as fuel for lamps or primus stoves and is often kept in an old squash or beer bottle. A child usually does not drink more than a mouthful because of the unpleasant taste.

from p. 22.2, *Child Health,* African Medical and Research Foundation

MORE APPROPRIATE—Letters are large and clear, lines short, sentences and words short, and the message is clear.

9. Do not break words at the ends of lines.

LESS APPROPRIATE	MORE APPROPRIATE
To make writing clearer for mar- ginal readers, try to avoid di- viding words at ends of lines.	To make writing clearer for marginal readers, try to avoid dividing words at ends of lines.

10. Make information easy to find and use.

- Include a clear and complete INDEX—perhaps on paper of a different color, as in *Where There Is No Doctor.*
- Include pictures that show the subjects covered on each page. That way readers can find what they want by flipping through the book.
- Arrange material under headings and subheadings (such as *Signs, Treatment,* and *Prevention*).
- Put related points of information in the form of a list. Mark each item with a number (1,2,3) or a bullet (•), as we have done with this list. (Inexperienced readers may at first have trouble with lists, but with a little practice they soon get used to them. Once they do, the lists make it easier and quicker to review information.)

11. Field testing. Before final production of a manual, or any teaching material, try it out with the people who will be using it. Get their responses to these questions:

- Can you understand everything easily?
- Can you find the subjects you are looking for?
- Does it answer your questions and provide the information you need?
- Do you find it so interesting and informative that you want to read more of it?
- How could it be improved?

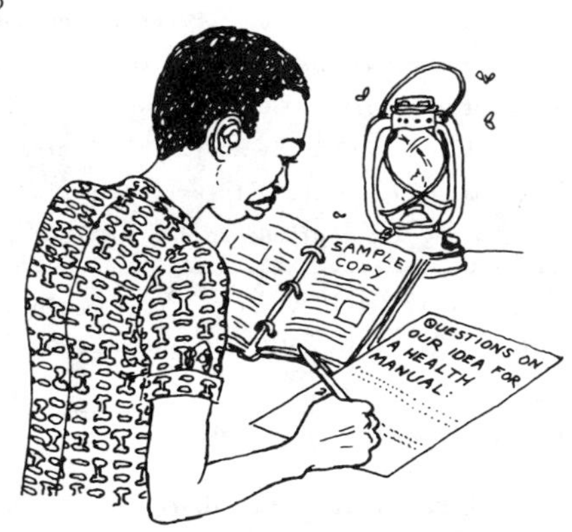

12. Show you care. The care you put into the preparation of teaching materials or manuals will inspire health workers to take equal care in their work. The care you take also reflects your appreciation and respect for the health workers and the people they serve.

CHAPTER 17

Solving Problems Step by Step (Scientific Method)

A health educator in Zaire, Africa writes:

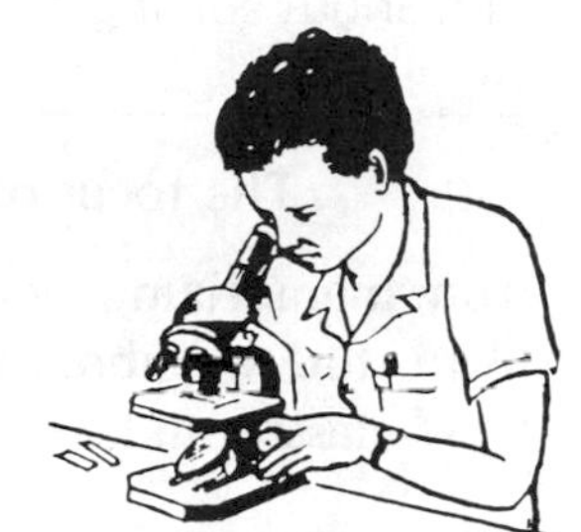

"We are wrestling with some very difficult problems in the education of auxiliary health workers . . . The frame of reference of the young people we train is so vastly different from our own. Ours is a physical, technical one; theirs is more traditional and spiritual . . .

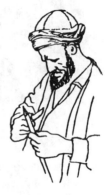

"Deductive [step-by-step] reasoning is a real problem for them. They can perceive cause-and-effect relationships within their traditional frame of reference, but only with great difficulty in the physical and technical frame of reference. Therefore, problem analysis and problem solving are very difficult . . .

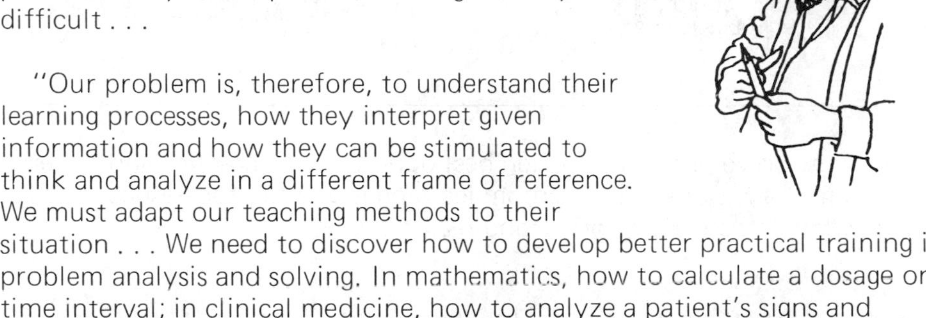

"Our problem is, therefore, to understand their learning processes, how they interpret given information and how they can be stimulated to think and analyze in a different frame of reference. We must adapt our teaching methods to their situation . . . We need to discover how to develop better practical training in problem analysis and solving. In mathematics, how to calculate a dosage or a time interval; in clinical medicine, how to analyze a patient's signs and symptoms in order to come up with a correct diagnosis; in health, how to approach the health and development problems of the community . . ."*

Problem-solving skills are among the most basic skills a health worker can master. By this we mean **the ability to look carefully at a situation, analyze what problems exist, and determine steps to improve the situation.**

The main focus of health worker training needs to be on learning problem-solving skills.

This means that, whatever the subject, instructors need always to **relate what students learn to the work they will do in their communities.** The main job of the health worker is to help people better understand and resolve their problems.

*From personal correspondence.

Too many training programs have students concentrate on memorizing facts or performing 'clearly defined tasks', rather than learning problem-solving skills. Even when problem solving is emphasized, often learning takes place mostly in the classroom, rather than where people's basic problems occur—the home, fields, water hole, clinic, jail, etc.

Today, many training programs are moving the focus of learning out of the classroom and into the village, the street, the home, and the clinic. From the first, students begin to work with real problems of real people. In this way, learning about solving problems becomes urgent and meaningful.

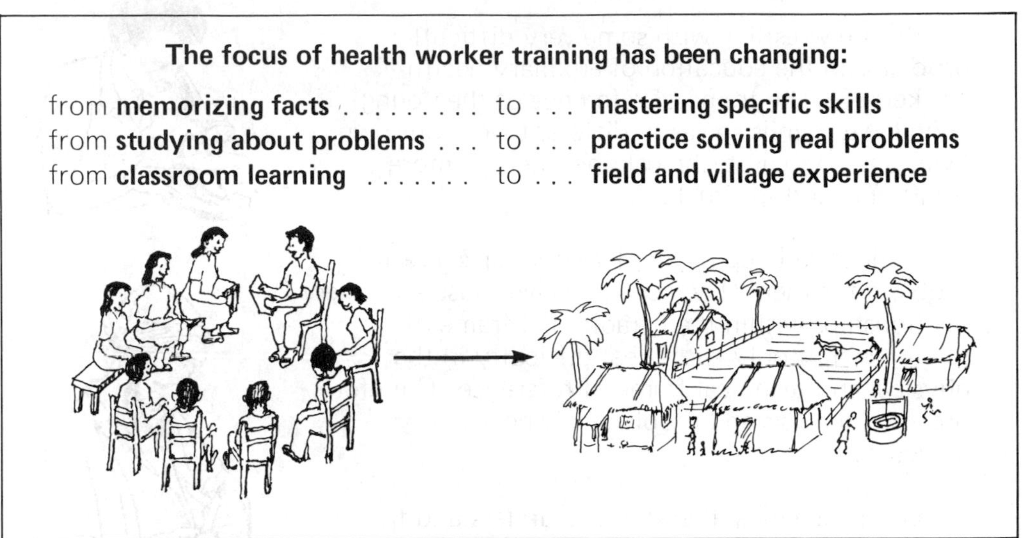

The focus of health worker training has been changing:
from **memorizing facts** . . . . to . . . **mastering specific skills**
from **studying about problems** . . . to . . . **practice solving real problems**
from **classroom learning** . . . . to . . . **field and village experience**

Learning to solve problems is often best done through practice and experience in the community. But some classroom learning is helpful, too—especially if approached in an active, exploring, and realistic way.

Suggestions for helping develop thinking and problem-solving skills in the classroom:

- Teach (even basic information) through **role plays and sociodramas** rather than through lectures. Have students act out lifelike problems and practice solving them in a lifelike way (see Ch. 14).
- **Invite people from the community into the classroom.** Farmers, mothers, children, experienced health workers, and others can talk with the students about their needs and problems.
- **Use a dialogue or discussion approach to learning.** Help students build on their own experience and put what they already know together in new ways—like pieces of a puzzle.
- Use teaching aids that do not simply demonstrate or show things, but that **invite students to figure out answers for themselves** (see p. **11**-13).
- Teach by asking questions (whether in discussions or in exams) that **encourage thinking and problem solving** related to needs in the students' communities (see p. **9**-3).

In the classroom, it is also a good idea to explore with health workers the steps involved in a scientific approach to solving problems. The group can compare how this scientific method differs from the traditional approaches to problem solving they have observed or practiced in their own communities.

In this chapter, we will look at ways of helping people with limited schooling to understand the process and purpose of scientific method. Once again, our job is to **relate learning to familiar experiences.**

SCIENTIFIC METHOD— A STEP-BY-STEP APPROACH TO PROBLEM SOLVING

A careful, step-by-step approach is essential to the accurate diagnosis and treatment of different illnesses. It is also useful for analyzing and dealing with other problems in a community.

To take a scientific approach, the health worker needs to **start by asking searching questions rather than by jumping to quick answers.** At first this may be difficult or confusing for a person whose experience has been mainly in traditional or folk medicine. Herb doctors and traditional healers generally depend on **faith, magic, and the power of suggestion** as a large part of their curative art. People's belief in the instant knowledge of the healer may be as important to their cure as the herbs or medication used. For this reason, the healer tries to show that he or she has immediate understanding of the illness, its cause, and its treatment.

But while the traditional healer tries to be certain about the illness from the first, **the scientific healer starts with uncertainty or doubt** about the nature of the illness.

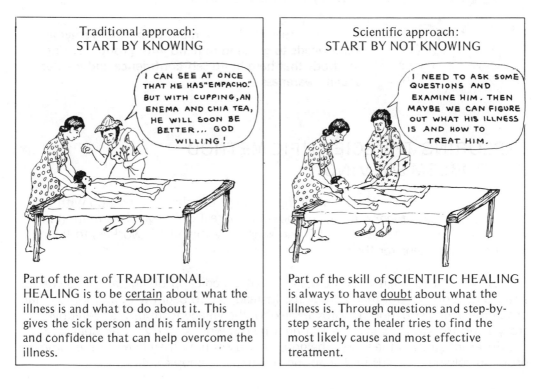

Traditional approach:
START BY KNOWING

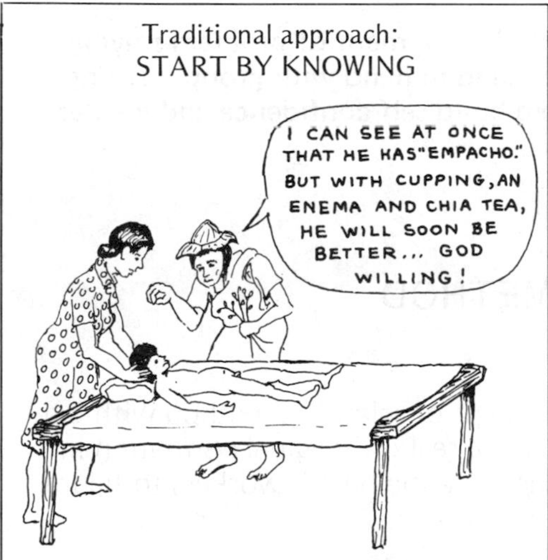

I CAN SEE AT ONCE THAT HE HAS "EMPACHO." BUT WITH CUPPING, AN ENEMA AND CHIA TEA, HE WILL SOON BE BETTER... GOD WILLING!

Part of the art of TRADITIONAL HEALING is to be <u>certain</u> about what the illness is and what to do about it. This gives the sick person and his family strength and confidence that can help overcome the illness.

Scientific approach:
START BY NOT KNOWING

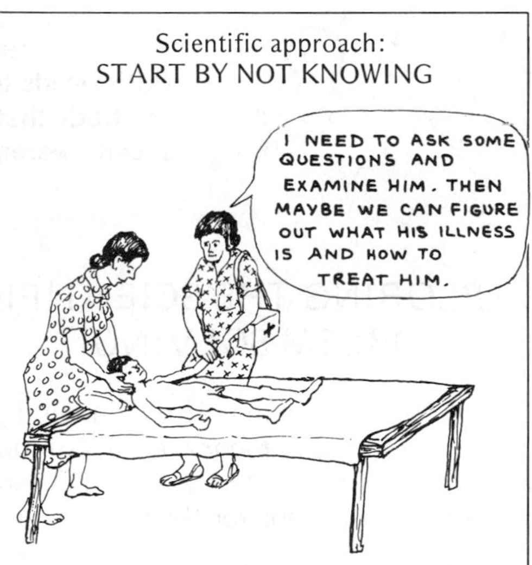

Part of the skill of SCIENTIFIC HEALING is always to have <u>doubt</u> about what the illness is. Through questions and step-by-step search, the healer tries to find the most likely cause and most effective treatment.

NOT THIS 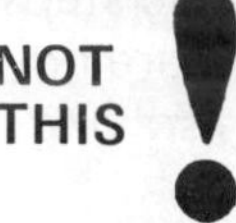

In scientific problem solving, it is important to start with <u>doubt</u> and then systematically gather information to figure out the most probable answer.

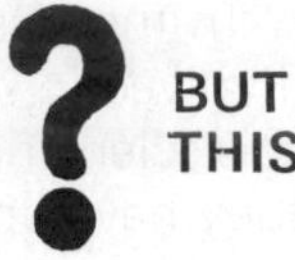 BUT THIS

Helping health workers learn to solve problems in a questioning, step-by-step way is not easy. Many find it difficult to accept uncertainty as a starting point. They may be ashamed or afraid to admit their uncertainties—even to themselves. Instead they may jump to 'obvious' answers, or even invent test results for things they have not understood. ***Appearing to have the answer*** somehow seems more acceptable than ***doubting and carefully searching for one.*** This is an attitude the health workers may have learned in school, where good grades tend to be valued more than useful knowledge.

This leap-before-you-look approach to problem solving, when mixed with modern medical science, can give poor or dangerous results. For this reason, some health professionals argue against teaching village health workers to use important medicines or take on major responsibilities.

However, **a reasoning, step-by-step approach to problem solving can be learned.** It can be learned by non-literate persons just as by medical students. One reason why it sometimes presents special problems for villagers is that, in a training situation, they often feel unsure of themselves. This is especially true when instructors are professionals from a 'higher' level of society, or use manners, dress, and language that make villagers feel inferior. Persons who feel unsure of themselves, understandably, may have greater difficulty admitting their uncertainties. They fear being laughed at or scorned for what they do not know. Afraid to ask questions, they may try to guess at answers.

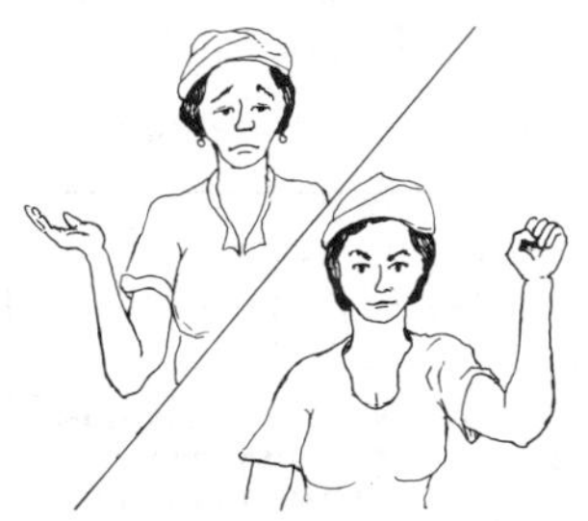

For this reason, **development of problem-solving skills needs to go hand in hand with group learning methods that help build self-confidence and greater social awareness.**

EXPLORING THE SCIENTIFIC METHOD OF PROBLEM SOLVING

Rather than starting off by explaining the steps of scientific method with big words (***hypothesis, theory,*** etc.), try looking at a real or imaginary situation in which the different steps are used. Then encourage the health workers to figure out the various steps for themselves.

It is best not to begin with the diagnosis of a medical problem, as this is still a strange new process for many students. Instead, try to begin with a more familiar problem-solving situation. In Ajoya, Mexico, the village team uses a 'detective story', and the students take part in figuring out who is guilty. After analyzing the different steps in the story, the group discusses how they can use the same problem-solving methods in diagnosing and treating people's illnesses.

A detective story: **"WHO STOLE THE GUALAMO JAM?"***

This story is used for helping health workers learn about the scientific method of problem solving. It is not simply told by one person; rather it is created together by the student group. You can use drawings to give it more life. The story will turn out somewhat differently with each group, but may develop something like this:

Instructor: Who knows what a detective is?

A student: Isn't it someone like a policeman who tries to figure out who committed a crime?

Instructor: Right! Well, this is a sort of 'detective story' that could take place in a village home. The mother is the detective.

Let us suppose that one morning Mama prepares a batch of *gualamo* jam for her husband's birthday.

Then she goes to the river to wash clothes.

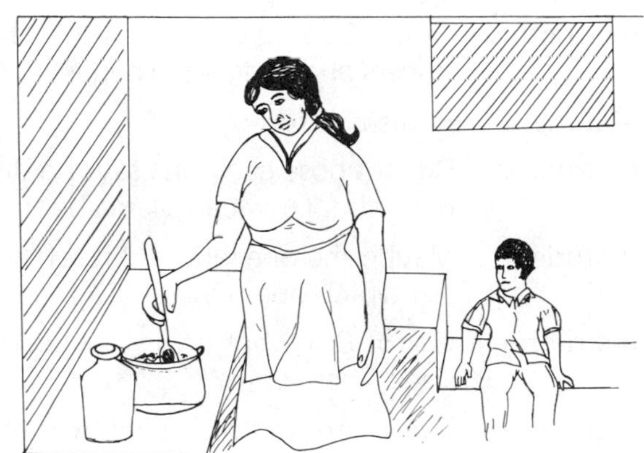

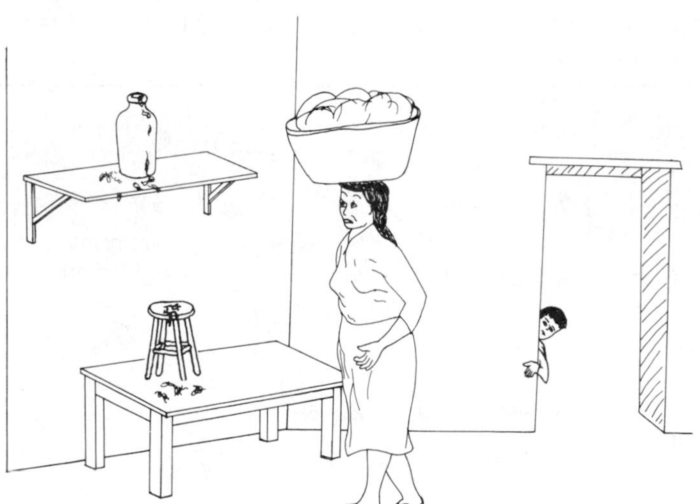

In the afternoon Mama comes back from the river. She sees that someone has been into the jam and made a big mess.

What is her first idea about how this happened?

**Gualamo* is a black, grape-like fruit that grows wild on trees in western Mexico.

Students: That one of her children stole the jam.

Instructor: How can she find out which of her 7 children did it?

A student: She could call all the children and ask them.

A student: But what if they don't tell?

A student: Or what if the one who did it lies and says someone else did it?

A student: She could find out what the children were doing while she was at the river. Maybe some were away so she can be sure they didn't steal the jam.

Instructor: Good! Let us suppose she finds that one of the children was away gathering firewood and has the wood to prove it. And that another was at her grandmother's house. But the others were all at home. How many possible culprits does that leave?

A student: Five.

A student: Why doesn't she look at their hands and mouths? Gualamo leaves a purple stain.

Instructor: Good! Suppose she finds that 3 of them have purple stains on their fingers and tongues. Then what?

A student: Punish all three!

Instructor: But suppose each one says he didn't steal the jam; that another gave it to him. How can Mama be sure which one actually stole it?

A student: Maybe the one who did it left handprints in the kitchen, so she can tell which one it was.

Instructor: Good! But what if the 3 children's hands are all about the same size? Then what?

A student: I've heard that real detectives take fingerprints. Maybe she could take their fingerprints with ink . . .

A student: . . . or with the jam itself! Then she could compare the prints of each child with the prints in the kitchen. That would be a good test!

If some students don't know about fingerprints, and if there is time, the instructor can have students actually take each other's fingerprints. They can use ink or jam and act out the 'test' to see which child stole the jam.

fingerprints of the three children

1. 

2. 

jam print in kitchen

3. 

Which child do you think stole the jam?

Instructor: Fine! Let's say the fingerprints are a little blurred, but that after doing the fingerprint test Mama is almost sure that one boy stole the jam. What should she do next?

Students: Punish him!

Instructor: And after punishing him, how can she tell if she was right about who did it, and if the punishment was effective?

A student: By seeing whether any more jam is stolen!

After the 'detective story' has been completed, the instructor helps the students analyze the various steps that Mama took to find out who stole the jam. The steps will be something like this:

1. Mama **becomes aware** of the problem.
2. She **is uncertain** about how it happened.
3. She **guesses** that one of her children is responsible.
4. She **notices** the details or 'evidence'.
5. She **asks questions.**
6. She **examines** her children's fingers.
7. She **considers all possibilities.**
8. She **conducts tests** to prove or disprove the different possibilities.
9. She **decides** who is probably guilty.
10. She **provides punishment.**
11. She **sees the results:** Whether or not punishment was effective.
12. She **starts over again** with step 1 if the punishment was not effective.

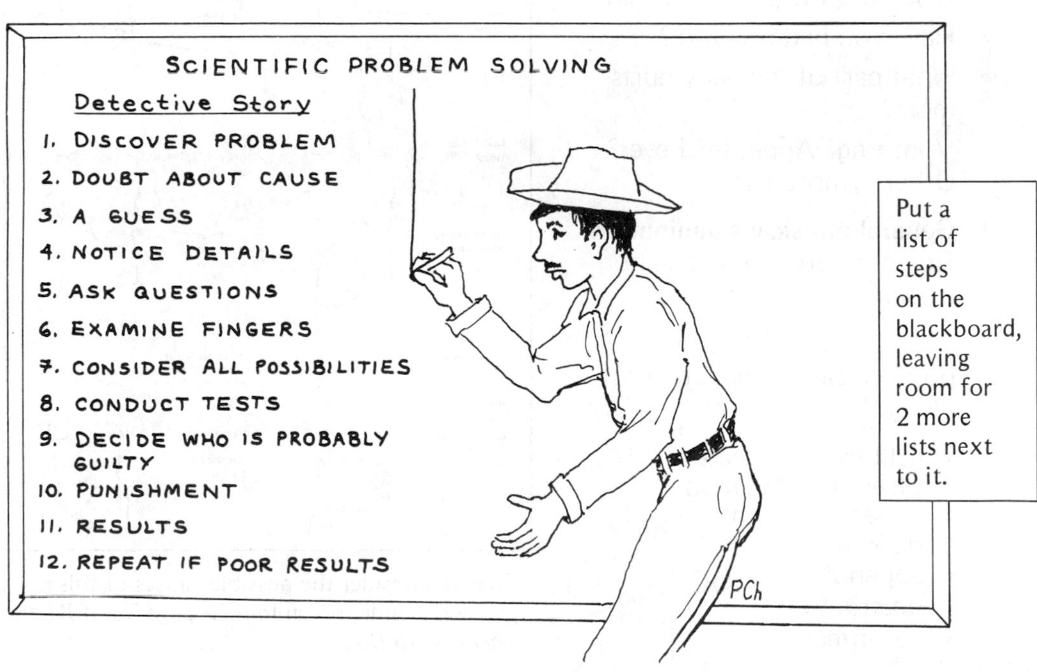

Put a list of steps on the blackboard, leaving room for 2 more lists next to it.

A second detective story: A HEALTH PROBLEM

After discussing the steps Mama took to solve the ***gualamo*** jam mystery, students can compare these with the steps in the diagnosis and treatment of a health problem. This can be more fun if done as a role play with a student or instructor pretending to be sick. For example:

A 40-year-old woman arrives complaining of severe pain in her belly. What steps might a health worker take to figure out the cause of the pain and what to do about it?

Following the general outline of steps Mama took in the first detective story, the learning group tries to diagnose the woman's problem. The steps they develop in this new story or role play might be as follows:

1. **Main complaint.** (What bothers the sick woman most?)
2. **Doubt or uncertainty** about the cause. (Start by **not** knowing.)
3. An **idea** or **guess** about the possible cause or causes. (This idea may change as more information is gathered.)
4. **Observation** of the person. (How ill she looks, skin color, etc.)
5. **Questions** (clinical history). For example:

   When did the problem begin?

   Have you had it before?

   What part of the belly hurts most?

   Vomiting? Appetite? Fever? Other symptoms?
6. **General physical examination** (temperature, pulse, location of pain, etc.).
7. Consider carefully all the **possible causes** that are most likely. For example:
   - gallbladder disease
   - ulcer or indigestion
   - hepatitis or other liver disease
   - appendicitis or gut obstruction
   - gut infection

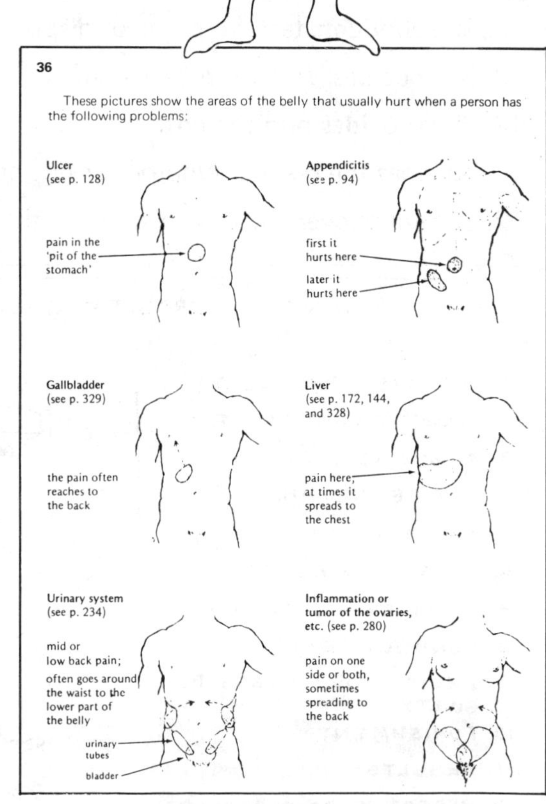
36
These pictures show the areas of the belly that usually hurt when a person has the following problems:
Ulcer
(see p. 128)
pain in the 'pit of the stomach'
Appendicitis
(see p. 94)
first it hurts here
later it hurts here
Gallbladder
(see p. 329)
the pain often reaches to the back
Liver
(see p. 172, 144, and 328)
pain here; at times it spreads to the chest
Urinary system
(see p. 234)
mid or low back pain; often goes around the waist to the lower part of the belly
urinary tubes
bladder
Inflammation or tumor of the ovaries, etc. (see p. 280)
pain on one side or both, sometimes spreading to the back

To help consider the possible causes of this problem, students can look at page 36 of *Where There Is No Doctor.*

8. **Specific tests and examinations, and more questions** to help find out which of the possibilities are most likely or unlikely to be the problem.

   Depending on the location, type, and duration of pain, and whether or not there is fever, diarrhea, or vomiting, some of the possible causes may be eliminated.

   For the possibilities that remain, sometimes specific tests can help. Examples are the 'rebound test' for appendicitis (see *WTND,* p. 95) or the 'urine foam test' for liver or gallbladder disease (p. **5**-15 to **5**-16 of this book). Even for less likely possibilities, it is wise to check using simple tests when you can.

   Sometimes health workers will not be able to perform necessary tests. In these cases they should consider sending the sick person to a clinic, laboratory, or hospital that can do what is needed. Be sure to discuss this.

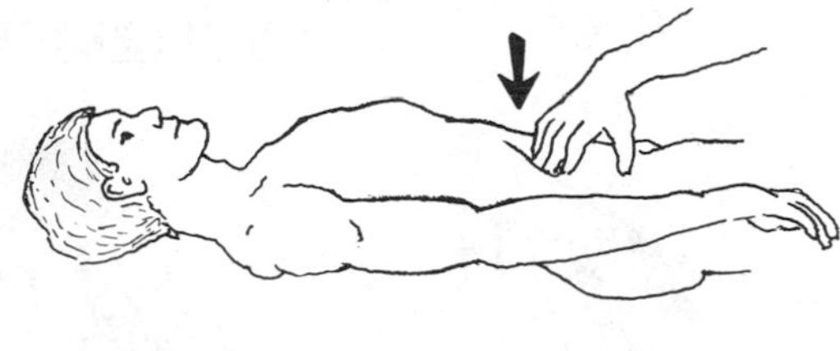

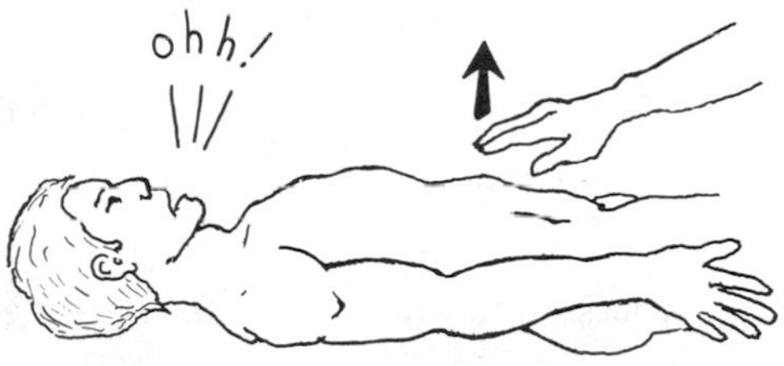

rebound test as shown in *WTND*

9. **Diagnosis.** Decide (if you can) which cause of the problem is most likely.

   It is important that the diagnosis not be considered a certainty, but rather a **strong probability based on all information and tests.** Be ready to reconsider the diagnosis whenever you get new information.

10. **Management or treatment.** Your decision to give treatment or to refer the person to a hospital or larger clinic will depend on:

    - how sure you are of the diagnosis,
    - how serious the problem seems, and
    - distance, economic considerations, personal factors, etc.

    Be sure to include **preventive information** and **health education** along with treatment, when appropriate.

11. **Results.** Carefully observe the results of management or treatment of the problem. If results are good, the diagnosis was probably correct.

12. **Repeat** the problem-solving process if treatment fails.

To make this diagnostic 'detective story' more real, the person pretending to be sick should supply a clinical history and test results typical for one of the possible causes of the woman's pain—gallbladder disease, for example. Then the students can actually follow the step-by-step method to diagnose her illness.

To clearly show the comparison between the *gualamo* jam story and the diagnosis, list the problem-solving steps of each on the blackboard (or on a mimeographed sheet). But please do not just copy the list below. Use one based on your group's suggestions. The steps may be fewer, more, or in a somewhat different order.

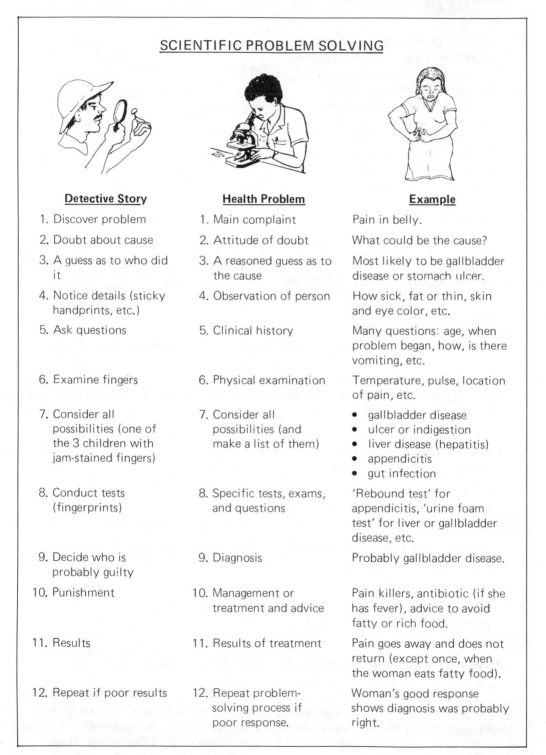

SCIENTIFIC PROBLEM SOLVING

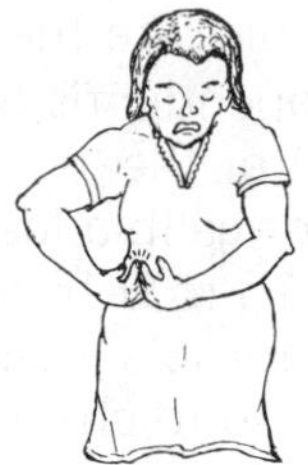

Detective Story	Health Problem	Example
1. Discover problem	1. Main complaint	Pain in belly.
2. Doubt about cause	2. Attitude of doubt	What could be the cause?
3. A guess as to who did it	3. A reasoned guess as to the cause	Most likely to be gallbladder disease or stomach ulcer.
4. Notice details (sticky handprints, etc.)	4. Observation of person	How sick, fat or thin, skin and eye color, etc.
5. Ask questions	5. Clinical history	Many questions: age, when problem began, how, is there vomiting, etc.
6. Examine fingers	6. Physical examination	Temperature, pulse, location of pain, etc.
7. Consider all possibilities (one of the 3 children with jam-stained fingers)	7. Consider all possibilities (and make a list of them)	• gallbladder disease • ulcer or indigestion • liver disease (hepatitis) • appendicitis • gut infection
8. Conduct tests (fingerprints)	8. Specific tests, exams, and questions	'Rebound test' for appendicitis, 'urine foam test' for liver or gallbladder disease, etc.
9. Decide who is probably guilty	9. Diagnosis	Probably gallbladder disease.
10. Punishment	10. Management or treatment and advice	Pain killers, antibiotic (if she has fever), advice to avoid fatty or rich food.
11. Results	11. Results of treatment	Pain goes away and does not return (except once, when the woman eats fatty food).
12. Repeat if poor results	12. Repeat problem-solving process if poor response.	Woman's good response shows diagnosis was probably right.

Follow-up to the two 'detective stories'

After the first class on scientific problem solving has been given, use every opportunity for students to try the new method. Several follow-up classes may also be helpful. The group can act out additional role plays to practice solving or diagnosing problems with the step-by-step approach.

Give special emphasis to step 7—**careful consideration of different possibilities.** Encourage students to make a habit of asking themselves, "What are all the possible causes of this problem?" Have them ask questions and do tests to find out which possibilities are most likely. **This process of systematically eliminating different possibilities is basic to the scientific method.**

Special emphasis should also be given to the importance of maintaining 'doubt throughout'. It is best to **never be absolutely sure** of a diagnosis; that would mean closing your mind to the possibility of error. The health worker should always be ready to consider new information and possibilities.

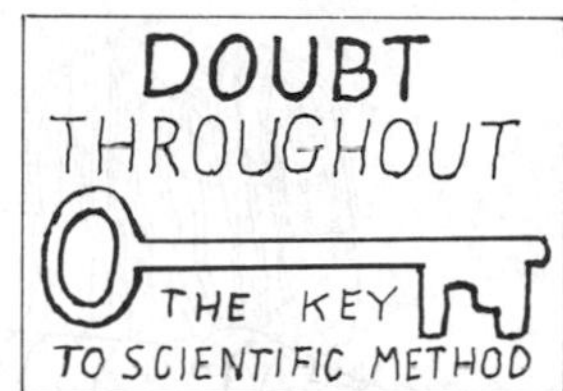
DOUBT
THROUGHOUT
THE KEY
TO SCIENTIFIC METHOD

Some of the best chances to practice step-by-step problem solving come during clinical practice and on home visits to sick persons. Instructors can reinforce the students' understanding and use of scientific method by making sure they **always follow the steps systematically.**

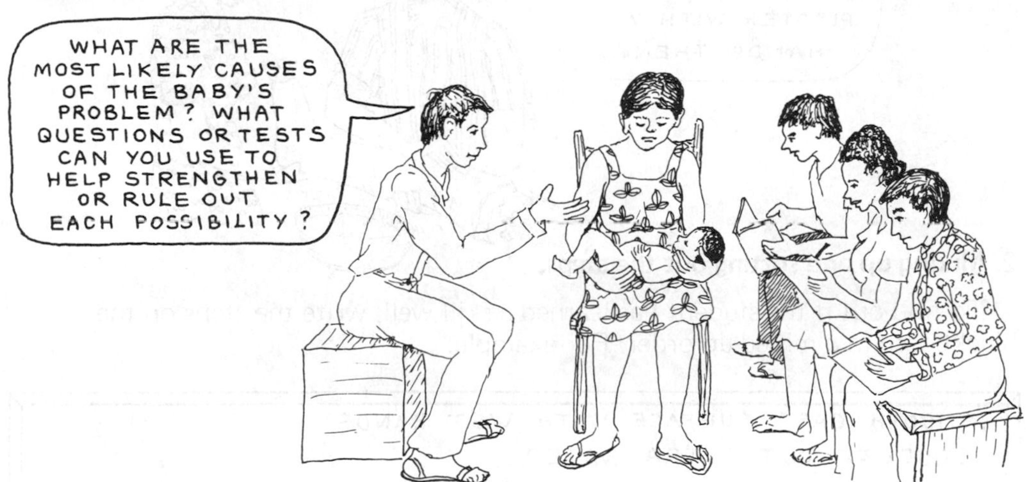
WHAT ARE THE MOST LIKELY CAUSES OF THE BABY'S PROBLEM? WHAT QUESTIONS OR TESTS CAN YOU USE TO HELP STRENGTHEN OR RULE OUT EACH POSSIBILITY?

The instructor can do much to help students develop a scientific approach to solving problems, both in clinical practice and in role plays. (See Chapter 21.)

The scientific approach to problem solving is especially important for diagnosing and treating health problems. But it has many other applications. If health workers are to help people find their own answers to the problems that most affect their lives, step-by-step problem solving is an essential tool.

For ideas on helping people analyze social problems, see Chapter 26.

SUGGESTIONS FOR HELPING STUDENTS LEARN STEP-BY-STEP SKILLS

Like scientific problem solving, many specific skills or procedures in health care involve a thoughtful, step-by-step approach. Here are suggestions for helping students learn such skills, and for testing to see if they have learned them well.

1. **I do and say—you do and say.**

First, show how to do it. As you demonstrate, **say what you are doing,** step by step.

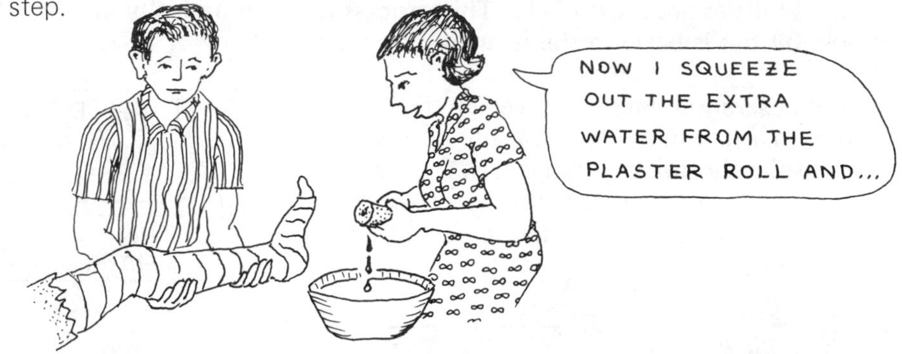

NOW I SQUEEZE OUT THE EXTRA WATER FROM THE PLASTER ROLL AND...

Then have the student do it. **Have the student also say each step as he does it.**

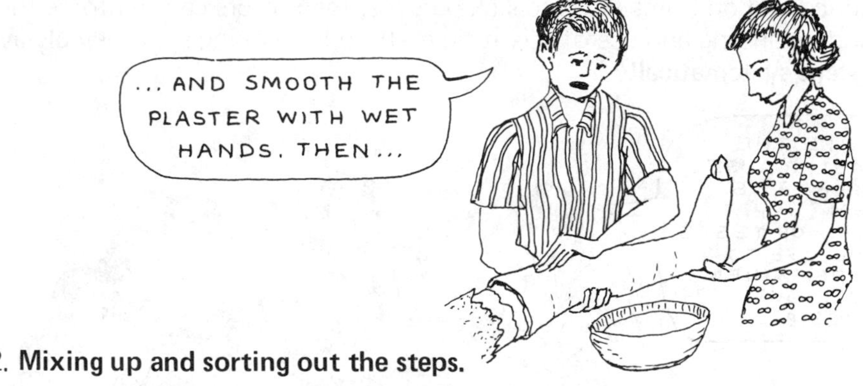

... AND SMOOTH THE PLASTER WITH WET HANDS. THEN...

2. **Mixing up and sorting out the steps.**

To find out if the student has learned a skill well, write the steps on the blackboard in a mixed-up order. For example:

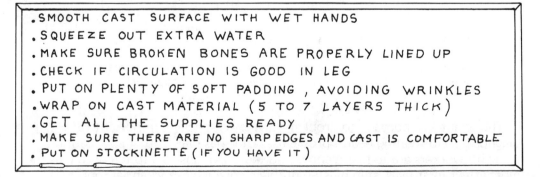

- SMOOTH CAST SURFACE WITH WET HANDS
- SQUEEZE OUT EXTRA WATER
- MAKE SURE BROKEN BONES ARE PROPERLY LINED UP
- CHECK IF CIRCULATION IS GOOD IN LEG
- PUT ON PLENTY OF SOFT PADDING, AVOIDING WRINKLES
- WRAP ON CAST MATERIAL (5 TO 7 LAYERS THICK)
- GET ALL THE SUPPLIES READY
- MAKE SURE THERE ARE NO SHARP EDGES AND CAST IS COMFORTABLE
- PUT ON STOCKINETTE (IF YOU HAVE IT)

Then ask the student to number the steps in the right order. If he can do it correctly, he probably has learned well (although more practice may still be needed).

RECOGNIZING THE HUMAN LIMITATIONS OF SCIENCE

Many people think that scientific knowledge is exact. But much of it is not. Some of what scientists and experts 'know' to be true today, in a few months or years will prove to be false. As our knowledge grows, it changes.

Especially in the science of nutrition, changes in knowledge have been rapid. This can be confusing both for health workers and for those whom they advise.

For example, a few years ago nutritionists placed strong emphasis on giving poorly nourished children more protein. Now we know that most underweight children need more high-energy food rather than more protein. The small amount of protein in their normal diet is usually enough, provided they get plenty of high-energy foods. (See p. **25**-40.)

An angry health worker in Africa complained, "First you told us that our traditional diet, high in energy foods, was not healthy for our children, that they needed more meat and eggs and fish. So we tried to change the traditional diet. Now you tell us what children really need most is more energy foods! What next?!"

Confusion also results when advice that works well in one part of the world is carried elsewhere. For example, some health programs advise giving orange juice to babies as young as 2 months. However, this advice comes from rich countries where many babies drink boiled or ***pasteurized*** cow's milk. Boiling destroys vitamin C; the orange juice replaces it. But in poor countries where breast feeding is more common, babies get enough vitamin C from breast milk. For these babies, orange juice at 2 months can do more harm than good. Because it is hard to keep it clean when preparing it, orange juice can actually increase the risk of infection. So now we advise mothers to **give babies nothing except breast milk during the first 4 months.**

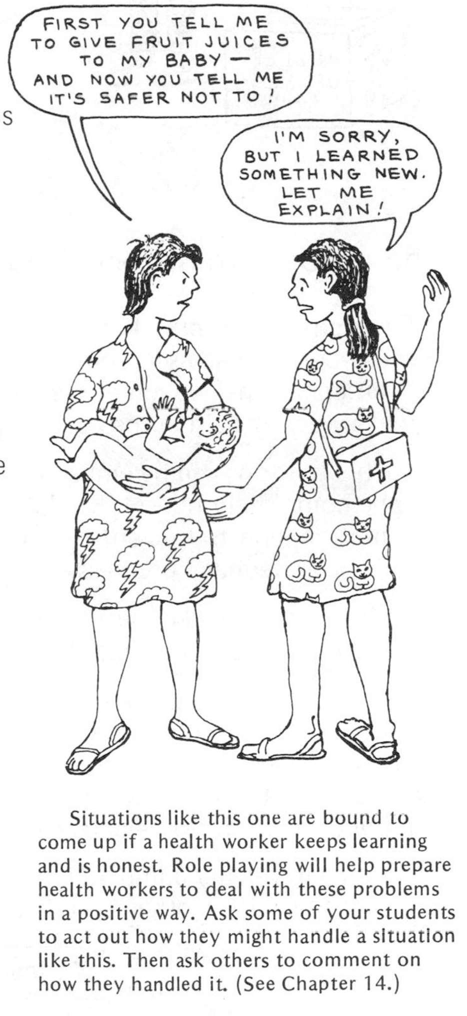

Situations like this one are bound to come up if a health worker keeps learning and is honest. Role playing will help prepare health workers to deal with these problems in a positive way. Ask some of your students to act out how they might handle a situation like this. Then ask others to comment on how they handled it. (See Chapter 14.)

Every area has examples of advice that later proved inappropriate or was suddenly changed by experts or advisers. Look for local examples and discuss these with fellow instructors and health workers.

It is important that health workers learn how to approach problem solving scientifically. But it is equally important that they recognize and help others to see the human limitations of science. What is 'right' today may be 'wrong' tomorrow.

To make the most of new 'scientific' approaches, it is important that instructors, health workers, and the people they work with learn to:

- Question advice or instructions that come from outside the area (and also advice that comes from inside).
- Try to understand the reasons behind the advice given.
- Modify advice or instructions to fit the local situation.
- When teaching or advising others, admit it openly if you find that advice you have given is wrong or needs to be changed.

It is essential for health workers to develop a critical, questioning attitude—especially when it comes to advice from outsiders.

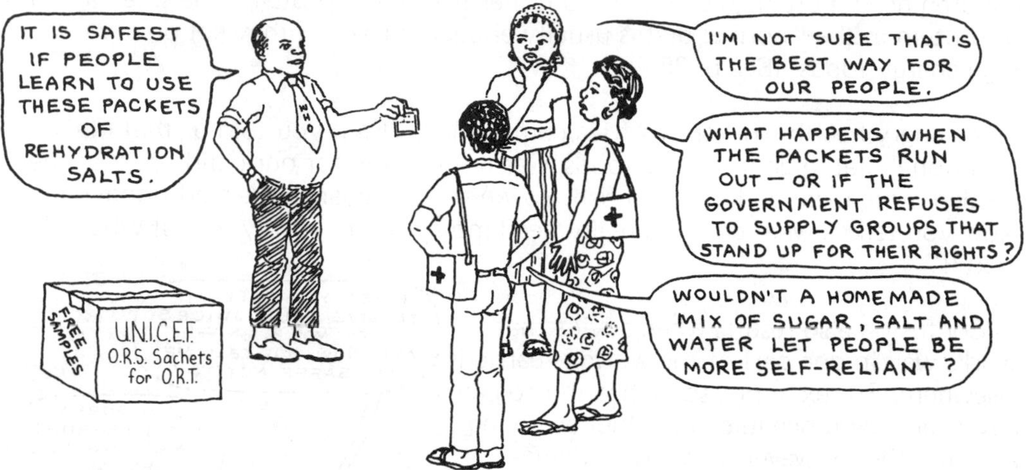
IT IS SAFEST IF PEOPLE LEARN TO USE THESE PACKETS OF REHYDRATION SALTS.
WHO
I'M NOT SURE THAT'S THE BEST WAY FOR OUR PEOPLE.
WHAT HAPPENS WHEN THE PACKETS RUN OUT — OR IF THE GOVERNMENT REFUSES TO SUPPLY GROUPS THAT STAND UP FOR THEIR RIGHTS?
WOULDN'T A HOMEMADE MIX OF SUGAR, SALT AND WATER LET PEOPLE BE MORE SELF-RELIANT?
FREE SAMPLES
U.N.I.C.E.F.
O.R.S. Sachets for O.R.T.

The need to be honest about mistakes and changes in knowledge

Everyone makes mistakes, including experts, instructors, and health workers. Because our own advisers sometimes change their minds about certain health recommendations, we sometimes find ourselves giving advice that is the opposite of what we have said in the past.

Such situations can be embarrassing. But usually the easiest way to handle them is to be completely honest. Explain to people that you have received new information, and that scientific knowledge is continually growing and changing. That is how we make progress.

By being open and honest about mistakes and changes in knowledge, you as an instructor can set an example for the student health workers.

There is another important reason for discussing changes in scientific knowledge with health workers during training. It helps take some of the magic out of what we teach and are taught. It helps us all to weigh everything new we are told against our own experience. This can be one of the most basic lessons health workers can learn—and teach!

Practice in openly admitting mistakes and explaining changes in advice should be a part of health worker training.

To learn is to question.

CHAPTER 18

Learning to Use Medicines Sensibly

Helping health workers learn to use medicines wisely is not easy. But this is not because the knowledge and skills needed are difficult. It is because the misuse and overuse of medicines is so common—among doctors and among people in general.

Even in wealthy countries, where there are stricter controls on the marketing and use of medications, **studies show that a great many doctors consistently misuse medicines.** Either they prescribe too many, give the wrong medicines for certain illnesses, or recommend expensive medicines when cheaper ones would work as well.

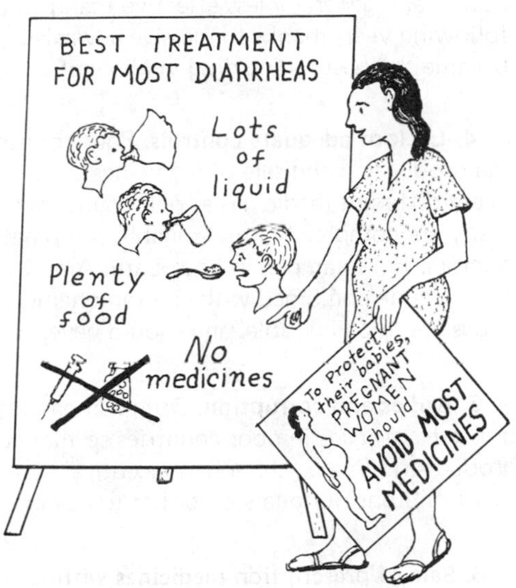

Because the overuse of medicine is such a big problem in many areas, health workers should place great emphasis on when <u>not</u> to use medicines.

Misprescribing of antibiotics is an especially common problem (see Chapter 19). For example, a study in the United States showed that up to 70% of doctors' prescriptions for tetracycline were for treating the common cold—for which no antibiotic does any good! (See *WTND,* p. 163 and 353.) In poorer countries, the misuse—and overuse—of medicines tends to be even greater.

SOME REASONS FOR THE WIDESPREAD MISUSE AND OVERUSE OF MEDICINES:

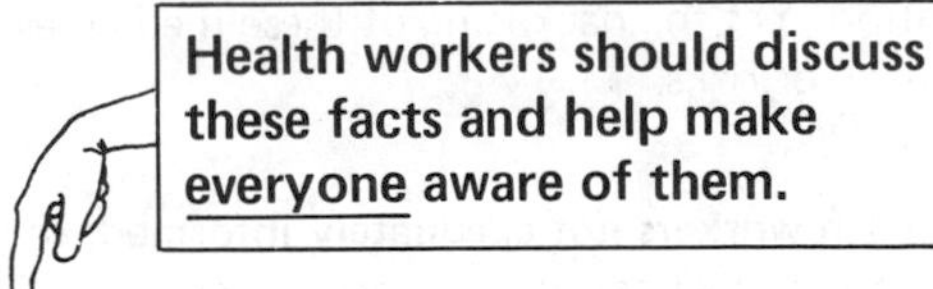

Health workers should discuss these facts and help make <u>everyone</u> aware of them.

1. Big business. The production and marketing of modern medicines is one of the biggest, most profitable businesses in the world. Drug companies are continually inventing new products to increase their sales and profits. Some of these medicines are useful. But **at least 90% of medicines on the market today are unnecessary.** Doctors prescribe them, and people buy them, because the drug companies spend millions on advertising.

2. False advertising. Especially in poor countries, much of the advertising, and even the information published in 'pharmaceutical indexes', is misleading or false. Information on dangerous side effects is often not included. Risky medicines are frequently recommended for illnesses less dangerous than the medicines. (For example, chloramphenicol has often been advertised as a treatment for minor diarrhea and respiratory infections—see *WTND,* p. 50.)

3. 'Dumping'. Drug companies in wealthy countries sometimes produce medicines that do not sell well in their homelands. Or the use of certain medicines is restricted or prohibited because they have been proved unsafe. It is a common practice for drug companies to 'dump' these medicines on poor countries—often with a great deal of false advertising. For example, several years ago the U.S. government restricted the use of ***Lincocin*** (lincomycin) because it proved more dangerous, more costly, and generally less effective than penicillin. The following year, thanks to massive advertising, ***Lincocin*** became the best selling drug in Mexico!

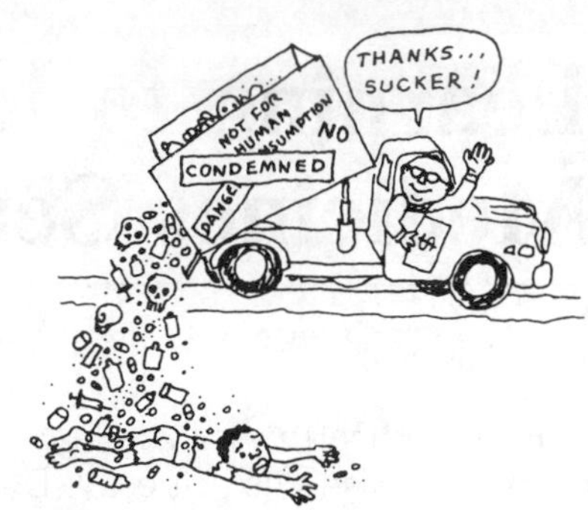

4. Lack of adequate controls. Poor countries, especially, have inadequate laws controlling the production and sale of medicines. As a result, many poor countries sell up to 3 times as many different medicines as rich countries do. Most of these medicines are a waste of money. Many are completely unreasonable combinations of drugs, yet they are widely prescribed by doctors. For example, in both Latin America and Asia, a popular injectable medicine is tetracycline combined with chloramphenicol. This is a senseless combination because the two drugs are 'incompatible' and should never be used together (see p. **19**-5).

5. Bribes and corruption. Drug companies in rich countries pay millions in bribes to officials in poor countries so that governments will buy their products. (A major U.S. pharmaceutical company recently admitted to having spent millions of dollars on bribes to advance its products in poor countries.)

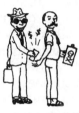

6. Sale of prescription medicines without prescriptions. This is common in many countries (partly because poor people cannot afford doctors' fees). Most people who 'self-medicate' try to use the medicines well, so they follow the patterns set by doctors. Unfortunately, this often leads to incorrect use. For example, in Latin America at least 95% of doctors' prescriptions for Vitamin B_{12} are incorrect and wasteful. Because villagers follow the doctors' example, vitamin B_{12} injections are among the most widely used self-prescribed medicines in Latin America—at a cost of millions to a people too poor to eat well!

7. People not adequately informed. Neither doctors nor the people are adequately informed about the correct use of medicines. Most doctors rely on the information given in misleading 'blurbs' supplied with sample medicines, while villagers who self-prescribe often receive no information at all. In Mexico, for example, up to 70% of prescription drugs are sold without prescription. Yet the packaging of these medicines generally contains no information about use, dosage, or risks.

8. Health workers not adequately informed. In spite of the tremendous amount of self-medication in most countries, many programs still do not teach health workers much about the use—or misuse—of commonly self-prescribed medicines. As a result, many health workers, to meet popular demand, secretly purchase and administer a wide range of medicines they know little about.

For more information on the unethical promotion of medicines and their abuse in developing countries, see: ***Pills, Profits and Politics,*** Philip Lee and Milton Silverman, and ***The Drugging of the Americas,*** Milton Silverman, University of California Press, Berkeley, California, USA; ***Hungry for Profits,*** Robert J. Ledogar, Corporate Interfaith Council, New York, USA; ***Who Needs the Drug Companies,*** a Haslemere Group, War on Want, and Third World First publication; and ***Poor Health, Rich Profits: Multinational Drug Companies and the Third World,*** Tom Heller, Spokesman Books, Nottingham, England.

9. Use of medicine to gain prestige and power. Another reason for medicine overuse is that many professionals use their ability to medicate as a sort of magic to make people grateful and dependent. This way they gain special privilege and power. In the same way, health workers may be tempted to give injections or expensive drugs when home remedies or kindly advice would cost less and do more good.

"ONLY I CAN CURE YOUR CHILD."

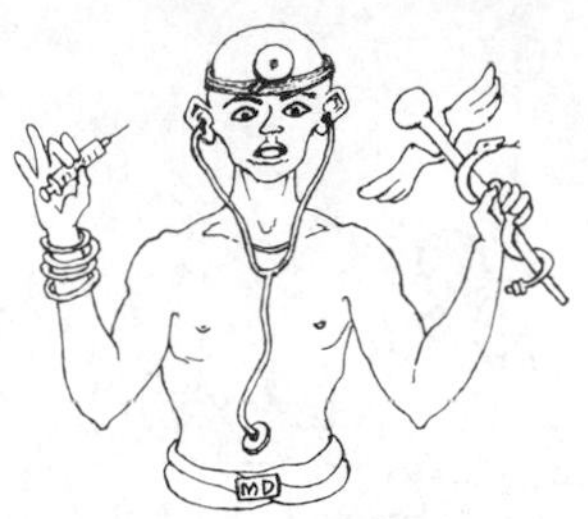

Modern healers, like witch doctors, too often use their medicines to gain power and create dependency.

Medication as a substitute for caring

Perhaps the biggest reason for overuse of medicines, however, is that doctors and health workers often find it easier to hand out medicine than to give the time and personal attention that people need.

About 4 out of 5 illnesses are *self-limiting.* This means people get well whether they take medicine or not. **Most health problems can be better managed without any medication. What often will help people most is friendly advice and understanding support.** (See Healing Without Medicines, *WTND,* p. 45.)

However, many doctors and health workers get into the habit of giving everyone medicine—for any and every problem they have. The less curable the problem, the more medicines they give!

At the same time, people have come to expect medicine every time they visit a doctor or health worker. They like to believe that "there is a medicine for everything." They are disappointed if the doctor or health worker does not give them any, even when medicines will do no good and the health worker carefully explains why.

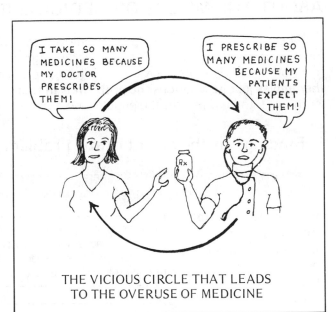

I TAKE SO MANY MEDICINES BECAUSE MY DOCTOR PRESCRIBES THEM!

I PRESCRIBE SO MANY MEDICINES BECAUSE MY PATIENTS EXPECT THEM!

Rx

THE VICIOUS CIRCLE THAT LEADS TO THE OVERUSE OF MEDICINE

So a 'vicious circle' results in which the doctor always gives medicine because the 'patient' always expects (or demands) it, because the doctor always gives it. **The prescribing of a medicine becomes both the symbol and the substitute for human caring.** This problem is especially common in places where doctors, nurses, and health workers are overworked. The result is not only a costly overuse of medicine, but a failure to meet human needs on human terms.

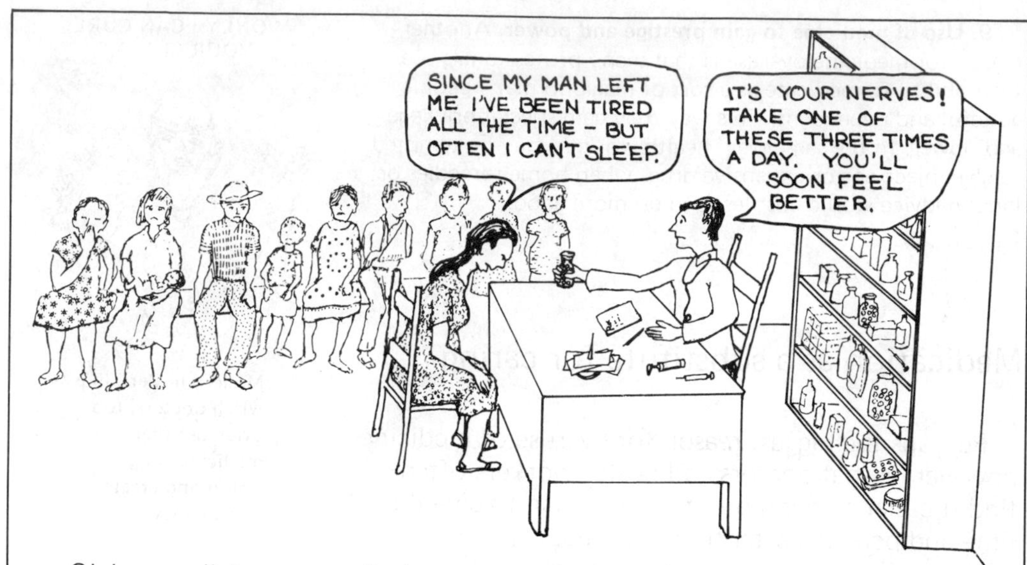
SINCE MY MAN LEFT ME I'VE BEEN TIRED ALL THE TIME – BUT OFTEN I CAN'T SLEEP.
IT'S YOUR NERVES! TAKE ONE OF THESE THREE TIMES A DAY. YOU'LL SOON FEEL BETTER.

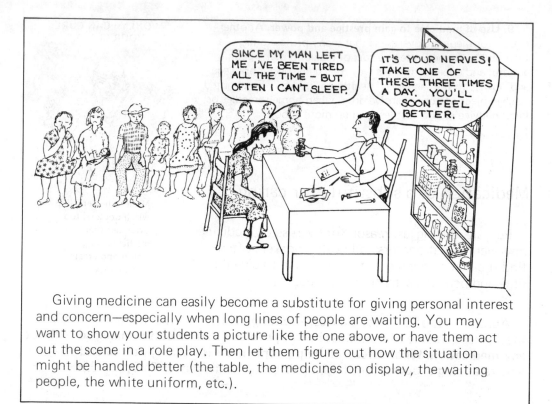

Giving medicine can easily become a substitute for giving personal interest and concern—especially when long lines of people are waiting. You may want to show your students a picture like the one above, or have them act out the scene in a role play. Then let them figure out how the situation might be handled better (the table, the medicines on display, the waiting people, the white uniform, etc.).

HELPING HEALTH WORKERS LEARN ABOUT THE MISUSE OF MEDICINE IN THEIR AREA

If health workers are to help stop the overuse and misuse of medicines, they must understand the problem clearly and recognize its cost to human health. But it is not enough simply to give them information. **They need to find out for themselves just how serious the problem is in their own area.** And they need to learn ways to help inform the people who come to them 'for medicine'.

1. Finding out the extent of the problem

Perhaps you can help health workers to compare their own experiences or take simple surveys. They can investigate questions like these:

How many prescription medicines do people in the community buy and use without a prescription?

In Mexico, a group of health workers-in-training made a survey in 5 pharmacies in a nearby city. They found that nearly 80% of prescription drugs were sold without prescription. Perhaps your students can conduct a similar survey.

How often do doctors prescribe too many medicines or the wrong medicine?

Often people come to a health center with prescriptions from doctors in other places. With the help of instructors, students can keep a record of how many prescriptions appear to be incorrect or overdone. (For most health problems, 1 or 2 medicines are enough.)

What evidence is there of physical harm caused to people by overuse or misuse of medicines?

Students can keep a record of problems—such as diarrhea or 'thrush'—caused by overuse of antibiotics, abscesses caused by unnecessary injections, deaths or harm to women and babies that may have been caused by medicines injected to speed up birth, etc.

What evidence is there of economic harm to people caused by the overuse and misuse of medicine?

Students can try to find out how much poor families spend on health care and medicines (both traditional and modern). Then try to estimate how much of this is spent on useless or harmful treatments. Is it worth it? Could health be improved if the money were spent differently?

How often do health workers, doctors, or instructors in the health center appear to give medicine simply to please people—not because it is necessary?

We all do it sometimes. Admit it! Discuss it. Is it ever right to give medicine when it is not needed? How does doing this create false beliefs, dependency, and mystification of medicine?

Many programs give out colorful cough syrup and anti-diarrhea medicine, both of which are unnecessary, in order to attract mothers to the under-fives clinic. Is this wise?

2. Looking at the causes of local misuse of medicines

The larger causes—national, international, commercial, and professional—are mostly out of the health workers' control. Yet health workers need to be aware of these causes and discuss how they affect the overuse and misuse of medicines in their own communities. Helping people become aware of the high profits and dishonesty of the medicine business may lead them to more careful and critical use.

The more immediate personal causes of misuse and overuse of medicines are things health workers can do more about.

Perhaps the biggest personal cause of medicine misuse by health workers is 'popular demand'. We know of health workers who feel they have to give at least 2 or 3 pills to every 'patient'—no matter what his problem. As a result, these health workers regularly use up their monthly supplies of chloroquine (for malaria) and sulfa in the first week or so. This means that many people who really need those medicines must go without!

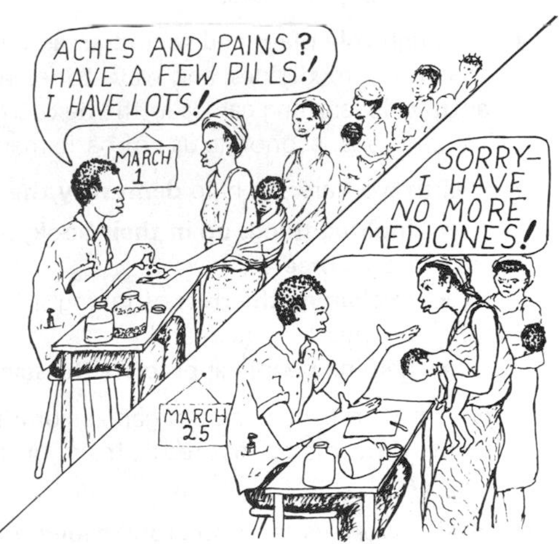
ACHES AND PAINS? HAVE A FEW PILLS! I HAVE LOTS!
MARCH 1
SORRY— I HAVE NO MORE MEDICINES!
MARCH 25

Overuse of medicines, where the supply is limited, causes increased illness and death.

Health workers need to look at these things carefully. Student health workers may not realize how great the temptation can be to give medicine needlessly. It helps to **invite experienced health workers to talk with those in training about the difficulties and obstacles they have run into.**

ONE OF THE HARDEST SITUATIONS I HAVE TO HANDLE IS WHEN A MOTHER BRINGS IN HER CHILD WITH A COLD AND INSISTS I INJECT HIM. I TRY TO EXPLAIN THAT IT WON'T DO ANY GOOD AND MAY HARM HIM. BUT THE MOTHER THINKS I JUST DON'T CARE ENOUGH ABOUT HER CHILD. I TRY MY BEST, BUT I FEEL I LOSE THE TRUST OF A LOT OF MOTHERS.
BUT I BET YOU WIN THE TRUST OF A LOT OF CHILDREN!

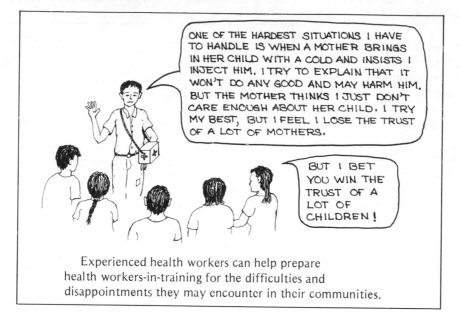

Experienced health workers can help prepare health workers-in-training for the difficulties and disappointments they may encounter in their communities.

3. Trying to solve the problem

During training, a number of steps can be taken to discourage the misuse and overuse of medicines:

- **Set a good example.** Program doctors, nurses, and instructors, when attending the sick, should take great care to use medicines only when needed. Encourage the use of helpful home remedies. Whenever anyone gives medicine as a substitute for caring, point this out and discuss it in class.
- Through **role plays and sociodramas,** students can explore the pressures and temptations to overuse medicines, and ways to resist them. **Imaginative teaching aids** (such as the antibiotic learning games in the next chapter) also help health workers discover the need for cautious, economic use of basic medicines.
- Health workers can help **demystify the use of modern medicine** by . . .
    - **looking things up in their book,** together with the sick person's family (see p. **Part Three**-4),
    - **explaining the risks** of taking specific medicines—especially for children and pregnant women, and
    - helping people **appreciate the scientific value of useful home remedies** (see Ch. 7).
- Health workers can help organize community groups to perform **short skits or plays** showing problems that result from local misuse of medicines (see examples on pages **27**-3 and **27**-14).
- Health workers can **visit storekeepers who sell medicines.** Help them learn more about these products. Encourage them not to sell harmful or overpriced medicines, to explain uses, dosages, and risks, and to suggest that people buy nutritious foods rather than costly vitamins, cold formulas, and cough syrups.
- **Help people to become aware of how much they spend on medicines and why, and to look for low-cost alternatives.** (For example, see *Where There Is No Doctor,* p. 46, Healing with Water.)

Health care as a cause of poor health—and what to do about it

An example from the Philippines:

In August, 1981, the authors and 4 village health workers from Central America visited the Philippines to exchange ideas with health workers there. On the edge of the city of Tacloban, we watched workers from the Makapawa Health Program and local mothers prepare an herbal cough syrup from ginger, tamarind leaves, bitter orange, and brown sugar. There was something exciting (almost magical—but not secret) about this process. Everyone took part. Men and children gathered dried palm fronds for the fire. Women stirred the boiling pot. Suddenly, as predicted, the dark brew changed into a fluffy white powder, double in volume. Finally, the bitter orange juice was added—after cooling, in order to protect the vitamin C.

This cough syrup—based on traditional herbal remedies—is now widely used in the area as a 'cure-all' for colds, coughs, stomach distress, and many minor problems. It is a useful, low-cost home remedy that prevents people from wasting so much money on commercial medicines. The health workers have also taught local families to prepare an herbal 'ABC Drink' (rehydration drink) for children with diarrhea. At the same time, they have helped people to learn about the misleading advertising of drug companies. As a result, families now spend less on doctors and costly medicines, and fewer children die.

Only when we sat down to talk with those present did we realize the impact on health of these inexpensive home remedies. The families told us the main problems affecting their health were **diarrhea, poor nutrition,** and **low wages.** But the health workers reported that far fewer children in the area are underweight today than when the program started 2 years ago. When we asked why, the health workers said it might be the nutrition education for mothers during the 'under-six' clinics. But the mothers said they had heard it all before—that the main reason for their children's hunger had been lack of money. Yet today's wages are as low as ever. So why has health improved?

We asked the mothers how much their families are now spending on health care—herbal remedies, modern medicines, travel to doctors, etc. The average turned out to be from 10% to 12% of their year's earnings. (This seemed remarkably low in comparison to Africa and Latin America, where poor families we have asked often figure they spend from 30% to 50% of their year's earnings on health care.) Then one mother said, "We don't spend nearly as much now as we used to." So we asked everyone what they used to spend on health care before the program was begun. The average worked out to be between 40% and 60% of people's earnings! The hungry children were always getting sick. So their families would spend money on a witch doctor, then on tonics and cough syrups, and finally on expensive trips to city doctors and hospitals. And sometimes on a funeral. Often they had gone into debt and fallen prey to 'loan sharks'. If their children recovered, they had no money left to feed them well, so the children soon fell ill again. **Costly health care had become a main cause of poor health!**

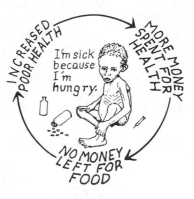

Vicious cycle of health care causing poor health

But today, thanks to the homemade herbal medicines and community organization to fight the 'loan sharks', the poor people's economy has improved. Spending less on health care, they can spend more on food for their children. The vicious cycle (of health care causing poor health) has been broken.

PAGES IN *WHERE THERE IS NO DOCTOR* THAT DISCUSS THE MISUSE, OVERUSE, AND CAREFUL USE OF MEDICINES

page

w18 to w19 . . . Sensible and limited use of medicines

45 to 48 . . . **Chapter 5,** Healing without medicines

49 to 53 . . . **Chapter 6,** Right and wrong uses of medicines, especially:
- 49 . . . . . Guidelines for the use of medicine
- 50 to 52 . . . . . The most dangerous misuse of medicine
- 53 . . . . . When should medicine not be taken?

55 to 58 . . . **Chapter 7,** Antibiotics: what they are and how to use them, especially:
- 56 . . . . . Guidelines for the use of all antibiotics
- 56 to 57 . . . . . Guidelines for the use of certain antibiotics
- 58 . . . . . Importance of limited use of antibiotics

59 to 64 . . . **Chapter 8,** How to measure and give medicine

65 to 73 . . . **Chapter 9,** Instructions and precautions for injections, especially:
- 65 . . . . . When to inject and when not to
- 65 . . . . . What to do when the doctor prescribes injections
- 67 . . . . . Medicines not to inject
- 68 to 69 . . . . . Risks and precautions
- 70 . . . . . Dangerous reactions from injecting certain medicines
- 71 . . . . . How to avoid serious reactions to a penicillin injection

119 . . . Where to get vitamins: in pills, injections, syrups—or in foods?
156 . . . Medicines not to use for diarrhea
247 . . . How to stay healthy during pregnancy—avoid taking medicines
266 . . . The correct use of oxytocics: ergonovine, oxytocin, *Pitocin,* etc.
272 . . . Care in giving medicines to the newborn
288 . . . Who should not take birth control pills?
338 . . . Words to the village storekeeper or pharmacist
Green Pages . . . Risks and precautions for each medicine are listed.

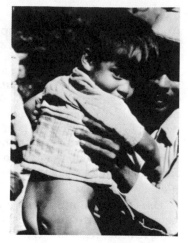

Boy with abscess from an unnecessary injection.

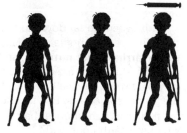

Today 1 of every 3 cases of crippling polio is caused by injections given to children. These children already have mild, undiagnosed polio, which is often mistaken for a severe cold. The injected medicine irritates the surrounding muscles, and can cause paralysis in the arm or leg.

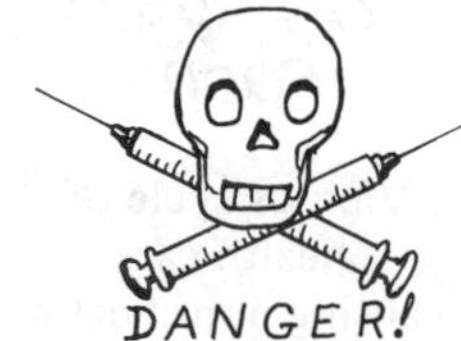

REMEMBER: Teaching health workers to help people use medications sensibly is a vital part of preventive medicine.

ANOTHER PROBLEM: USING THE WRONG DOSAGE

In addition to the problem of medicines being used when they are not needed, it is a common mistake to use the wrong dosage. Using too little medicine may make treatment ineffective, and increase the resistance of infections to the medicine. Using too much may cause serious side effects, especially in small babies and children. Their bodies often cannot tolerate more than the recommended amount.

Mistakes in dosage are common for several reasons: In many countries, dosage information is not included with each medicine sold in the pharmacies. A person may hear about a medicine from a friend or neighbor, and give the adult dose used by the friend to a small child. Sometimes a person forgets what his doctor or pharmacist said about how much medicine to take and how often. Or perhaps the doctor or health worker does not explain the dosage clearly, or writes it in **handwriting that is impossible to read.** Maybe the sick person cannot read well. And even if he or she tries to look up the dosage in a 'pharmaceutical index', **the big medical words are hard to understand.**

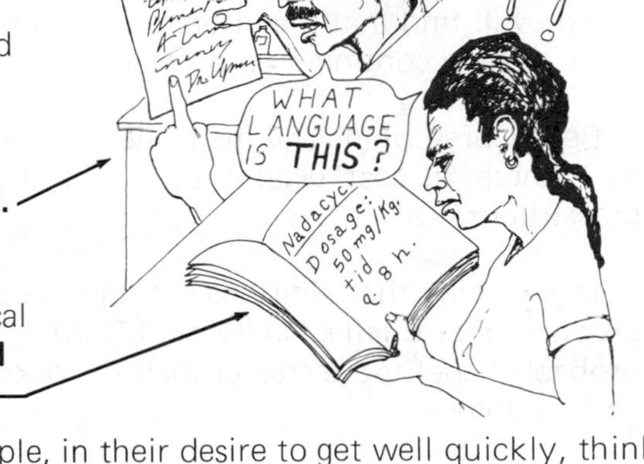
PHARMACY
PRESCRIPTION
WHAT LANGUAGE IS THIS?
Dosage: 50 mg/Kg. tid q 8 h.

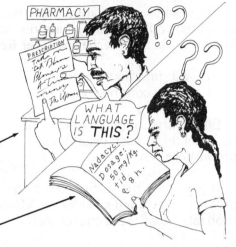

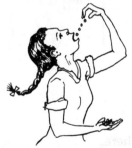

Some sick people, in their desire to get well quickly, think that, "If one pill is good, more are better." So they take 2 or 3 pills (or spoonfuls or injections) when only one is recommended.

In other cases, sick persons cannot afford to buy a full prescription of a costly medicine. So they buy only a part, and take less than is needed.

Health workers, too, may make mistakes if they lack practice in looking up dosages and explaining them carefully. During training it is important that they learn to use the correct dosage for any medicine that they might be recommending. The health program can make this easier by taking some basic precautions:

- **Decide on a short list of basic medicines** that can effectively deal with the everyday problems and serious emergencies that are common in the area. This way health workers are not burdened with too wide a range of medicines, or the temptation to prescribe something for every problem. For a list of basic medicines needed in rural areas, see *WTND,* p. 334 to 337.
- **Always provide each medicine in the same standard strength.** This saves health workers from having to deal with the same medicine in 250 mg. capsules one week, 500 mg. capsules the next week, and 125 mg. spoonfuls after that. Avoid accepting a wide assortment of donated sample medicines.
- **Teach health workers (through example and practice) to look up dosages** in a book like *Where There Is No Doctor* or *Primary Child Care,* each time they use or recommend a medicine.

Learning to look up medicine dosages

In *Where There Is No Doctor* it is easy to find the uses, dosage, and precautions for most basic medicines. Look in the **Green Pages.**

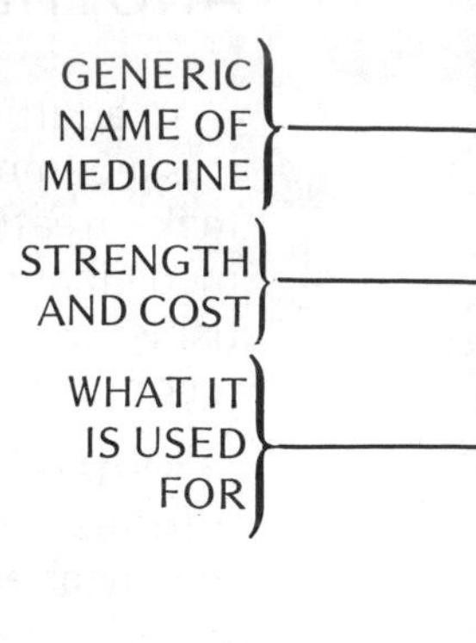

To find the medicine you are looking for, check the List of Medicines (*WTND,* p. 341) or the Index of Medicines (*WTND,* p. 345). These lists show which pages have information about each medicine.

For example, pretend that Mrs. Babalama has asked you about the correct dosage of **aspirin** for her **4-year-old son,** Edafi. He has a **headache and fever from a cold.**

You will find that the information about aspirin begins on page 365 and continues on page 366.

Before prescribing any medicine, read all about it. Find out its strength, its cost, what it is used for, its risks and precautions.

If you think that aspirin is the right medicine for the problem, that Edafi's family can afford it, and that the probable benefits are greater than the risks, then look for the correct dosage.

Make sure that the dosage listed is for the problem you want to treat. (Some medicines have more than one use, and different dosages for different uses. For example, see the dosage of aspirin for severe arthritis or rheumatic fever.)

Now check the strength of the aspirin you have.

ASPIRIN 300 mg. (5 grain)

If you have 300 mg. (5 grain) tablets, read here.

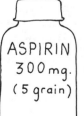

How often the boy should take the medicine.

How much he should take each time.

½ tablet

CHILDREN'S ASPIRIN 75 mg.

If you have 75 mg. 'children's aspirin', read here.

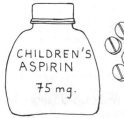

How often he should take the medicine.

How much he should take each time.

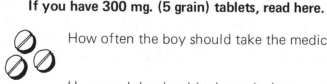

2 to 3 tablets

from *WTND,* pages 379 and 380

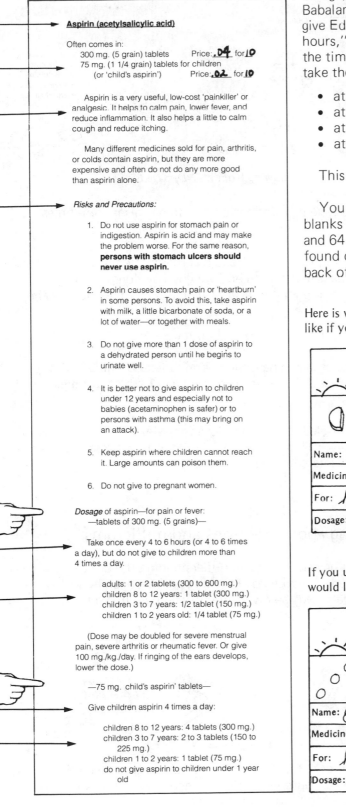

Aspirin (acetylsalicylic acid)

Often comes in:
300 mg. (5 grain) tablets Price: .04 for 10
75 mg. (1 1/4 grain) tablets for children (or 'child's aspirin') Price: .02 for 10

Aspirin is a very useful, low-cost 'painkiller' or analgesic. It helps to calm pain, lower fever, and reduce inflammation. It also helps a little to calm cough and reduce itching.

Many different medicines sold for pain, arthritis, or colds contain aspirin, but they are more expensive and often do not do any more good than aspirin alone.

Risks and Precautions:

1. Do not use aspirin for stomach pain or indigestion. Aspirin is acid and may make the problem worse. For the same reason, **persons with stomach ulcers should never use aspirin.**
2. Aspirin causes stomach pain or 'heartburn' in some persons. To avoid this, take aspirin with milk, a little bicarbonate of soda, or a lot of water—or together with meals.
3. Do not give more than 1 dose of aspirin to a dehydrated person until he begins to urinate well.
4. It is better not to give aspirin to children under 12 years and especially not to babies (acetaminophen is safer) or to persons with asthma (this may bring on an attack).
5. Keep aspirin where children cannot reach it. Large amounts can poison them.
6. Do not give to pregnant women.

Dosage of aspirin—for pain or fever:
—tablets of 300 mg. (5 grains)—

Take once every 4 to 6 hours (or 4 to 6 times a day), but do not give to children more than 4 times a day.

adults: 1 or 2 tablets (300 to 600 mg.)
children 8 to 12 years: 1 tablet (300 mg.)
children 3 to 7 years: 1/2 tablet (150 mg.)
children 1 to 2 years old: 1/4 tablet (75 mg.)

(Dose may be doubled for severe menstrual pain, severe arthritis or rheumatic fever. Or give 100 mg./kg./day. If ringing of the ears develops, lower the dose.)

—75 mg. child's aspirin' tablets—

Give children aspirin 4 times a day:

children 8 to 12 years: 4 tablets (300 mg.)
children 3 to 7 years: 2 to 3 tablets (150 to 225 mg.)
children 1 to 2 years: 1 tablet (75 mg.)
do not give aspirin to children under 1 year old

Once you have found the correct dosage, explain it carefully to Mrs. Babalama. Instead of telling her to give Edafi the medicine "every 4 to 6 hours," it may be better to tell her the times of day when Edafi should take the aspirin:

- at sunrise
- at noon
- at sunset
- at night, before going to sleep

This is about every 6 hours.

You may want to use the dosage blanks that are explained on pages 63 and 64 of ***WTND.*** Extra copies can be found on the last yellow page in the back of the book.

Here is what Edafi's dosage blank would look like if you used 300 mg. tablets.

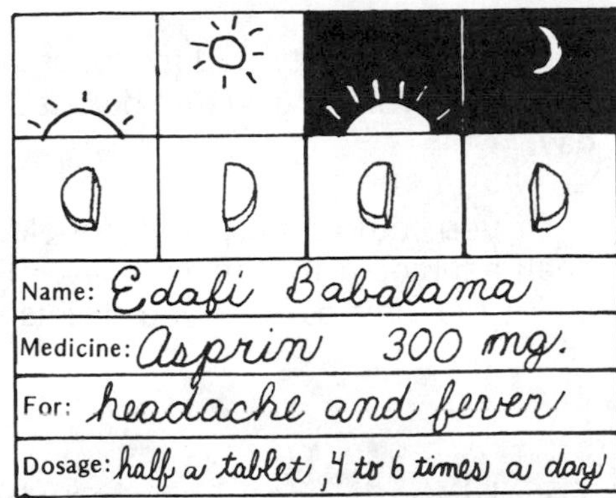

Name: Edafi Babalama
Medicine: Child's asprin 75mg.
Medicine: Asprin 300 mg.
For: headache and fever
Dosage: 2 or 3 tablets, 4 times a day
Dosage: half a tablet, 4 to 6 times a day

If you used 75 mg. 'children's aspirin', it would look like this.

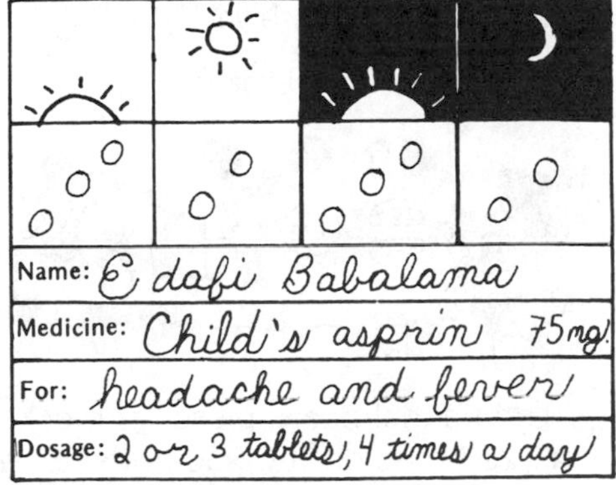

Calculating the dosage

In the **Green Pages** of ***Where There Is No Doctor,*** most of the dosage instructions are given according to age—so that children get smaller doses than adults.

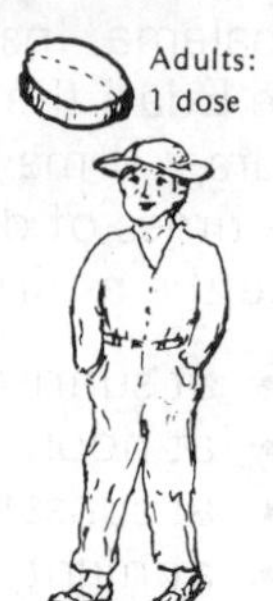
Adults:
1 dose

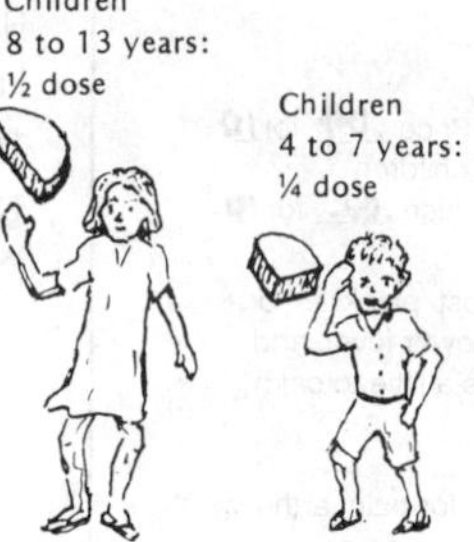
Children
8 to 13 years:
½ dose
Children
4 to 7 years:
¼ dose

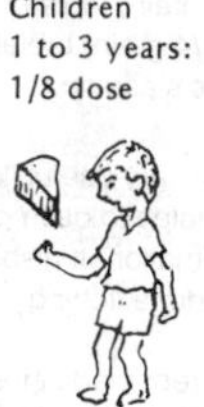
Children
1 to 3 years:
1/8 dose

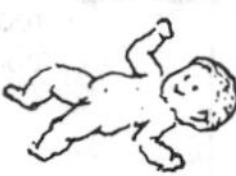
Give a child
under 1 year
old the dose
for a child of
1 year, but ask
medical advice
when possible.

drawing from *WTND,* page 62

However, it is sometimes more accurate to determine dosage according to a person's weight. Information for doing this is sometimes included in parentheses ( ) for health workers who have scales.

For example, suppose Mrs. Abu's daughter Irene has rheumatic fever. What dose of aspirin should she take? Irene is 4 years old and weighs 15 kilograms. The recommended dose of aspirin for rheumatic fever is 100 mg./kg./day—double the normal dose.

Multiply 100 mg. x 15 = 1500 mg.

Irene should get 1500 mg. of aspirin a day. Since one tablet contains 300 mg. of aspirin, 1500 mg. would be 5 tablets. So Irene should get **1 tablet, 5 times a day.**

Or you could simply have doubled the normal dose for a 4-year-old, which was "half a tablet, 4 to 6 times a day." That would be **1 tablet, 4 to 6 times a day**—about the same as what you calculated based on Irene's weight!

Teaching aids for learning about fractions and milligrams

Many health workers at first have difficulty in understanding the use of fractions and milligrams for medicine dosages. Teaching aids that can help them to 'see' what fractions mean are shown below. Students can help make these teaching aids themselves.

a flannel-board

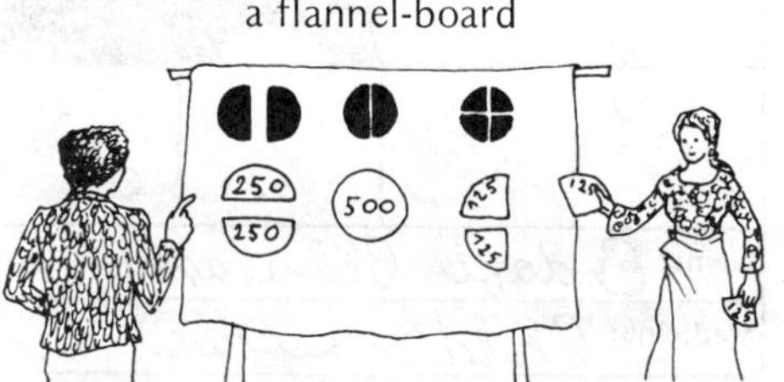
250
250
500
125
125

a set of blocks

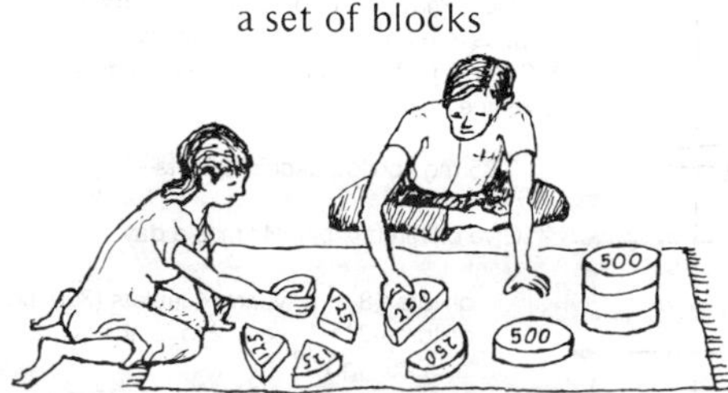
500
500
250

The flannel-board pieces or blocks that stand for tablets can be labeled 500 mg., 250 mg., or 400,000 units, to represent different medicines. Then students can practice figuring out dosages for adults and children.

If your program has a few old, outdated pills, it is good practice for health workers to actually cut some into halves and quarters. That way they can see the doses that should be given to children of different ages.

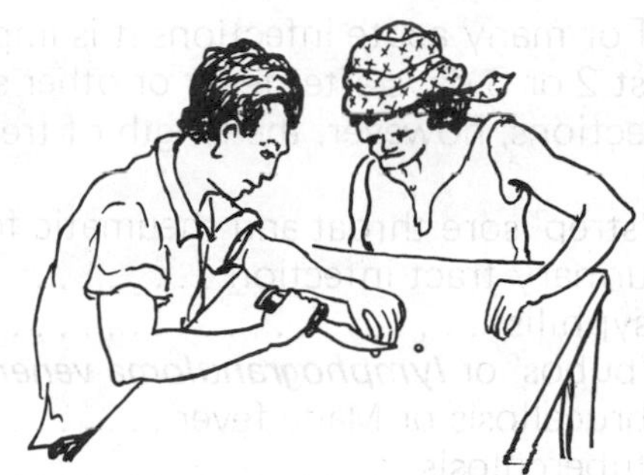

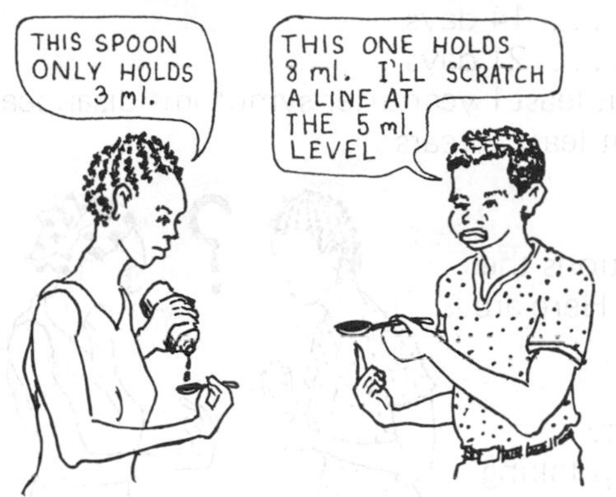
THIS SPOON ONLY HOLDS 3 ml.
THIS ONE HOLDS 8 ml. I'LL SCRATCH A LINE AT THE 5 ml. LEVEL

It is also a good idea to have students check how much liquid medicine local spoons will hold. Ways of doing this are described on page 61 of ***WTND.*** **A standard teaspoon should measure 5 ml.,** but spoons will vary greatly.

Practice in giving medicines to people

Students can practice in class with role plays about imaginary health problems. They can practice looking up medicines, figuring out the dosage, and then explaining the medicine's use to the 'sick person'. Experience shows that a great deal of practice is needed if health workers are to reliably give the right medicines in the right dosage. But with enough practice, they can do so.

Many mistakes in using medicines can be avoided if there is good communication between the health worker and the sick person. So it is important that students' role plays explore all of the points at which misunderstandings could arise. Make sure that health workers explain things carefully, and that the sick person clearly understands . . .

- How often to take the medicine
  - at what times of day
  - before or after eating (when this matters).
- How many days to continue taking the medicine, and when to expect to feel better. (Some persons expect to get well after having only a few pills or one injection.)

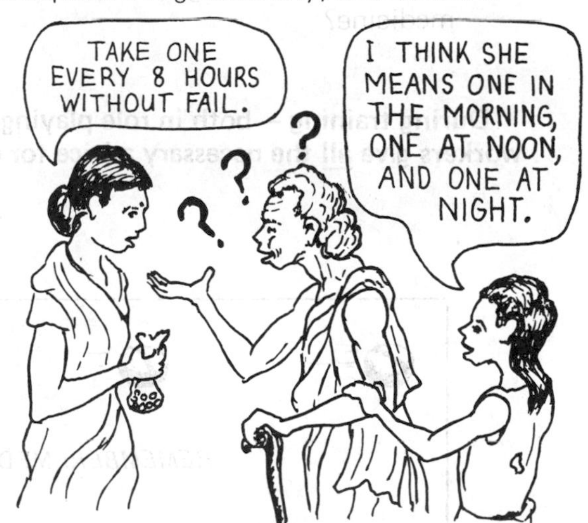
TAKE ONE EVERY 8 HOURS WITHOUT FAIL.
I THINK SHE MEANS ONE IN THE MORNING, ONE AT NOON, AND ONE AT NIGHT.
?
?
?

Many persons will take their medicine only until they feel better, and then stop. This may do no harm in cases where the problem gets better by itself and the medicine serves only to calm symptoms like mild pain, fever, or itching. But for serious chronic problems, like tuberculosis, epilepsy, diabetes, and high blood pressure, to stop taking the medicine could be a serious mistake.

For many acute infections it is important to keep taking the medicine for at least 2 or 3 days after fever or other signs of infection are gone. For some infections, however, the length of treatment is longer:

'strep' sore throat and rheumatic fever	10 days
urinary tract infection	10 days or more
syphilis	12 days
'bubos' or *lymphogranuloma venereum*	14 days
brucellosis or Malta fever	21 days
tuberculosis	at least 1 year after symptoms disappear
leprosy	at least 2 years

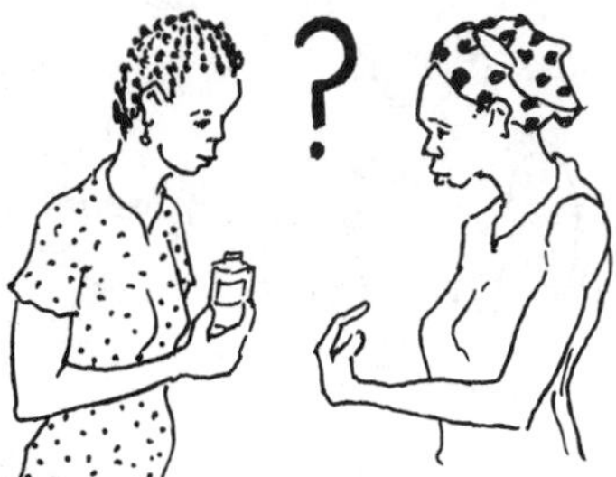
?

It is also important to clear up any questions the sick person may have about her treatment. Here are some questions or doubts she might have:

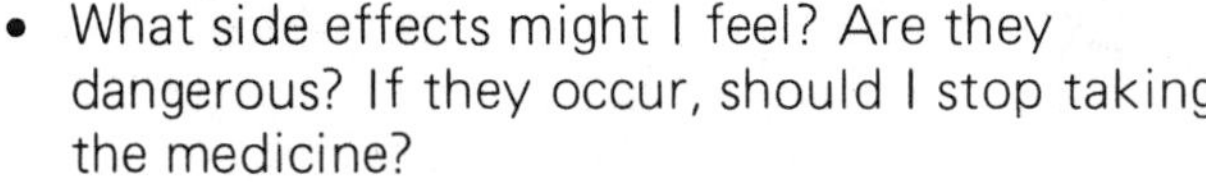

- What side effects might I feel? Are they dangerous? If they occur, should I stop taking the medicine?
- I am pregnant. Will this medicine harm my baby? (Try to give no medicines during pregnancy, if possible.)
- I am breast feeding. Will the medicine enter the milk and harm my baby?
- Is it all right to use this medicine along with other medication I am taking for a different health problem?
- What foods should I avoid when taking this medicine? What foods should I eat?
- What about drinking alcoholic beverages or smoking while I am taking this medicine?

During training — both in role playing and in clinical practice—be sure health workers give <u>all</u> the necessary advice for each medicine they recommend.

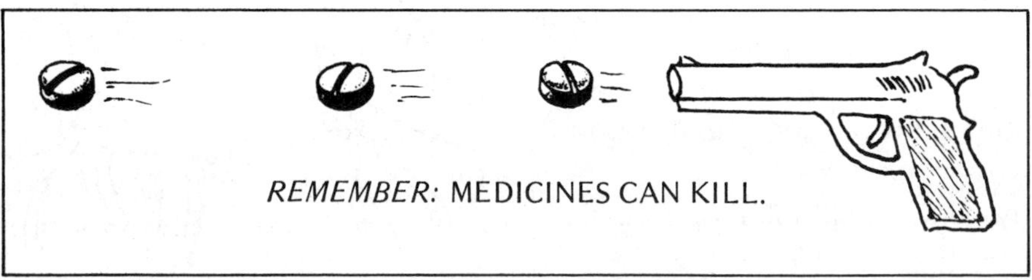
REMEMBER: MEDICINES CAN KILL.

BUT IF USED SENSIBLY, SOME MEDICINES
CAN PREVENT SUFFERING AND SAVE LIVES.

CHAPTER 19

Aids for Learning to Use Medicines and Equipment

In this chapter we look at two fairly unrelated areas of medical skill: **the use of antibiotics** and **the measurement of blood pressure.**

What these two topics have in common is that the training health workers receive about them is frequently inadequate—even dangerously so. We have, therefore, chosen these two subjects for a detailed exploration of learning methods. In each case, imaginative teaching aids can help health workers discover and grasp the basic principles. This, in turn, leads to safer, more capable practice.

LEARNING TO USE ANTIBIOTICS WISELY

In Chapter 18 we discussed the misuse of medicines. The misuse and overuse of antibiotics is an especially common and dangerous problem. It leads to unnecessary suffering and death, due to harmful side effects. It creates resistant forms of infection (see *WTND,* p. 58). It wastes millions that could be better spent for health. And it leads to countless cases of incorrect, inadequate treatment.

Teaching health workers to use antibiotics correctly is a special challenge. Even among doctors and health authorities, there is a great deal of misuse and misunderstanding of these important medicines.* Some programs decide not to permit health workers to use antibiotics at all. But in many areas this simply results in health workers using antibiotics without permission, and without any training in their use.

Yet we have found that **after a few days of appropriate training and practice, village health workers can select and use common antibiotics more wisely than the average doctor.**

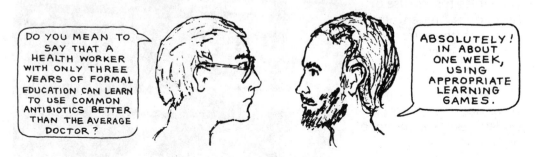

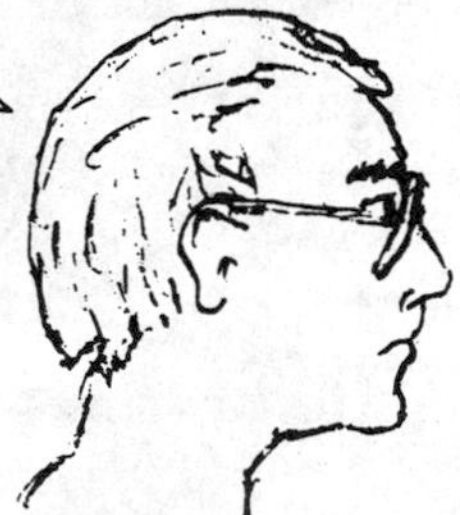
DO YOU MEAN TO SAY THAT A HEALTH WORKER WITH ONLY THREE YEARS OF FORMAL EDUCATION CAN LEARN TO USE COMMON ANTIBIOTICS BETTER THAN THE AVERAGE DOCTOR?

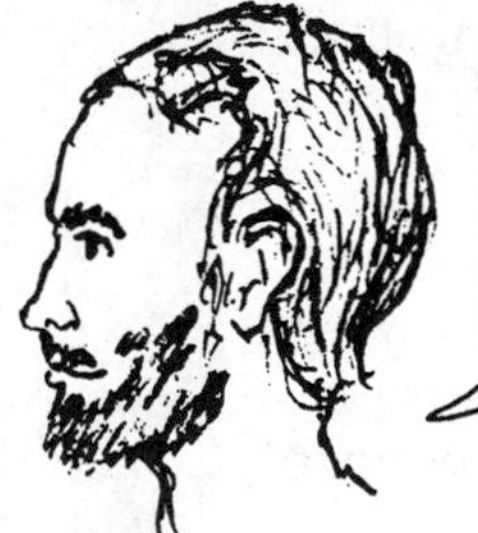
ABSOLUTELY! IN ABOUT ONE WEEK, USING APPROPRIATE LEARNING GAMES.

*For example, neomycin has been shown to make diarrhea, dehydration, and nutritional losses worse. Yet it is still produced by drug companies and prescribed by many doctors for diarrhea. The money spent by one Central American ministry of health in 1 year for neomycin-kaolin-pectin medicines could have paid for 3 million packets of oral rehydration salts—enough to treat all the cases of diarrhea in children under two for 16 months.

THE TEACHING METHODS AND AIDS

It is important not to use medicines when they are not needed. But for certain infections caused by bacteria, the correct use of antibiotics is of great benefit and can even save lives. Health workers need to have a clear understanding of . . .

- when antibiotics are needed
- when they are not needed or are likely to be harmful
- which of the common antibiotics to use for different infections and why
- the relative advantages and disadvantages of different antibiotics (effectiveness, risks, side effects, and cost)
- how to give them and with what advice

On the following pages, we describe a set of teaching aids that has been used very successfully for learning games about antibiotics. They help health workers understand the basic principles behind the proper use of these medicines. The aids were developed by Project Piaxtla, in Mexico, and can be made by the students themselves (although this takes a good deal of time and is perhaps best done in advance).

Two learning games have been developed. The second follows from the first. Both require sets of cards and figures, which can be made by following the patterns we show on these pages. Or you can adapt them by using local symbols. If you prepare the figures for use on a large flannel-board, everyone will be able to see them clearly.

A set of color slides showing these teaching aids will soon be available from TALC or the Hesperian Foundation (see p. **Back**-3). It is possible that TALC will also distribute a flannel sheet on which the figures for the games are printed, ready to cut out.

After using these games to learn the basic principles for the use of antibiotics, students can play with the games to test each other.

The first learning game helps health workers understand how common antibiotics work and what their effects are—both beneficial and harmful. These different effects are summarized on the next page.

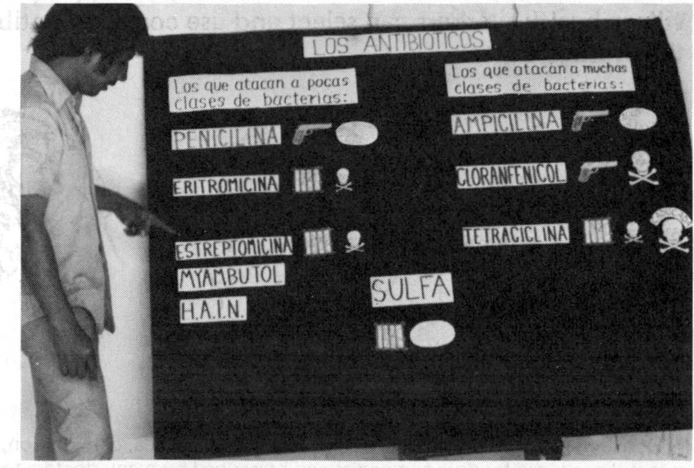

THE FIRST ANTIBIOTIC LEARNING GAME—
demonstrated by Pablo Chavez of Ajoya, Mexico

Beneficial effects

Different antibiotics fight infections in different ways:

1. Some antibiotics attack relatively few kinds of bacteria. Others attack many different kinds. So, as a start, students learn to divide commonly used antibiotics into 2 groups, which they list on the flannel-board under cut-out signs like these:

ANTIBIOTICS THAT ATTACK FEW KINDS OF BACTERIA:	ANTIBIOTICS THAT ATTACK MANY KINDS OF BACTERIA:
(NARROW-RANGE ANTIBIOTICS)	(BROAD-RANGE ANTIBIOTICS)

2. Also, some antibiotics are 'stronger' than others:

Some antibiotics **kill** bacteria.

Other antibiotics only **capture** them or slow them down.

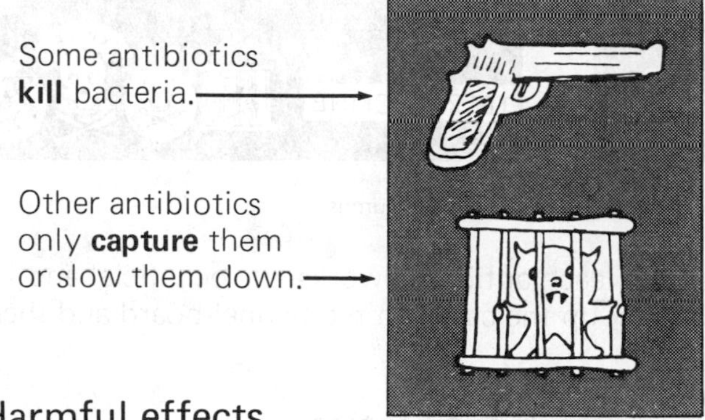

Students can use cut-out figures like these to represent antibiotics that kill bacteria

and

antibiotics that only capture them.

Color the pistol black and the cage white (or yellow).

Harmful effects

Possible harmful effects also differ with different antibiotics:

1. Some antibiotics cause **allergic reactions** in certain persons. Reaction does not depend on the amount of medicine taken, but on whether the person is allergic. (See ***WTND,*** p. 351)
2. Some antibiotics cause **poisoning or 'toxic' reactions**—especially if more than the recommended amount is used. (See *WTND,* p. 58.)
3. Broad-range antibiotics sometimes cause **diarrhea, 'thrush', and other problems.** This is because they attack 'good' bacteria along with the bad. (See *WTND,* p. 58.)

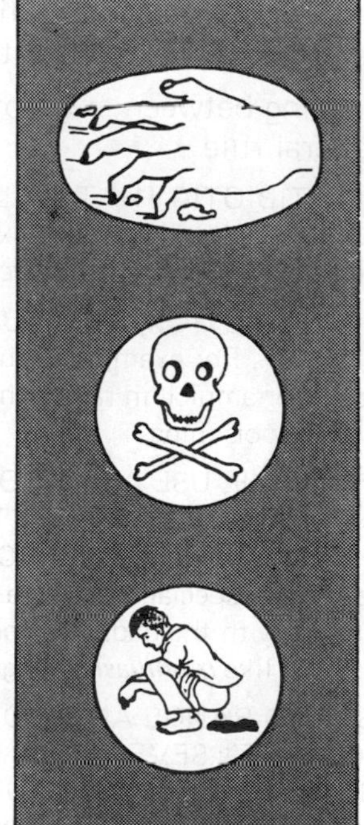

A scratching hand represents allergic reactions because itching is the most common sign.

A skull represents a poisonous reaction. Different sizes of skulls can be used to show greater or lesser danger.

A person with diarrhea represents problems that result from attacking good bacteria as well as bad.

THE FIRST LEARNING GAME

The students read from their books, discuss, and tell of their own experiences with the beneficial and harmful effects of different antibiotics. As they do this, they can begin to group the antibiotics in 2 columns and place the cut-out symbols where they belong.

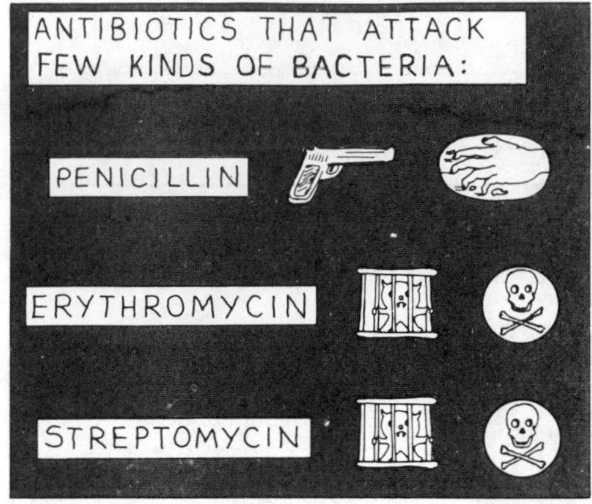

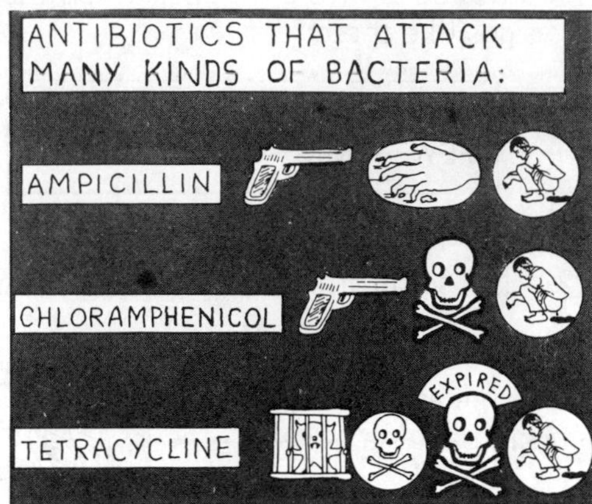

Note: Sulfas, if included, probably fall midway between these 2 columns.

To help themselves remember how each antibiotic works—its beneficial and harmful effects—the students can mix up the cards on the flannel-board and then take turns grouping them correctly.

Developing guidelines for choosing antibiotics

Students must first realize that **certain antibiotics work only for certain kinds of infections,** and that for any specific infection **some will work better than others.** The instructor can then use the information on the flannel-board to help develop a set of guidelines on which antibiotics to use for specific infections.

First guidelines: When choosing between antibiotics known to fight a particular illness or infection, as a general rule . . .

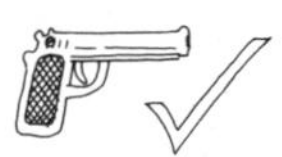

1. USE AN ANTIBIOTIC THAT KILLS BACTERIA RATHER THAN ONE THAT JUST SLOWS THEM DOWN. This usually gives quicker results and prevents the infection from becoming resistant to treatment.

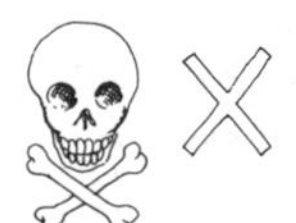

2. USE AN ANTIBIOTIC THAT CAUSES FEWER SIDE EFFECTS AND IS LESS RISKY. For example, if the person is not allergic, it is safer to use penicillin or ampicillin rather than an antibiotic like erythromycin that can cause poisoning.

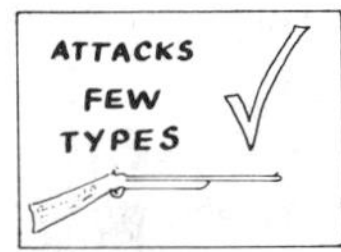

3. WHEN POSSIBLE, USE A NARROW-RANGE ANTIBIOTIC THAT ATTACKS THE SPECIFIC INFECTION RATHER THAN ONE THAT ATTACKS MANY KINDS OF BACTERIA. Broad-range antibiotics cause more problems—especially diarrhea and thrush—because they attack good bacteria along with the bad. The good bacteria prevent the growth of harmful things like *moniliasis* (fungus that can cause diarrhea, thrush, etc.).

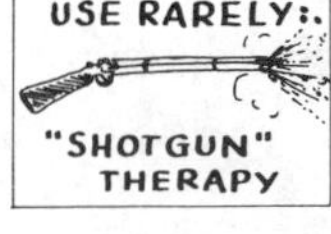

4. USE A BROAD-RANGE ANTIBIOTIC ONLY WHEN NO OTHER WILL WORK, OR WHEN SEVERAL KINDS OF BACTERIA MAY BE CAUSING THE INFECTION (as with infections of the gut, peritonitis, appendicitis, some urinary infections, etc.).

Additional guidelines for further learning:

> Take care not to burden students with too much at once. These additional guidelines can be introduced little by little when playing the games and discussing the uses of different antibiotics.

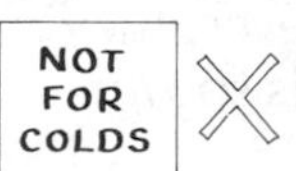

5. USE ANTIBIOTICS ONLY FOR BACTERIAL INFECTIONS! Do not use them for viral infections, because **antibiotics do nothing against viruses** (common cold, measles, chicken pox, etc.).

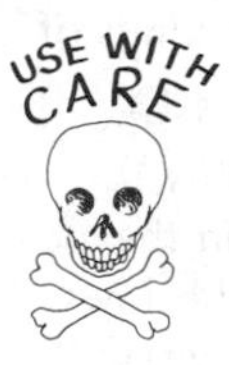

6. BE CAREFUL NEVER TO GIVE MORE THAN THE RECOMMENDED DOSE OF A TOXIC (POISONOUS) ANTIBIOTIC. However, it is usually not dangerous to give higher doses of an antibiotic that is not poisonous (penicillin or ampicillin). For example, it is all right to use penicillin for months or even years after it has expired, and to increase the dose to allow for any loss of strength. (But **tetracycline becomes more poisonous when old. It should never be used beyond the expiration date or in more than the recommended dose.)**

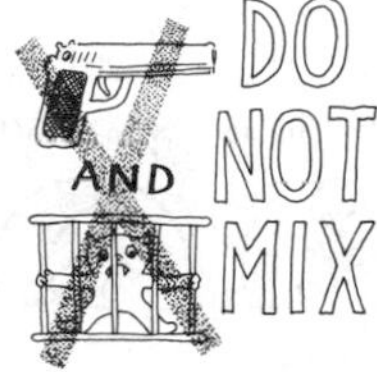

7. DO NOT USE AN ANTIBIOTIC THAT SLOWS DOWN BACTERIA TOGETHER WITH AN ANTIBIOTIC THAT KILLS THEM. The combination is often less effective than one alone. (Once the bacteria are captured or slowed, they stay hidden where the other antibiotics cannot kill them.) For example, never use tetracycline in combination with chloramphenicol.

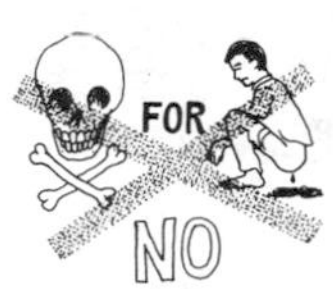

8. WHENEVER POSSIBLE, AVOID USING A TOXIC MEDICINE FOR A PERSON WITH DIARRHEA OR DEHYDRATION. A dehydrated person's body cannot get rid of poisons as quickly in the urine. Even normal doses of a toxic medicine may build up and poison the person. (Sulfas are especially risky for treating diarrhea. Unless the person is making a lot of urine, sulfa can form crystals in the kidneys and cause damage.)

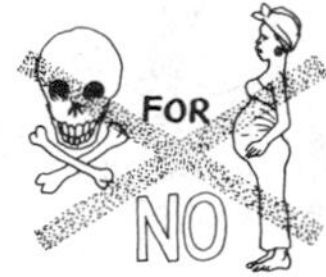

9. DO NOT USE TOXIC MEDICINES DURING PREGNANCY— ESPECIALLY DURING THE FIRST 3 MONTHS. Some medicines can cause severe birth defects.

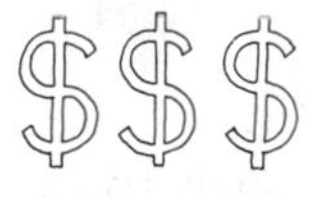

10. USE A MEDICINE THE FAMILY CAN AFFORD. When choosing between medicines, always consider the relative cost, and weigh this with other advantages and disadvantages.

THE SECOND LEARNING GAME

This game helps students use the guidelines from the first learning game to practice choosing antibiotics for specific infections.

This photo of the second antibiotic learning game was taken in Ajoya, Mexico. The game is discussed in detail on the pages to follow.

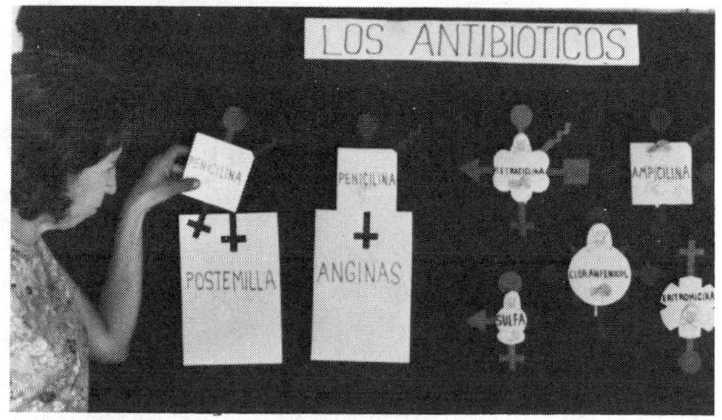

THE SECOND ANTIBIOTIC LEARNING GAME

1. THE ANTIBIOTICS: First make a series of cardboard figures representing the different antibiotics. Each figure has a number of strange shapes that stick out from it. These represent 'weapons' for attacking specific kinds of bacteria. (The shapes of these projecting 'weapons' have no special meaning. However, they must match appropriately with the cut-out parts of the disease cards shown below.)

If there are few weapons sticking out, it is a narrow-range antibiotic that attacks few kinds of bacteria.

Black weapons mean the antibiotic kills the bacteria.

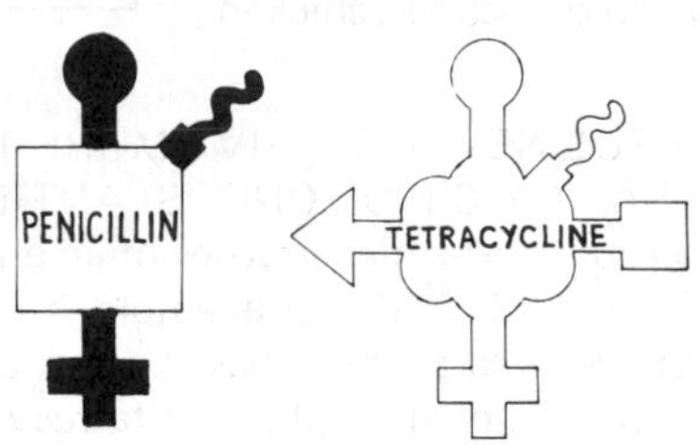

If there are many weapons, it is a broad-range antibiotic that attacks many kinds of bacteria.

White (or yellow) weapons mean the antibiotic only slows down the bacteria.

Make small tabs like these to represent the various side effects and reactions. These tabs fit into small cuts in the antibiotic figures.

allergy | poisonous (toxic) | very poisonous | diarrhea & thrush

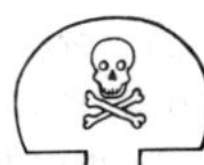

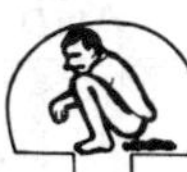

Another tab can be used for tetracycline, to show that it can stain the teeth of young (or unborn) children.

Students put together the side effect tabs and antibiotic figures, using what they learned in the first game.

For example, ampicillin, a broad-range antibiotic, can cause allergic reactions or diarrhea.

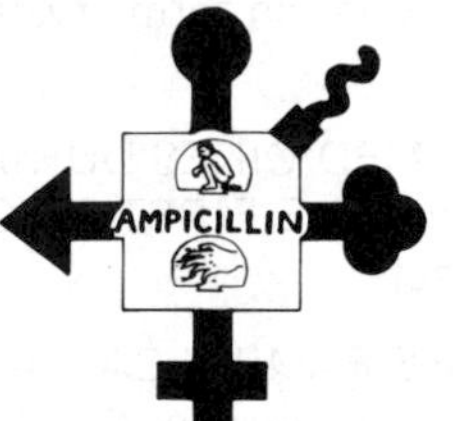

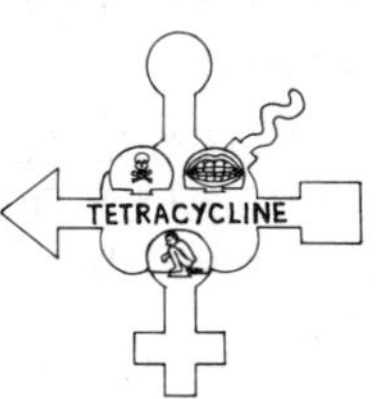

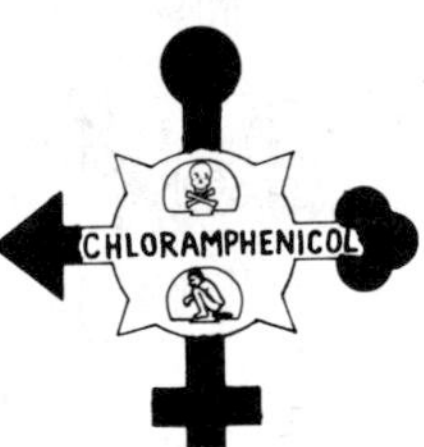

2. THE INFECTIONS: After preparing the antibiotic figures, make cards to represent infections found in your area. For each card, cut out shapes to match the 'weapons' of the antibiotics that can fight that infection.

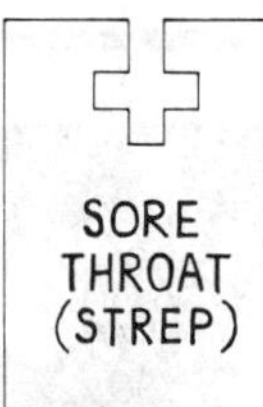

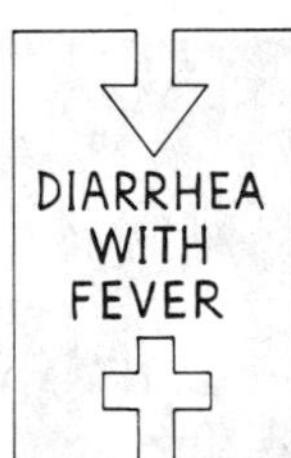

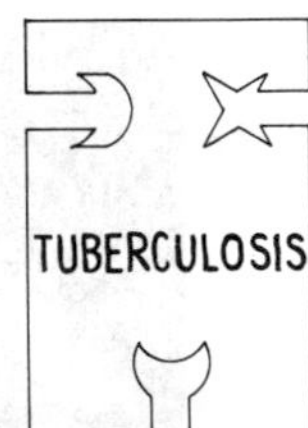

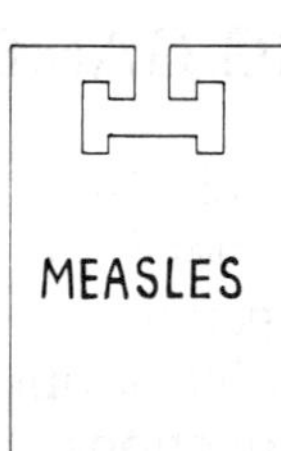

In this way, the 'weapons' of antibiotics that attack certain diseases will fit into them like pieces of a jigsaw puzzle.

A wide selection of figures and cards for this learning game are shown on page **19**-11. Use the ones that are appropriate for your area, or make up new ones as needed.

Choosing the most appropriate antibiotic

Students can now play a 'game of choice', deciding which antibiotics are the best choices for specific infections. Here are several examples.

THE PROBLEMS

TOOTH ABSCESS	SORE THROAT (STREP)

EXAMPLE 1: Suppose someone has a tooth abscess or 'strep' throat.

The students can see that any of the antibiotics below will fight these problems. (They all have the weapon shape that fits the cut-out part of the disease cards.)

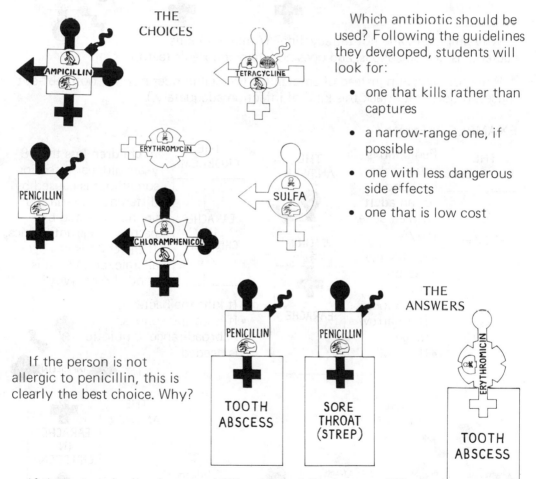

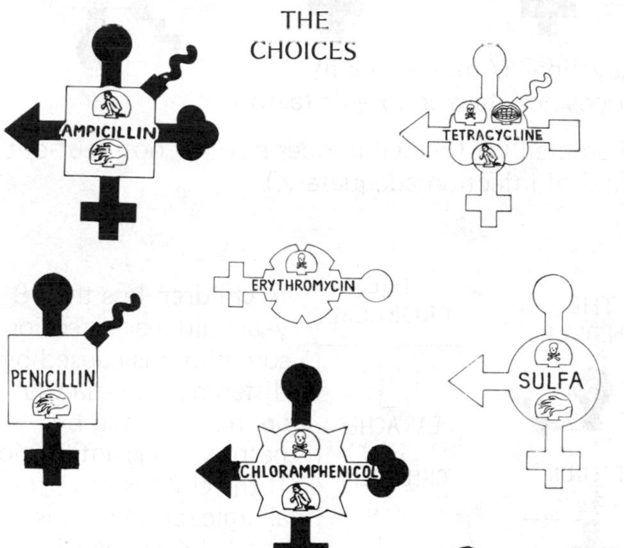

Which antibiotic should be used? Following the guidelines they developed, students will look for:

- one that kills rather than captures
- a narrow-range one, if possible
- one with less dangerous side effects
- one that is low cost

THE ANSWERS

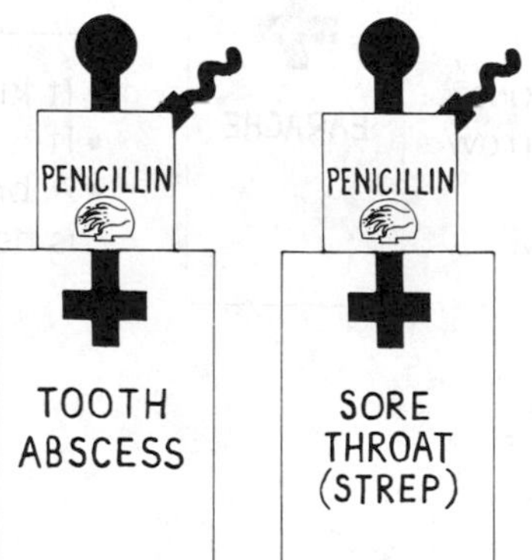

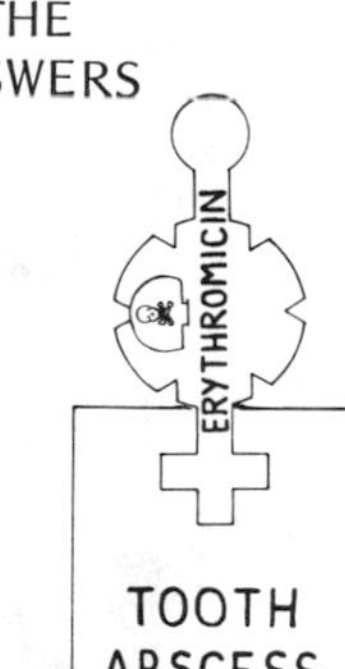

If the person is not allergic to penicillin, this is clearly the best choice. Why?

If the person is allergic to penicillin, the decision is more difficult. But erythromycin is probably a good choice. Why?

Why not ampicillin? (Because persons allergic to penicillin are also allergic to ampicillin.) Why not chloramphenicol? (Because it is broad-range and because it is too poisonous. The treatment could be worse than the illness!) If the person is allergic to penicillin and you do not have erythromycin (or it is too expensive), what is the next best choice? Why?

EXAMPLE 2: Suppose a 4-year-old child has acute diarrhea, with blood and mucus and high fever. She is **not** allergic to penicillin. What antibiotic would you choose?

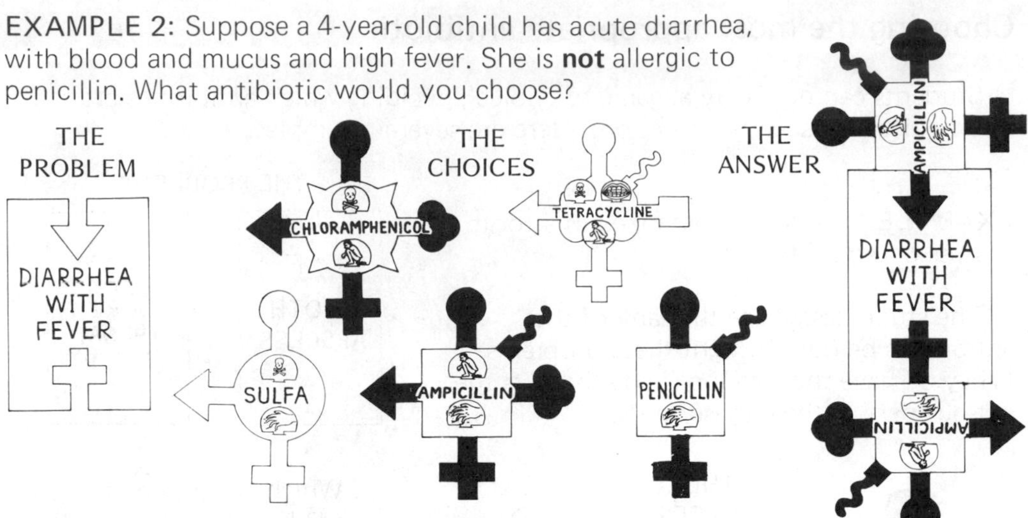

Why ampicillin and not tetracycline? (Ampicillin kills bacteria, is not poisonous, and does not stain children's teeth.)

Why not penicillin instead of ampicillin? (Penicillin does not 'fit' both cut-out spaces; it does not attack this kind of infection adequately.)

EXAMPLE 3: Earache

THE PROBLEM

EARACHE

Penicillin is usually the best choice for an **adult** with earache. Why?

- It kills the bacteria.
- It is not poisonous.
- It is narrow range.
- It is low cost.

THE ANSWER

PENICILLIN

EARACHE

THE PROBLEM

EARACHE IN CHILDREN

In **children** less than 8 years old, ear infection sometimes is caused by different bacteria that are not affected by narrow-range antibiotics. If the child is not allergic, ampicillin is a good choice. Why?

- It kills the bacteria.
- It is not poisonous.
- A broad-range antibiotic is needed.

THE CHOICES

AMPICILLIN

TETRACYCLINE

CHLORAMPHENICOL

SULFA

ERYTHROMYCIN

THE ANSWER

AMPICILLIN

EARACHE IN CHILDREN

AMPICILLIN

If the child is allergic to penicillin, what would you give him instead? Why?

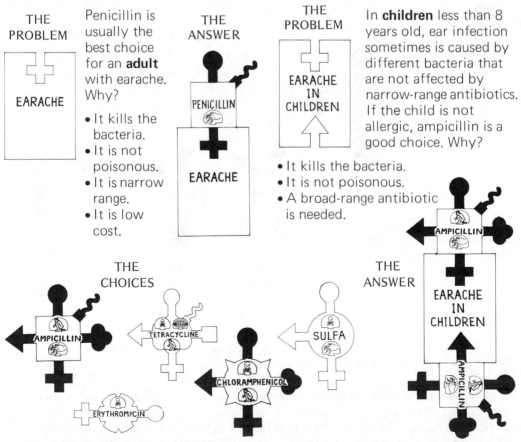

Antibiotics with special uses

Some antibiotics are especially effective for particular illnesses:

Tetracycline works for brucellosis (and also for gallbladder infections).

Ampicillin is best for typhoid fever. (Use chloramphenicol if ampicillin does not work or is not available.)

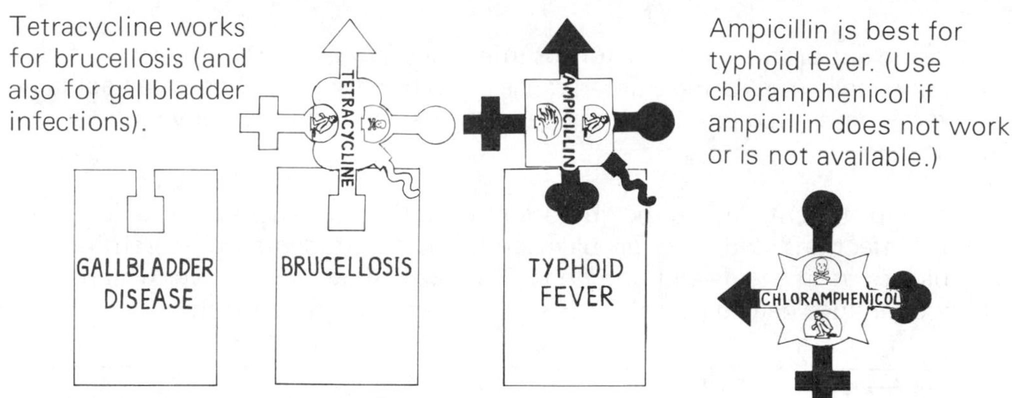

Three medicines together are needed to fight tuberculosis.

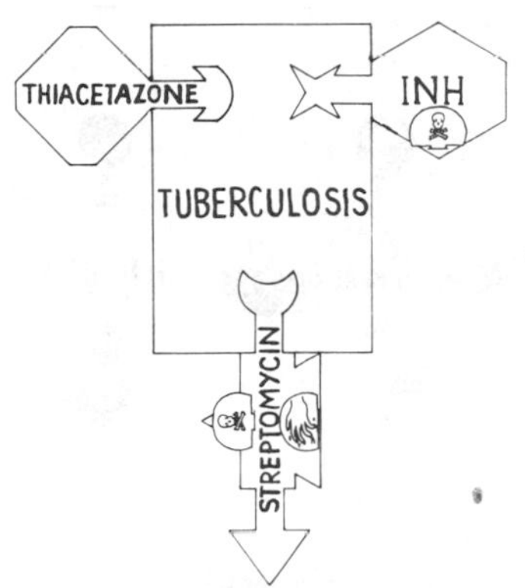

(Include whichever TB medicines are commonly used in your area.)

A sulfa drug is best for most minor bladder and urinary tract infections. It is low cost and has a narrower range than other choices. However, if the infection is severe or has gone into the kidneys, ampicillin may be a better choice. Why?

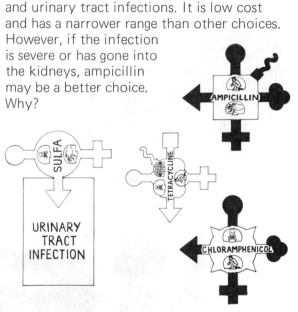

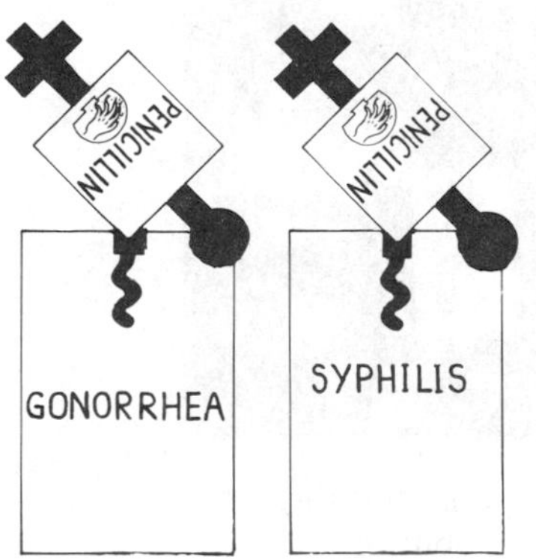

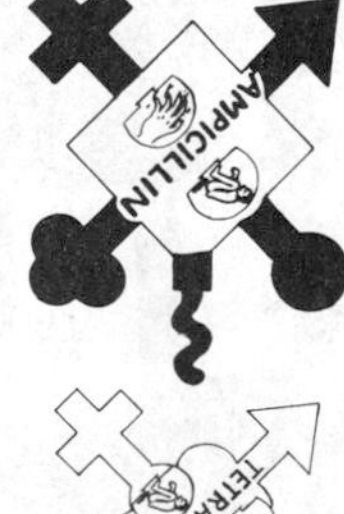

If the person is not allergic, penicillin is often best for gonorrhea and syphilis because:

- It kills the bacteria.
- It is not poisonous.
- It has a narrow range.

Note: In some areas, ampicillin may work better for gonorrhea and syphilis. In other areas, gonorrhea has become resistant to penicillin, ampicillin, and some other antibiotics. Tetracycline is not usually recommended to treat syphilis, unless the person is allergic to penicillin.

When not to use antibiotics

No antibiotic helps the common cold or measles, as these infections are caused by viruses.

Nor do antibiotics work for fungus infections (thrush or moniliasis). In fact, the opposite is true. Using a broad-range antibiotic for several days can actually cause a fungus infection. If this happens, the person should usually stop using the antibiotic.

To help students realize the limitations of antibiotics, include cards for viruses, fungus infections, and other problems in the game. Students will search for antibiotics to fit them—and find none. That way, they will discover which diseases are not helped by antibiotics. This is an important lesson!

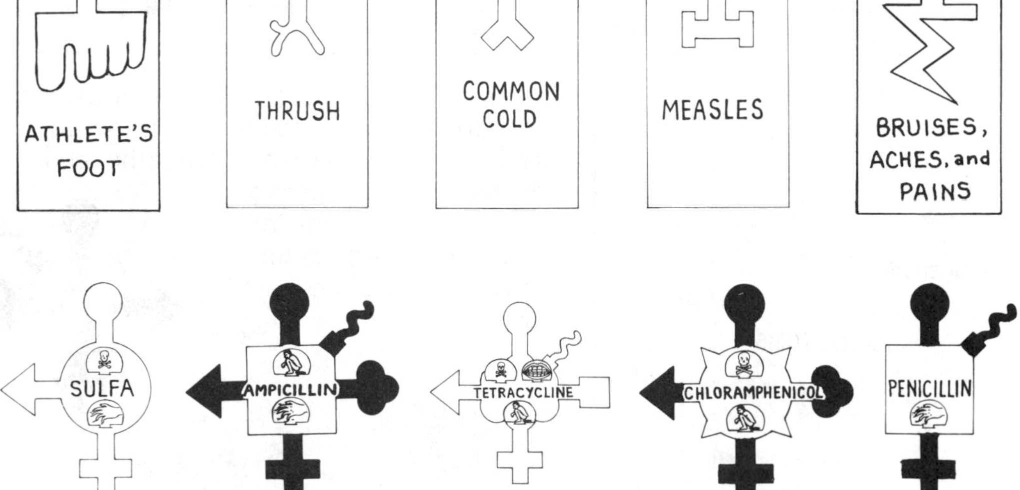

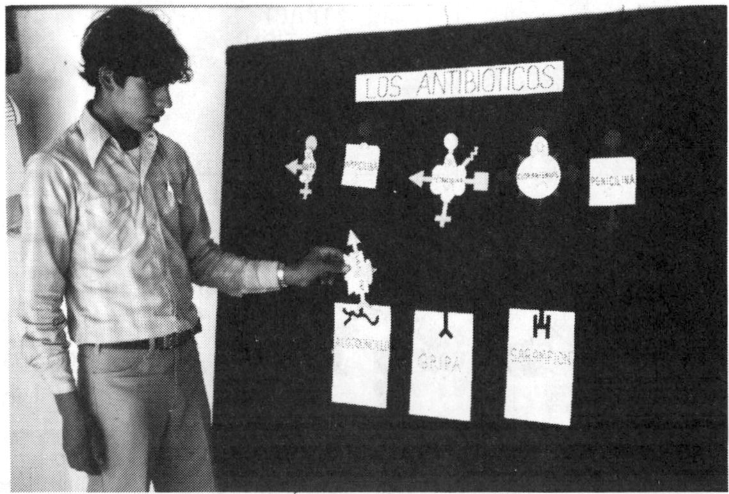

A student tries to find an antibiotic that will work for 'thrush'.
At last he gives up—because there is none.

PIECES NEEDED FOR THE SECOND ANTIBIOTIC LEARNING GAME

Use the pieces appropriate for your area and program. Add new pieces as needed for other antibiotics or diseases.

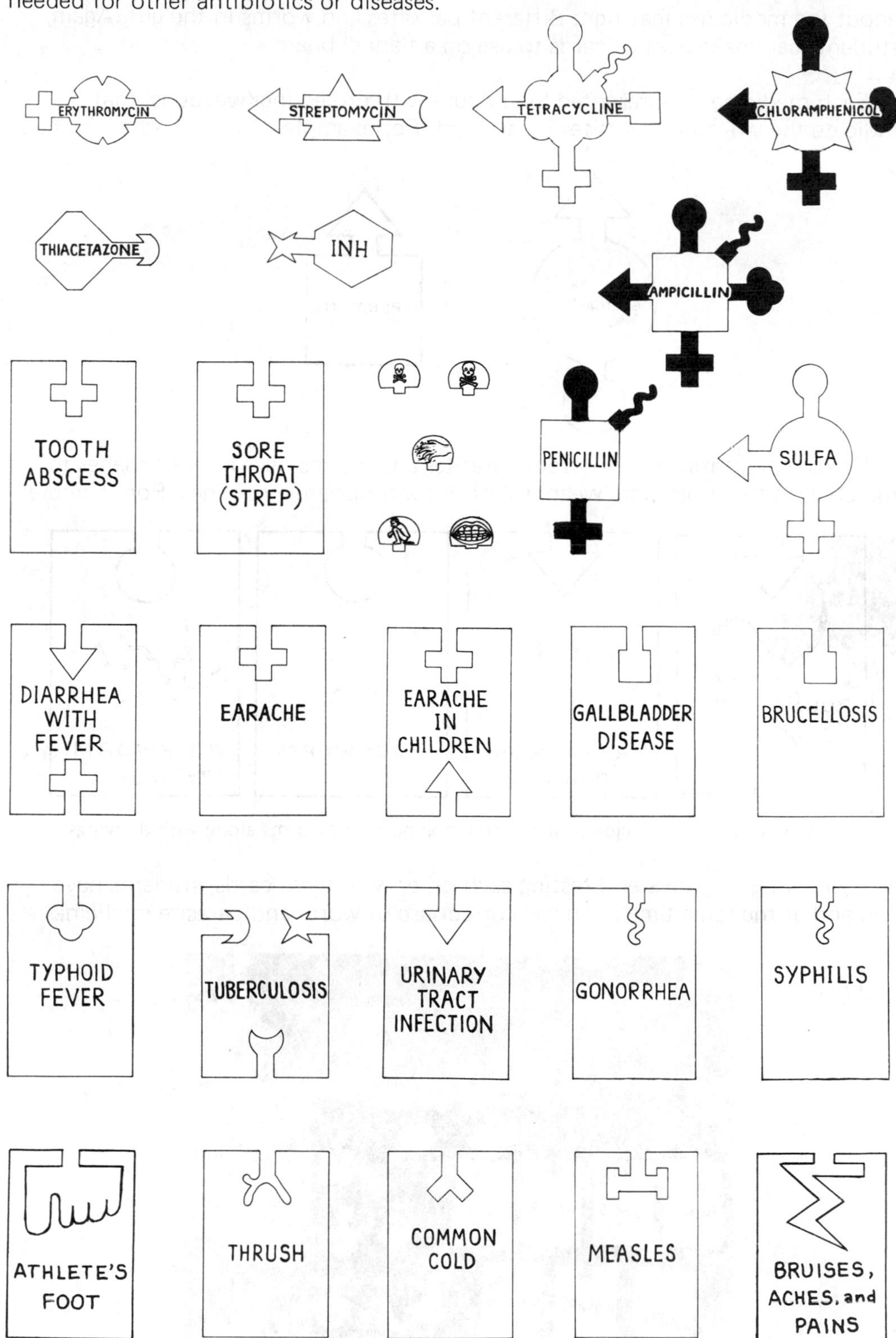

THE USE OF MEDICINES FOR WORMS AND PARASITES

Teaching aids like the second antibiotic game can also be used for learning about the medicines that fight different parasites and worms in the gut. Again, students can make a set of cards to use on a flannel-board.

Each medicine is represented by a figure with projecting 'weapons' that indicate the worms or parasites it can fight. For example:

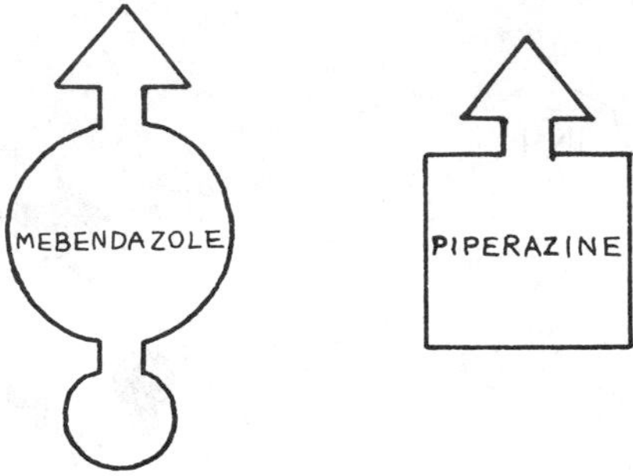

Cards representing the different parasites and worms have cut-out shapes to match with the projecting 'weapons' of the appropriate medicines. For example:

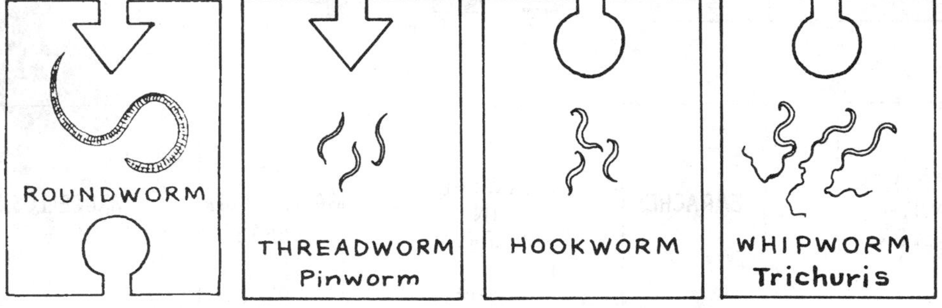

To be sure things are clear, use the common names of worms along with drawings.

By making up games and testing each other with these cards, students have fun and at the same time learn the correct use of worm and parasite medicines.

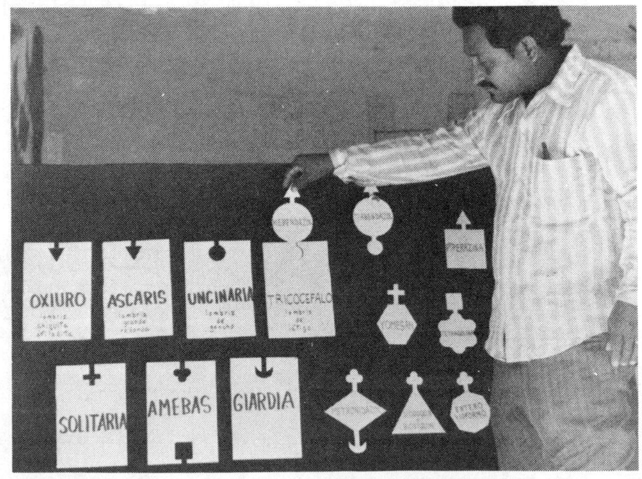

LEARNING TO MEASURE BLOOD PRESSURE

Some health programs choose not to teach health workers how to measure blood pressure. Others cannot afford the necessary equipment. But blood pressure measurement can be an important skill—especially in communities where high blood pressure and related diseases are common. It is also a valuable skill for midwives and others who regularly check women's health during pregnancy—because high blood pressure increases the risk for the mother during childbirth. Also, a marked increase in blood pressure late in pregnancy may be a sign of toxemia of pregnancy (see *WTND,* p. 249).

Anyone who knows how to count can learn to measure blood pressure.

Health workers learn more easily how to take blood pressure when they **understand the principles behind it.** For this reason, it helps if they learn with the older type of mercury *sphygmomanometer,* or at least see one demonstrated.

With this older kind of blood pressure instrument, learners can actually see the pressure lift the mercury in the tube. Blood pressure is measured in millimeters (mm.) of mercury.

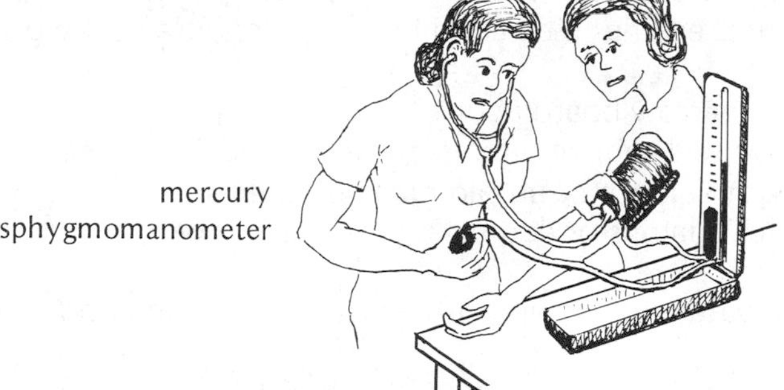

mercury sphygmomanometer

To help a health worker realize how much pressure is in the blood stream, have him try to lift a column of mercury by blowing, like this.

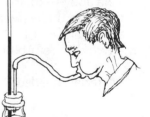

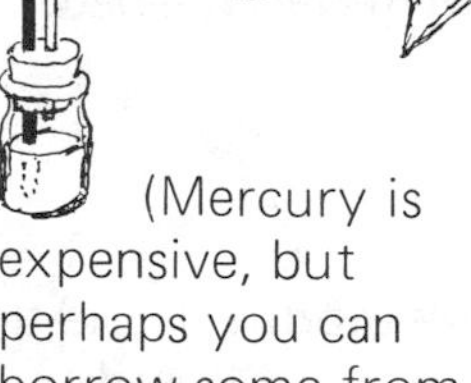

(Mercury is expensive, but perhaps you can borrow some from a dental clinic.)

To measure blood pressure:

- **Explain what you are going to do,** so the person will not be alarmed.
- **Fasten the pressure cuff** around the person's bare upper arm.
- **Close the valve** on the rubber bulb by turning the screw clockwise.
- **Pump the pressure up** to more than 200 millimeters of mercury.
- **Place the stethoscope over the artery** on the inner side of the person's elbow.
- **Very slowly, release the pressure** in the cuff by loosening the screw on the rubber bulb.
- **With the stethoscope, listen carefully for the pulse** as you continue letting the air out of the cuff. As the needle of the gauge (or the level of mercury) slowly drops, **take two readings:**

1. **Take the first reading the moment you begin to hear the soft thumping of the pulse.** This happens when the pressure in the cuff drops to the highest pressure in the artery (*systolic* or 'top' pressure). This top pressure is reached each time the heart contracts and forces the blood through the arteries. In a normal person, this top pressure reading is usually around 110-120 mm.

2. Continue to slowly release the pressure while listening carefully. **Take the second reading when the sound of the pulse begins to fade or disappear.** This happens when the pressure in the cuff drops to the lowest pressure in the artery (***diastolic*** or 'bottom' pressure). This bottom pressure occurs when the heart relaxes between pulses. It is normally around 60 to 80 mm.

When you record a person's blood pressure, always write both the top and bottom arterial pressure readings. We say that an adult's normal blood pressure (BP) is "120 over 80," and write it like this:

BP $\frac{120}{80}$ or BP 120/80

120 is the top (systolic) reading.
80 is the bottom (diastolic) reading.

For health workers, it may be better to speak of the "top" and "bottom" numbers (TN and BN), rather than use confusing words like ***systolic*** and ***diastolic.***

A SIMPLE AID FOR LEARNING ABOUT BLOOD PRESSURE

The above explanation of the top and bottom blood pressure numbers is difficult to understand when explained with words alone. However, a simple teaching aid that the health workers themselves can make, clearly shows what the two different blood pressure readings mean and how the pressure cuff works.

Materials needed:
1 thick, narrow board about ½ meter long
1 thin-walled rubber tube (surgical tubing 2 to 3 cm. wide, or a piece of an old bicycle inner tube)
2 surgical clamps or equivalent (string will work)

Method: Fill the tube with water and clamp both ends. Put the tube under the board.

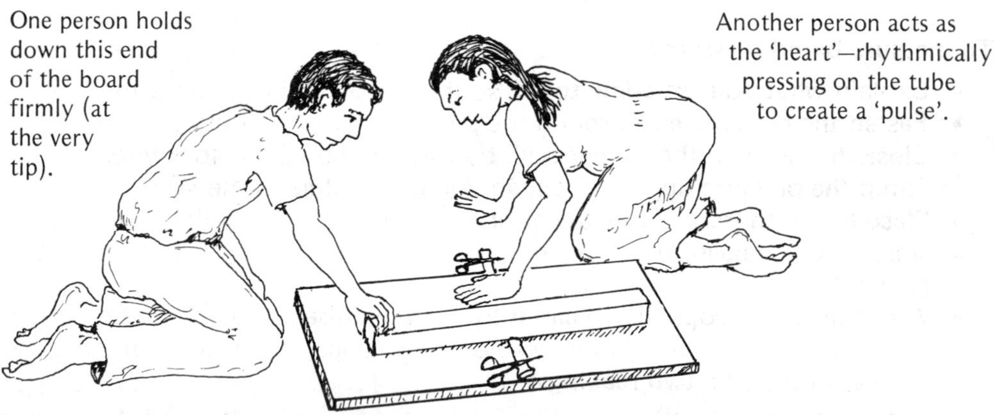
One person holds down this end of the board firmly (at the very tip).
Another person acts as the 'heart'—rhythmically pressing on the tube to create a 'pulse'.

This should be done on a hard, smooth floor or on a flat board.

Each 'pulse' or 'heartbeat' will lift the piece of wood off the floor. Between pulses it will drop back with a loud thump. (You may have to add more water or let some out for the thumping to occur.)

To understand how a pressure cuff works, start with the tube near the end of the board that is being held down.

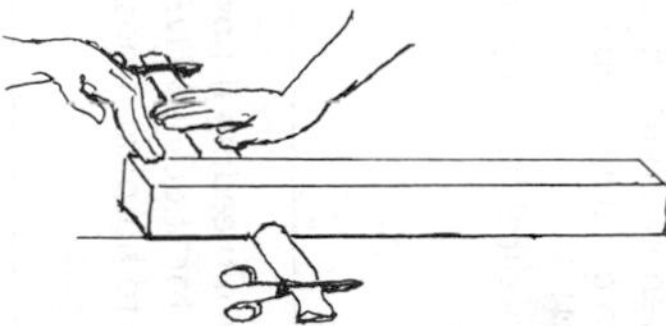

DOES NOT LIFT

There the weight, or pressure, will be so great that the 'pulse' will not lift the board and no thump will occur.

Slowly move the board backward until it begins to lift and thump.

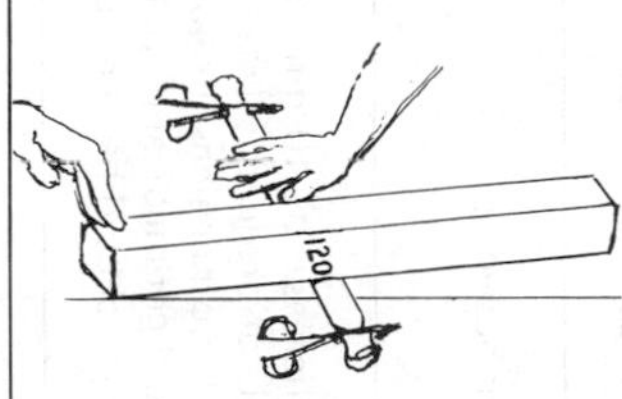

LIFTS WHEN TUBE IS PRESSED

This is the top pressure reading. Mark the board "120" at this spot.

Keep sliding the board back until it stops thumping the floor and stays lifted between pulses.

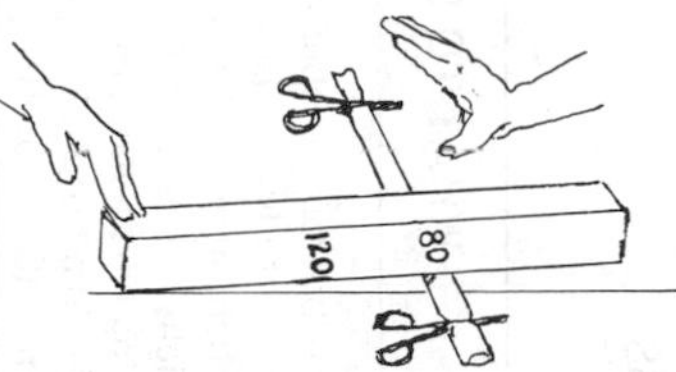

STAYS LIFTED

This is the bottom pressure reading. Mark the board "80" at this spot.

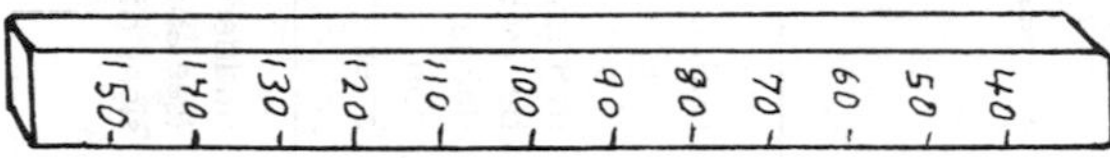

After marking the positions of 80 and 120 on the stick, students can add other numbers to form a scale.

By taking water out of the tube or adding more water (or by changing the positions of the clamps) they can make the pressure higher and lower, and practice measuring it. This provides a good opportunity to discuss some of the causes of **low blood pressure** that relate to lowering the volume of blood (shock, severe blood loss, etc.).

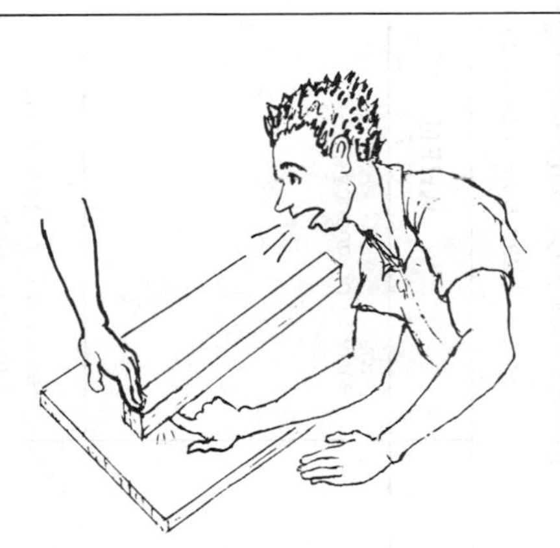

If someone doubts that the pressure is greater near the end of the board that is held down, have him put his finger under it instead of the tube!

Note: In another part of this book, we discuss reasons for not starting a course by teaching 'anatomy and physiology' (see p. **5**-13). Instead, we suggest including information on the body and how it works whenever needed to help explain specific problems or practical activities. This demonstration for learning about blood pressure and its measurement is a good example. Here, students learn about the heart and blood vessels in an active way that relates to and helps explain a basic skill (measuring blood pressure).

WHEN TO TAKE BLOOD PRESSURE AND WHAT TO DO ABOUT YOUR FINDINGS

(This list can be expanded or shortened, according to the local situation.)

WHO	WHEN	WHAT TO LOOK FOR	WHAT TO DO
PREGNANT WOMEN	early in pregnancy	• Possible high blood pressure (BP). • What is normal BP for the woman.	• If high—bottom number (BN) over 100—watch carefully. Advise her not to eat too much fatty food and energy foods—especially if she is fat. Consider referring her to a doctor. Childbirth will be safer in a hospital. • If normal (60 to 95 BN), record BP to use for comparison later.
	regularly during pregnancy (every 2 months or so)	Changed or high blood pressure.	Same as above.
	more often late in pregnancy (last 2 to 3 months—especially during ninth month or if there are problems)	Increase in blood pressure.	If BP increases by 10 mm. or more, suspect toxemia of pregnancy (see ***WTND,*** p. 249). Check for other signs. Follow advice in book and get medical help if possible. Childbirth should be in hospital.
MOTHERS AT CHILDBIRTH	during childbirth (or abortion), and in hours or days following—especially when there is blood loss (but even when there is little visible bleeding, as lost blood may be trapped in the womb)	Sudden drop in BP with signs of shock (see ***WTND,*** p. 77). If bottom number (BN) drops more than 20 mm. or falls below 50 mm., she is in danger. (Some drop in BP is normal as the woman relaxes after childbirth.)	• Treat for shock (lots of liquid if conscious, intravenous solution if possible, etc.). • Try to control bleeding (see ***WTND,*** p. 264). • Get medical help if possible, or rush to hospital.
ANYONE	if the person may be losing blood from any part of the body, inside or out	Sudden or marked drop in BP (see above). Look for other signs of shock (***WTND,*** p. 77).	• Control bleeding if possible. • Treat for shock (***WTND,*** p. 77). • Rush to hospital if possible.

ANYONE	if the person might be in shock (***WTND,*** p. 77), including allergic shock (***WTND,*** p. 70). If the person is not yet in shock, but there is danger of it, take blood pressure often and watch for drop.	Same as above.	• Control bleeding, if any. • Treat for shock (***WTND,*** p. 77). • Rush to hospital if possible.
PEOPLE OVER 40 FAT PEOPLE PEOPLE WITH SIGNS OF: • heart trouble • stroke • difficulty breathing • frequent headaches • swelling • diabetes • chronic urinary problems • swollen or painful veins	each time you see them, as they are especially likely to have high BP	• High blood pressure (bottom number over 100). • Signs of related disease. • Wide difference (over 80 mm.) between top and bottom numbers (possible sign of hardening of the arteries), and other abnormalties in BP. • Little difference between top and bottom numbers may mean a kidney problem. Get medical help.	• If BN over 100 mm. but under 110, give advice on diet (***WTND,*** p. 126). Encourage fat person to lose weight. • If BN over 110 mm., give same advice on diet and, if possible, have the person get medicine for lowering BP. • If the underlying problem is known and can be treated, see that the person gets treatment if she wants it.
PERSONS KNOWN TO HAVE HIGH BLOOD PRESSURE	at regular intervals (once a month or every few months), but more often . . . • at first • when beginning to use blood pressure medicine or changing dosage • if BP is very high or changes often	• How BP compares with the last reading you took. • Related problems such as heart trouble, stroke, diabetes, chronic urinary problems, or painful veins.	• Follow the advice in the square above and in ***WTND,*** p. 126. • If BN drops below 100 mm. with diet alone, congratulate the person and tell him to continue the diet. • If BN does not drop below 100 or gets higher (over 110), try to see that the person gets medicine to lower his blood pressure. • Continue to check BP regularly.
WOMEN TAKING BIRTH CONTROL PILLS	before beginning, and then every six months	High or rising BP.	If BN is over 100 mm., it is safer not to use the pill. Recommend another method to avoid pregnancy.

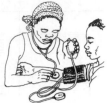

Points to cover when teaching about blood pressure:

- Before health workers begin to measure blood pressure, be sure they know how to use a stethoscope. Have them listen to each other's heartbeats to become familiar with the sound of the pulse.

- Caution each health worker against using either the stethoscope or pressure cuff as 'magic medicine' to make people think he has special powers or knowledge. Use these instruments as tools, and only when necessary—never for show or prestige.

- Measure blood pressure when the person is 'at rest'. Recent exercise (running, walking, or working), anger, worry, fear, or nervousness can make pressure rise and give a falsely high reading. In a doctor's office the most common problem is nervousness, especially if the patient is a woman and the doctor is a man. Ask the health workers why they think this is so. Discuss with them what can be done to make the person as comfortable and relaxed as possible before taking their blood pressure.

- Always take a person's blood pressure 2 or 3 times to be sure your readings are about the same.

NORMAL

- Normal blood pressure for an adult at rest is usually around 120/80, but this varies a lot. Anything from 100/60 to 140/90 can be considered normal. Older people usually have somewhat higher blood pressure than young people.

- Of the two readings, top (systolic) and bottom (diastolic), it is usually the bottom number that tells us more about a person's health. For example, if a person's blood pressure is 140/85, there is not much need for concern. But if it is 135/110, he has seriously high blood pressure and should lose weight (if fat) or get treatment. It is generally agreed that a bottom number (BN) of over 100 means the blood pressure is high enough to require attention (diet and perhaps medicine).

TOO HIGH

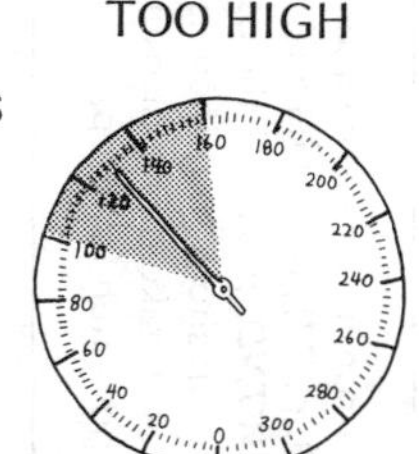

- Advise health workers that they usually do not have to worry when a person regularly has low blood pressure. In fact, blood pressure on the low side of normal, 90/60 to 110/70, means a person is likely to live long and is less likely to suffer from heart trouble or stroke. Many normal, healthy village people, especially in Latin America, have blood pressure as low as 90/60.

- A sudden or marked drop in blood pressure is a danger sign (blood loss, shock), especially if it falls below 60/40. Health workers should watch for any sudden drop in the blood pressure of persons who are losing blood or at risk of shock. However, some drop in pressure may happen normally when a woman relaxes after giving birth or a person calms down after an accident. Always look for other signs of shock besides a drop in blood pressure. (See the test for shock on p. **16**-9.)

TOO LOW

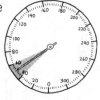

Note: References to blood pressure in ***Where There Is No Doctor*** are: Shock, p. 70 and 77 (also see Index); Fat People, p. 126; Heart Trouble, p. 325; High Blood Pressure, p. 125 and 326; Stroke, p. 327; Pregnancy, p. 249, 251, and 253; Toxemia of Pregnancy, p. 249; Childbirth (blood loss), p. 265; and Birth Control Pills, p. 289.

PART THREE

LEARNING TO USE THE BOOK, *WHERE THERE IS NO DOCTOR*

A book on basic health care is a tool for sharing ideas and knowledge. If clearly and simply written, it can be used by anyone who knows how to read. However, if persons are given suggestions and guided practice in use of the book, it will usually serve them better.

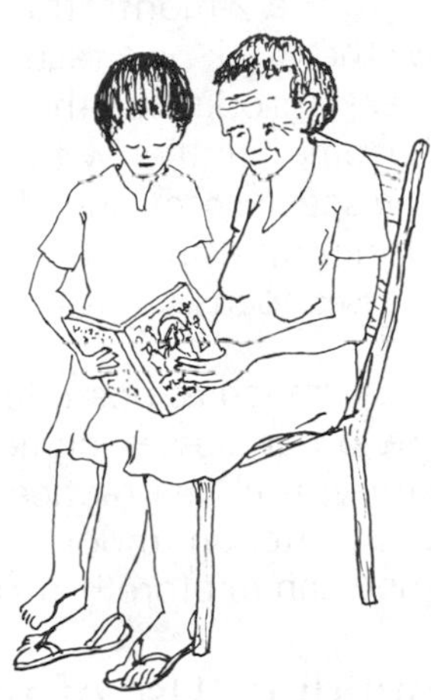

We know an old folk healer who cannot read. But she has her 8-year-old granddaughter read to her from *WTND* while she studies the pictures.

In Part Three of this book, we give many suggestions for helping people learn to use the village health care handbook, ***Where There Is No Doctor (WTND).*** But many of these suggestions apply to any health or 'how-to-do-it' manual.

'Book learning' for health workers has two objectives:

- To help health workers themselves learn to use their books effectively.
- To help health workers learn how to help others use the book, or to use the ideas and information it contains.

Instruction in 'use of the book' can take place in many ways. It may be a key part of a 2- or 3-month health worker training course. It may take place in weekly meetings of village mothers, led by a health worker. Or it may be only a brief explanation given by a health worker to a folk healer or midwife from a distant village.

LEARNING TO USE BOOKS RATHER THAN RELYING ON MEMORY:

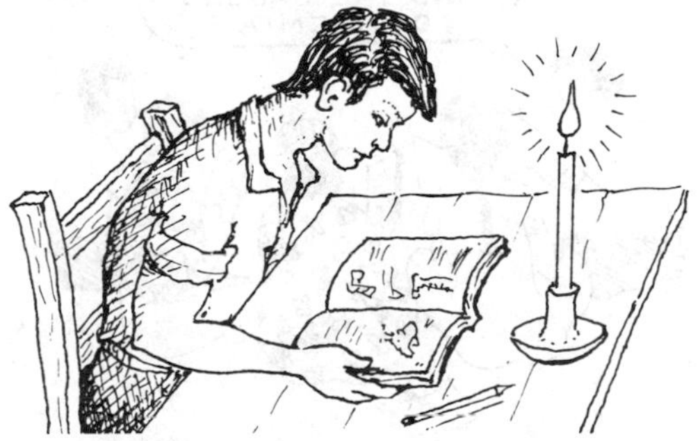

If training helps health workers learn to use reference books effectively, they will continue to learn and study long after the course is over.

A community health worker needs to know how to do many things. A wide range of information and skills are needed in his work. But he cannot be expected to keep all the necessary information in his head. Therefore . . .

Training should not focus on memorizing a lot of information, but on LEARNING HOW TO LOOK THINGS UP.

Combining literacy training with health skills: Because being able to look things up is such an important skill, some programs—especially in Africa—link learning to read with practice in solving health problems. Student health workers who can already read and write help teach those who are learning. Thus, a book like *Where There Is No Doctor* in the local language helps people learn health skills and literacy skills at the same time. (For more ideas on combining literacy training with health skills and critical awareness, see Chapter 26.)

SCHEDULED CLASSES ON 'USE OF THE BOOK' DURING HEALTH WORKER TRAINING

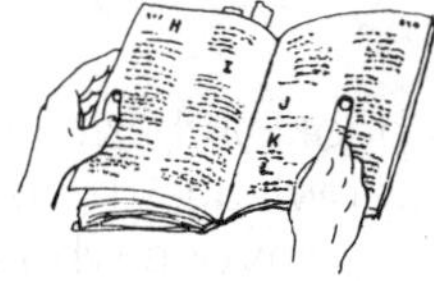

In the 2-month training course in Ajoya, Mexico, 'Use of the Book' is a regular class that takes place twice a week throughout the course. The first classes help students become familiar with what is in each chapter and each of the special sections of the book. They practice looking things up using the INDEX, list of CONTENTS, charts, and page references. Later classes focus on using the book to help solve problems acted out in role plays.

As much as possible, these classes on 'Use of the Book' are coordinated with the other classes, clinical practice, and community visits. They provide related study, lifelike practice, and review. Scheduling is kept flexible so that if students encounter an important problem in clinical practice or community activities, they can explore it further in their next 'Use of the Book' class.

Building 'Use of the Book' into other classes and activities

It is important that learning to use the book not be limited to specific classes. Practice in looking things up and using the book as a tool needs to be built into many areas of study and learning. This means that . . .

During any class, if you have a choice between telling students something or having them find and read it out loud from their books, have them read it from their books!

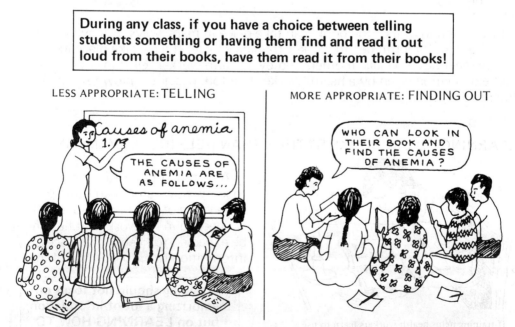

LESS APPROPRIATE: TELLING

MORE APPROPRIATE: FINDING OUT

WHO CAN LOOK IN THEIR BOOK AND FIND THE CAUSES OF ANEMIA ?

Do not tell the students things that they can learn to look up for themselves.

WAYS HEALTH WORKERS CAN USE THEIR BOOK

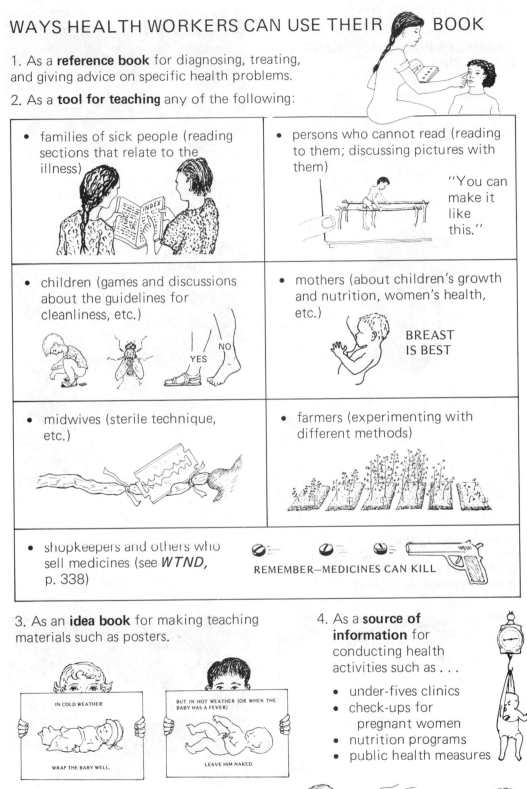

1. As a **reference book** for diagnosing, treating, and giving advice on specific health problems.
2. As a **tool for teaching** any of the following:

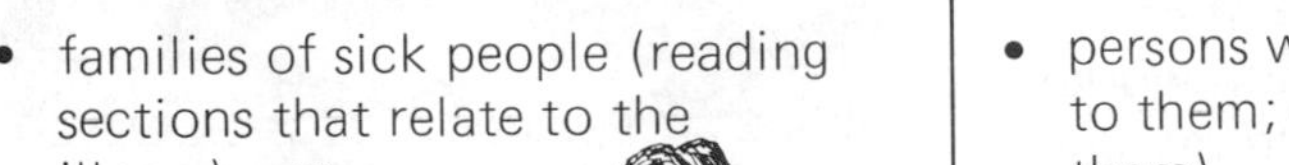

- families of sick people (reading sections that relate to the illness)

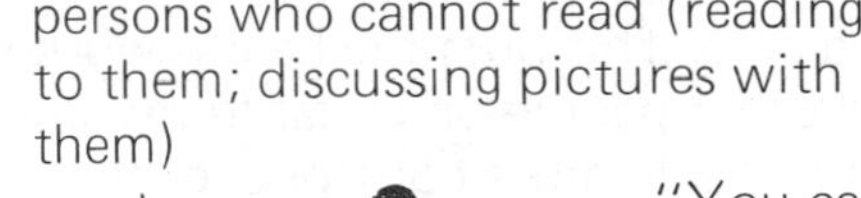

- persons who cannot read (reading to them; discussing pictures with them)

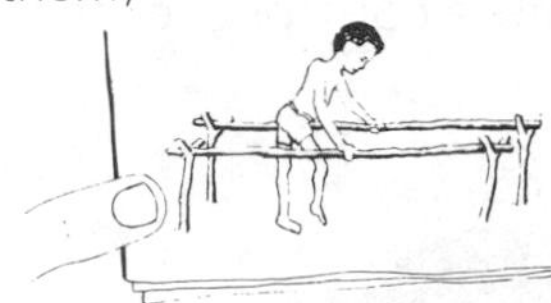
"You can make it like this."

- children (games and discussions about the guidelines for cleanliness, etc.)

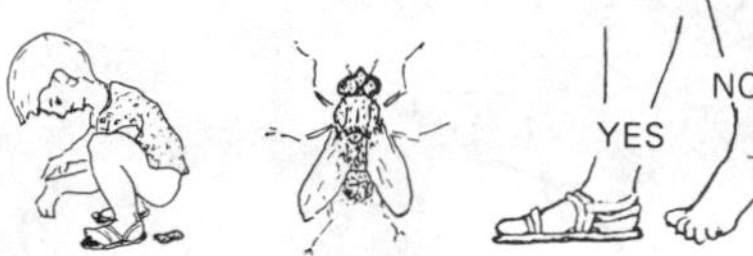

- mothers (about children's growth and nutrition, women's health, etc.)

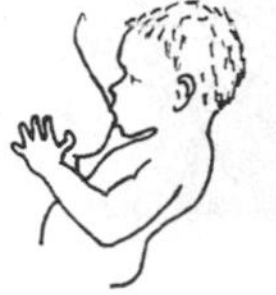
BREAST IS BEST

- midwives (sterile technique, etc.)

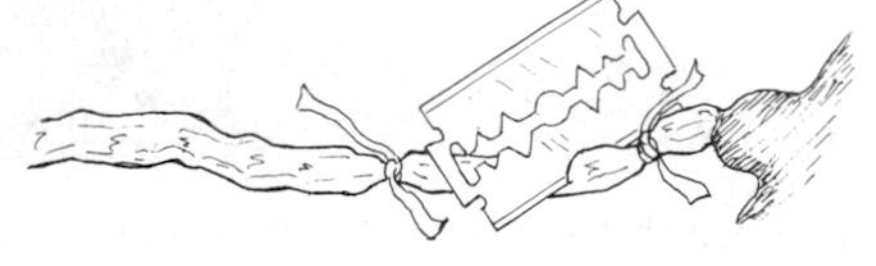

- farmers (experimenting with different methods)

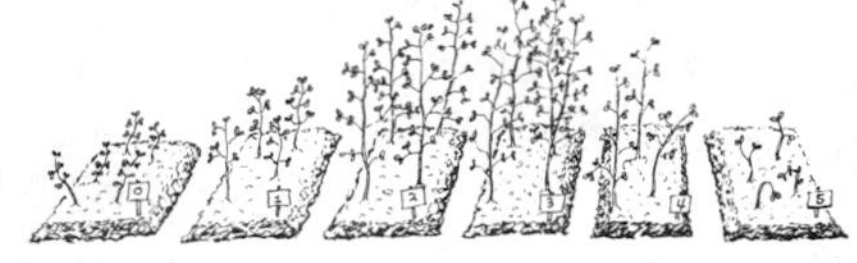

- shopkeepers and others who sell medicines (see *WTND,* p. 338)

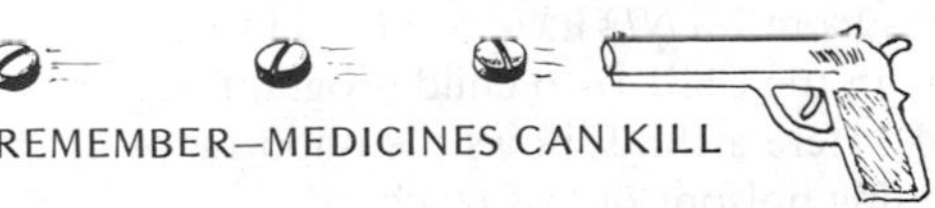

3. As an **idea book** for making teaching materials such as posters.

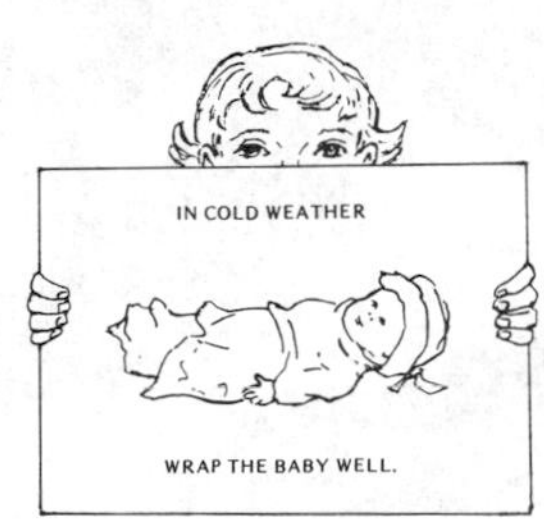
IN COLD WEATHER
WRAP THE BABY WELL.

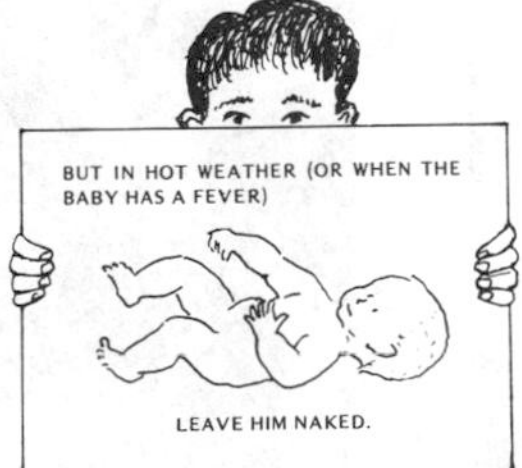

BUT IN HOT WEATHER (OR WHEN THE BABY HAS A FEVER)
LEAVE HIM NAKED.

4. As a **source of information** for conducting health activities such as . . .
   - under-fives clinics
   - check-ups for pregnant women
   - nutrition programs
   - public health measures

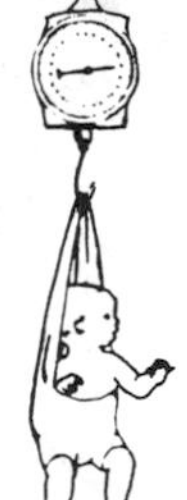

5. As a **guide** for discussing and exploring traditional forms of healing.

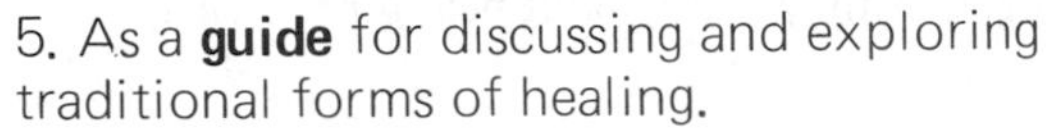
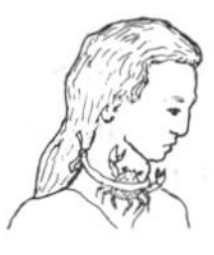
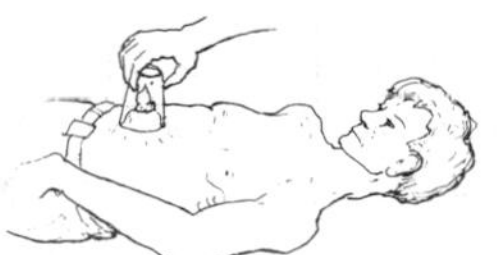
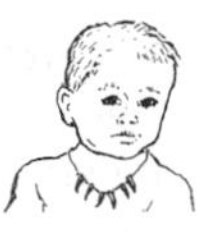

SHARING THE BOOK:

EXAMPLES FROM DIFFERENT COUNTRIES

By looking things up in her book together with people, a health worker takes some of the mystery out of medicine. This puts the health worker and other people on equal terms, and gives people more control over their own health.

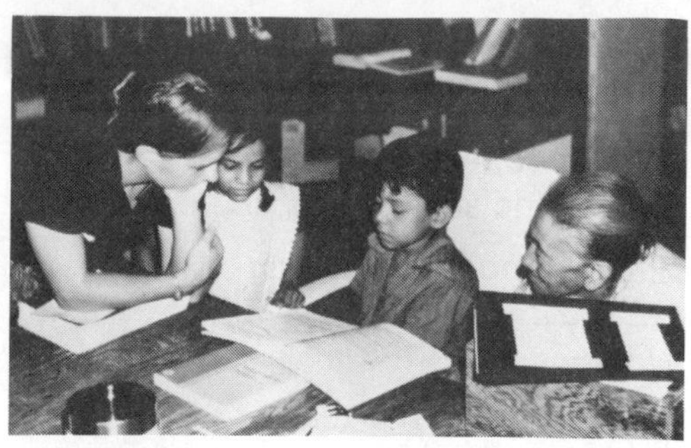

A health worker in Ajoya, Mexico shows two children the pictures of worms in *WTND* and asks them what kind they have.

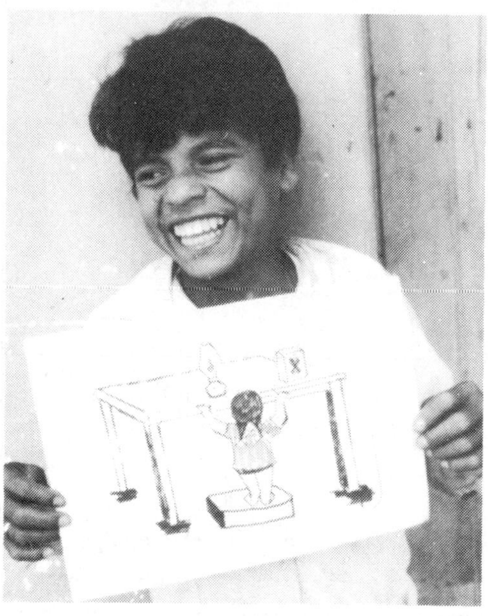

Pictures from *WTND* have been used for posters in the CHILD-to-child program (see Ch. 24). Here a child shows the importance of keeping poisons out of reach.

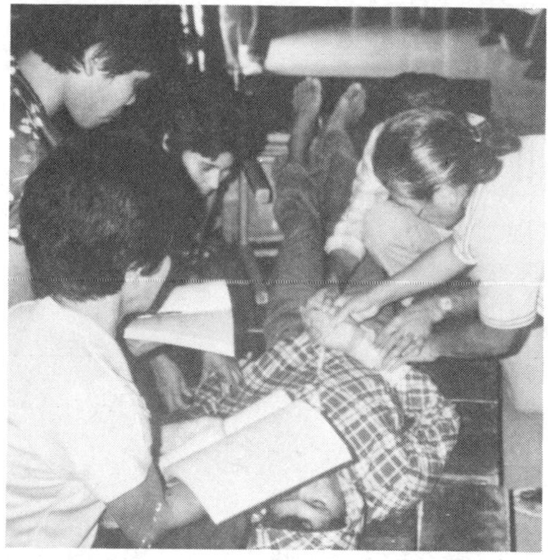

Here health workers in the Philippines use *WTND* to learn about fractures, bleeding, and shock in a role play.

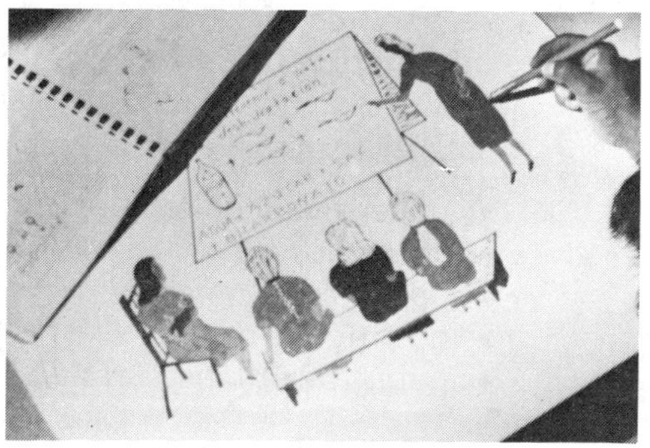

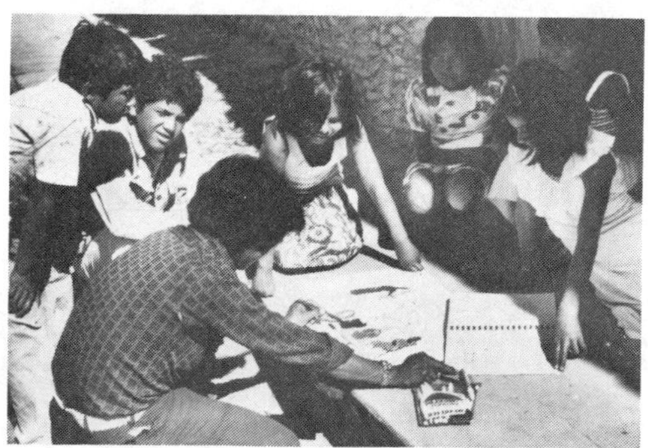

A health worker from Guatemala uses his book in preparing a poster about 'oral rehydration'. A group of curious school children look on. Together they learn about health problems, drawing, teaching, and sharing of ideas.

HELPING OTHERS LEARN TO USE THE BOOK

Where There Is No Doctor was not originally written for trained health workers, but for villagers who need information to care for the health of their families and neighbors. In areas the book has reached, it has served this purpose fairly well. Time and again, we have found that in villages where only one or two persons know how to read, these persons have become important health resources for the village. Their neighbors ask them to look in the book for information about medicines, health problems, and other concerns.

Seeing how often *Where There Is No Doctor* was used as a manual for health workers, after several years we added the introductory section called "Words to the Village Health Worker." However, we still feel that **the book is a tool for anyone who can read and is interested in health.**

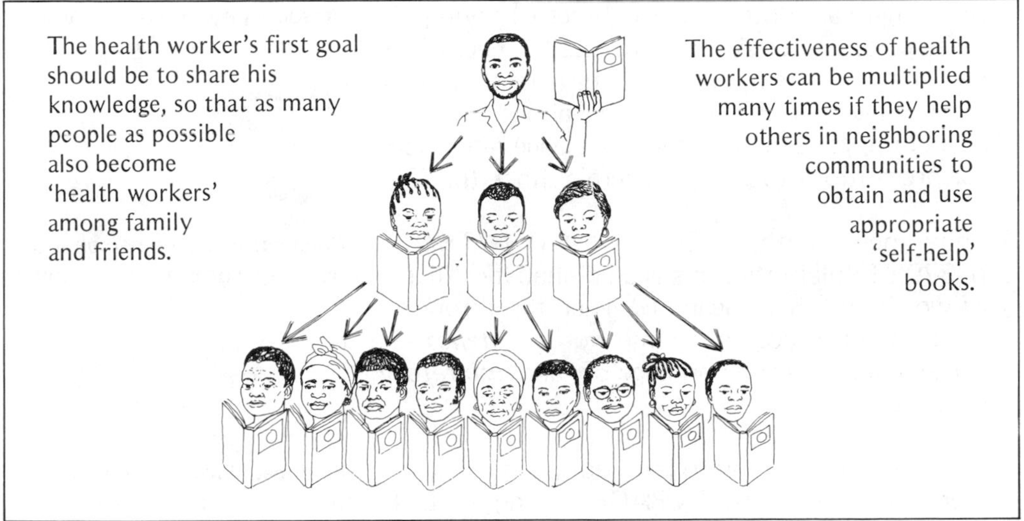

The health worker's first goal should be to share his knowledge, so that as many people as possible also become 'health workers' among family and friends.
The effectiveness of health workers can be multiplied many times if they help others in neighboring communities to obtain and use appropriate 'self-help' books.

Giving brief instructions on how to use the book

Health workers can help others use *Where There Is No Doctor* more effectively if they explain certain features of the book to them. They can point out the different reference sections—the Contents, Index, and Green Pages—and help persons to practice looking up topics that interest them. Even 10 or 15 minutes of such practice can be a big help. Sometimes a health worker can bring small groups together to learn about using the book.

Here we give 12 suggestions for helping others learn how to use *Where There Is No Doctor.* Many of these will be developed more fully in the next 2 chapters.

1. Show the person the inside of the front cover, and read the suggestions for HOW TO USE THIS BOOK.

2. Next, review the CONTENTS briefly, so the person gets an idea of what is in each chapter. Explain that she can look in the Contents for the chapter most likely to include the topic she wants. Then she can read the subheadings under the chapter title to see what page to turn to. Help her to practice doing this.

3. Now turn to the INDEX (yellow pages). Show how the subjects are listed in alphabetical order.

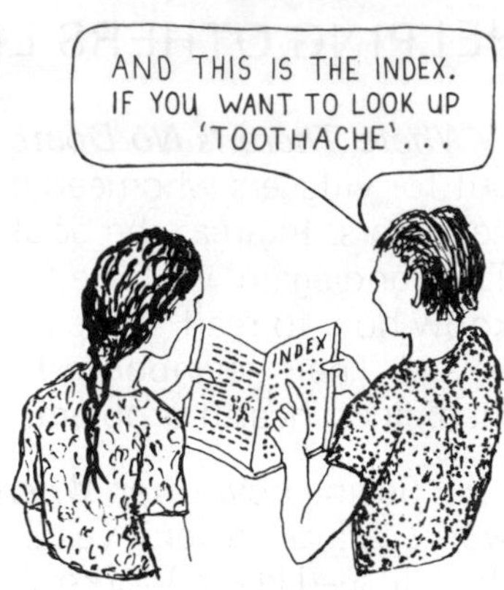
AND THIS IS THE INDEX. IF YOU WANT TO LOOK UP 'TOOTHACHE'...
INDEX

Practice: Ask the person to name a health problem that concerns her. Suppose she says "toothache." First have her flip through the book looking for pictures of teeth. (This is the way most people look for things first.) Next, show her how to find "Toothache" in the CONTENTS, then in the INDEX.

Now have her pick another subject, such as snakebite. Let her try to find it herself, first by flipping through the book, then by using the CONTENTS and the INDEX. Have her turn to the right page and read what it says.

4. **Page references.** Point out that throughout the book there are notes in parentheses ( ) saying "(see p.____)" or simply "(p.____)." These give the numbers of pages that have related information. On the second page about snakebite, for example, there is a page reference for precautions to prevent allergic shock (p. 70).

Practice: Have the person look up some page references and read the relevant parts.

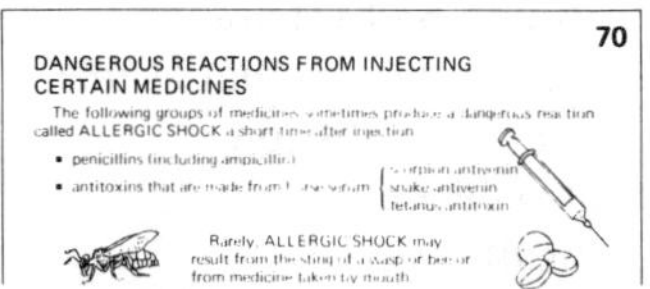
70

DANGEROUS REACTIONS FROM INJECTING CERTAIN MEDICINES

The following groups of medicines sometimes produce a dangerous reaction called ALLERGIC SHOCK a short time after injection

- penicillins (including ampicillin)
- antitoxins that are made from [illegible] serum: scorpion antivenin, snake antivenin, tetanus antitoxin

Rarely, ALLERGIC SHOCK may result from the sting of a wasp or bee or from medicine taken by mouth

5. Show the person the VOCABULARY *(WTND,* p. 379). Explain that this is an alphabetical list of words and their meanings. Then flip through the book until you spot some words in *italics*— for example, *bacteria* on page 55, and *respiratory* on page 57.

Practice: Have the person look up these words in the vocabulary.

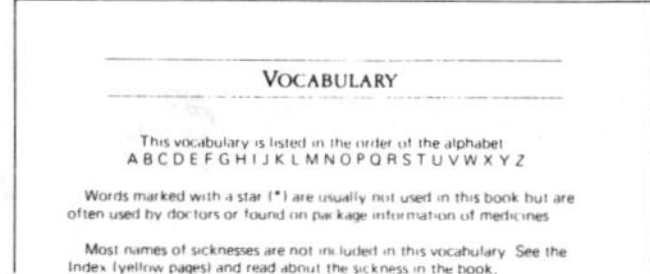
VOCABULARY

This vocabulary is listed in the order of the alphabet
A B C D E F G H I J K L M N O P Q R S T U V W X Y Z

Words marked with a star (*) are usually not used in this book but are often used by doctors or found on package information of medicines

Most names of sicknesses are not included in this vocabulary. See the Index (yellow pages) and read about the sickness in the book.

6. Show the person how to look up specific medicines in the GREEN PAGES, using the List of Medicines on page 341 and the Index of Medicines on page 345.

339

THE GREEN PAGES

THE USES, DOSAGE, AND PRECAUTIONS FOR THE MEDICINES REFERRED TO IN THIS BOOK

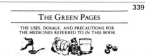

Practice: Have her look up a common medicine, such as aspirin, and read about it. Point out the importance of correct use, correct dosage, and always reading and following the precautions.

7. **Finding out about a health problem when you are not sure just what it is.** Have the person look in the book under the general kind of problem (skin problem, eye problem, old person's problem, etc.). Or look under the most important symptom or sign—for example, 'cough' or 'fever'.

Point out that in many parts of the book there are guides to help you decide which illness a person probably has. For example:

- Guide to Identification of Skin Problems, p. 196
- Different Illnesses that Cause Fever, p. 26
- Different Kinds of Cough, p. 168

For a more complete list of these guides and a discussion of how to use them, see Chapter 21 of this book.

8. **Avoiding mistakes.** Point out the first 8 chapters of ***Where There Is No Doctor,*** being sure to show the person Chapter 2, "Sicknesses that are Often Confused," and Chapter 6, "Right and Wrong Uses of Medicines." Look especially at the parts that deal with problems and beliefs common in your area. You may want to mark these pages in the book, so the person can read them later. For example, if people in your area tend to overuse and misuse injections, mark the first 6 pages of Chapter 9 (pages 65-70) for special reading.

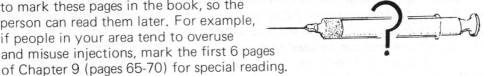

9. If the person will be providing care for sick or injured persons, encourage her to carefully study Chapter 3, "How to Examine a Sick Person," and Chapter 4, "How to Take Care of a Sick Person." If there is time, teach the person some of the basic aspects of history taking and physical examination.

10. **Prevention.** People's first interest in a book like ***Where There Is No Doctor*** usually has to do with curative medicine. But this interest can serve as a doorway to learning about prevention. Point out how, in discussing nearly any health problem, advice about prevention can be included. Look, for example, at Scabies on p. 199. Stress the importance of preventive advice.

    Also encourage the person to read Chapters 11 and 12, on "Nutrition" and "Prevention." Consider putting markers at pages describing preventive action that is especially needed in your area. For example, if blindness due to lack of vitamin A is common in your community, mark page 226. Encourage the person to follow the advice on that page, and to help others to do the same.

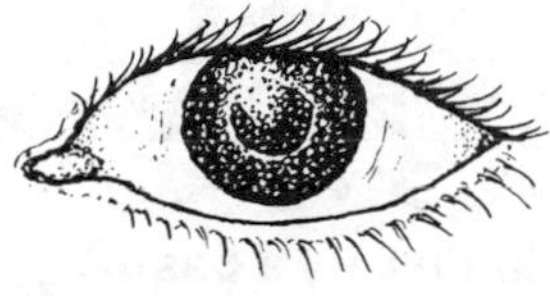

11. Point out the chapters and sections that are of special importance to the reader. For example, if she is a mother, show her the chapter on children's health problems. Ask if any of her children has an illness at the moment. See if she can find it in the book. Have her read about it. Then discuss it with her to make sure she understands the information.

12. **Knowing when to seek help.** In making suggestions on how to use the book, emphasize that the person needs to recognize her limitations. Help her to realize that sometimes she will need to seek help from a health worker or doctor. Show her the following pages:
    - p. 42, Signs of Dangerous Illness
    - p. 159, When to Seek Medical Help in Cases of Diarrhea
    - p. 256, Signs of Special Risk that Make It Important that a Doctor or Skilled Midwife Attend the Birth—if Possible in a Hospital

---

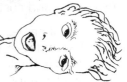

By focusing on the 12 points presented here, a person can gain some understanding of how to use the book in as little as 2 or 3 hours. However, these guidelines are only a beginning. There may be other parts of the book that are especially useful for your area. And a great deal of practice is needed to use the book really well. The next 2 chapters suggest ways of providing such practice in a training course.

ADAPTING *WHERE THERE IS NO DOCTOR* TO THE LOCAL SITUATION

The original Spanish edition of ***Where There Is No Doctor*** was written specifically for use in the mountain area of Western Mexico. In the English version, we tried to make the book so it could be used in many different countries. But clearly, a book that can be used in many areas will not be completely appropriate to any single place. Therefore, some of the information and ideas in the book will apply to your area. Others will not. And some basic information will certainly be missing.

Health workers should recognize the limitations of the book and never use it as their 'bible'. (Unfortunately, this has happened in some health programs.)

Ideally, ***Where There Is No Doctor*** (or any reference book) should be adapted or rewritten for each area. This has already been done in some parts of the world.

SENEGAL
(French)

TANZANIA
(Swahili)

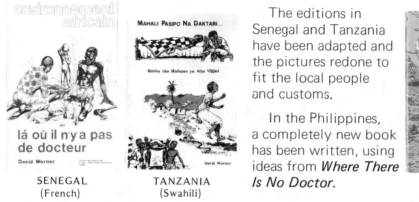

The editions in Senegal and Tanzania have been adapted and the pictures redone to fit the local people and customs.

In the Philippines, a completely new book has been written, using ideas from ***Where There Is No Doctor.***

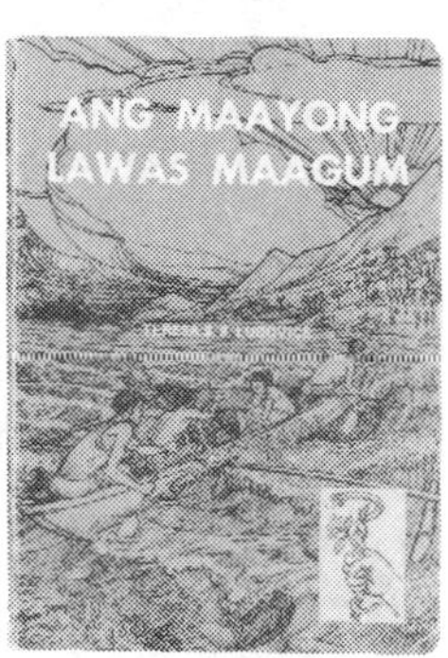

PHILIPPINES
(Ilonggo)

Unfortunately, not every area will have the time and money to write their own villager's health care handbook, or to adapt the whole of ***Where There Is No Doctor.*** Where complete adaptations are not possible, we suggest that training programs produce mimeographed sheets or pamphlets to be used along with the book. These can cover additional information that relates to local needs, problems, and customs. Such information sheets might include:

- Local names of illnesses, and ways of looking at sickness and health.
- Examples of traditional forms of healing: beneficial and harmful.
- Names (including brand names and comparative prices) of medicines that are available locally. Or at least have students write this information into the Green Pages of their books.
- A list of commonly misused medicines and mistaken medical practices in your area, with explanations and warnings.
- Information about the diagnosis, treatment, and prevention of health problems that are important in your area but are not included in ***Where There Is No Doctor.***

Discuss with your students which parts of their books are appropriate to your area and which are not. Encourage them to question the truth or usefulness of anything they read.

CHAPTER 20

Using the Contents, Index, Page References, and Vocabulary

Note: Some instructors may feel that certain things explained in this chapter are very obvious. They may think that to teach them would be a waste of time, or even an insult to the students. But skills in using an index and looking up page references should not be taken for granted. **If you allow time for explaining and helping students master these basic skills, it can make a big difference in their problem-solving abilities.**

LEARNING HOW TO LOOK THINGS UP

Persons who have not done much reading may find it difficult to use an information book effectively. In addition to reading slowly, they may also have difficulty finding what they are looking for. Sometimes they try to find things by flipping through the book, looking at the pictures. But this can be slow, and they may miss important information.

Early in the training course, **take time to show students how to use their books.** Instructors and more experienced students can guide others in practicing how to look things up.* The following are some points you may want to explain.

Page numbering

The pages are numbered in order: 1,2,3,4,5,6,7,8,9,10 . . . 20 . . . 30 . . . 100 . . . 200, and so on. So if you want to find page 168 to read about 'Cough', do not start at the beginning of the book and go through it page by page. Instead . . .

Open the book somewhere in the middle— for instance to pages 198 and 199.

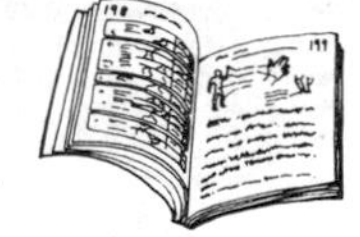

That is too far forward, so turn back some, say to page 184 and then to 166.

Now you are very close. Turn the page to 168.

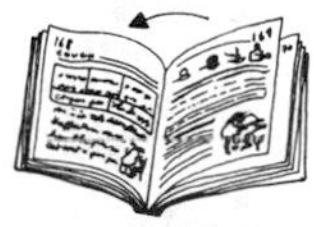

*It is a good idea, in the first days of the course, to check each person's reading ability, knowledge of alphabetical order, and basic arithmetic skills. Provide special practice for those who need it. But be sure these students are not made to feel ashamed because they have had less schooling. Include them in all regular classes and help them feel free to participate.

Alphabetical lists

Where There Is No Doctor has several reference sections, or lists where you can look things up. Three of these are arranged in alphabetical order:

- The **INDEX** (the yellow pages at the end of the book)—where you can look up the page or pages with information about almost anything in the book.
- The **INDEX OF MEDICINES** in the GREEN PAGES—to help you find the page with the uses, dosage, and precautions for the medicine you want to know about.
- The **VOCABULARY**—where you can look up the meanings of words written in *italics* in the main part of the book.

In each of these lists, the words are arranged so that their first letters are in the order of the alphabet: A,B,C,D,E, and so on until Z.

Suppose you want to look up 'Vomiting'. Depending on whether you are interested in **medicines,** a **definition,** or a **full discussion** on vomiting, you can look it up in the GREEN PAGES, the VOCABULARY, or the INDEX.

First, **look for the large dark letters** in the center of each column. **V** will be near the end of the lists because it is near the end of the alphabet.

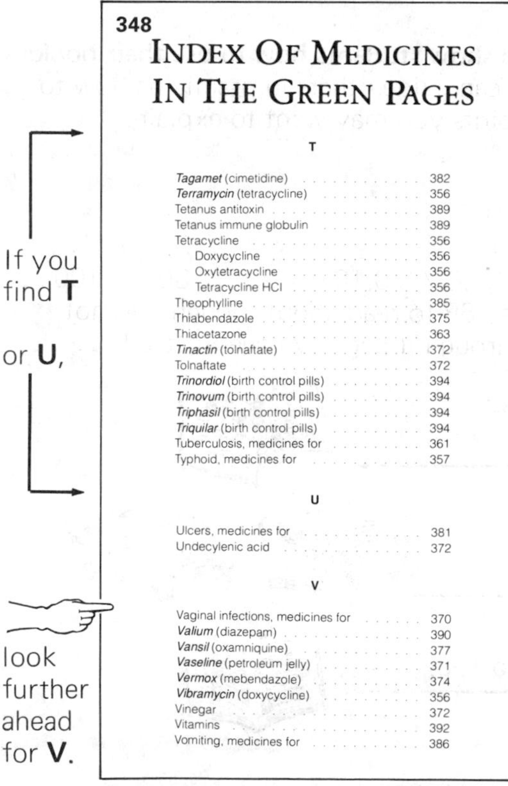
If you find **T**
or **U**,
look further ahead for **V**.

348

INDEX OF MEDICINES IN THE GREEN PAGES

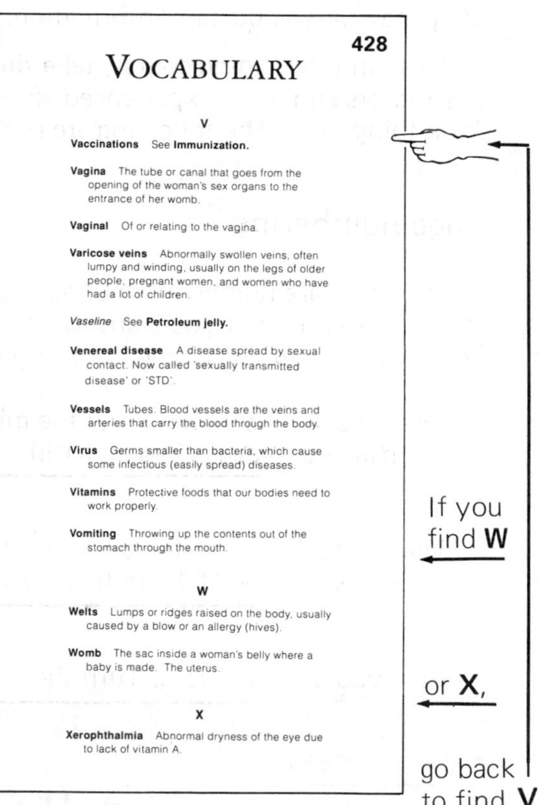
If you find **W**
or **X**,
go back to find **V**.

428

VOCABULARY

V

Vaccinations See **Immunization.**

Vagina The tube or canal that goes from the opening of the woman's sex organs to the entrance of her womb.

Vaginal Of or relating to the vagina.

Varicose veins Abnormally swollen veins, often lumpy and winding, usually on the legs of older people, pregnant women, and women who have had a lot of children.

Vaseline See **Petroleum jelly.**

Venereal disease A disease spread by sexual contact. Now called 'sexually transmitted disease' or 'STD'.

Vessels Tubes. Blood vessels are the veins and arteries that carry the blood through the body.

Virus Germs smaller than bacteria, which cause some infectious (easily spread) diseases.

Vitamins Protective foods that our bodies need to work properly.

Vomiting Throwing up the contents out of the stomach through the mouth.

W

Welts Lumps or ridges raised on the body, usually caused by a blow or an allergy (hives).

Womb The sac inside a woman's belly where a baby is made. The uterus.

X

Xerophthalmia Abnormal dryness of the eye due to lack of vitamin A.

After you find **V,** start looking for '**Vo**miting'—after '**Va**ccinations' and '**Vi**tamins'.

Using the INDEX (yellow pages) of *Where There Is No Doctor*

When you find a word in the index followed by several page numbers, the **dark number** indicates the page that has the most information. For example,

page **147** for 'Vaccinations',

pages **241-242** for 'Vaginal discharge',

and

page **175** under 'Varicose veins'.

What others do you find in this list?

If you find several words listed in lighter letters under the main word, these are subheadings related to the main topic or idea. For example, 'with diarrhea' refers to **'Vomiting** with diarrhea'.

If you do not find the subject you want in the INDEX, try looking for it under another name. For example, you might look first for 'Upset stomach'. If that is not listed, look up other words that mean the same thing: 'Puking', 'Throwing up', or 'Vomiting'. Usually the most widely known word is listed.

Practice at finding things in alphabetical lists will make it easier for health workers to use the INDEX and VOCABULARY.

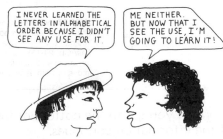

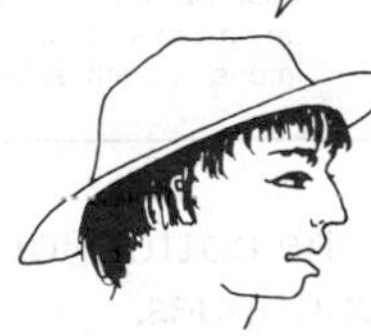

I NEVER LEARNED THE LETTERS IN ALPHABETICAL ORDER BECAUSE I DIDN'T SEE ANY USE FOR IT.

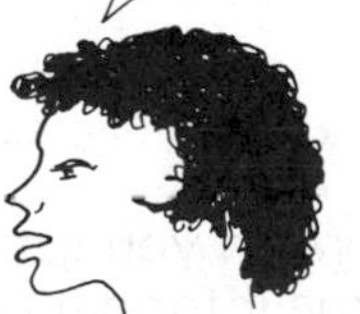

ME NEITHER. BUT NOW THAT I SEE THE USE, I'M GOING TO LEARN IT!

Finding what you are looking for on a page

After you have looked something up in the INDEX and have turned to the page with the topic you want, take a moment to **look over the whole page.** Do not just start reading from the top. First notice what part of the page has the information you are looking for.

For example: Suppose some neighbors have a baby who is cross-eyed, and you want to discuss with them what can be done to correct the problem. You look in the INDEX (or the CONTENTS) and find that the main reference to cross-eyes is page 223. But **where on page 223 should you read?** Here are some clues:

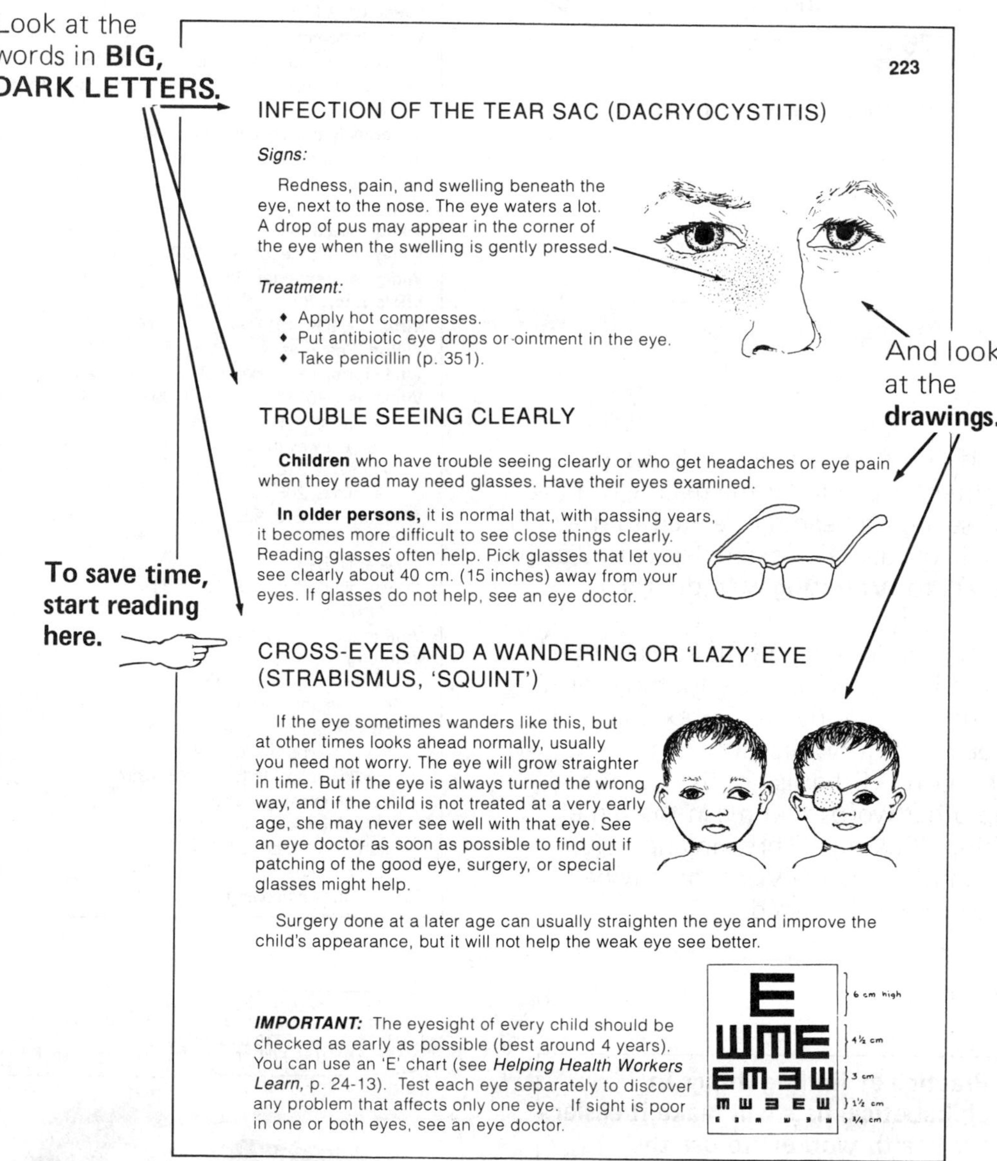

Look at the words in BIG, DARK LETTERS.
And look at the drawings.
To save time, start reading here.
223
INFECTION OF THE TEAR SAC (DACRYOCYSTITIS)
Signs:
Redness, pain, and swelling beneath the eye, next to the nose. The eye waters a lot. A drop of pus may appear in the corner of the eye when the swelling is gently pressed.
Treatment:
♦ Apply hot compresses.
♦ Put antibiotic eye drops or ointment in the eye.
♦ Take penicillin (p. 351).
TROUBLE SEEING CLEARLY
Children who have trouble seeing clearly or who get headaches or eye pain when they read may need glasses. Have their eyes examined.
In older persons, it is normal that, with passing years, it becomes more difficult to see close things clearly. Reading glasses often help. Pick glasses that let you see clearly about 40 cm. (15 inches) away from your eyes. If glasses do not help, see an eye doctor.
CROSS-EYES AND A WANDERING OR 'LAZY' EYE (STRABISMUS, 'SQUINT')
If the eye sometimes wanders like this, but at other times looks ahead normally, usually you need not worry. The eye will grow straighter in time. But if the eye is always turned the wrong way, and if the child is not treated at a very early age, she may never see well with that eye. See an eye doctor as soon as possible to find out if patching of the good eye, surgery, or special glasses might help.
Surgery done at a later age can usually straighten the eye and improve the child's appearance, but it will not help the weak eye see better.
IMPORTANT: The eyesight of every child should be checked as early as possible (best around 4 years). You can use an 'E' chart (see Helping Health Workers Learn, p. 24-13). Test each eye separately to discover any problem that affects only one eye. If sight is poor in one or both eyes, see an eye doctor.
6 cm high
4½ cm
3 cm
1½ cm
¾ cm

When you get to the bottom of the page, be sure to check the next page to see if the information continues.

Looking up page references

Once you have read about the topic you looked up, you may want to turn also to other pages mentioned in the text. These are often referred to in parentheses (inside curved lines like these)—for example, "(see p. 140)," or simply "(p. 125)." On these pages you will find additional information, such as:

- another disease that may be a cause of the problem you are interested in
- danger signs you should watch for
- how the same disease can affect another part of the body or another person
- medicines recommended for treatment, their dosage and precautions
- other recommended treatments
- how to prevent the problem you are reading about

Page 307 of *Where There Is No Doctor* refers you to various causes of anemia in children.

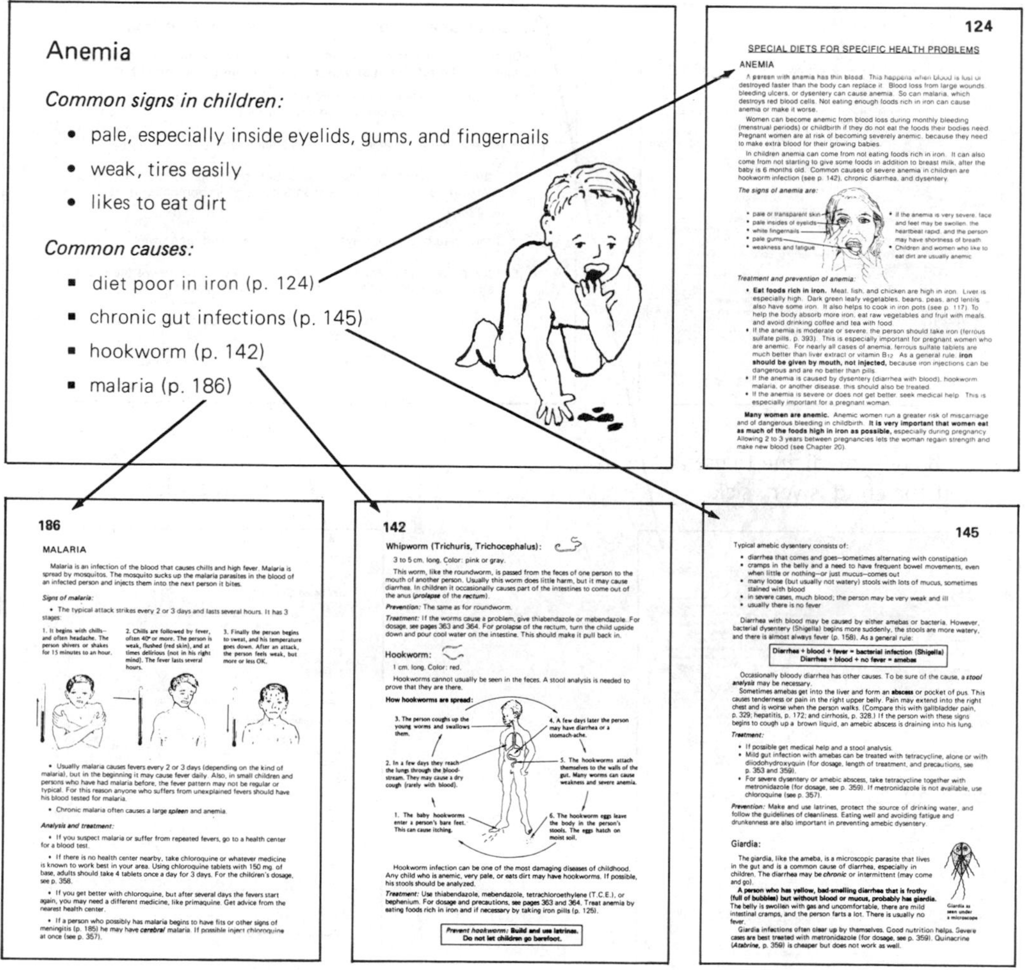

Anemia

Common signs in children:

- pale, especially inside eyelids, gums, and fingernails
- weak, tires easily
- likes to eat dirt

Common causes:

- diet poor in iron (p. 124)
- chronic gut infections (p. 145)
- hookworm (p. 142)
- malaria (p. 186)

124

SPECIAL DIETS FOR SPECIFIC HEALTH PROBLEMS

ANEMIA

A person with anemia has thin blood. This happens when blood is lost or destroyed faster than the body can replace it. Blood loss from large wounds, bleeding ulcers, or dysentery can cause anemia. So can malaria, which destroys red blood cells. Not eating enough foods rich in iron can cause anemia or make it worse.

Women can become anemic from blood loss during monthly bleeding (menstrual periods) or childbirth if they do not eat the foods their bodies need. Pregnant women are at risk of becoming severely anemic, because they need to make extra blood for their growing babies.

In children anemia can come from not eating foods rich in iron. It can also come from not starting to give some foods in addition to breast milk, after the baby is 6 months old. Common causes of severe anemia in children are hookworm infection (see p. 142), chronic diarrhea, and dysentery.

The signs of anemia are:

- pale or transparent skin
- pale insides of eyelids
- white fingernails
- pale gums
- weakness and fatigue

- If the anemia is very severe, face and feet may be swollen, the heartbeat rapid, and the person may have shortness of breath.
- Children and women who like to eat dirt are usually anemic.

Treatment and prevention of anemia:

- **Eat foods rich in iron.** Meat, fish, and chicken are high in iron. Liver is especially high. Dark green leafy vegetables, beans, peas, and lentils also have some iron. It also helps to cook in iron pots (see p. 117). To help the body absorb more iron, eat raw vegetables and fruit with meals and avoid drinking coffee and tea with food.
- If the anemia is moderate or severe, the person should take iron (ferrous sulfate pills, p. 393). This is especially important for pregnant women who are anemic. For nearly all cases of anemia, ferrous sulfate tablets are much better than liver extract or vitamin B_{12}. As a general rule, **iron should be given by mouth, not injected,** because iron injections can be dangerous and are no better than pills.
- If the anemia is caused by dysentery (diarrhea with blood), hookworm, malaria, or another disease, this should also be treated.
- If the anemia is severe or does not get better, seek medical help. This is especially important for a pregnant woman.

Many women are anemic. Anemic women run a greater risk of miscarriage and of dangerous bleeding in childbirth. **It is very important that women eat as much of the foods high in iron as possible,** especially during pregnancy. Allowing 2 to 3 years between pregnancies lets the woman regain strength and make new blood (see Chapter 20).

186

MALARIA

Malaria is an infection of the blood that causes chills and high fever. Malaria is spread by mosquitos. The mosquito sucks up the malaria parasites in the blood of an infected person and injects them into the next person it bites.

Signs of malaria:

- The typical attack strikes every 2 or 3 days and lasts several hours. It has 3 stages:

1. It begins with chills—and often headache. The person shivers or shakes for 15 minutes to an hour.
2. Chills are followed by fever, often 40° or more. The person is weak, flushed (red skin), and at times delirious (not in his right mind). The fever lasts several hours.
3. Finally the person begins to sweat, and his temperature goes down. After an attack, the person feels weak, but more or less OK.

- Usually malaria causes fevers every 2 or 3 days (depending on the kind of malaria), but in the beginning it may cause fever daily. Also, in small children and persons who have had malaria before, the fever pattern may not be regular or typical. For this reason anyone who suffers from unexplained fevers should have his blood tested for malaria.
- Chronic malaria often causes a large ***spleen*** and anemia.

Analysis and treatment:

- If you suspect malaria or suffer from repeated fevers, go to a health center for a blood test.
- If there is no health center nearby, take chloroquine or whatever medicine is known to work best in your area. Using chloroquine tablets with 150 mg. of base, adults should take 4 tablets once a day for 3 days. For the children's dosage, see p. 358.
- If you get better with chloroquine, but after several days the fevers start again, you may need a different medicine, like primaquine. Get advice from the nearest health center.
- If a person who possibly has malaria begins to have fits or other signs of meningitis (p. 185) he may have ***cerebral*** malaria. If possible inject chloroquine at once (see p. 357).

142

Whipworm (Trichuris, Trichocephalus):

3 to 5 cm. long. Color: pink or gray.

This worm, like the roundworm, is passed from the feces of one person to the mouth of another person. Usually this worm does little harm, but it may cause diarrhea. In children it occasionally causes part of the intestines to come out of the anus (***prolapse*** of the ***rectum***).

Prevention: The same as for roundworm.

Treatment: If the worms cause a problem, give thiabendazole or mebendazole. For dosage, see pages 363 and 364. For prolapse of the rectum, turn the child upside down and pour cool water on the intestine. This should make it pull back in.

Hookworm:

1 cm. long. Color: red.

Hookworms cannot usually be seen in the feces. A stool analysis is needed to prove that they are there.

How hookworms are spread:

1. The baby hookworms enter a person's bare feet. This can cause itching.
2. In a few days they reach the lungs through the blood-stream. They may cause a dry cough (rarely with blood).
3. The person coughs up the young worms and swallows them.
4. A few days later the person may have diarrhea or a stomach-ache.
5. The hookworms attach themselves to the walls of the gut. Many worms can cause weakness and severe anemia.
6. The hookworm eggs leave the body in the person's stools. The eggs hatch on moist soil.

Hookworm infection can be one of the most damaging diseases of childhood. Any child who is anemic, very pale, or eats dirt may have hookworms. If possible, his stools should be analyzed.

Treatment: Use thiabendazole, mebendazole, tetrachloroethylene (T.C.E.), or bephenium. For dosage and precautions, see pages 363 and 364. Treat anemia by eating foods rich in iron and if necessary by taking iron pills (p. 125).

Prevent hookworm: **Build and use latrines. Do not let children go barefoot.**

145

Typical amebic dysentery consists of:

- diarrhea that comes and goes—sometimes alternating with constipation
- cramps in the belly and a need to have frequent bowel movements, even when little or nothing—or just mucus—comes out
- many loose (but usually not watery) stools with lots of mucus, sometimes stained with blood
- in severe cases, much blood; the person may be very weak and ill
- usually there is no fever

Diarrhea with blood may be caused by either amebas or bacteria. However, bacterial dysentery (Shigella) begins more suddenly, the stools are more watery, and there is almost always fever (p. 158). As a general rule:

Diarrhea + blood + fever = bacterial infection (Shigella)
Diarrhea + blood + no fever = amebas

Occasionally bloody diarrhea has other causes. To be sure of the cause, a ***stool analysis*** may be necessary.

Sometimes amebas get into the liver and form an **abscess** or pocket of pus. This causes tenderness or pain in the right upper belly. Pain may extend into the right chest and is worse when the person walks. (Compare this with gallbladder pain, p. 329; hepatitis, p. 172; and cirrhosis, p. 328.) If the person with these signs begins to cough up a brown liquid, an amebic abscess is draining into his lung.

Treatment:

- If possible get medical help and a stool analysis.
- Mild gut infection with amebas can be treated with tetracycline, alone or with diiodohydroxyquin (for dosage, length of treatment, and precautions, see p. 353 and 359).
- For severe dysentery or amebic abscess, take tetracycline together with metronidazole (for dosage, see p. 359). If metronidazole is not available, use chloroquine (see p. 357).

Prevention: Make and use latrines, protect the source of drinking water, and follow the guidelines of cleanliness. Eating well and avoiding fatigue and drunkenness are also important in preventing amebic dysentery.

Giardia:

The giardia, like the ameba, is a microscopic parasite that lives in the gut and is a common cause of diarrhea, especially in children. The diarrhea may be ***chronic*** or intermittent (may come and go).

A person who has yellow, bad-smelling diarrhea that is frothy (full of bubbles) but without blood or mucus, probably has giardia. The belly is swollen with gas and uncomfortable, there are mild intestinal cramps, and the person farts a lot. There is usually no fever.

Giardia as seen under a microscope

Giardia infections often clear up by themselves. Good nutrition helps. Severe cases are best treated with metronidazole (for dosage, see p. 359). Quinacrine (***Atabrine***, p. 359) is cheaper but does not work as well.

Also point out how arrows are used in the book to join writing with pictures (as on page 124 above) or to show which direction to read (page 142 above). Check students' ability to follow the arrows.

Page 159 of *Where There Is No Doctor* refers you to several pages with more information about . . .

159

Care of Babies with Diarrhea

Diarrhea is especially dangerous in babies and small children. Often no medicine is needed, but special care must be taken because a baby can die very quickly of dehydration.

GIVE HIM BREAST MILK

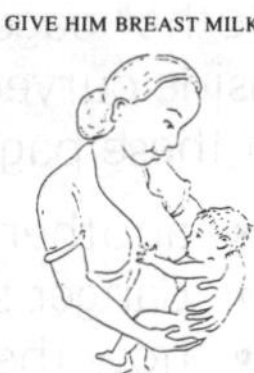

- **Continue breast feeding** and also give sips of **Rehydration Drink.**
- If vomiting is a problem, give breast milk often, but only a little at a time. Also give Rehydration Drink in small sips every 5 to 10 minutes (see Vomiting, p. 161).
- If there is no breast milk, try giving frequent small feedings of some other milk or milk substitute (like milk made from soybeans) **mixed to half normal strength with boiled water.** If milk seems to make the diarrhea worse, give some other protein (mashed chicken, eggs, lean meat, or skinned mashed beans, mixed with sugar or well-cooked rice or another carbohydrate, and boiled water).

AND ALSO REHYDRATION DRINK

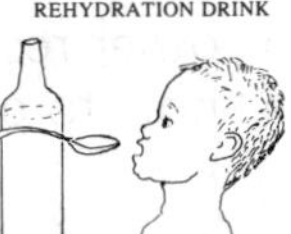

- If the child is younger than 1 month, try to find a health worker before giving any medicine. If there is no health worker and the child is very sick, give him an 'infant syrup' that contains ampicillin: half a teaspoon 4 times daily (see p. 353). It is better not to use other antibiotics.

When to Seek Medical Help in Cases of Diarrhea

Diarrhea and dysentery can be very dangerous—especially in small children. **In the following situations you should get medical help:**

- if diarrhea lasts more than 4 days and is not getting better—or more than 1 day in a small child with severe diarrhea
- if the person shows signs of dehydration and is getting worse
- if the child vomits everything he drinks, or drinks nothing, or if frequent vomiting continues for more than 3 hours after beginning Rehydration Drink
- if the child begins to have fits, or if the feet and face swell
- if the person was very sick, weak, or malnourished before the diarrhea began (especially a little child or a very old person)
- if there is much blood in the stools. This can be dangerous even if there is only very little diarrhea (see gut obstruction, p. 94).

special treatment if vomiting is a problem

161

VOMITING

Many people, especially children, have an occasional 'stomach upset' with vomiting. Often no cause can be found. There may be mild stomach or gut ache or fever. This kind of simple vomiting usually is not serious and clears up by itself.

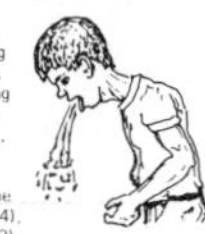

Vomiting is one of the signs of many different problems, some minor and some quite serious, so it is important to examine the person carefully. Vomiting often comes from a problem in the stomach or guts, such as: an infection (see diarrhea, p. 153), poisoning from spoiled food (p. 135), or 'acute abdomen' (for example, appendicitis or something blocking the gut, p. 94). Also, almost any sickness with high fever or severe pain may cause vomiting, especially malaria (p. 186), hepatitis (p. 172), tonsillitis (p. 309), earache (p. 309), meningitis (p. 185), urinary infection (p. 234), gallbladder pain (p. 329) or migraine headache (p. 162).

Danger signs with vomiting—seek medical help quickly!

- dehydration that increases and that you cannot control, (p. 152)
- severe vomiting that lasts more than 24 hours
- violent vomiting, especially if vomit is dark green, brown, or smells like feces (signs of obstruction, p. 94)
- constant pain in the gut, especially if the person cannot defecate (shit) or if you cannot hear gurgles when you put your ear to the belly (see acute abdomen: obstruction, appendicitis, p. 94)
- vomiting of blood (ulcer, p. 128, cirrhosis, p. 328)

To help control simple vomiting:

- Eat nothing while vomiting is severe.
- Sip a cola drink or ginger ale. Some herbal teas, like camomile, may also help.
- For dehydration give small frequent sips of cola, tea, or Rehydration Drink (p. 152).
- If vomiting does not stop soon, use a vomit control medicine like promethazine (p. 371), diphenhydramine (p. 371), or phenobarbital (p. 373).

Most of these come in pills, syrups, injections, and suppositories (soft pills you push up the ***anus***). Tablets or syrup can also be put up the anus. Grind up the tablet in a little water. Put it in with an enema set or syringe without a needle.

When taken by mouth, the medicine should be swallowed with very little water and nothing else should be swallowed for 5 minutes. Never give more than the recommended dose. Do not give a second dose until dehydration has been corrected and the person has begun to urinate. If severe vomiting and diarrhea make medication by mouth or anus impossible, give an injection of 1 of these vomit control medicines. Promethazine may work best. Take care not to give too much.

the best medicine to use if the child is very sick

353

Dosage of procaine penicillin—for moderately severe infections:

Give **1** injection a day.

With each injection give:

adults: 600,000 to 1,200,000 U.
children age 8 to 12: 600,000 U.
children age 3 to 7: 300,000 U.
children under 3: 150,000 U.
newborn babies: DO NOT USE unless no other penicillin or ampicillin is available. In emergencies, 75,000 U.

For very severe infections, give twice the above dose. However, it is better to use a short-acting penicillin.

The dosage for procaine penicillin combined with a short-acting penicillin is the same as for procaine penicillin alone.

For treatment of gonorrhea and syphilis, procaine penicillin is best. Very high doses are needed. For dosage, see pages 237 and 238.

Benzathine penicillin (long-acting)

Name ________________ price ______ for ___

Often comes in: vials of 1,200,000 or 2,400,000 U.

Dosage of benzathine penicillin—for mild to moderately severe infections:

Give 1 injection every 4 days. For mild infections, 1 injection may be enough.

adults: 1,200,000 U.
children age 8 to 12: 600,000 U.
children age 3 to 8: 300,000 U.
children under 3 years: 150,000 U.

To prevent return infection in persons who have had rheumatic fever, give twice the above dose once every 3 or 4 weeks (see p. 310).

AMPICILLIN: A WIDE-RANGE (BROAD-SPECTRUM PENICILLIN)

Ampicillin

Name ________________

Often comes in solutions,

125 or 250 mg./tsp. price: ______ for ___
capsules, 250 mg. price: ______ for ___
injections, 250 mg. price: ______ for ___

Ampicillin is a ***broad-spectrum*** (wide-range) penicillin that kills many more kinds of bacteria than are killed by other penicillins. It is safer than other broad-spectrum antibiotics and is especially useful for babies and small children.

Because it is expensive, and sometimes causes diarrhea or 'thrush', ampicillin should not be used when regular penicillin is likely to do the job as well.

Ampicillin works well when taken by mouth. Injections should only be used for severe illnesses such as meningitis, peritonitis, and appendicitis, or when the sick person vomits or cannot swallow the medicine.

Ampicillin is especially useful in treating the following:

septicemia and unexplained illness in the newborn
pneumonia or ear infections of children under 6 years
severe diarrhea or dysentery **with fever**
meningitis
peritonitis and appendicitis
severe urinary tract infections
typhoid fever (after illness has been controlled with chloramphenicol or if it is resistant to chloramphenicol)

Persons allergic to penicillin should not take ampicillin. See ***Risks and Precautions*** for penicillin, page 349.

Dosage for ampicillin:

By mouth: (25 to 50 mg./kg./day)
capsules of 250 mg., syrup with 125 mg. per teaspoon (5 ml.)

Give 4 doses a day.

In each dose give:

adults: 2 capsules or 4 teaspoons (500 mg.)
children age 8 to 12: 1 capsule or 2 teaspoons (250 mg.)
children 3 to 7: ½ capsule or 1 teaspoon (125 mg.)
children under 3: ¼ capsule or ½ teaspoon (62 mg.)
newborn babies: same as for children under 3 years

By injection, for severe infections—(50 to 100 mg./kg./day - up to 300 mg./kg./day for meningitis)
vials of 250 mg.

Give 4 doses a day, once every 6 hours.

a sign of danger

94

Obstructed Gut

An acute abdomen may be caused by something that blocks or 'obstructs' a part of the gut, so that food and stools cannot pass. More common causes are:

- a ball or knot of roundworms (Ascaris, p. 140)
- a loop of gut that is pinched in a hernia (p. 177)
- a part of the gut that slips inside the part below it (intussusception)

Almost any kind of acute abdomen may show some signs of obstruction. Because it hurts the damaged gut to move, it stops moving.

Signs of an obstructed gut:

Steady, severe pain in the belly.

This child's belly is swollen, hard, and very tender. It hurts more when you touch it. He tries to protect his belly and keeps his legs doubled up. His belly is often 'silent'. (When you put your ear to it, you hear no sound of normal gurgles.)

Sudden vomiting with great force! The vomit may shoot out a meter or more. It may have green bile in it or smell and look like feces.

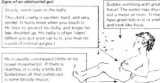

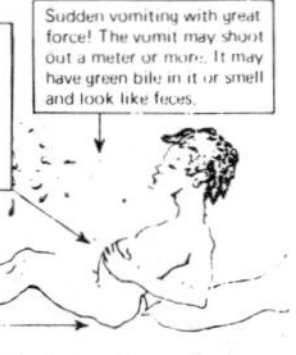

He is usually constipated (little or no bowel movements). If there is diarrhea, it is only a little bit. Sometimes all that comes out is some bloody mucus.

Get this person to a hospital **at once.** His life is in danger and surgery may be needed.

Appendicitis, Peritonitis

These dangerous conditions often require surgery. Seek medical help fast.

Appendicitis is an infection of the ***appendix***, a finger shaped sac attached to the large intestine in the lower right-hand part of the belly. An infected appendix sometimes bursts open, causing ***peritonitis***.

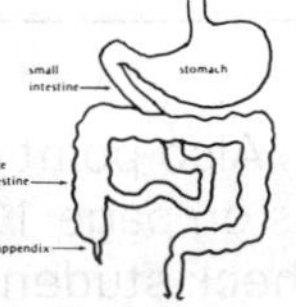

Peritonitis is an acute, serious infection of the lining of the cavity or bag that holds the gut. It results when the appendix or another part of the gut bursts or is torn.

Looking up related information—even when page references are not given

Usually a book gives only the most important page references, to save you time in looking things up. But sometimes you will want to look up related information, or something you are unsure about—even though no page reference is given.

Read this information about measles from pages 311 and 312 of *Where There Is No Doctor:*

> **Measles**
>
> This severe virus infection is **especially dangerous in children** who are **poorly nourished** or have **tuberculosis.** Ten days after being near a person with measles, it begins with signs of a cold—fever, runny nose, red sore eyes, and cough.
>
> The child becomes increasingly ill. The mouth may become very sore and he may develop diarrhea.
>
> After 2 or 3 days a few tiny white spots like salt grains appear in the mouth. A day or 2 later the rash appears—first behind the ears and on the neck, then on the face and body, and last on the arms and legs. After the rash appears, the child usually begins to get better. The rash lasts about 5 days. Sometimes there are scattered black spots caused by bleeding into the skin ('black measles'). This means the attack is very severe. Get medical help.
>
> *Treatment:*
>
> - The child should stay in bed, drink lots of liquids, and be given nutritious food. If she cannot swallow solid food, give her liquids like soup. If a baby cannot breast feed, give breast milk in a spoon (see p. 120).
> - If possible, give vitamin A to prevent eye damage (p. 392).
> - For fever and discomfort, give acetaminophen (or aspirin).
> - If earache develops, give an antibiotic (p. 351).
> - If signs of pneumonia, meningitis, or severe pain in the ear or stomach develop, get medical help.
> - If the child has diarrhea, give Rehydration Drink (p. 152).
>
> *Prevention of measles:*
>
> Children with measles should keep far away from other children, even from brothers and sisters. Especially try to protect children who are poorly nourished or who have tuberculosis or other chronic illnesses. Children from other families should not go into a house where there is measles. If children in a family where there is measles have not yet had measles themselves, they should not go to school or into stores or other public places for 10 days.
>
> **To prevent measles from killing children, make sure all children are well nourished. Have your children vaccinated against measles when they are 8 to 14 months of age.**

Do you know what a *virus* is? If not, look it up in the VOCABULARY.

What foods are *nutritious?* Look in the INDEX, the VOCABULARY, or Chapter 11 on Nutrition.

This is an exact page reference. Turn to page 120.

What are the dosages, risks, and precautions for these medicines? Look them up in the GREEN PAGES.

What is an antibiotic? You can turn to p. 351, as suggested. But for more information, look in the INDEX or the GREEN PAGES.

What are the signs of *pneumonia* and *meningitis?* How can you check for *severe pain in the ear or stomach?* If you are uncertain, look these up in the INDEX or the CONTENTS.

What are *vaccinations?* You can look in the VOCABULARY. Where can you find out more about them? Look in the INDEX or the CONTENTS. You might also try looking under 'Prevention'.

Be sure students practice looking up page references and reading the related information. They should keep practicing this until they can do it easily. The group can play a game by following references from page to page. They will find that almost everything in health care is related!

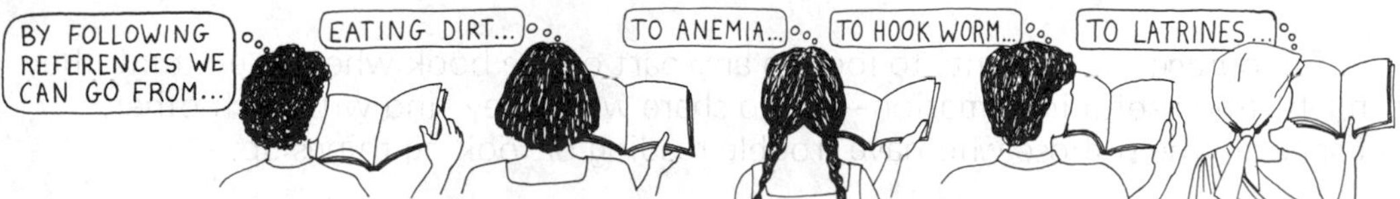

BY FOLLOWING REFERENCES WE CAN GO FROM...
EATING DIRT...
TO ANEMIA...
TO HOOK WORM...
TO LATRINES...

PRACTICE IN READING AND USING THE BOOK

Role-playing exercises can give students a good chance to develop skill in using *Where There Is No Doctor*—especially the CONTENTS, the INDEX, and the page references.

For example, one person can pretend he is sick with a very bad cough, in this case pneumonia. (But do not tell the students what the illness is. Let them find out through their own investigation and use of their books.) The person says his sickness began a few days ago like a cold or the flu—with a headache and sore throat. But now he feels much worse.

The students must ask questions to get more information. The 'sick person' can complain of chills or chest pain. To make it more realistic, he breathes with rapid, shallow breaths (as described in this book on page **14**-11). A pretend thermometer can be used to show that he has a fever (see page **14**-4).

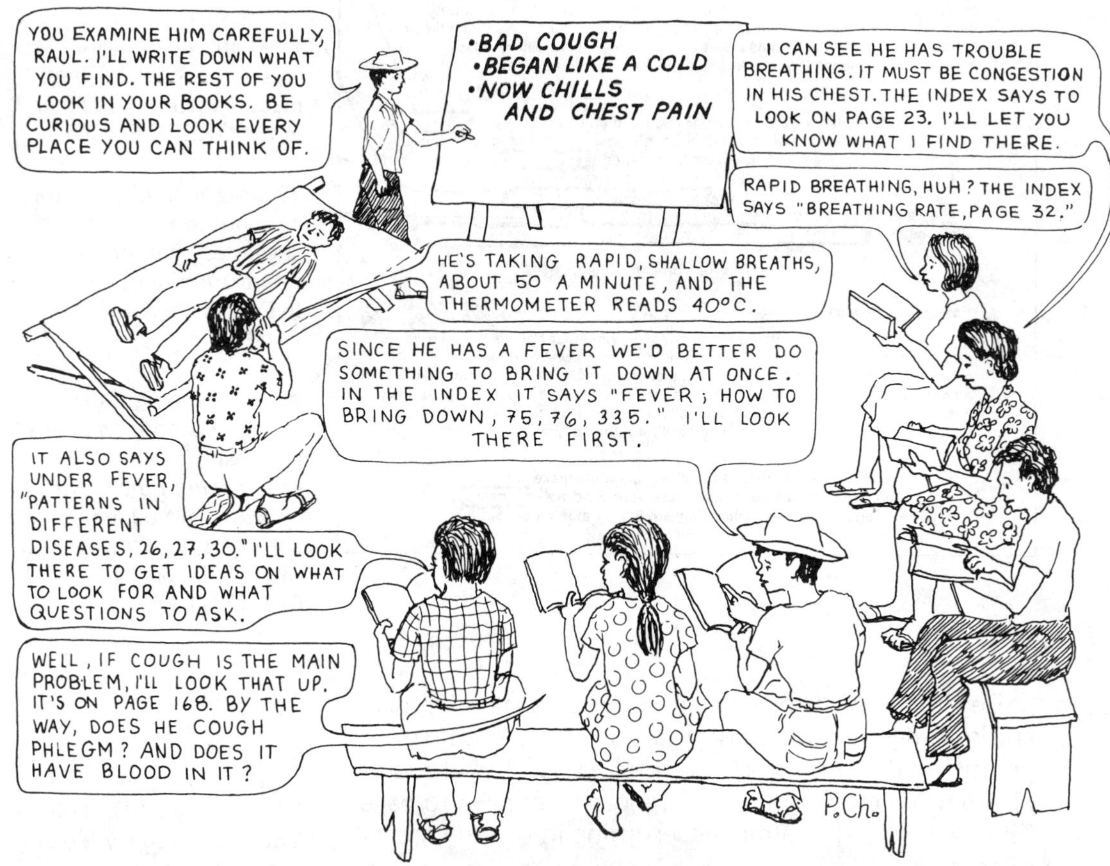
YOU EXAMINE HIM CAREFULLY, RAUL. I'LL WRITE DOWN WHAT YOU FIND. THE REST OF YOU LOOK IN YOUR BOOKS. BE CURIOUS AND LOOK EVERY PLACE YOU CAN THINK OF.
•BAD COUGH •BEGAN LIKE A COLD •NOW CHILLS AND CHEST PAIN
I CAN SEE HE HAS TROUBLE BREATHING. IT MUST BE CONGESTION IN HIS CHEST. THE INDEX SAYS TO LOOK ON PAGE 23. I'LL LET YOU KNOW WHAT I FIND THERE.
RAPID BREATHING, HUH? THE INDEX SAYS "BREATHING RATE, PAGE 32."
HE'S TAKING RAPID, SHALLOW BREATHS, ABOUT 50 A MINUTE, AND THE THERMOMETER READS 40°C.
SINCE HE HAS A FEVER WE'D BETTER DO SOMETHING TO BRING IT DOWN AT ONCE. IN THE INDEX IT SAYS "FEVER; HOW TO BRING DOWN, 75, 76, 335." I'LL LOOK THERE FIRST.
IT ALSO SAYS UNDER FEVER, "PATTERNS IN DIFFERENT DISEASES, 26, 27, 30." I'LL LOOK THERE TO GET IDEAS ON WHAT TO LOOK FOR AND WHAT QUESTIONS TO ASK.
WELL, IF COUGH IS THE MAIN PROBLEM, I'LL LOOK THAT UP. IT'S ON PAGE 168. BY THE WAY, DOES HE COUGH PHLEGM? AND DOES IT HAVE BLOOD IN IT?
P.Ch.

Encourage the students to look in any part of the book where they think they might find useful information—and to share what they find with each other. Especially help those who have trouble reading or looking things up.

If the group decides that the person in the role play probably has pneumonia, be sure that everyone looks up the references mentioned in the treatment section on page 171.

171

PNEUMONIA

Pneumonia is an *acute* infection of the lungs. It often occurs after another respiratory illness such as measles, whooping cough, flu, bronchitis, asthma—or any very serious illness, especially in babies and old people. Also, persons with AIDS may develop pneumonia.

Signs:

- Sudden chills and then high fever.
- Rapid, shallow breathing, with little grunts or sometimes wheezing. The nostrils may spread with each breath.
- Fever (sometimes newborns and old or very weak persons have severe pneumonia with little or no fever).
- Cough (often with yellow, greenish, rust-colored, or slightly bloody mucus).
- Chest pain (sometimes).
- The person looks very ill.
- Cold sores often appear on the face or lips (p. 232).

A very sick child who takes more than 50 **shallow** breaths a minute probably has pneumonia.

(If breathing is rapid and **deep,** check for dehydration, p. 151, or hyperventilation, p. 24.)

Treatment:

- For pneumonia, treatment with antibiotics can make the difference between life and death. Give penicillin (p. 351), co-trimoxazole (p. 358), or erythromycin (p. 355). In serious cases, inject procaine penicillin (p. 353), adults: 400,000 units (250 mg.) 2 or 3 times a day, or give ampicillin by mouth (p. 353), 500 mg., 4 times a day. Give small children 1/4 to 1/2 the adult dose. For children under 6, ampicillin is usually best.
- Give aspirin (p. 379) or acetaminophen (p. 380) to lower the temperature and lessen the pain.
- Give plenty of liquids. If the person will not eat, give him liquid foods or Rehydration Drink (see p. 152).
- Ease the cough and loosen the mucus by giving the person plenty of water and having him breathe hot water vapors (see p. 168). Postural drainage may also help (see p. 169).
- If the person is wheezing, an anti-asthma medicine with theophylline or ephedrine may help.

the correct medicines to fight the infection

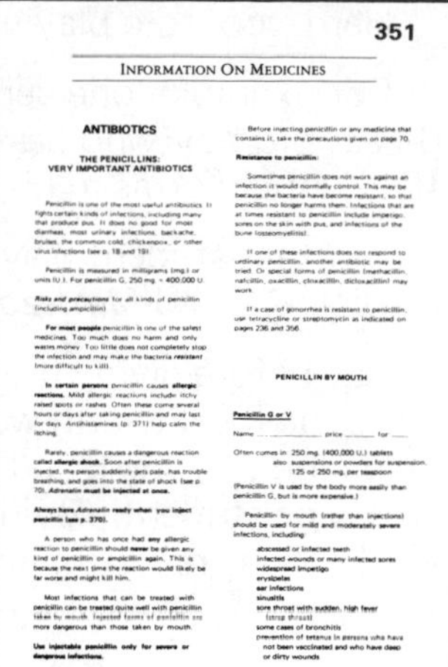

351

INFORMATION ON MEDICINES

ANTIBIOTICS

THE PENICILLINS: VERY IMPORTANT ANTIBIOTICS

Penicillin is one of the most useful antibiotics. It fights certain kinds of infections, including many that produce pus. It does no good for most diarrheas, most urinary infections, backache, bruises, the common cold, chickenpox, or other virus infections (see p. 18 and 19).

Penicillin is measured in milligrams (mg.) or units (U.). For penicillin G, 250 mg. = 400,000 U.

Risks and precautions for all kinds of penicillin (including ampicillin):

For most people penicillin is one of the safest medicines. Too much does no harm and only wastes money. Too little does not completely stop the infection and may make the bacteria ***resistant*** (more difficult to kill).

In certain persons penicillin causes **allergic reactions.** Mild allergic reactions include itchy raised spots or rashes. Often these come several hours or days after taking penicillin and may last for days. Antihistamines (p. 371) help calm the itching.

Rarely, penicillin causes a dangerous reaction called **allergic shock.** Soon after penicillin is injected, the person suddenly gets pale, has trouble breathing, and goes into the state of shock (see p. 70). ***Adrenalin must be injected at once.***

Always have *Adrenalin* ready when you inject penicillin (see p. 370).

A person who has once had **any** allergic reaction to penicillin should **never** be given any kind of penicillin or ampicillin again. This is because the next time the reaction would likely be far worse and might kill him.

Most infections that can be treated with penicillin can be treated quite well with penicillin taken by mouth. Injected forms of penicillin are more dangerous than those taken by mouth.

Use injectable penicillin only for severe or dangerous infections.

Before injecting penicillin or any medicine that contains it, take the precautions given on page 70.

Resistance to penicillin:

Sometimes penicillin does not work against an infection it would normally control. This may be because the bacteria have become resistant, so that penicillin no longer harms them. Infections that are at times resistant to penicillin include impetigo, sores on the skin with pus, and infections of the bone (osteomyelitis).

If one of these infections does not respond to ordinary penicillin, another antibiotic may be tried. Or special forms of penicillin (methacillin, nafcillin, oxacillin, cloxacillin, dicloxacillin) may work.

If a case of gonorrhea is resistant to penicillin, use tetracycline or streptomycin as indicated on pages 236 and 356.

PENICILLIN BY MOUTH

Penicillin G or V

Name ________ price ______ for ____

Often comes in: 250 mg. (400,000 U.) tablets
also: suspensions or powders for suspension, 125 or 250 mg. per teaspoon

(Penicillin V is used by the body more easily than penicillin G, but is more expensive.)

Penicillin by mouth (rather than injections) should be used for mild and moderately **severe** infections, including:

abscessed or infected teeth
infected wounds or many infected sores
widespread impetigo
erysipelas
ear infections
sinusitis
sore throat with sudden, high fever (strep throat)
some cases of bronchitis
prevention of tetanus in persons who have not been vaccinated and who have deep or dirty wounds

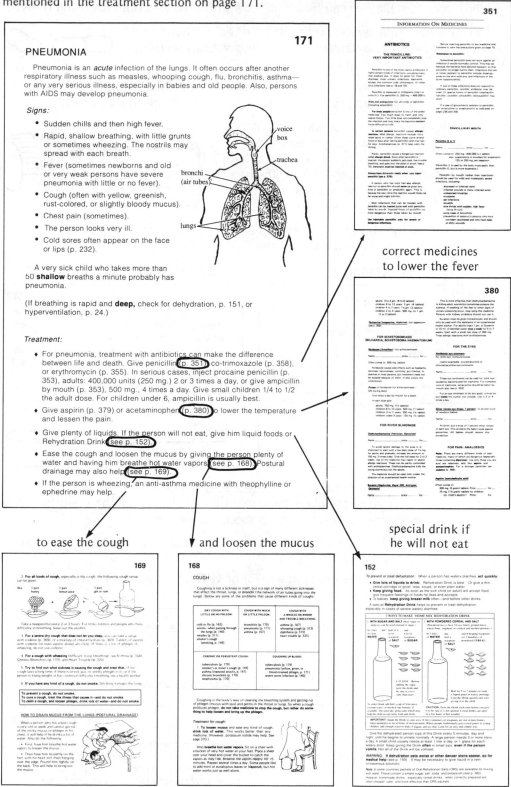

correct medicines to lower the fever

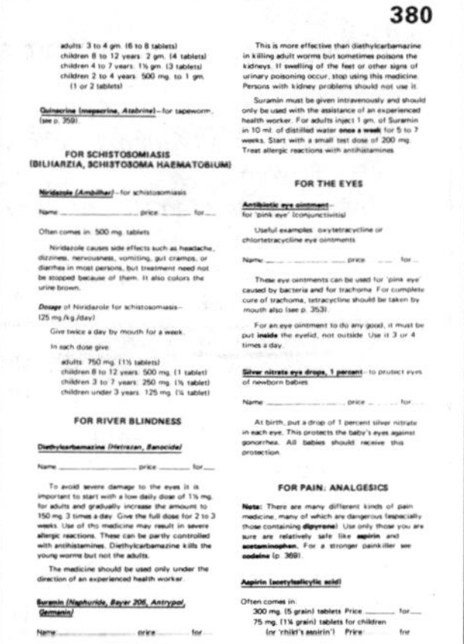

380

adults: 3 to 4 gm. (6 to 8 tablets)
children 8 to 12 years: 2 gm. (4 tablets)
children 4 to 7 years: 1½ gm. (3 tablets)
children 2 to 4 years: 500 mg. to 1 gm. (1 or 2 tablets)

Quinacrine (*mepacrine, Atabrine*)—for tapeworm, (see p. 359).

FOR SCHISTOSOMIASIS (BILHARZIA, SCHISTOSOMA HAEMATOBIUM)

Niridazole (*Ambilhar*)—for schistosomiasis

Name ________ price ______ for ____

Often comes in: 500 mg. tablets

Niridazole causes side effects such as headache, dizziness, nervousness, vomiting, gut cramps, or diarrhea in most persons, but treatment need not be stopped because of them. It also colors the urine brown.

Dosage of Niridazole for schistosomiasis—(25 mg./kg./day)

Give twice a day by mouth for a week.

In each dose give:

adults: 750 mg. (1½ tablets)
children 8 to 12 years: 500 mg. (1 tablet)
children 3 to 7 years: 250 mg. (½ tablet)
children under 3 years: 125 mg. (¼ tablet)

FOR RIVER BLINDNESS

Diethylcarbamazine (*Hetrazan, Banocide*)

Name ________ price ______ for ____

To avoid severe damage to the eyes it is important to start with a low daily dose of 1½ mg. for adults and gradually increase the amount to 150 mg. 3 times a day. Give the full dose for 2 to 3 weeks. Use of this medicine may result in severe allergic reactions. These can be partly controlled with antihistamines. Diethylcarbamazine kills the young worms but not the adults.

The medicine should be used only under the direction of an experienced health worker.

Suramin (*Naphuride, Bayer 205, Antrypol, Germanin*)

Name ________ price ______ for ____

This is more effective than diethylcarbamazine in killing adult worms but sometimes poisons the kidneys. If swelling of the feet or other signs of urinary poisoning occur, stop using this medicine. Persons with kidney problems should not use it.

Suramin must be given intravenously and should only be used with the assistance of an experienced health worker. For adults inject 1 gm. of Suramin in 10 ml. of distilled water **once a week** for 5 to 7 weeks. Start with a small test dose of 200 mg. Treat allergic reactions with antihistamines.

FOR THE EYES

Antibiotic eye ointment—for 'pink eye' (conjunctivitis)

Useful examples: oxytetracycline or chlortetracycline eye ointments

Name ________ price ______ for ____

These eye ointments can be used for 'pink eye' caused by bacteria and for trachoma. For complete cure of trachoma, tetracycline should be taken by mouth also (see p. 353).

For an eye ointment to do any good, it must be put **inside** the eyelid, not outside. Use it 3 or 4 times a day.

Silver nitrate eye drops, 1 percent—to protect eyes of newborn babies

Name ________ price ______ for ____

At birth, put a drop of 1 percent silver nitrate in each eye. This protects the baby's eyes against gonorrhea. All babies should receive this protection.

FOR PAIN: ANALGESICS

Note: There are many different kinds of pain medicine, many of which are dangerous (especially those containing **dipyrone**). Use only those you are sure are relatively safe like **aspirin** and **acetaminophen.** For a stronger painkiller see **codeine** (p. 369).

Aspirin (acetylsalicylic acid)

Often comes in:
300 mg. (5 grain) tablets Price ______ for ____
75 mg. (1¼ grain) tablets for children (or 'child's aspirin') Price ______ for ____

special drink if he will not eat

to ease the cough

169

2. **For all kinds of cough,** especially a dry cough, the following cough syrup can be given:

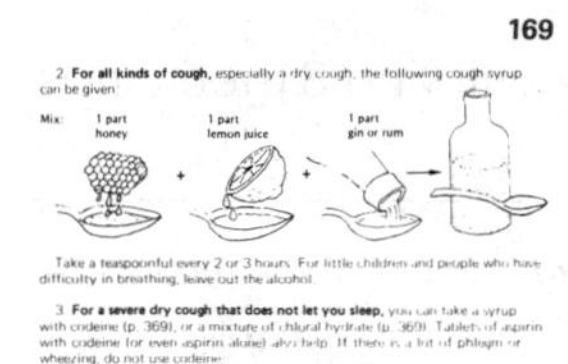

Take a teaspoonful every 2 or 3 hours. For little children and people who have difficulty in breathing, leave out the alcohol.

3. **For a severe dry cough that does not let you sleep,** you can take a syrup with codeine (p. 369), or a mixture of chloral hydrate (p. 369). Tablets of aspirin with codeine (or even aspirin alone) also help. If there is a lot of phlegm or wheezing, do not use codeine.

4. **For a cough with wheezing** (difficult, noisy breathing), see Asthma (p. 164), Chronic Bronchitis (p. 170), and Heart Trouble (p. 325).

5. **Try to find out what sickness is causing the cough and treat that.** If the cough lasts a long time, if there is blood, pus, or smelly phlegm in it, or if the person is losing weight or has continual difficulty breathing, see a health worker.

6. **If you have any kind of a cough, do not smoke.** Smoking damages the lungs.

To prevent a cough, do not smoke.
To cure a cough, treat the illness that causes it—and do not smoke.
To calm a cough, and loosen phlegm, drink lots of water—and do not smoke.

HOW TO DRAIN MUCUS FROM THE LUNGS (POSTURAL DRAINAGE):

When a person who has a bad cough is very old or weak and cannot get rid of the sticky mucus or phlegm in his chest, it will help if he drinks a lot of water. Also do the following:

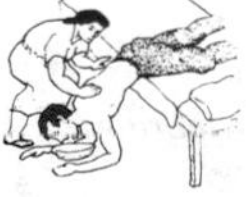

- First, have him breathe hot water vapors to loosen the mucus.
- Then have him lie partly on the bed, with his head and chest hanging over the edge. Pound him lightly on the back. This will help to bring out the mucus.

and loosen the mucus

168

COUGH

Coughing is not a sickness in itself, but is a sign of many different sicknesses that affect the throat, lungs, or ***bronchi*** (the network of air tubes going into the lungs). Below are some of the problems that cause different kinds of coughs:

DRY COUGH WITH LITTLE OR NO PHLEGM:	COUGH WITH MUCH OR LITTLE PHLEGM:	COUGH WITH A WHEEZE OR WHOOP AND TROUBLE BREATHING:
cold or flu (p. 163) worms—when passing through the lungs (p. 140) measles (p. 311) smoker's cough (smoking, p. 149)	bronchitis (p. 170) pneumonia (p. 171) asthma (p. 167)	asthma (p. 167) whooping cough (p. 313) diphtheria (p. 313) heart trouble (p. 325)

CHRONIC OR PERSISTENT COUGH:	COUGHING UP BLOOD:
tuberculosis (p. 179) smoker's or miner's cough (p. 149) asthma (repeated attacks, p. 167) chronic bronchitis (p. 170) emphysema (p. 170)	tuberculosis (p. 179) pneumonia (yellow, green, or blood-streaked phlegm, p. 171) severe worm infection (p. 140)

Coughing is the body's way of cleaning the breathing system and getting rid of phlegm (mucus with pus) and germs in the throat or lungs. So when a cough produces phlegm, **do not take medicine to stop the cough, but rather do something to help loosen and bring up the phlegm.**

Treatment for cough:

1. **To loosen mucus** and ease any kind of cough, **drink lots of water.** This works better than any medicine. (However, potassium iodide may help. See page 370.)

Also **breathe hot water vapors.** Sit on a chair with a bucket of very hot water at your feet. Place a sheet over your head and cover the bucket to catch the vapors as they rise. Breathe the vapors deeply for 15 minutes. Repeat several times a day. Some people like to add mint or eucalyptus leaves or ***Vaporub,*** but hot water works just as well alone.

152

To prevent or treat dehydration: When a person has watery diarrhea, **act quickly:**

- **Give lots of liquids to drink:** Rehydration Drink is best. Or give a thin cereal porridge or gruel, teas, soups, or even plain water.
- **Keep giving food.** As soon as the sick child (or adult) will accept food, give frequent feedings of foods he likes and accepts.
- To babies, **keep giving breast milk** often—and before other drinks.

A special **Rehydration Drink** helps to prevent or treat dehydration, especially in cases of severe watery diarrhea:

2 WAYS TO MAKE 'HOME MIX' REHYDRATION DRINK

1. **WITH SUGAR AND SALT** (Raw sugar or molasses can be used instead of sugar.)

In 1 liter of clean **WATER** put half of a level teaspoon of **SALT** and 8 level teaspoons of **SUGAR**.

CAUTION: Before adding the sugar, taste the drink and be sure it is less salty than tears.

To either Drink add half a cup of fruit juice, coconut water, or mashed ripe banana, if available. This provides potassium which may help the child accept more food and drink.

2. **WITH POWDERED CEREAL AND SALT** (Powdered rice is best. Or use finely ground maize, wheat flour, sorghum, or cooked and mashed potatoes.)

In 1 liter of **WATER** put half a teaspoon of **SALT** and 8 heaping teaspoons (or 2 handfuls) of powdered **CEREAL**.

Boil for 5 to 7 minutes to form a liquid gruel or watery porridge. Cool the Drink quickly and start giving it to the child.

CAUTION: Taste the Drink each time before you give it to be sure it is not spoiled. Cereal drinks can spoil in a few hours in hot weather.

IMPORTANT: Adapt the Drink to your area. If liter containers or teaspoons are not in most homes, adjust quantities to local forms of measurement. Where people traditionally give cereal gruels to young children, add enough water to make it liquid, and use that. Look for an easy and simple way.

Give the dehydrated person sips of this Drink every 5 minutes, day and night, until he begins to urinate normally. A large person needs 3 or more liters a day. A small child usually needs at least 1 liter a day, or 1 glass for each watery stool. Keep giving the Drink **often** in small sips, **even if the person vomits.** Not all of the Drink will be vomited.

WARNING: **If dehydration gets worse or other danger signs appear, go for medical help** (see p. 159). It may be necessary to give liquid in a vein (intravenous solution).

Note: In some countries packets of Oral Rehydration Salts (ORS) are available for mixing with water. These contain a simple sugar, salt, soda, and potassium (see p. 382). However, homemade drinks, especially cereal drinks, when correctly prepared are often cheaper, safer, and more effective than ORS packets.

Using the GREEN PAGES to find information about medicines

Here, too, role playing can be a realistic and fun way to practice using ***WTND.***

For example, one person pretends to be the mother of a 6-year-old boy who has tapeworm. She says she has seen little flat, white worms in his shit.

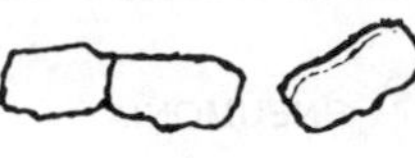

Another student plays the role of the local store owner. He sells the mother a medicine called ***Mintezol,*** saying that it is "good for all kinds of worms."

But before giving it to her son, the mother visits the local health worker to ask if the medicine will work and how much she should give. The student playing the role of the health worker first reads the fine print on the side of the bottle:

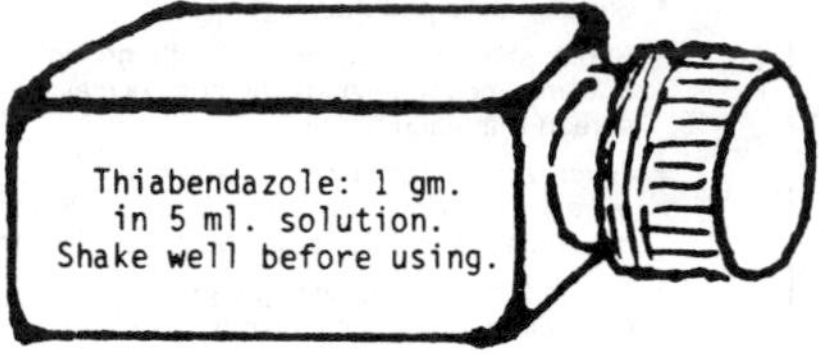

Then he and the rest of the class help each other to look up 'Thiabendazole' in either of the lists at the beginning of the GREEN PAGES.

LIST OF MEDICINES

INDEX OF MEDICINES

Both lists say to turn to page 375. Together, the 'health worker' and the 'mother' (and the rest of the class) read what the medicine can be used for. They notice that the description says nothing about tapeworm.

So the health worker tells the mother that ***Mintezol*** would probably not be useful for her son's tapeworm.

If the class looks at the next page (376) of ***WTND,*** they will find 3 medicines that do work for tapeworm: niclosamide **(Yomesan),** praziquantel **(Biltricide, Droncit),** and quinacrine (mepacrine, **Atabrine).** They can read about the risks and precautions, and compare the prices and availability of the different medications. The students will need to have already written in the prices of products in their area. Or the instructor can provide this information during the role play. Be sure all students write it into their books.

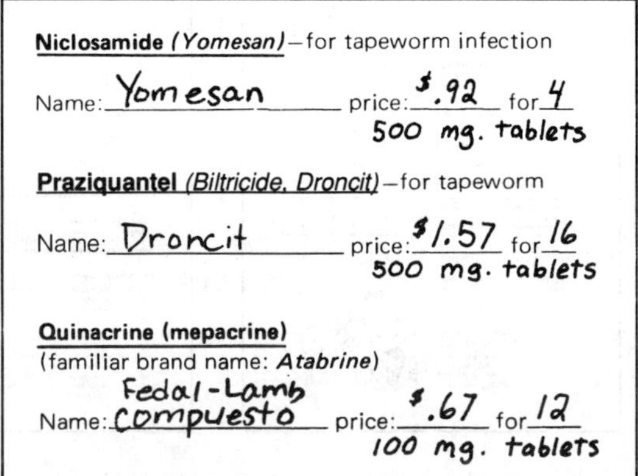

Niclosamide *(Yomesan)*—for tapeworm infection

Name: Yomesan price: $.92 for 4 500 mg. tablets

Praziquantel *(Biltricide, Droncit)*—for tapeworm

Name: Droncit price: $1.57 for 16 500 mg. tablets

Quinacrine (mepacrine)
(familiar brand name: ***Atabrine***)

Name: Fedal-Lamb compuesto price: $.67 for 12 100 mg. tablets

The students can now decide with the 'mother' which medicine may work best at a price she can afford. The health worker then reads or figures out the exact dosage for the child, writes it down, and explains it to the mother. If she cannot read, the health worker can use a dosage blank with pictures (see page 64 of *Where There Is No Doctor).* **Practice in finding and explaining the right dosage is extremely important.** (See page **18**-10.)

It is also important that health workers read all they can about a problem before recommending medicines. So, during the role play, be sure students look up 'Tapeworm' in the INDEX or CONTENTS of ***Where There Is No Doctor,*** and turn to page 143.

> *Prevention:* **Be careful that all meat is well cooked, especially pork.** Make sure no parts in the center of roasted meat are still raw.
>
> **Effect on health:** Tapeworms in the intestines sometimes cause mild stomach-aches, but few other problems.
>
> The greatest danger exists when the ***cysts*** (small sacs containing baby worms) get into a person's brain. This happens when the eggs pass from his stools to his mouth. For this reason, **anyone with tapeworms must follow the guidelines of cleanliness carefully—and get treatment as soon as possible.**

The students can use the pictures in the book to help explain to the 'mother' and her 'son' about tapeworms and how to avoid them. They may also want to look up the 'Guidelines of Cleanliness' referred to in the discussion of tapeworm prevention. (See especially p. 133 of ***WTND.)***

Depending on your local situation, the role play can be developed in various ways. For example, the mother might complain that her son will not swallow pills. What should she do? The health worker and mother can look in the INDEX or CONTENTS, and will be guided to page 62.

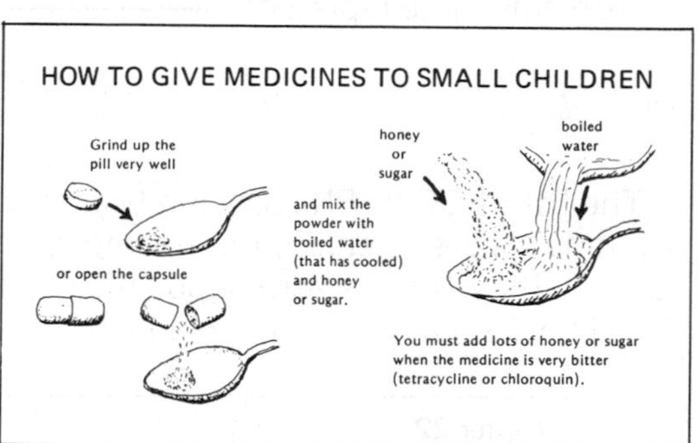

Grind up the pill very well
or open the capsule
and mix the powder with boiled water (that has cooled) and honey or sugar.
honey or sugar

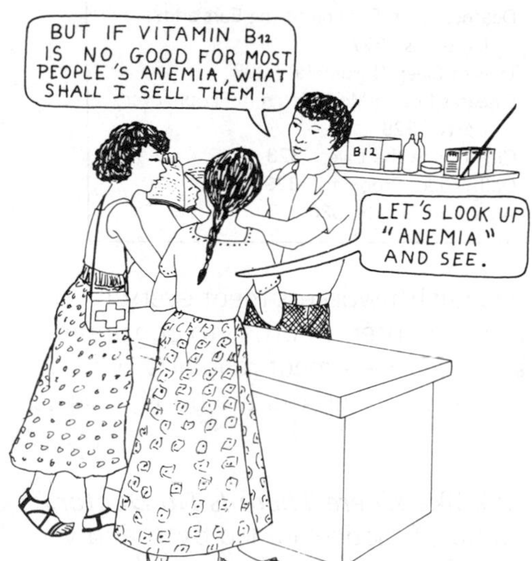
BUT IF VITAMIN B12 IS NO GOOD FOR MOST PEOPLE'S ANEMIA, WHAT SHALL I SELL THEM!
B12
LET'S LOOK UP "ANEMIA" AND SEE.

Or the health worker might go with the mother to return the unused medicine and buy one that is effective against tapeworm. To interest the store owner in learning more about the medicines he buys and sells, the health worker might show him the 'Words to the Village Storekeeper (or Pharmacist)' on page 338 of ***Where There Is No Doctor.***

Using the INDEX or CONTENTS to plan classes or for independent study

The INDEX (yellow pages) is a good source of ideas for independent or group study because it lists all the pages that have information about a specific subject. For example:

These pages listed in the INDEX can give you ideas for what to teach.

If health workers want to refresh their knowledge about how to ***examine*** someone: →

If mothers have already learned the importance of giving ***Rehydration Drink*** to children with diarrhea, and want to learn about other uses for it: →

If health workers need to review the possible changes in appearance of the ***urine,*** and what problems these represent: →

The list of CONTENTS at the beginning of the book can also be useful for planning classes or study. For example, if a group of concerned persons in the community wants to learn about the special problems of old people, the list of CONTENTS may help them plan what to study.

In several health programs we know, village health workers meet every month or so to review a chapter of ***WTND,*** or part of a chapter, in order to continue learning. In other programs, health workers and teachers meet regularly with parents, school children, or mothers' clubs to read and discuss the book, chapter by chapter.

There are many ways people can use a book like ***Where There Is No Doctor.*** But to use it fully and well takes a lot of practice. Practice guided by friendly persons who have experience in using reference books is especially helpful.

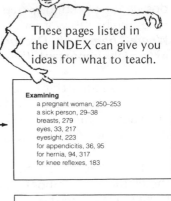

CHAPTER 21

Practice in Using Guides, Charts, and Record Sheets

GUIDES AND CHARTS THAT HELP TELL DIFFERENT PROBLEMS APART

Many illnesses look similar and can easily be confused. And sometimes similar-looking illnesses are called by the same traditional name. Yet they may have different causes and require very different treatments. Health workers need to know what to ask and what to look for, so they can systematically consider the different possibilities. (See Chapter 17 on Solving Problems Step by Step.)

The process of considering several possible diseases that may be causing a person's problem, and figuring out which is the most likely, we will call *comparative diagnosis.*

A health handbook like *Where There Is No Doctor* can be a useful tool for comparative diagnosis. But to learn to use it well takes considerable practice.

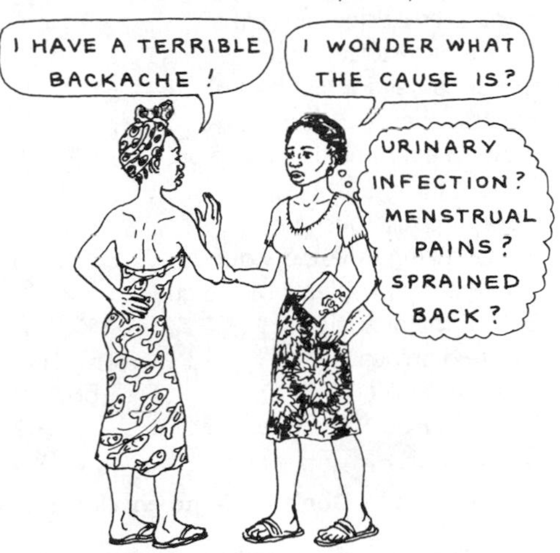

I HAVE A TERRIBLE BACKACHE !
I WONDER WHAT THE CAUSE IS?
URINARY INFECTION? MENSTRUAL PAINS? SPRAINED BACK?

A problem like back pain can have many different causes.

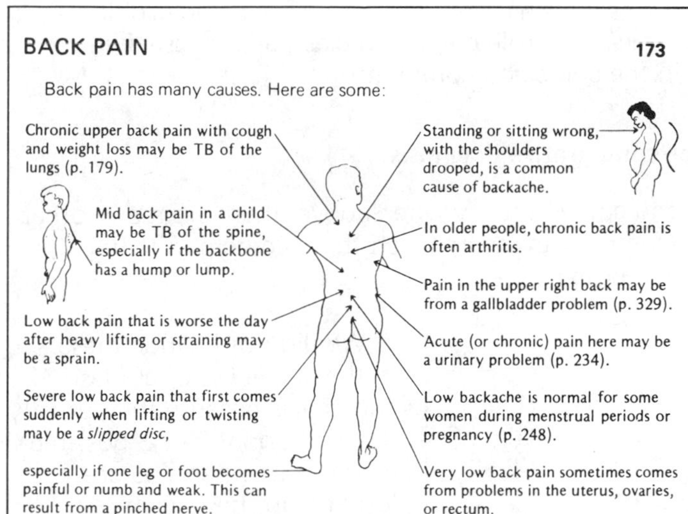
BACK PAIN 173

Back pain has many causes. Here are some:

Chronic upper back pain with cough and weight loss may be TB of the lungs (p. 179).

Mid back pain in a child may be TB of the spine, especially if the backbone has a hump or lump.

Low back pain that is worse the day after heavy lifting or straining may be a sprain.

Severe low back pain that first comes suddenly when lifting or twisting may be a *slipped disc,*

especially if one leg or foot becomes painful or numb and weak. This can result from a pinched nerve.

Standing or sitting wrong, with the shoulders drooped, is a common cause of backache.

In older people, chronic back pain is often arthritis.

Pain in the upper right back may be from a gallbladder problem (p. 329).

Acute (or chronic) pain here may be a urinary problem (p. 234).

Low backache is normal for some women during menstrual periods or pregnancy (p. 248).

Very low back pain sometimes comes from problems in the uterus, ovaries, or rectum.

This diagram on page 173 of *Where There Is No Doctor* shows common causes of pain in different parts of the back. After finding out exactly where the person feels pain, look up and read about each possible cause of his problem.

Learning to use diagnostic guides and charts:

Where There Is No Doctor contains several guides and charts that can help you tell similar health problems apart. These charts usually list one or two important signs for each problem. If the person you are examining has any of these signs, turn to the page number shown on the chart for more information. Compare the signs and symptoms of each problem to determine which is most likely.

When helping persons learn to use *Where There Is No Doctor,* be sure to **review the various diagnostic charts and guides, and explain how to use them.** Some of the guides and charts show drawings or give details to make it easier to tell one problem from another. Others just list possible causes for readers to look up for themselves. It can be more fun and realistic if you invent problems and act out situations to help the students use their books as guides for comparative diagnosis.

USEFUL INFORMATION, GUIDES, AND CHARTS FOR TELLING HEALTH PROBLEMS APART

(page numbers in *Where There Is No Doctor)*

	page		**page**
Examples of sicknesses that are hard to tell apart	20	Back pain	173
Local names for sicknesses	21-27	Swelling of the feet	176
Severe fever	26-27	Fits (convulsions)	178
How to examine a sick person	29-38	Skin problems	196-198
Belly pain	35-36	Red, painful eyes	219
Loss of consciousness	78	Eye problems	224-225
Recognizing infected wounds	88	White patches or spots in the mouth	232
Emergency problems of the gut	93	Urinary tract problems	234
Severe malnutrition	112,114	Vaginal discharge	241-242
Acute diarrhea	153,157, 158,160	Pain in the lower part of a woman's belly	243
Vomiting	161	Infertility	244
Cough	168	Illnesses of the newborn	272-275

Don't forget to check the INDEX 433-440

We have found it helpful to practice using one or two of these guides each week during training. Choose those that relate to the health problems the students are learning about that week. This way, as they increase their knowledge of health problems, they also develop skills in using the book and in scientific problem solving. They can practice by means of role playing in class, as well as when helping attend sick persons in the clinic and community.

Other information useful for comparative diagnosis:

In addition to the charts and guides already listed above, there are many other pages in *Where There Is No Doctor* with information that can help in telling one health problem from another. For example:

Information	**page**
Emergencies caused by heat	81
Snakebite	104
Difficulty passing urine	234-236
Different kinds of breast lumps	279
Lumps or growths in the lower part of the belly	280
A 'swollen testicle'	317
Paralysis of the face	327

We did not include these in the above list of guides and charts because they usually deal with only 2 or 3 possible causes. But when you are looking up these health problems, the comparisons of signs and histories will help you tell one cause from another.

LEARNING TO TELL SIMILAR PROBLEMS APART

A good way to introduce the idea of ***comparative diagnosis*** is to have students turn to page 20 of ***Where There Is No Doctor.***

There they will find 2 examples showing similar-looking problems that can be caused by many different diseases.

The students can take turns role playing each of the possible causes. Each person who acts out a particular problem should be sure to look up the signs and history ahead of time. In the role play, everyone asks him questions and examines him to figure out which possibility is most likely. See Chapter 14 of this book for ideas on how to make role playing more effective and fun.

20

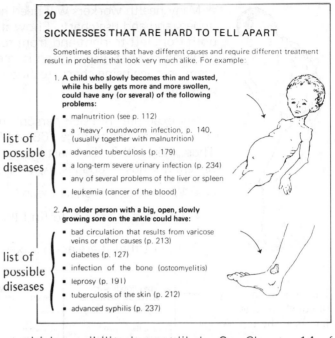

SICKNESSES THAT ARE HARD TO TELL APART

Sometimes diseases that have different causes and require different treatment result in problems that look very much alike. For example:

1. **A child who slowly becomes thin and wasted, while his belly gets more and more swollen, could have any (or several) of the following problems:**

list of possible diseases

- malnutrition (see p. 112)
- a 'heavy' roundworm infection, p. 140, (usually together with malnutrition)
- advanced tuberculosis (p. 179)
- a long-term severe urinary infection (p. 234)
- any of several problems of the liver or spleen
- leukemia (cancer of the blood)

2. **An older person with a big, open, slowly growing sore on the ankle could have:**

list of possible diseases

- bad circulation that results from varicose veins or other causes (p. 213)
- diabetes (p. 127)
- infection of the bone (osteomyelitis)
- leprosy (p. 191)
- tuberculosis of the skin (p. 212)
- advanced syphilis (p. 237)

During each role play, students can **list the possible causes of the problem on the blackboard.** Then write any reasons that make each one more or less likely.

If someone pretends that an open sore painted on her ankle is caused by diabetes, the blackboard might look like this after role playing.

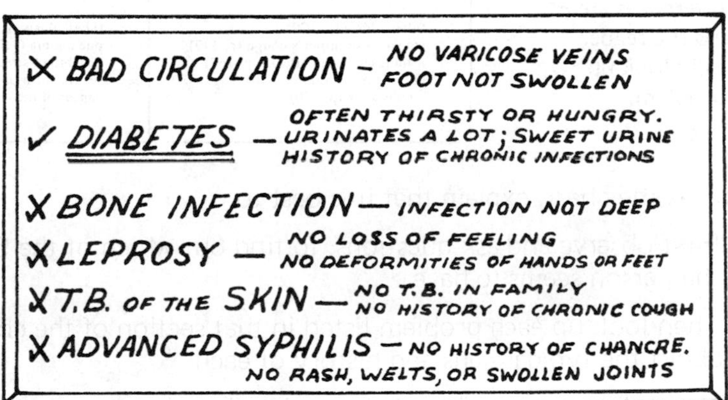

X BAD CIRCULATION – NO VARICOSE VEINS FOOT NOT SWOLLEN
✓ DIABETES – OFTEN THIRSTY OR HUNGRY. URINATES A LOT; SWEET URINE HISTORY OF CHRONIC INFECTIONS
X BONE INFECTION — INFECTION NOT DEEP
X LEPROSY — NO LOSS OF FEELING NO DEFORMITIES OF HANDS OR FEET
X T.B. OF THE SKIN — NO T.B. IN FAMILY NO HISTORY OF CHRONIC COUGH
X ADVANCED SYPHILIS – NO HISTORY OF CHANCRE. NO RASH, WELTS, OR SWOLLEN JOINTS

Make a check (✔) beside each possible cause, after the group has asked questions about it and examined the person for signs. If the illness proves unlikely, make a cross through the check mark (✘).

The same system of listing problems and checking them off can be used when the health workers are learning to attend sick people in the clinic or community. Each person can keep track of his or her questions, tests, findings, and diagnoses in a notebook or on a record sheet. That way, if the problem is discussed afterward in class, each student will have a written record of what he thought and asked.

LEARNING TO READ CHARTS

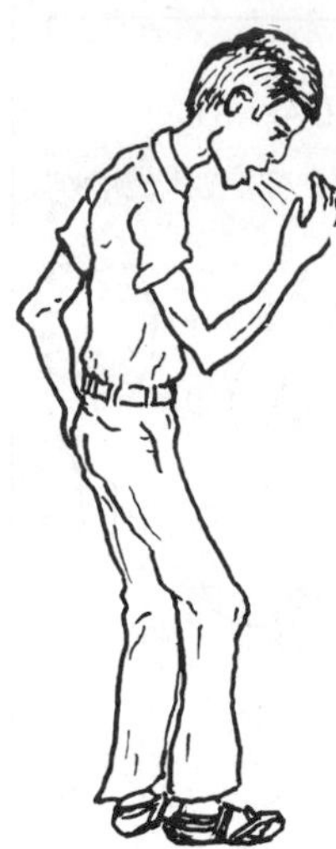

Many health workers will need help, at first, in learning to understand and use charts. Show students how to read them—both from left to right and from top to bottom. Help them understand what information is in each column or box. Have them practice using charts to find the most likely cause of a problem.

For example: If a sick person's main complaint is a cough, students can turn to page 168 of ***Where There Is No Doctor.*** There they will find a chart listing the problems that cause different kinds of coughs. Ask the students:

- What does this chart mean?
- How can it help us to find the cause of the person's cough?

Point out that there are 5 boxes.

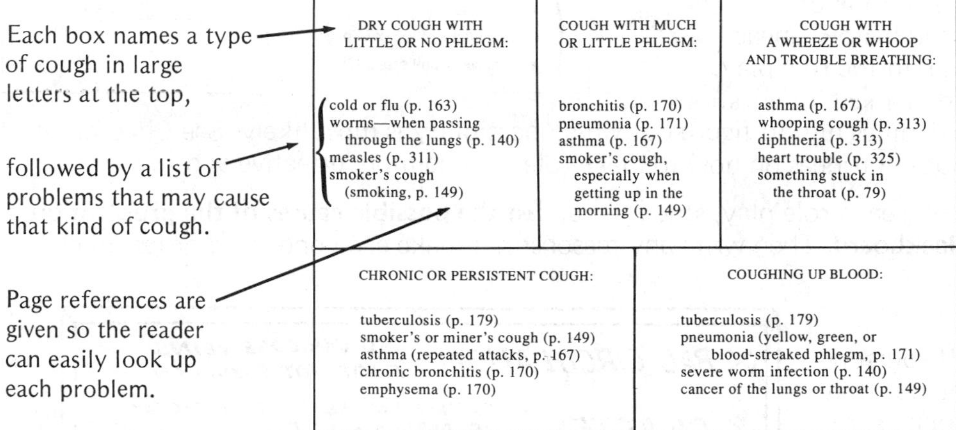

DRY COUGH WITH LITTLE OR NO PHLEGM:	COUGH WITH MUCH OR LITTLE PHLEGM:	COUGH WITH A WHEEZE OR WHOOP AND TROUBLE BREATHING:
cold or flu (p. 163) worms—when passing through the lungs (p. 140) measles (p. 311) smoker's cough (smoking, p. 149)	bronchitis (p. 170) pneumonia (p. 171) asthma (p. 167) smoker's cough, especially when getting up in the morning (p. 149)	asthma (p. 167) whooping cough (p. 313) diphtheria (p. 313) heart trouble (p. 325) something stuck in the throat (p. 79)

CHRONIC OR PERSISTENT COUGH:	COUGHING UP BLOOD:
tuberculosis (p. 179) smoker's or miner's cough (p. 149) asthma (repeated attacks, p. 167) chronic bronchitis (p. 170) emphysema (p. 170)	tuberculosis (p. 179) pneumonia (yellow, green, or blood-streaked phlegm, p. 171) severe worm infection (p. 140) cancer of the lungs or throat (p. 149)

To use the chart, explain that it is best to:

- First observe and ask questions, to find out which of the 5 types of cough the person seems to have.
- Then look up each problem listed in that section of the chart. Read more about the typical signs and history of each.
- Now ask more questions and examine the person to determine which cause is most likely. Use the step-by-step approach to problem solving (Chapter 17).
- At each step be sure to **consider all of the possibilities.** Do not make the diagnosis until you have made sure that other causes are less likely.

Note: Remind students that their book does not include every possible cause of a problem, but only the more common causes. If the diagnosis is unclear or the signs are confusing, they should try to get more experienced medical help.

AN EXAMPLE OF HOW TO LOOK SOMETHING UP, USING CHARTS OR THE INDEX:

Suppose someone has swollen glands (swollen lymph nodes) and you want to know the possible causes. There are 3 places in your book where you might look.

1. **The Guide to Identification of Skin Problems**—pages 196 to 198 of ***Where There Is No Doctor.*** This has drawings and descriptions of various skin problems. You can see what each problem looks like up close, and where it usually occurs on the body. The possible causes are named, and page references are given.

To make the best use of this guide, health workers need to understand how the information is organized.

Problems that look similar are grouped in the same box.

There is a box for each of the following signs:

- small sores
- large open sores
- lumps
- swollen lymph nodes
- spots or patches
- warts
- rings
- welts or hives
- blisters
- rash

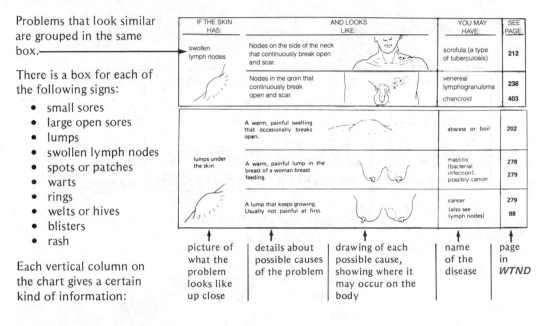

IF THE SKIN HAS:	AND LOOKS LIKE:	YOU MAY HAVE:	SEE PAGE:
swollen lymph nodes	Nodes on the side of the neck that continuously break open and scar.	scrofula (a type of tuberculosis)	212
	Nodes in the groin that continuously break open and scar.	venereal lymphogranuloma chancroid	238 403
lumps under the skin	A warm, painful swelling that occasionally breaks open.	abscess or boil	202
	A warm, painful lump in the breast of a woman breast feeding.	mastitis (bacterial infection), possibly cancer	278 279
	A lump that keeps growing. Usually not painful at first.	cancer (also see lymph nodes)	279 88

Each vertical column on the chart gives a certain kind of information:

picture of what the problem looks like up close	details about possible causes of the problem	drawing of each possible cause, showing where it may occur on the body	name of the disease	page in *WTND*

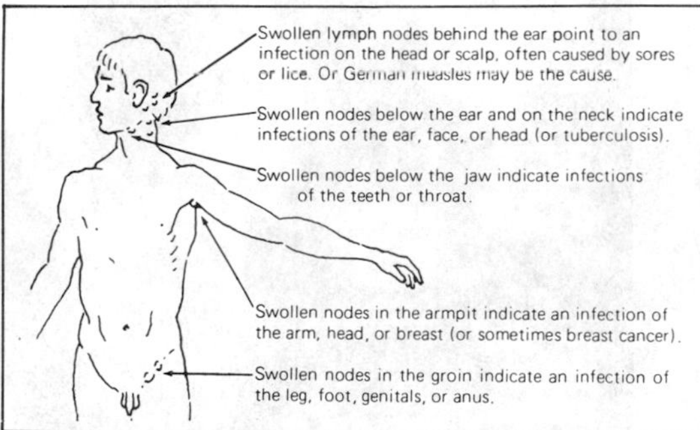

Swollen lymph nodes behind the ear point to an infection on the head or scalp, often caused by sores or lice. Or German measles may be the cause.
Swollen nodes below the ear and on the neck indicate infections of the ear, face, or head (or tuberculosis).
Swollen nodes below the jaw indicate infections of the teeth or throat.
Swollen nodes in the armpit indicate an infection of the arm, head, or breast (or sometimes breast cancer).
Swollen nodes in the groin indicate an infection of the leg, foot, genitals, or anus.

2. **Discussion of swollen lymph nodes**—page 88 of *WTND.* This has a picture showing places on the body where swollen lymph nodes can appear with different problems. But no page references are given. You have to look up possible causes in the index.

3. **The INDEX** (yellow pages) of ***WTND*** also can be used as a guide to possible causes of health problems. It does not provide any details, but it lists the pages on which you can find more information. When in doubt about the cause of a problem, be sure you **check all of the page references.** Some may be more helpful than others.

from the INDEX of ***WTND***

Lymph nodes, swollen, 88, 317, 424
caused by an abscess, 202
in the groin, 238, 403
signs of infection, 194
TB of, 212
with AIDS, 400
with breast cancer, 279
with brucellosis, 188 or typhus, 190
with German measles, 312
with scabies or lice, 199, 200

BASING TEACHING MATERIALS ON CHARTS OR GUIDES

Many of the charts and guides in *Where There Is No Doctor* can provide ideas for teaching aids that help health workers to practice comparative diagnosis. Here are two examples from Project Piaxtla in Mexico.

Example 1: Swollen lymph nodes

During one training course, health workers made a flannel-board puzzle to help themselves review the different kinds of swollen lymph nodes. The puzzle is based on information from pages 88, 196, and 197 of *Where There Is No Doctor.*

First they made puzzle cards showing on one half the signs of a problem causing swollen lymph nodes, and on the other half the name of the problem that most often causes those signs.

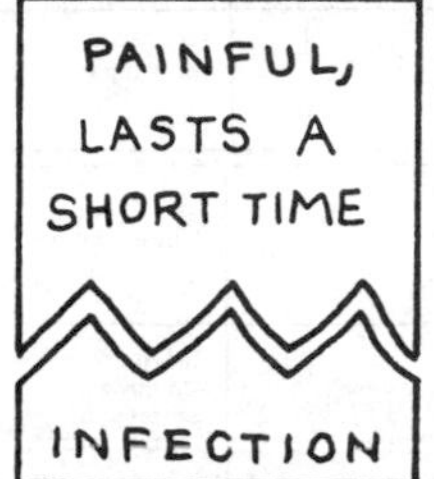

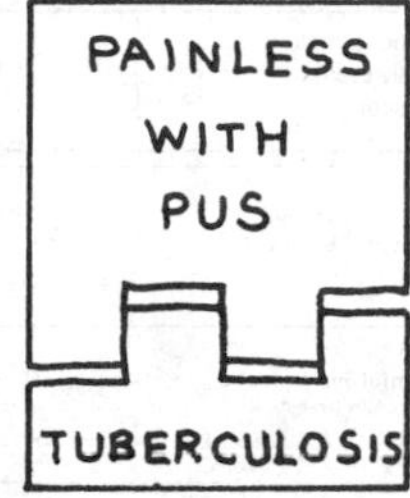

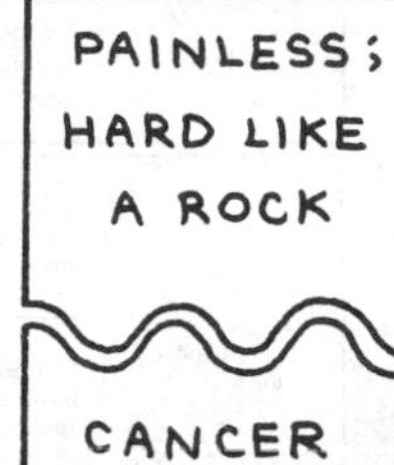

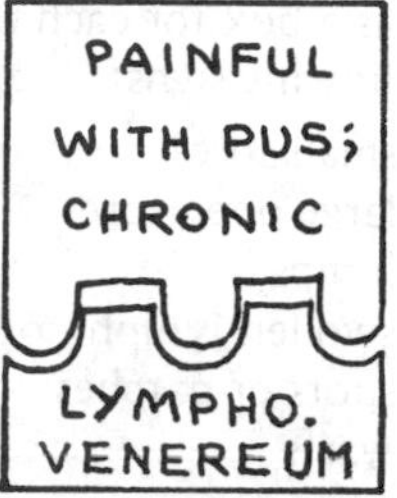

They chose 3 colors to represent signs of different kinds of swollen lymph nodes:

RED = PAINFUL BLUE = PAINLESS YELLOW = WITH PUS

Then the students made a figure of a man, with slits cut in the neck and other places where swollen lymph nodes occur.

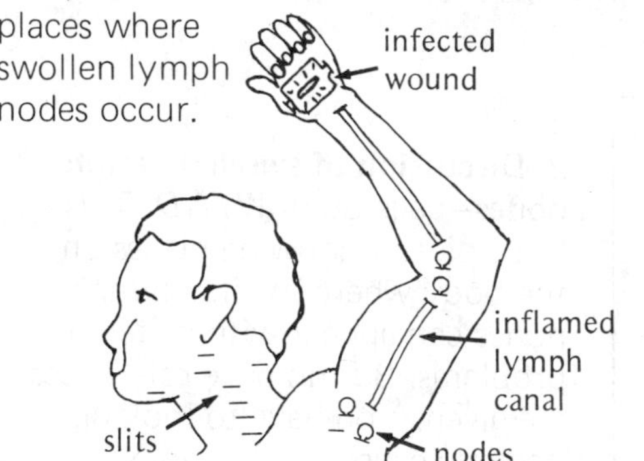

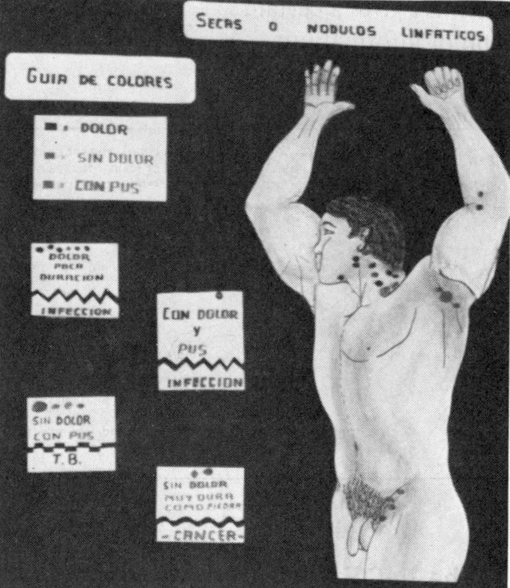

Next they cut out and colored 4 kinds of cardboard lymph nodes:

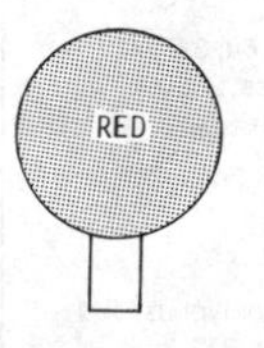

PAINFUL

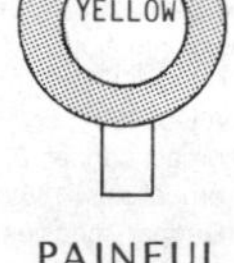

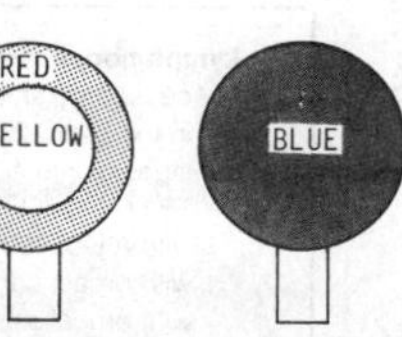

PAINFUL WITH PUS

PAINLESS

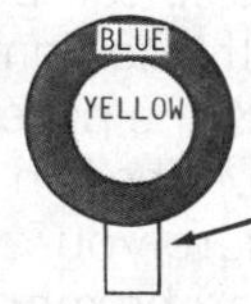

PAINLESS WITH PUS

The 'nodes' have tabs that fit into the slits in the cardboard man.

The student health workers first practice with the puzzle cards to learn the signs of each problem. Then they use the big drawing of the man to review the different problems and where on the body they appear.

The students take turns placing the colored nodes, wound, and lymph canal pieces on the cardboard man to show the signs of problems described in ***Where There Is No Doctor.*** They challenge each other to correctly identify and find the treatment and prevention for each problem they create.

Test yourself. Can you name the probable causes of the swollen lymph nodes shown in these photos?

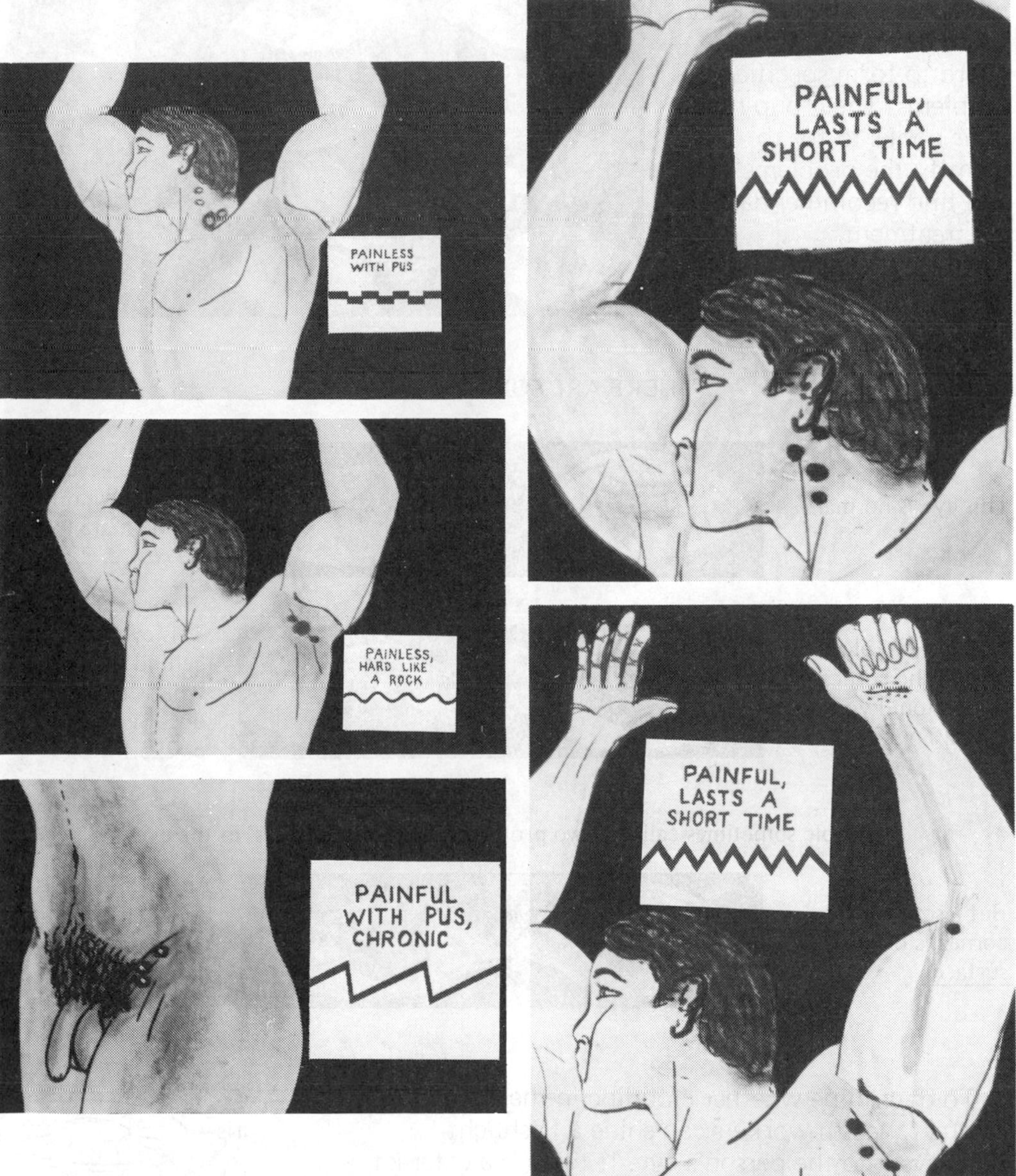

By making these teaching materials themselves and testing each other with the puzzle cards, health workers soon learn to recognize the different problems.

Example 2: Eye problems

During another Project Piaxtla training course, the student health workers made a flannel-board puzzle for eye problems. It includes most of the problems described in Chapter 16 of ***Where There Is No Doctor.*** The students cut out and colored cardboard pieces to represent the whites of the eyes, irises, and lenses. They also made cut-outs of blood clots, Bitot's spots, corneal scars, fleshy growths ***(pterygia),*** pus, and so on. One 'white of an eye' they colored yellow to represent jaundice.

Then the students took turns putting the pieces together on the flannel-board to form specific problems. The group used their books to try to identify the problems and find recommendations for treatment.

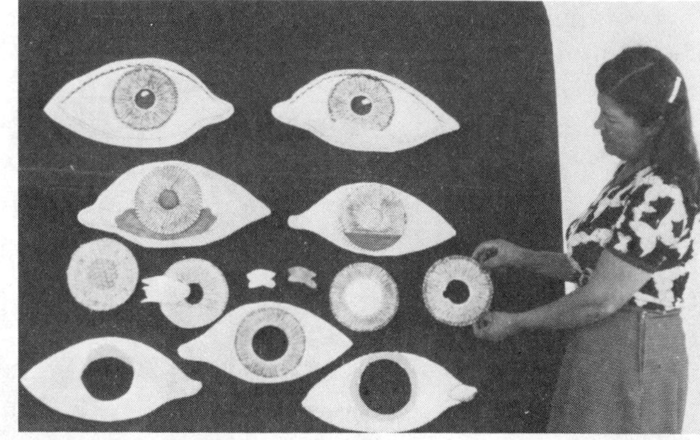

HERE ARE SOME EXAMPLES:

This eye is normal.

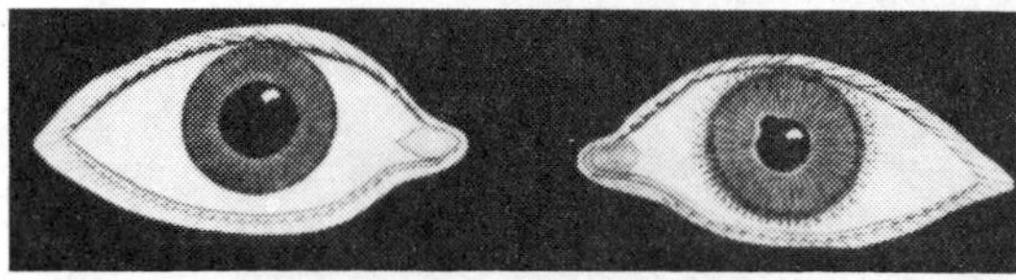

This eye is very painful. What is the problem? (See *WTND,* p. 221.)

This eye has bleeding behind the cornea. What should you do? (See *WTND,* p. 225.)

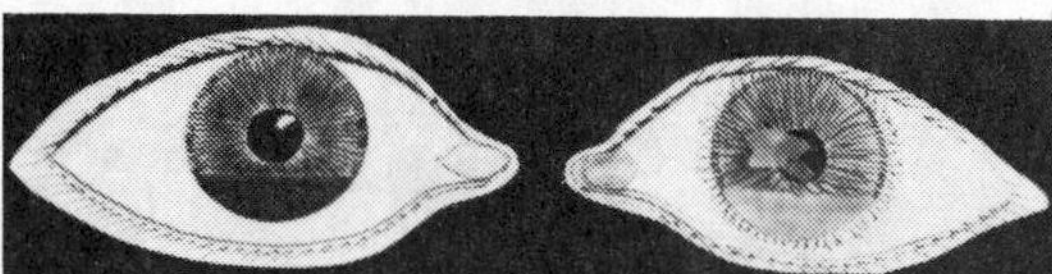

This eye has pus behind the cornea. What should you do? (See *WTND,* p. 225.)

People sometimes call the two problems below 'cloudiness' in the eye.

But a scar on the cornea is on the surface.

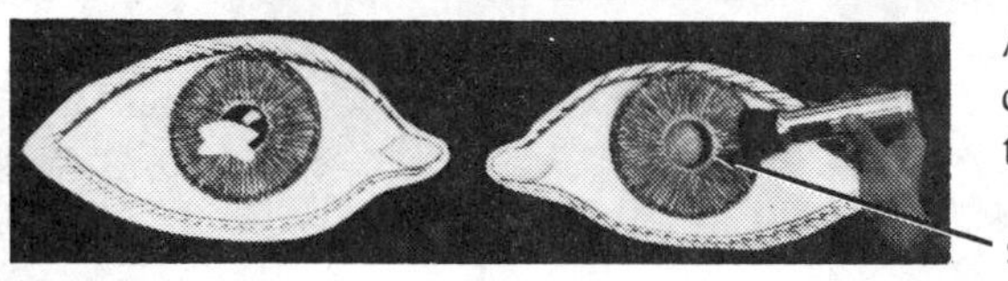

And a cataract is a cloudy lens behind the pupil.

To determine whether clouding in the pupil is a cataract, health workers can shine a flashlight sideways into the person's eye. If there is a cataract, a moon-shaped shadow is seen on the clouded lens. To get the same effect in the teaching aid, put a ring of thick cardboard between the iris and the lens.

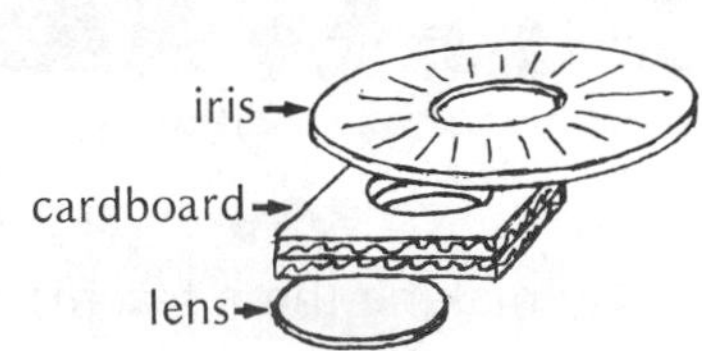

GUIDES AND CHARTS THAT TEACH SAFE LIMITS

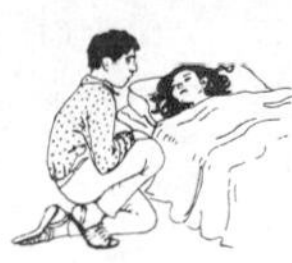

An essential part of training is to help health workers learn to recognize their limits: "Which sick persons can I safely treat in the community?" "Which should I send to a clinic or hospital for more specialized medical care?"

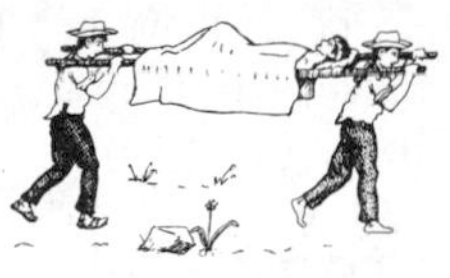

The answers to these questions will be different for each health program. They will also differ from one health worker to another and from village to village. When considering limits of what health workers should be taught or encouraged to do, several factors need to be taken into account:

- How common are the different serious problems in your area?
- How much curative medicine has the health worker learned?
- How much practice has he had in careful, step-by-step problem solving?
- What medicines and supplies are likely to be available?
- How long, difficult, or dangerous is the journey to the closest clinic or hospital?
- How much would doctors be likely to do to help the sick person?
- Can the family afford the emergency trip and the cost of reliable professional treatment?
- What do local people believe or fear about doctors and hospitals?

Clearly, community health workers should be trained to take certain essential emergency measures—even when they are able to refer the sick person to a hospital. Correct early treatment for a serious illness can often make the difference between life and death.

Where There Is No Doctor has several guides and charts to help identify serious illnesses that require medical care beyond the limits of most health workers. In some cases, immediate emergency treatment is also indicated.

GUIDES AND CHARTS INDICATING NEED FOR SPECIAL CARE

During training, health workers can learn to use these charts and guides through story telling, role plays, and actual clinical practice. Almost everyone has had experiences with emergencies in his own village. These can be told or acted out by the group. Students can use the guides and charts in their books to decide how to handle the different emergencies, and to determine when they would have to refer persons to a hospital or clinic.

Stories that help students to explore limits and use charts

To follow are two examples of how story telling can help students to practice using their health manuals. As a story is told, have students look things up in their books and discuss what they might have done.

STORY 1: A child with severe pneumonia

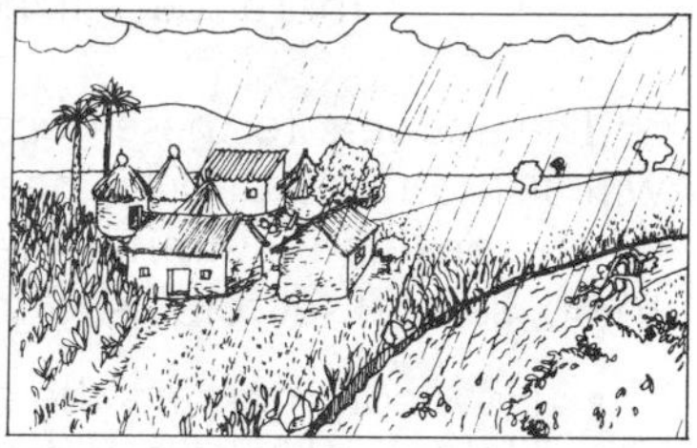

In a village in the *llanos* (plains) of Colombia, a young child got severe pneumonia during the rainy season. Although it would have been easy to make the 2-hour trip to the hospital during dry weather, now the river was high and the trip was impossible.

Luisa, the local health worker, looked in her copy of ***Where There Is No Doctor*** and found this on the chart on page 66.

> **66**
>
> **EMERGENCIES WHEN IT IS IMPORTANT TO GIVE INJECTIONS**
>
> In case of the following sicknesses, get medical help as fast as you can. If there will be any delay in getting help or in taking the sick person to a health center, inject the appropriate medicine as soon as possible. For details of the doses, consult the pages listed below. Before injecting, know the possible side effects and take the needed precautions.
>
> | For these sicknesses | Inject these medicines |
> |---|---|
> | Severe pneumonia (p. 171)
Infections after childbirth (p. 276)
Gangrene (p. 213) | penicillin in high doses (p. 350) |

Her training had not covered injecting of antibiotics, and she had no penicillin among her supplies. The program leaders had decided that it was "too risky" for health workers to treat serious infections like pneumonia. So all health workers had been instructed to refer anyone with pneumonia to the hospital.

Since they were unable to cross the river, Luisa took the family to the local storekeeper. He sold them the penicillin and agreed to give the injections himself. Luisa also helped the family to follow the other steps for treatment of pneumonia, described on p. 171 of ***WTND.*** The child soon got well.

After telling the story, start a discussion with questions like these:

- Do problems like this happen in your area?
- Was the health worker correct in going to the storekeeper for help?
- What would you have done?
- Had the program leaders thought about the village's isolation during the rainy season when they planned the training course?
- If so, why do you suppose they did not teach the health workers emergency measures for life-threatening problems? Who were these leaders trying to protect? (The sick? The health workers? Themselves?)
- How might the program leaders have handled the training differently?

STORY 2: A childbirth emergency

In the mountains of Mexico, a village health worker named Esteban was called in the middle of the night to help Doña Mercedes, a local midwife. A woman whose baby she had delivered was bleeding dangerously. Only part of the placenta had come out. By the time Esteban arrived, 4 sheets and several towels were soaked with blood and the woman, Carmelita, was bleeding faster. She was in danger of going into shock.

Esteban looked on page 42 of ***Where There Is No Doctor.*** He found this.

> **42**
>
> SIGNS OF DANGEROUS ILLNESS
>
> A person who has one or more of the following signs is probably too sick to be treated at home without skilled medical help. His life may be in danger. **Seek medical help as soon as possible.** Until help comes, follow the instructions on the pages indicated.
>
> **page**
>
> 1. Loss of large amounts of blood from anywhere in the body 82, 264, 281

Turning to page 264, Esteban and Doña Mercedes read about how to stop the bleeding. First they put the baby to Carmelita's breast. Then Doña Mercedes massaged the womb as shown in the pictures on page 265, while Esteban prepared an injection of oxytocin. They also gave Carmelita some hot tea, and began to treat her for shock. Together they managed to stop the bleeding.

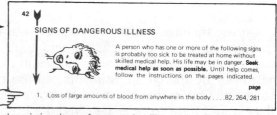

Esteban recommended that they take Carmelita to a hospital at once. Her husband made a stretcher, and he and some neighbors began the 8-hour journey to the nearest road. Esteban went, too. He made sure that Carmelita kept warm and drank plenty of liquids. He massaged her womb every time it began to get soft, and gave her injections of oxytocin every 3 hours.

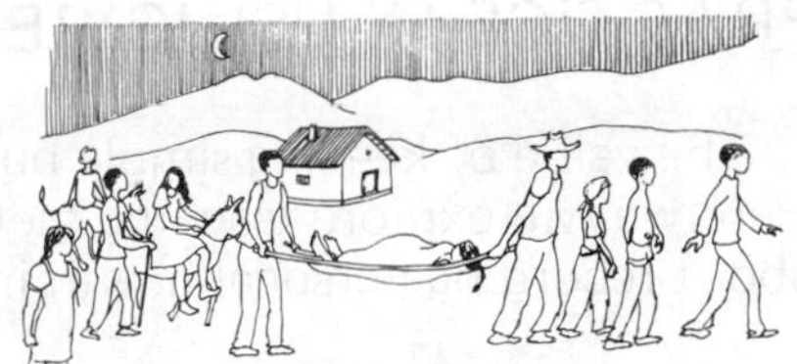

Esteban took Carmelita to a hospital where there was a doctor he trusted. She needed a blood transfusion and a simple operation. In a few days she was out of danger, though still very weak. The doctor praised the quick action by Doña Mercedes and Esteban, saying that their emergency treatment had saved Carmelita's life.

After returning to her village, Carmelita was still very pale from losing so much blood. So Esteban showed her the pages on anemia in ***Where There Is No Doctor*** (p. 124). She began eating ***quelite*** (wild spinach) and other foods rich in iron. She and her husband discussed with Doña Mercedes and Esteban how they might plan their family to give her body time to recover strength and make new blood between births.

Two years later, Carmelita became pregnant again. Doña Mercedes visited her and her husband to talk about the coming birth. Together, they looked on page 256 of *Where There Is No Doctor.*

One warning sign definitely applied to Carmelita: "If she has had serious trouble or severe bleeding with other births." Carmelita's husband agreed to take her to stay with her cousin in the city at least a month before the baby was due.

Signs of Special Risk that Make It Important that a Doctor or Skilled Midwife Attend the Birth—If Possible in a Hospital:

- If regular labor pains begin more than 3 weeks before the baby is expected.
- If the woman begins to bleed before labor.
- If there are signs of toxemia of pregnancy (see p. 249).
- If the woman is suffering from a chronic or acute illness.
- If the woman is very anemic, or if her blood does not clot normally (when she cuts herself).
- If she is under 15, over 40, or over 35 at her first pregnancy.
- If she has had more than 5 or 6 babies.
- If she is especially short or has narrow hips (p. 267).
- If she has had serious trouble or severe bleeding with other births.
- If she has diabetes or heart trouble.
- If she has a hernia.
- If it looks like she will have twins (see p. 269).
- If it seems the baby is not in a normal position in the womb.
- If the bag of waters breaks and labor does not begin within a few hours. (The danger is even greater if there is fever.)
- If the baby is still not born 2 weeks after 9 months of pregnancy.

Discussion questions:

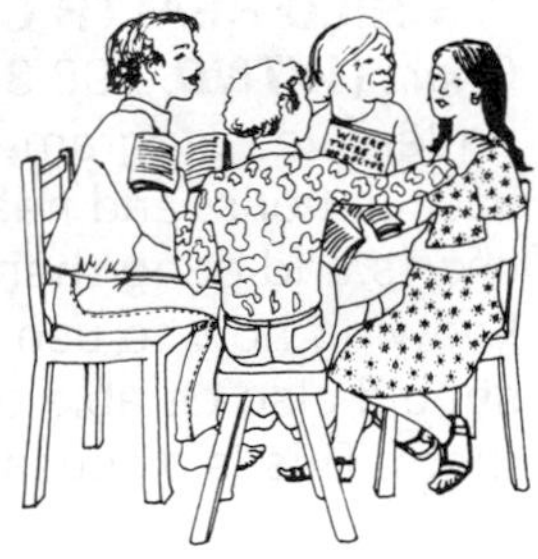

- Do you know of women who have had problems like Carmelita's? What happened?
- What would you have done as a health worker in Esteban's position?
- Did Esteban work within his limits?
- How were his limits determined? By whom? Were they reasonable?
- If Esteban had been within ten minutes of a doctor, should he have done the same thing? Why or why not?
- In general, what are the factors that should determine a health worker's limits (how much he should or should not do)?
- Should the limits be the same for all health workers with the same training? Who should decide?

Note to instructors: Rather than reading these stories to a group of health workers, you may prefer to tell stories from your own area. Also, instead of stating the page numbers of charts and information from ***Where There Is No Doctor,*** you may want to interrupt the story by asking students, "Where would you look in your books to find out about this?"

PRACTICE IN USING RECORD SHEETS

The value of keeping simple but effective records is discussed on page **10**-8. Here we will explore teaching methods and aids that help health workers learn about recording personal health information.

Where There Is No Doctor contains 4 different forms for recording health information:

PATIENT* REPORT *(WTND,* p. 44). This is intended for use by sick persons or their families when sending for medical help. But health workers can also use this form to keep a record of a person's illness, or to pass on information if the person is referred to a hospital or clinic.

DOSAGE BLANKS *(WTND,* p. 63-64). These are used for giving written instructions on how to take medicines. If carefully explained, they can be understood even by persons who cannot read. A copy of this information should also be kept with the health worker's own records.

Name:	Johnny Brown
Medicine:	Piperazine 500mg. tablets
For:	threadworm
Dosage:	take 2 tablets twice a day

RECORD OF PRENATAL CARE *(WTND,* p. 253). This is an important tool for keeping track of a woman's health during pregnancy. Health workers can use the form as part of a program of regular prenatal check-ups. Or they can assist local midwives in organizing a prenatal program and keeping records. (Methods of childbirth record keeping for midwives who cannot read are discussed on page **22**-7 of this book.)

CHILD HEALTH CHART, formerly called Road to Health Chart **(*WTND,*** 298-304). This form, an important part of an under-fives program, is used to record the monthly weighing, vaccinations, and health of small children. Parents keep the charts and bring them to each weighing. In addition to knowing how to use the charts themselves, health workers should also be able to teach parents to use and understand them. This is discussed in the next chapter, on page **22**-15.

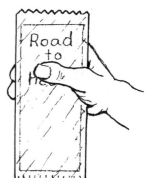

Health workers need practice in using—and teaching others to use—forms and record sheets like the ones described on this page. The use of these forms can be brought to life through role playing and practice in the community or clinic. On the following pages we give two examples of ways to introduce record sheets and forms. You will think of other ways yourself.

---

*Normally in this book and in our health work, we try not to use the word 'patient'. We prefer to say 'sick person', keeping in mind the whole person, who (like all of us from time to time) happens to be sick.

LEARNING RECORD KEEPING THROUGH ROLE PLAYS

To sit down with a group of students and tell them how to fill out record sheets can be boring for everyone. This is because such a lesson does not immediately relate to real problems or real life. Students are likely to pay little attention and to end up using the record forms incorrectly, carelessly, or not at all.

It is far more interesting for health workers to learn to fill in records while actually attending a sick person, weighing a baby, or checking the health of a pregnant woman. But in fairness to everyone, some classroom preparation should be done in advance.

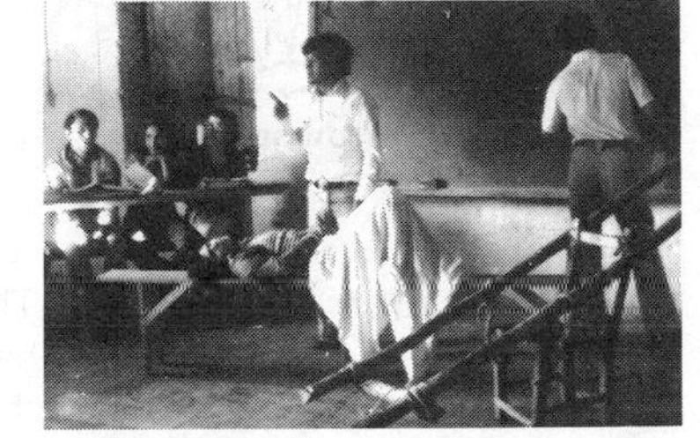

A role play about an injured person who was carried in on this stretcher the day before. (Mexico)

To make the classroom learning more realistic, whenever possible try to base it on situations that students have just experienced in the clinic or community. These may be emergencies, consultations, or health problems seen in prenatal check-ups or under-fives clinics. Students can report what they have seen to the rest of the group, perhaps in a role play. At the same time, the rest of the class practices recording the information on the suitable form. This way, everyone learns from the experience of a few students. Even those who were actually involved benefit from the suggestions and criticism of the group.

Example: Using the record form for prenatal care

Some student health workers in Mexico saw a pregnant woman at one of her regular prenatal check-ups. Her main complaint was swollen feet. Otherwise she felt fine. This is what was written on her RECORD OF PRENATAL CARE:

RECORD OF PRENATAL CARE

NAME JUANA GARCIA AGE 28 NUMBER OF CHILDREN 6 AGES ______ DATE OF LAST CHILDBIRTH MARCH 1, '79

DATE OF LAST MENSTRUAL PERIOD JULY 17, '79 PROBABLE DATE FOR BIRTH APRIL 24, '80 PROBLEMS WITH OTHER BIRTHS ONE BREECH

MONTH	DATE OF VISIT	WHAT OFTEN HAPPENS	GENERAL HEALTH AND MINOR PROBLEMS	ANEMIA (how severe)?	DANGER SIGNS (see p. 249)	SWELLING (where? how much?)	PULSE	TEMP. C.	WEIGHT (estimate or measure)	BLOOD PRESSURE *	PROTEIN IN URINE *	SUGAR IN URINE *	POSITION OF BABY IN WOMB	SIZE OF WOMB (how many fingers above (+) or below (-) the navel?)		
1 Aug.														-		
2 Sept.	15	tiredness, nausea, and morning sickness	tired vomiting	NO	NONE	NO	68	37	51 kg.	110/70	NO	NO		-		
3 Oct.														-		
4 Nov.	12	womb at level of the navel	O.K.	"	"	"	68	36.9	52.5 kg.	112/70	"	"		0		
5 Dec.	8	baby heartbeat & 1st movements	O.K.	"	"	"	70	37	53 kg.	108/68	"	"		+ 1	TETANUS VACCINE	
6 Jan.	10		O.K.	"	"	"	72	36.9	54 kg.	110/70	"	"		+ 3	1st	✓
7 Feb.	15	some swelling of feet	Swelling of feet	"	"	Feet ++	70	36.9	55.5 kg.	112/74	"	"	8	+ 5	2nd or booster	✓
8 March		constipation												+	3rd	
9 April 1st week		heartburn												+		
2nd week		varicose veins, shortness of breath												+		
3rd week		frequent urination												+		
4th week		baby moves lower in belly												+		
														+		
BIRTH																

The students made a copy of the record form, leaving the line for the 7th month blank. The next day they organized the following role play for their fellow students. (See next page.)

The instructor helped the students make a pretend baby:

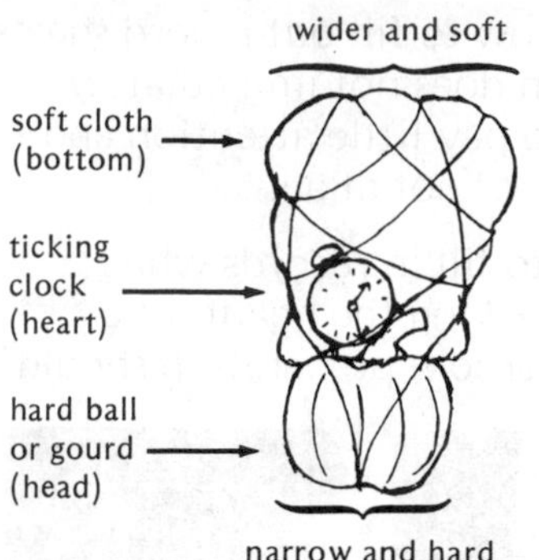

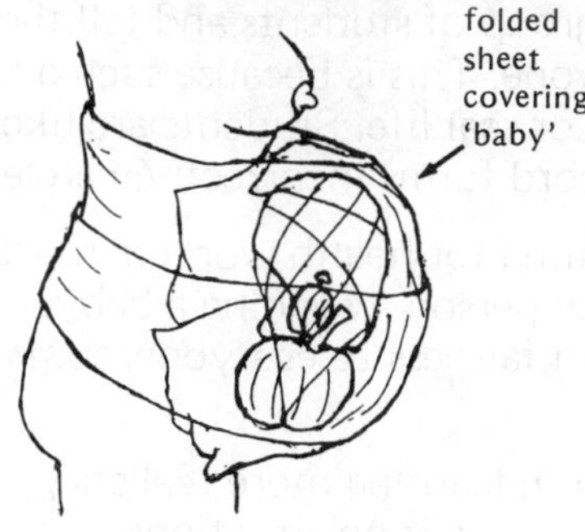

Note: Most clocks make about 240 ticks —or 120 ticktocks— per minute. The normal heartbeat of an unborn baby is 160. Below 140 or over 180 is a sign of trouble. This can be discussed with the students. Practice in timing a rapid prenatal heartbeat is important.

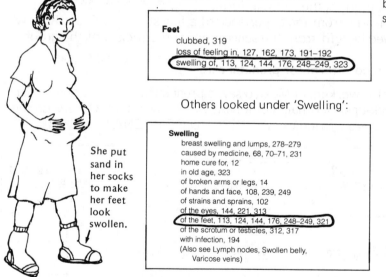

One student put the 'baby' under her dress and pretended that she was about 7 months pregnant.

She put sand in her socks to make her feet look swollen.

The other students asked her about her problem and then looked in the INDEX of ***WTND.***

Some looked under 'Feet':

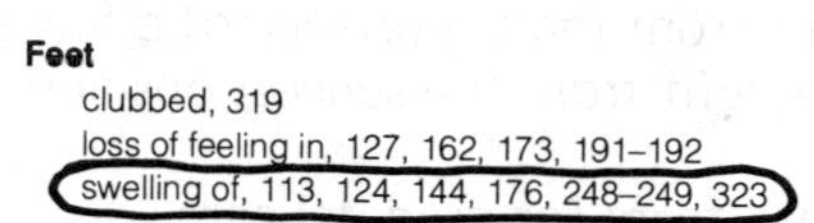

Feet
clubbed, 319
loss of feeling in, 127, 162, 173, 191–192
swelling of, 113, 124, 144, 176, 248–249, 323

Others looked under 'Swelling':

Swelling
breast swelling and lumps, 278–279
caused by medicine, 68, 70–71, 231
home cure for, 12
in old age, 323
of broken arms or legs, 14
of hands and face, 108, 239, 249
of strains and sprains, 102
of the eyes, 144, 221, 313
of the feet, 113, 124, 144, 176, 248–249, 321
of the scrotum or testicles, 312, 317
with infection, 194
(Also see Lymph nodes, Swollen belly, Varicose veins)

They found the same page references listed under both headings. Look up these page references in your own book to see what the students found:

Wet malnutrition (kwashiorkor), 113

Anemia (severe), 124

Trichinosis, 144

Swelling of the feet (several causes), 176

Minor problems and danger signs during pregnancy, 248-249

Swelling of the feet in older people, 323

The students then asked the 'pregnant woman' about what she had been eating and what other problems she had. They examined her for swelling of the face and hands, paleness of the gums and fingernails, and other signs of the possible causes of swollen feet. They took care to explain what they were looking for and why, so the woman would learn about her problem and also feel more relaxed.

Following the suggestions for prenatal care in ***Where There Is No Doctor,*** the health workers measured the woman's pulse, temperature, weight, and blood pressure. Since they had just learned how to use a small plastic 'dipstick' to check protein and sugar in the urine, they did that also. Last, they checked the size of the 'womb', felt for the position of the baby, and listened for its heartbeat. To their surprise (since the student was not really pregnant), they were able to determine all three!

This is how the blackboard looked after the health workers had finished figuring out the most likely cause of the woman's swollen feet:

	PROBLEM	WHAT WE FOUND
✗	MALNUTRITION –	SHE HAS BEEN EATING WELL
✗	ANEMIA –	SHE HAS BEEN EATING WELL NO SIGNS OF ANEMIA
✗	TRICHINOSIS –	HAS NOT EATEN PORK RECENTLY
✓	POOR CIRCULATION –	PROBABLY DUE TO PRESSURE OF CHILD IN WOMB
✗	TOXEMIA OF PREGNANCY –	NO SWELLING OF HANDS OR FACE; BLOOD PRESSURE O.K.; URINE O.K.
✗	HEART TROUBLE –	NO SIGNS
✗	KIDNEY DISEASE –	FREQUENT URINATION PROBABLY DUE TO PRESSURE OF CHILD; OTHERWISE NO SIGNS

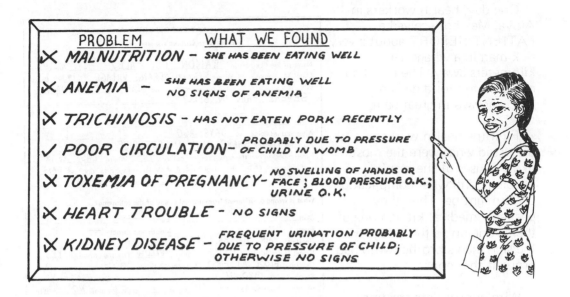

Luckily for the woman, the swelling was probably due to the pressure of the baby in her womb causing poor blood circulation in her legs. This is a common but minor problem during the last months of pregnancy. (The other possible causes are all serious health problems.)

The group reassured the woman that her problem did not seem to be dangerous. They suggested that she rest with her feet up as often as possible. They advised her to keep eating nutritious food, but with relatively little salt. And they also suggested that she drink a tea made from maize silk (see *Where There Is No Doctor,* page 12). Then they explained the signs of toxemia of pregnancy, warned her to watch for them, and asked her to come back immediately if any danger signs appeared.

The role play might have ended there. But the health workers who had actually seen the pregnant woman reminded their fellow students to think more about prevention and about other minor problems common in the last months of pregnancy. With this in mind, the students checked their books and decided they should give the woman a second tetanus vaccination. (According to her chart, she had been given the first at 6 months.) And some students offered her advice about other minor problems she might expect in the coming weeks: constipation, heartburn, varicose veins, shortness of breath, and frequent urination. Last of all, they recorded the information on the line opposite the 7th month on the RECORD OF PRENATAL CARE.

Note: When students do role plays or actual consultations, try having them use the CHECKLIST FOR EVALUATING A CONSULTATION (page **8**-10 of this book) to see how well they have done.

USING RECORD SHEETS AND TEACHING AIDS TO HELP STUDENTS UNDERSTAND SPECIFIC TREATMENTS

One day, health workers in Ajoya, Mexico received a PATIENT REPORT about a very sick man in a village 19 kilometers away. The man had not urinated for a day and a half, and was in great pain.

First the health workers discussed what were the most likely causes of the man's problem, and what complications there might be. Then they packed a medical kit and one of them rode up to the village with the sick man's brother, who had brought the report.

With appropriate treatment and advice, the man's condition soon improved.

During the next training course, the health workers decided to use that same PATIENT REPORT as the basis for a class on urinary problems. One person pretended to be the sick man, while someone else led the students in figuring out the cause of the problem and how to treat it.

PATIENT REPORT

TO USE WHEN SENDING FOR MEDICAL HELP.

Name of the sick person: RAMON GONZALEZ Age: 43

Male X Female ___ Where is he (she)? VERANO VILLAGE - 19 km away

What is the main sickness or problem right now? CAN NOT URINATE, SEVERE PAIN IN BELLY

When did it begin? 2 DAYS AGO

How did it begin? SHARP PAIN IN LEFT SIDE

Has the person had the same problem before? YES When? LAST YEAR

Is there fever? YES How high? 38.8 ° When and for how long? 2 DAYS

Pain? YES Where? LOWER BELLY What kind? SEVERE

What is wrong or different from normal in any of the following?

Skin: — **Ears:** —

Eyes: — **Mouth and throat:** —

Genitals: PAIN AT BASE OF PENIS

Urine: Much or little? LITTLE Color? YELLOW Trouble urinating? YES

Describe: BLOOD AT FIRST Times in 24 hours: 0 Times at night: 0

Stools: Color? BROWN Blood or mucus? — Diarrhea? —

Number of times a day: — Cramps? ___ Dehydration? NO Mild or severe? — Worms? NO What kind? —

Breathing: Breaths per minute: 20 Deep, shallow, or normal? NORMAL

Difficulty breathing (describe): NO Cough (describe): —

Wheezing? — Mucus? — With blood? —

Does the person have any of the SIGNS OF DANGEROUS ILLNESS listed on page 42? YES Which? (give details) 7. A DAY OR MORE WITHOUT BEING ABLE TO URINATE 17. BLOOD IN URINE

Other signs: SWELLING OF BLADDER, PASSED A STONE IN URINE

Is the person taking medicine? YES What? SULFATHIAZONE

Has the person ever used medicine that has caused hives (or bumps) with itching, or other allergic reactions? NO What? —

The state of the sick person is: Not very serious: ___ Serious: ___ Very serious: X

On the back of this form write any other information you think may be important.

Students were shown the original PATIENT REPORT. Then they were asked to look in their books and try to answer the following questions:

- What are the possible causes of the man's problem?
- Does the report contain enough information to show which cause is most likely?
- What should you look for and ask in order to find out which cause is most likely?
- Is it a serious problem?
- What would you recommend to help the man urinate?
- What about the fever? Is it a sign of infection?
- Is the man taking a safe medicine?
- What other treatments or medicines would be helpful?
- What would you have done if you had gone to the village to treat him?

To learn about the urinary system, how it works, and what could have caused the man to stop urinating, the health workers and students made a large cardboard model, based on the drawing on page 233 of ***Where There Is No Doctor.*** They used a large paper cup, a balloon, and some old tubing to form the different parts. The model shows how two different problems can block the urine in the bladder. To read about the signs and treatments of these problems, see *WTND,* pages 234-235.

An **enlarged prostate gland** can cause difficulty in urinating and even block urination completely if it swells and presses against the urinary tube.

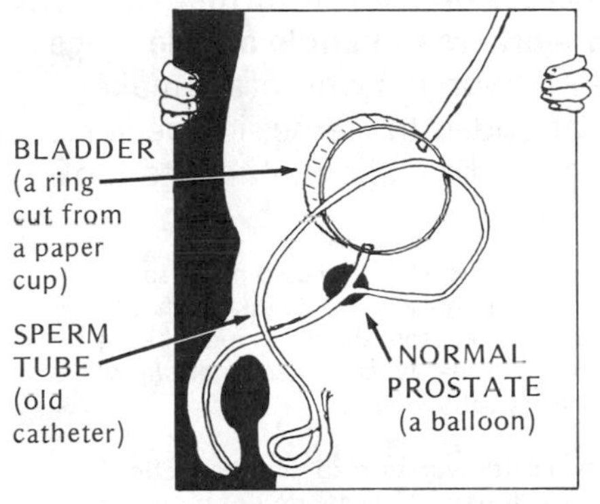

A balloon is used to represent the prostate gland.

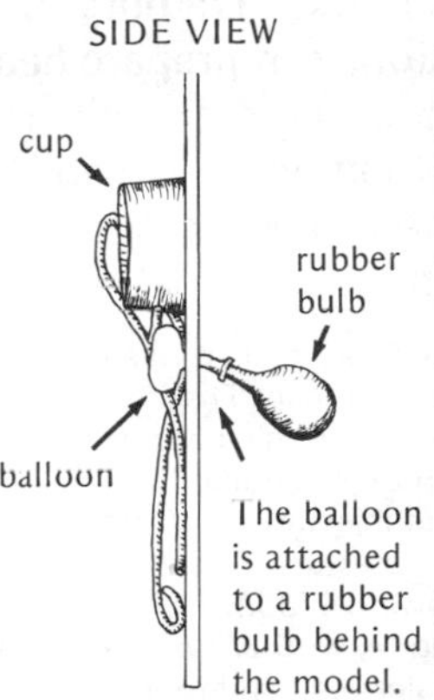

The balloon is attached to a rubber bulb behind the model.

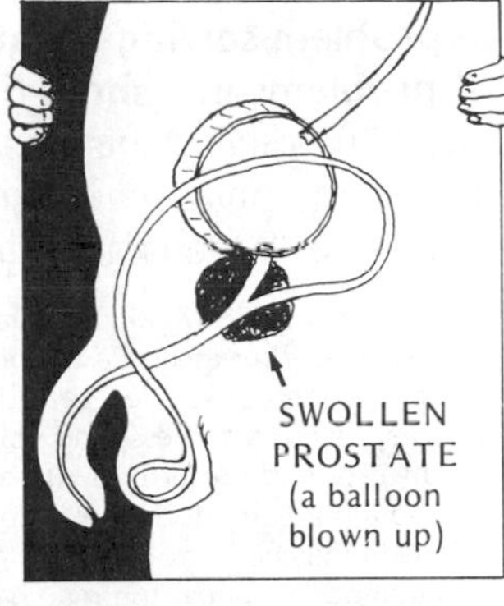

By squeezing the bulb, students can blow up the balloon to show a 'swollen prostate'.

A **bladder stone** can also block the urinary tube so that the person has difficulty passing urine—or cannot pass any at all. The students were asked, "What can be done in a case like this?"

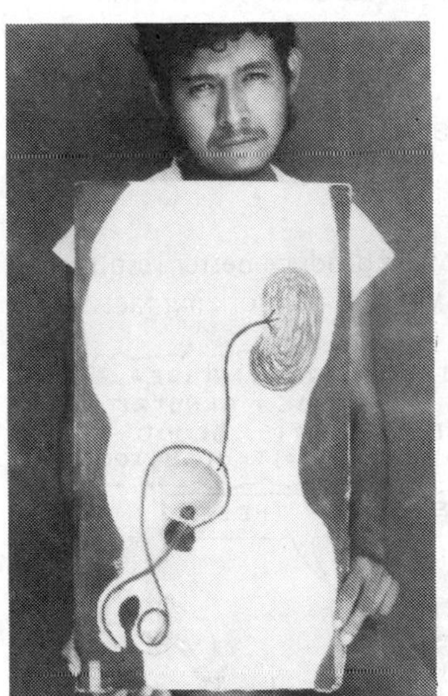

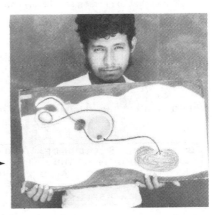

After thinking for a while, one student suggested that if the person would lie down, maybe the stone would roll back and free the opening to the urinary tube, like this:——→

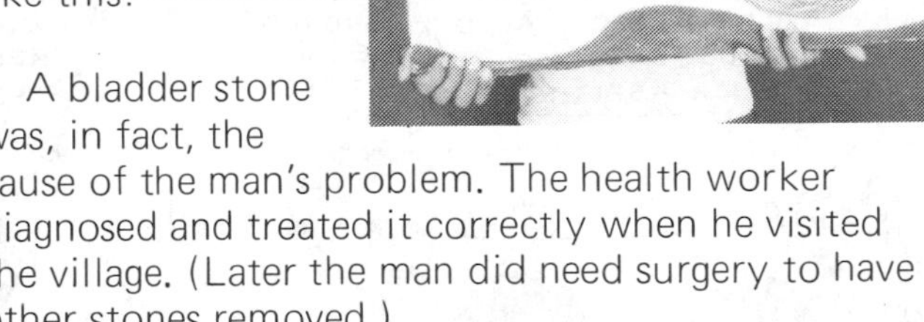

A bladder stone was, in fact, the cause of the man's problem. The health worker diagnosed and treated it correctly when he visited the village. (Later the man did need surgery to have other stones removed.)

Using their books, the student group tried to figure out answers to the questions at the bottom of page **21**-16. The use of a real PATIENT REPORT together with the teaching aid made the class more effective.

CAREFUL USE OF A REFERENCE BOOK CAN EQUAL YEARS OF TRAINING

In a short training course, you cannot teach great amounts of detailed information about a wide range of health problems. If you try to do this, students will forget or confuse important points, and end up making many mistakes. On the other hand, if health workers learn to manage only a few health problems, they will have trouble winning their communities' confidence. How, then, can health workers be trained in 2 or 3 months to deal effectively with a range of local health problems?

The answer, in part, is books. **Training that focuses on using informative books in problem-solving situations can prepare health workers to handle a wide range of problems in a short time.** We know village health workers who often make better medical decisions than doctors who have attended the same sick persons. This is mainly because the village workers have learned to take the time to look things up. Here is an example:

Recently in Mexico, I (David) watched a village health worker attend a 50-year-old man. The man complained of sudden periods with ringing of the ears, severe dizziness, and vomiting. A doctor in the city had prescribed vitamin injections, antacids, and a medicine to lower blood pressure. But these medicines had not helped. However, following a neighbor's advice, the man had taken ***Dramamine*** (an antihistamine for motion sickness) and found temporary relief. But the problem kept returning.

The health worker found the man's blood pressure and other vital signs normal. He looked in the INDEX of ***WTND*** under 'Dizziness', and then turned to page 327, 'Deafness with Ringing of the Ears and Dizziness'. There he read about Ménière's disease, noting that antihistamines often help and that the person should have no salt in his food.

He asked the man if he used much salt. "Yes, lots!" said the man. He asked what the man had eaten before the dizzy spells began. The man said that twice he had eaten ***suero salado*** (very salty whey).

The health worker read him the section on Ménière's disease. "So why don't you try eating your food without salt? And don't touch salty foods like ***suero salado*** and pork cracklings." "Okay, I'll try!" said the man.

Two weeks later, the man returned. "I'm well!" he said joyously. "You cured me—and the doctor couldn't!"

"You cured yourself," said the health worker, "after we read about your problem together."

In this case, the health worker was able to help treat a problem he had never heard of before—Ménière's disease— because he had learned how to find and use information in ***Where There Is No Doctor.***

Two months' training in use of the book . . . . can often produce better results than years of memorizing facts.

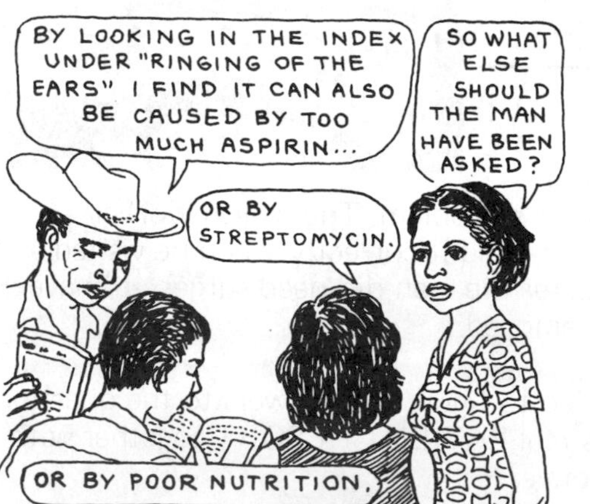

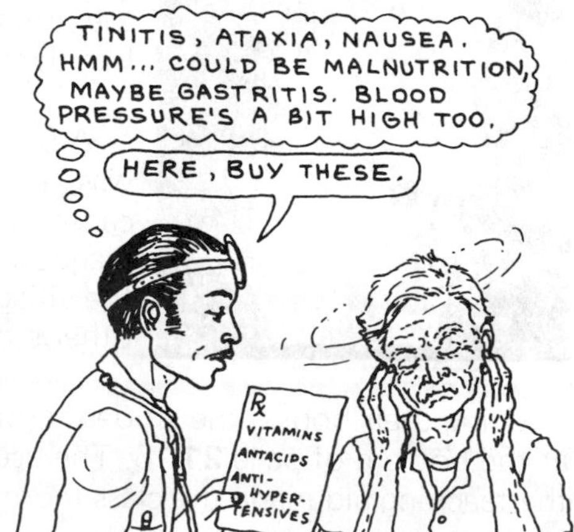

Learning like this . . . . helps prevent errors like this.

PART FOUR

ACTIVITIES WITH MOTHERS AND CHILDREN

Most trainers of health workers agree that activities with mothers and children are the most important part of health work in a community. This is because . . .

- Women and children make up more than half the people (up to 75%).
- The health needs of mothers and children are especially great.
- Mothers and older children are the main providers of care for babies and younger children, whose needs are greatest of all.

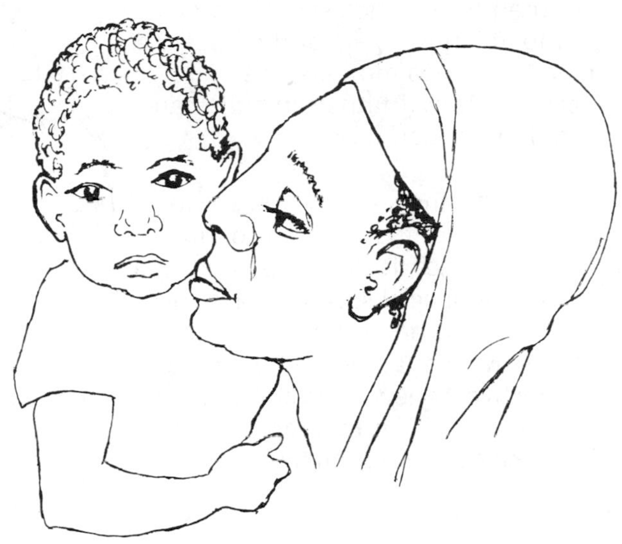

Part Four of this book has three chapters:

In **Chapter 22,** we consider activities that help safeguard the health of pregnant women, mothers, and small children. We discuss the role of health workers in coordinating prenatal and 'under-fives' programs. But we also stress the importance of having local mothers and midwives take leadership in running these activities. Baby weighing is discussed. We explore creative teaching aids that help mothers understand Road to Health charts. Finally, we look at women's special strengths.

In **Chapter 23,** we examine family planning. We include this as a separate chapter, not because we feel birth control should be separated from the rest of mother and child health care. Rather, we do this because of the confusing politics and abuses connected with family planning. Too often, in the many arguments concerning birth control, the interests of the poor are forgotten. In this chapter, we discuss the conflicts of interest that often exist, and consider ways in which health workers can help people plan their families on their own terms.

Chapter 24 is about "Children as Health Workers." The material in this chapter is based on the CHILD-to-child Program. Many of the original CHILD-to-child activities were field tested by health workers and school teachers in Ajoya, Mexico. They include simple teaching aids and exciting approaches that help children discover things for themselves. The program attempts to bring schooling closer to children's lives and needs, and to place the focus of education on helping one another. The health worker can play an important role in this process.

THE ROLE OF FATHERS IN CHILD CARE

Traditionally, in most areas, it is the mother who takes the main responsibility for small children. But fathers are also responsible—or should be. In some societies, fathers share part of the child care or even take the children to the under-fives clinic. Although in this part of the book we mainly refer to mothers, the participation of fathers in child care should be encouraged.

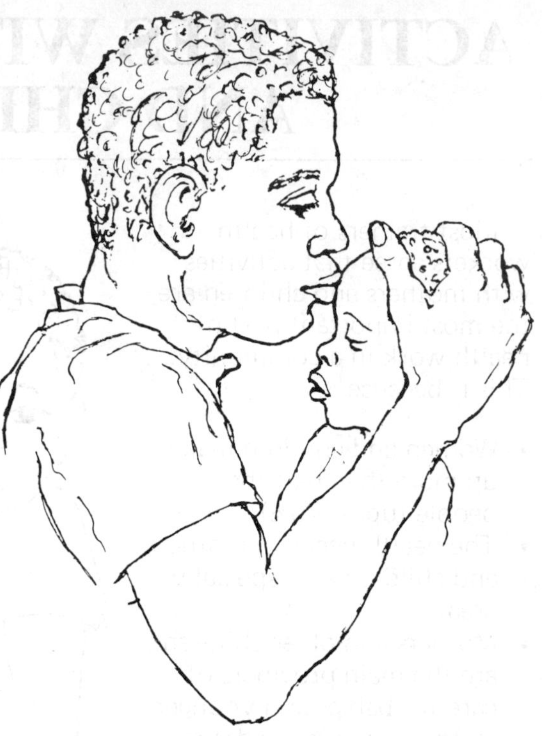

Since mothers are the ones who generally take the children to 'under-fives' activities, it may be a good idea to arrange special sessions for fathers, or for fathers and mothers together. That way, the fathers will be more supportive of new ideas about child care and nutrition that mothers learn in the under-fives program.

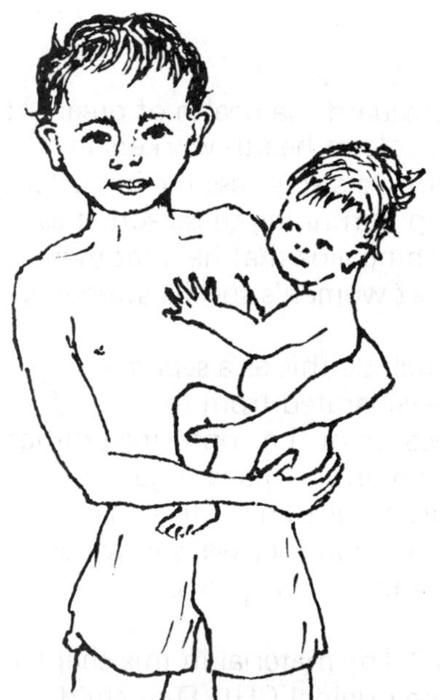

Not only mothers and fathers, but also older brothers and sisters have a very important role in the care of small children. This is the subject of Chapter 24.

CHAPTER 22

Pregnant Women, Mothers, and Young Children

To help improve mothers' and children's health, health workers need to lead or organize activities in the following areas:

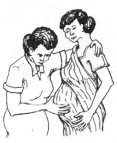

1. **Prenatal care** (for pregnant women)
   - history and check-ups for problems
   - health education with emphasis on nutrition and safety (and medicines that could harm the baby)
   - tetanus vaccinations and other precautions (iron supplements when needed)
2. **Birth**—special care for 'high-risk' mothers and babies
   - cooperation and learning with local midwives
   - special precautions to prevent infection and hemorrhage
   - referral to hospital for high-risk deliveries and complications
   - care of the newborn
3. **Mothers and young children**
   - observation of children's growth and health
   - health education with a focus on nutrition, cleanliness, safety measures, and activities that help children's bodies and minds to grow strong and active
   - oral rehydration
   - vaccinations
   - diagnosis and treatment of common health problems
   - care and attention for children who have special problems

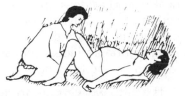

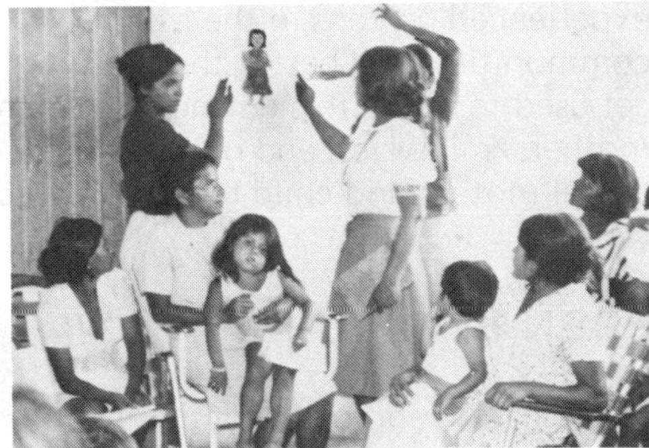

Health workers in Ajoya, Mexico leading mothers in a discussion about nutrition.

4. **Child spacing or family planning**

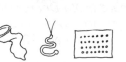

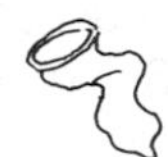

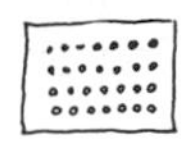

In this chapter, we do not go into the details of each of these areas. They are discussed in ***Where There Is No Doctor*** and in many other books on mother and child health.* Instead, we look at common difficulties that health workers encounter in promoting mother and child health activities. We explore approaches to training that help avoid or overcome some of these difficulties. And we give examples of methods and aids that health workers can use to help mothers learn about the health needs of their children.

---

*See, for example, ***Practical Mother and Child Health in Developing Countries,*** by G. J. Ebrahim, available through TALC (see p. **Back**-3).

Getting started: Have mothers and midwives take the lead

Health workers, especially if young, single, and from the village where they work, often have difficulty in promoting prenatal and mother and child activities. For them to be advising older women about pregnancy, birth, and child care may seem ridiculous or even insulting.

In such cases, it is a good idea for the young health worker to explain her problem to some of the respected older women, including local midwives. Rather than trying to tell these older women what to do (which might offend them), the health worker can ask them for their advice and help in organizing and running the prenatal or mother and child program. That way the young health worker does not lead the activities, but stays in the background, sharing the information and ideas that she learned during training.

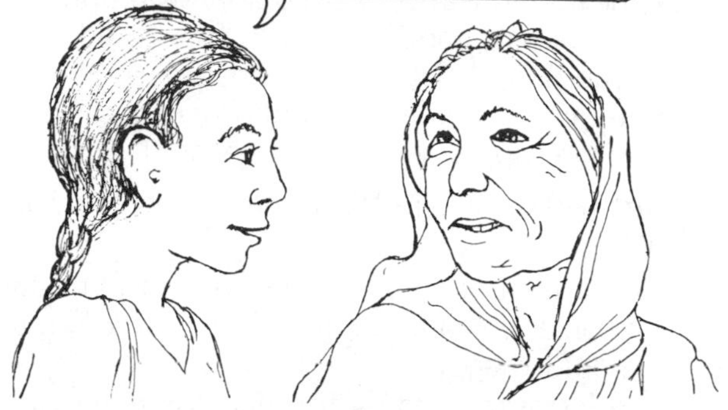

DOÑA MARIA, I'M HAVING TROUBLE GETTING A MOTHER AND CHILD PROGRAM STARTED. THE PEOPLE TRUST AND LISTEN MORE TO *YOU*. CAN YOU HELP ME?

Asking people's help is the best way to win their cooperation.

If health workers are to seek advice and leadership from more experienced persons in their communities, it is best if they get used to doing this during their training. Encourage students to invite local mothers, midwives, and other experienced persons to take part in classes and in actual mother and child health activities conducted during the training course.

PRENATAL CARE

Education and health activities with pregnant women are among the most important areas of mother and child care.

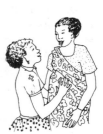

You will find information concerning prenatal care on pages 250 to 253 of *Where There Is No Doctor.* Ideas for adapting prenatal advice about nutrition to local customs and beliefs are found in the story beginning on page **13**-1 of this book.

Holding special prenatal clinics at a separate time or place from the children's clinic usually does not make sense. Most pregnant women already have small children, so it is more convenient (for them) if you **include prenatal care as part of an under-fives program. This can combine education, preventive care, and treatment for both women and children.**

Young women who are pregnant for the first time often will not come to any kind of clinic. But since first pregnancies involve more risk, special care is called for. Health workers can visit the homes of these women and win their trust and cooperation.

During their training, students may be able to visit pregnant women in the community, and help them take care of their needs. The women will feel better about this if the instructor or local midwife first asks them to help 'teach' the students. They can discuss their experiences of pregnancy and help the students learn to ask questions and give advice in ways that most women will appreciate.

Before beginning visits to pregnant women, it also helps if students practice with role plays in class. On page **21**-13 there is an example of a role play of a prenatal check-up. In it, students act out how to examine a woman, and practice filling out the RECORD OF PRENATAL CARE.

Note: In a mixed group of students, the girls or women may be shy about role plays involving pregnancy or birth, especially if these involve physical examination. In such cases, encourage the male students to dress up and play the role. This not only makes the class more fun, it is also a valuable lesson for the male health workers to experience—if only in make believe—what a woman goes through during pregnancy, prenatal exams, and childbirth.

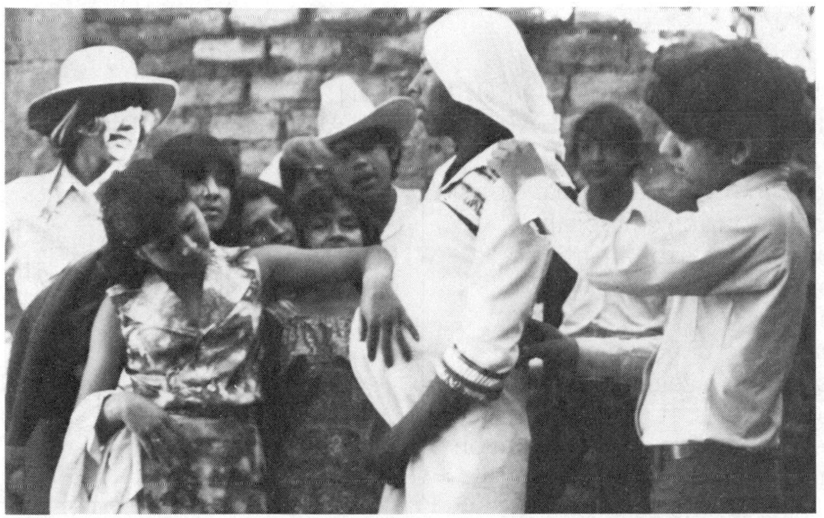

Here a male health worker in Ajoya, Mexico plays the role of a pregnant woman, complete with mask of pregnancy and swollen ankles. Other students ask questions and examine 'her'.

LEARNING ABOUT BIRTH

In a 2-month training course, health workers may not gain enough experience to be able to attend births alone (except in emergencies). Therefore . . .

Prepare health workers to assist, learn from, and share ideas with local midwives or birth attendants.

A good way to do this is to **invite local birth attendants to take part in the classes on childbirth.** (See the next page.)

One of the most exciting classes we have seen took place when an old midwife from a neighboring village came to the Ajoya clinic. She had come with some questions of her own about 'modern methods' of midwifery. So one of the instructors invited her to a childbirth class for new health workers. Together, the students and the midwife explored what they knew, what she knew, and what each still wanted to learn. Together they drew up lists of information and ideas that they could share with each other (see below).

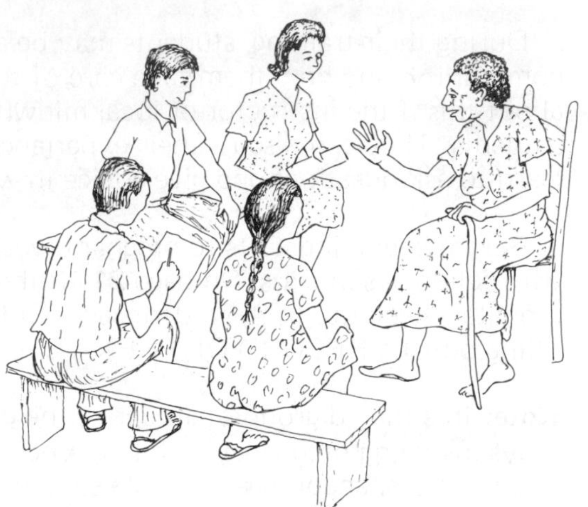

Not surprisingly, their ideas were not always in agreement. But each showed respect for the other. The midwife invited the students to attend births with her. And the students invited her to future classes.

EXAMPLES OF IDEAS AND INFORMATION THAT HEALTH WORKERS CAN SHARE WITH TRADITIONAL MIDWIVES:

- Foods that will help make women stronger during childbirth.
- How to check for anemia and other danger signs during pregnancy.
- When to refer a woman to a hospital to give birth (before trouble starts, if possible).
- The importance of **not** sitting on the mother or pushing on her belly to get the baby out.

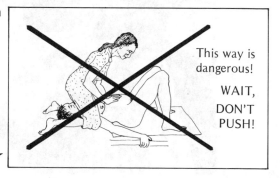

This way is dangerous!
WAIT, DON'T PUSH!

- The proper use of oxytocics (to control bleeding after birth, not to speed up labor!).
- How to prevent tetanus of the newborn (with special emphasis on helpful and harmful local traditions—see p. 184 of ***WTND,*** and p. **22**-6 of this book).
- The need to hold the baby below the level of the mother until the cord is tied (this provides the baby with extra blood and makes him stronger).
- The importance of putting the baby to the breast right after birth (to help control bleeding and push out the placenta).
- The value of ***colostrum*** (the mother's first milk) for the baby.
- The importance of urging mothers to **breast feed,** not bottle feed their children.
- Signs of danger and aspects of care for the newborn.
- The importance of the mother eating a variety of nutritious foods following birth (and the danger of avoiding eggs, beans, meat, and fruit, as is the tradition in some places).
- Ways for midwives who cannot read to keep records and to send information with mothers or babies they refer to hospitals (see examples on page **22**-7).

EXAMPLES OF INFORMATION AND EXPERIENCES THAT TRADITIONAL MIDWIVES CAN SHARE WITH HEALTH WORKERS:

- Personal experiences and insights from many years of attending births.
- How to respond to the common questions and concerns of pregnant women in terms of the local culture and language (see the story of Janaki and Saraswati, p. **13**-1).
- How to feel the position and size of the unborn baby; doing this in a friendly, confidence-building way.
- Safe ways to help make labor easier and shorter:
  - — Allow the woman in labor to eat a little, if she feels hungry.
  - — Give her herbal teas and other drinks.
  - — Permit the woman to get up and walk around, or to change to any position that is comfortable.
  - — Show her real babies or pictures of babies happily nursing. The warm feeling this produces in the mother helps her womb contract strongly. If labor slows down, let a baby or caring person suck the woman's breasts.
- Ways to give comfort and to calm the fears that can slow or stop labor:
  - — Avoid letting the room get too crowded with friends and relatives.
  - — Avoid having those present discuss cases of death or misfortune in childbirth.
  - — Reassure the woman, hold her, massage her, and comfort her. Let her feel your confidence that all is progressing well.
- The need of the woman in labor to have a kind and sympathetic person stay close to her and offer support. This person could be the midwife, or the woman's sister, mother, or close friend—or, if acceptable, her husband.*
- Knowledge of local beliefs and traditions relating to childbirth.

  In Mexico, for example, some village women believe it is essential to take the following preventive measures:

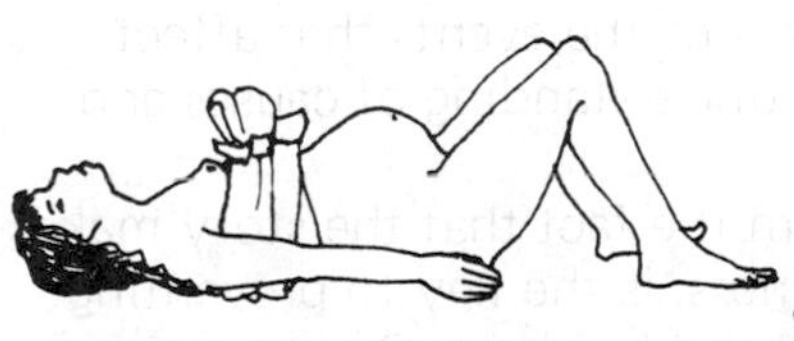

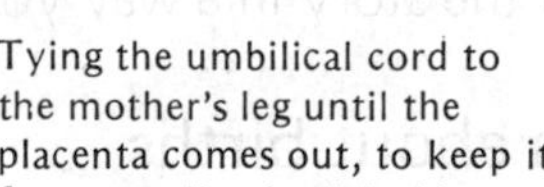

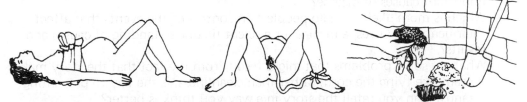

Using a 'belly band' to prevent the baby from trying to come out through the mother's mouth.

Tying the umbilical cord to the mother's leg until the placenta comes out, to keep it from crawling back inside.

Burying the placenta in a corner of the room to protect the mother's spirit.

Traditional midwives can tell health workers about common local beliefs and discuss ways to respect them when attending births. If a belief is helpful, health workers can encourage it. If harmless, they can go along with the custom to help the family feel more confident and comfortable. If it is harmful, they should help people understand why. Or they may be able to build on local beliefs to help explain new and healthier ways. (See the story from Nigeria on the next page.)

---

*A recent study in the ***New England Journal of Medicine*** shows the importance of having a familiar, loving person present at childbirth. The average length of labor for first births in a Guatemalan hospital was 8.8 hours for mothers accompanied by a sympathetic woman, and 19.3 hours for women who were attended only by nurses and doctors. Also, those with companions had fewer birth complications and felt more warmly toward their new babies. Does this speak in favor of home births?

Adapting new ideas to old beliefs

In Lardin Gabas, Nigeria, health workers learn to teach new ideas through the local tradition of story telling (see p. **13**-5). They also learn to adapt their health advice to local beliefs.

An example is a story they tell to help mothers and midwives learn about the prevention of tetanus in newborn babies. Midwives in Lardin Gabas traditionally rub dry dirt or cow dung into the end of a baby's cut cord to prevent bleeding. The result is that babies often die of tetanus from the infection that enters through the cord. But people think the illness is caused by a certain kind of bird that lands above the baby. They believe that when the bird sings, the spirit of the baby flows out through the cord, causing the baby's body to stiffen with spasms.

The story the health workers tell describes how a village midwife learned to prevent this form of infant death. After carefully washing her hands, she would tightly tie the baby's cord with clean strips of cloth, then cut it with a boiled bamboo knife. Later, when the bird landed over the baby and sang, the baby's spirit could not escape because the cord was tightly tied.

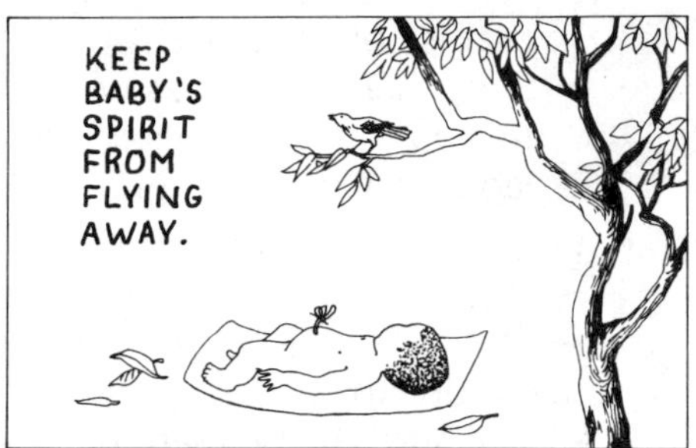
KEEP
BABY'S
SPIRIT
FROM
FLYING
AWAY.

Questions for discussion:

If you tell this story to a group of health workers-in-training, have them discuss its strengths and weaknesses. Ask questions like these:

- In what ways does this story help mothers and midwives gain greater understanding and learn healthier practices?
- In what ways does the story mislead people or block their understanding of important causes of disease?
- Which is more likely to help people gain control of the events that affect their health and lives, a magical or a scientific understanding of causes and results?
- What are some problems that might result from the fact that the story makes it seem like tying the cord, rather than cleanliness, is the key to preventing tetanus? Can you retell the story in a way you think is better?

Reporting information about births

Keeping records of prenatal care and providing accurate information when referring emergency births or complications to a hospital is an important part of any birth attendant's job. On page **10**-8, we discuss the need to keep such forms simple and useful. Health workers and midwives who can read may want to use the RECORD OF PRENATAL CARE (***WTND,*** p. 253). But for those who cannot read, other solutions are needed.

Health workers in Ecuador have developed a reporting system for midwives, using different colored cards. Local midwives learn to associate each color with a specific problem: red if the mother is hemorrhaging, white if she is very ***anemic*** (pale), blue if the baby has delayed or difficult breathing, and yellow if he is ***jaundiced*** (yellow).

In Indonesia, a birth report form using pictures was developed for midwives who cannot read. The form was later adapted for use in Egypt, with the help of a group of traditional midwives. Here are some of the changes they suggested.

The Egyptian midwives found these drawings on the Indonesian form too abstract.

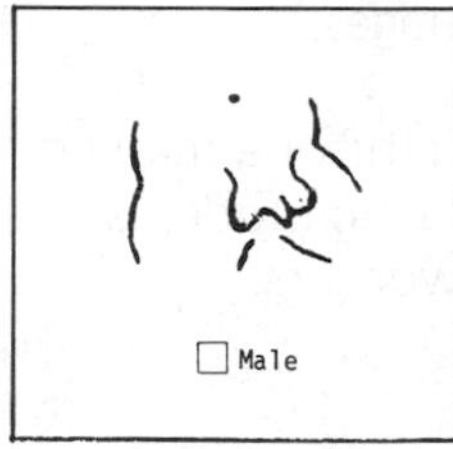

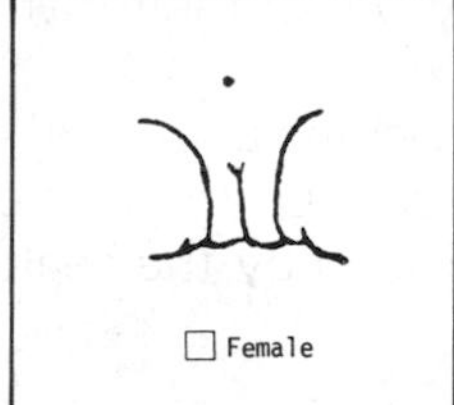

They said it would be better to draw the whole baby, with an earring for the girl (since all baby girls in Egypt are given earrings).

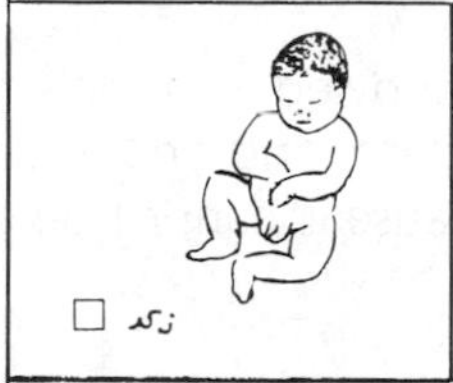

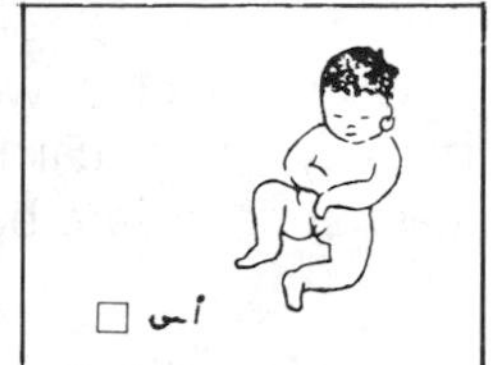

They thought this Indonesian drawing of a dead baby looked more like a sweet wrapped in paper.

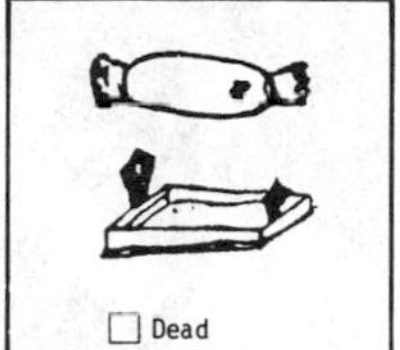

They suggested that the dead baby be shown wrapped like a mummy, as is often done in Egypt.

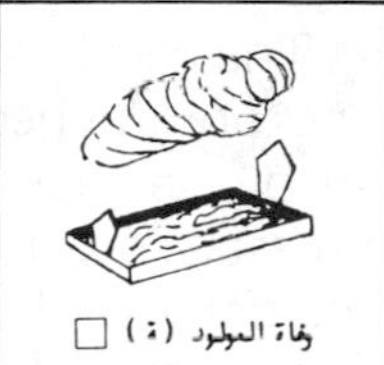

And they suggested changing the red cross on the ambulance

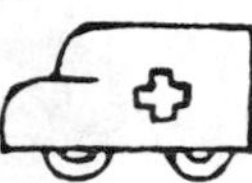

to the red crescent used on Egyptian ambulances.

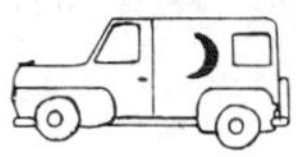

The revised Egyptian form is shown below. Read it from right to left. start here

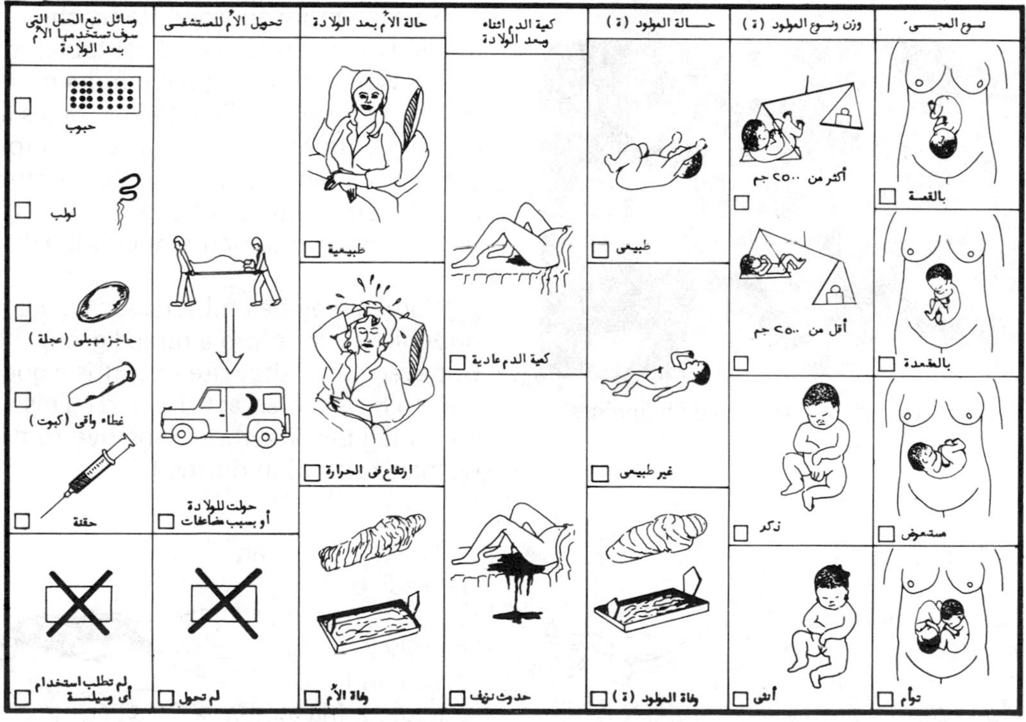

Reporting form for traditional birth attendants in Egypt,
adapted from an Indonesian form with the help of local midwives.

(Taken from *Salubritas,* American Public Health Association, July, 1980.)

TEACHING AIDS FOR LEARNING ABOUT BIRTH

In a short training course in a village setting, health workers usually do not have a chance to attend many births. Good teaching aids are therefore essential. The more lifelike they are, the better. But it is important that the aids used be ones that the students can make themselves at low cost. That way they can use them for health education with mothers and midwives in their own villages.

On page **11**-3, we showed 3 models for teaching about childbirth: one made of plastic, one of cardboard, and one a real person. Of these, the plastic model is least appropriate because it cannot be duplicated by the health workers.

The cardboard box model is appropriate because of its simplicity. Also, the back flap can be cut to form breasts, so students can practice putting the baby to the breast right after birth. This is important because it helps to prevent hemorrhage and to push out the placenta.

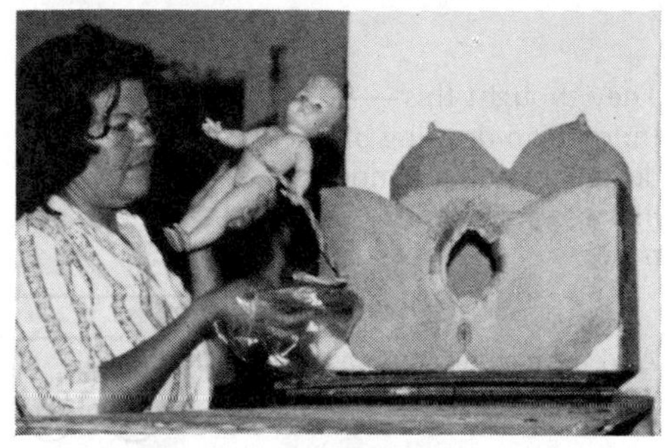

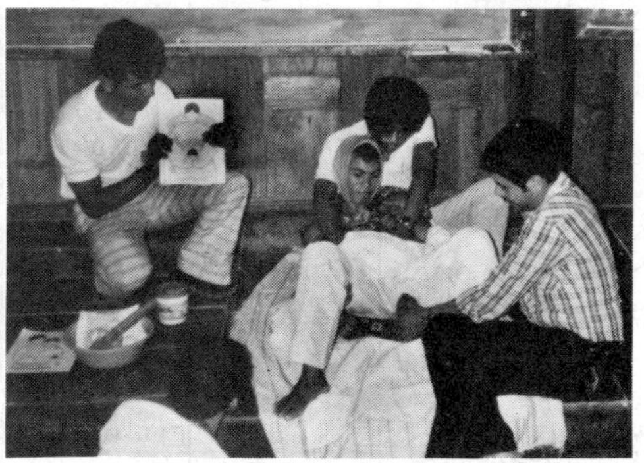

A male health worker in the Philippines 'delivers a baby'.

An even more appropriate teaching model (where culturally acceptable) is a real person with a doll baby hidden inside her clothing. The person wears a pair of pants with the crotch cut to form a 'birth opening'. This way, the 'mother' and the birth attendant can act out all the emotions and events of childbirth.

Women may be embarrassed to act out childbirth before a mixed group. But even when they are not, it is a good idea to have a man act the part! This way, men become more sensitive to the woman's situation during labor.

Babies for these demonstrations can be made of cloth stuffed with rags or straw, or children's dolls can be used.

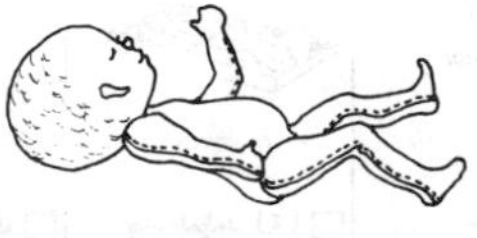

The placenta can be made of red cloth sewn so that the lobes can be spread and inspected. Make the membrane of thin plastic (cellophane).

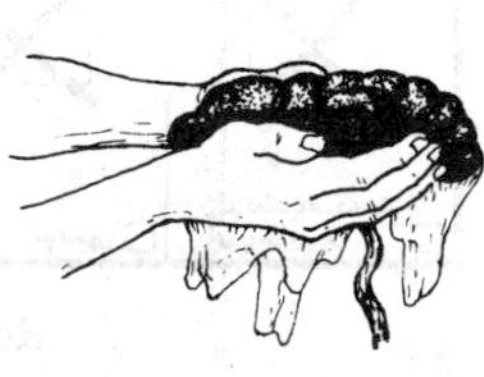

If having a real person act out childbirth is not culturally acceptable in your area, try using the cardboard 'birth box' instead. To make the demonstration more lifelike, you can put the box on a cot, and have a person lie underneath.

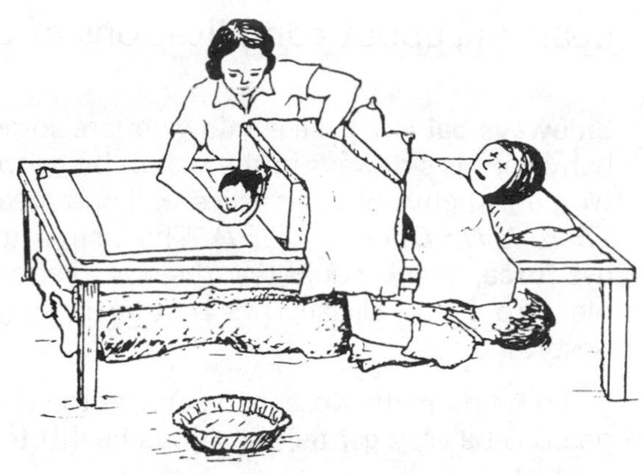

The person underneath can push on the box to show contractions of the womb, and make panting and groaning sounds and talk as the 'woman' gives birth.

A teaching aid to help health workers and mothers see the position of the baby inside the womb was invented by Pablo Chavez, the village health worker who has done some of the drawings for this book.

Pablo made a cardboard figure of a woman's body, with a window cut out to show the inside of the womb. This he covered with a clean piece of old X-ray film to form a transparent pocket.

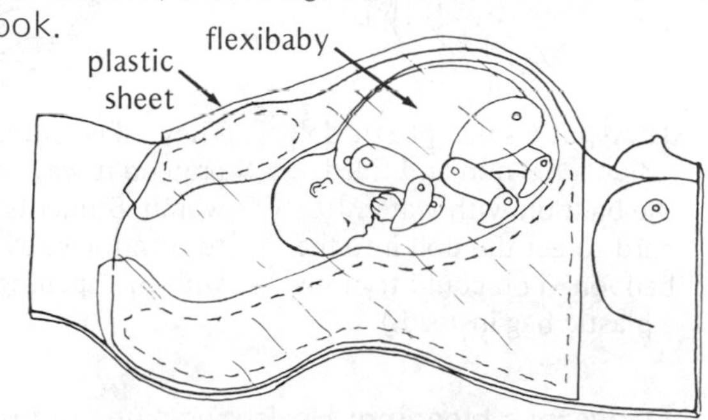

He also made a flexible baby model from pieces of cardboard and some rivets.

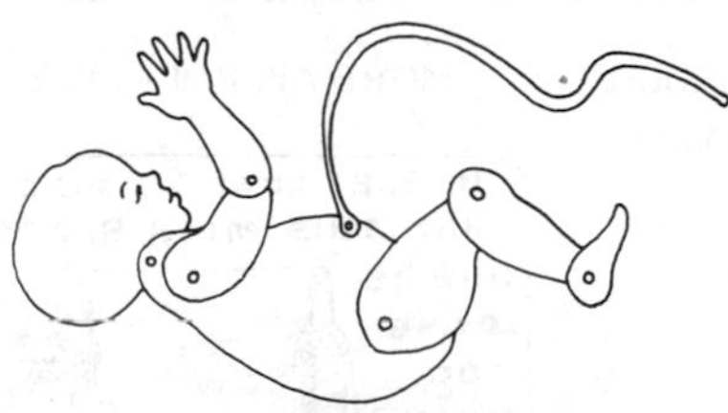

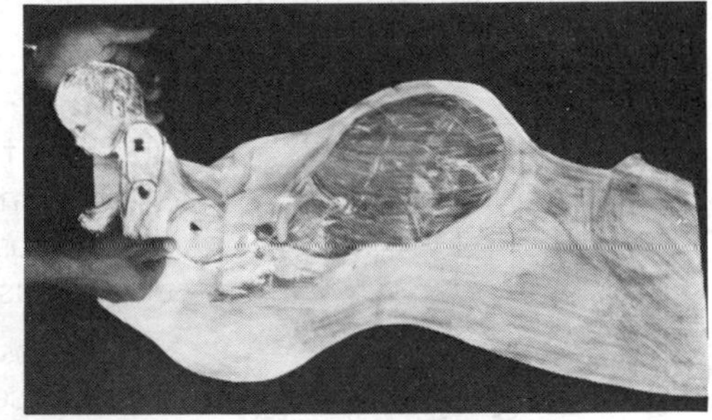

The 'flexibaby' can be placed in the 'womb' in any position, and then used to demonstrate the different presentations of birth (head first, butt first, foot or hand, etc.).

Another way to show the different birth positions is to use a real baby together with a drawing of a woman giving birth. A mother holds her baby in front of the picture, and shows how it would be delivered in various positions. (See also p. **12**-7.)

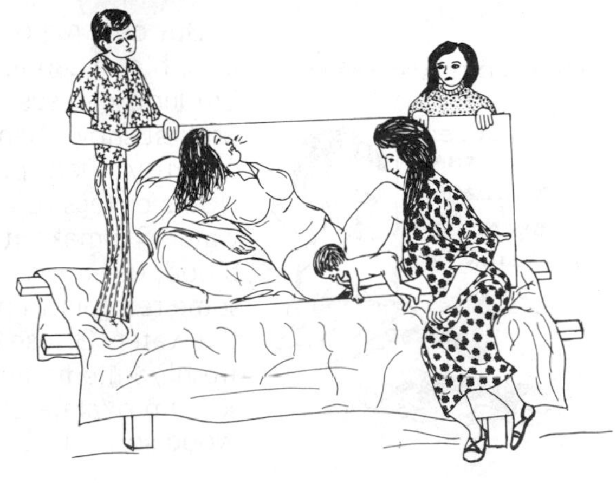

Learning about complications of childbirth

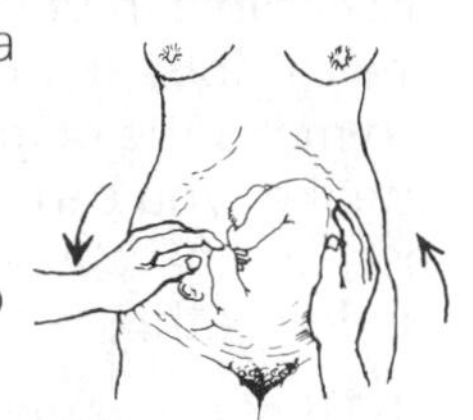

Sideways babies: Village midwives are sometimes able to turn a baby that is sideways in the womb by ***gently*** handling the woman's belly. But this takes skill and great care (see *Where There Is No Doctor,* p. 267). The birth attendant must **never use force,** as this could tear the womb and cause the mother to bleed to death. Usually it is best to try to get the mother to a hospital.

To help health workers recognize the danger in trying to turn the baby, and the need to be very gentle, the Ajoya health team invented this teaching aid:

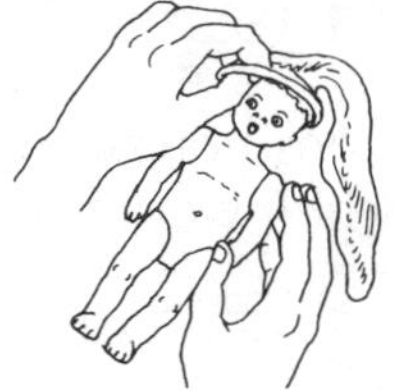

They put a small plastic doll inside a balloon and filled the balloon with water. (It is hard to get the doll into the balloon. You could try using a plastic bag instead.)

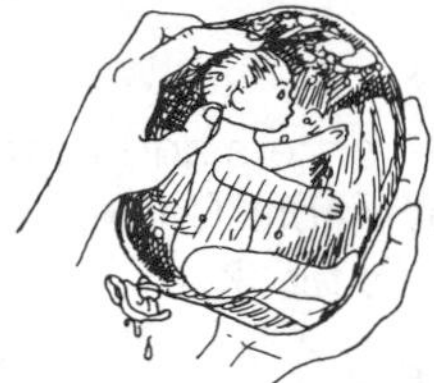

They asked students to pretend it was a baby in a womb. Students then tried to turn the baby to line it up with the opening.

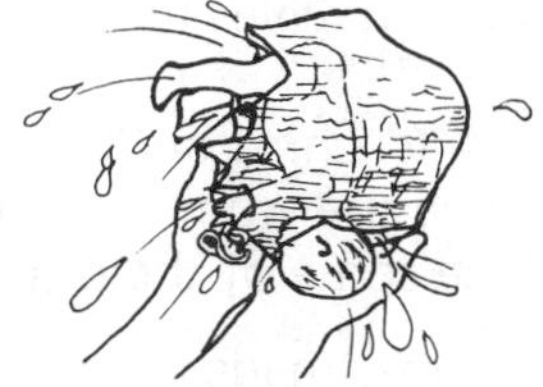

Although they were careful, the balloon popped! So they learned that the womb, like the balloon, can tear easily if not handled with extreme care.

Dangerous bleeding: Health workers and midwives need to be able to tell the difference between normal bleeding after childbirth and dangerous blood loss.

LESS APPROPRIATE

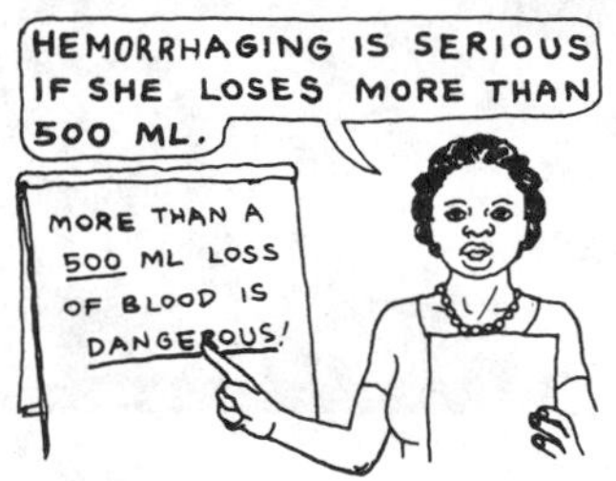

MORE THAN A 500 ML LOSS OF BLOOD IS DANGEROUS!

Instructors often teach that it is normal to lose up to half a liter of blood after giving birth, but that to lose more is dangerous.

It helps if students actually see the quantity of blood.

MORE APPROPRIATE

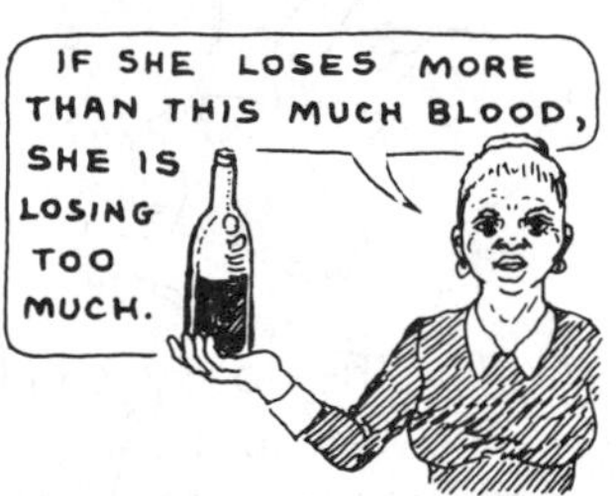

IF SHE LOSES MORE THAN THIS MUCH BLOOD, SHE IS LOSING TOO MUCH.

EVEN MORE APPROPRIATE

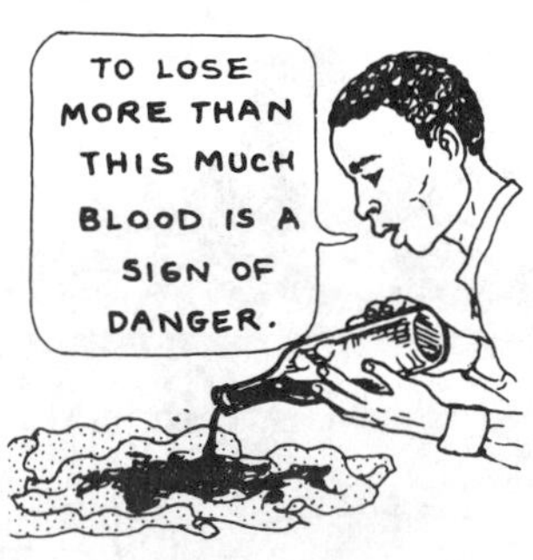

TO LOSE MORE THAN THIS MUCH BLOOD IS A SIGN OF DANGER.

But on a rag or sheets, a little blood can look like a lot. Students can easily misjudge. So first show them the quantity, then spill it over cloths or rags. Use red-colored water. To make it thick like blood, use tomato juice or mix some red gelatin powder into the water. Or use blood from a freshly killed animal. (Add sodium oxalate or juice of wood sorrel to delay clotting.)

MOST APPROPRIATE

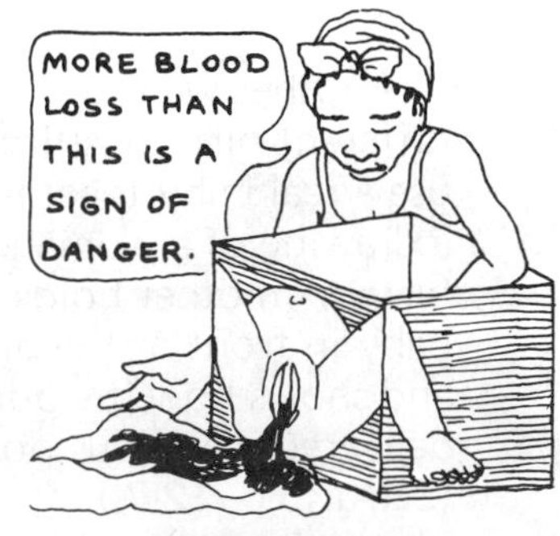

MORE BLOOD LOSS THAN THIS IS A SIGN OF DANGER.

USE OF THEATER TO CORRECT HARMFUL PRACTICES

Many traditional midwives are more skilled at some aspects of childbirth than are many modern doctors. Some, for example, can successfully turn babies that are sideways or butt first (see p. **22**-10).

Unfortunately, however, a few commonly accepted practices by midwives are harmful. For example, in Latin America many midwives now use injections of ***pituitrin*** or ***ergotrate*** to speed up labor and "give the mother strength." This can cause the womb to tear and the mother to quickly bleed to death. Or it can cause the blood vessels in the womb to contract so much that the baby suffers brain damage or dies from lack of oxygen.

This new custom is hard to change. Both midwives and mothers believe it is right and modern to use the injections. Midwives argue that if they do not use them, mothers will go to another midwife who does.

To make people aware of the dangers of misusing these strong injections during childbirth, village health workers in Ajoya staged a short skit before the whole community.

In the first scene, Maria begins to have labor pains. She is about to send for her favorite midwife. But a gossipy neighbor tells her that the midwife is old-fashioned. She convinces Maria to call for a modern midwife who uses injections. The modern midwife attends the birth and injects Maria with ***pituitrin*** to speed things up. The baby is born blue and never breathes.

In the second scene, one year later, Maria is in labor again. But this time she calls her favorite, trusted midwife, Doña Julia. When Maria feels exhausted during the long labor, she begs for an injection "to give me strength." But Julia explains why that would not be safe. She helps Maria to relax. Soon the baby is born healthy and 'pink'. Everyone is glad that Julia did not use the medicine.

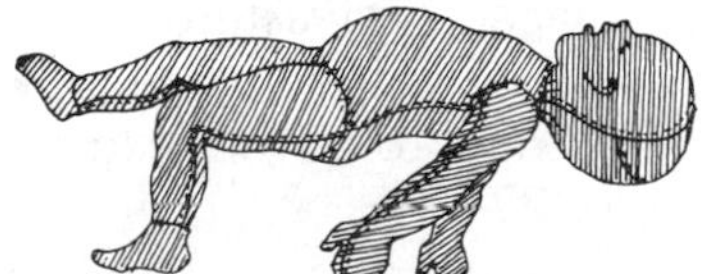

The baby born dead.
(Made of blue cloth.)

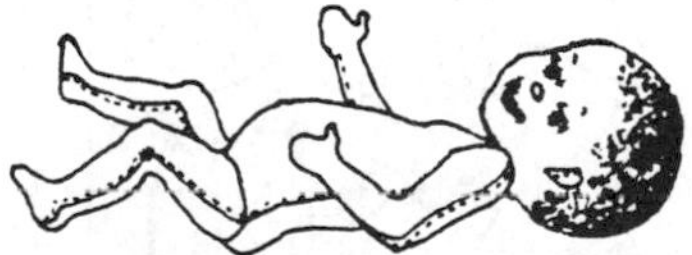

The baby born healthy.
(They used a child's doll.)

At the end of the play, a health worker holds up both dolls and repeats the message:

THERE IS NO SAFE MEDICINE FOR GIVING STRENGTH TO THE MOTHER OR FOR MAKING THE BIRTH QUICKER AND EASIER.

IF YOU WANT TO HAVE STRENGTH DURING CHILDBIRTH, EAT GOOD FOODS DURING PREGNANCY: BEANS, GROUNDNUTS, DARK GREEN LEAFY VEGETABLES, EGGS, AND CHICKEN.

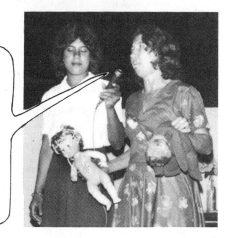

MOTHERS AND YOUNG CHILDREN—'UNDER-FIVES' CLINIC

The first years of life are when a child's health is most delicate and when good nutrition, cleanliness, and other protective measures are critical. For this reason, many health programs conduct special 'under-fives' clinics. But as with any other health activities, unless the approach is adapted to the local situation, problems are likely to occur.

Two common mistakes:

1. Some under-fives programs focus only on baby weighing, health education, and preventive measures such as vaccination. For curative care, mothers must bring their babies back on a different day. This separation of prevention and cure is unfortunate. Most mothers are busy or have to come a long way to the health center. For many, it is difficult to bring their babies one day for weighing and another day for treatment.

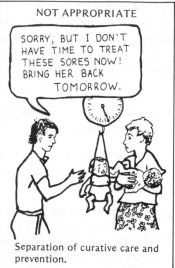

NOT APPROPRIATE
I SEE YOU BROUGHT A BOTTLE FOR MORE COUGH MEDICINE TO GIVE JOHNNY. I'LL FILL IT RIGHT AWAY.

SORRY, BUT I DON'T HAVE TIME TO TREAT THESE SORES NOW! BRING HER BACK TOMORROW.

Separation of curative care and prevention.

2. Other under-fives programs use curative medicine as a 'magnet'. They attract mothers to monthly baby weighings by giving away colorful cough syrups, diarrhea 'plugs', or other unnecessary medicines. To get the free medicines, mothers sometimes tell health workers that their babies have a cough or diarrhea—even when they do not. This use of 'medicine as a magnet' is wasteful, dishonest, and creates dependency. (Giving out free milk is even worse. It leads mothers to bottle feed rather than breast feed. See p. **27**-31.)

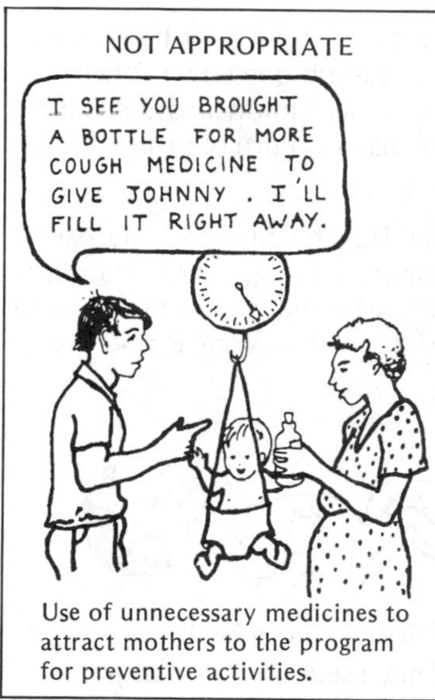

Use of unnecessary medicines to attract mothers to the program for preventive activities.

To avoid these mistakes, help health workers learn to organize under-fives activities in an appropriate way:

- **Deal with preventive, curative, and educational needs at the same place and time.**
- If there are more children than you could attend on one day, divide them into 2 or more groups and have them come on different days.
- **Do not use either medicine or food giveaways to attract mothers.** Instead, make the educational activities so exciting that mothers will not want to miss them.

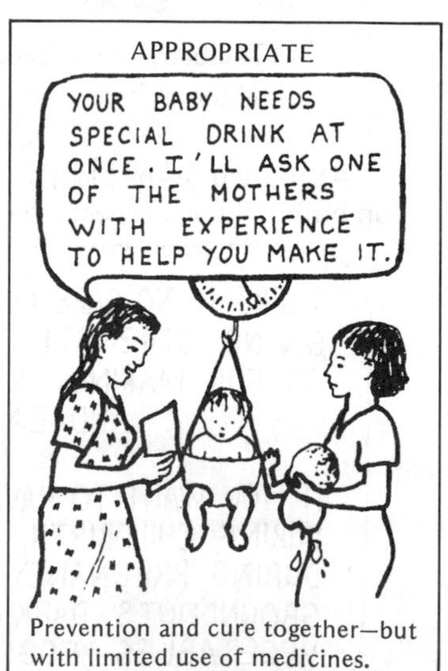

APPROPRIATE
YOUR BABY NEEDS SPECIAL DRINK AT ONCE. I'LL ASK ONE OF THE MOTHERS WITH EXPERIENCE TO HELP YOU MAKE IT.

Prevention and cure together—but with limited use of medicines.

WEIGHING BABIES—WHAT PURPOSE DOES IT SERVE?

The periodic weighing of babies has become a standard feature of many health programs. But the purpose it actually serves differs greatly from program to program. Instructors and health workers would do well to ask themselves questions like the following:

WHOSE PURPOSE DOES OUR BABY-WEIGHING PROGRAM SERVE?
M.O.H.
epidemiologist
etc.

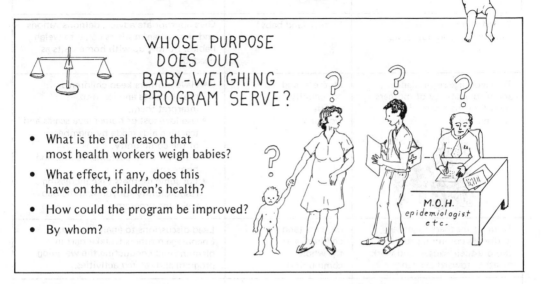

- What is the real reason that most health workers weigh babies?
- What effect, if any, does this have on the children's health?
- How could the program be improved?
- By whom?

At best, baby weighing serves a valuable purpose. It helps health workers and mothers to discover problems in children's growth and correct them before they become too severe. So **baby weighing helps to protect and improve children's health.**

But in many health programs we have visited, there is little evidence that baby weighing has any real effect on children's health. The purposes it serves may be quite different.

- In some programs, baby weighing has become a mysterious ritual. Or it is done only to fulfill a requirement or impress the supervisors. Little use is made of the weights that are so religiously (and often inaccurately) recorded.
- In other programs, the main purpose of baby weighing seems to be to provide statistics for the health authorities. If babies are only weighed once every 3 or 4 months, statistics are generally the only purpose served. To be of much benefit to the mothers and children, weighing needs to be done more often. About once a month is best.
- In some programs, the chief purpose of the baby-weighing ceremony seems to be social. It gives mothers a chance to come together and talk. (This can be a valuable function of a baby-weighing program, but should not be its only purpose.)

Weighing babies can serve many purposes. But its main goal should be to help meet the health needs of the children. On the next page is an outline of appropriate reasons for weighing babies and how health workers can help achieve the goals they set.

ASPECTS OF AN APPROPRIATE BABY-WEIGHING PROGRAM

Purposes	Who is Most Served	How It Is Done
To find which babies are underweight, and to help mothers correct the underlying problem in time.	Baby (and mother)	Weigh each baby every month. Explain the weight and what it means to the mother. Seek out and invite 'high-risk' mothers and babies.
To teach mothers about child health and nutrition.	Mother (and baby)	Give appropriate advice, demonstrations, and skits when mothers come to weigh babies. Follow up with home visits as needed.
To encourage self-reliance and responsibility of mothers and other members of the community.	Mothers (and community health workers)	• Have mothers keep children's health charts and learn to interpret them. • Use low-cost or homemade scales and teaching aids made by members of the community. • Build on local customs, values, and home care. • Let some mothers take increasing responsibility for running the baby-weighing program.
To bring mothers together to discuss common problems, explore their causes, and work together toward change.	Mothers (and children, and the whole community)	Lead discussions to analyze needs. Encourage mothers to take part in planning and conducting the weighing program and related activities.
Information or ***data*** collection, for determining nutritional needs in community and evaluating progress.	Health team (and community, and health authorities)	Carefully record and periodically analyze the weight records of all children in the community (every 6 months or each year).
To provide an occasion for related preventive and curative activities.	Children and mothers	If possible, provide at the same time and place: • vaccinations • early identification and treatment of health problems • prenatal care • opportunity for family planning

As with almost any aspect of health care, **the way health workers learn about baby weighing during their training will affect how they approach it in their communities.** At worst, a baby-weighing program can be a meaningless and humiliating experience for mothers. At best, it can help bring people—especially mothers—together to better understand and solve their common problems. It can help strengthen their capacity for working together toward change.

The teaching methods used for helping health workers learn about weighing babies will serve a double purpose. Health workers can later use these same methods to explain growth charts to mothers in their villages.

The following ideas for learning about baby weighing and the use of growth charts have been developed by village workers in western Mexico. They have proven especially useful in that region, but may need to be adapted for use in other areas.

LEARNING TO USE AND UNDERSTAND GROWTH CHARTS

Health workers who are not used to reading charts and graphs may at first have difficulty recording babies' weights accurately or interpreting what they mean. But with appropriate teaching methods, health workers can quickly learn to understand and use weight charts. They also can learn to teach non-literate mothers to follow the growth of their children on the 'Road to Health'.

Choosing an appropriate chart

Different types of age-weight charts are used by different programs. We prefer David Morley's 'Child Health Chart' because of its simplicity (see page **25**-9 or ***Where There Is No Doctor,*** p. 299). But others prefer more complex charts.

Preferred by mothers and those who work with mothers

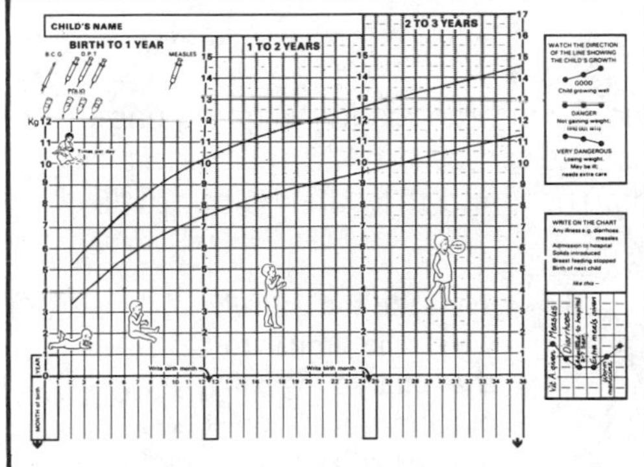

Morley's Child Health Chart has only two curved lines. The lines clearly form a 'road', the 'Road to Health'. Even mothers who cannot read can learn to see whether their children are growing well or falling below the 'Road to Health'.

Preferred by health authorities and data experts

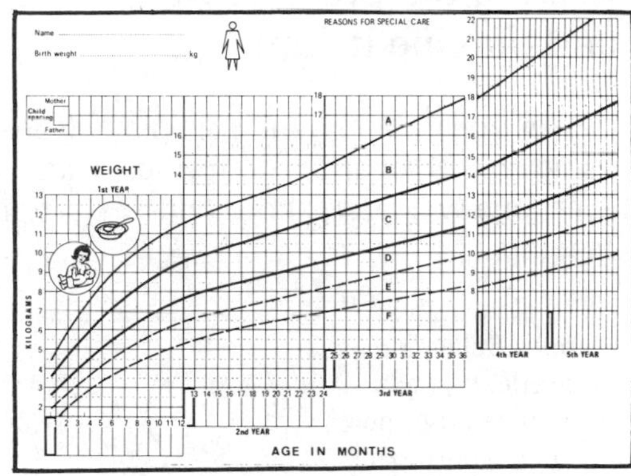

Other charts have additional lines for estimating different degrees of malnutrition. Although perhaps more useful for conducting large surveys, these charts are often confusing to mothers.

Charts for teaching

The basic teaching aid for learning to use a growth chart is the chart itself. **Practice charts** can be mimeographed or silkscreened at relatively low cost. Prepared mimeograph stencils of the 'Road to Health' chart are available from TALC (see p. **Back**-3). TALC also sells low-cost practice charts on inexpensive paper.

A large flannel-board chart is particularly useful for group practice. These can be purchased from TALC—or better still, they can be made by the student health workers or a mothers' group.

If students are not used to drawing, but have experience in sewing, they can make the chart by sewing strings and ribbons onto a flannel cloth. That way they build on skills they already have, rather than struggling with an activity that is foreign to them. (This idea was discussed on page **11**-4.)

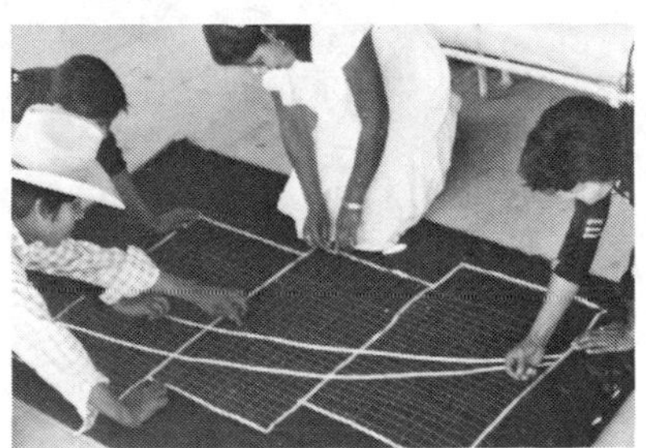

Sewing a 'Road to Health' chart. (Ajoya, Mexico)

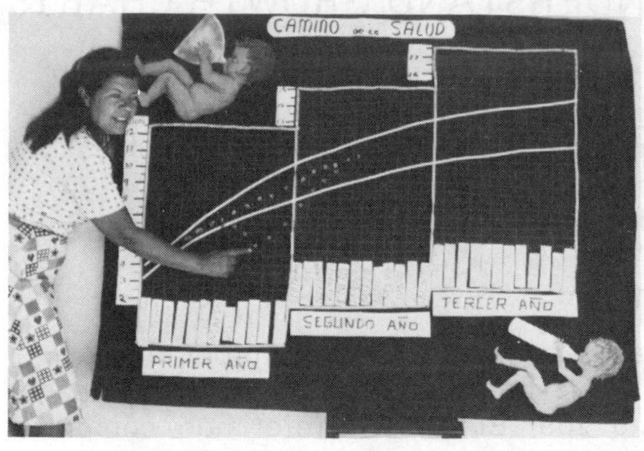

On the large flannel-board Road to Health chart, students can take turns placing small flannel spots representing the ages and weights of children. Use different colored spots to show the growth patterns of different children.

The flannel-board chart in this photo compares the growth patterns of a breast-fed baby and a bottle-fed baby. (See *WTND,* p. 304.)

Making the practice weighing and use of charts seem real—and making it fun!

If model 'babies' and role playing are used, then practice in weighing babies, using growth charts, and giving advice to parents can be fun. At the same time, everyone will learn about child nutrition, diarrhea, and the dangers of bottle feeding.

Make a 'baby' out of clay, a plastic bottle, or a gourd. You can use the same 'gourd baby' used for teaching mothers and children about dehydration (see page **24**-18).

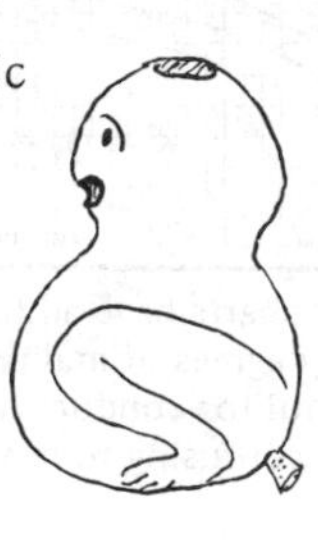

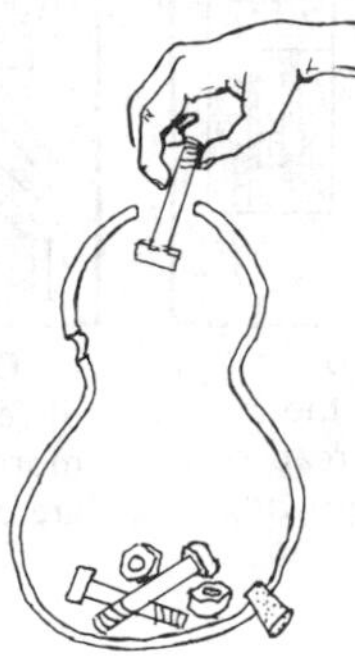

To make the gourd's weight be similar to that of a young baby, put some heavy objects in it. The 'baby' can actually be made to gain weight each 'month'. Simply add increasing amounts of water between weighings.

To make practice more realistic and fun, make a life-size model of a breast-feeding 'mother'. You can use a cardboard carton and a plastic bottle filled with water.

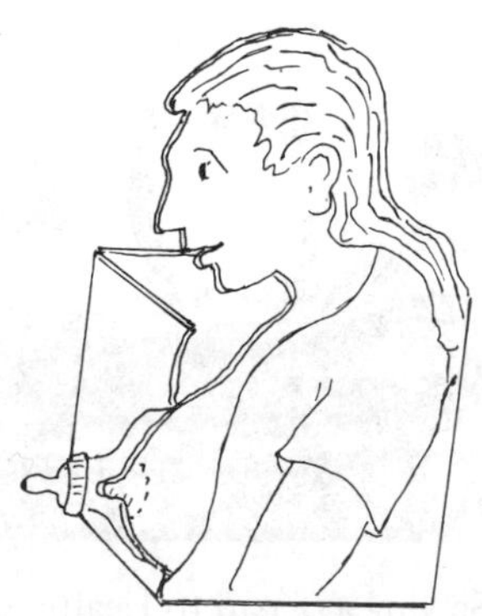

Attach a baby-bottle nipple so that the 'mother' can actually breast feed the gourd baby.

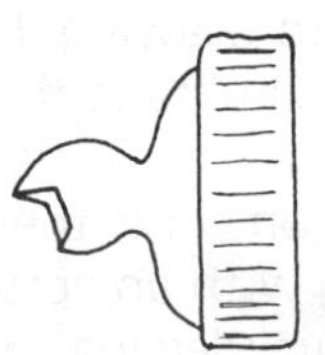

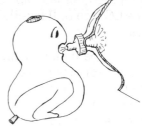

In order to let the 'milk' run quickly into the gourd baby, cut a large hole in the rubber nipple.

Using these teaching aids, the students (or mothers) practice the monthly weighing of the 'baby'. Between weighings, the 'mother' breast feeds the gourd baby so that it gains weight each time.

It helps to hang a calendar on the wall and change it to the next month before each weighing. This helps everyone understand that the skit represents a period of several months.

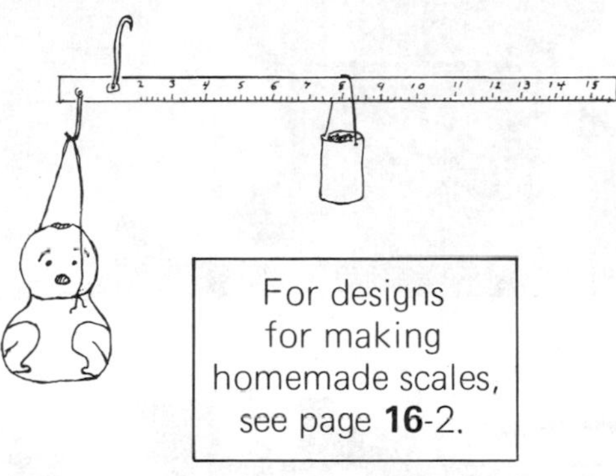

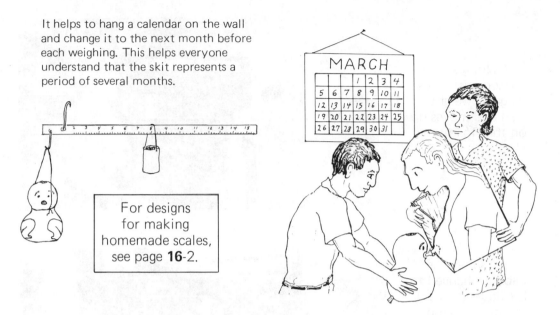

For designs for making homemade scales, see page **16**-2.

Each 'month', as the baby is weighed, the health workers or mothers take turns recording the baby's age and weight on the flannel-board Road to Health chart.

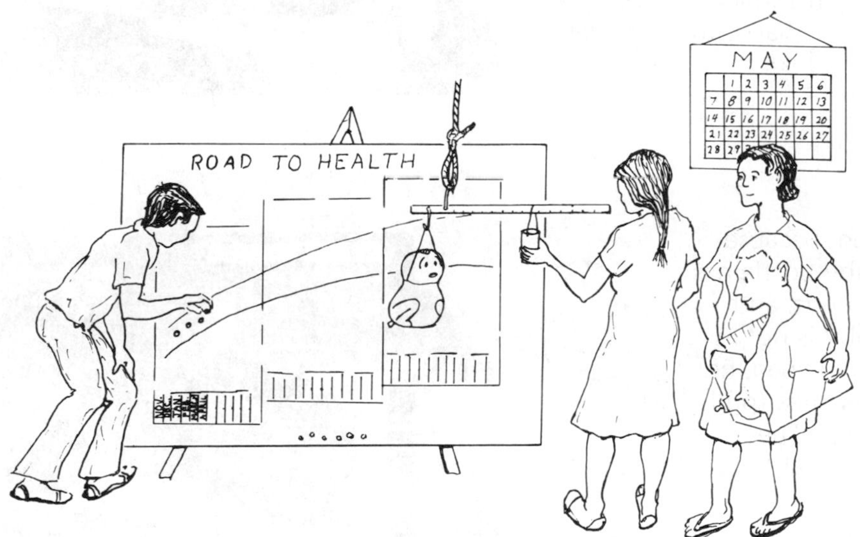

In this way, everyone sees how the baby's weight goes up each month, and how the baby advances along the Road to Health.

The group can also act out various nutritional or health problems that could affect the baby's weight, and show how these appear on the chart.

For example, have the group act out what can happen when a baby is changed from breast to bottle feeding.

As long as the baby breast feeds, he gains weight well and moves up on the Road to Health.

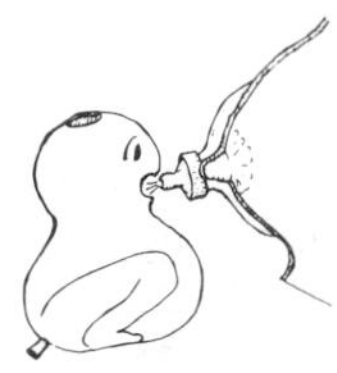

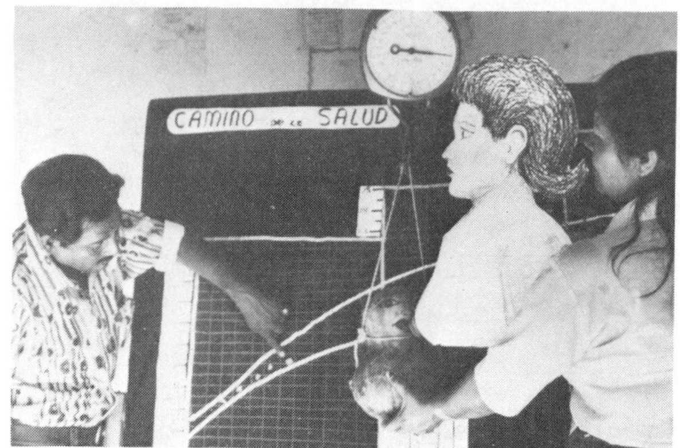

But when the baby is changed to bottle feeding at 6 months, he stops gaining weight. (Plug the nipple of the bottle so that liquid comes out very slowly.) The dots showing his weight on the Road to Health chart stay at the same level.

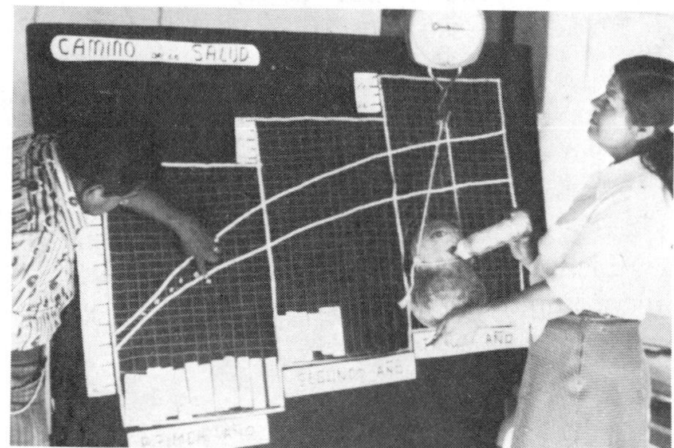

Then, because the baby bottle has germs on it, and the baby is not as well nourished, he gets diarrhea (pull the plug). The baby's weight goes down.

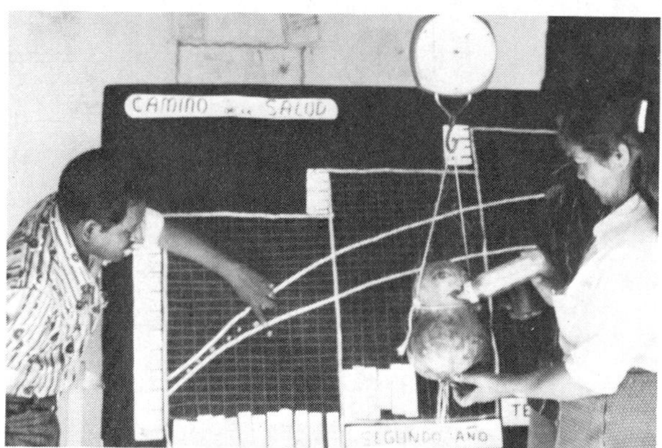

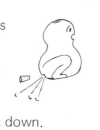

Note: The use of the gourd baby and cardboard mother is only one idea for teaching the use of weight charts. It was developed by village instructors and students during a training program, and that was part of what made it a success. We hope you and your students will think of new and even better teaching ideas.

Follow-up discussions and further learning

Flannel-board Road to Health charts can be used to start many lively discussions, and to help health workers or mothers learn to interpret the charts correctly. Here are two examples:

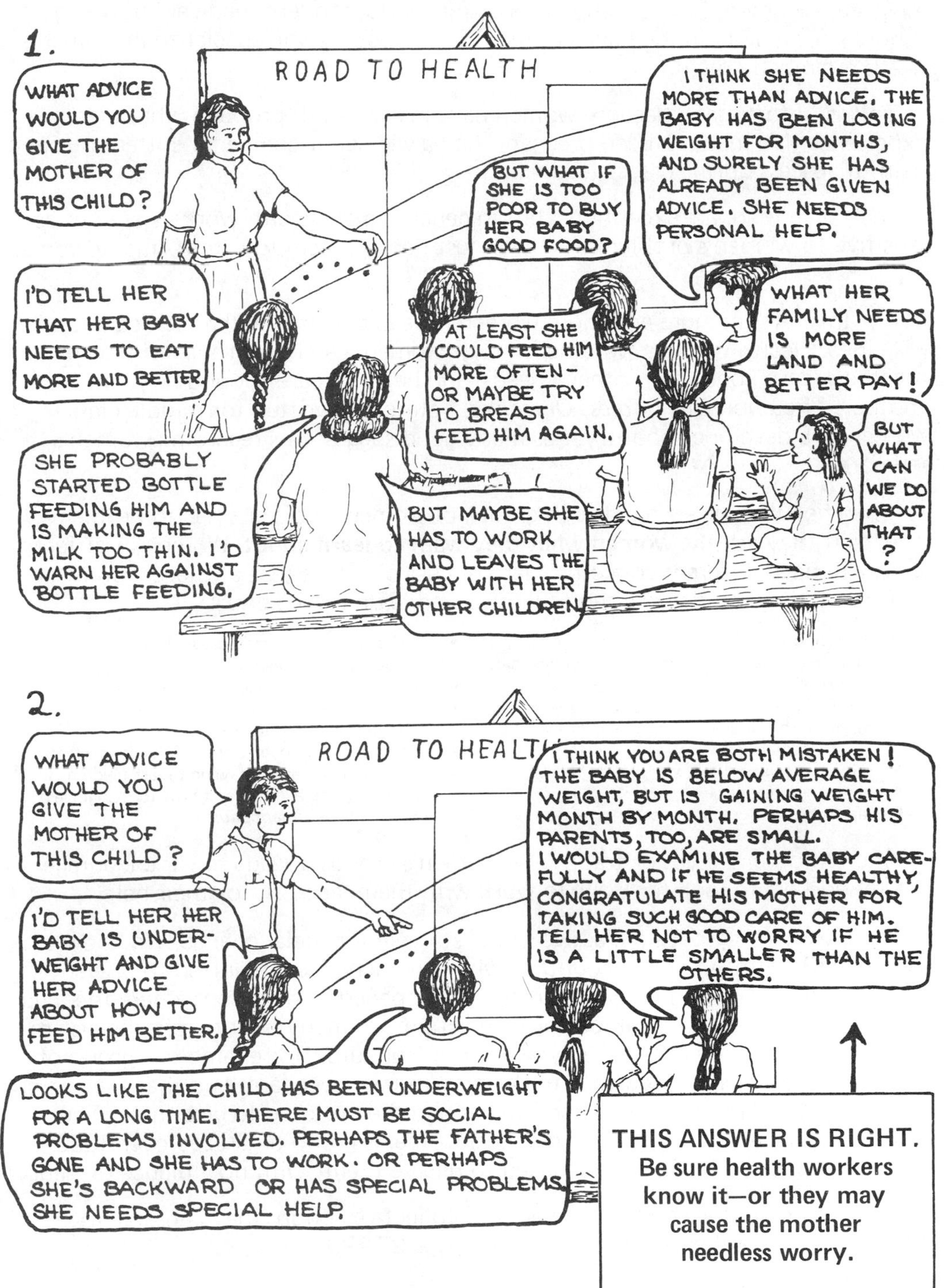

WOMEN'S HEALTH—AND STRENGTHS

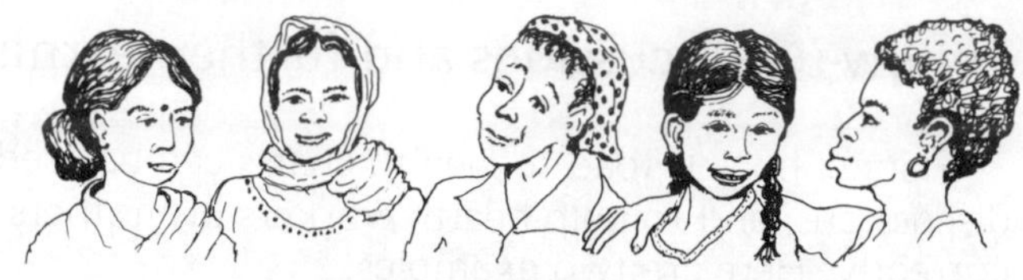

Traditionally, childbirth and women's health problems have been attended to mostly by women. But in many parts of the world, modern medical knowledge is now kept mainly in the hands of men. Even doctors who specialize in women's needs are mostly men!

This is unfortunate, because women have many health problems that men never experience. No man has been pregnant, had a vaginal discharge, or suffered from a painful abscess during breast feeding.

Of course there are exceptions, but in general, male health workers are not as sensitive to women's problems. "A man just doesn't seem to listen," many women say.

For this reason, more and more women have begun to feel that self-care is a wise idea. Health workers, whether men or women, can help groups of women get together, learn about each other's needs, and begin to care for and help one another. The book ***Our Bodies, Ourselves,**** although written for middle class women in a developed country, has many good suggestions regarding women's self-care.

When health workers meet with groups of women to discuss health problems, it helps if they **ask the women what they want to learn about.** Women in different areas will have different concerns. Here is a list of topics that a village women's group in Latin America wanted to discuss and learn more about:

- 'bad blood' (venereal disease) and infertility
- 'burning urine' and other urinary and vaginal problems
- a girl's first bleeding and related problems
- failure to bleed every month, and other menstrual problems
- miscarriage and abortion
- pain when having sex
- rape, abuses by men, and self-protection
- how to avoid unwanted pregnancy
- diet during pregnancy and following childbirth
- causes of 'eclipsed' babies (birth defects)
- specific problems and 'modern practices' related to childbirth
- care of newborn babies and young children
- breast pain and abscess when breast feeding
- cancer, how to avoid it and how to recognize it
- 'change of life' ***(menopause)***

Where mother's clubs or traditional women's groups already exist, encourage health workers to look for ways to work with them, and ask for their help.

Some women's groups are active in the struggle for social change. We know of villages in 3 Latin American countries where women have organized to prevent abuses by local authorities. Sometimes this happened in situations where the men were too frightened to speak out or take action. (In many countries, officials are less likely to use violence against women.) In Honduras, for example, a group of teen-age boys was jailed recently for helping to take over farmland that the government had promised to poor families and then refused to give them. The boys' fathers were afraid to act, so a local women's group organized over 4000 women, stormed the jail, and managed to release them—with no violence or injury!

When women awaken to their power of collective action, they can do a lot! (See the women's theater presentation on page **27**-19.)

---

*Written by the Boston Women's Health Book Collective, Box 192, Somerville, MA 02144, USA.

CHAPTER 23

The Politics of Family Planning

Voluntary family planning is an important health measure. Availability of fair and trustworthy services makes a big difference to the health of women, families, communities, and nations.

It is relatively easy to instruct health workers on how to use or explain family planning methods. (See Chapter 20 of ***Where There Is No Doctor.)*** But it is far more difficult to help them gain an understanding of the many complex attitudes about birth control. No other area in health care has become more confused and abused by conflicting political interests. On all sides, the real needs and wishes of the people—especially of women—are often ignored or forgotten.

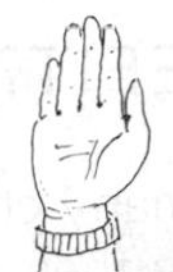

Many who represent the economically powerful see the 'population explosion' (rapidly growing number of people) as the main cause of poverty and hunger in the world. They say the answer lies in making sure that the poor have smaller families. By blaming the poor for having too many children (rather than the rich for having more than their share of land, food, and resources), these persons avoid facing the need for social change. They focus on the 'population problem' to avoid looking closely at the 'distribution problem'.

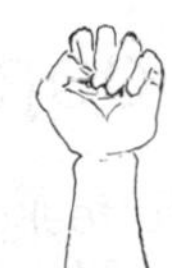

Many social leaders say birth control is a weapon used by the powerful to control and regulate the poor. They insist that large families are a response to poverty, not the cause of it. There is some truth in what they say. But unfortunately, social leaders sometimes make it appear that all family planning works against the interests of the poor. This is not true. 'Child spacing' can be very important to family health—when it is the parents' informed decision. It can also help women gain greater freedom and equality.

Dishonesty occurs on both sides. **Those who promote population control often do not inform people adequately about the risks.** For example, *Depo-Provera* has been promoted as an injectable contraceptive in poor countries, by persons from rich countries where its use to prevent pregnancy is prohibited. On the other hand, **those who oppose population control often exaggerate the risks.** Even those who object to certain family planning methods for religious reasons sometimes find it easier to influence people with the fear of cancer than with the fear of God.

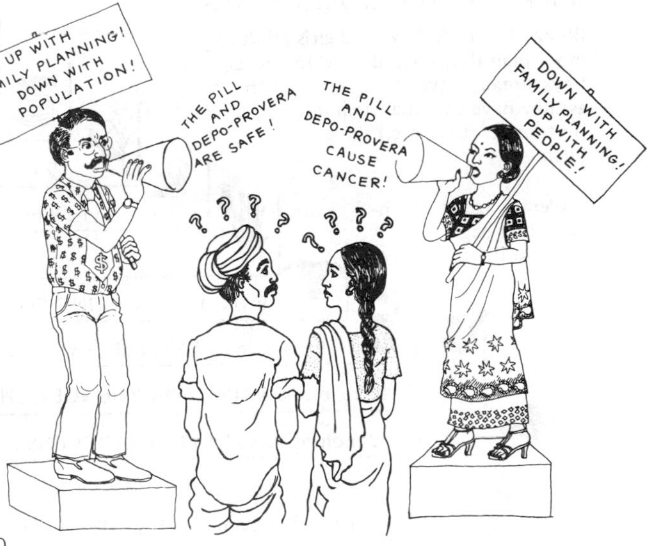
UP WITH FAMILY PLANNING! DOWN WITH POPULATION!
THE PILL AND DEPO-PROVERA ARE SAFE!
THE PILL AND DEPO-PROVERA CAUSE CANCER!
DOWN WITH FAMILY PLANNING! UP WITH PEOPLE!

In the political battle over birth control, the wishes of the poor are often forgotten.

To add to the confusion, women's rights groups in rich countries sometimes protest that birth control pills are too dangerous to use. Yet in poor countries, the risks related to childbirth itself are often so high that 'the pill' may be one of the cheapest, surest ways to help save women's lives. The fear that well-intending groups spread about 'the pill', and about birth control in general, may actually result in more deaths—of both mothers and babies!

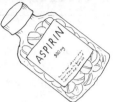

In considering family planning methods, health workers must help people remember that all medicines have some risks. **For each person, the risks need to be weighed against the benefits.** Even aspirin, which is considered harmless enough to sell without prescription, causes ulcers and even fatal bleeding in some persons. In fact, aspirin probably causes more deaths than 'the pill'. Yet nobody protests the huge sales promotion of aspirin, because it is not a political, religious, or women's rights issue.

Aspirin probably harms more people than birth control pills. But no one protests, because it is not a political issue.

CHILDREN OF THE POOR—A BURDEN OR A BENEFIT?

The poor are often made to feel guilty or irresponsible for having many children. Posters and radios tell people, *The small family lives better,* and advise them to *Have only the number of children you can afford.*

Yet **for many poor families, to have many children is an economic necessity.** For rural families, especially, children are a valuable source of low-cost labor. This study from Java (adapted from *Population and Development Review,* September, 1977) shows how much children can do.

WHY THE POOR NEED CHILDREN

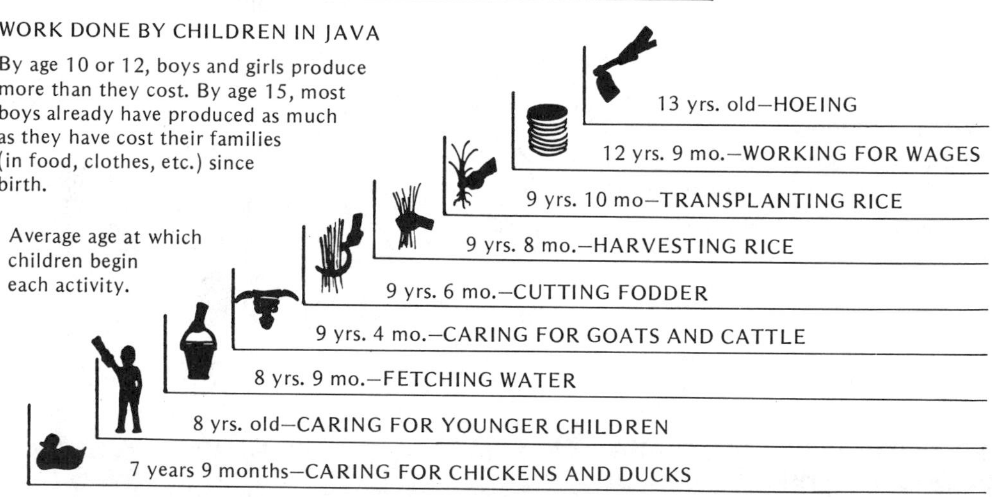
WORK DONE BY CHILDREN IN JAVA
By age 10 or 12, boys and girls produce more than they cost. By age 15, most boys already have produced as much as they have cost their families (in food, clothes, etc.) since birth.
Average age at which children begin each activity.
13 yrs. old—HOEING
12 yrs. 9 mo.—WORKING FOR WAGES
9 yrs. 10 mo—TRANSPLANTING RICE
9 yrs. 8 mo.—HARVESTING RICE
9 yrs. 6 mo.—CUTTING FODDER
9 yrs. 4 mo.—CARING FOR GOATS AND CATTLE
8 yrs. 9 mo.—FETCHING WATER
8 yrs. old—CARING FOR YOUNGER CHILDREN
7 years 9 months—CARING FOR CHICKENS AND DUCKS

Even in some cities, by working, begging, and stealing in the streets, children sometimes earn more than their parents, who are underpaid and often unemployed. Especially as parents grow old, become ill, and can no longer work hard themselves, having many children may be their best guarantee for getting enough to eat.

In many cases, having a small family is a privilege that only persons with a certain amount of economic security can afford. In wealthy countries, most men and women choose to have few children. By contrast, in those poor countries where poor people have few guarantees, family size usually remains large—in spite of millions spent on family planning. But studies have shown that **in poor countries where resources have been more fairly distributed, and where employment, housing, and care for the sick and old are guaranteed, people usually choose to have smaller families.*** Also, where women have equal access to educational opportunities and jobs, they see their future as more than just producing babies. In Cuba, for example, the birth rate has decreased remarkably, even though the Cuban government does not emphasize family planning.**

Most people will choose to have small families only when they have a basic amount of economic security.

SELLING FAMILY PLANNING TO THE POOR

Governments and foreign agencies have tried many tricks to get the poor to have fewer children. These have included the use of 'incentives' (gifts of food or money) to family planning 'accepters'. **But the use of incentives invites abuse.** In some countries, women sign up for 'pills' at several different centers in order to collect more gifts. A report from Bangladesh claims that so many birth control pills have been thrown into a stream that the fish population has dropped!

In some countries, a negative incentive or punishment is used. Tax credits or free schooling may be refused to families that have more than 3 or 4 children. In other countries, commercial marketing techniques are used, including songs on the radio and the distribution of bright-colored condoms.

Some tricks used to promote family planning are insulting or offensive. But others are very clever or amusing, and help take the mystery and embarrassment out of family planning.

Many couples who want to avoid pregnancy are too shy to ask a health worker or druggist for contraceptives. To remove this embarrassment, health planners in Thailand have tried to 'put a smile into family planning'. Large signs in stores advertise ***CABBAGES AND CONDOMS.*** Police are given free contraceptives in a campaign known as ***COPS AND RUBBERS.*** Contests are held in which boys blow up condoms like balloons. (He who blows the biggest wins a free pack for his father!)

As a result of these efforts, Thailand reports the biggest drop in birth rate in Asia (except for China). But each country needs to evaluate how these methods relate to people's traditions and dignity.

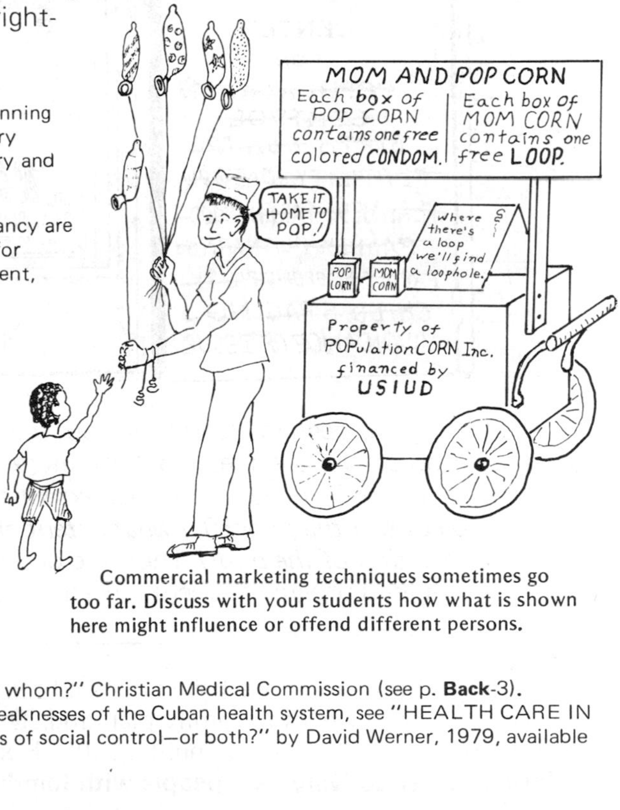

Commercial marketing techniques sometimes go too far. Discuss with your students how what is shown here might influence or offend different persons.

*See ***Contact*** 30, "Family planning to benefit whom?" Christian Medical Commission (see p. **Back**-3).

**For more discussion of the strengths and weaknesses of the Cuban health system, see "HEALTH CARE IN CUBA TODAY: A model service or a means of social control—or both?" by David Werner, 1979, available from the Hesperian Foundation.

The quota system—and the problems it creates

To meet their goals for 'number of couples controlled' by a family planning campaign, many health ministries have introduced a ***quota system.*** Every month, each medical officer or health worker is required to recruit a certain number of new birth control 'accepters'.

Such quotas frequently lead to abuses. People are seen as numbers. Couples are often pressured into planning their families against their will. In Latin America, mothers have been refused medical care for their sick babies until they agree to use contraceptives. In Asia, young women and teenage boys have been sterilized by force so that authorities could meet their quotas!

Trying to force, bribe, or shame people into 'planning' breeds anger and distrust. Many women who do not want another child end up getting pregnant because they do not trust family planning programs. In Mexico, Project Piaxtla had a voluntary birth control program long before the government approved family planning. Many couples were interested and became involved. But since the government started its family planning campaign, the number of couples planning their families in the Piaxtla area has dropped to less than half. People have grown distrustful.

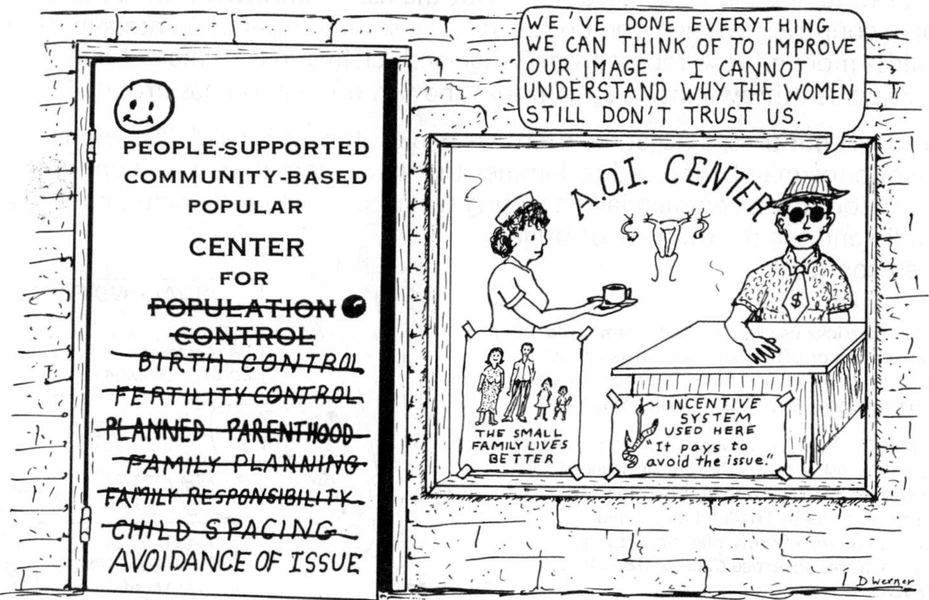
WE'VE DONE EVERYTHING WE CAN THINK OF TO IMPROVE OUR IMAGE. I CANNOT UNDERSTAND WHY THE WOMEN STILL DON'T TRUST US.
PEOPLE-SUPPORTED COMMUNITY-BASED POPULAR CENTER FOR
~~POPULATION CONTROL~~
~~BIRTH CONTROL~~
~~FERTILITY CONTROL~~
~~PLANNED PARENTHOOD~~
~~FAMILY PLANNING~~
~~FAMILY RESPONSIBILITY~~
~~CHILD SPACING~~
AVOIDANCE OF ISSUE
A.O.I. CENTER
THE SMALL FAMILY LIVES BETTER
INCENTIVE SYSTEM USED HERE
"It pays to avoid the issue."
D Werner

An attempt has been made to 'clean up' the image of population programs, to make their objectives seem less political, more personal, and more health oriented. But the big questions remain: ***To what extent are family planning efforts an attempt to control the poor? To what extent are they an attempt to strengthen the social position of the poor?*** These are questions that health workers in community-based programs urgently need to consider and discuss.

So far in this chapter, we have discussed the abuses and problems connected with certain approaches to family planning. The distrust that has resulted can only be overcome by uncovering the truth. **Health workers need to be well informed to effectively help people with family planning.**

FAMILY PLANNING ON THE PEOPLE'S TERMS

It is important that health workers recognize and discuss the various ways that birth control—as a tool of a well-informed people—can help meet the needs of the poor and strengthen their social position. The facts are these:

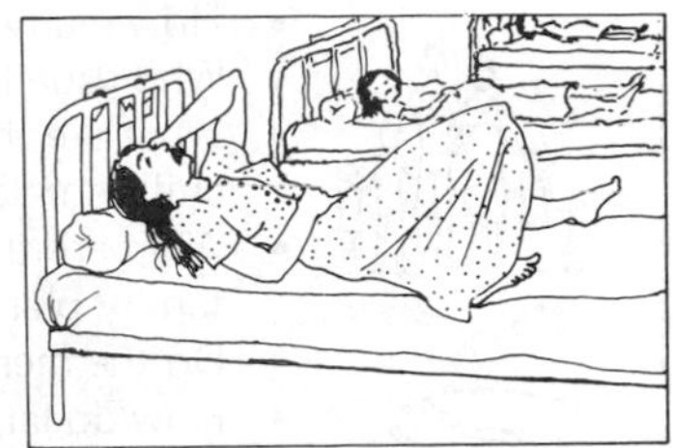

- Many women desperately want to avoid another pregnancy. The large number of illegal abortions in most countries is proof of this. In Bogota, Colombia, for example, over half the women in public maternity hospitals are there because of complications from illegal abortions. Many of these women die. To prevent these deaths, abortion must be legalized. But most important, family planning services must be such that people trust and use them.
- For many women, the constant cycle of pregnancy, birth, and infant care drains their energy and health. Child spacing can not only help protect the health of mothers and children, it can free women to do other things: to work, study, organize, and eventually gain greater equality with men.
- Although many poor families feel they want and need as many as 4, 5, or 6 children, most also agree that a very large number of children can create hardships. They want a family that is neither too small nor too large, and welcome family planning on their terms.
- Today, with modern medicine and health services, fewer children die, families are larger, and populations grow rapidly. In some countries the population doubles every 20 years. Although population growth is not the main cause of poverty and hunger, in some areas it is a contributing factor. As numbers of people increase, available land will become scarcer and more costly. Even in some parts of Africa that seem 'underpopulated', the growing number of people means too many trees are being cut for firewood. As a result, forests and farmland are being turned into deserts. Too many people destroys the balance between man and nature.

The population problem is not usually discussed with the poor because planners generally say that the poor think only of their immediate needs and are not concerned with the future needs of society. But isn't this because there is so little opportunity for the poor to take part in the decisions that shape the social order? History has shown, however, that when the poor begin to organize and gain control, they often become deeply concerned with planning ahead for a healthier society. Thus, if the poor are to cooperate with goals to limit population growth, they must also have a strong role in policy and decision making for the future.

Group discussion about population control and family planning

The challenge to both instructors and health workers is this: ***How can we help people to understand the issues surrounding birth control and to plan their families effectively ON THEIR OWN TERMS?***

It is essential that health workers try to understand the ideas and feelings of those who are most affected. Perhaps they can lead discussions with women or couples about their concerns and experiences related to family planning.

On the next page is a list of questions to help start a discussion. But they are only suggestions. Think of your own questions to fit the situation in your area.

KEY QUESTIONS FOR DISCUSSION ABOUT FAMILY PLANNING

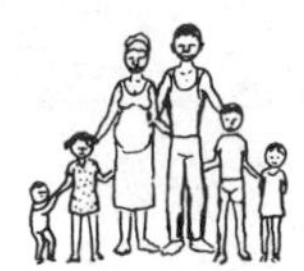

- How many children does the average couple have in our community?
- Who usually have more children—rich families or poor ones? Why?
- What are the advantages of having many children? Of having few children? If you are rich? If you are poor?
- What are the attitudes of most of the people in our community toward family planning? Why?

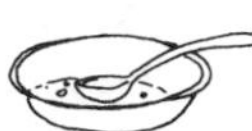

- Do the men often have different attitudes than the women? Why?
- How do large families affect the population (number of people)?
- Is the number of people in our village or community growing? Is there enough land (or work or food) for everybody? Are things getting better or worse? Why?

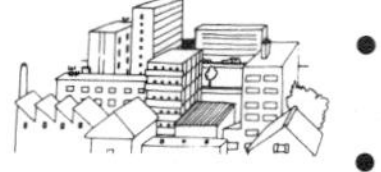

- Do some persons or families leave the village to move to the city or another country? Why? What sort of life do they lead there?
- Do you think that the growing number of people is partly responsible for the hunger or hardship of the poor? What else do you think is responsible?

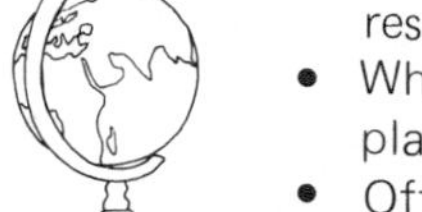

- What does the government do about these other causes? About family planning? Why? Where does the money for this come from?
- Official announcements tell people they should plan their families in order to protect the health of mothers and children. What other reasons do you think the officials might have?

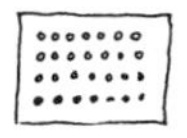

- What doubts or fears do you (or mothers, or people in general) have about different family planning methods? Why? Where can you get truthful information?

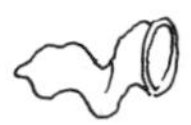

- In what ways do family planning programs meet people's needs? In what ways do they abuse people? What have you yourself experienced?
- Do you think family planning workers should be required to sign up a certain number of new users each month? Why? How would this requirement affect the way health workers relate to people?

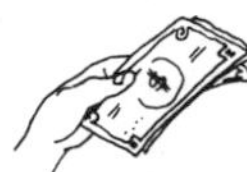

- Should parents be rewarded (given 'incentives') for planning their families? Why or why not? How does the incentive system affect people's attitudes about family planning? About the government? About themselves?

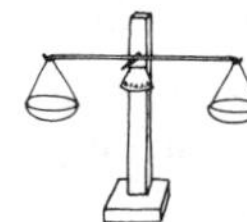

- In many countries, illegal abortion is the most common form of 'family planning'. Why? What are the results?
- Is it better to abort or to bring an unwanted child into the world?
- Is it just and fair for men to make the laws about abortion and other issues concerning women's health and lives?
- Is family planning important? For whom and in what way?

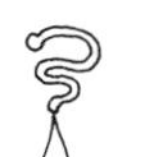

- Should a health worker encourage parents to plan their families? All parents? Only some parents? Which? Should a health worker bring up the subject of family planning when mothers come for medical care or bring their children? Should she discuss it with them only when they express interest? Or should this depend on the problems and needs of the individual family?

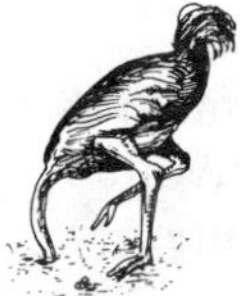

- Whose needs does family planning presently meet in your area?
- How could it better meet the needs of the poor?
- What can we do about it? What will happen to us if we speak out or take action? Is it worth it?

ADAPTING FAMILY PLANNING TO LOCAL CIRCUMSTANCES

Which family planning methods are appropriate in your area, and which are not? This will depend on local circumstances, beliefs, and customs, including . . .

RELIGION: In some areas, religion influences people's attitudes about family planning, and may dictate which methods (if any) are acceptable. It is important that health workers respect people's religious beliefs. At the same time, it is important for them to realize that some religious leaders and the beliefs they teach help to ***perpetuate**** a social order that keeps a few privileged people on top and the poor on the bottom.

Within the same religion, some leaders may be rigid and resistant to change, while others may be more open and flexible. Some may believe in doing things just the way they have always been done. Others consider the people's present needs, and interpret the scriptures so as to best serve their modern reality.

Among Catholic leaders, for example, there has been a great deal of argument about family planning. Some say that artificial contraception is a sin, and only approve of 'natural ways', such as the rhythm and mucus (Billings) methods. Others argue that if family planning can help protect health or improve the quality of life for a family, then the method most likely to give the desired results should be used. The choice, they feel, should be left to the conscience of each family. They point out that the high failure (pregnancy) rate with the rhythm and mucus methods makes the teaching of only these methods unrealistic and—in some cases—harmful.**

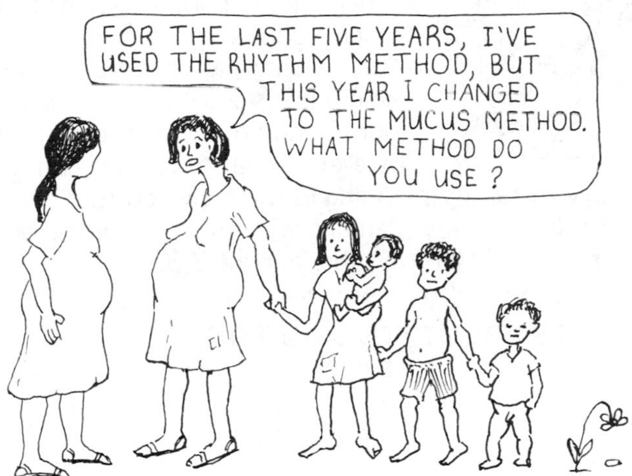

FOR THE LAST FIVE YEARS, I'VE USED THE RHYTHM METHOD, BUT THIS YEAR I CHANGED TO THE MUCUS METHOD. WHAT METHOD DO YOU USE ?

Some religious leaders defend family planning on the grounds that it helps prevent unwanted pregnancies and lowers the high rate of intentional abortions. In fact, a study in one city (Boston) showed that the rate of intentional abortion is highest among women whose religions forbid artificial birth control—even though those religions also forbid abortion!

In places where religion strongly influences attitudes toward family planning, these matters can be discussed among health workers and community people. But the health workers will need skill in leading such discussions and in raising delicate questions without causing great offense. Holding practice discussions during training may help prepare them. It also may help to invite a religious leader or someone from a birth control program to take part in, or lead, the discussion. If possible, this should be a person who respects and defends the rights of the poor and who works toward social change.

Perpetuate: To make something last or continue.

**Reports of high success rates with rhythm and mucus methods are based on idealized studies using only those women who 'do it right' and whose husbands cooperate. In poor communities where they have been tried, these methods have often led to unwanted pregnancies.

LOCAL CUSTOMS: In many parts of the world, villagers use 'home remedies' to prevent or interrupt pregnancy. Some of these work fairly well and are relatively safe (see the Sponge Method on page 294 of ***WTND***). Others do not work well, or are dangerous. (In Mexico, some women have tried to prevent pregnancy by inserting bones or pieces of dead cats into their vaginas!) The existence of these methods is a sign of women's desire for birth control.

Newer methods have also appeared in some areas. Women have occasionally tried taking several birth control pills or injections at once, in order to 'bring on their menstrual period' and interrupt an unwanted pregnancy. Sometimes this has cost women's lives or caused birth defects. During health worker training, discuss local methods of birth control with students, local midwives, and healers. It is important that where such methods are still used, health workers be familiar with them and be able to give sensible advice.

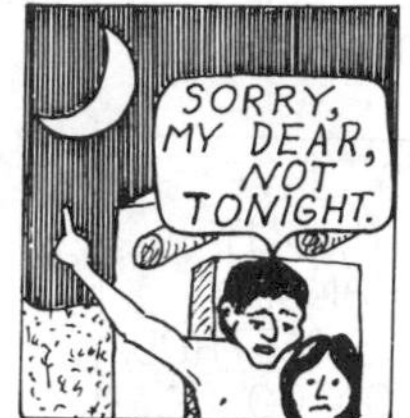
SORRY, MY DEAR, NOT TONIGHT.

Sometimes local customs serve as a form of birth control, although many people may not realize it. In parts of Africa women traditionally did not sleep with their husbands while breast feeding—often for 2 years or longer. In Mexico, Indian men did not sleep with their wives during certain phases of the moon. Today many of these old traditions are breaking down. However, if health workers can help people understand the history of family planning in their own culture, this will help them look at modern methods of family planning with more insight. (See the discussion on family planning traditions in Liberia, page **7**-3.)

BELIEFS ABOUT FOOD AND DIET: In some areas, there are food customs or beliefs that affect the way people use—or misuse—modern contraceptives.

For example, in parts of Latin America, people believe that they should not take any medicine on days when they eat pork. So a woman may stop taking birth control pills for a few days whenever a pig is killed and she eats the meat.

In such places, the health worker can help to prevent unwanted pregnancies by giving careful advice. Each time she explains the use of birth control pills to a woman, she can say, "You need to take one pill each day, even when you eat pork. It does you no harm to take it on days you eat pork. And if you stop taking it, you may become pregnant."

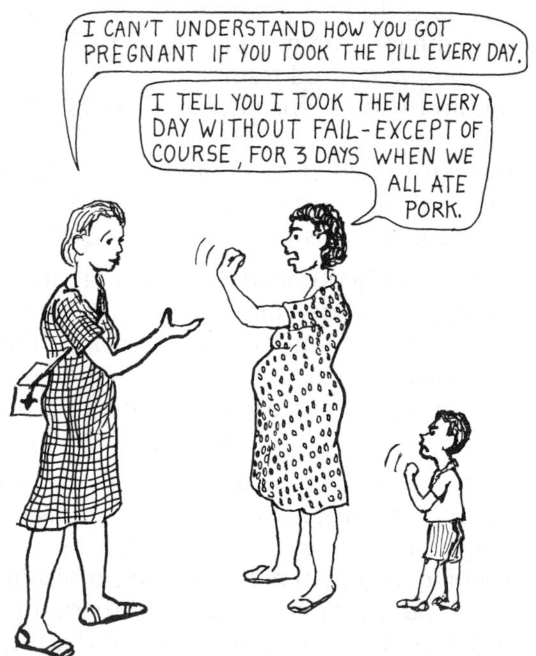
I CAN'T UNDERSTAND HOW YOU GOT PREGNANT IF YOU TOOK THE PILL EVERY DAY.
I TELL YOU I TOOK THEM EVERY DAY WITHOUT FAIL-EXCEPT OF COURSE, FOR 3 DAYS WHEN WE ALL ATE PORK.

In other places, people may have different customs or beliefs that create problems or misunderstandings. Health workers need to take these into account when discussing family planning with people in their communities.

MEN WHO DO NOT LET THEIR WIVES USE CONTRACEPTIVES: In countries where society encourages equality for women, family planning is usually well accepted. But conflicts often arise where male domination is strong. Health workers may ask, "What do I do when a woman wants or needs to avoid another pregnancy, but her husband will not agree to let her use contraceptives?"

From our own experience in Latin America, where this problem is common, we have found that husbands are usually more considerate if an effort is made to discuss the issues with them from the first. When possible, **include men as well as women in discussions about family planning.**

Family planning is far more likely to be successful when both parents make the decision together and share the responsibility.

There are many ways that a man can share the responsibility for family planning. He can remind his wife to take the pill each day, or check to make sure that she has put in her diaphragm. Or he can take even greater responsibility by buying and using condoms—or choosing to have a *vasectomy* (male sterilization).

Nevertheless, sometimes a man may refuse to let his wife take steps to avoid pregnancy. The woman may come to the health worker asking that her use of contraceptives be kept secret from her husband. In some parts of the world, this problem provides one of the strongest arguments for injectable contraceptives like *Depo-Provera*—in spite of uncertainty about their safety. Many women insist that the injection, given once every 3 months, is the form of birth control that is easiest to keep secret from their husbands. They consider the risks of the injections to be small compared to the danger to them if their husbands find out.

These situations must be handled with sensitivity. How health workers deal with them will depend on local factors and, in each case, the individual couple's relationship.

There are no easy answers. But it is easy to make mistakes. For example, a health worker might try to talk a husband into cooperating, but by revealing the wife's intention to use birth control, cause her to be severely beaten. We have seen this happen.

Exploring some of the possibilities through group discussion and role playing will help prepare health workers for these difficult situations—some of which are sure to arise.

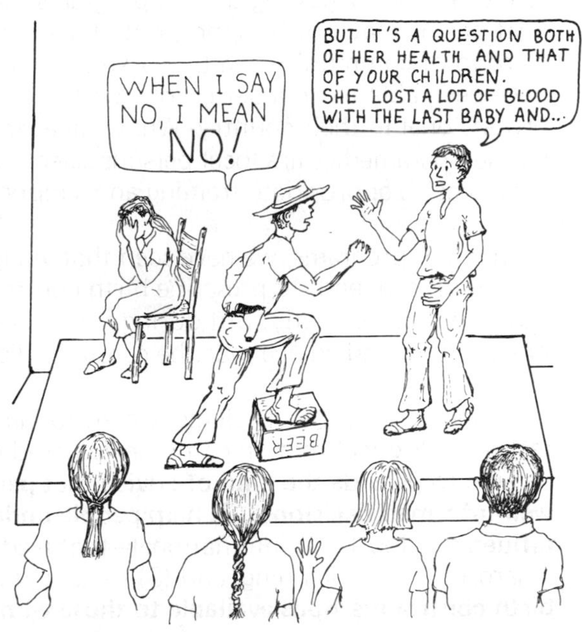
WHEN I SAY NO, I MEAN NO!
BUT IT'S A QUESTION BOTH OF HER HEALTH AND THAT OF YOUR CHILDREN. SHE LOST A LOT OF BLOOD WITH THE LAST BABY AND...
BEER

Role plays or sociodramas help prepare health workers to handle difficult problems in their communities.

How much responsibility should health workers be given?

In different programs, health workers play very different roles with respect to family planning.

• Many larger government programs instruct health workers to encourage people to plan their families. Most of these health workers simply refer interested women to a family planning clinic. However, an increasing number of programs now supply health workers with condoms and birth control pills to distribute.

• Some programs train special 'community nurses' to work mainly in family planning. The nurses learn just enough other health skills so that it does not look as though they are there only to promote family planning.

• By contrast, many community programs train health workers in a wide range of health skills, family planning included. Quite wisely, family planning services are often linked with under-fives activities.

GO HOME AND THINK ABOUT IT. BUT REMEMBER, AFTER THE OPERATION YOU CAN NEVER HAVE MORE CHILDREN.

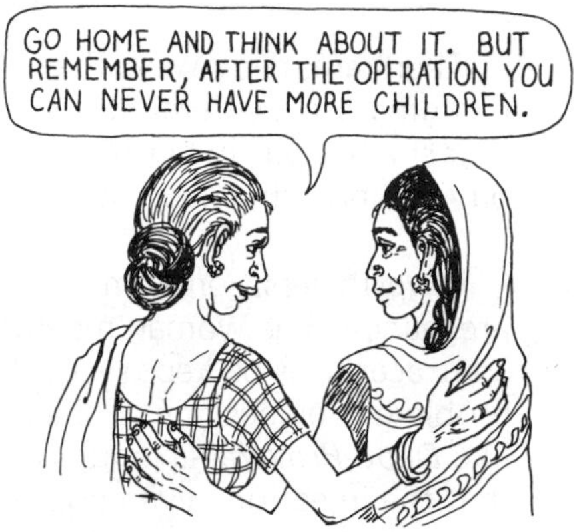

• Some community-based programs even train local health workers to do sterilization operations. In Gonoshasthaya Kendra, in Bangladesh, village women 'paramedics' have skillfully performed hundreds of **tubal ligations** (female sterilizations, see ***WTND,*** p. 293). The incidence of infection from their operations is lower than the national average for doctors. Furthermore, the percentage of women who have chosen sterilization is much higher in the program area than in the rest of the country. This is probably because the operations are performed only when asked for, by local women whom the others know and trust.

We are not suggesting that all programs teach health workers to perform tubal ligations. It may not be appropriate for your area. We are only pointing out that a group of community health workers, some of whom have never attended school, have been able to do a better job—both technically and socially— than the average professional in their country. What makes the difference is the fact that these women paramedics are local persons selected for their human concern, and that they receive appropriate training and support.

In many programs, we have seen that village health workers with little formal education can learn to prescribe birth control pills and other contraceptives carefully and correctly. But during training, the basic information about selection, precautions, and advice must be carefully discussed and clearly presented.

In conclusion, the problems related to family planning are more human than technical. We feel that, in community-based programs, health workers should (1) be able to **provide the kind of advice that permits people to make intelligent, well-informed decisions,** (2) **help people understand the political and religious influences**—local and international—that lead to misinformation and abuse with regard to family planning, and (3) be taught and permitted to **make appropriate birth control methods available to those who want them.**

It is women's right to control their own bodies.

CHAPTER 24

Children as Health Workers

In villages and communities throughout the world, **young children are often cared for by their older brothers and sisters.** These young 'child-minders' not only play with their smaller brothers and sisters, but carry them about and even bathe, change, and feed them. It is not unusual for a small child to spend more time under the care of an older sister or brother than with his mother or father.

In some areas, children—especially girls—do not attend school regularly because they are needed at home to watch the smaller children while their mothers work.

If children can learn more about how to protect the health of their younger brothers and sisters, they can make a big difference in the well-being and development of young children in their communities.

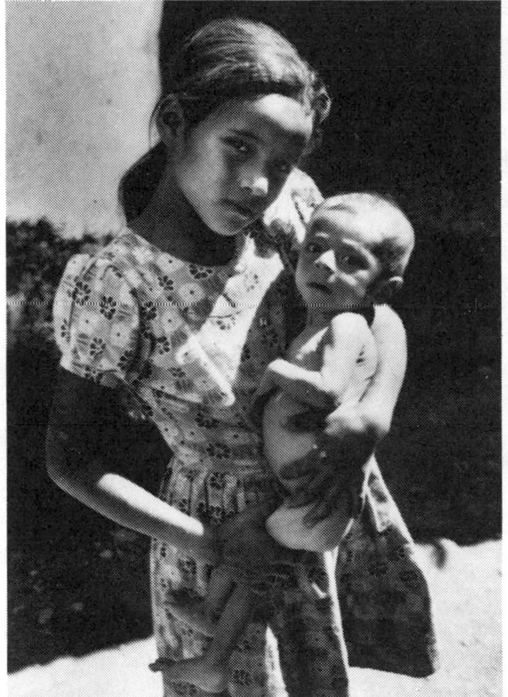

After their mother died, this young girl did her best to care for her baby brother. If she had known more about his needs and how to care for him, perhaps he would be healthier.

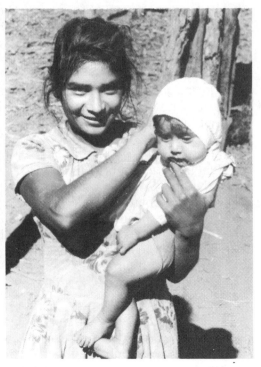

This girl is doing a good job of caring for her baby brother. If health workers can help children to learn more about meeting the needs of their smaller brothers and sisters, this will do much to improve children's health.

CHILD-to-child

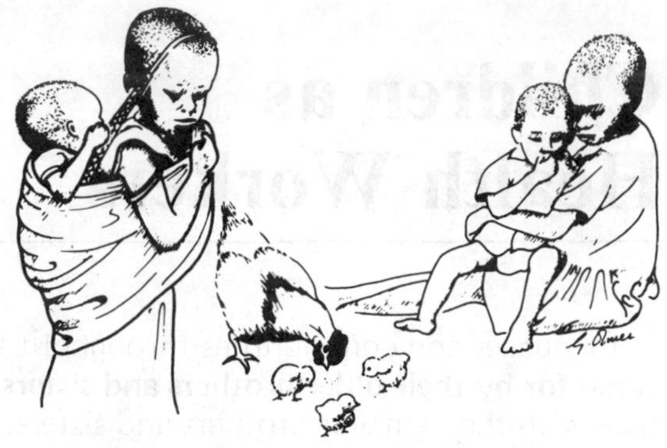

Some of the best ideas for teaching and involving children in health care have been developed through the CHILD-to-child Program.

CHILD-to-child is an international program designed to teach and encourage school-aged children to concern themselves with the health of their younger brothers and sisters. The children learn simple preventive and curative measures appropriate for their communities. They pass on what they learn to other children and to their families.

The CHILD-to-child Program first began in preparation for the International Year of the Child, 1979. David Morley (author of ***Paediatric Priorities in the Developing World*** and ***See How They Grow***) brought together a group of health workers and educators from many countries. This international group designed an experimental series of 'activity sheets' for children, to be tried out by teachers and health workers. The activity sheets are not intended as step-by-step instructions. Rather, they are suggestions for helping teach children about important health-related subjects.

CHILD-to-child activity sheets have been written on the following themes:

- How do we know if our children get enough food?
- Healthier foods for babies and children*
- Care of children with diarrhea*
- Accidents*
- Our neighborhood—making it better*
- Let's find out how well children see and hear
- Looking after eyes
- Our teeth
- Health scouts*
- Playing with younger children*
- Toys and games for young children
- A place to play
- Children's theater—and stories about safety and health
- Understanding children with special problems
- Understanding children's feelings
- Early signs of illness
- Caring for children who are sick*
- Better health habits*

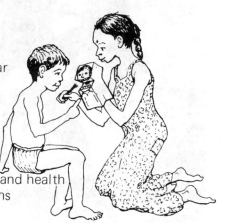

These activity sheets are available in several languages from TALC (see page **Back**-3). TALC also distributes a 104-page book entitled ***CHILD-to-child,*** by Aarons and Hawes, published by Macmillan Press in England. The book contains 8 of the activities, but does not include all of the ideas from the original sheets. The more complete versions of the 4 CHILD-to-child activities in this chapter are available in English or Spanish from The Hesperian Foundation.

It should be clearly understood that the activity sheets, written for use in many countries, must be adapted to local situations.

---

*Included in the book, ***CHILD-to-child.***

THE SOCIAL AND EDUCATIONAL VISION BEHIND CHILD-to-child

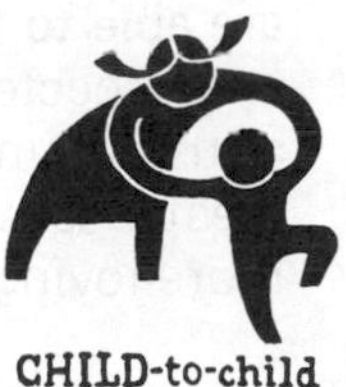

Some of us involved in CHILD-to-child see far more possible value in it than simply teaching children about the health needs of their younger brothers and sisters. The educational process that it encourages is equally important.

These are some of the social and educational principles behind CHILD-to-child:

- Children are not only a first priority for health work, but also an enormous resource as enthusiastic health care providers. With a little assistance, **children could soon do more to improve the well-being of their younger brothers and sisters than all doctors and health workers put together**—and at far lower cost.
- Through learning in an active, practical way about health care when young, children will become better parents. They will be more likely to meet the needs of their own children.
- CHILD-to-child can help introduce a liberating learning process into schools. It can help bring schooling closer to the needs of the children, their families, and their communities.
- It can also make children more aware of their own ability to change and improve their situation, through sharing and helping each other.

There are several ways that CHILD-to-child activities can help change or transform the schools:

- CHILD-to-child introduces into the classroom information and skills that children can use right away, in their homes, to benefit their younger brothers and sisters. Both children and teachers can discover the excitement of learning that has immediate value to families and the community. So a seed of change is sown.
- In CHILD-to-child, children learn to work together and help each other. Older grades organize to help teach younger grades. Younger grades conduct activities (story telling, puppet shows, seeing and hearing tests, etc.) with pre-school children. Everybody teaches and everybody learns from each other.
- There is no competition for grades, because in CHILD-to-child no grades are given (we hope!). **The children learn the importance of trying to help each other** rather than trying to end up on top of others. So another seed of change is sown.
- CHILD-to-child emphasizes **learning through experience.** Rather than simply being told things, **the children conduct their own surveys, perform their own experiments, and discover answers for themselves.** They are encouraged to **think,** to **observe,** to **explore,** and to **invent.** This makes learning adventurous and fun. It helps the children develop ways of looking critically and openly at life. It encourages the independence of thought that helps form leaders in the process of change. And so another seed is sown.

- Most important of all, CHILD-to-child is founded on the belief that **children are able to take on a responsible role in family health.** This means children are respected and trusted. They are valued not simply as future adults, but as useful, important persons in their own right. In this way, children gain a greater sense of personal worth and direction. They may grow up to be more loving human beings.

Through CHILD-to-child, at least part of the children's education will help them to help each other—so that everyone can move forward together. At least the seed will be sown.

THE ROLE OF HEALTH WORKERS IN CHILD-to-child

CHILD-to-child activities can be led by health workers, school teachers, parents, or anyone who likes working with children. But health workers can play an especially important role in promoting and developing CHILD-to-child and similar activities with children.

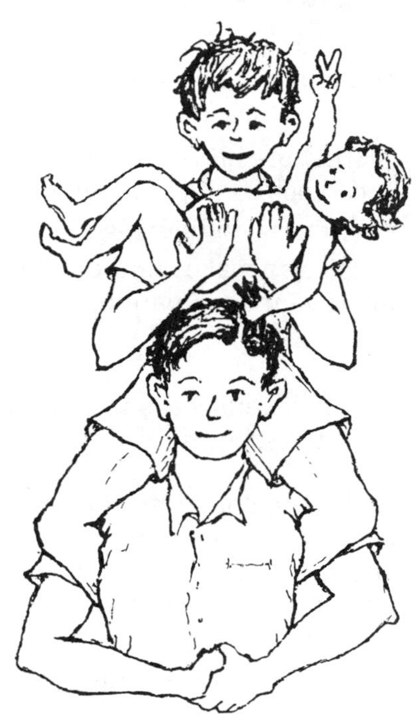

In Mexico, some 'health promoters' have done this in several ways:

- They organize CHILD-to-child activities with children in the primary school (with the teacher's permission).
- They interest school teachers in conducting CHILD-to-child activities with their classes.
- They meet at the health post with children who do not attend school, so they, too, can take part in CHILD-to-child activities.

Health workers may also be able to work with children through local clubs and organizations (for example, Girl Guides or Boy Scouts).

In some countries, CHILD-to-child activities have been included in the official curriculum (study plan) for primary schools. Where this is the case, health workers can offer to work with the teachers. They can help both in developing the activities with the children and in adapting them to the needs of the community.

The health worker's role can be of great value. For in the process of fitting CHILD-to-child into the school study plan, some of the social and educational principles can easily be lost. The big challenge is to **help the teacher understand and use educational methods based on equality, experience, discovery, and sharing.**

INVOLVING THE NON-SCHOOL CHILD

Some children often miss school because they are needed at home to care for younger brothers and sisters. Other children have to work to help their families earn a living. Health workers need to look for ways to reach these children who do not attend school. After all, they are the children who can benefit most from CHILD-to-child.

Encourage these children to come to the health post with their baby brothers and sisters, especially on days of baby weighing, 'under-fives' clinic, or child nutrition programs. Or try to set up special meetings to involve them in CHILD-to-child activities. Invite parents and school children to help.

Some health programs have helped start 'day care' centers for babies of working mothers. Such centers free more of the older children to attend school. Some of those who still cannot go to school may be able to help care for their younger brothers and sisters at the day care center. There they can be involved in CHILD-to-child activities.

Sometimes, **school children themselves can become the 'teachers' of those who do not attend school.** If a health worker can help this to happen, he will not only be acting to solve immediate health problems. He will also be preparing children to help build a healthier community as they grow up.

To help children learn about each other's health . . .

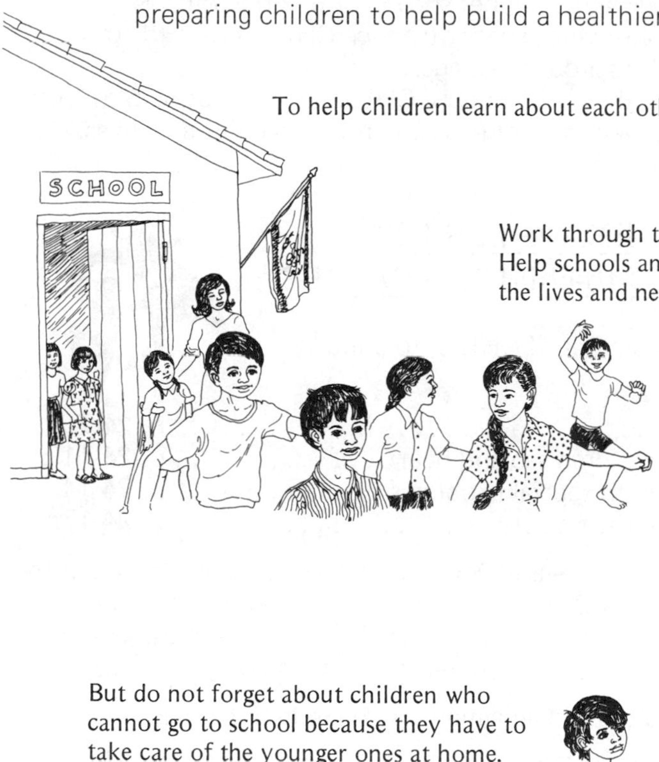

SCHOOL

Work through the schools when possible. Help schools and teachers relate more to the lives and needs of the children.

But do not forget about children who cannot go to school because they have to take care of the younger ones at home.

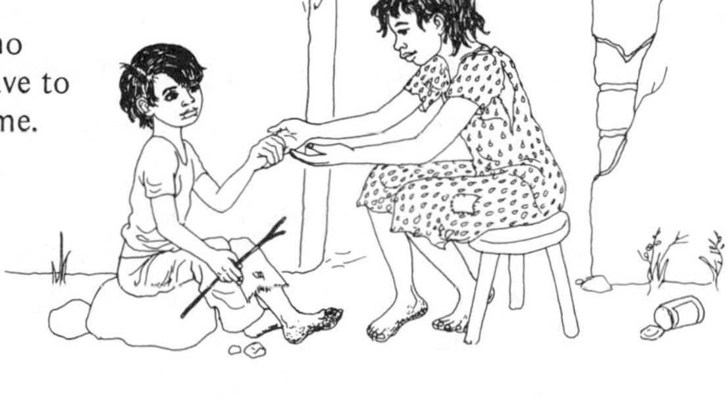

TIPS FOR TRYING OUT CHILD-to-child ACTIVITIES:

- Choose a place that is not too noisy or distracting.
- Start small, if possible with no more than 20 children.
- Allow enough time, so you do not have to rush.
- Have all materials ready ahead of time. Try to have enough so that all children can take part actively, instead of just watching.
- Use words familiar to the children. Avoid big scientific terms.
- Do not try to do too much at once. One activity sheet may have enough ideas to help you plan several meetings with the children.
- Before doing activities in a school, speak with the headmaster or teachers. Try to get their interest, understanding, and cooperation.
- Also discuss the activities with parents, so they will be more accepting of the children's new ideas. Perhaps some parents will want to help.

POSSIBILITIES FOR FOLLOWING UP CHILD-to-child ACTIVITIES:

- Older school children can lead activities with younger grades.
- School children can lead activities with pre-school and non-school children.
- Children can report back to the group about ways they have used their new knowledge at home and with younger children.
- Children's surveys can be repeated to check for improvements.
- Children can put on public skits, puppet shows, or demonstrations.
- Children from one school or village can introduce CHILD-to-child to children in another nearby school or village.
- Teachers can discuss how they might apply CHILD-to-child principles to the rest of their teaching, to make schooling relate more to children's lives.

EXAMPLES OF CHILD-to-child ACTIVITIES

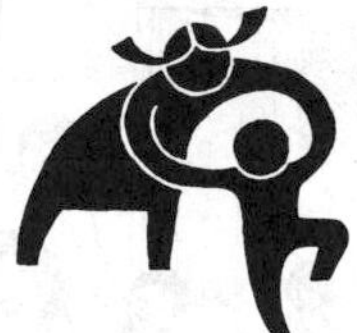

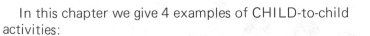

In this chapter we give 4 examples of CHILD-to-child activities:

These activities are expanded or revised versions of those available through the CHILD-to-child Program and TALC. We also have included photographs and observations on how the activities worked in Ajoya, Mexico, where the village health team and local school teachers conducted some of the original trials.

References to 4 other Child-to-child activities are made in this book:

We hope that, as you review these CHILD-to-child activities, you will get a clearer idea of how they can be translated into exciting and rewarding action.

CHILD-to-child ACCIDENTS

THE IDEA

In some villages or neighborhoods, several children die each year because of accidents, and many more are injured. Many of these accidents could be prevented.

This activity is to help children prevent as many accidents as possible. Different sorts of accidents happen in towns and in rural areas. This activity sheet gives advice about only the most common accidents.

In order to do something about accidents, children need to know . . .

- what the most common dangers are
- how those dangers can be avoided
- what to do if an accident does happen

THE ACTIVITY

What accidents happen to children?

To get children interested, have them tell about accidents that have happened in their homes or their village. Have them list these on the blackboard.

BAD ACCIDENTS IN OUR FAMILIES

	BABIES	OLDER CHILDREN	GROWN-UPS
BURNS	////	/	
CUTS AND FALLS	/	///	/
ROAD ACCIDENTS		//	///
SWALLOWING BAD THINGS	///	/	

Ask why the accidents happened. If children can find out why, they will be better able to prevent them.

Preventing accidents

Together, children can decide what they might do to help prevent accidents. For example:

To prevent accidents in the road, they can . . .

- teach young children to stop, listen, and look both ways before crossing
- build bumps across the road at the edge of town and in front of the school so that fast drivers slow down
- write letters to newspapers and authorities about the worst accident spots

To prevent burns, they can . . .

- take care to see that their younger brothers and sisters do not go too close to the cooking fire

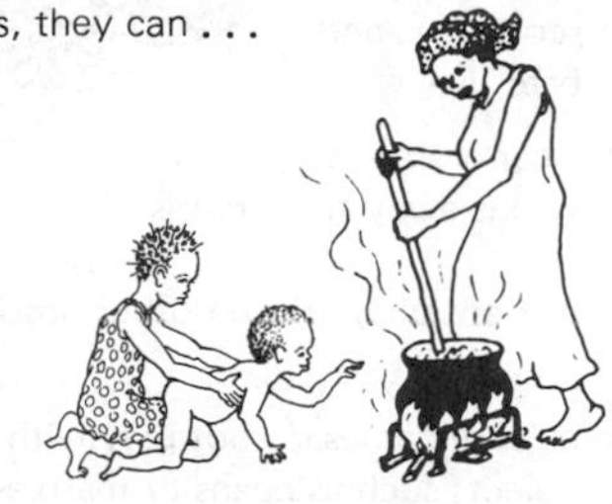

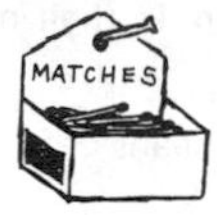

- keep matches out of the reach of small children (they can even make a small basket or shelf for matches to be stored high on the wall)

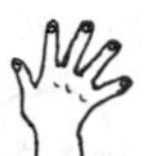

- be sure that handles of pans are turned so that they do not get knocked over

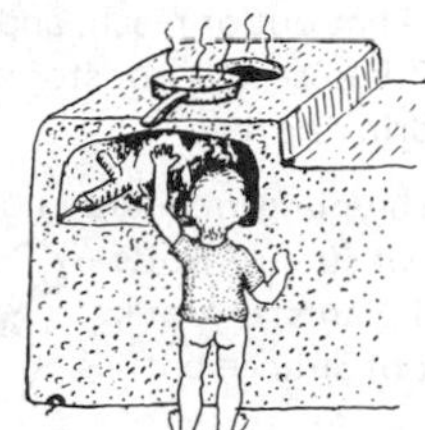

To make play safer, they can . . .

- warn others about the dangers of climbing dead trees, throwing stones, swimming in swift-flowing rivers, running when chewing sticks, etc.
- pick up broken glass, sharp stones, and garbage from streets and play areas

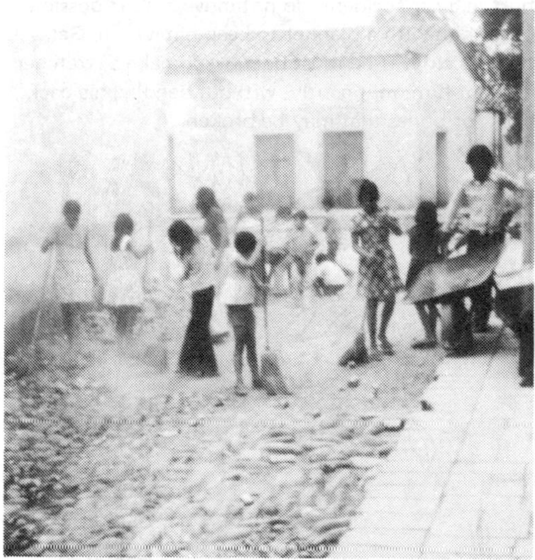

Children in Mexico cleaning up broken glass and garbage from the street.

To prevent bites and stings, they can . . .

- warn younger children about where snakes, scorpions, and bees live

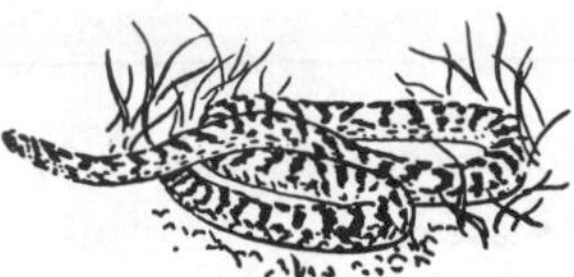

- clear grass and weeds away from paths

To prevent choking and other problems, they can . . .

- be sure babies do not play with small round objects such as beans or marbles (babies could easily choke on these, or put them in their noses or ears)
- mash foods like groundnuts and beans before feeding them to babies
- give teething babies large, clean objects to chew
- make sure poisons such as medicines and insecticides are kept out of reach, and that kerosene is not stored in drink bottles

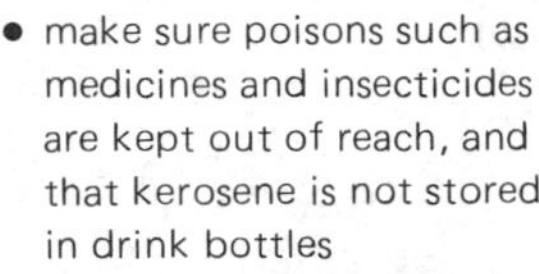

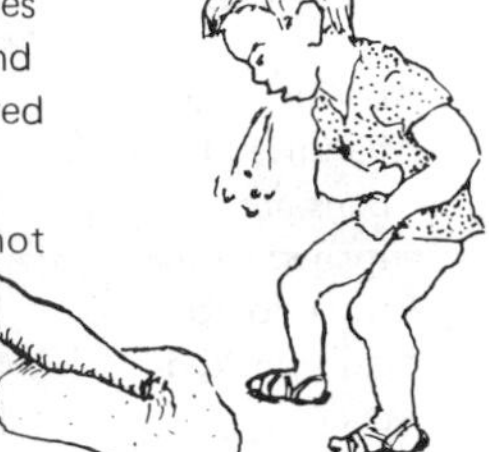

- warn younger children not to eat strange fruits and plants, or drink out of strange bottles

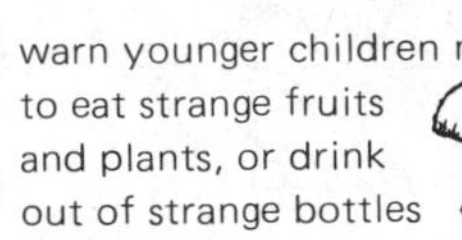

If an accident happens . . .

There are many basic treatments children can learn. Here are a few suggestions:

Accidents

If someone has a bad fall from a tree or gets badly hurt in a car accident, do not move him. If possible, cover him with a blanket to keep him warm. **Get help quickly.** If he must be moved, make a stretcher and put him on it gently, without bending his back, neck, or bones that may be broken.

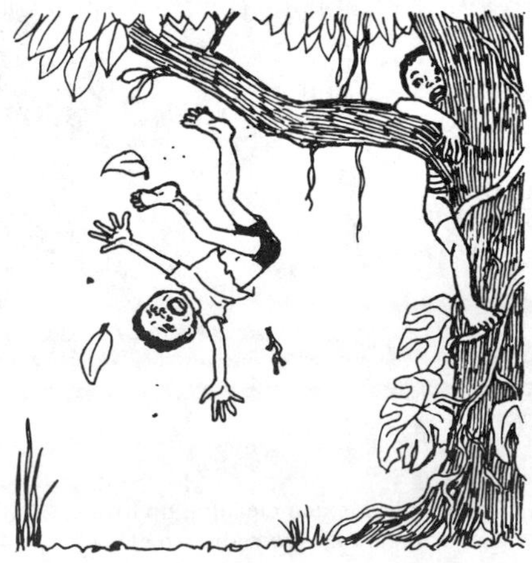

Snakebite

Learn to tell the bite of a poisonous snake from that of a non-poisonous one. If someone gets a poisonous bite, move him as little as possible. Moving will spread the poison around the body. **Get help fast.**

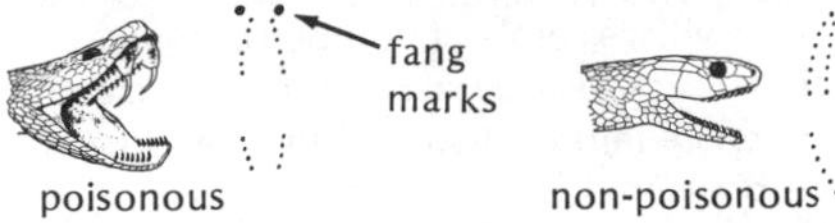

Burns

Put in cold water ***at once.*** If the burn is bad, cover loosely with a clean cloth. Give Special Drink. **Get help quickly.** *Never* use grease or butter on burns. Keep burns clean. Small burns are best left uncovered.

Cuts and wounds

When possible, wash cuts with soap and water that has been boiled and cooled. Wounds left dirty get infected. Do not put mud, iodine, or merthiolate on open cuts. Only use bandages if they are very clean.

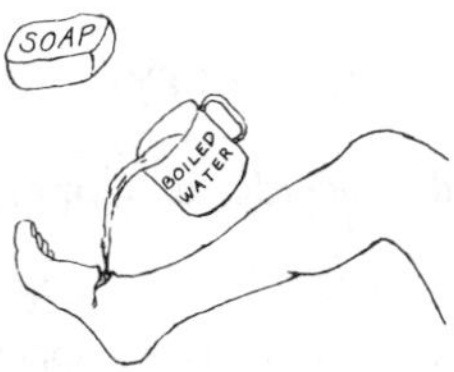

FINDING OUT HOW WELL THE ACTIVITY WORKED

- Children can compare the number of accidents before and after they take specific actions.
- They can talk about accidents they have prevented and others that still happen.

OTHER ACTIVITIES FOR CHILDREN

- Children at school can organize their own first-aid clinic for treating simple cuts and wounds.
- Each older child can 'adopt' a younger child to see that he crosses the road safely on the way to and from school.

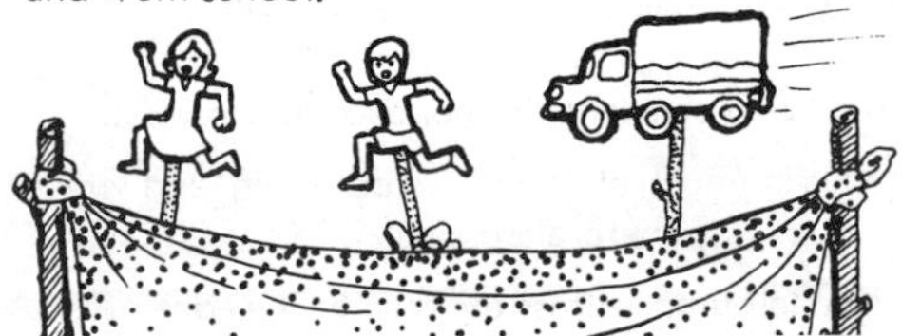

- Children can make plays and puppets to teach about accident prevention. They can show these to others at school, waiting at clinics, and at village meetings.

How teachers and health workers presented the Accidents Activity

Many of the CHILD-to-child activity sheets were first tried out in the small Mexican village of Ajoya. In order to learn if they were useful, both the village health team and the primary school teachers were given the sheets, with very little additional information or assistance.

It is interesting to compare the teaching methods used by the school teachers with those used by the health workers.

The health workers in Ajoya have found it important to bring learning as close to real life as possible. For teaching aids, they try to **use real objects rather than just drawings.** People learn best from what they can touch and handle.

Whereas the teachers made excellent posters to help the children learn about accidents, the health workers figured out ways to use real objects and lifelike situations to teach the same ideas.

For example: **Injuries from falls**

APPROPRIATE

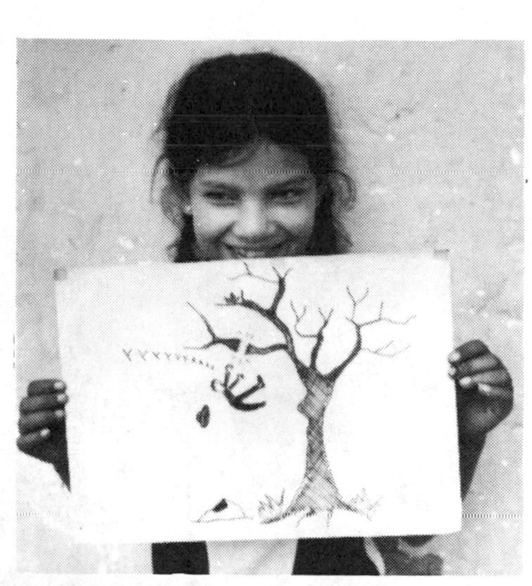

The teacher made this poster to get the children thinking and talking about accidents from falls.

MORE APPROPRIATE

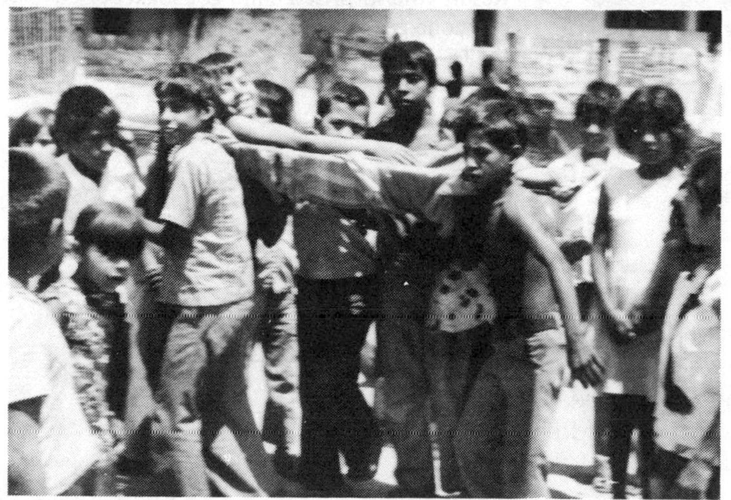

The health workers, however, had the children pretend one of them had fallen. The children then figured out how to build a stretcher using brooms and their shirts.

Another example: **Burns from hot food**

APPROPRIATE

To help children understand that it is important to turn handles of pots so small children cannot reach them, the teacher copied this drawing from the activity sheet.

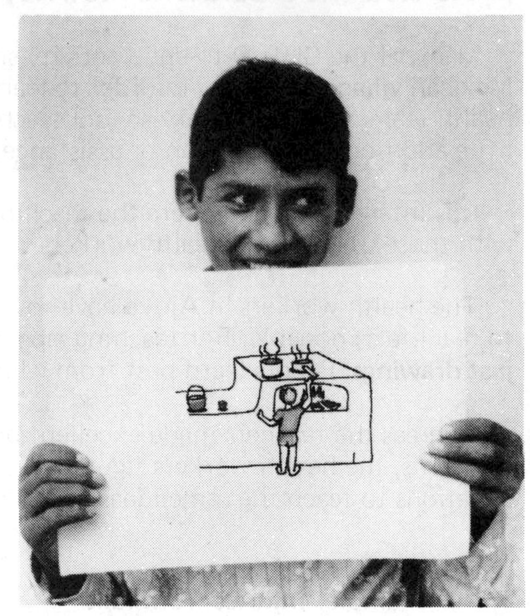

MORE APPROPRIATE

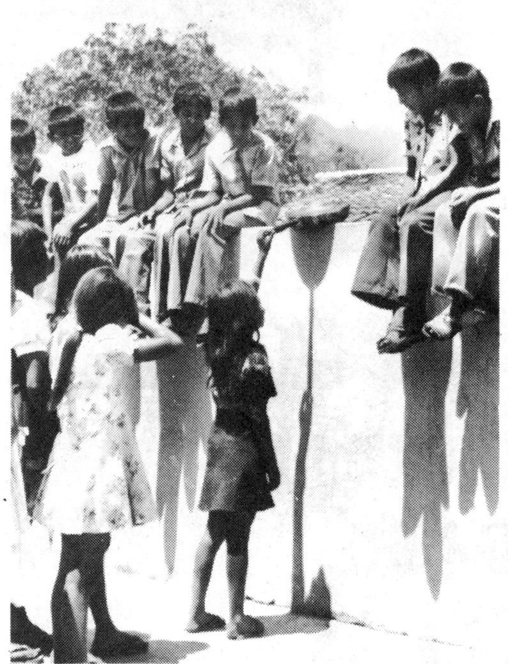

To teach the same idea, the health worker brought a big pan to school. He filled it with water and had a child (who did not know it had water in it) demonstrate how a baby might reach up and spill hot food on her head.

Result: the surprised child got soaked, everyone got a laugh, and no one forgot the lesson!

In a similar way, instead of drawing the tooth marks of poisonous and non-poisonous snakes on a poster, the health worker drew them right on the children's arms. (For photos and discussion of this example, see p. **11**-6.)

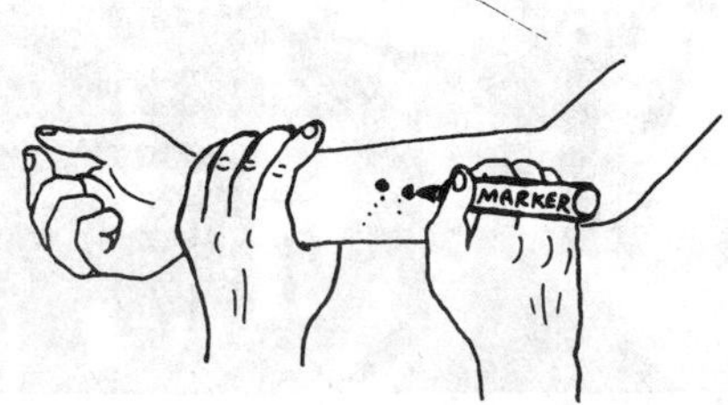

CHILD-to-child LET'S FIND OUT HOW WELL CHILDREN SEE AND HEAR

BACKGROUND DISCUSSION

Some children cannot see or hear as well as other children. Often we do not know about this and the child says nothing. But because the child does not hear the teacher or see the blackboard, he may not learn as quickly as others. So he may try to hide in a corner. **We can help him by letting him sit close to the teacher.**

Also, babies who cannot hear well do not learn to talk or understand as early as others.

In this activity, the school children try to find out which small children and babies need help.

HELPING CHILDREN UNDERSTAND THE PROBLEM

One way to get children thinking about problems of seeing and hearing is to ask questions like these:

- Do you know anybody who does not see or hear well?
- Do you act differently with these people? Why?
- How would you feel if you did not see well? Or hear well?

You can help children understand these things better through games. For example:

Game 1. One child plugs his ears while another tells a funny story to the group. Then one of the children plays 'teacher' and asks everyone, including the child who has his ears plugged, to answer questions about the story. Finally they ask him what it felt like, not being able to hear the story well.

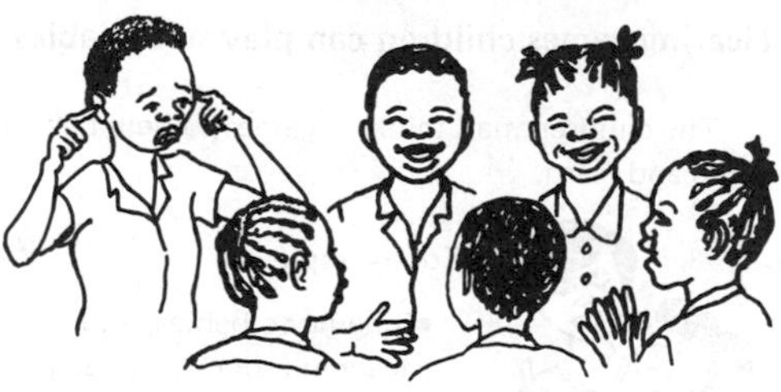

Game 2. The children form a circle. One child stands in the middle with her eyes covered. Around her feet are small stones, nuts, or other small objects.

The other children, one by one, try to creep up and steal these things.

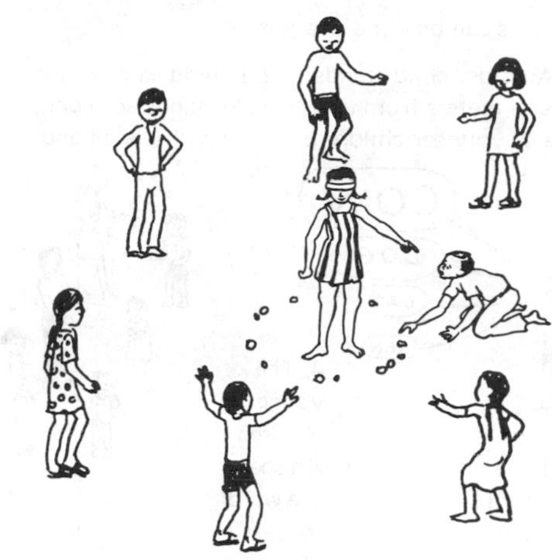

If the child in the middle hears the 'thief', she points to him and that one is out of the game.

The goal is to steal the most objects without being heard.

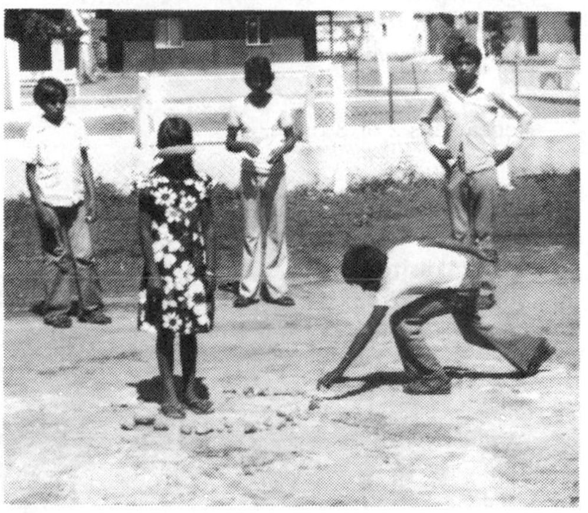

Children in Mexico playing the 'hearing game'.

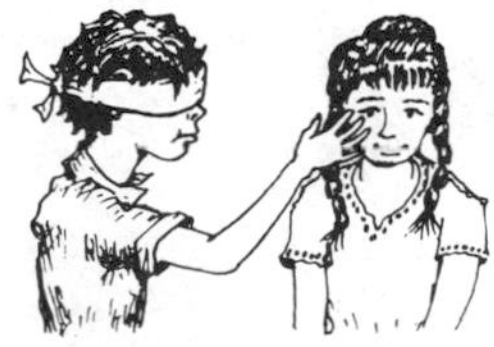

These games help children realize how important hearing is. They can invent other games to learn the difficulties of children who cannot see well. For example, they could play a game in which one child is blindfolded. He then tries to recognize his friends by feeling them.

FINDING OUT WHICH CHILDREN HAVE THESE PROBLEMS

Testing children's hearing

This can be done as a game:

1. An older child stands several meters from a line of younger children.

2. Behind each young child stands an older child with pencil and paper.

3. The first child calls the name of an animal, VERY LOUDLY.

4. The young children whisper the word to their older partners.

5. And the older children write it down.

Then the first child names other animals, each in a softer and softer voice, until at last he is whispering.

After about 10 animals have been named, and the words that the younger children heard have been written down, compare the different lists.

Repeat this 2 or 3 times.

Any child who has not heard nearly as many words as the others probably has a hearing problem. Let this child sit at the front of the class. If possible, he should be examined by a health worker—especially if he has pus in an ear or frequent earache.

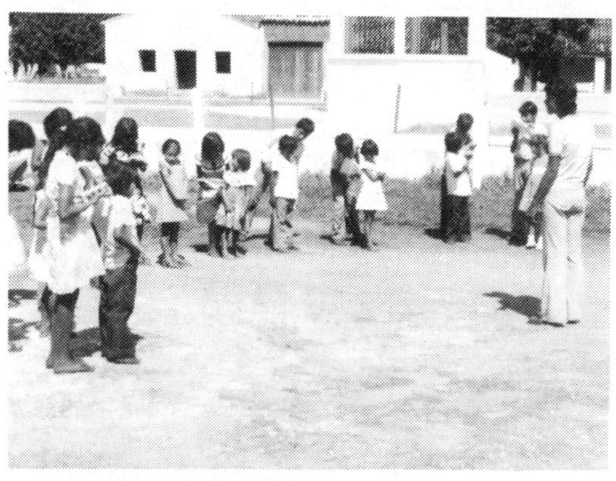

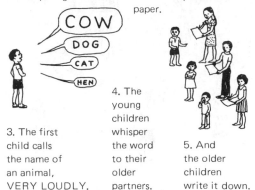

Children testing hearing in Mexico.

Testing the hearing of babies

What can children do to find out how well the babies in their families can hear?

- They can make a rattle from seeds or small stones, creep up and shake it behind the baby's head, and see if the baby is surprised.

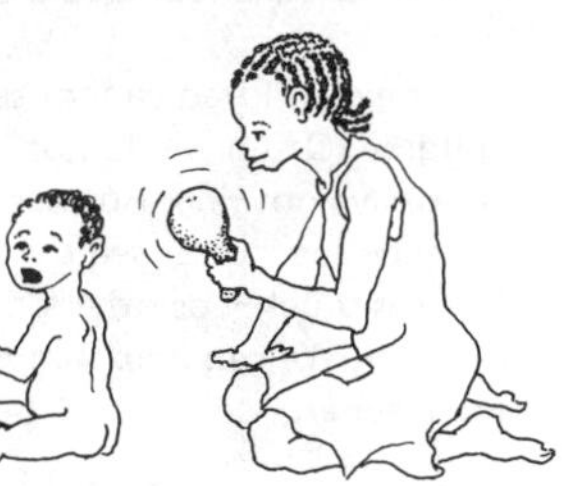

- Or they can call out the baby's name from different places in the room, and see if the baby responds.

If the baby is not surprised at the sudden noise, or does not turn his head when his name is called, he probably does not hear well. The baby may need to be taken to a health worker to have his hearing checked.

How can children help look after the ears of their brothers and sisters?

They can regularly look in their ears to see that there is no pus or small object inside. If they see anything wrong they should tell an older person, who should take the child to a health worker for help.

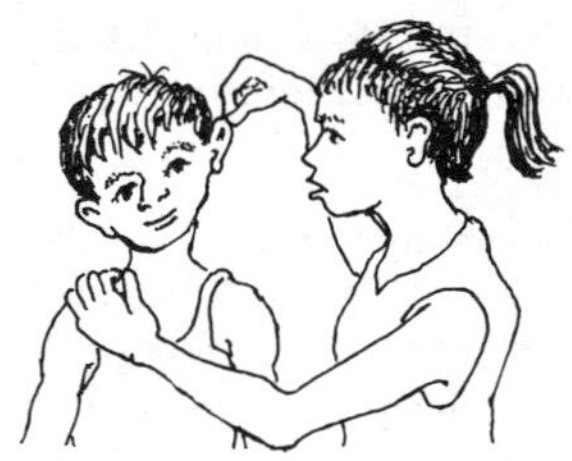

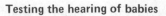

Hearing games children can play with babies

The children may think of games to help babies listen and learn.

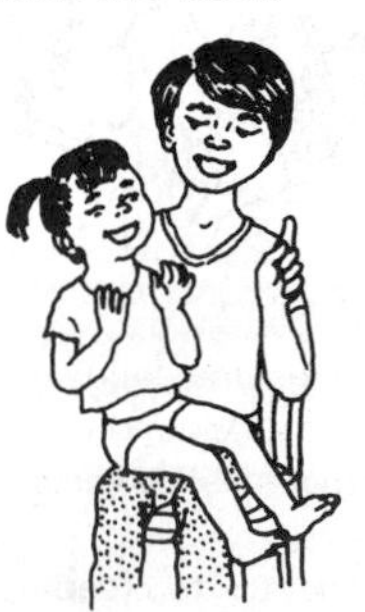

For example:

- Singing to babies, and teaching songs to young children.
- Telling stories and changing voices to sound like different people in the story—loud, soft, angry.

Testing children's eyesight

Older children can make their own eye chart. They can cut out black 'E's of different sizes and paste them on white cardboard.

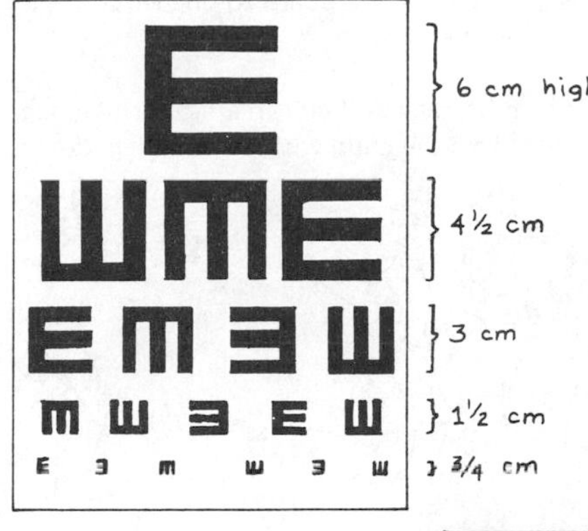

Also make a large 'E' shape out of cardboard or other material.→

First let the children test each other. Hang the chart in a place where the light is good. Then make a line about 6 meters from the chart. The child to be tested stands behind the line, holding the cut-out 'E'. Another child points at different letters, starting from the top.

The child being tested is asked to hold the cut-out 'E' in the same direction as the letter pointed to on the chart. Test each eye by covering the other.

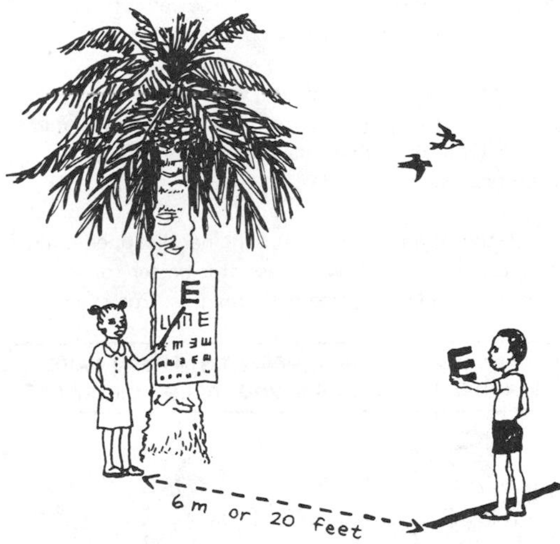

If the child can easily see the 'E's on the bottom line, he sees well. **If he has trouble seeing the second or third line, he sees poorly and needs to sit up front.** If possible, the child should go to a health worker for further tests. He may need glasses.

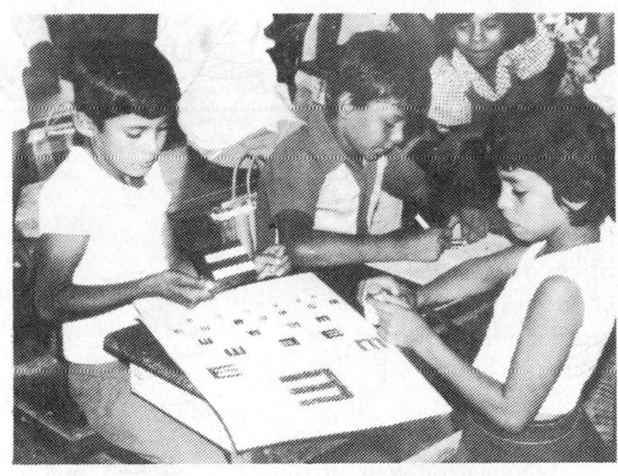

Children making an eye chart.

After the children practice testing each other, they can test the eyesight of those in the younger grades and the children who will be starting school soon.

Looking at each other's eyes

Start with questions to get the children interested. For example:

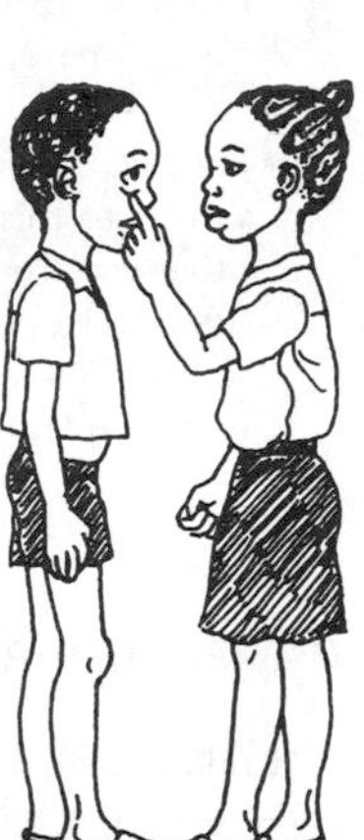

- Are your eyes the same as your classmates'? Shiny? Clear?
- How about the eyes of your younger brothers and sisters? Can they see well in the dark? Or do they often stumble at night?
- Do their eyes look dull? Are there any unusual spots or wrinkles? If so, something may be wrong.

Many children in different parts of the world become blind because they do not eat foods that make their eyes healthy. **Eating yellow and green fruits and vegetables helps protect the eyes.** Some extra cooking oil added to food also helps.

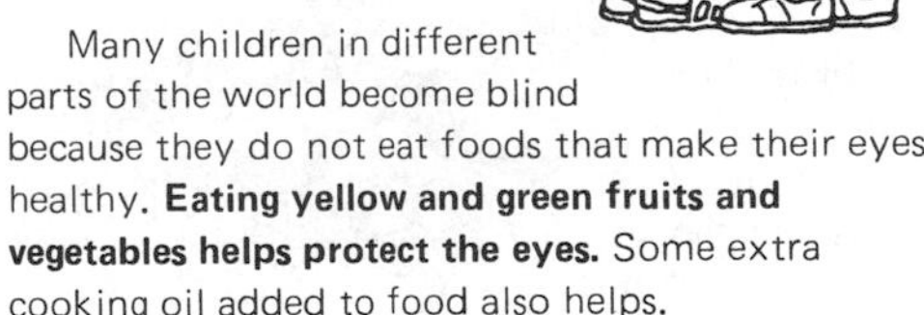

If children's eyes are red or sore, you can suggest that they wash them often with clean water with a little salt in it (no saltier than tears). This may help eyes get better and keep the flies away. If they do not get better soon, see a local health worker.

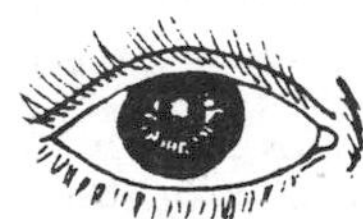

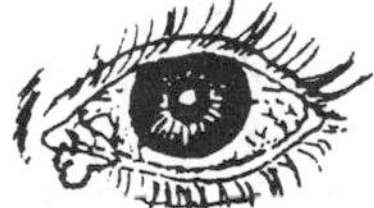

CHILD-to-child UNDERSTANDING CHILDREN WITH SPECIAL PROBLEMS

GROUP DISCUSSION

Encourage a class or group of children to talk about children who have some special problem or 'handicap'. Ask questions like:

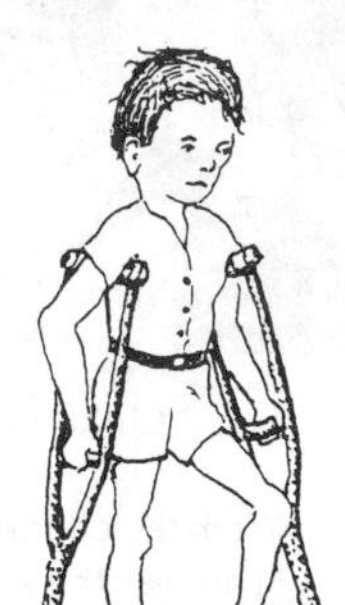

- Do you know any child who cannot walk or run or talk or play like other children?
- Why can't this child do everything the same as you can?
- Is the child to blame?
- How do other children treat this child? Are they kind to him? Are they mean? Do they make fun of him? Do they include him in their games?
- How would you feel if you had a problem similar to this child's? How would you want other children to treat you? Would you like them to laugh at you? To pay no attention to you? To feel sorry for you? To do things with you and become your friend?

GAMES AND ROLE PLAYING

Children will better understand the child with a special problem if they can 'put themselves in his shoes'. They can **play a game in which one child pretends to have a handicap.**

The other children act out different ways of behaving toward the 'handicapped' child. Some are friendly. Some ignore him. Some make fun of him. Some help him. Some include him in their games. Let the children come up with their own ideas and act them out.

After several minutes, another child can pretend to have the handicap. Let several children have a turn with a handicap. Try to make the pretend handicap seem real.

For example, to pretend one child is lame, the others can tie a pole or board to one leg so the child cannot bend it.

Then have the children run a race or play tag. How well does the child with the 'bad leg' do?

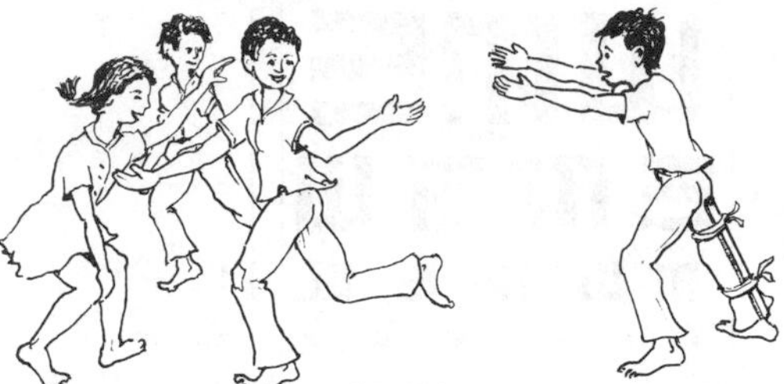

After several children have played different handicapped roles, have each of them discuss his experience with the others: what it was like, what he felt, and why.

REMEMBER: Children are usually kind to a child with a very severe handicap. They are often more cruel to a child with a less severe problem, such as a limp.

THINGS THAT HANDICAPPED CHILDREN DO WELL

A handicapped child cannot do ***everything*** as well as other children. But often there are ***some things*** she can do as well, or even better. Try to have the children think of examples.

A child with crippled legs, who has to walk with crutches, often develops very strong arms and hands. Or a blind child may develop unusually keen hearing.

Rather than feel sorry for the handicapped child and look only at her weakness, it is better to recognize and encourage her strengths. For example:

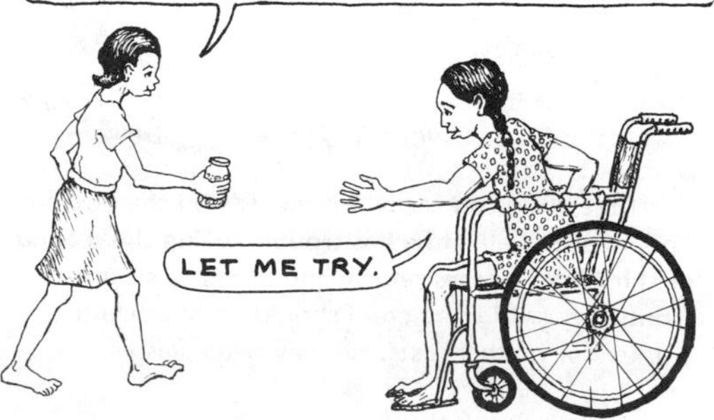

MARCELA, I CAN'T OPEN THIS. YOU HAVE STRONG HANDS. CAN YOU OPEN IT, PLEASE?
LET ME TRY.

Play with a handicapped child

Children, try to include the handicapped child in your games and adventures. Let him do as much for himself as he can, and help him only when he needs it. But remember, he cannot do everything you can. Protect him from danger . . . but do not protect him too much! Too much protection is dangerous to any child's health. Children need adventure for their minds to grow, just as they need food for their bodies to grow.

Swimming

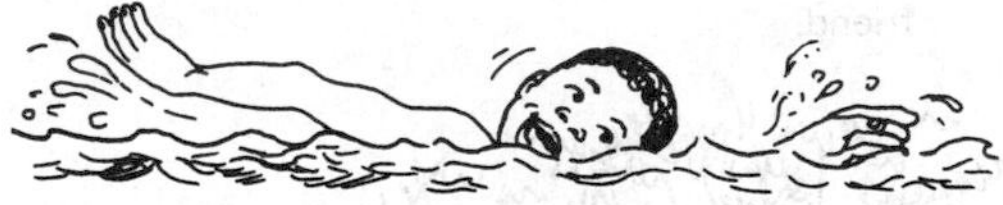

Many children with crippled legs can learn to swim well. Their arms become unusually strong from using crutches, and in the water they easily keep up with other children. But sometimes they have trouble getting to the water, or the other children forget to invite them . . .

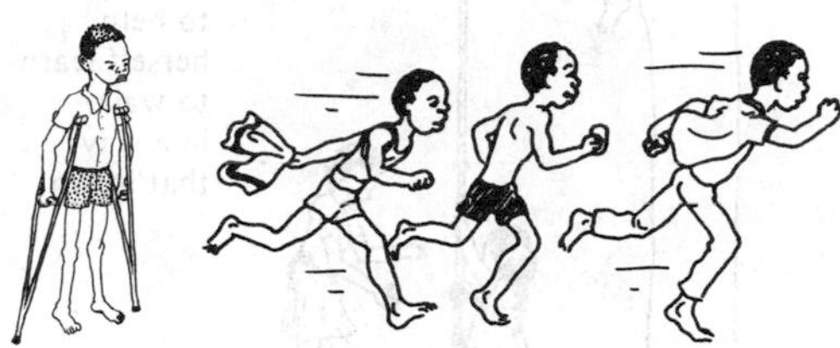

A friendly word of welcome to include the child with a special problem, or a little extra time or attention given to him, can make a big difference— and can make everyone feel good.

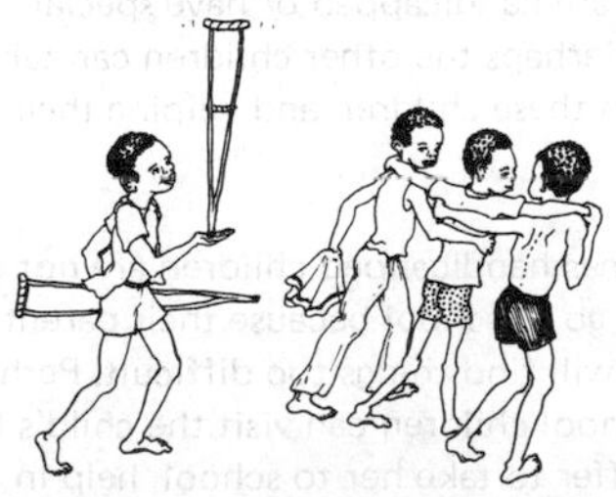

To help children see how much it matters to the handicapped child to be included in their fun, perhaps they can act out the pictures above.

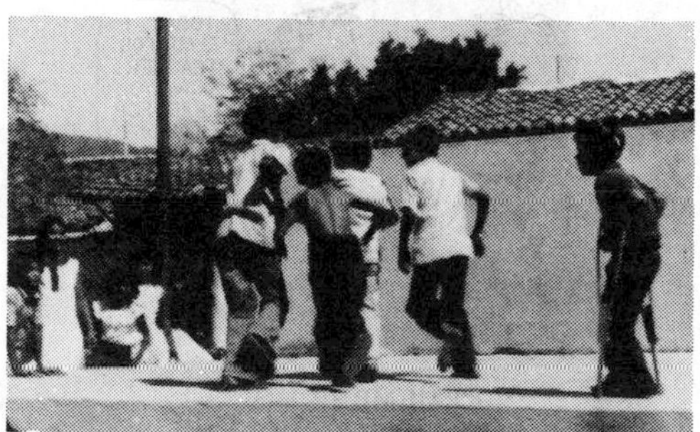

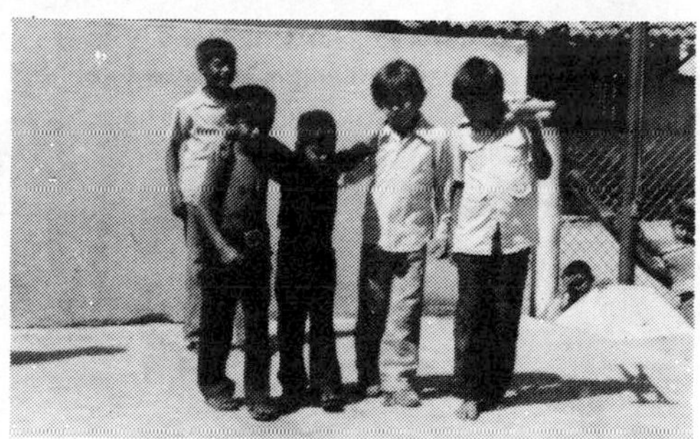

Photos from Ajoya, Mexico

CHILDREN WITH VERY BAD HANDICAPS

Some children have very bad handicaps. They cannot swim or play many games. But sometimes these children can learn to play marbles, cards, or guessing games.

It is especially difficult for a child who cannot speak or think as easily as other children. This child may be very lonely. Sometimes a child who cannot speak, understands a lot more than people think he does. If there is such a child in your neighborhood, perhaps children could take turns visiting him, to talk or play with him. Let him know you care.

BABIES WITH PROBLEMS

Sometimes a baby has problems that make it very hard for him to learn to sit or crawl or walk. The muscles in his back or legs may be too weak, or may make jerky movements the child cannot control.

A child like this needs special help. Often there are things that older brothers and sisters can do to help the child learn to use both his mind and his body better.

For example: If a child has trouble learning to crawl, perhaps his older brothers and sisters, or other children, can play 'crawling games' with him.

Two children can hold up part of the baby's weight as he tries to crawl. Another child encourages the baby to crawl by holding out a fruit or toy.

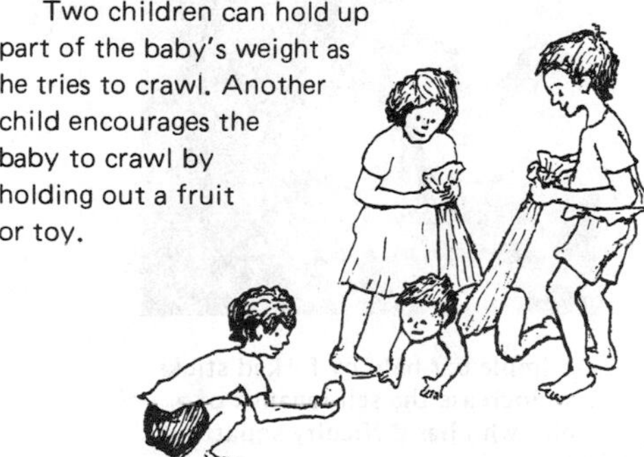

Play the game every day. As the baby grows stronger, less of his weight will need to be held up. In time he may be able to crawl without help.

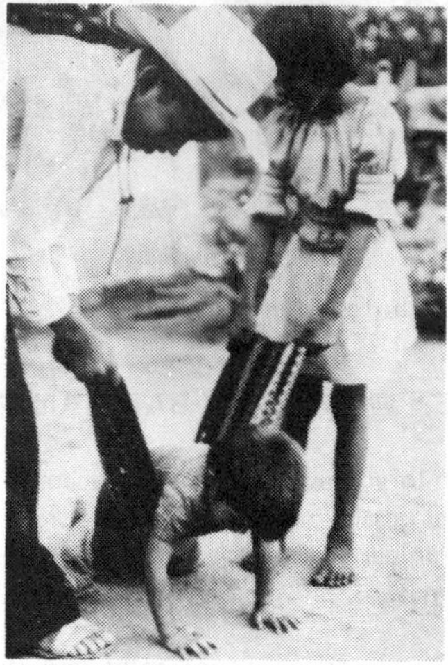

Children in Mexico playing a 'crawling game'.

HOW CHILDREN CAN HELP A HANDICAPPED CHILD

There are many ways that children can help a baby or young child with a special problem to learn to do new things. Here are some ideas:

- **Make it fun!** If exercises can be turned into games, the child will learn faster and everyone will enjoy it more.
- **Self-help.** Help the handicapped child only as much as he needs. Encourage him to do as much as he can for himself and by himself.

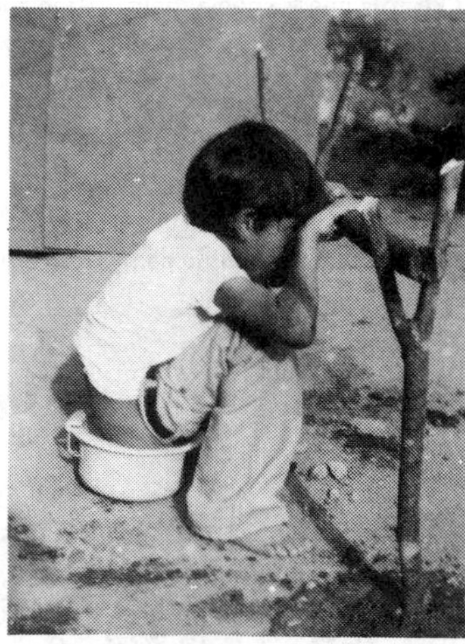

A simple bar held by forked sticks can increase the self-reliance of a child who has difficulty squatting to shit.

- **Little by little.** But remember, some things are especially difficult for the handicapped child. Encourage her to do a little more than she already does—and then a little more. If you have her try to do too much, she may get discouraged and stop trying.
- **Show you care.** Show the child how glad you are when she learns to do new things.
- **Mind over body.** Play often with the child, in ways that help her develop not only her body but also her mind. Talk with her and tell her stories. Carry her about. Become her friend.

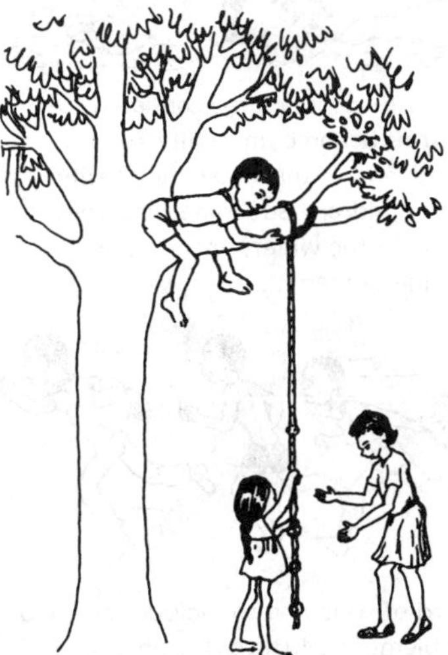

A rope swing like this can help a child who is lame to help herself learn to walk—in a way that is fun!

Are there any babies or young children in your village who are handicapped or have special problems? Perhaps the other children can take turns playing with these children and helping their families.

Sometimes handicapped children are not given a chance to go to school because their parents are afraid they will find things too difficult. Perhaps a group of school children can visit the child's family. They can offer to take her to school, help in whatever way they can, and be her friend. This could make a big difference in that child's life. CHILD-to-child!

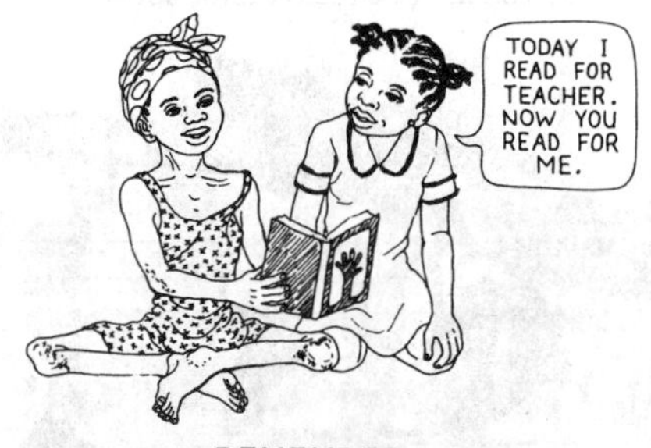

REMEMBER—
ALWAYS BE FRIENDLY!

CHILD-to-child CARE OF CHILDREN WITH DIARRHEA

BACKGROUND INFORMATION

Diarrhea means frequent, watery stools (shit). Often children with diarrhea also have vomiting and a swollen belly with cramps. The stools may smell worse than usual.

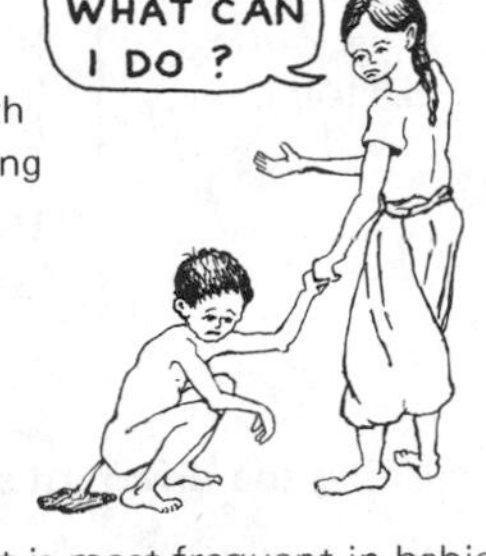

In many areas, diarrhea is the most common cause of death in small children. It is most frequent in babies between 6 months and 2 years. It is more common and more dangerous in children who are malnourished. **Bottle-fed babies have diarrhea 5 to 6 times more often than breast-fed babies.** Diarrhea is less common where there is piped water in the houses.

A lot of diarrhea can be prevented if we . . .

- breast feed babies for as long as possible
- see that children get enough good food
- take care with cleanliness and use piped water wherever possible

Children who die from diarrhea usually die because their bodies lose too much water. This loss of water is called ***dehydration.*** Therefore, the most important part of treatment is to replace the water lost through diarrhea and vomiting. For most diarrheas, medicines are not very effective. What do help are drinks that put liquid back into the child: water, breast milk, soups, herbal teas, etc. Also, children with diarrhea should be given food as soon as they can take it. Food gives their bodies strength to fight the sickness.

Even better than plain water or herbal teas is 'Special Drink' (often called 'Rehydration Drink'). This is water with some sugar and salt dissolved in it. Children can easily learn how to make the drink and give it to their baby brothers and sisters when they have diarrhea.

To sum up, children with diarrhea . . .

- must be given lots to drink, and
- must be encouraged to eat as soon as they are able.

In treating diarrhea, liquids and food are more important than medicines.

Who can introduce this activity?

Teachers, health workers, or anyone who is interested.

HELPING CHILDREN UNDERSTAND THE PROBLEM

How common and how dangerous is diarrhea?

To discover this, the children can make a simple survey. They can ask their mothers how many times during the last year their younger brothers and sisters had diarrhea. For each pre-school child they can find out:

- his **age**
- how he is fed **(breast** or **bottle)**
- **how many times he had diarrhea in the last year** (or during the last rainy season, or since some big fiesta, if people do not think in terms of years)
- **how many children died because of diarrhea** in the last year

When the children return to school, they write their findings on the blackboard.

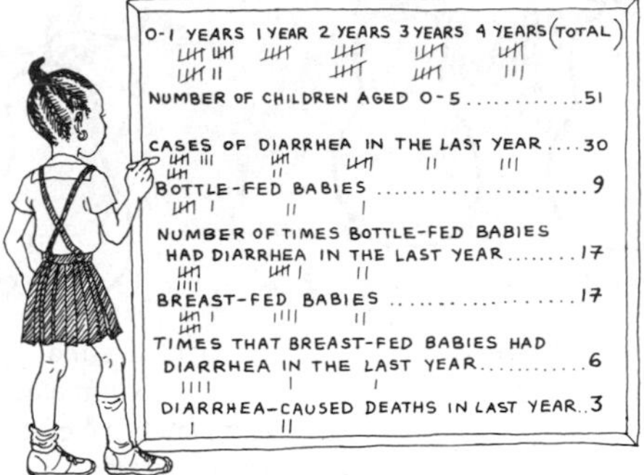

In this way, the children can see at what ages diarrhea is most common. Probably they will also discover that the breast-fed babies do not get diarrhea as often as the babies who are bottle fed.

The children may want to make posters like these to help everyone know the importance of breast feeding:

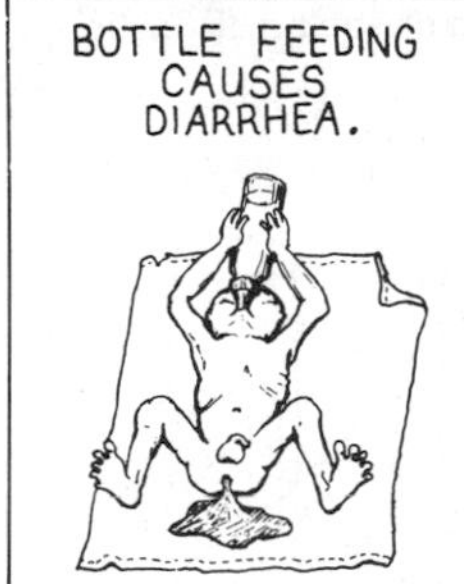

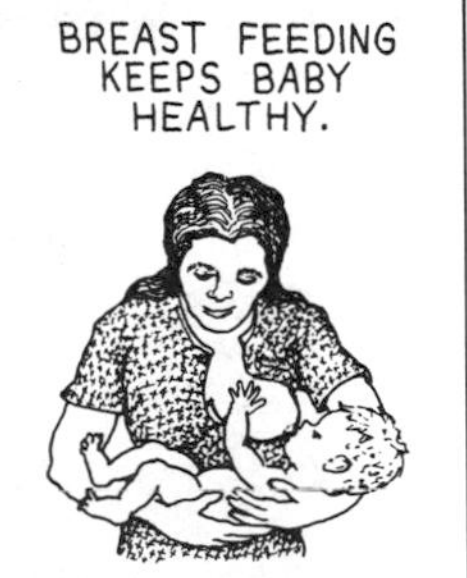

The information the children gather not only helps them to learn about the situation in their village. They can also use it later to find out if their health activities have made a difference.

What is dehydration?

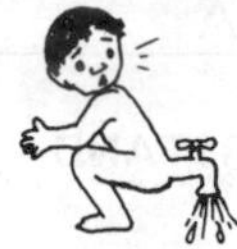

It is the loss of too much water!

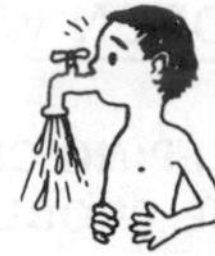

To look at the problem of dehydration, **start by talking about something familiar to the children.**

For example, in Latin America and parts of Africa, people associate diarrhea with sinking in of the soft spot (fontanel) on the top of a baby's head. People believe the brains have slipped down and this has caused the baby's diarrhea. Help the children see for themselves that the sinking of the soft spot results from the loss of water in the baby's body (dehydration).

The children may want to make drawings or posters like this one so that other persons can learn, too.

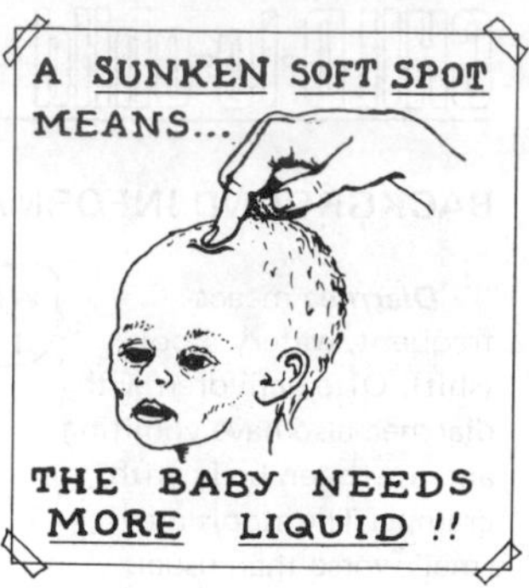

To learn about dehydration, the children can conduct their own experiment by making a 'gourd baby' like this one:

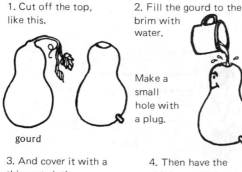

1. Cut off the top, like this.

gourd

2. Fill the gourd to the brim with water.

Make a small hole with a plug.

3. And cover it with a thin wet cloth.

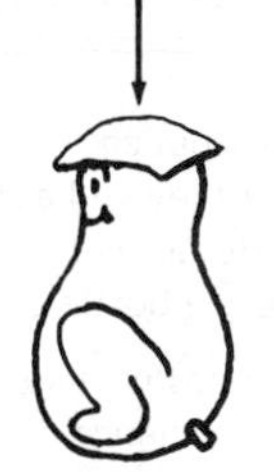

4. Then have the children pull the plug and watch the cloth (soft spot) sink in!

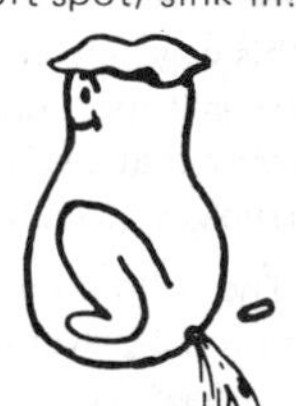

If you do not have gourds, a plastic bottle or tin can will do.

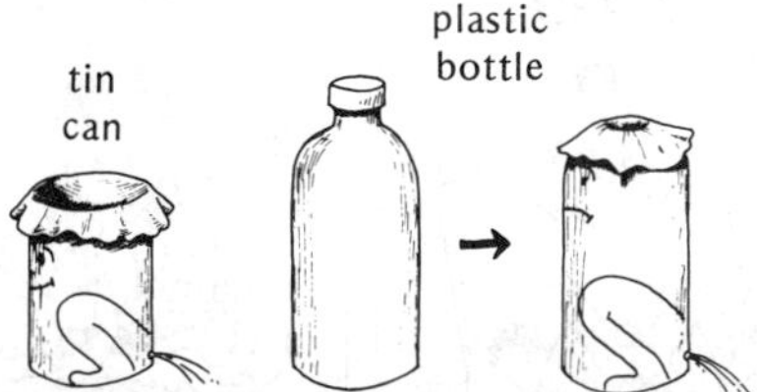

Ask the children: "Why did the cloth sink in? What does the baby need to make the soft spot rise again?" In this way **the children find out for themselves that a sunken soft spot in a baby is a sign of dehydration.**

Learning the different signs of dehydration

The children have already discovered that a sunken soft spot is a sign of dehydration. By putting additional holes in the 'gourd baby', they can experiment to learn other signs of dehydration.

When a baby has enough water, he pees well.

When he has lost a lot of liquid, he no longer passes urine (although the diarrhea continues).

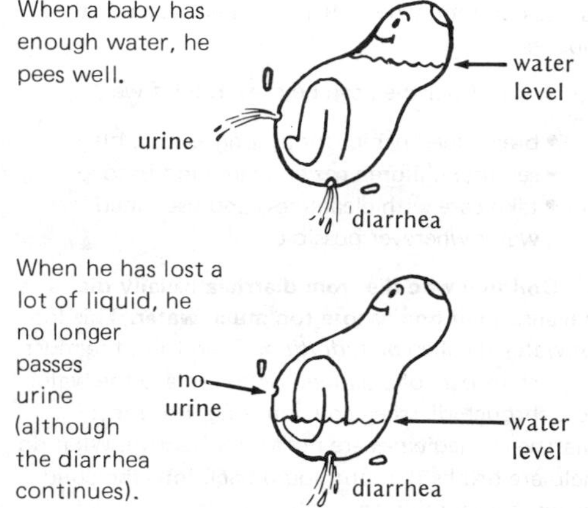

In this way, the children discover that **a child who passes little or no urine is probably dehydrated.**

By putting a small hole at the corner of each eye, the children can notice that tears no longer form when a baby is dehydrated.

When the gourd is full of water, it forms tears.

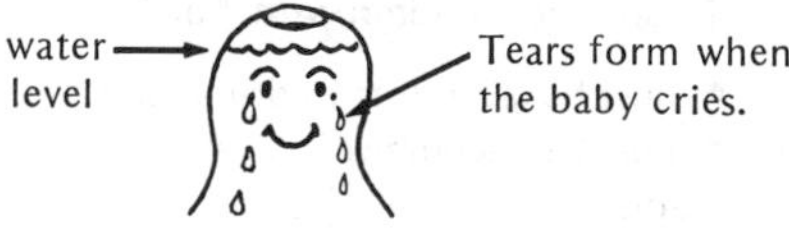

water
level
Tears form when
the baby cries.

When water is lost, tears no longer form.

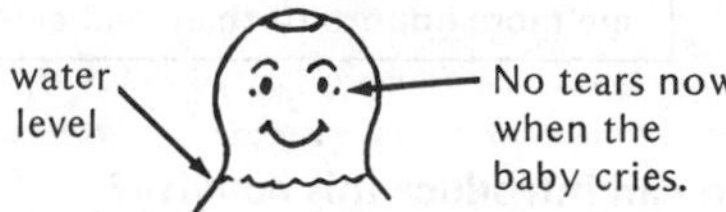

So the children learn that **if a baby does not form tears when he cries, he is probably dehydrated.**

To find out what happens when a child has vomiting as well as diarrhea, the children can do the following:

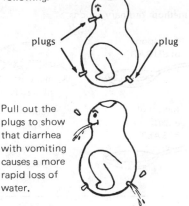

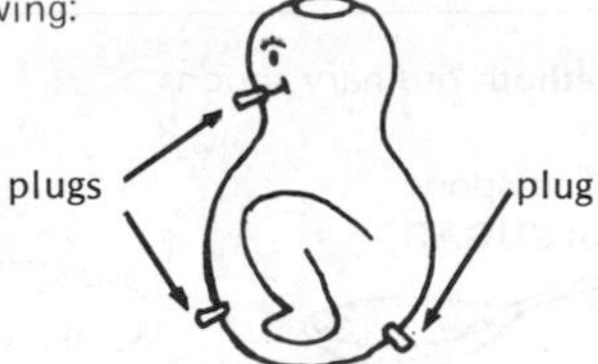
plugs
plug

Pull out the plugs to show that diarrhea with vomiting causes a more rapid loss of water.

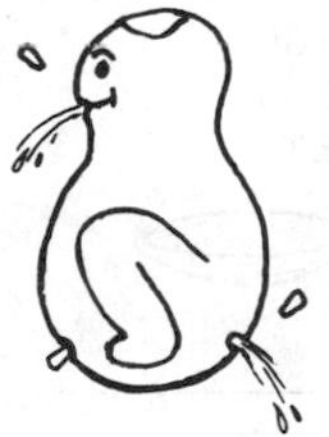

In this way, the children find that **dehydration comes more quickly and is more dangerous when a child with diarrhea also has vomiting.**

What happens when a child loses too much water?

The children can experiment to see how dangerous dehydration is to a baby.

For example: They can pick 2 flowers, put one in water, and keep the other without water. They will see that one lives while the other wilts and dies. Ask them why this happens.

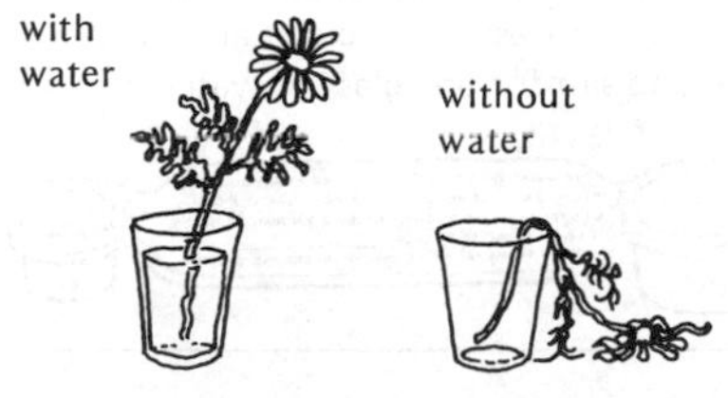
with water
without water

Let the children compare this to a child with diarrhea.

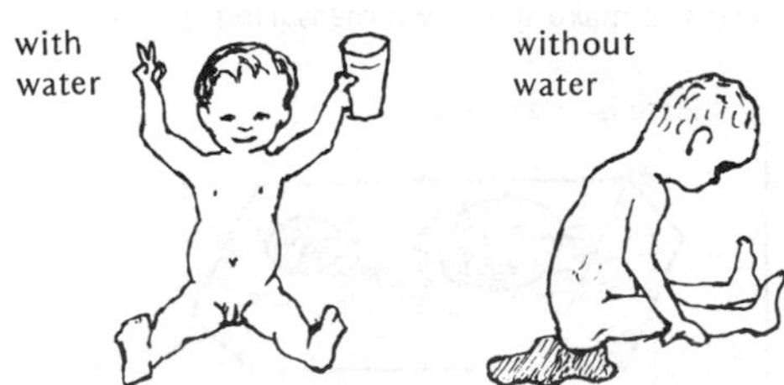
with water
without water

Ask the children, "What does a baby with diarrhea need so it will not wilt and die?"

Or the children can put a fruit like a plum or guava in the hot sun to see what happens to it.

Fresh fruit full of water.

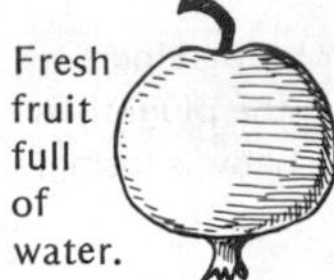

Fruit after it dries in the sun.

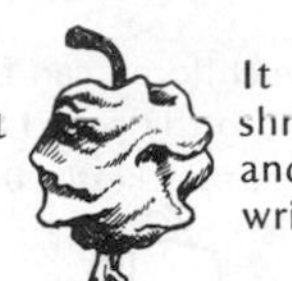

It shrinks and wrinkles.

Ask the children what they think happens to a baby when he dries out. Right! He loses weight and can even become wrinkled.

Often you will not see the wrinkles of a dehydrated child at once. But children can learn to do the following 'belly wrinkle test':

Lift the skin of the belly between two fingers, like this.

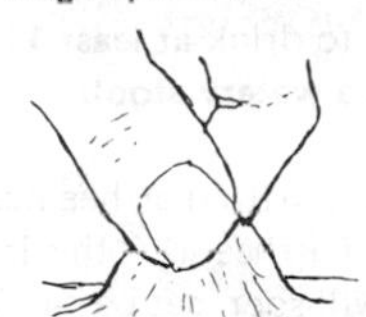

Then let go. If the skin does not spring right back to normal, the child is dehydrated.

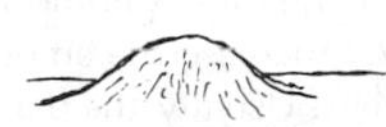

Children can practice this test by pinching the skin on the back of an adult's hand. To make it seem more real, the children can make a simple doll baby like this from an old sock.

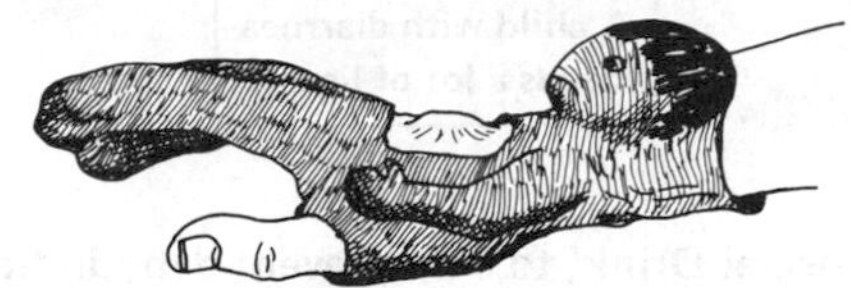

After the children find out the different signs of dehydration from their experiments, they can write the list of signs on the blackboard or on a poster.

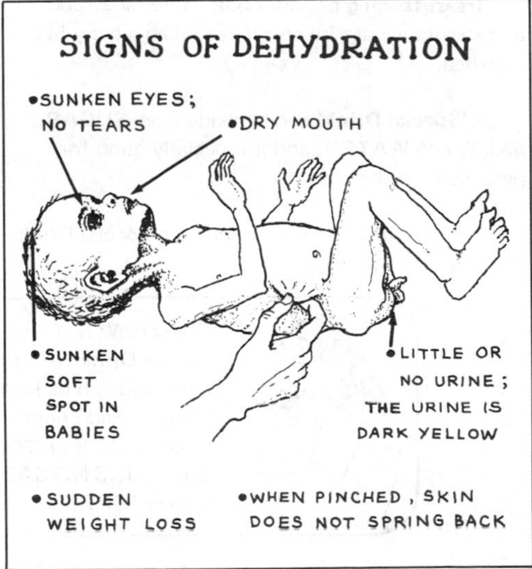
SIGNS OF DEHYDRATION
•SUNKEN EYES; NO TEARS
•DRY MOUTH
•SUNKEN SOFT SPOT IN BABIES
•LITTLE OR NO URINE; THE URINE IS DARK YELLOW
•SUDDEN WEIGHT LOSS
•WHEN PINCHED, SKIN DOES NOT SPRING BACK

How can dehydration from diarrhea be prevented?

The children can find the answer by playing a game with the gourd baby. They pull the plug, then try to put back as much water as the baby is losing, like this:

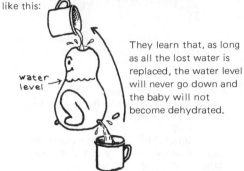

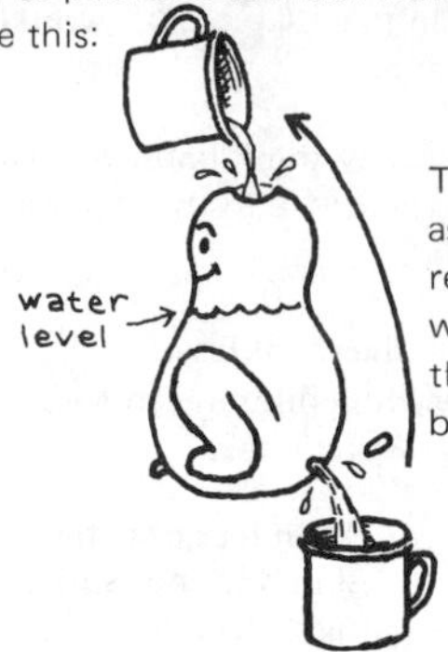

They learn that, as long as all the lost water is replaced, the water level will never go down and the baby will not become dehydrated.

A child with diarrhea needs to drink **at least 1 glass of liquid each time he has a watery stool.**

Giving lots of liquid to a baby with diarrhea may at first increase the amount of diarrhea. But this is all right. Usually the diarrhea will soon get better. The important thing is to **be sure that the child drinks as much liquid as he loses.**

The children have now found out that:

A child with diarrhea needs a lot of liquid.

A 'Special Drink' to help prevent dehydration

Many of the **herbal teas and soups** that mothers give to children with diarrhea do a lot of good, because they help to get water back into the child.

Breast feeding provides both water and food, and should always be continued when a baby has diarrhea.

A **'Special Drink'** can be made from **SUGAR, SALT,** and **WATER,** and is especially good for persons with diarrhea.

The children can learn to prepare Special Drink in any of several ways.

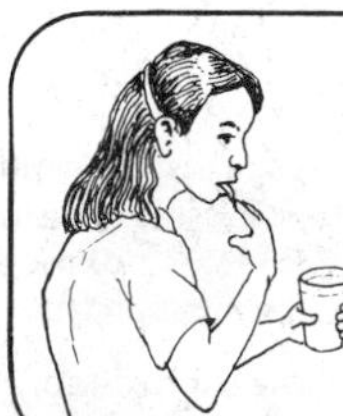

CAUTION: Making Special Drink with too much salt can be harmful. So before adding the sugar, TASTE IT TO BE SURE IT IS NO SALTIER THAN TEARS.

Ways to prepare Special Drink

First method: ordinary spoons

Mix 1 teaspoon of **SUGAR**

+ the tip of a teaspoon of **SALT**

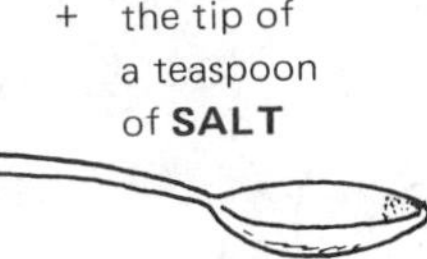

in a glass of water (about 1/3 of a liter)

Second method: by hand

Mix about this much **SUGAR**

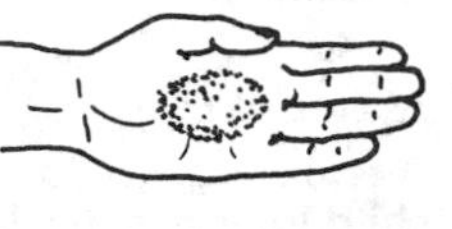

+ a pinch of **SALT**

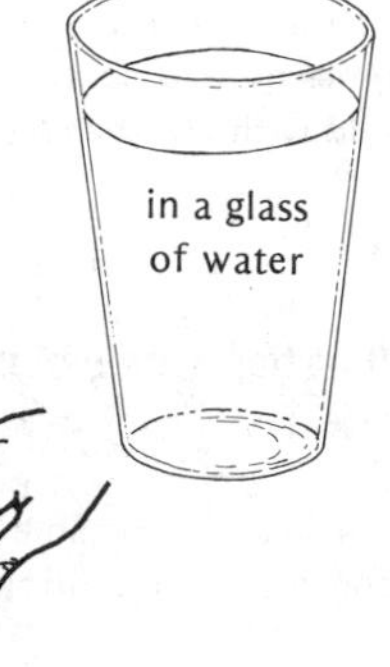

Third method: plastic measuring spoons

In some places, special plastic spoons are available to measure the exact amounts of sugar and salt for one glass of water.

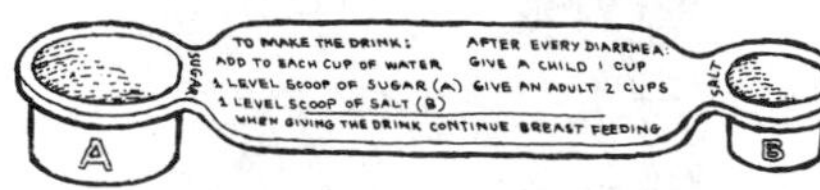

Fourth method: homemade spoons

Rather than depend on plastic spoons that can get lost or broken, the children can learn to make their own measuring spoons.

Here is one example.

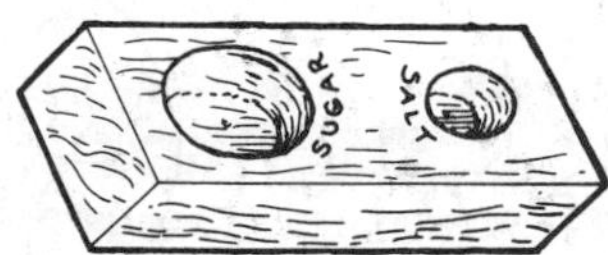

For another example, see the next page.

A WAY TO MAKE MEASURING SPOONS FOR PREPARING SPECIAL DRINK

Children can make measuring spoons from many things. But it is important that they measure roughly the right amounts of sugar and salt.

Here is one way to make spoons, using things that have been thrown away.

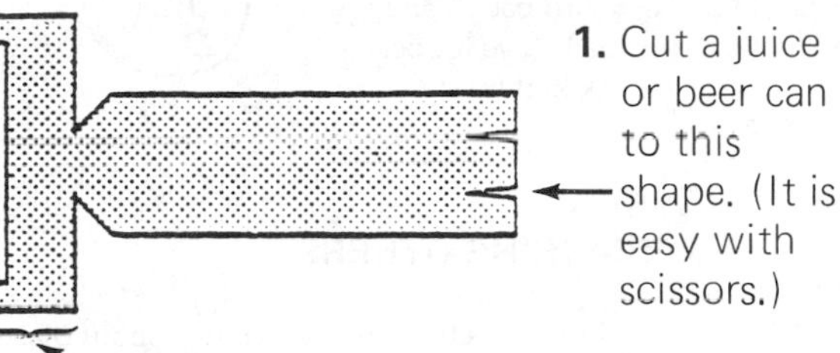

1. Cut a juice or beer can to this shape. (It is easy with scissors.)

Make this part as wide as a pencil is thick.

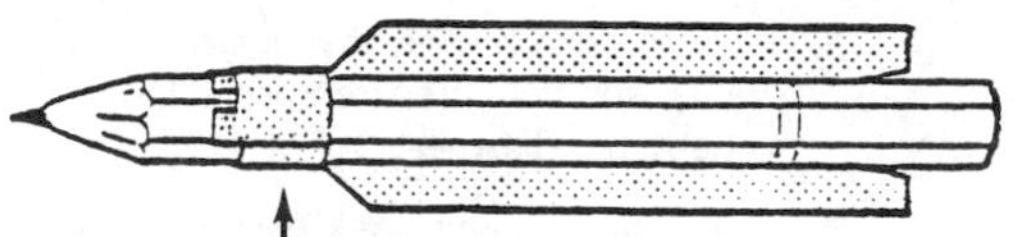

2. Wrap this part tightly around a pencil.

3. In the middle of a bottle cap make a small cut.

4. Join the pieces and bend over the tabs.

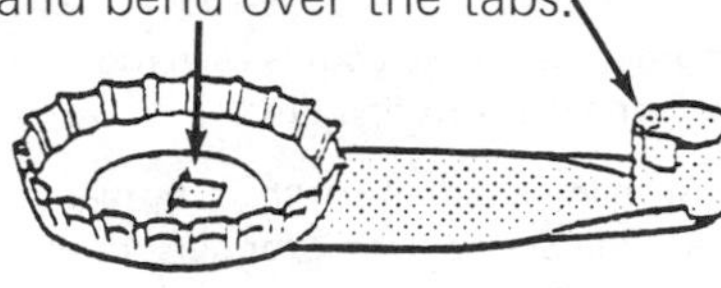

Give the child 1 glass of SPECIAL DRINK for each time he makes diarrhea.

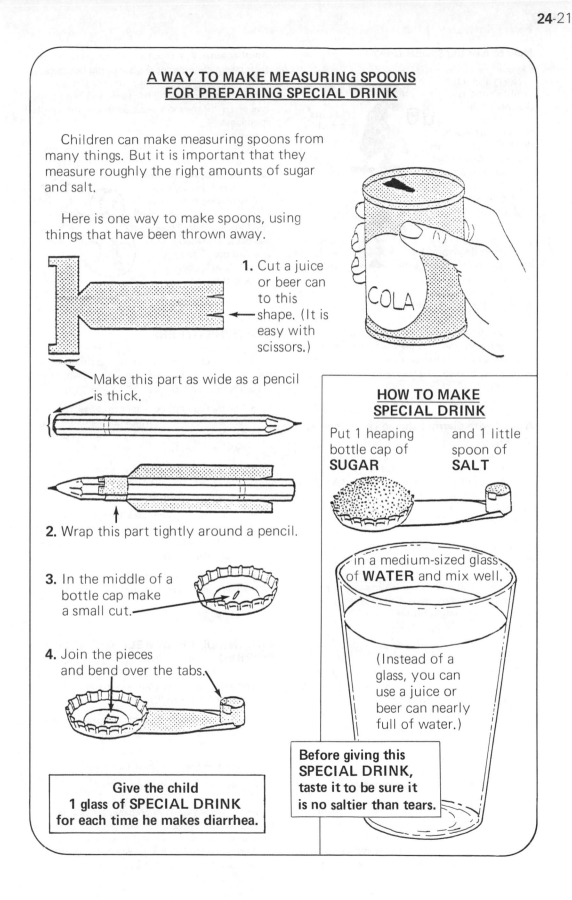

HOW TO MAKE SPECIAL DRINK

Put 1 heaping bottle cap of **SUGAR** and 1 little spoon of **SALT**

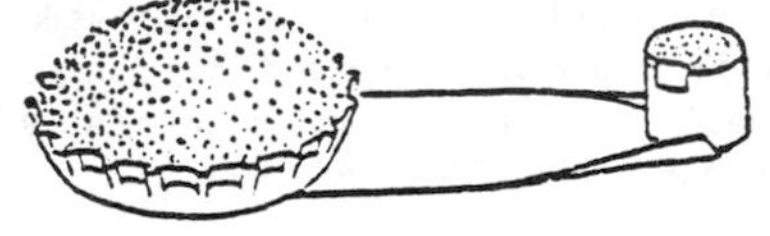

in a medium-sized glass of **WATER** and mix well.

(Instead of a glass, you can use a juice or beer can nearly full of water.)

Before giving this SPECIAL DRINK, taste it to be sure it is no saltier than tears.

How to give the Special Drink

Start giving the drink as soon as diarrhea begins.

An adult should drink at least 2 glasses of Special Drink after each watery stool.

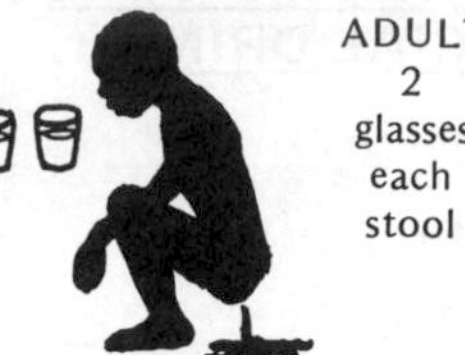

A child should drink at least 1 glass of Special Drink after each watery stool.

CHILD
1
glass
each
stool

If the child vomits the drink, give him more. A little will stay in him. Give sips every 2 or 3 minutes. If the child does not want to drink, gently insist that he do so.

Keep giving the drink every 2 or 3 minutes, day and night, until the child pees normally (every 2 or 3 hours). Older children and their parents can take turns giving the drink all through the night.

A child with diarrhea should eat as soon as he can.

Many people still believe that persons with diarrhea should not eat. This is a big mistake. A sick person must eat well in order to overcome the sickness. A child with diarrhea should eat as soon as he is able.

To help children understand why this is important, ask if any of the children has ever missed a meal or spent a day without food. How did they feel? Weak? This way, the children can realize that a child with diarrhea needs food in order to be strong enough to fight off the illness.

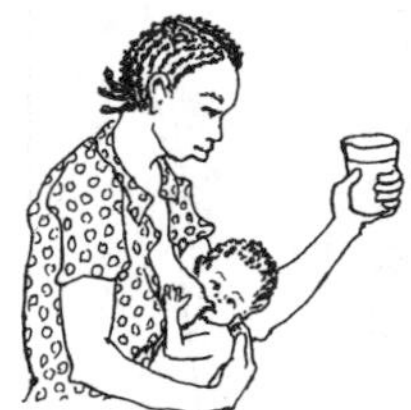

When a breast-feeding baby gets diarrhea, KEEP GIVING BREAST MILK, BUT GIVE SPECIAL DRINK, TOO.

Helping to make learning more real

A game: Give the children the plastic spoon, salt, sugar, and water. Do not tell them how much to use. See if they can mix the drink correctly by following the instructions on the spoon. **It is important that they learn to make the drink correctly.**

Another game: Ask children to invent ways to make their own measuring spoons out of old bottle caps, juice cans, or whatever. Make sure the finished spoons hold about the correct amounts. You can give prizes for the most accurate spoon, the simplest spoon, etc.

Skits, puppets, role playing: Children can use puppets or role playing to act out what to do when a younger child has diarrhea. They can cut a large mouth in a 'gourd baby', and actually give it Special Drink and food.

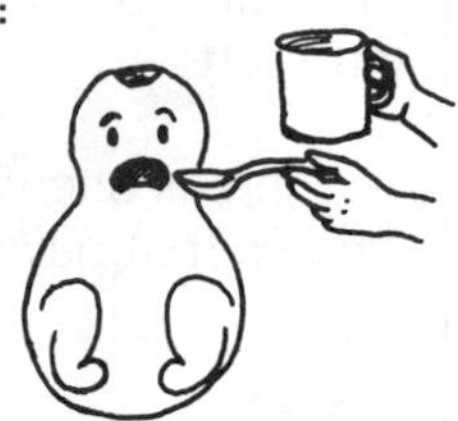

TEACHING OTHERS

After the children have learned about diarrhea and dehydration, they can help teach others. Here are a few possibilities:

- Children can put on demonstrations, plays, or puppet shows to convince people that giving liquids and Special Drink can save children's lives.
- They can discuss what they learn with their parents, and help prepare Special Drink when the baby has diarrhea.
- School children who took part in this activity can teach children who do not go to school because they have to care for younger brothers and sisters.
- Children from older grades can help teach these ideas to children in the younger grades.

FINDING OUT HOW WELL THE ACTIVITY WORKED

The group can make counts each month (or after 6 months or a year) to find out:

- How many children (or their mothers) have made the Special Drink for persons with diarrhea?
- How many children have had diarrhea?
- How many (if any) died?

Ask any child who has prepared the Special Drink for a brother or sister with diarrhea to tell his story at school. He can explain how he (or his mother) made the Drink and used it, any problems he had, and if it seemed to help.

MORE IDEAS FOR HELPING CHILDREN LEARN AND TEACH

Avoiding parent-child conflict over new ideas

One big doubt often raised about the CHILD-to-child Program is this:

People, including parents, often have very fixed ideas about managing common illnesses. **Is it fair to ask children to take home new ideas that may conflict with the beliefs and customs of their parents?** Could this weaken children's respect for their parents or for local traditions? Or will it make parents angry with the children and, perhaps, with the school?

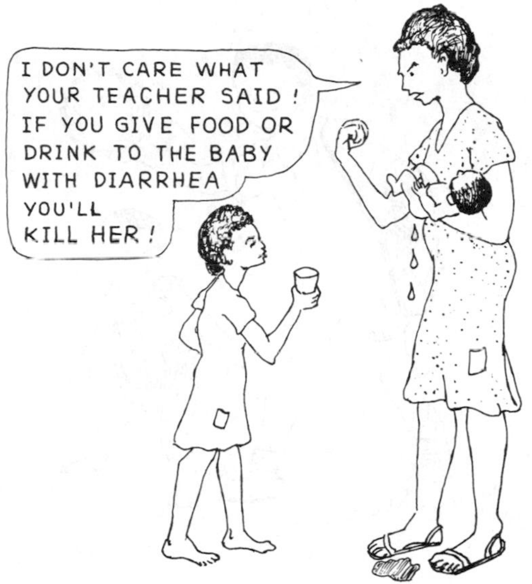
I DON'T CARE WHAT YOUR TEACHER SAID ! IF YOU GIVE FOOD OR DRINK TO THE BABY WITH DIARRHEA YOU'LL KILL HER !

Will the new ideas children learn from CHILD-to-child get them in trouble at home?

These are valid questions. In many areas, for example, parents believe it is harmful to give a child with diarrhea anything to eat or drink. They argue from experience that giving food or drink to the child may make him have another watery stool more quickly. How, then, can a boy or girl convince parents that, even though the sick child continues to have diarrhea or to vomit, it is very important to give lots of liquid and also food?

There are no easy answers to these questions, but one thing is clear. In a program such as CHILD-to-child, **it is not enough to work only with the children.** Health workers and teachers need to work with the parents and the community as well. There are ways they can help families become more open to the new ideas children bring home from school. These include discussion groups, mimeographed sheets (where enough people know how to read), and evenings of entertainment with role plays and skits.

It is best when both children and adults take part. A good way to win community acceptance is to involve parents and opinion leaders from the first. Ask the help of parents or the local health committee in planning CHILD-to-child activities and explaining them to other parents.

It is important that teachers and health workers show respect for the ideas and traditions of the children's parents. At the same time, **try to prepare the children for some of the difficulties that may arise** when they introduce their new ideas at home. Role playing and story telling are good ways to do this.

To follow is an example of a story that can be used to help children learn and teach about diarrhea, dehydration, and Special Drink.

ABDUL AND SERI

A CHILDREN'S STORY FROM INDONESIA*

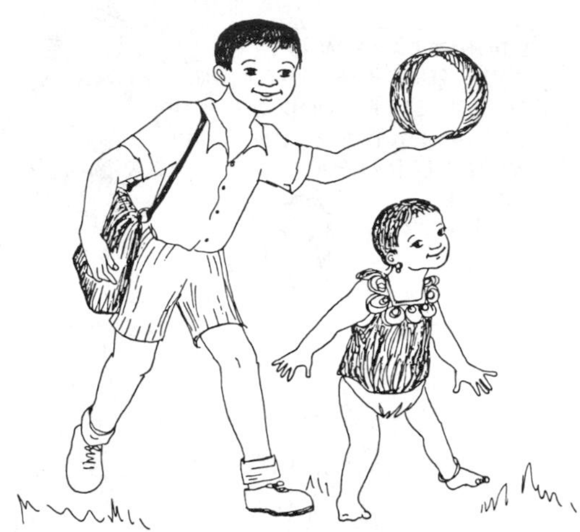

Abdul ran home from school almost as fast as on the day his sister Seri had been born. As soon as he saw her in the court-yard, his eyes lit up, for although Abdul was already 8 years old, he loved to play with his little sister.

Seri was only one and a half years old. She would clap her hands in delight when he made funny faces at her, or giggle when he counted her toes. He had helped her with her first steps, picking her up gently when she tumbled.

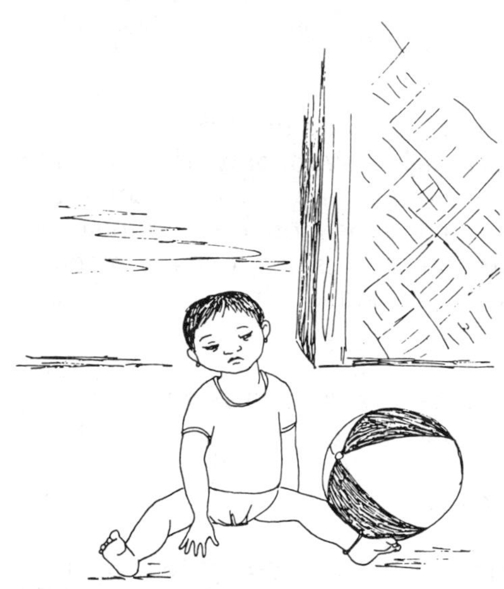

But what was wrong today? Usually Seri toddled straight for her favorite Abdul with her arms outstretched. But now she just sat on the porch and gazed at him with dull eyes. Quickly he lifted her up to his hip. He noticed that she must not have had her usual bath before he came home, because she had an unpleasant smell about her.

Their grandma greeted him with a tired voice. Worried, Abdul asked her, "Is Seri sick? Why does she act like this?" "She's had several watery bowel movements today," answered Grandma, "and she's been very fussy, Abdul. You must not let her have any food or drink so that the diarrhea will stop and she will get better."

***Note:** This story and its pictures are reproduced with permission from John Rohde, M.D. This or similar stories should be adapted to fit the situation and language of children in your area.

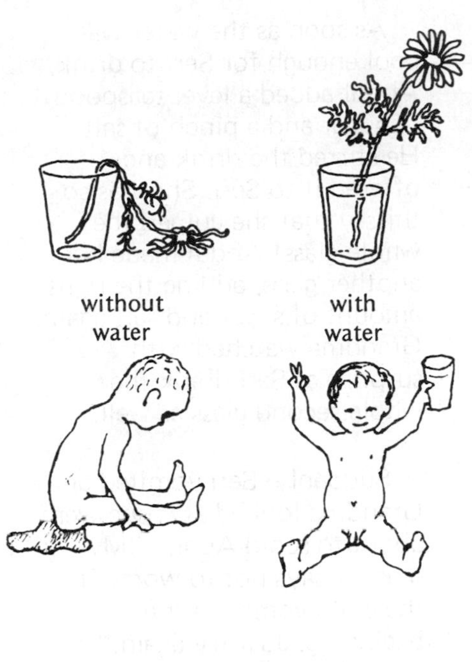

Abdul thought for a moment, and then he took a deep breath. "But Grandma," he cried out, "my teacher told me that a watery stool can be very dangerous. If the body loses water, it's like a plant that isn't watered. First it gets weak, and then it dies! We have to give Seri enough to drink so she won't be weak like this."

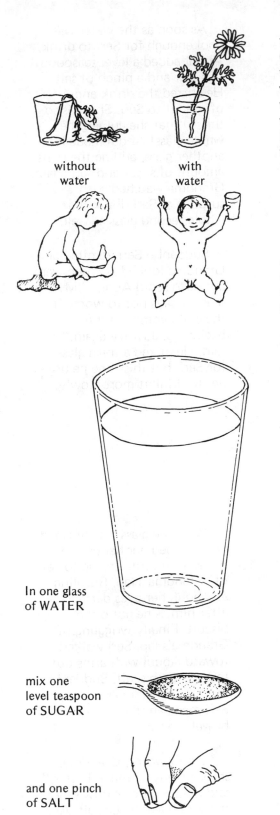

Grandma could feel how much Abdul believed in what he was saying, and she was very proud that her grandchild had a chance to go to school and learn new things. But still, no one had ever given any food or drink to a child with watery stools as long as she could remember. Then, while Abdul looked at her with pleading eyes and waited for her response, she thought of one of her own dear children she had lost after only 2 days of watery stools. And what about little Tini next door, who had died the same way? Grandma sighed and said gently to Abdul, "Perhaps your teacher is right. Maybe we should try a new way. What does she say we ought to do?"

In one glass of WATER

mix one level teaspoon of SUGAR

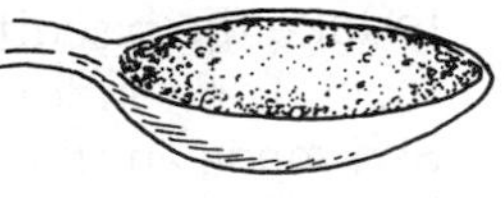

and one pinch of SALT

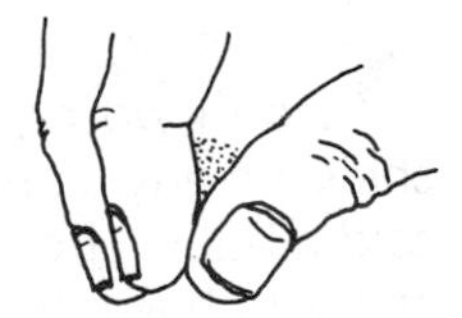

Abdul looked at his grandmother with new respect, put Seri into her arms, and urged her to follow him. Quickly, he put some water on to boil* and afterwards (while they waited for it to cool) he told Grandma the simple recipe that would help Seri. Grandma could hardly believe that one level teaspoon of sugar and a pinch of salt in a glass of boiled water would be the right thing to give Seri, but she was determined to let Abdul try.

*The delay caused by boiling may not be wise. See the discussion on p. **15**-3. (Editor's note.)

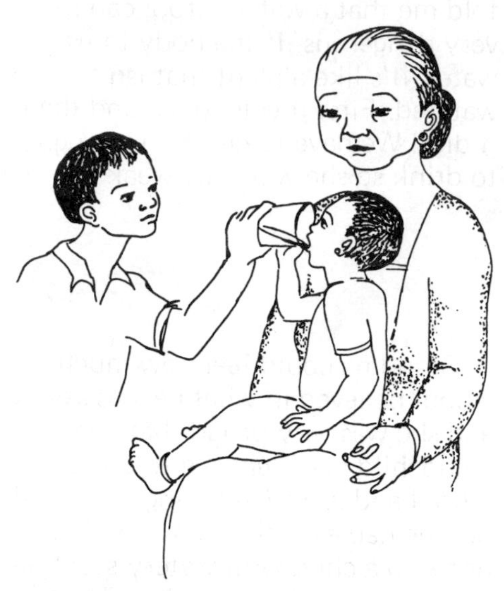

As soon as the water was cool enough for Seri to drink, Abdul added a level teaspoon of sugar and a pinch of salt. He stirred the drink and offered it to Seri. She was so thirsty that she gulped the whole glass! Abdul made her another glass, adding the right amount of sugar and salt again. Grandma watched with surprise as Seri drank the whole second glass as well.

Suddenly, Seri vomited and Grandma looked as if she were about to scold Abdul. "My teacher says not to worry if the child vomits in the beginning. Just try again," he said. He mixed a third glass for Seri, but this time he urged her to drink it more slowly.

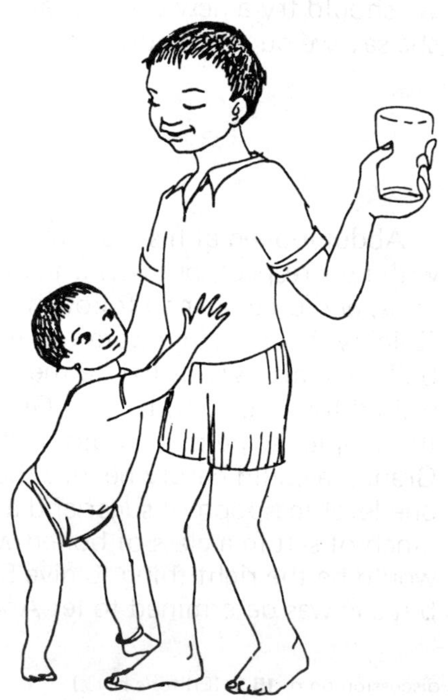

When the glass was finished, Seri clapped her hands and began to squirm, trying to get off Grandma's lap. Burbling at Abdul, her eyes darted after him as he got out a biscuit. Finally wriggling off Grandma's lap, Seri walked toward Abdul with arms out to take the biscuit. Suddenly, much to Grandma's dismay, Seri made another watery bowel movement.

"Don't worry, Grandma, she's already so much better," said Abdul. "Look how eager she is to have the biscuit. And she's still thirsty! She's trying to reach the glass."

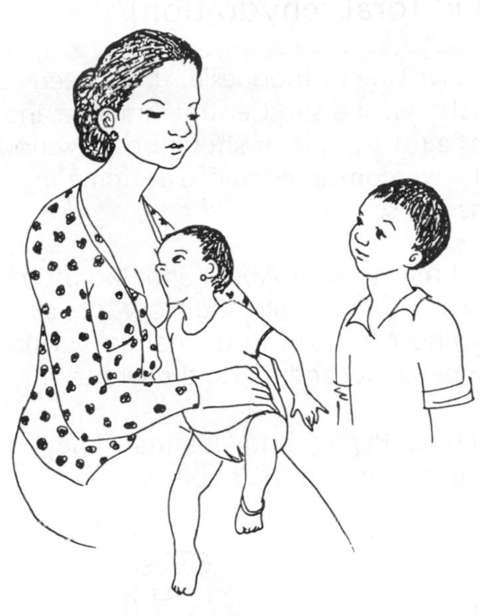

Abdul had just helped Seri finish another glass of the Special Drink, when his mother arrived home from her trip to the market. "How is Seri?" she asked Grandma anxiously. Seri moved toward her mother's voice, her eyes bright with recognition. "Why, she's much better, I see. I'm so relieved. Not giving her anything to eat or drink must have helped her."

"Oh, no," said Grandma, smiling at Abdul. "We've tried a new way, and look how Seri has changed since this morning. Abdul, tell your mother what you've given Seri."

"I'll wait till you nurse her, Mother. She'll be even happier then," answered Abdul.

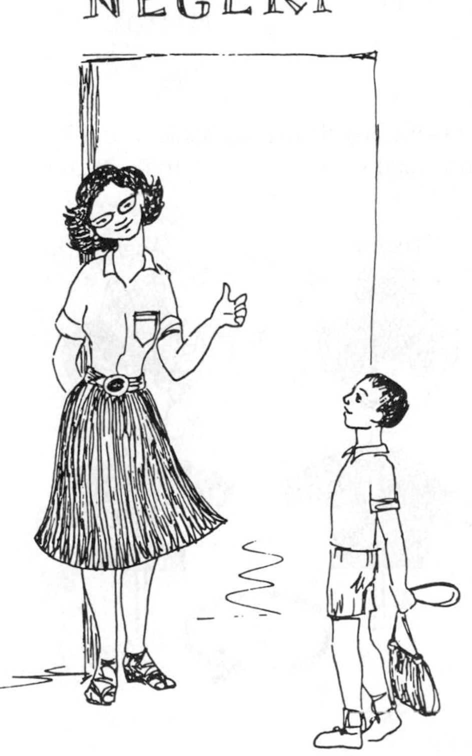

The next day, Abdul got to school early. He shyly told his teacher that he had tried the recipe she had taught the class to use in case anybody in their families had watery stools. His teacher was very happy that Abdul had remembered to use 1 level teaspoon of sugar and a pinch of salt in the glass of boiled water. She was even happier to know that, although Seri had had a watery stool two more times that day, today the diarrhea had stopped completely.

"Make sure she keeps drinking and eats some extra meals so she'll be just as strong as she was before," the teacher cautioned Abdul. "You've really learned well."

Abdul glowed inside. When school was over that day, he ran home with a happy heart to find Seri wanting to play, her arms outstretched and her eyes shining, waiting for a new game.

A puppet show about 'Special Drink' (oral rehydration)

Although the story of Abdul and Seri was written in Indonesia, it has been used with school children in Mexico and with health workers in Central America and Africa. Everyone enjoys the story and learns a lot from it. It shows how a school child—through love, concern, and good will—overcomes resistance at home in order to put into practice a 'new way' learned in school.

The school children in Ajoya, Mexico read the story of Abdul and Seri after doing the CHILD-to-child activity on diarrhea. They thought the story was so important that everyone in the village should hear it. So with the help of a village health worker, they decided to put on a puppet show and invite the whole village.

They changed the names of Abdul and Seri to 'Pepito' and 'Juanita'. They even changed the story somewhat, to seem more like things in their village.

They made simple stick puppets like this one.

Perhaps the health workers you train can help children in their villages to do the same.

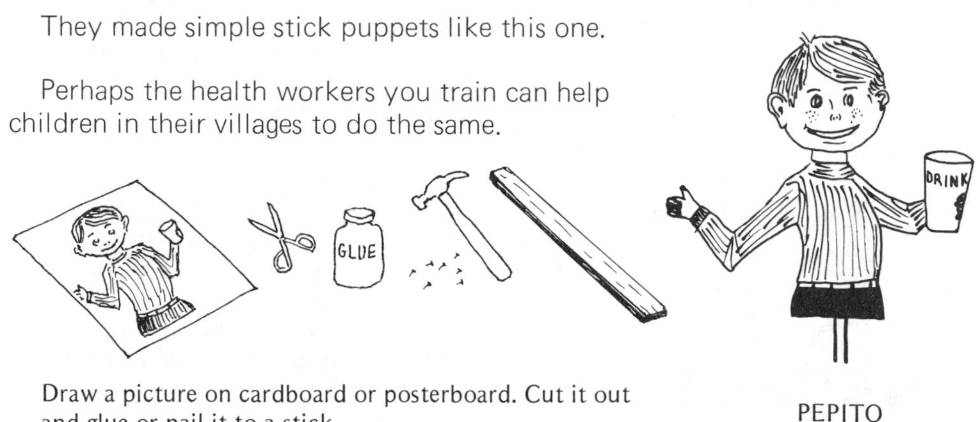

Draw a picture on cardboard or posterboard. Cut it out and glue or nail it to a stick.

PEPITO

If the puppet needs 2 expressions, put 2 cardboard drawings back to back. During the show, turn the puppet to show the face you want. (To make a puppet with 4 different expressions, see p. **27**-36.)

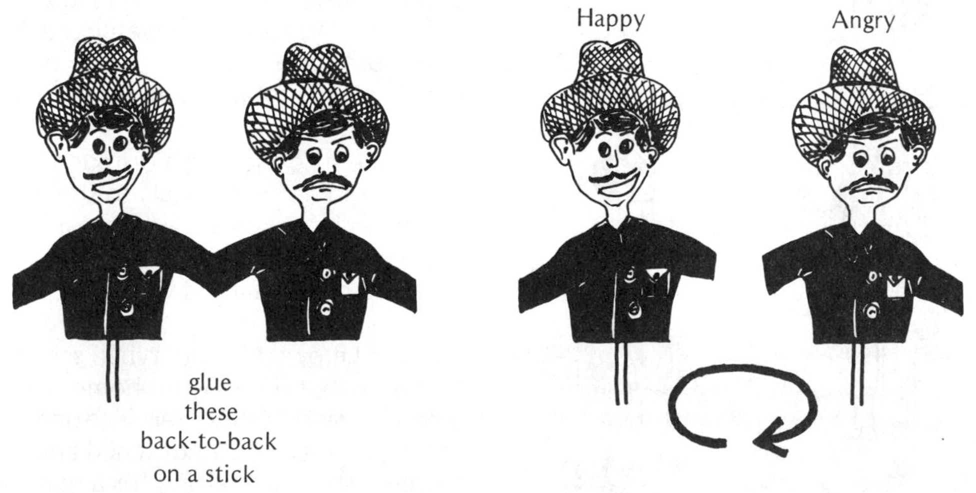

PEPITO'S FATHER

The children's puppet show in Ajoya was a huge success. Here are some photos from their performance.

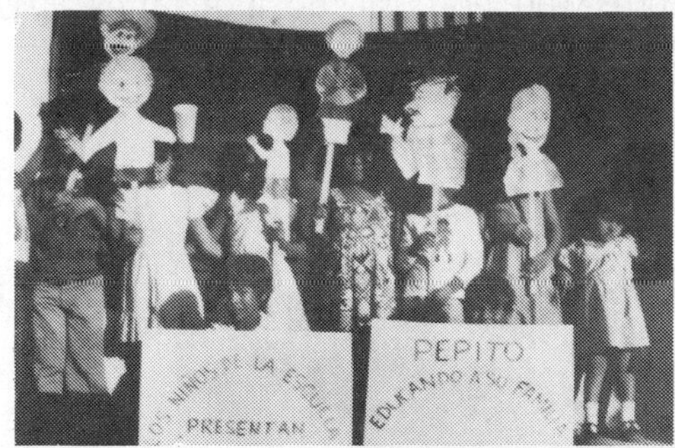

Here the children greet the audience before the puppet show begins. The sign in Spanish says, THE SCHOOL CHILDREN PRESENT: "PEPITO TEACHES HIS FAMILY."

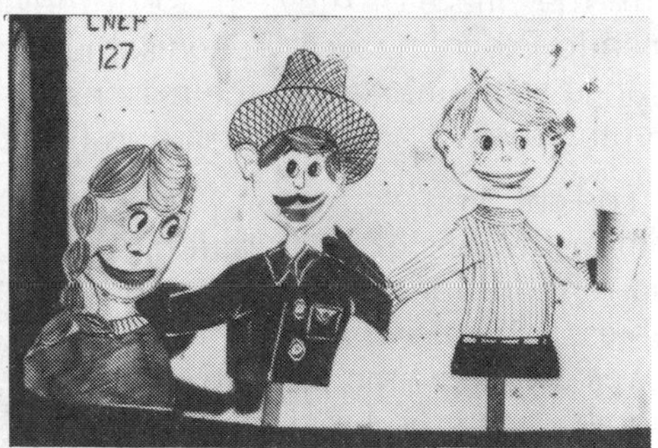

Here is Pepito, explaining to his parents how to make 'Special Drink' for his baby sister who has diarrhea.

Children can make the puppet show even more exciting by using a 'gourd baby' with water in it—so the baby can actually have diarrhea and vomit.

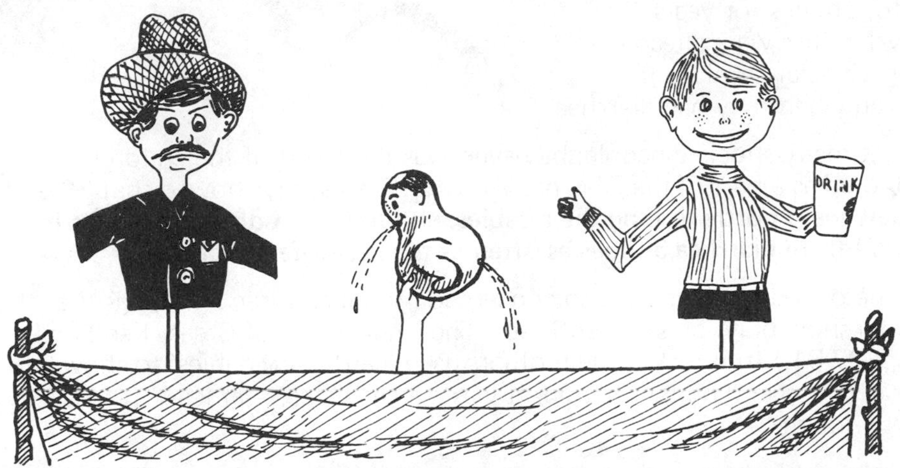

Or they can make a puppet with some rubber or plastic tubes attached to jars of muddy water. When a child blows into the jar, the puppet 'vomits' or has 'diarrhea'.

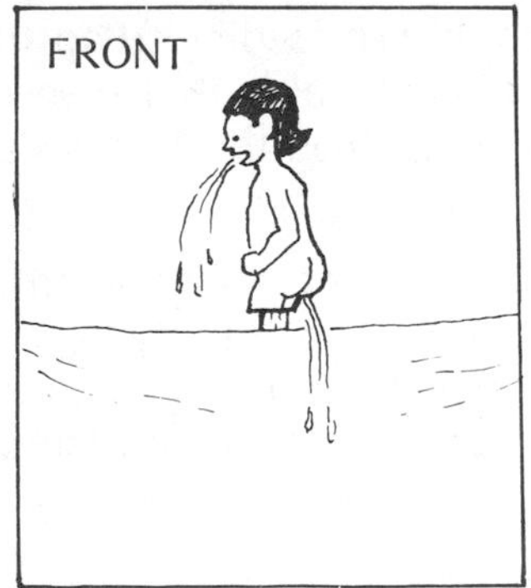

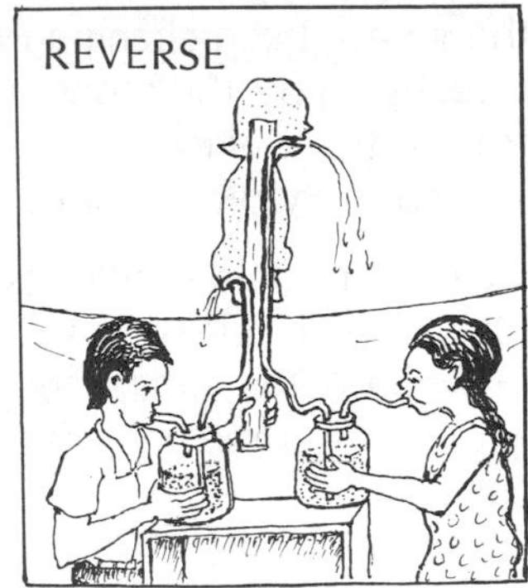

Color slides or filmstrip with a script of the play, "Pepito Teaches His Family," are available from the Hesperian Foundation.

PARENTS' RESPONSE TO CHILD-to-child

In the village of Ajoya, most of the parents were enthusiastic about the CHILD-to-child Program, even though some of the new ways of doing things seemed strange to them. Among the reasons for the community's acceptance were the evening theater and puppet shows (including "Pepito"*).

The children also gave demonstrations of dehydration and rehydration using the 'gourd babies', which everyone loved! It was the first time that most people understood that the sunken soft spot is caused by water loss from diarrhea.

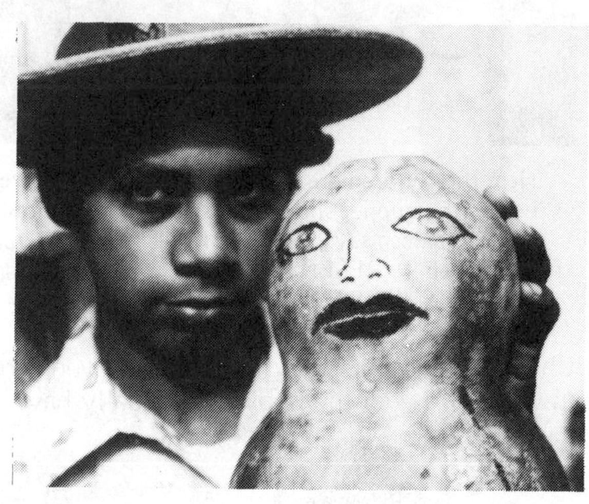

In Ajoya, the boys and girls found that most of their parents accepted the idea of giving Special Drink to children with diarrhea. The local health workers had been explaining this to families for years. So many families were already giving Special Drink to their children when they had diarrhea.

What really shocked people, however, was the result of the children's survey conducted as a part of the Diarrhea Activity. This study showed that **70% of mothers were bottle feeding their babies,** and that **the bottle-fed babies in Ajoya suffered from diarrhea 5 times as often as the breast-fed babies!**

Some of the mothers were so concerned by the children's findings that they staged a short play, or 'skit', entitled "The Importance of Breast Feeding." (See p. **27**-31.) In this skit, the mothers used 'cardboard babies' to show various stages of good and poor nutrition. It was a great success—at least in terms of entertainment.

It is hard to say how much influence the children's study and the skit have had on the way village mothers feed their babies. Throughout Latin America, many mothers have been changing from breast feeding to bottle feeding, in part because of advertising by the producers of artificial milk. However, we have talked to several mothers who decided to breast feed their babies as a result of the children's study and the women's skit.

Apart from measurable results, however, the cooperation, concern, and fun that have come out of this CHILD-to-child activity have made it enormously worthwhile. What final effect it may have on the children themselves, when they grow up to become parents and perhaps leaders in their communities, we may never know.

---

*Besides the puppet show on using Special Drink, the children later presented a puppet show about "Care of the Teeth" (see p. **27**-37). These children's shows were performed on the same nights that villagers and health workers-in-training presented Village Theater productions.

PART FIVE

HEALTH IN RELATION TO FOOD, LAND, AND SOCIAL PROBLEMS

Part Five of this book focuses on ways in which health is influenced by human relationships. This has been a theme throughout this book. But here we look more closely at the problems that result from greed, unfair distribution of land and resources, and a social structure that favors the few at the expense of the many. We explore ways in which health workers can learn about these problems and help people to gain the awareness, self-confidence, and skills necessary to work together to change their situation.

In **Chapter 25** we examine the causes of malnutrition. We point out that hunger is usually caused, not by an overall shortage of farmland or food, but by unfair distribution. We explore ways to find out if children and other persons are well nourished or too thin. Then we consider ways that health workers can help people analyze their food problems and better meet their needs. Finally, we look at an alternative way to teach about 'food groups', focusing on the main foods in the local diet.

In **Chapter 26** we explore ways to help people look at the different causes of their problems, especially the human or social causes (cultural, economic, and political). We examine methods of helping people gain self-confidence and greater social awareness. We discuss both the possibilities and the pitfalls of applying popular 'conscientization' methods to health education. And we give examples of how these methods have helped villagers to improve health and overcome forms of exploitation at the community level.

Chapter 27 is about using popular theater as a means of raising people's awareness. We place this chapter at the end of the book (rather than with the chapter on role plays) because of the strong social content of the skits, plays, and puppet shows it gives as examples. These theater presentations, which deal with local problems affecting health, were put on in Mexico by village mothers, school children, and student health workers. They demonstrate two different possibilities for community involvement. First, the preparations and performances brought about greater awareness through the participation of both the actors and the audience. Second, the skits presented ways that poor families can join together to overcome the causes of their suffering and poor health. Most of the stories are based on true events.

These people's theater presentations show how people in some communities have struggled to find answers to their biggest problems. We believe they will provide both ideas and hope to others.

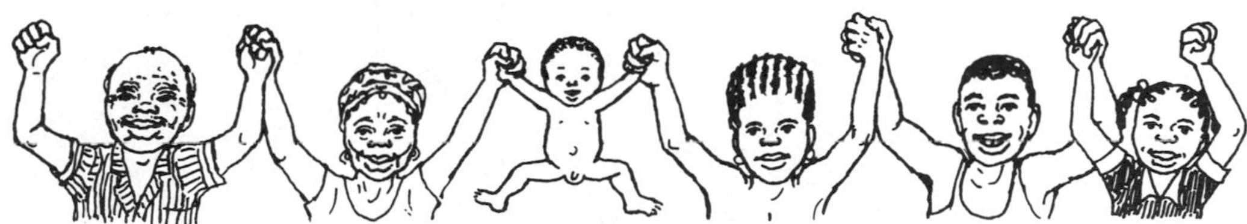

THE KEY TO HEALTH LIES IN THE PEOPLE THEMSELVES.

"Primary health care is generally only lacking when other rights are also being denied. Usually it is only lacking where the greed of some goes unchecked and unrecognized (or unacknowledged) as being the cause. Once primary health is accepted as a human right, then the primary health worker becomes, first and foremost, a political figure, involved in the life of the community in its integrity. With a sensitivity to the villagers and the community as a whole, he will be better able to diagnose and prescribe. Basically, though, he will bring about the health that is the birthright of the community by facing the more comprehensive political problems of oppression and injustice, ignorance, apathy, and misguided good will."

—Zafrullah Chowdhury, of Gonoshasthaya Kendra, a community-based health program in Bangladesh

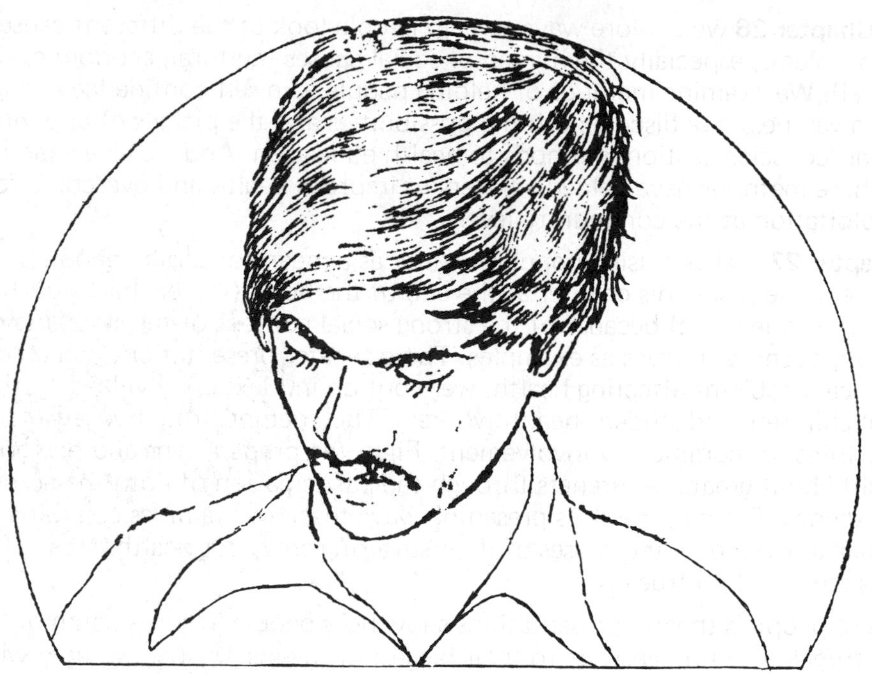

CHAPTER 25

Food First

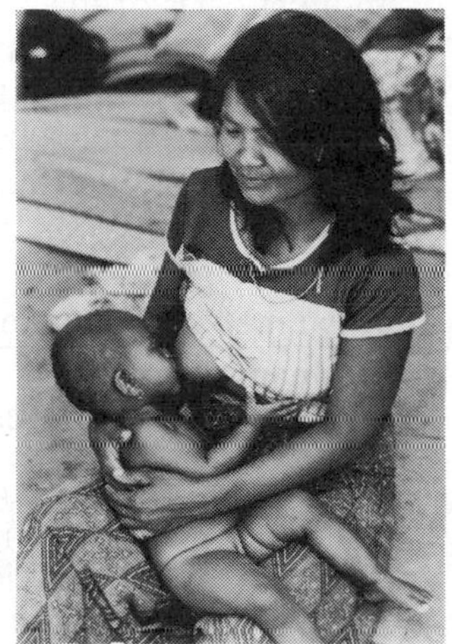

Good health depends on many things, but above all on getting enough to eat. A person who does not eat enough of the foods his body needs becomes thin and weak. He has trouble resisting infections and other illnesses. Also, disability and death from many diseases—especially diarrhea, measles, and tuberculosis—are more frequent in persons who are malnourished. Poor nutrition, with its related illnesses, is responsible for more deaths than any other problem, and is an especially great danger to young children.

Food must be a first concern for health work in a community where people are hungry or many children are malnourished.

LOOKING AT THE PROBLEM OF POOR NUTRITION

Before health workers begin specific nutrition activities, it is important for them to look at their people's food problems as a whole. Planners and experts have tried many approaches to combatting hunger and malnutrition. But in spite of billions spent on agricultural extension, the Green Revolution, irrigation systems, development projects, food supplements, and nutrition centers, **there are more malnourished children today than ever before in human history.**

One reason why so many approaches fail is that they are usually designed by persons who have never suffered from hunger or malnutrition themselves. Planners and scientists often are blind to important social factors that are painfully clear to the poor. As a result, new methods and technologies intended to reduce malnutrition repeatedly end up benefiting the well fed at the expense of the hungry. Health workers who unquestioningly follow the plans of outside experts can easily make similar mistakes.

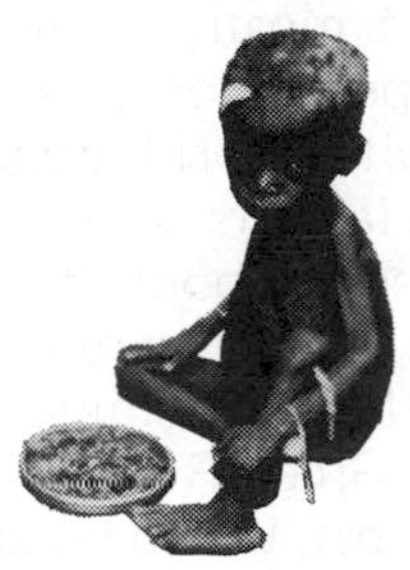

It is important, therefore, that health workers and their instructors not simply accept the standard approaches to working with nutritional problems. They need to critically examine the suggestions of outsiders and to use only what fits the needs of the people in their own area.

Any nutrition plan a health worker uses should be designed or adapted with the help of the people it is intended to serve.

The following discussion is based largely on our experience in Latin America, where unfair distribution (of land, resources, and power) is a main cause of malnutrition. Of course, the situation is different in each country and each village. Let your students decide how much or how little of this discussion applies to their own communities.

Poor nutrition and poverty

In most parts of the world, poor nutrition is closely linked with poverty. This is so obvious that it might not seem necessary to say. Yet a surprising number of programs do not look directly at poverty and its causes when they teach about health and nutrition. If health workers are to help people get at the root of their problems, however, the causes of hunger and poverty need to be carefully explored.

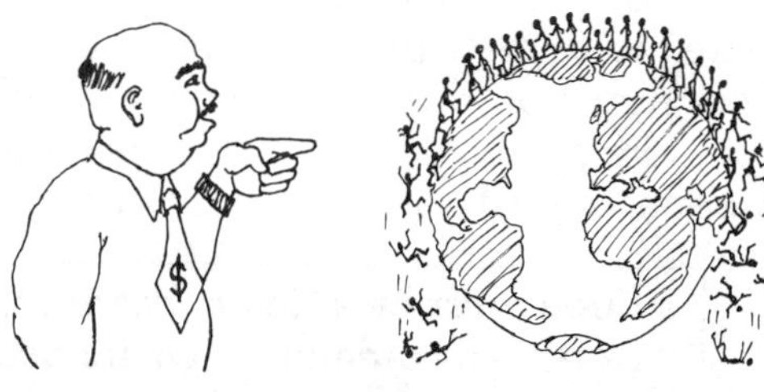

The rich man's explanation of hunger:

too many people,
too little land and resources.

The common explanation for the increasing amount of hunger in the world is that the population is growing too fast: there are too many people and not enough land, food, and resources to go around. Therefore, efforts to overcome hunger have focused on 1) population control, 2) increasing the productivity of existing farmland by using irrigation, high-yield crops, fertilizers, and other Green Revolution methods, 3) opening up new farmland by using dams and irrigation systems, and 4) massive foreign aid and food supplements in times of famine.

All these activities combined, however, have not led to less hunger in the world. Each has failed for a variety of reasons—but mainly because none combats the underlying social causes of hunger.

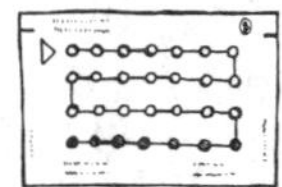

1. Population control efforts have not had much success because people with little economic security often cannot afford to have small families (see p. **23**-2).

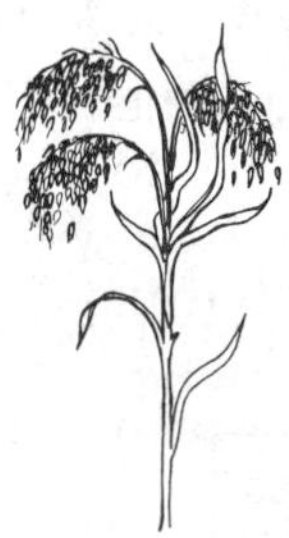

2. The Green Revolution actually made the problem of malnutrition worse in many areas. High-yield ***hybrids*** (artificially bred varieties of grain) require expensive fertilizers, insecticides, and irrigation. Persons who ended up growing these hybrids were mostly the more fortunate farmers who could afford the extra expenses, or who qualified for loans. Their increased production with hybrids gave them an even greater advantage over the poorest farmers. Also, it temporarily pushed down grain prices. This forced the poorest farmers to sell their land to those growing the hybrids. The result: more landless, underpaid farmworkers and more hungry families. More food may have been produced through the Green Revolution, but it was not available to those who needed it most. World hunger increased.

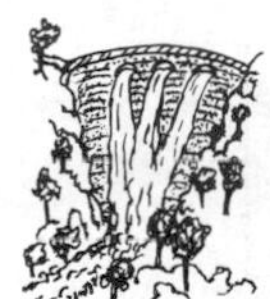

3. In a similar way, new dams that were designed to open more farmland through irrigation have actually flooded many poor farmers off their land. Meanwhile, the newly irrigated lands typically end up in the hands of wealthier farmers.

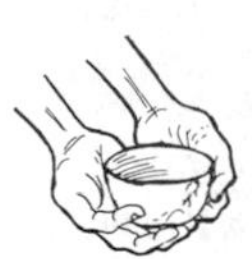

4. Unfortunately, foreign aid and food supplements in times of famine have tended to increase the poverty and dependency of poor countries and poor families. Foreign food aid has often pushed down local grain prices, causing the ruin of struggling small farmers. In any case, much of the food sent as aid ends up in the hands of the rich, not the hungry.

The poor people's explanation of hunger: unfair distribution of land and resources, too much in the hands of too few.

Studies by various groups, including the U.N. Food and Agriculture Organization, the *New Internationalist,* the Institute for Food and Development Policy, and the Human Needs/Global Development Program have shown that:

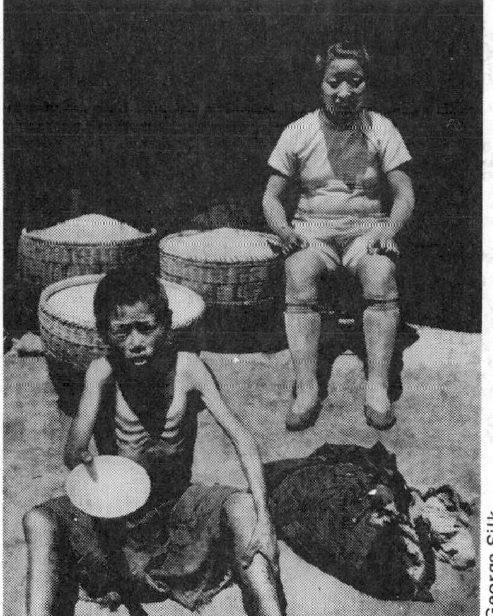

The problem of hunger is not caused by shortages, but by unfair distribution. Or as Mahatma Gandhi put it, "There is enough for every man's need, but not for every man's greed."

- There is plenty of food in the world today to feed all people adequately.
- There is enough farmland to feed 2 to 3 times the present world population. However, much of the land held by big property owners is unused or poorly used.
- For the world's 3 major grain crops (rice, wheat, and maize), the most productive systems are those organized on the basis of small-owner operations. The most productive landlord system yields less than half as much per hectare as most small-owner systems.
- In all the major famines of the 1970's, there was enough food stored within the affected countries to feed all the people adequately. But the price of food rose too high for people to afford. Many of those with extra food hoarded it instead of sharing it with the starving.
- There is no scarcity of total resources, but rather a tremendous misuse of them. In the course of 2 weeks, the world's governments spend $4,000,000,000 on weapons of war—enough to feed everyone on earth for an entire year!
- Increased agricultural assistance has never brought lasting increases in food production in any country with a big-landowner/tenant-farmer system.

World hunger is not a technical, but rather a social problem. It exists not so much because of shortage of land, food, or wealth, but because these are very unequally distributed.

Where distribution is most unfair and the rights of the working people most limited, the problem of hunger is greatest:

IN THE WHOLE WORLD:

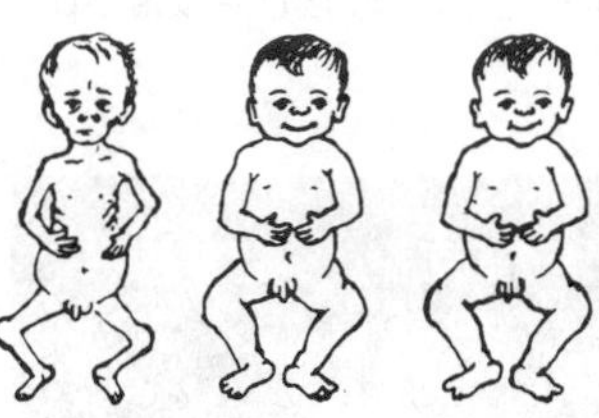

1 OUT OF 3

One out of three children in the world is undernourished. But in some countries, more than two out of three children are undernourished. These are usually the countries where the differences between rich and poor are most striking. These are the places where a small, powerful group has control over most of the land and resources. Wages are low. Production of 'cash crops' for export is high. Often foreign companies and governments have considerable control over the economy. And the people's right to organize or take part in planning and decision making is severely limited.

IN COUNTRIES WITH WORST SOCIAL INJUSTICE:

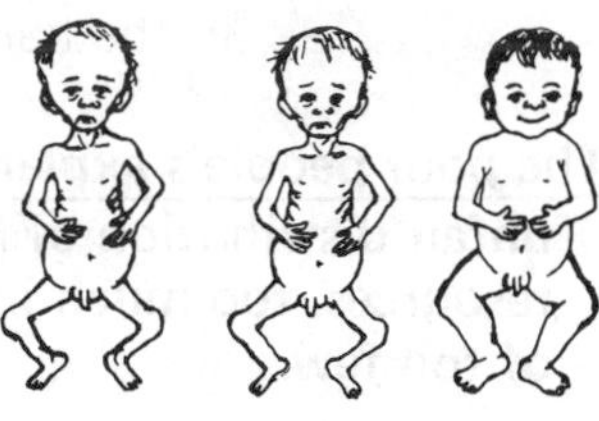

2 OUT OF 3

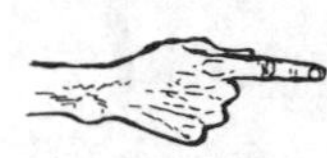

The number of hungry children in a country or community may be one of the most accurate measures of social justice and human rights.

Poverty, the root cause of poor nutrition and hunger, results from an unequal distribution of wealth, land, and decision-making power. In the world today . . .

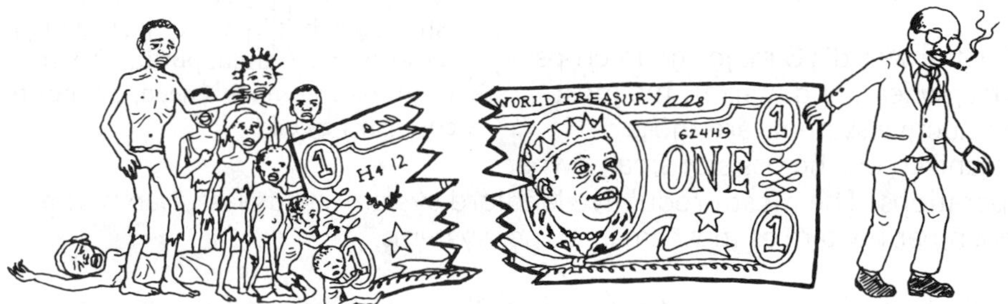

50% of the people try to survive on 10% of the wealth and resources,

while the richest 10% control over 50% of the wealth and resources.

This unequal division exists between rich and poor countries. It also exists between the rich and poor within many countries, even within villages. In areas where unfair distribution affects health, nutrition programs that do not help the poor deal with this problem are only treating, and not really trying to prevent, hunger and related illnesses.

WHAT ARE REALISTIC ANSWERS TO HUNGER?

Meaningful answers must come from those who do the work to produce the food. Leaders of the poor point out that **in places where unfair distribution is a cause of malnutrition, lasting solutions can only come through fairer distribution**—of land, resources, and decision making. In many countries this will require major social change, with the formation of new governments that fairly represent the working people.

Clearly, however, small community-based programs and village health workers are not in a position to combat national problems singlehandedly. In countries where the rights of the poor are severely restricted, they even may have to be careful of how and with whom they discuss these questions. (See 'A call for courage and caution', page **Back**-1.)

But whether or not the problem of unfair distribution is openly discussed and combatted, community-based programs need to keep it in mind. People can be helped to look at their food problems and carry out nutrition activities in ways that develop their self-confidence, determination, and cooperative spirit. This will help prepare them to work for far-reaching changes when the time is right.

We cannot wait for the big changes that may put an end to hunger. In whatever ways they can, large and small, health workers need to make sure the children in their communities get enough to eat. **The children who are hungry need food now.**

We are guilty of many errors and many faults,
but our worst crime is abandoning the children,
neglecting the fountain of life.
Many of the things we need can wait.
The child cannot.
Right now is the time his bones are being formed,
his blood is being made,
and his senses are being developed.
To him we cannot answer 'Tomorrow'.
His name is 'Today'.

—Gabriela Mistral, of Chile

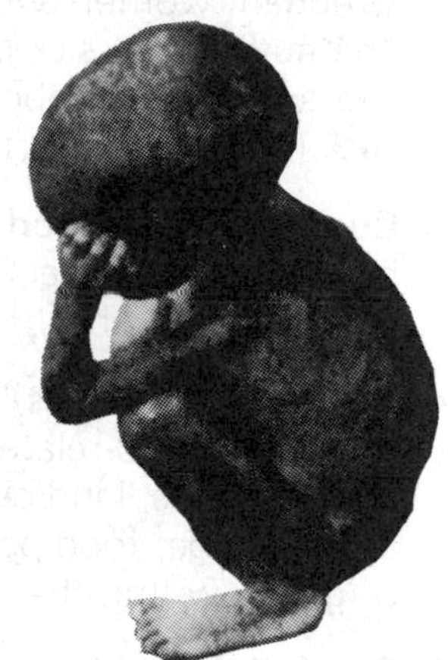

His name is 'Today'.

Far-reaching change—which is the only final answer to hunger—will take time and well-organized preparation. But sometimes, within their local areas, health programs or health workers can help people achieve greater fairness or more control of land, food, marketing, or specific resources. This can mean more food for the poor—through greater self-reliance. These possibilities will be discussed later in this chapter, and in the rest of Part Five.

SOLVING NUTRITION PROBLEMS IN THE COMMUNITY

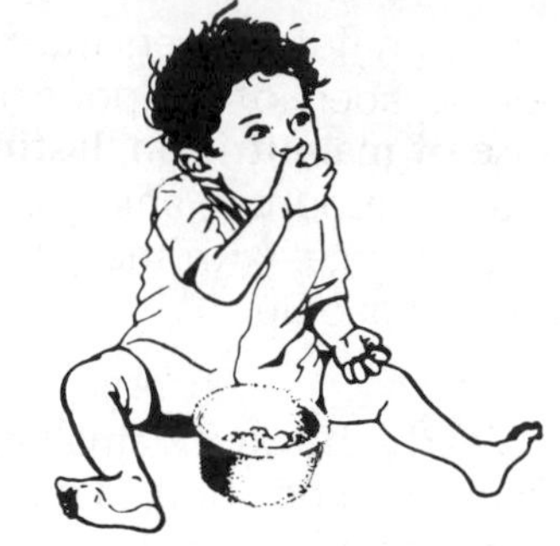

In helping health workers learn about food needs in their communities and what to do about them, it makes sense to use a problem-solving approach. Health workers will be better prepared to put their learning into practice if they **learn by actually working with people and their needs.** This means moving the focus of learning out of the classroom and into the community.

To follow is a list of steps that health workers may find useful in approaching the nutritional and food problems in their communities. Although it may help to discuss the steps first, they can best be learned through practice. (Chapter 6 gives additional ideas for ways to make 'field work' in nearby communities a basic part of the training program.)

Suggested steps for approaching food problems in a community:

1. **Know (or get to know) the people well.** Try to understand their attitudes, beliefs, traditions, and fears, especially those that relate to food. (See Chapter 7.)

2. Try to **find out how much malnutrition there is in your community and who is most affected.** Often children suffer most from malnutrition, then pregnant women and nursing mothers, and then old people. Be sure to check the nutrition of sick persons. This is often a big problem because of traditional fears and beliefs about what people should or should not eat and drink when sick (or after childbirth—see ***Where There Is No Doctor,*** page 123).

3. **Consider which food and nutrition problems are most important**—in terms of how the people feel about them (felt needs) and in terms of how much they affect people's health and well-being (real needs).

4. **Look for the causes** (often a combination or chain of causes) of malnutrition and other food-related problems. These causes may include people's habits and attitudes, land ownership, farming practices, water shortages, storage and spoilage, food prices, marketing, and wages. Try to separate causes that originate within the community from those that come from outside.

5. **Carefully consider the obstacles** that you might meet in trying to solve specific problems. (Many nutrition projects have failed because of obstacles that were not considered ahead of time.)

6. Together with the community, **decide which problems to attack first.** Try to be sure that . . .
   - the people recognize the importance of the problems they choose and are interested in working together to solve them, and
   - the first problems chosen are fairly easy to combat, and that action taken is likely to give quick, obviously beneficial results.

TAKING A SURVEY TO FIND OUT ABOUT NUTRITION NEEDS IN YOUR COMMUNITY

Some food and nutrition problems tend to go unnoticed, even by those who live in the village or neighborhood where they exist. A good way to find out about these problems is to take a simple nutrition survey. As we discussed in Chapter 6, surveys ***of*** people often reduce their sense of dignity and control over their lives. However, surveys ***by*** the people in a community at times can help increase their understanding and control of the factors affecting their health. The health worker can serve as the survey coordinator or ***facilitator*** (someone who makes it easier).

A simple community survey to check for nutritional problems can perform at least 4 functions:

1. It can help people determine **how many** persons in their area are poorly nourished. If more than 1 out of every 7 children (15%) is underweight or too thin, then the community probably has a serious food problem.
2. It can help show **which children and which families** have the greatest need and deserve special care and concern.
3. The health worker can use the survey to help **interest, inform, and involve** various groups in the community—mothers, fathers, school children, and community leaders.
4. The survey can provide a **basis for comparison** at a later date. People will be able to see if the action they have taken to improve nutrition in their village has been successful.

Different groups from the community can be involved in different aspects of a survey. For example:

- School children might check to see whether their younger sisters and brothers are well nourished or too thin.
- Midwives could help in reviewing the nutrition of pregnant women.
- Mothers could find out how many babies are breast fed or bottle fed, and how this affects the babies' health.
- Fathers might do a study on how the drinking habits of men affect the nutrition of different families.

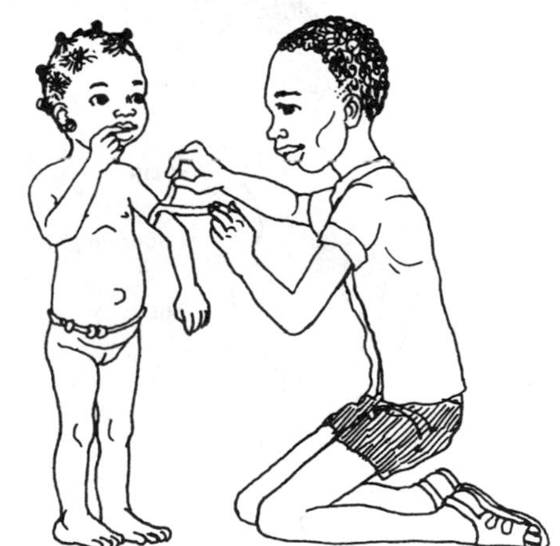

By helping to conduct their own survey, the villagers become more aware of the problems and the need for action to combat them.

However, **if surveys are to be conducted by untrained people, they should be simple, quick and interesting.** On the following pages we explore a variety of survey methods.

Finding out about the nutrition of children in a community

We can usually recognize children who are severely malnourished without taking measurements. Here are two examples from ***Where There Is No Doctor,*** pages 112 and 113:

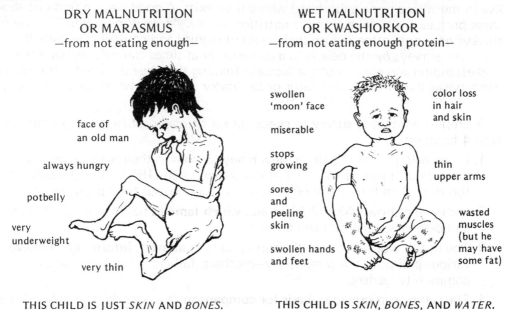

DRY MALNUTRITION OR MARASMUS
—from not eating enough—

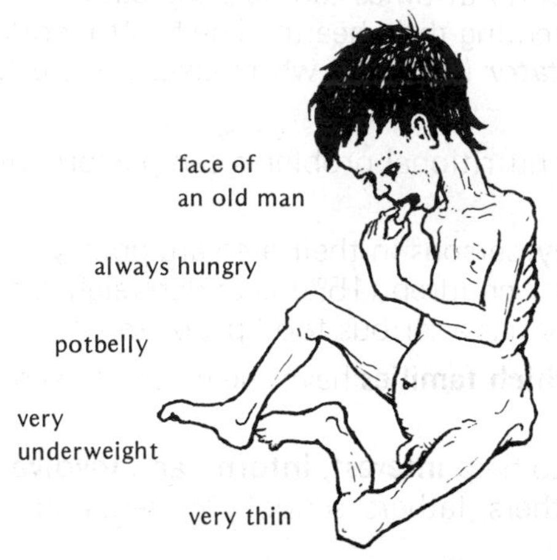

THIS CHILD IS JUST *SKIN* AND *BONES.*

WET MALNUTRITION OR KWASHIORKOR
—from not eating enough protein—

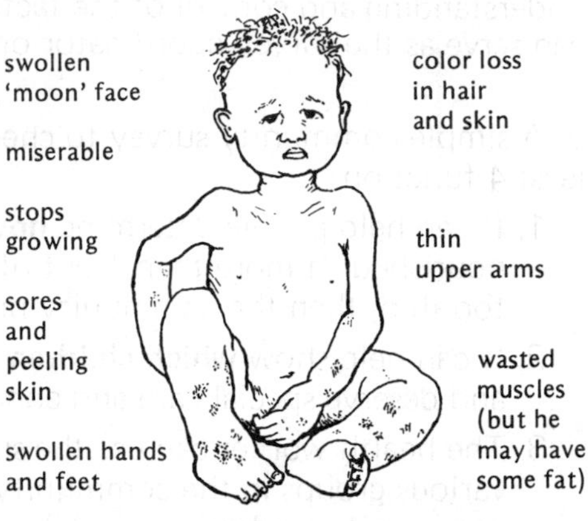

THIS CHILD IS *SKIN, BONES,* AND *WATER.*

But **for every child who is seriously malnourished like the two above, there are usually many others who are less severely malnourished,** like this:

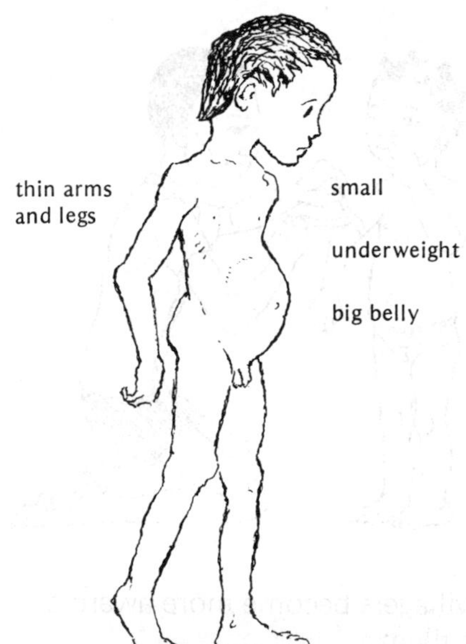

This more common form of malnutrition is not always obvious. The child simply does not grow or gain weight as fast as a well-nourished child. Although he may appear rather small and thin, he usually does not look sick. However, because he is poorly nourished, he may lack the strength ***(resistance)*** to fight infections. So he tends to get sick more frequently than a well-nourished child.

Children with this form of malnutrition suffer from more diarrhea and more colds. Their colds usually last longer and are more likely to turn into pneumonia. Measles, tuberculosis, and many other infectious diseases are far more dangerous for these malnourished children. More of them die.

It is important to find children like this and make sure they get the special care and food they need before they become seriously ill. Because it is not always obvious which children are growing well and which are not, some form of measurement is often helpful.

Measuring to find which children are too thin or not growing well

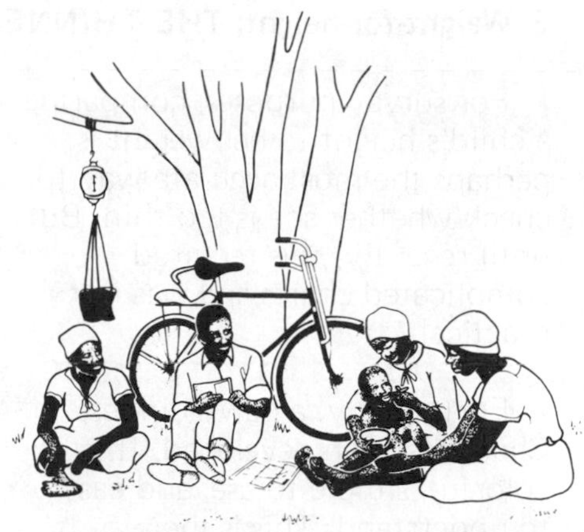

In Zimbabwe, 'health scouts' cycle from village to village weighing children, recording weights, and encouraging mothers to attend under-fives clinics.

Parents often do not take their underweight children to the health post until they are seriously ill. By then it may be too late. Even if health workers ask mothers to bring all children under five each month, the sickest or weakest are sometimes left at home. It is therefore important that health workers visit all homes and try to identify those children who are too thin or need special care.

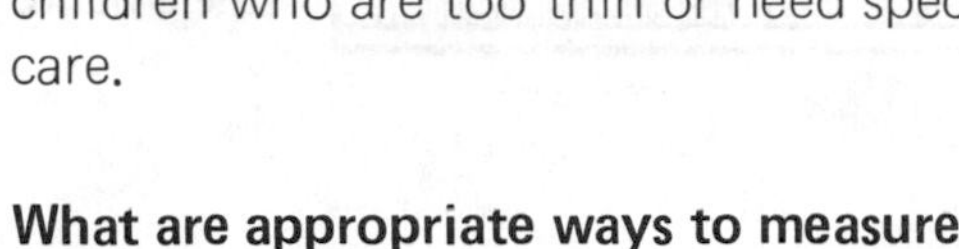

What are appropriate ways to measure thinness of children under five?

We will discuss three useful methods: 1) weight-for-age, 2) weight-for-height, and 3) arm thickness. The method you choose will depend on local resources, needs, and who does the measuring.

1. Weight-for-age: THE CHILD HEALTH CHART

The use of the Child Health Chart for individual children is explained in ***Where There Is No Doctor,*** (pages 297-304); and in much greater detail in David Morley's book, **See How They Grow.** Methods for teaching health workers and mothers to use the charts this way are on pages **22**-15 to **22**-19 of this book.

For the purpose of a nutrition survey, however, a single weighing of all children under five can be recorded on one chart.

Below are examples of survey charts for two different villages. Each dot on the charts represents the age and weight of a different child.

BREASTVILLE

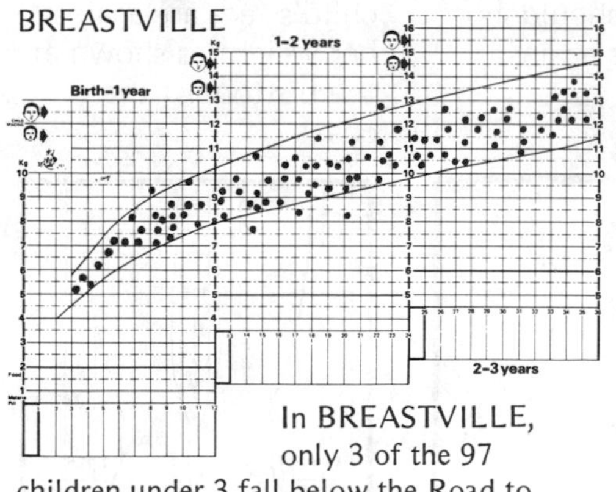

In BREASTVILLE, only 3 of the 97 children under 3 fall below the Road to Health (below the two curved lines). Malnutrition in young children is not a big problem in this village.

BOTTLEBURGH

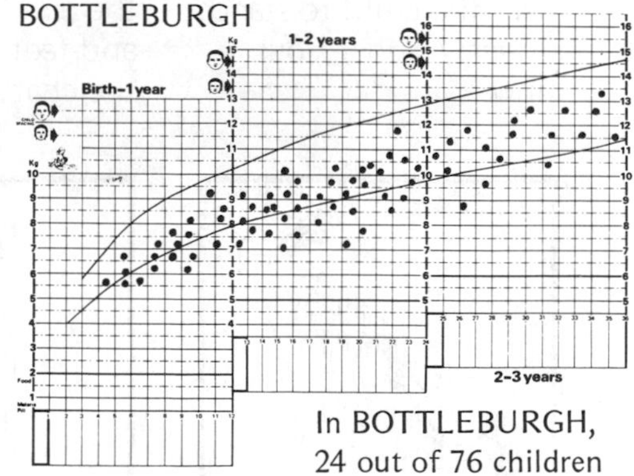

In BOTTLEBURGH, 24 out of 76 children are below the Road to Health. This village has a serious problem with the nutrition of young children. (What do you think might explain the big difference between the two villages?)

2. Weight-for-height: THE THINNESS CHART

For survey purposes, comparing a child's height to her weight is perhaps the most accurate way to check whether she is too thin. But until recently, this required complicated charts and was not practical.

Fortunately, a new Thinness Chart has been developed. It is colorful, simple to use, and easy to understand. This is the way it is used:

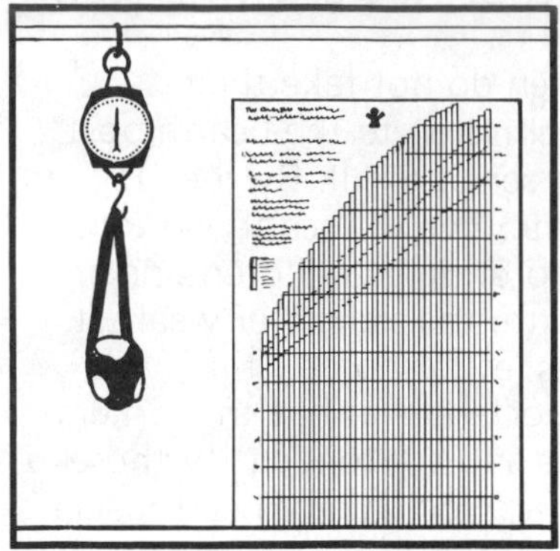

Hang the chart on a wall near the scales.

Be sure the bottom edge of it touches the ground.

1. Weigh the child.

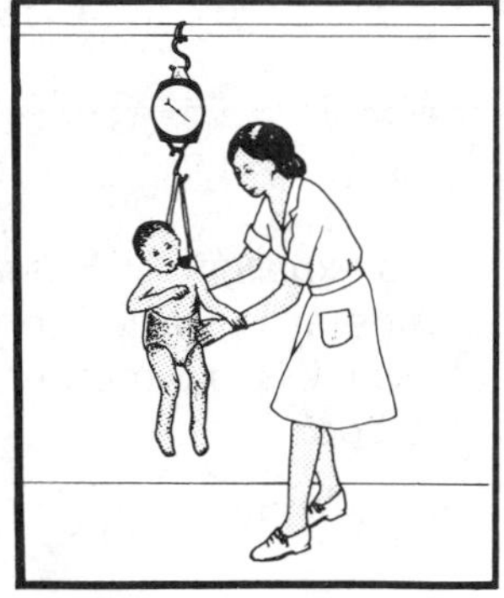

2. Note the weight.

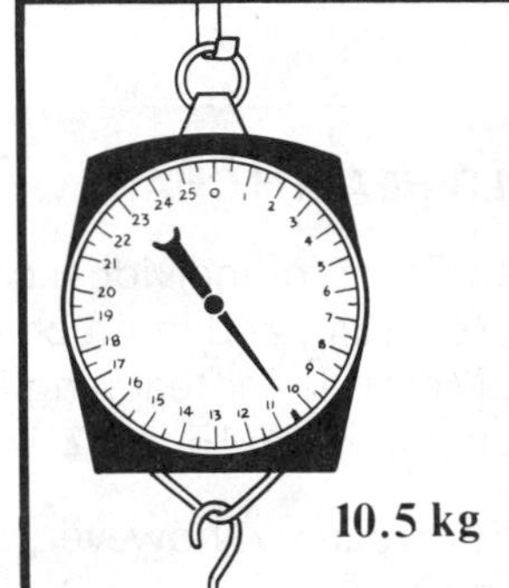

3. Find the weight on the chart with your finger.

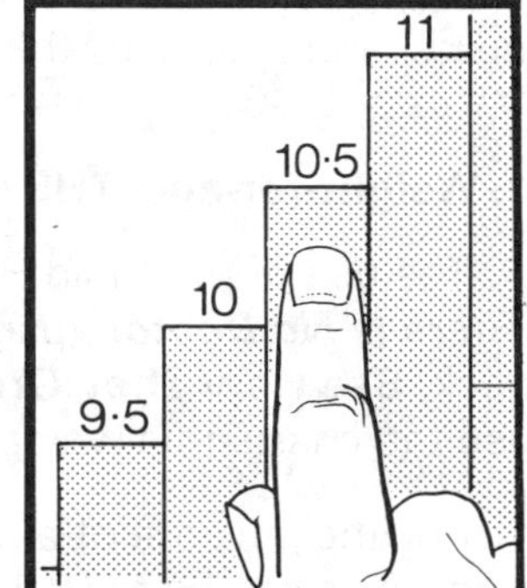

4. Have the mother help the child to stand directly under your finger.

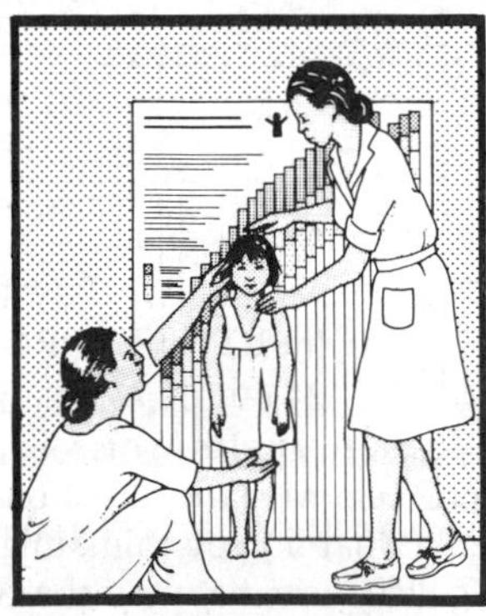

5. Check to see that the child's shoulders and feet are against the chart.

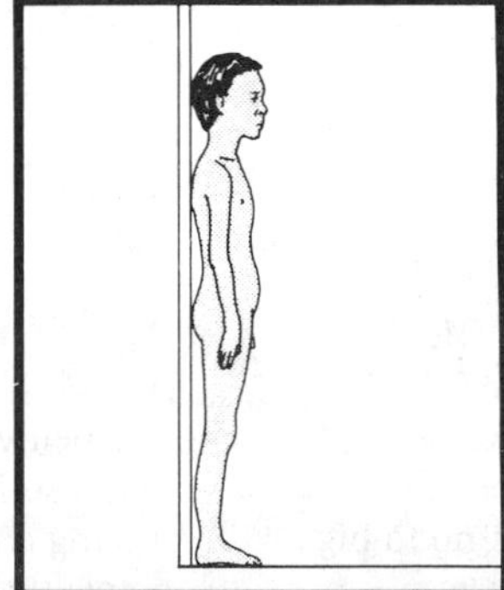

6. Make sure that the child's feet are against her weight as shown at the bottom of the chart.

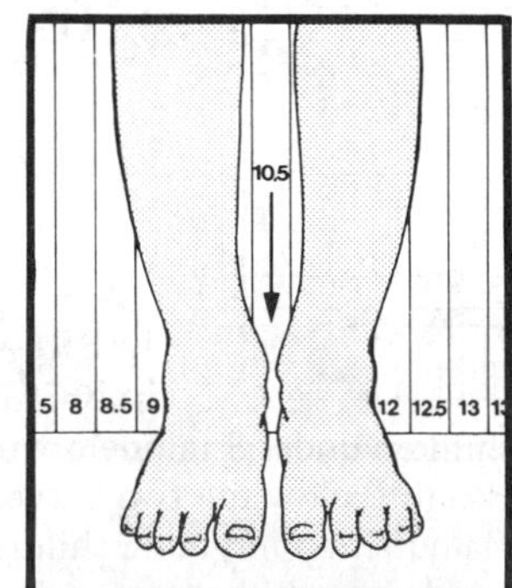

7. Now put your hand flat on the child's head. **Which color does your finger touch?**

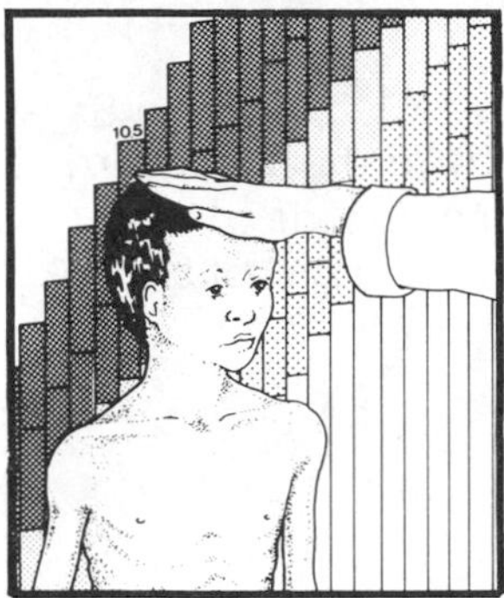

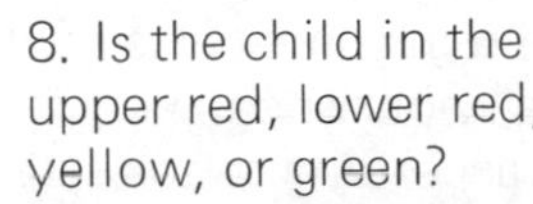

8. Is the child in the upper red, lower red, yellow, or green?

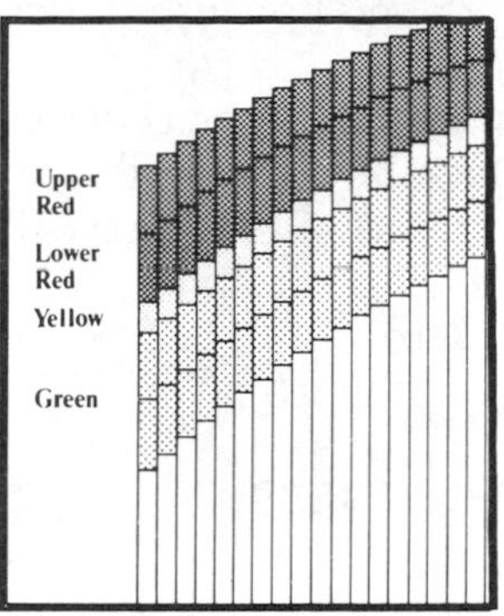

9. If the child is in the **upper red,** he is dangerously thin and needs **more food urgently.**

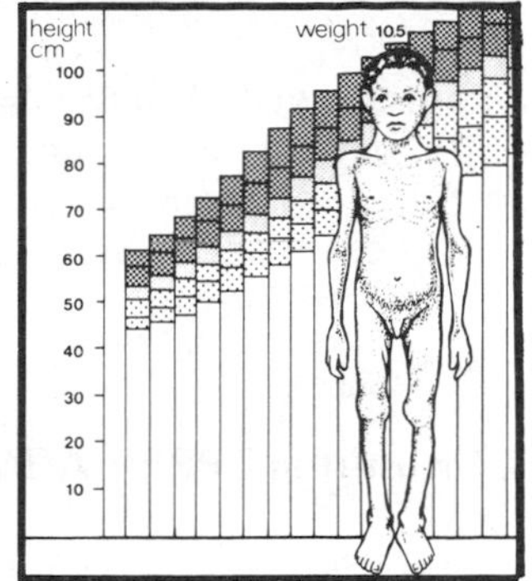

10. If the child is in the **lower red,** he is very thin and needs **more food at once.**

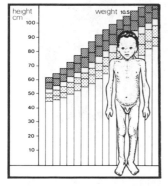

11. If the child is in the **yellow,** he is thin and **may need more food.** Check him regularly.

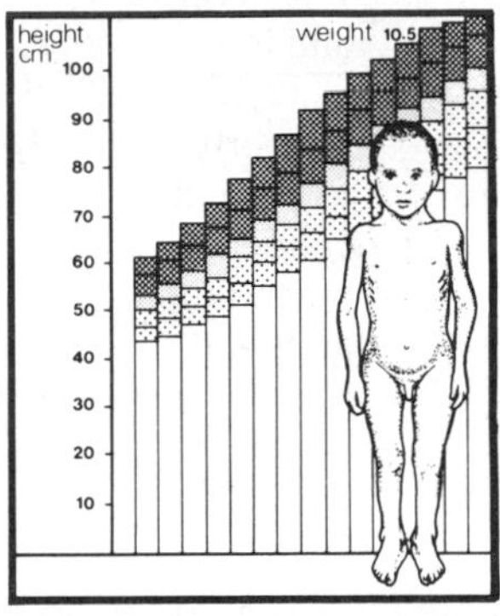

12. If the child is in the **green,** he is well nourished. **Three cheers!**

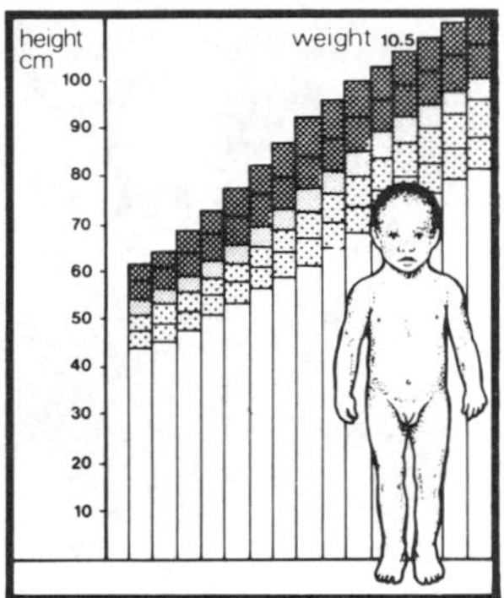

(Notice that the younger, smaller, well-nourished child on the right weighs as much as the older, very thin child on the left.)

The Thinness Chart is especially useful when children are measured only once—as in a survey. But it can also be used together with the Road to Health chart. It lets you know whether a child who measures below the Road to Health is too thin, or is simply smaller than average. If a child is too thin according to the Thinness Chart, this can be noted on the Road to Health chart. Simply put a RED CIRCLE around the dot on the chart, like this:

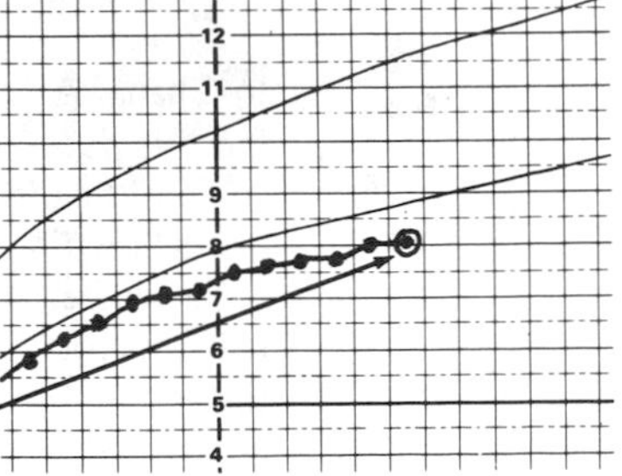

PRECAUTION: At first the Thinness Chart may confuse persons who have used the Road to Health chart. This is because on the Road to Health chart, the thin child appears ***below*** the level of the well-fed child. But on the Thinness Chart, the thin child appears ***higher*** on the chart than a well-fed child of the same weight. This difference needs to be carefully explained.

Also keep in mind that children in some parts of the world have relatively thin bones and bodies, even when well nourished. You may have to adapt the Thinness Chart (raise or lower it slightly) according to the size of well-nourished children in your area. These charts are new and still being tried out. If you try them, please let us know how well they work and how useful you find them.

Where to get Thinness Charts: These can be ordered from TALC, or from Save the Children Federation (see p. **Back**-3). An easy-to-use weight-for-height record card (also in color) comes with the Chart. TALC also offers a color slide of the Thinness Chart. To make a wall chart from it, project the slide against a blank wall and trace over it (see p. **12**-16).

3. Measuring UPPER ARM THICKNESS

The thickness of a child's upper arms or legs is usually a good indicator of how well nourished he is.

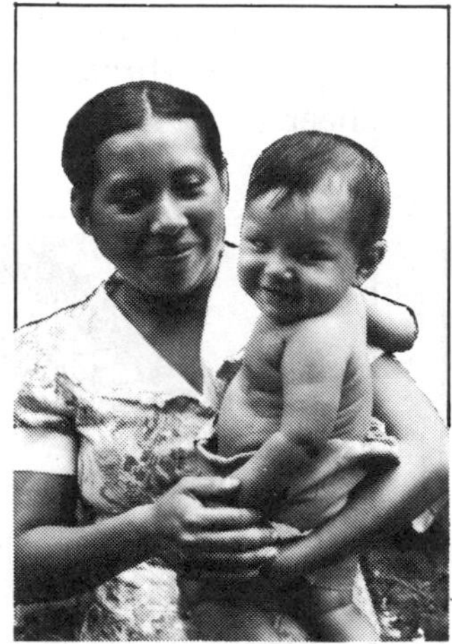

A well-nourished child usually has fairly thick arms and legs.

A poorly nourished child has much thinner arms and legs.

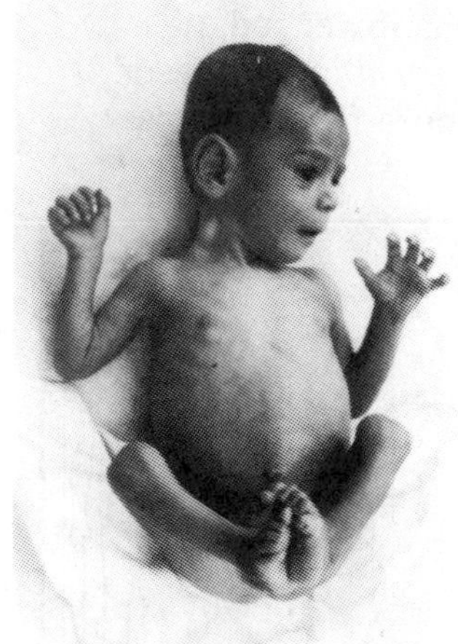

Measuring arm or leg thickness has recently been recognized as one of the easiest and best methods for checking to see whether children are well nourished. In parts of Africa and Asia, such measurements have been village traditions for many years.

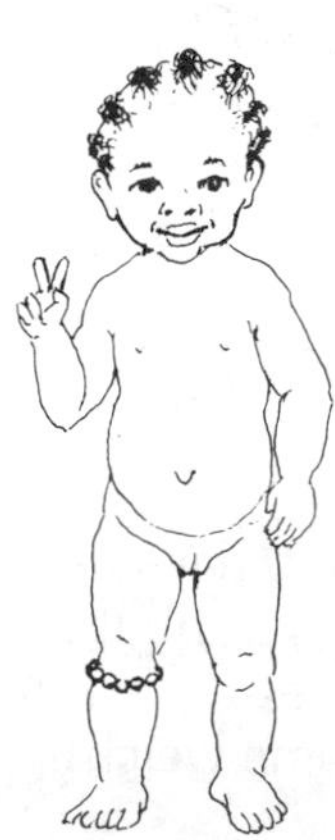

In Ghana, Africa, families put a chain of beads just below the baby's knee. If it gets too tight, they are pleased.

If it slips down, they become worried.

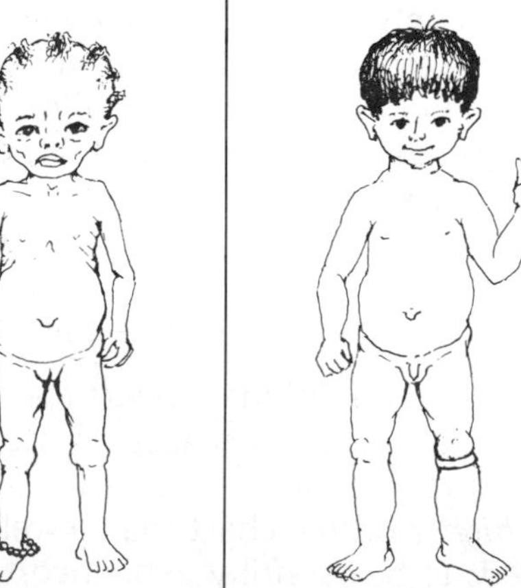

In Kerala, India, mothers put a metal ring below the baby's knee. If the ring slips down, they say that "the devil is sucking out the baby's juices." (This could refer to either malnutrition or dehydration.)

THE BRACELET:

From age 1 to 5, the thickness of a child's upper arm does not normally change much. But a well-nourished child has a thicker arm than a poorly nourished child. By measuring the distance around children's arms, we can tell if they are well fed or too thin.

One way to measure the thickness of a child's arm is with a bracelet like this:

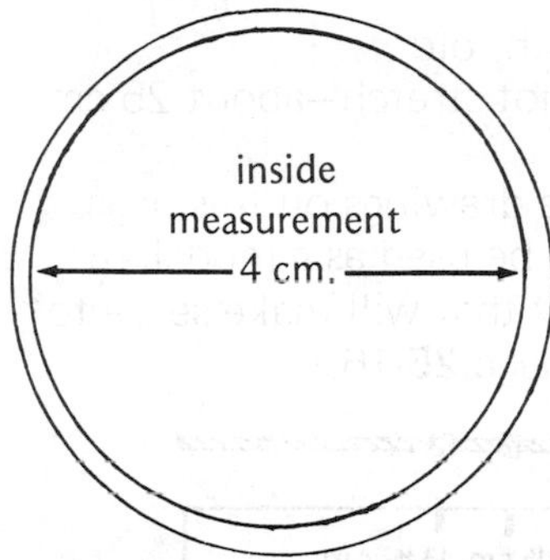

If the bracelet will not slide past the elbow, the child is well nourished.

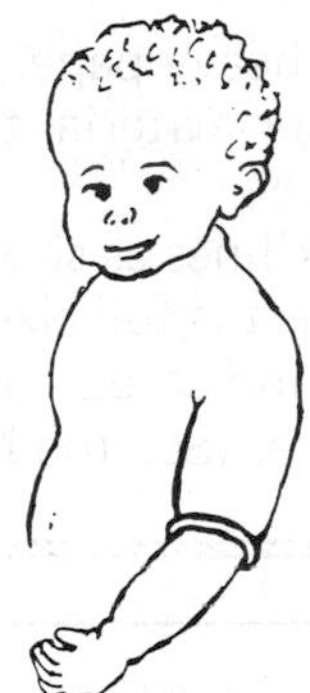

If the bracelet slides easily onto the upper arm, the child is poorly nourished.

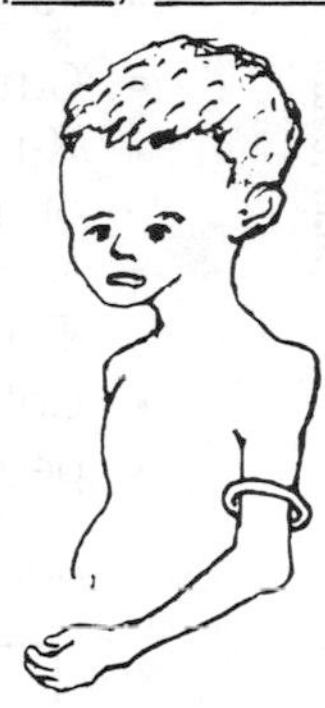

Brown

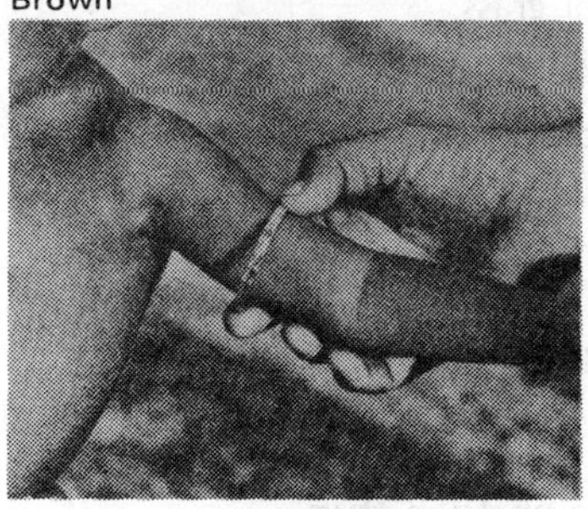

The photo at left shows how the upper arm is measured with a bracelet. This child's arm is too thin. She is malnourished.

Bracelets like this are commonly used in some countries as wrist ornaments for women. Be sure to check that the inside measurement is right.

The bracelet can also be made of twisted grass, rattan, or wire.

This method is simple to use and easy to understand. It may be especially useful for village thinness surveys because health workers can involve persons with little or no formal education. Any child, mother, father, or midwife who wants to can take part in and understand the survey.

Persons who cannot read can record their findings on a simple card with drawings, like this.

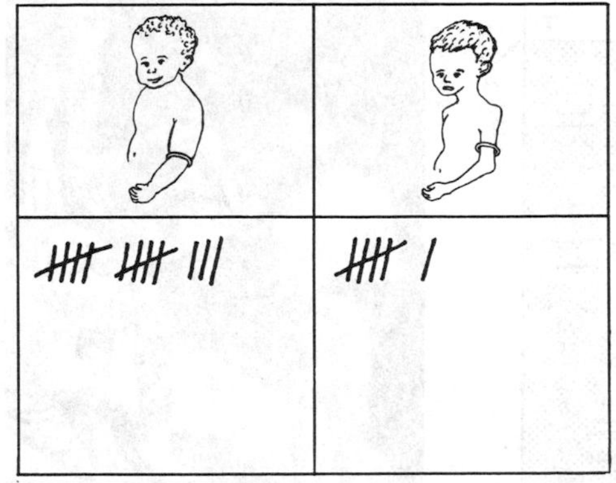

CAUTION: Unfortunately, some health workers have reported difficulties in getting the bracelets over the elbows of even very thin children. We suspect that this method may work better where most people are thin boned (India, the Philippines, etc.) and less well where they have thicker bones (parts of Africa and Latin America, etc.). If you try this method, please let us know how it works in your area.

measure from here →

0 cm. (begin measurement here)

RED (too thin)

12½ cm.

YELLOW

13½ cm.

GREEN (growing well)

THE STRIP:

This easy method is ideal for community thinness surveys conducted by parents or school children.* Even the measuring instrument, or strip, can be made by young children. While this method is a little more complex than the bracelet, it is more accurate and is useful anywhere.

Making the strips:

- Cut thin strips of heavy paper, firm cloth, old X-ray film, or other material that will not stretch—about 25 cm. or 10 inches long.
- Measure and mark lines as shown in the drawings on this page. The strip on the left is full size and can be used as a model.
- Color the strip as indicated—or in a way that will make sense to people in your area. (See the **Note** on page **25**-16.)

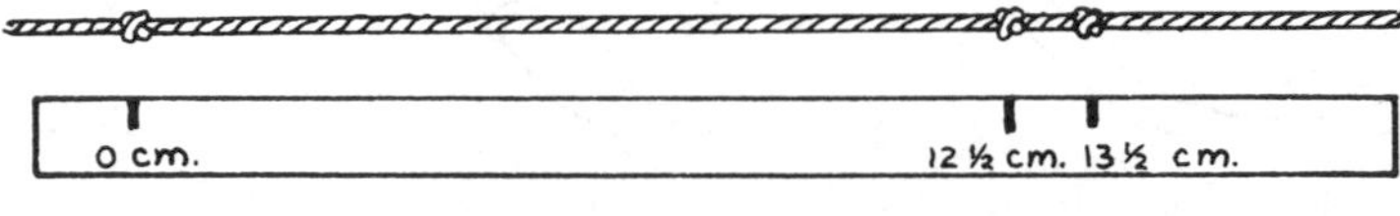

Strips can be made of string or grass.
Put knots at the correct distances.

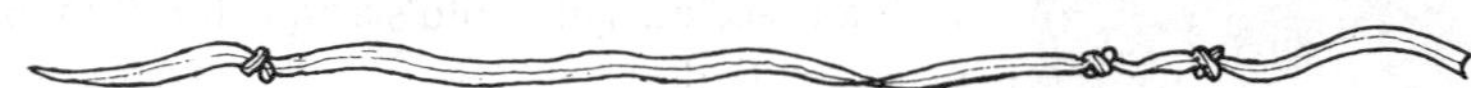

Measuring the children:

- Measure the arms of children between 1 and 5 years old.
- If a child measures in the **green** (over 13½ cm.), he is **well nourished.**
- If in the **yellow** (12½ to 13½ cm.), the child is **thin.**
- If in the **red** (below 12½ cm.), the child is **too thin.**

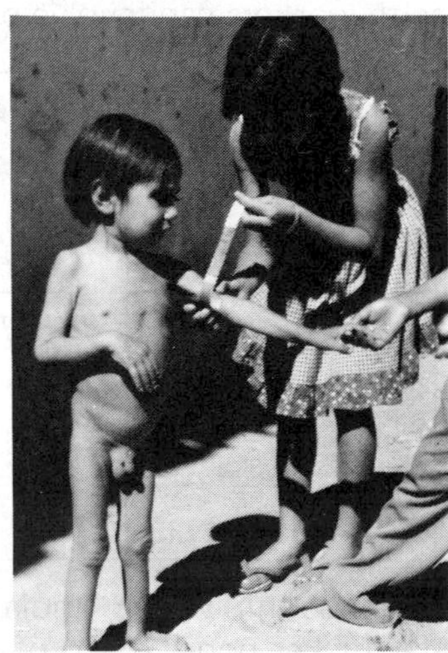

Measuring a child who is too thin.

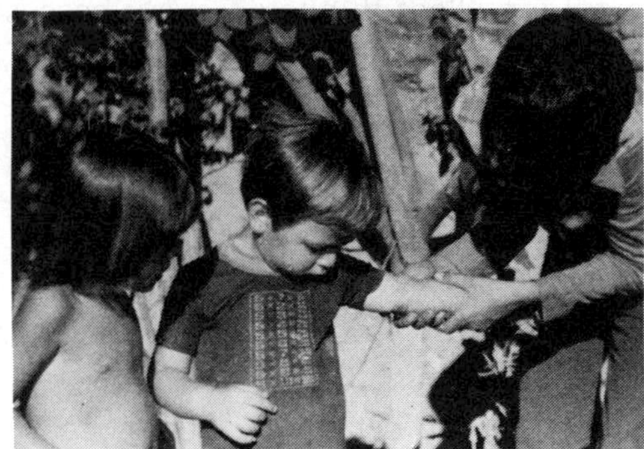

Measuring a child who is growing well.

*A CHILD-to-child activity that uses the 'strip' is available from TALC or the Hesperian Foundation. It is titled "How do we know if our children get enough food?"

Practice measuring:

Before measuring children's arms, the health workers, parents, or children can practice on pieces of wood cut from the branch of a tree, or on rolled cardboard or newsprint. Use pieces that vary in thickness from 11 to 15 cm. Write a child's name on each one. Then play games, pretending that the pieces of wood or cardboard are different children's arms. See who can discover which children are healthy and which are too thin. Practice giving advice on nutrition. Make sure everyone measures correctly.

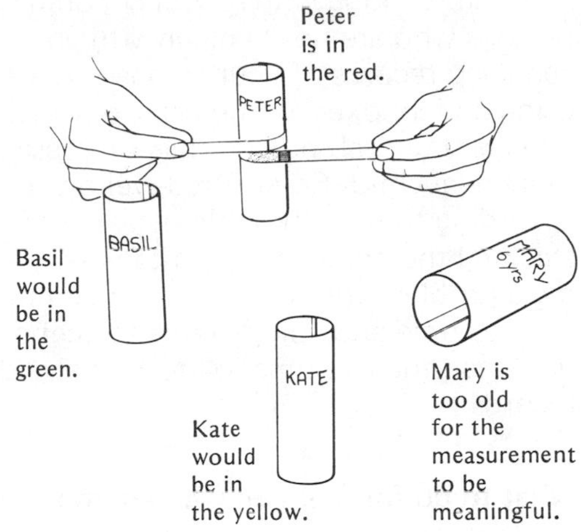

Peter is in the red.
PETER
BASIL
Basil would be in the green.
MARY 6yrs
KATE
Kate would be in the yellow.
Mary is too old for the measurement to be meaningful.

With practice, health workers can learn to measure for thinness using only their fingers. This can become a standard part of their physical examination of young children.

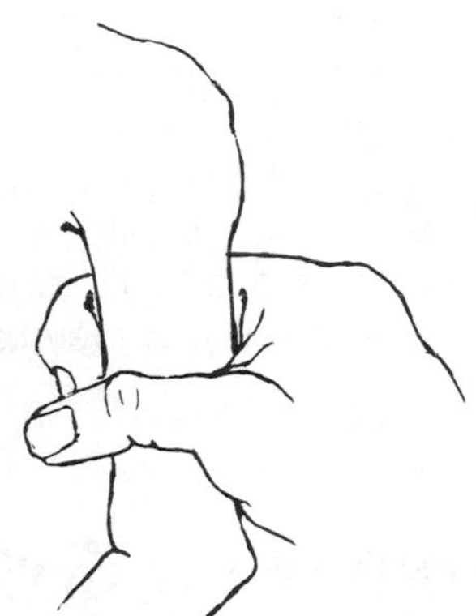

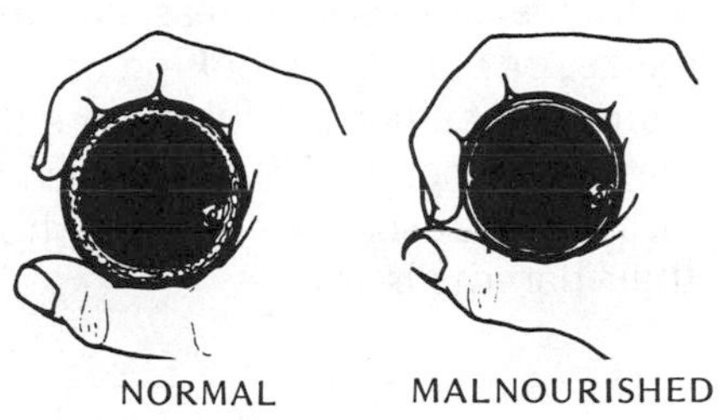

Note: These drawings are just an example and not true for everyone, since the sizes of our hands vary.

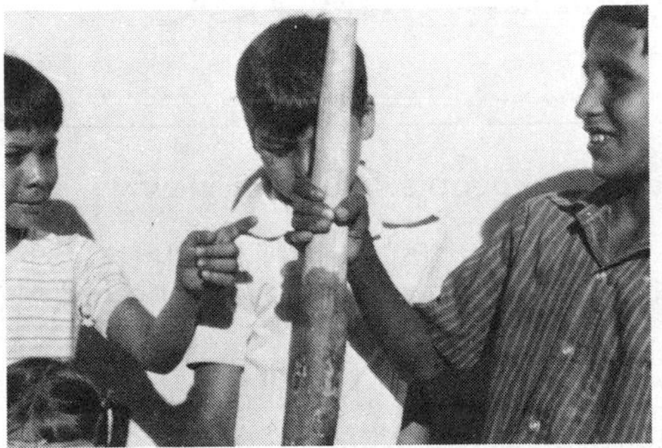

Here school children learn to judge the thinness of a child's arm by practicing on a stick of variable thickness. (Ajoya, Mexico)

A learning game:

Put different-sized rolls of wood or newsprint in a bag. Have the students tell by feel which are too thin.

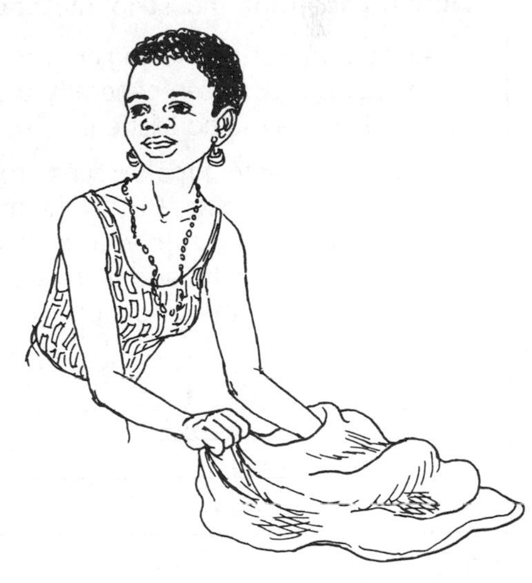

Recording the results of the thinness survey:

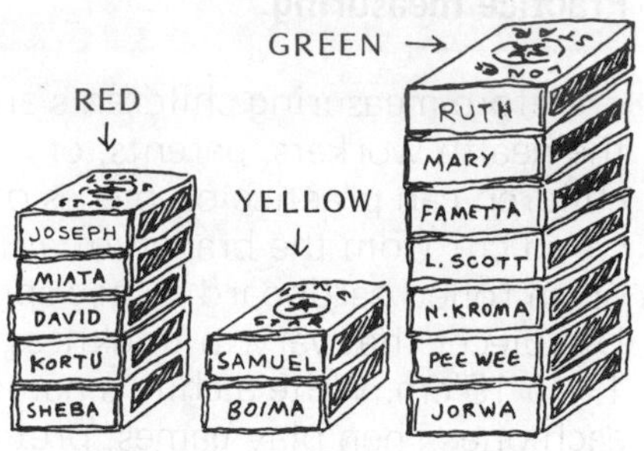

When working with school children or persons who are not familiar with graphs, you can keep records of your thinness survey by using matchboxes, bottle caps, or other objects. Let each box or object represent an individual child. Color it red, yellow, or green, according to how the child measures. By stacking the boxes, children can easily see how big a problem thinness is in their community. They can repeat the survey from time to time and compare the matchbox stacks to see if fewer children are too thin than the last time. (Also see page **25**-13 for another way to keep thinness records.)

What to do for children who are too thin?

Children who are too thin need more and better food. But poor nutrition can be a complex problem, the solutions to which vary from one community or family to the next. In some areas, children of poor families eat mostly foods like cassava, maize, or plantain (cooking banana). These contain so much water and fiber that children's bellies get full before they have eaten enough calories (energy food) to meet their needs. These children need to eat more often. Therefore, the simplest message that school children who have made a thinness survey can take home to their parents is this:

If a child measures . . .

Green . . . give the child at least **3 meals a day.**

Yellow . . give the child at least **4 meals a day.**

Red . . . . give the child at least **5 meals a day.**

Note on adapting the 'strip' method to the local people's point of view:

Armbands for measuring children's thinness are often colored green, yellow, and red. Green generally means healthy, yellow in between, and red means danger—malnourished.

This color system makes sense to city persons used to the 'stop' and 'go' colors of traffic lights. But in the mountain villages of India, it confused people. To them, a child who is redder has good blood and is healthy, a yellow child is sickly, and a greenish child is very sick! So the local health workers reversed the colors on the armbands. Then no one was confused.

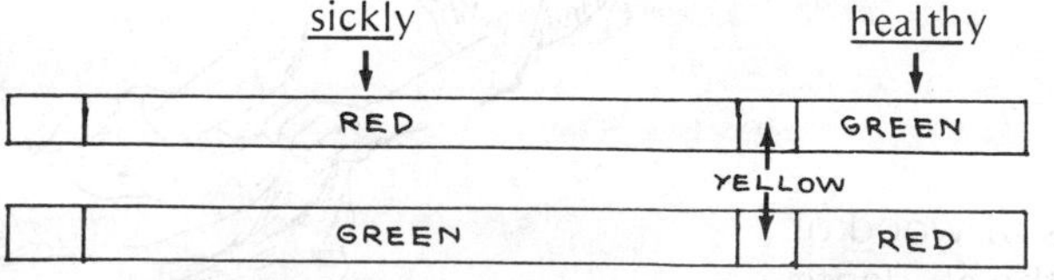

for city folk used to traffic lights

for country folk used to children

A GAME TO HELP CHILDREN LOOK AT THE CAUSES OF THINNESS

To help a group of school children explore the question, *"Why do some children not get enough to eat?"* you can have them play a game called *"Another One!"* (Compare with *"But why . . .?"* on page **26**-4.)

In this game, the health worker or teacher tells a story or shows a picture, and asks a question like, *"Why is this child too thin?"* The children think first of one answer, and then "another one," and "another one." Perhaps each child can think of a different possible answer.

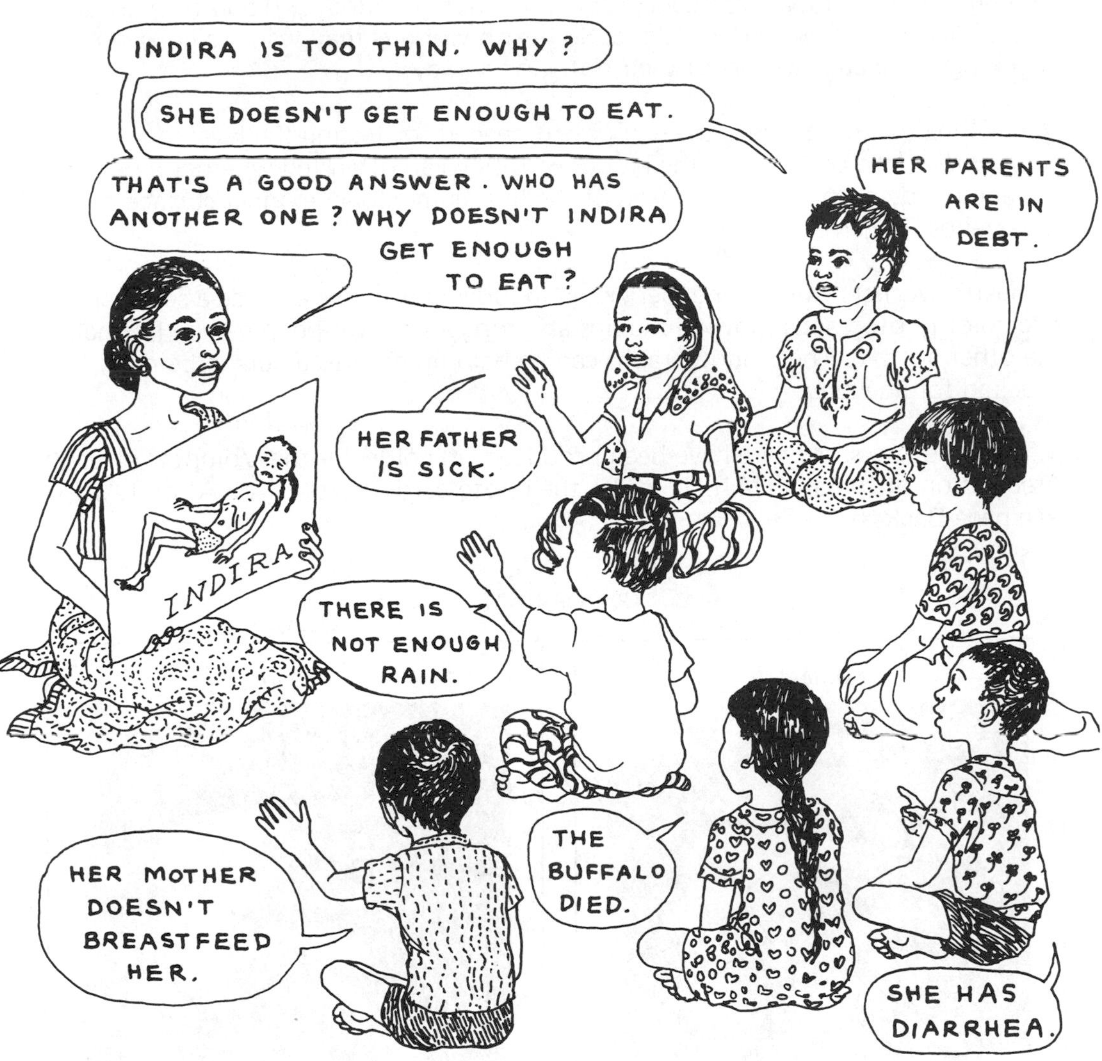
INDIRA IS TOO THIN. WHY?
SHE DOESN'T GET ENOUGH TO EAT.
THAT'S A GOOD ANSWER. WHO HAS ANOTHER ONE? WHY DOESN'T INDIRA GET ENOUGH TO EAT?
HER PARENTS ARE IN DEBT.
HER FATHER IS SICK.
INDIRA
THERE IS NOT ENOUGH RAIN.
HER MOTHER DOESN'T BREASTFEED HER.
THE BUFFALO DIED.
SHE HAS DIARRHEA.

This way, the children begin to think about the many related causes of hunger and poor nutrition.

Similar games can be played with health workers-in-training. Health workers can play them with groups of children, mothers, fathers, and others in the community.

Finding out about the nutrition of persons other than children

In conducting a nutrition survey, the main focus should usually be on the children. But other persons may also have nutrition problems—especially women, old people, and sick people.

Checking for anemia:

Anemia is one of the most common problems for pregnant women and breast-feeding mothers. It may also be a problem for both children and adults in areas where there is hookworm or malaria. So health workers may want to consider checking for anemia as part of their nutrition survey.

Few health workers have the equipment needed for testing the level of ***hemoglobin*** (red coloring) in the blood. But they can often tell whether a person has anemia by checking for paleness of the lips, gums, tongue, inner surface of the eyelids, fingernails, or palms.

Health workers who are inexperienced in judging paleness can use a set of life-size color photographs showing the lips and tongues of two people—one normal, the other anemic. These photographs can be held up next to a person being checked for anemia.

The cards we show here have been produced (in color) by the Voluntary Health Association of India (VHAI). To order the photo cards, write to VHAI or TALC (see page **Back**-3).

APPROPRIATE

NORMAL

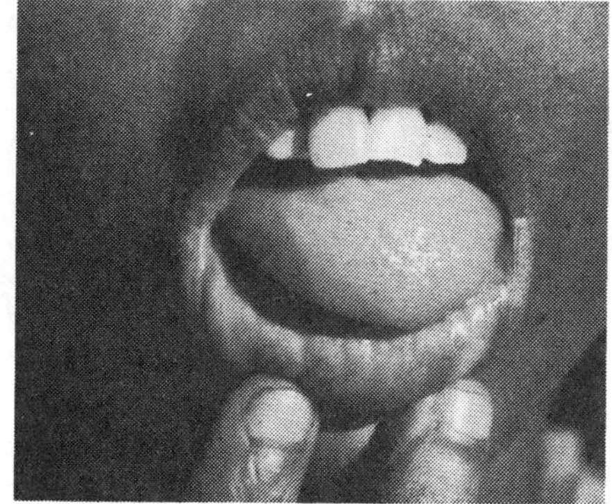

This woman does not have anaemia. She has red and healthy lips and tongue. After one month of treatment the anaemic person should look like this. She should feel stronger. Continue treatment for another month. If she still looks pale after the first month of treatment, refer the patient to a health centre. Iron tablets cost a few paise each, but are free from Government health centres.

ANEMIA

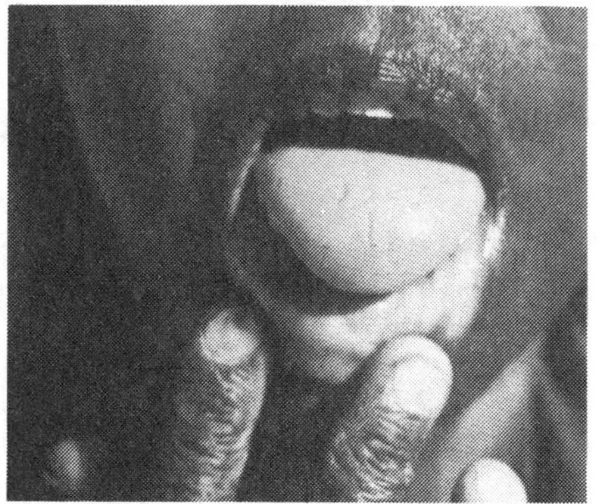

This woman's lips and tongue are very pale. She has severe anaemia. This is dangerous. She needs treatment with 2 iron tablets taken with food 3 times a day. If the patient has pale lips and tongue, but not as pale as in this picture, give 1 iron tablet three times a day with food. Small children who have anaemia need 1 iron tablet daily with food.

An even better way may be to ask a healthy person to stand beside the person being checked for anemia, so that their tongues, lips, and palms can be compared.

Try to choose someone whose normal skin color is as dark or light as that of the person being tested.

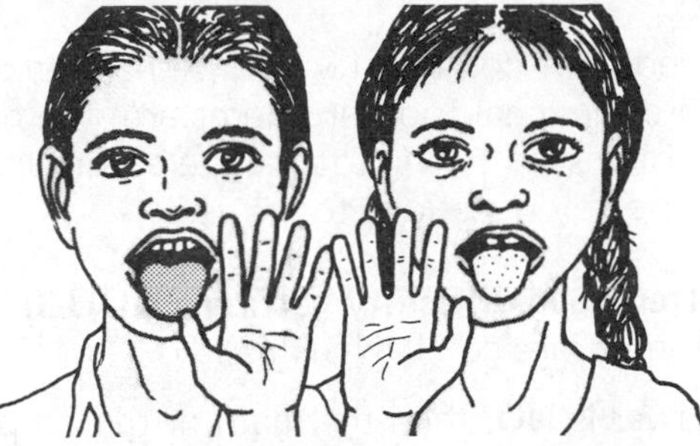

MORE APPROPRIATE

This method uses an important local resource: people.

CAUTION: Some persons object that comparing paleness is not a reliable test for anemia, especially where natural skin color differs greatly from person to person. We realize that sometimes even experienced persons can be fooled. But in trials we have made, we have found that most health workers can spot serious anemias by this method. These trials were done in Mexico, where there is considerable variation in skin color. We would appreciate hearing from you about your experiences with this method.

Here is another way to check for anemia:

Have the person stretch her hand, like this:

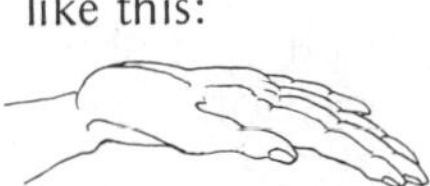

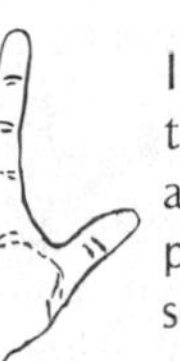

If the lines in the hand are red and clear, the person is not severely anemic.

If the lines disappear or are very pale, the person is severely anemic.

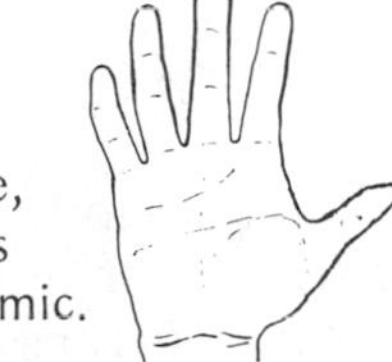

Still another way:

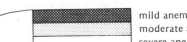

From Bombay, India and WHO comes the so-called 'anemiometer'—a strip of paper with 3 bands in different shades of red. The strip is held up to a person's inner eyelid, and the color matched. Tests show that the degree of anemia can be determined in 4 out of 5 cases.

Color bands represent:

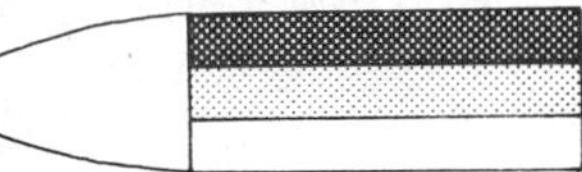

Food problems in old people and sick people:

These two groups often suffer from special nutrition problems:

- Old people may not be strong enough to work in order to grow or buy the food they need. Or they may lack teeth, energy, interest, or—sometimes—love. Help health workers to be sensitive to their special needs.
- Sick people sometimes feel too ill to eat. Yet it is important that they eat well as soon as they can. Also, they may be given little or no food because of cultural beliefs about what sick persons should or should not eat. This *dangerous custom of starving the sick* is discussed on page **25**-38.

Keeping your eyes and ears open

Some helpful information about people's eating habits and their beliefs about foods can perhaps be gathered through a community survey. But one of the best ways you can learn about these things is to keep your eyes and ears open—while you work, while you relax, and, of course, at meal time!

Health workers need to learn to observe people carefully.

LOOKING AT DIFFERENT FOOD PROBLEMS AND THEIR CAUSES

After you have observed your community and perhaps taken a simple survey to help determine how severe the local food problems are, the next step is to find out the causes of the problems. In trying to analyze community food problems and their causes, one of the key questions to ask is:

Do families often have difficulty getting ENOUGH FOOD?
(Do families sometimes go HUNGRY?)

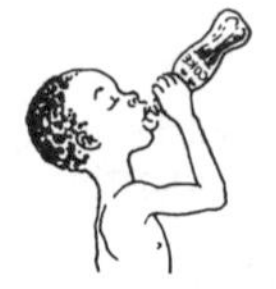

- If the answer is **NO,** then the main nutrition problems probably result from people's eating habits. These can be considered ***cultural problems*** because they are related to people's customs, beliefs, and attitudes.

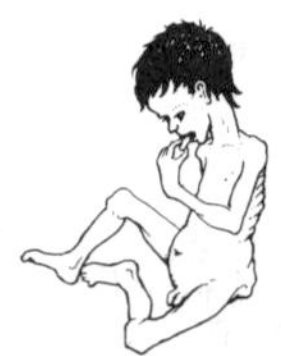

- If the answer is **YES,** then the people's main problems probably have to do with the growing, producing, storing, or buying of food. These are mostly ***economic, technical, and political problems*** (the problems of poverty). However, people's eating habits may also be a factor.

To help in finding the causes of children's food problems, Judith and Richard Brown (nutrition workers in Zaire, Africa) have developed a checklist of basic questions. These are grouped according to 3 problem areas: PRODUCING FOOD, BUYING FOOD, and FEEDING CHILDREN. Nearly all the 'yes' answers on the checklist are ***danger signs*** that indicate food problems in the community. With the Browns' permission, we reproduce the list here.*

WHAT ARE THE CAUSES OF FOOD PROBLEMS IN YOUR COMMUNITY?

A CHECKLIST OF QUESTIONS

	YES	NO
A. DO FAMILIES OFTEN LACK FOOD? (DO SOME PEOPLE GO HUNGRY?) If YES, go to B-1. If NO, go to D-1.		
B. PRODUCING FOOD		
B-1 Can the families produce some of their own food? . . . . If YES, go to B-2. If NO, go to C-1.		
B-2 Are the family fields too small?		
B-3 Are there too few adults who do farm work?		
B-4 Could the families improve their farming methods cheaply and easily?		
B-5 Could the families choose better crops?		
B-6 Do the families raise things to sell, instead of food to eat?		
B-7 Do the families fail to keep enough seed for the next year's planting? . . .		

*From ***Finding the Causes of Child Malnutrition,*** by Judith and Richard Brown, available from TALC (p. **Back**-3) or from Task Force on World Hunger, 341 Ponce de Leon N.E., Atlanta, GA 30308 USA.

		YES	NO
B-8	Do insects, animals, or diseases attack the plants in the field?		
B-9	Do the plants lack water (rain, irrigation)?		
B-10	Do the families lack good places to store food?		
B-11	Could the families raise small animals for food?		
B-12	Do serious diseases attack the animals?		
B-13	Could the families gather more wild foods, or could they hunt or fish?		
B-14	Do the families sell their food instead of feeding it to the children?		

C. BUYING FOOD

		YES	NO
C-1	Do the families buy some of their food? If YES, go to C-2. If NO, go to D-1.		
C-2	Do shops and markets often lack important foods?		
C-3	Do the families lack money to buy the foods for sale?		
C-4	Does food cost too much because transporters and shopkeepers raise the prices?		
C-5	Do the workers lack regular jobs?		
C-6	Do men working far away fail to send money to their families?		
C-7	Do the families have trouble selling their handicrafts or their extra animals and crops?		
C-8	Do the families buy the wrong foods (such as soft drinks, alcohol, powdered baby formulas, and expensive meats)?		

D. FEEDING THE CHILDREN

		YES	NO
D-1	Do the mothers choose not to breast feed their babies, or do they stop breast feeding too soon?		
D-2	Are the mothers malnourished so they do not have enough breast milk for their babies?		
D-3	Do the mothers stop breast feeding their children suddenly or too harshly?		
D-4	Do the mothers get pregnant again too soon?		
D-5	Do the families feed babies tinned milk or instant formulas?		
D-6	Do the babies start getting solid foods at the wrong age?		
D-7	Do the mothers leave their babies with people who do not feed them well?		
D-8	Are the children poorly fed because their families are separated (by jobs, illness, divorce, death)?		
D-9	Do the little children eat only 1 or 2 times a day?		
D-10	Do the families fill the children's stomachs with bulky foods (like cassava) that have few proteins or calories?		
D-11	Are the adult foods hard for little children to eat and digest?		
D-12	Do the adults and older children eat most of the food before the little children get any?		
D-13	Do traditions keep mothers and young children from eating important foods?		

Adapting the checklist for use in your area

The Browns' checklist is designed to help health workers look mainly at the food problems of children. To look at the food problems of other persons in the community, such as pregnant women, mothers, or sick persons, additional questions will need to be asked. Also, for many parts of the world the checklist will need to be revised to include other important causes of hunger. There may be **other useful questions for your particular area or situation** that you or your health workers would want to include in your own checklist.

Notice that in the Browns' checklist some of the more sensitive political and economic questions have not been directly asked—questions such as:

- Is most of the good farmland owned by only a few people?
- Are wages so low that people have trouble feeding their families?
- Do landholders and merchants bribe local authorities in order to illegally maintain large land holdings, high food prices, or exploitative interest rates on loans of grain or money?
- Do village shopkeepers stock alcoholic or fizzy drinks, vitamin tonics, or expensive canned foods, rather than badly needed low-cost foods?

In some places, care must be taken about asking questions such as these. The solutions to them are never quick or easy. Yet in many communities, these issues have more to do with malnutrition than all of the other questions put together. Although the social causes of poor nutrition must be approached with caution and careful timing, we cannot afford to close our eyes to them.

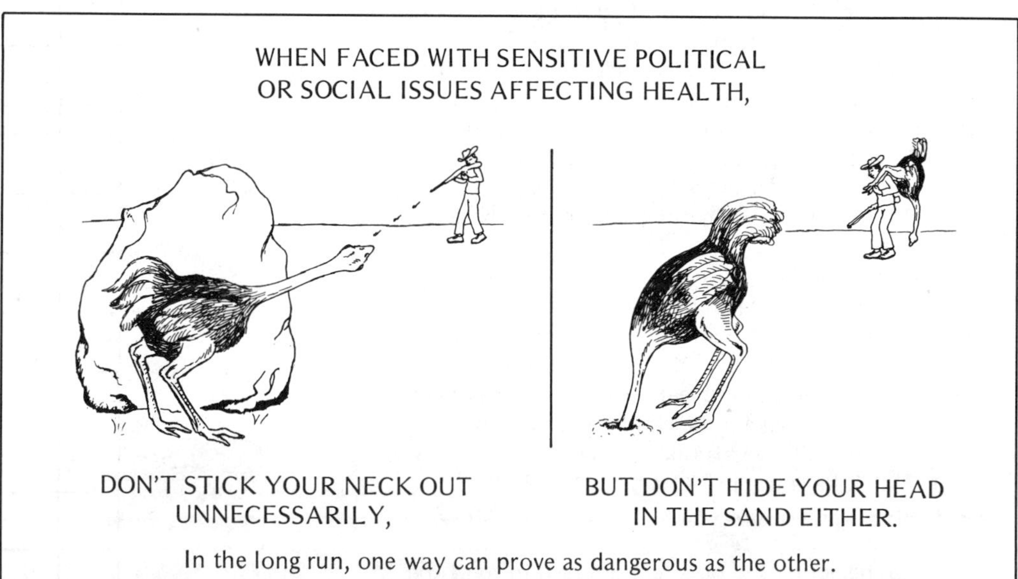

WHEN FACED WITH SENSITIVE POLITICAL OR SOCIAL ISSUES AFFECTING HEALTH,
DON'T STICK YOUR NECK OUT UNNECESSARILY,
BUT DON'T HIDE YOUR HEAD IN THE SAND EITHER.

In the long run, one way can prove as dangerous as the other.

Making survey and discussion questions specific—not general

The Browns point out the need to be very specific when asking people questions. Do not ask big, general questions that may be difficult to answer. **Ask people questions about themselves.** The Browns give the following examples:

LESS APPROPRIATE QUESTIONS	MORE APPROPRIATE QUESTIONS
Do the people in your village raise small animals?	How many chickens does your family have this year? How many goats? How many rabbits?
What foods are usually given to little children?	What foods do you give your child? What did your child eat today?
At what age do children stop getting their mother's milk?	At what age did your child stop getting your milk? (If the mother doesn't know, ask more questions: Did the child have teeth then? Could the child walk?)
What does your family usually eat?	What did you eat since this hour yesterday? What did your husband eat? What did your little children eat? What did your older children eat?

LESS APPROPRIATE

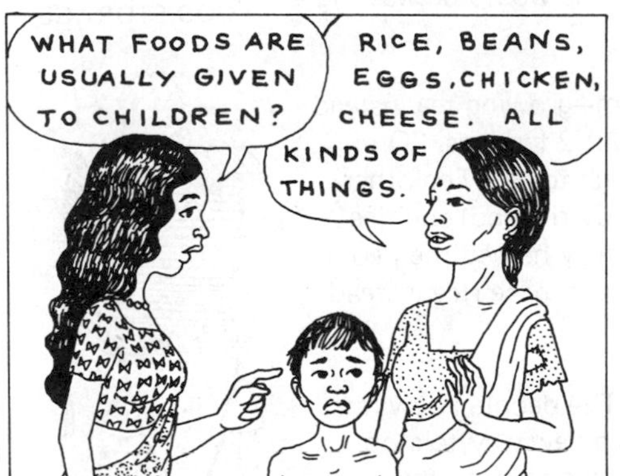
WHAT FOODS ARE USUALLY GIVEN TO CHILDREN?
RICE, BEANS, EGGS, CHICKEN, CHEESE. ALL KINDS OF THINGS.

MORE APPROPRIATE

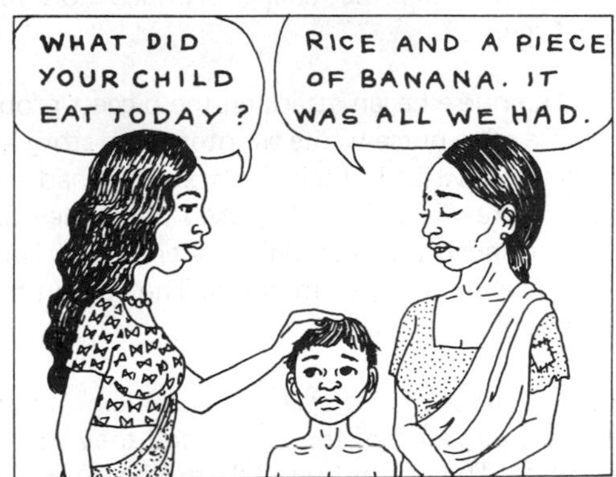
WHAT DID YOUR CHILD EAT TODAY?
RICE AND A PIECE OF BANANA. IT WAS ALL WE HAD.

Making questions specific helps people give answers that are closer to their day-to-day reality.

CHOOSING WHICH PROBLEMS TO ATTACK AND HOW (A COMMUNITY NUTRITION PLAN)

A checklist like the Browns' may help identify many food problems. But 'yes' and 'no' answers alone are not enough. Before deciding which problems to attack first and how, discuss in detail with members of the community all the problems answered 'yes'. Try to write a few words about each problem, telling exactly what is wrong as people see it. The Browns give this example:

EXAMPLE: Here is the list written by a nurse in a place called Tonaville.

A. **DO THE FAMILIES LACK FOOD?**
YES, families lack rice from August to December every year. They have to buy or borrow rice from shops, and it is very expensive during these months.

B. **PROBLEMS OF PRODUCING FOOD**
B-6 Do the families raise things to sell, instead of food to eat?
YES, many families grow a lot of tea to sell, but only a little rice to eat.
B-10 Do the families lack good places to store food?
YES, they store rice in small houses built on poles, but rats get in and eat the rice.

D. **PROBLEMS OF FEEDING CHILDREN**
D-12 Do the adults and older children eat most of the food before the little children get any?
YES, the father of the family always eats first. Then all the children get their food in one bowl. The big children fight for the food, and they don't leave enough for the little children.

The Tonaville nurse wanted to choose a nutrition plan to attack the most important problems. Should he attack the problems of producing food or the problems of feeding the children? What sort of plan should he choose?

The nurse knew it wouldn't help to just tell parents to give their children enough food. In Tonaville, nobody had enough food. Everyone was hungry. The biggest problem was producing enough food. That was the problem the nurse had to attack. If he didn't help the families produce more food, he would be wasting his time.

BETTER FOOD STORAGE

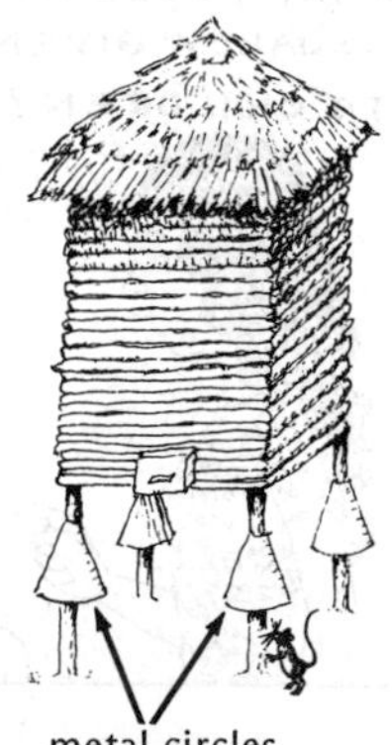

The nurse began attacking the biggest problem—growing tea instead of rice. The nurse wrote an interesting story about 2 families. "One family grew rice in their fields, so they had enough to eat. The other family grew tea. Then they used the money to buy rice, but the rice cost so much they couldn't buy enough." This story helped the people of Tonaville see their mistakes. They began to plant more rice instead of tea.

The nurse also attacked the problem of rats. The people knew rats were eating a lot of their food, and they wanted a new way to stop the rats. The nurse showed them how to put metal circles on the posts under the rice houses to keep the rats from climbing up to the rice. Many of the Tonaville families began to use the metal circles.

CONSIDERING OBSTACLES TO SOLVING NUTRITION PROBLEMS

Some obstacles, or difficulties that may prevent success, are similar in health work everywhere. Others differ from area to area. They will be recognized through observation and experience—or through trial and error.

In deciding which nutrition problems to attack, health workers need to carefully consider possible obstacles. During training, encourage them to discuss the special obstacles that may exist in their own communities. To get people thinking, it may help to tell them a story about obstacles encountered by health workers in other places. For example, here is Bushra Jabre's story of her experience with a rural nutrition program in the South Pacific:*

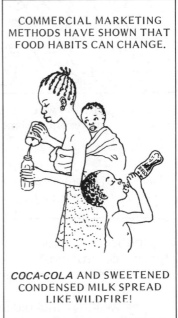

> "However good the intentions of introducing changes in nutrition, the difficulties preventing success are likely to persist. Yet we know from commercial marketing methods that food habits can change. *Coca-Cola* and sweetened condensed milk spread like fire. The changes that occur have nothing to do with nutrition but more to do with prestige. A vague promise of better health is a poor inducement to change food habits. Before we venture into 'selling' new habits, we have to take into consideration several factors. First of all the economic factors: can the people afford the change—and is the new alternative available in adequate quantities?
>
> "It was also found in the New Hebrides that there are several things besides ignorance which prevent a mother from preparing supplementary food for her baby: she spends all day in the garden; she goes to evening Mass; she has no utensils to prepare the food.
>
> "We cannot limit our efforts to educating young mothers. Experience shows that the grandmother has the say in what the baby eats. At well-baby clinics, cooking demonstrations, and mothers' classes, the child is brought by a different family member each time. What about the fathers? Who decides what to buy? Who controls the money? In the Pacific, men do cook, and yet schools exclude boys from home economics courses. Women do the gardening, and yet schools exclude them from agricultural and gardening courses."

COMMERCIAL MARKETING METHODS HAVE SHOWN THAT FOOD HABITS CAN CHANGE.

COCA-COLA AND SWEETENED CONDENSED MILK SPREAD LIKE WILDFIRE!

Bushra Jabre also points to some of the obstacles preventing acceptance of locally trained nutrition workers:

> "Young women are usually trained, but in Melanesia, the women do not have status. And in Polynesia, young people are not accepted as advice givers."

How do your health workers-in-training think these obstacles compare with the ones they may have to deal with in their own communities?

---

*From "Potentials and Pitfalls of Nutrition Education," by Bushra Jabre, in ***Teaching Nutrition in Developing Countries,*** Meals for Millions Foundation, 1800 Olympic Blvd., P.O. Box 680, Sta. Monica, CA 90406 USA.

DEALING WITH OBSTACLES

Health workers need to help people develop a community nutrition plan that takes into account their various strengths and resources. But they must also allow for any obstacles that exist or may arise, and consider how to deal with them.

Obstacles can be handled in different ways:

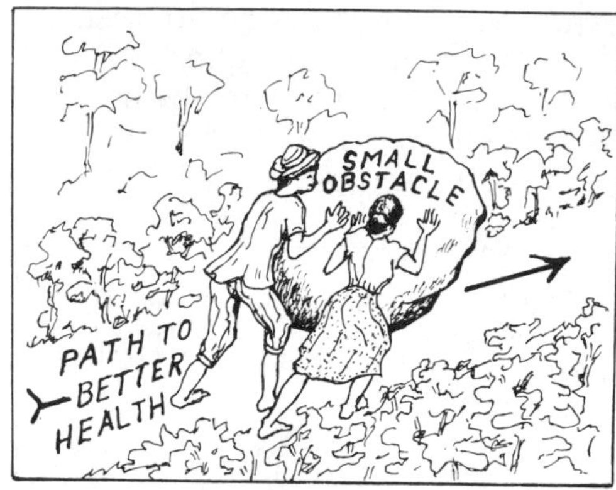

Smaller obstacles we can sometimes remove, or overcome.

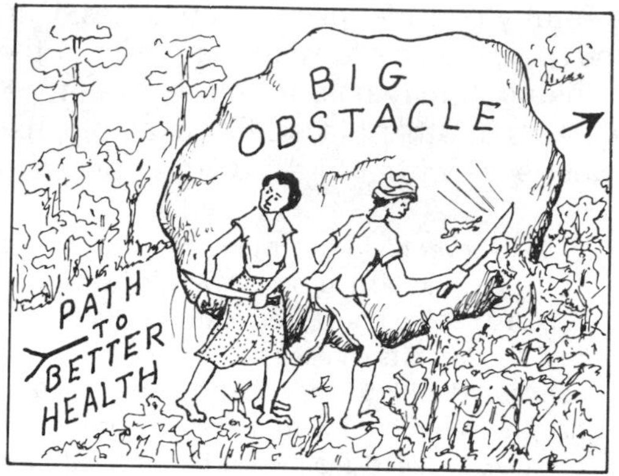

But larger obstacles we may need to work around—at least at first.

Here is an example of how a group of village health workers in Mexico were able to work around a large obstacle to good nutrition in their community.

In the health workers' village, land ownership is a big problem. A few people control most of the good farmland, not legally, but because they bribe the government engineers from the Land Reform Program.

The wealthy landholders lend maize (corn) to the poor farmers at planting time. Then at harvest time, the farmers must pay back three times as much maize as they were loaned. As a result, the families of the poor farmers sometimes do not have enough to eat. (See story, page **Front**-4, and village theater example, p. **27**-27.) Some have had to sell everything to pay their debt, and have been forced to move to the slums of the cities.

The basic problem is that poor farmers do not have a chance to keep and eat the food they grow. The cause of their problem lies in unjust—and illegal—possession of the best farmland by a few wealthy landholders.

The just solution will someday be redistribution of the land. But the obstacles to achieving this are, for the present, too big for the poor farmers to overcome. Instead, the local health workers have helped organize the poor farmers to start a cooperative corn bank, which lends maize to families at very low interest rates.

To permit such low interest rates, the maize had to be well protected from insects and rats. So the health workers built low-cost sheet metal bins to store the maize.

Now that people can borrow maize at low interest rates, they are able to keep and eat most of the food they grow.

Nobody pretends that the problem is completely solved. A few families still illegally possess most of the land. However, the success the people have had in overcoming at least a part of the problem has given them courage and hope to keep moving forward together—until the day comes when the bigger problems can be solved.

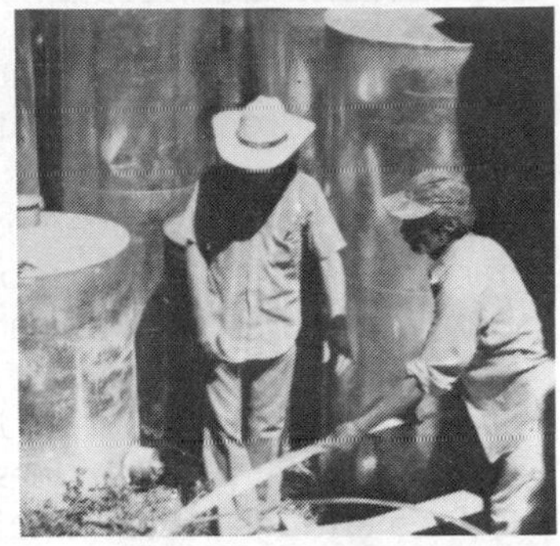

Making maize storage bins.

ATTACKING THE RIGHT PROBLEM

Each village or community has its own food problems that must be studied and analyzed carefully to design a nutrition plan that is likely to work.

Here are more examples from the Browns' book, *Finding the Causes of Child Malnutrition.* These stories can be read and discussed during health worker training. They will help people recognize **the importance of getting a clear understanding of food problems before trying to solve them.** But it will be better if you or the health workers can give similar examples based on your own experiences.

EXAMPLE 1: In Bulape Village, the families grew a lot of maize, groundnuts, and cassava in their fields. A farming teacher visited Bulape and told the people about several ways to improve their farming. "You should put your cassava plants in rows," he said. "You should plant soybeans instead of cowpeas, because soybeans grow faster. You should raise rabbits and pigeons, too."

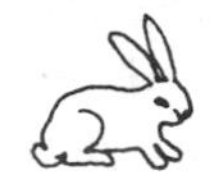

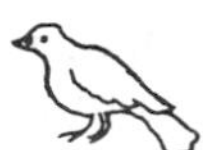

These were all good ideas. They probably would have helped the families grow more food. But Bulape families already had enough food, so producing food was not their real problem. The farming teacher's plan was not good for Bulape.

The real problems were that mothers became pregnant too soon, stopped breast feeding their babies, and then fed them only cassava porridge. The health team at Bulape started several nutrition centers. In the centers, the families practiced mixing maize and groundnuts in a porridge for the babies. Mothers also learned ways to keep from getting pregnant too soon, so they could give each child breast milk until he was 2 or 3 years old.

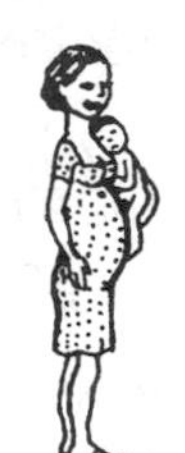

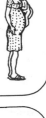

EXAMPLE 2: In Eta City, the health team chose the wrong nutrition plan. They started nutrition classes to show the mothers how to pound dried fish and how to add it to the babies' porridge. But the plan was no good, because the mothers didn't have enough money to buy dried fish in the market. These mothers really needed to sell their handmade baskets. They also needed to join together to buy fish more cheaply. In Eta City, **the problems were in buying food.** A good nutrition plan had to attack those problems.

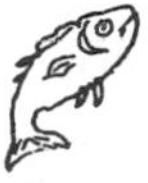

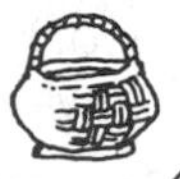

EXAMPLE 3: In Lo Thana, mothers believed that young children should not eat goat meat. The school teacher believed that goat meat was a good food, so she tried to teach the mothers to feed goat meat to the children. But after a year, the same number of children were still malnourished. Then the teacher learned that no one in Lo Thana ate meat very often. Animals were killed for meat only on special occasions. Usually people ate wheat or beans. **The real problem was that the family fields did not produce enough wheat and beans.** Lo Thana really needed help with farming, not lessons on feeding children goat meat.

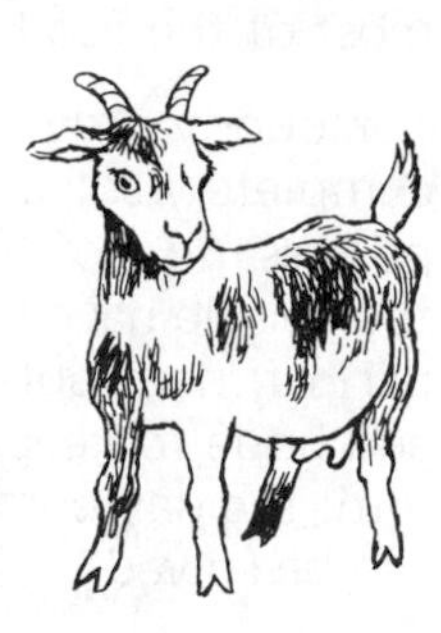

These 3 stories tell about problems that could be solved *inside the community.* However, in some areas the causes of the biggest food problem come from *outside the community.* Here are examples from the Browns:

EXAMPLE 4: On the edge of a large city was a poor neighborhood called Tintown. There was no space for gardens, so people bought all their food in markets and stores. But **food prices were so high that the families were never able to buy enough. The main cause of the high prices was middlemen.** The middlemen were people between the farmers in the country who raised the food and the families in Tintown who ate it.

Here is how maize meal got to the families of Tintown. Out in the country, women grew maize in their fields. When the maize was dry, they put it into sacks. A young man bought the sacks of maize and took them to a shed in the village. The owner of the shed bought the sacks and kept them in his shed. A truck came, and the truck driver picked up the sacks and took them to the mill. The mill owner ground the maize into meal and put it back into sacks. Another truck driver took the sacks to the big market. A young man bought a sack of maize meal and took it on a bus to Tintown. There he opened the sack and sold the meal to 6 market women. The market women took the maize to the Tintown market and sold it to the mothers.

All these people between the farm women and the Tintown mothers were middlemen. Every time the maize passed from one person to another, the price went up. The Tintown people needed to avoid some of these middlemen. So they found a man with a small truck who would bring sacks of maize from the farms directly to Tintown. The families could buy sacks of maize at a lower cost, and the women themselves pounded it into maize meal. The problem for Tintown families was really outside Tintown. By working together, they found a way to attack the problem.

EXAMPLE 5: In Silva Valley, the big problem is outside the community. Most of the Silva Valley land belongs to 3 rich families who live far away. The rich landholders have big farms that raise cattle and sheep to sell in the cities. The landholders do not allow anyone else to grow food on their land, not even the land that is not being used. The families in Silva Valley have only their own small gardens in which to grow food, and they cannot grow enough. **The real problem is that a few people own most of the land, while the rest of the people do not have enough land to grow food.**

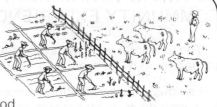

The people of Silva Valley must attack this big problem, for it is causing malnutrition in their children. But they cannot attack it alone. They must get help from important people. So they joined together to write a letter to the government to ask for help. The government is now trying to force the landholders to let the poorer families use some of their land. But the landholders are rich and powerful. They have not yet agreed to give up their land.

This last story, with its discouraging ending, is typical for much of the world. So is the government's failure to take effective action. As millions of landless villagers can testify, government 'land reform' often consists of promises only. Each year more of the land ends up in the hands of a few rich families.

In many countries, it is a deception to teach poor people that the government defends their land interests. Too often, government sides with the rich and powerful. After all, many government officials are rich landholders themselves.

Community-based programs in many parts of Asia and Latin America have learned to expect little help from "important people" over questions of land and justice. Nevertheless, a few programs have found ways to bring about small land reforms in a peaceful way, with or without government help.

In Guatemala, for example, the Chimaltenango Development Program has set up a 'land fund'. This fund lends money to organized groups of landless Indians so they can buy unused farmland. The program teaches the Indian farmers ways to improve soil and crops, so that in a few years they can pay back their loans. The same money is then loaned to other groups to buy more land.

In a similar way, the health team in Ajoya, Mexico has set up a 'fence fund'. Poor farmers can borrow money from the fund in order to fence their plots of farmland. Before this fund existed, poor farmers had to borrow from the rich to fence their land. The interest rates were so high that they could never pay back the loans. This allowed the rich landholders to claim grazing rights on the harvested fields, year after year. But now the poor farmers are able to sell grazing rights to the rich. This means they have more money for food.*

*__Note:__ The 2 funds we have just described were started with 'seed money' from international non-government organizations. These are examples of how foreign aid, when directed to self-help programs organized by the poor, can actually do more good than harm. (Foreign aid that is channeled through oppressive governments often ends up strengthening the rich and weakening the poor. See ***Aid as Obstacle,*** by Lappe, Collins, and Kinley, Institute for Food and Development Policy, 2588 Mission Street, San Francisco, CA 94110, U.S.A.)

NUTRITION TRAINING THROUGH COMMUNITY EXPERIENCE

The examples we have given show that food problems, their causes, and ways of solving them differ from area to area, and even from village to village.

For this reason, nutrition courses designed at the national or international level may do as much harm as good in individual villages. **Instead of learning from standardized plans, health workers need a flexible learning situation that helps them to observe, analyze, and adapt.**

More and more programs are making community practice the focus of nutrition training. A 10-day nutrition course in Indonesia bases training on 8 small-group 'field activities' in neighboring villages. Three of the activities involve observation of ongoing community programs, and 5 are practical working sessions with members of a selected village.

These 5 are:

1. General evening meetings in the village to get acquainted, discuss aims, and plan activities.
2. An evening session of nutrition training for a small group of villagers who will become nutrition volunteers ***(kaders)*** in the selected village.
3. Shopping in the market, then cooking and serving a noon meal to selected children.
4. Conducting a nutrition survey of all children under age 5, filling out weight charts, and visiting homes of malnourished children.
5. Final evening meeting to discuss results of activities and discuss future steps.*

Perhaps the most important part of this experience-based approach is that it brings learning down to earth. Real problems in real villages often are very different from the way they seem when studied in class. As the Indonesian program instructors point out:

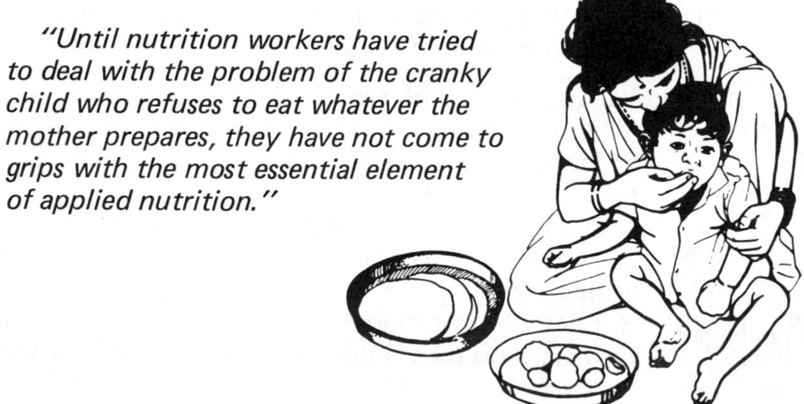
"Until nutrition workers have tried to deal with the problem of the cranky child who refuses to eat whatever the mother prepares, they have not come to grips with the most essential element of applied nutrition."

*From "Training Course for Village Nutrition Program," J.E. Rohde, D. Ishmail, and others in ***Tropical Pediatrics and Environmental Child Health,*** vol. 25, number 4, August, 1979.

POSSIBLE AREAS TO COVER IN A NUTRITION COURSE—BASED ON SHORT-TERM AND LONG-TERM PROBLEM SOLVING:

Emergency problems
- starving children
- poorest families lack food
- parents do not give sick children enough liquid or food (starving the sick)
- natural disasters

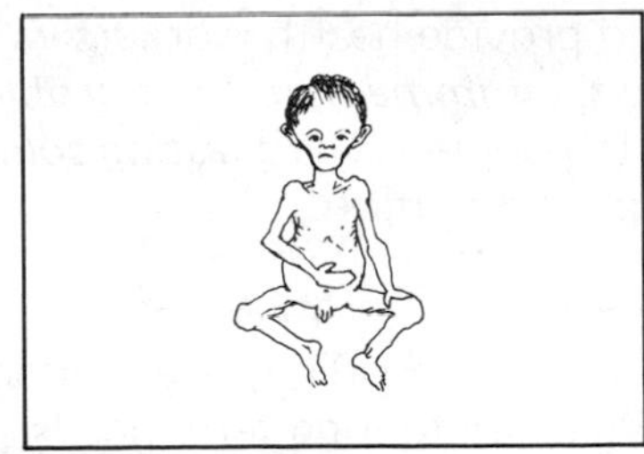

Emergency measures
- food supplements
- centers for feeding malnourished children
- oral rehydration
- full, normal feeding for children with diarrhea or other illness

Major problems
- underweight children
- loss of healthy customs (such as breast feeding)
- certain unhealthy or mistaken customs (new and old)
- lack of knowledge about healthy foods

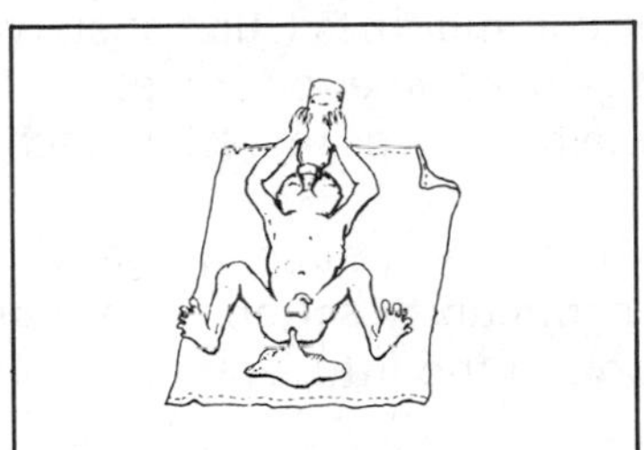

Solutions to major problems
- under-fives clinics
- baby weighing
- nutrition classes for mothers
- CHILD-to-child activities
- child spacing
- better eating habits
- looking for what is best in both old and new ways

Ongoing needs
- more and better foods
- greater self-reliance
- fairer distribution of land and resources

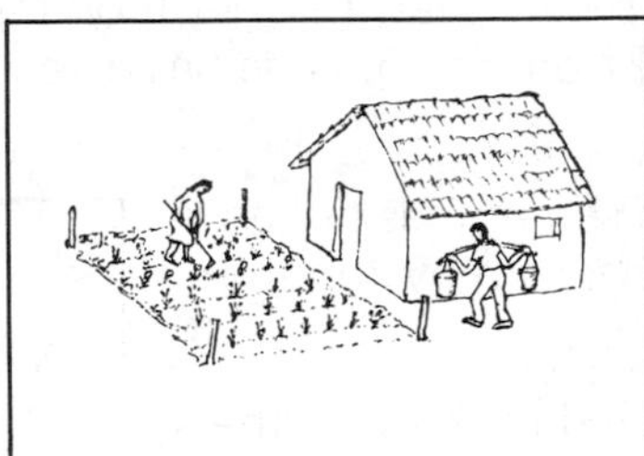

Partial solutions
- family gardens
- improved farming methods
- improved storage
- food crops, not cash crops
- mothers and children as nutrition workers
- more jobs (cottage industry, etc.)
- rotating loan program allowing poor families to buy their own land

Underlying needs
- equal opportunity for everyone
- more control by people over their lives and their health
- honest leaders
- social justice

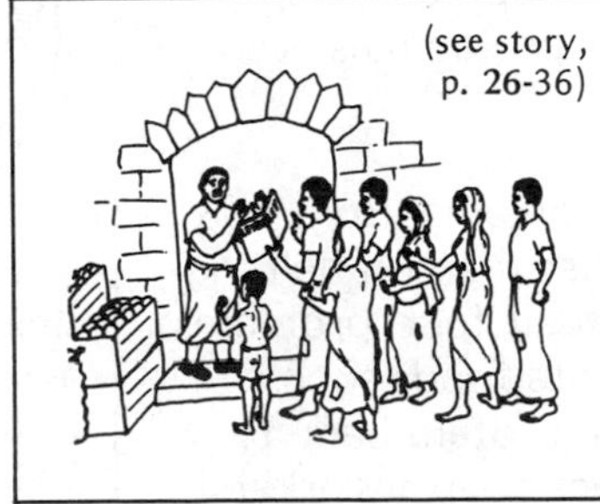

(see story, p. 26-36)

Toward long-term solutions
- raising awareness
- community organization
- change toward people-supportive government
- redistribution of land
- relevant education
- fairer wages
- restriction on advertising and profiteering by big business
- fairer representation and bargaining power for the poor

TRAINING FOR SHORT-TERM AND LONG-TERM PROBLEM SOLVING

Training in nutrition should provide health workers with skills, methods, and ideas for helping people solve their *immediate food problems.* But it also needs to prepare them for working with people toward *lasting solutions* to the underlying problems that contribute to poor nutrition.

On page **25**-31 we show some of the problem-solving activities that might be covered in a training course on nutrition. They are grouped into 4 categories, ranging from short-term emergencies to long-term needs.

Clearly, health workers should respond at once to any immediate, life-threatening problems in their communities (such as starvation of children). But as people work together and gain a deeper awareness of their underlying needs, the health worker can help them look for more far-reaching answers.

The health or nutrition worker's biggest challenge will be to see how fast he can **move the main focus of community action from short-term to long-term needs.** He can help people look to the future and plan ahead.

WARNING ABOUT FOOD SUPPLEMENTS:

When people are starving, seeing that they get food must be the first priority. However, free food provided from the outside has often created more problems than it has solved:

- Food supplements have sometimes driven poor farmers to economic ruin by forcing down prices of local crops.
- Provision of free powdered milk to mothers has caused increased bottle feeding, costing the health and lives of many babies.
- Instead of helping people become more self-reliant, food supplements often increase their dependency on outside help. Studies in several countries show that after long periods of receiving food supplements, poor nutrition is as big a problem as ever —or bigger.

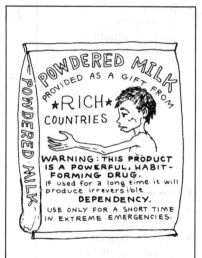

Free food supplements should carry the same warnings as dangerous, habit-forming medicines. Their use should be limited to short-term emergencies only.

Unfortunately, some relief organizations still focus on giving free food rather than on helping people correct the causes of their food problems. Some organizations even donate foods such as candies or chocolate-flavored 'protein bars' to health programs training village health workers! **Discuss with health workers the dangers of accepting such gifts.**

Self-help instead of handouts:

Fortunately, more and more volunteer and relief organizations are changing their focus of assistance from food supplements to self-help activities at the village level.

Rather than provide powdered milk and other outside foods, many health programs now try to **use only locally available foods** at nutrition centers.

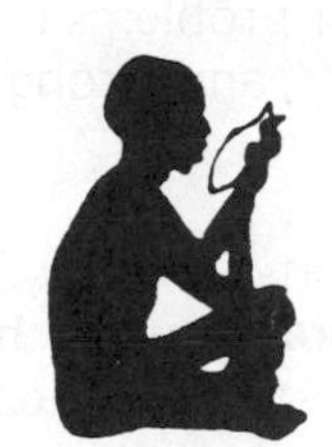

GIVE A MAN A FISH . . . AND YOU FEED HIM FOR A DAY.

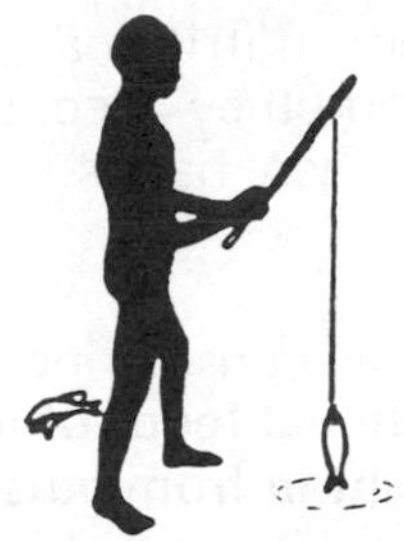

TEACH A MAN TO FISH . . . AND HE'LL FEED HIMSELF FOR LIFE.

For example, in the Indonesian training program described on page **25**-30, students go to the local market to buy low-cost foods for their child-feeding program. Thus, mothers learn about preparing nutritious low-cost meals from local foods, rather than growing dependent on outside gifts.

In Mexico, the Project Piaxtla health team also has moved increasingly toward community self-reliance to solve food problems. Several years ago, a limited quantity of donated powdered milk was made available as an emergency food supplement for severely malnourished children. But now no donated milk is used or needed. Far fewer severely malnourished children are seen in the area today. When a malnourished child is brought to the health center, **if the family is not able to provide adequate food, different families in the village will cooperate in supplying food and even in helping to prepare it for the child.**

In some areas, when a malnourished child cannot breast feed from his own mother, other women in the village help by contributing breast milk.

LESS APPROPRIATE

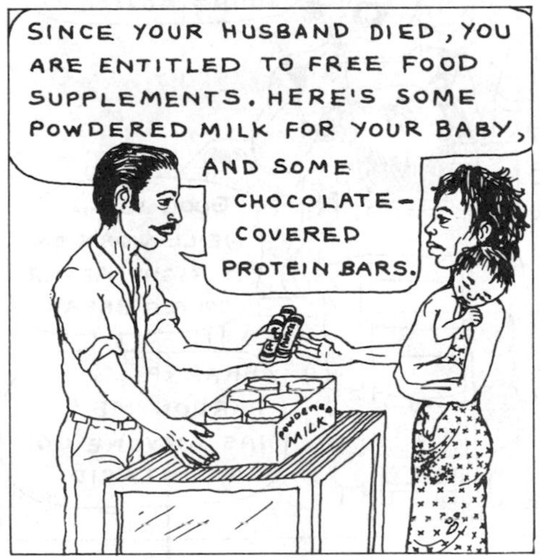

SINCE YOUR HUSBAND DIED, YOU ARE ENTITLED TO FREE FOOD SUPPLEMENTS. HERE'S SOME POWDERED MILK FOR YOUR BABY,
AND SOME CHOCOLATE-COVERED PROTEIN BARS.
POWDERED MILK

MORE APPROPRIATE

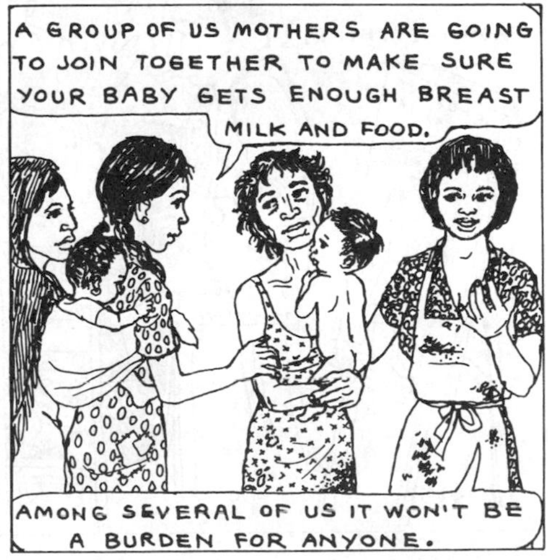

A GROUP OF US MOTHERS ARE GOING TO JOIN TOGETHER TO MAKE SURE YOUR BABY GETS ENOUGH BREAST MILK AND FOOD.
AMONG SEVERAL OF US IT WON'T BE A BURDEN FOR ANYONE.

WORKING WITH PEOPLE'S FOOD HABITS

Some nutritional problems exist because families are too poor to buy or grow the food they need. But other problems come from people's food habits. People everywhere have strong beliefs, and strong likes and dislikes, when it comes to food.

When considering food habits, it is very important to remember that **often the traditional foods of an area are (or were) healthier than many of the newer foods brought in from outside.** Breast milk is healthier than bottle feeding. Fresh or dried fruit is healthier than fizzy drinks. Millet, a traditional food of Africa, is healthier than cassava, introduced from Latin America. In Chapter 7 we give many other examples.

We health workers and nutritionists often fall into the trap of looking mainly at people's harmful habits and customs. We pay too little attention to their habits and customs that are healthy. This is unfortunate. People respond more eagerly when we emphasize their beneficial customs, and build on those.

Community-based nutrition education should not focus on changing people's bad habits. Rather, it should try to recognize and strengthen those food habits and traditions that are healthy.

A common mistake: We often talk about changing other people's attitudes and habits, but do not think of changing our own.

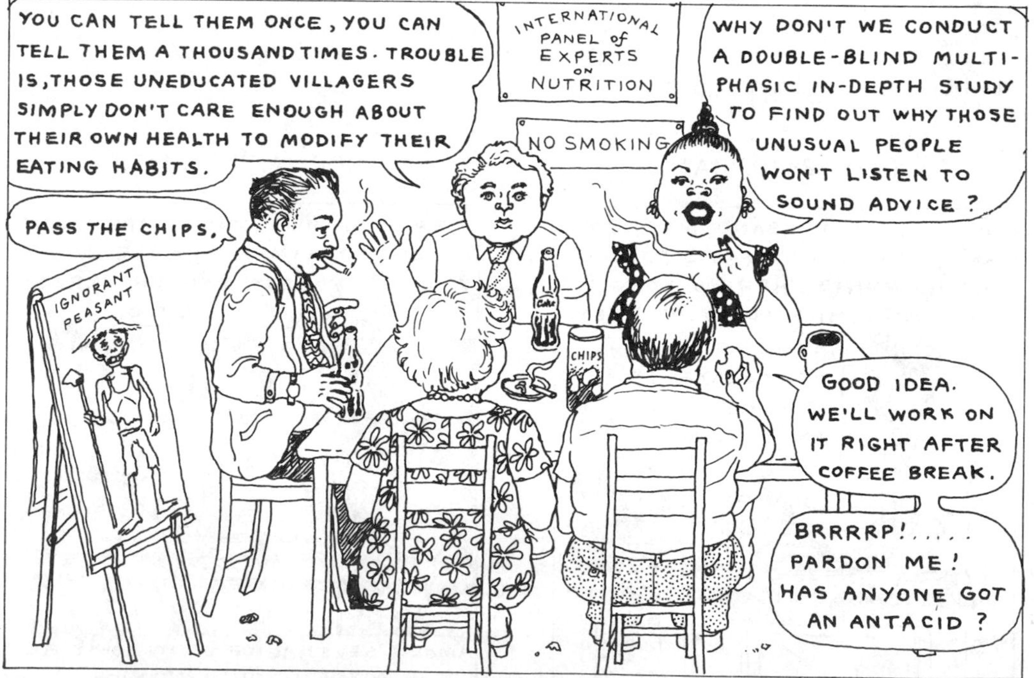
YOU CAN TELL THEM ONCE, YOU CAN TELL THEM A THOUSAND TIMES. TROUBLE IS, THOSE UNEDUCATED VILLAGERS SIMPLY DON'T CARE ENOUGH ABOUT THEIR OWN HEALTH TO MODIFY THEIR EATING HABITS.
INTERNATIONAL PANEL of EXPERTS ON NUTRITION
WHY DON'T WE CONDUCT A DOUBLE-BLIND MULTI-PHASIC IN-DEPTH STUDY TO FIND OUT WHY THOSE UNUSUAL PEOPLE WON'T LISTEN TO SOUND ADVICE ?
NO SMOKING
PASS THE CHIPS.
IGNORANT PEASANT
CHIPS
GOOD IDEA. WE'LL WORK ON IT RIGHT AFTER COFFEE BREAK.
BRRRRP!..... PARDON ME! HAS ANYONE GOT AN ANTACID ?

IDEAS AND METHODS FOR TEACHING NUTRITION

Many training programs still teach health workers to give standard nutrition talks to mothers, children, and anyone else who will sit through them. The lesson plans and teaching materials have often been designed by outsiders—even foreigners. A dialogue approach, flip charts, or flannel-board foods may be used. But information and advice still travel mostly one way: from an unseen expert through the health worker to the listeners. The results from such pre-packaged nutrition talks are often disappointing:

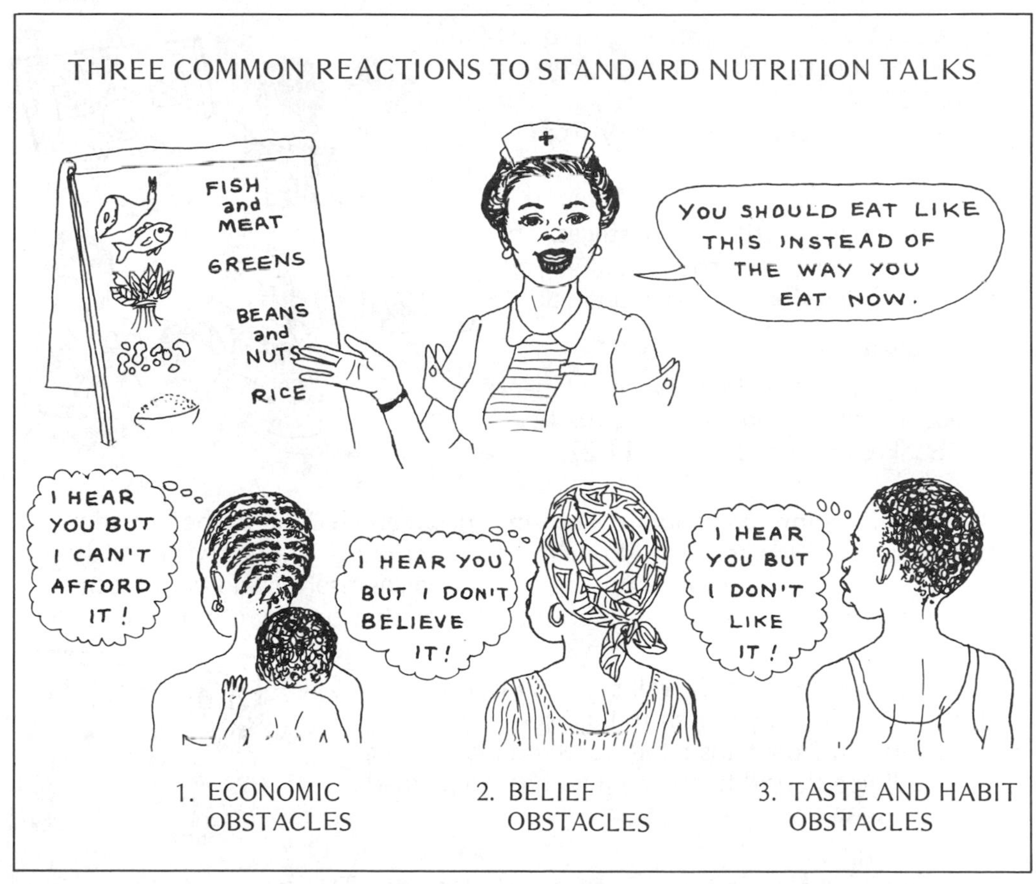
THREE COMMON REACTIONS TO STANDARD NUTRITION TALKS
FISH and MEAT
GREENS
BEANS and NUTS
RICE
YOU SHOULD EAT LIKE THIS INSTEAD OF THE WAY YOU EAT NOW.
I HEAR YOU BUT I CAN'T AFFORD IT!
I HEAR YOU BUT I DON'T BELIEVE IT!
I HEAR YOU BUT I DON'T LIKE IT!
1. ECONOMIC OBSTACLES
2. BELIEF OBSTACLES
3. TASTE AND HABIT OBSTACLES

If people are to learn to meet their food needs better, the educational approach needs to be active and should deal with real problems in a real way. It needs to be **a process in which the health workers and the people learn and explore new possibilities together.**

On the next 2 pages is a list of some of the methods and ideas that have been used to help health workers learn about food problems. Most can also be used by health workers to teach persons in the community. Examples for a few methods are given in this chapter, but many are included in other chapters. We refer you to the pages where they can be found.

SUMMARY OF WAYS TO TEACH AND LEARN ABOUT NUTRITION— FOR HEALTH WORKERS, MOTHERS, SCHOOL CHILDREN, AND OTHERS

1. Stories that help people to think about their problems and look for solutions. These are best in small groups, with the group taking part or discussing the stories afterwards. Flashcards or drawings can help to illustrate the stories and encourage discussions. You can also use open-ended stories that everyone helps to tell.

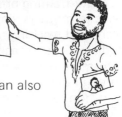

Examples of stories related to nutrition:

- The story of Abdul and Seri, on p. **24**-24
- Indian villagers get back their fruit trees, p. **26**-36
- Janaki and Saraswati—a story from India, p. **13**-1

2. Games with nutritional messages. These are best if they involve problem solving and are based on decisions, rather than luck.

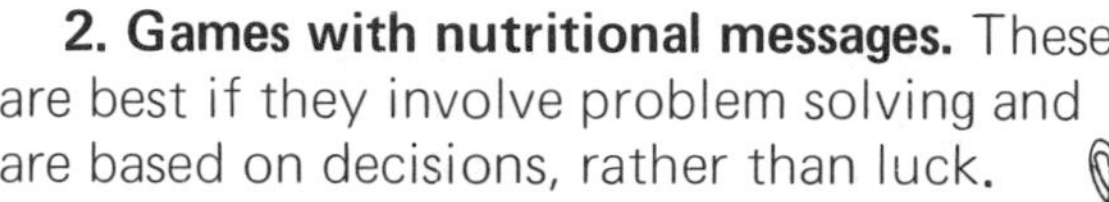

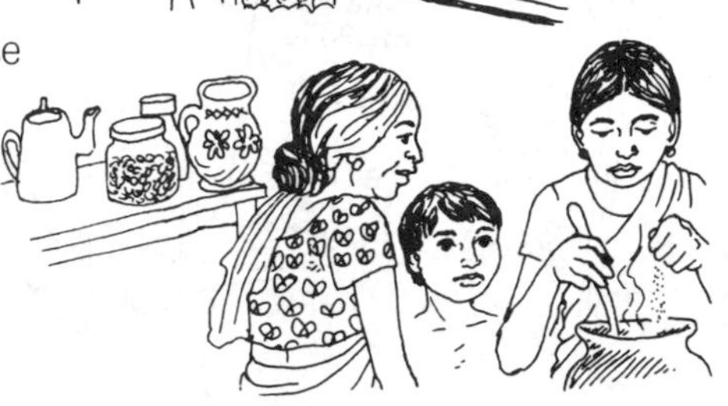

Examples:

- Card game on building balanced meals according to food groups, p. **25**-42
- "Snakes and Ladders," p. **11**-27

3. Demonstrations on food preparation. These can be done in the nutrition center. But it is often better to do them in the homes of families with poorly nourished children. Let mothers prepare the food themselves and help teach others. Use foods that are available in the local market or grown in family gardens.

4. Under-fives programs (well-baby clinics) with monthly weighing of children to help spot problems early. Chapter 22 contains many teaching ideas you can use, including a flannel-board weight chart to be made by mothers.

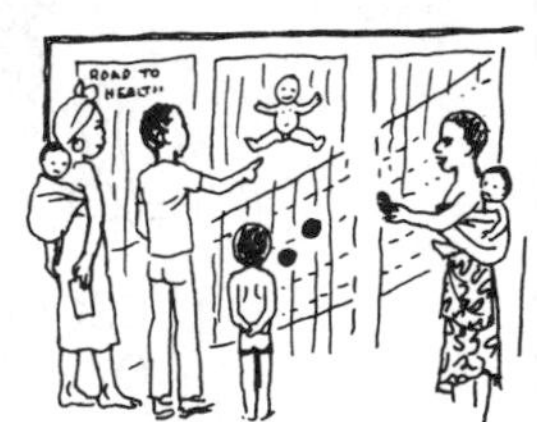

5. Role playing, sociodrama, mothers' theater, etc. Theater is excellent for getting people to think about ideas that require changes in the accepted way of doing things. Everyone can take part, or a group of villagers (or health workers) can perform. Follow up the performance with a discussion.

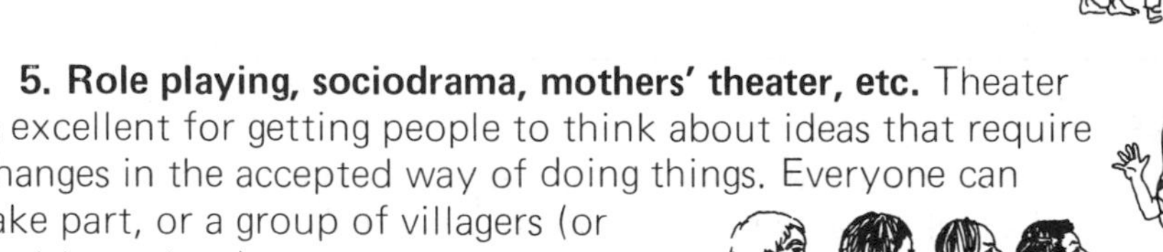

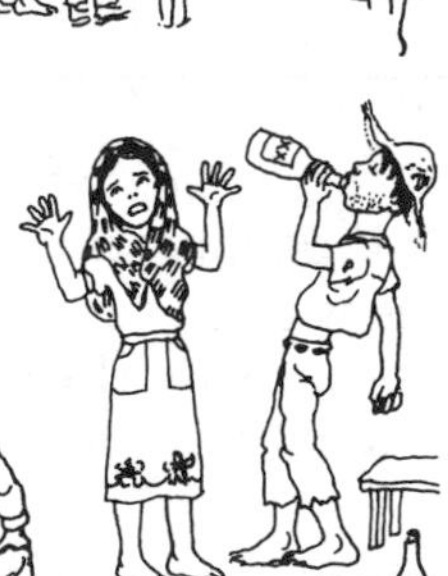

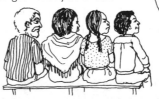

Examples:

- "Sensible Treatment of the Common Cold," p. **27**-3
- "Useless Medicines that Sometimes Kill," p. **27**-14
- "The Women Unite to Overcome Drunkenness," p. **27**-19
- "The Small Farmers Unite to Overcome Exploitation," p. **27**-27
- "The Importance of Breast Feeding," p. **27**-31

6. Puppet shows are especially fun and useful for children's groups. It is best if the children make puppets and conduct the show themselves.

Examples:

- Oral rehydration: Story of Pepito, p. **24**-28
- How to take care of your teeth, p. **27**-37

7. Small-group discussions and learning sessions with mothers, fathers, young people, etc. It is best if the talk about different foods is brought to life by having everyone bring real foods, rather than using flannel ones. (That way you will be sure to teach about foods that are available locally.) Use a dialogue approach and appropriate teaching aids (see Chapter 11).

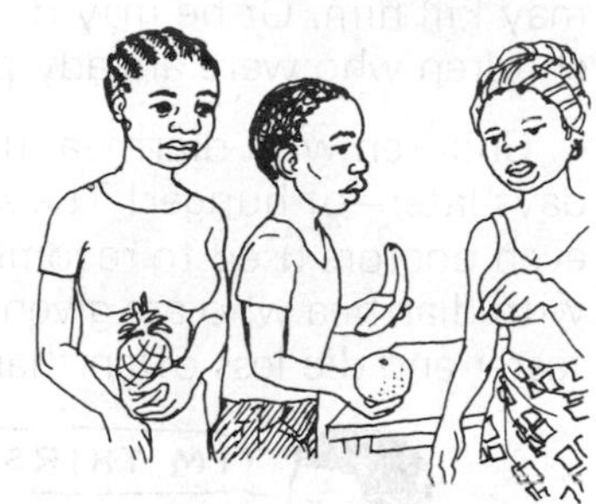

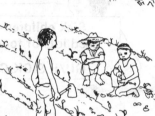

8. Garden and agricultural projects. Actual practice is the best way to learn about these.

Examples:

- Family or school gardens
- Better grain storage: making storage bins, pages **11**-1 and **25**-27
- Other possibilities for improved food production (see ***Where There Is No Doctor,*** p. w13 and w14)

9. Filmstrips, slides, films. It is a good idea to use methods health workers can later use for teaching in their villages. This means battery-operated projectors with filmstrips or slides rather than moving pictures, unless health workers will have access to movie projectors and electricity in their communities. Many groups distribute filmstrips and slides on nutrition. (See **Back**-3; also ***WTND,*** p. 429.)

10. CHILD-to-child activities help children to understand and meet the health needs of their younger sisters and brothers. Try to have children teach other children.

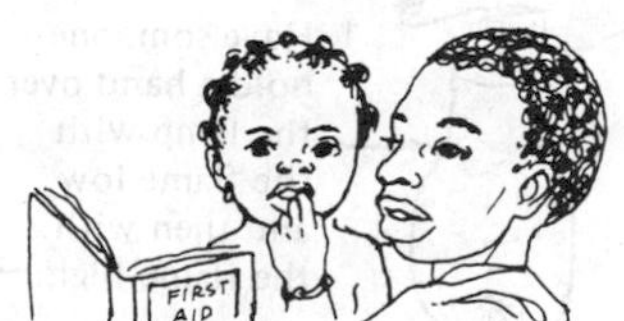

Examples related to nutrition:

- Learning about diarrhea: children discover through their own survey the importance of breast feeding, oral rehydration, and giving food to children with diarrhea, p. **24**-17
- Measuring to find which children are too thin: children make arm bands and measure younger children, p. **25**-14

11. Community practice and experience. As much as possible, health workers should have a chance during their training to practice all these different activities and teaching methods with people in a real village or community.

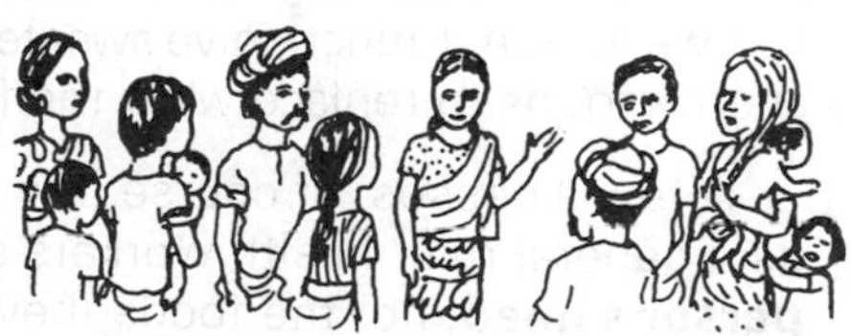

A TEACHING IDEA TO COMBAT THE DANGEROUS CUSTOM OF STARVING THE SICK

In many areas, people believe they should give little or no food or drink to sick persons. This custom contributes to many deaths—especially in children. When a sick child does not get enough food, he becomes so weak that his illness may kill him. Or he may die from malnutrition itself. The danger is greatest for children who were already poorly nourished before they became ill.

Children with diarrhea, if they do not die first of dehydration, often die a few days later—of hunger! The starving of children with diarrhea is a practice that even doctors used to recommend. (Some still do!) But studies show that children with diarrhea who are given a full, normal diet as soon as they can eat, get well faster and die less often than children who are given little or no food.

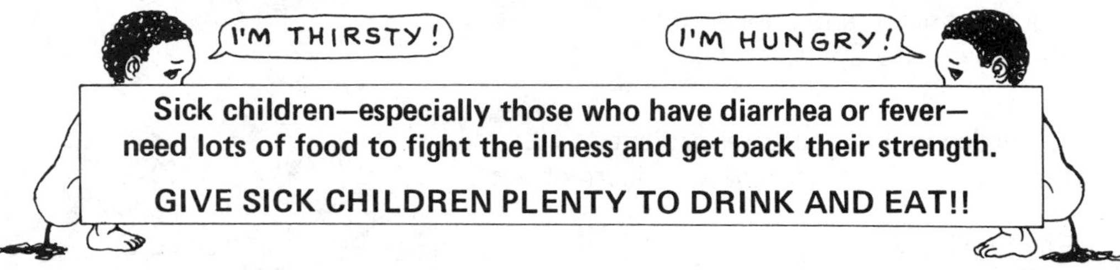

Sick children—especially those who have diarrhea or fever—need lots of food to fight the illness and get back their strength.
GIVE SICK CHILDREN PLENTY TO DRINK AND EAT!!

This is one of the most important lessons a health worker can teach people. But how? One way is to **compare fever with fire.**

High fever, like a hot fire, uses up a lot of fuel (energy foods). In one 3-hour attack of malaria, a person burns up as much energy as a farm worker needs for 8 hours of hard work! The sick person needs to eat enough energy foods (sugars, fats, and starchy foods) to replace what gets burned up by the fever. If not, the fever will begin to burn up the sick person's body, causing him to lose weight rapidly and grow very weak.

To help people understand this, you can use an oil lamp.

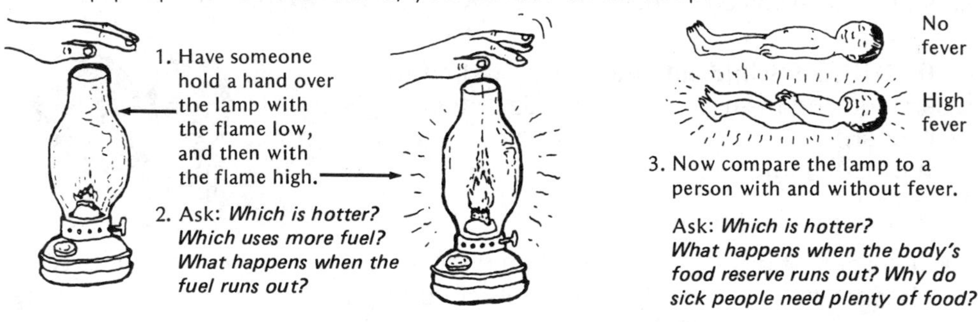

1. Have someone hold a hand over the lamp with the flame low, and then with the flame high.
2. Ask: *Which is hotter? Which uses more fuel? What happens when the fuel runs out?*
No fever
High fever
3. Now compare the lamp to a person with and without fever.
Ask: *Which is hotter? What happens when the body's food reserve runs out? Why do sick people need plenty of food?*

To fight infection and repair damage done by the illness, a sick person needs a balance of good foods (see Chapter 11 of ***Where There Is No Doctor***). If the person is too weak to chew, give him soups, broths, and mashed or liquid foods. If he is too weak to eat much, give sweetened drinks and juices. Be sure he gets enough energy foods to replace what the fever burns up.

A few illnesses, of course, require special diets (see ***WTND,*** p. 124 to 130). But as a general rule, health workers should **place emphasis on the foods sick persons need,** not the foods they should avoid.

A NEW WAY OF LOOKING AT FOOD GROUPS*

The typical food groups

To teach about nutritional needs, instructors often organize common foods into several groups. These food groups range in number from 3 or 4 to as many as 12, depending on whom you choose to listen to and where they come from.

The Food and Agriculture Organization (FAO) suggests 3 groups:

- *Body-building foods* (rich in proteins)
- *Protective foods* (rich in vitamins and minerals)
- *Energy foods* (starches and sugars, or carbohydrates; and fats)

In *Where There Is No Doctor* we use similar groups, but have divided energy foods into two groups: carbohydrates and fats.

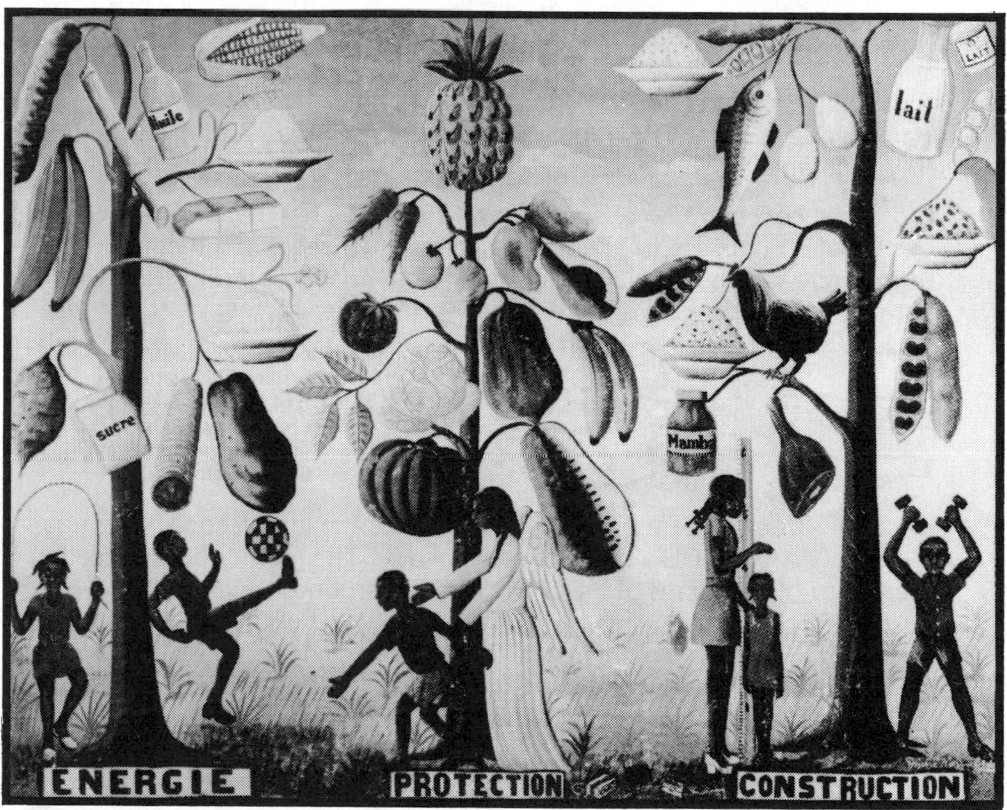

An imaginative poster for teaching typical food groups. (By Adeline Andre, from cover of *Teaching Nutrition in Developing Countries.)*

---

*Many of the ideas here are adapted from "Food Classification System for Developing Countries," by Abrahamsson and Velarde, in ***Teaching Nutrition in Developing Countries,*** Meals for Millions, 1800 Olympic Blvd., P.O. Box 680, Sta. Monica, CA 90406 USA.

The new food groups

The food groups as commonly taught reflect the food habits and training of people in wealthy countries. Too much emphasis is put on the ***kinds*** of foods that should be eaten. And not enough emphasis is placed on ***making sure children get enough to eat.*** We now know that in most places where malnutrition is common, **the main problem is not lack of protein, but lack of enough energy foods.**

In most parts of the world, one main low-cost energy food is eaten with almost every meal. Depending on the area, this may be rice, maize, millet, wheat, cassava, potato, breadfruit, or banana. In the typical food groups, this main food is simply listed with other energy foods. But, in addition to energy, **the main food usually provides half or more of the body's needed protein and vitamins.** It is the central or 'super' food in the local diet.

However, the MAIN FOOD alone is not enough to keep a person healthy, especially a growing child. HELPER FOODS are also needed. These include:

- Additional ***body-building foods.*** When eaten together with the main food, these help complete the body's protein needs. Examples are beans when eaten with maize ***tortillas*** in Latin America, and lentils or ***dahl*** when eaten with wheat ***chapatis*** in India.
- Additional ***protective foods.*** These help complete the body's need for vitamins and minerals. Examples are oranges, tomatoes, and dark green leafy vegetables.
- Additional ***concentrated energy foods.*** These include fats, oils, sugars, and foods that contain them. These are especially needed when the main food—for example, cassava or plantain—contains so much water and fiber (bulk) that it fills a child's belly before he gets enough energy supply (calories).

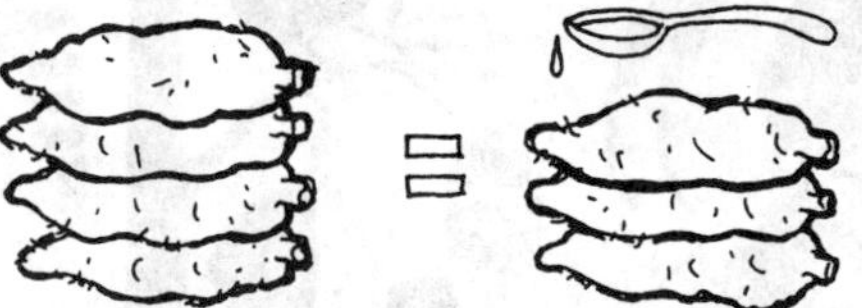

A spoonful of cooking oil added to a child's food means he only has to eat about ¾ as much of the local main food in order to meet his energy needs. The added oil helps make sure he gets enough calories by the time his belly is full.

A new way of looking at food groups emphasizes the importance of getting enough of the MAIN FOOD that people eat locally. The main food is placed in the center, with the 3 groups of HELPER FOODS around it.

The HELPER FOODS—which are the old groups of energy foods, body-building foods, and protective foods—can be called GO FOODS, GROW FOODS, and GLOW FOODS. These short names are fun and easier to remember. Remind students that:

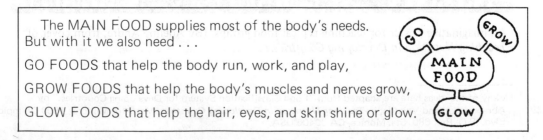

> The MAIN FOOD supplies most of the body's needs.
> But with it we also need . . .
>
> GO FOODS that help the body run, work, and play,
>
> GROW FOODS that help the body's muscles and nerves grow,
>
> GLOW FOODS that help the hair, eyes, and skin shine or glow.

A MORE APPROPRIATE WAY OF LOOKING AT FOOD GROUPS

GROW FOODS

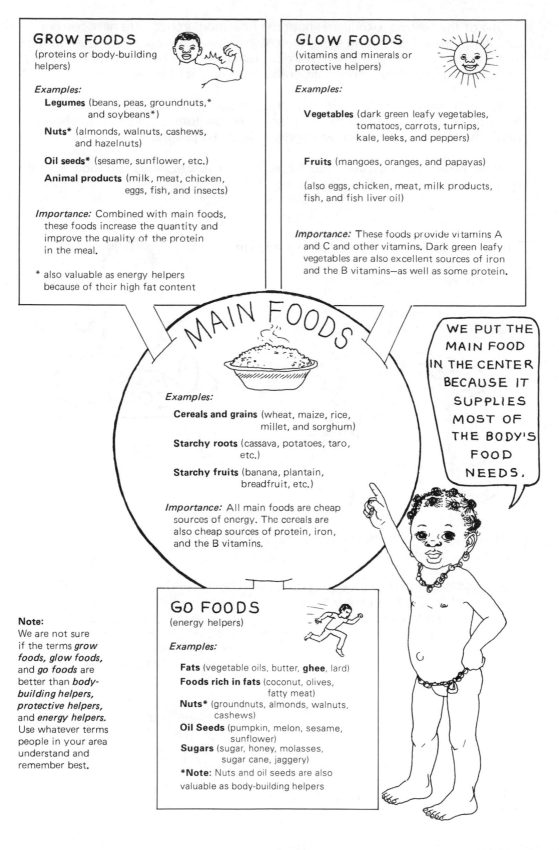

(proteins or body-building helpers)

Examples:

Legumes (beans, peas, groundnuts,* and soybeans*)

Nuts* (almonds, walnuts, cashews, and hazelnuts)

Oil seeds* (sesame, sunflower, etc.)

Animal products (milk, meat, chicken, eggs, fish, and insects)

Importance: Combined with main foods, these foods increase the quantity and improve the quality of the protein in the meal.

* also valuable as energy helpers because of their high fat content

GLOW FOODS

(vitamins and minerals or protective helpers)

Examples:

Vegetables (dark green leafy vegetables, tomatoes, carrots, turnips, kale, leeks, and peppers)

Fruits (mangoes, oranges, and papayas)

(also eggs, chicken, meat, milk products, fish, and fish liver oil)

Importance: These foods provide vitamins A and C and other vitamins. Dark green leafy vegetables are also excellent sources of iron and the B vitamins—as well as some protein.

MAIN FOODS

Examples:

Cereals and grains (wheat, maize, rice, millet, and sorghum)

Starchy roots (cassava, potatoes, taro, etc.)

Starchy fruits (banana, plantain, breadfruit, etc.)

Importance: All main foods are cheap sources of energy. The cereals are also cheap sources of protein, iron, and the B vitamins.

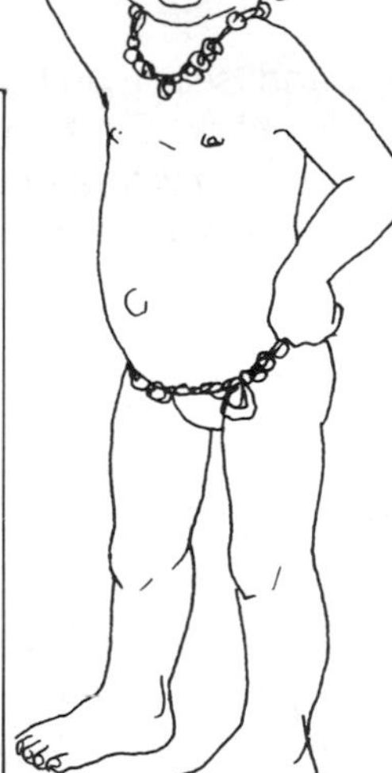

WE PUT THE MAIN FOOD IN THE CENTER BECAUSE IT SUPPLIES MOST OF THE BODY'S FOOD NEEDS.

GO FOODS

(energy helpers)

Examples:

Fats (vegetable oils, butter, **ghee**, lard)

Foods rich in fats (coconut, olives, fatty meat)

Nuts* (groundnuts, almonds, walnuts, cashews)

Oil Seeds (pumpkin, melon, sesame, sunflower)

Sugars (sugar, honey, molasses, sugar cane, jaggery)

***Note:** Nuts and oil seeds are also valuable as body-building helpers

Note:
We are not sure if the terms ***grow foods, glow foods,*** and ***go foods*** are better than ***body-building helpers, protective helpers,*** and ***energy helpers.*** Use whatever terms people in your area understand and remember best.

TEACHING IDEAS USING THE NEW FOOD GROUPS

One of the best ways to learn about the new food groups is to have persons actually prepare meals using foods they have grown themselves or bought in the local market. Even for classroom learning, real foods can be brought by students and arranged in different combinations to form balanced meals.

However, some local foods may not be available at all times of the year, so flannel-board foods or other pretend foods may be useful. Take care to **choose foods that are local, low-cost, and acceptable to the people.**

In whatever learning games you use, remember to keep the main food central. Here is an example of a teaching aid that does this:

The 3-legged stool for healthy eating

The seat of the stool is the MAIN FOOD and the 3 legs are formed by GROW FOODS, GO FOODS, and GLOW FOODS.

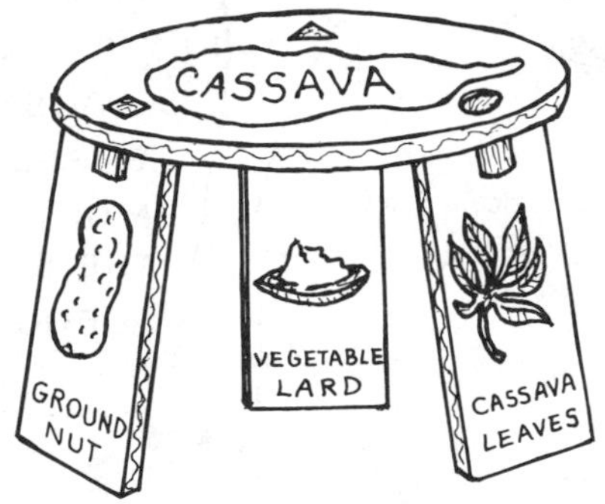

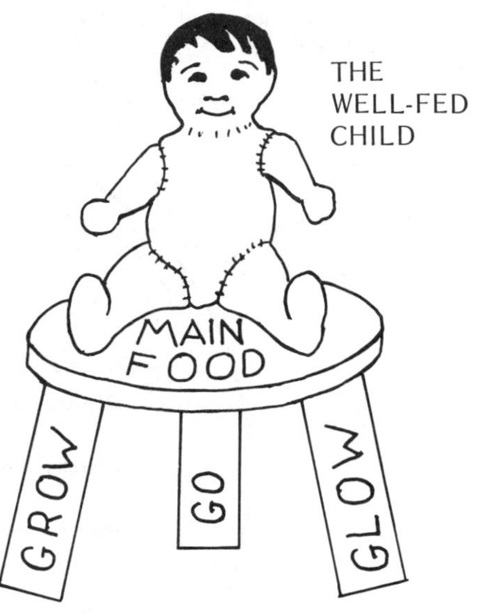

Have students make the doll and the stool themselves.

The round 'seat' can be made of cardboard, wood, or bark. Or if you live where the main food is ***tortilla*** or ***chapati*** (flat cakes of maize or wheat), use one of these, stale or toasted until stiff.

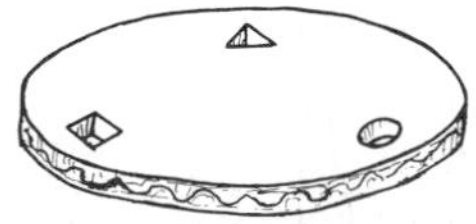

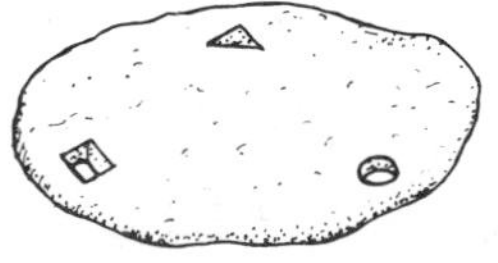

Make holes for the legs to fit into. You may want to use different-shaped holes for matching with the different food groups.

Using cardboard, fiberboard, wood, or pieces of tin cans, have students prepare cards with drawings of local foods on them. Include common GO FOODS, GROW FOODS, and GLOW FOODS. Use local names.

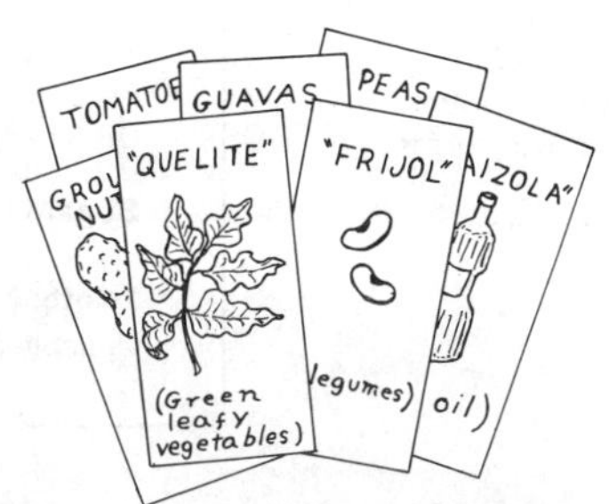

Figure out some way for the cards to fit into the stool seat as legs.

You could use different-shaped bits of wood with slots to grip the cards.

Or cut tabs on the tops of the cards to match slots in the seat.

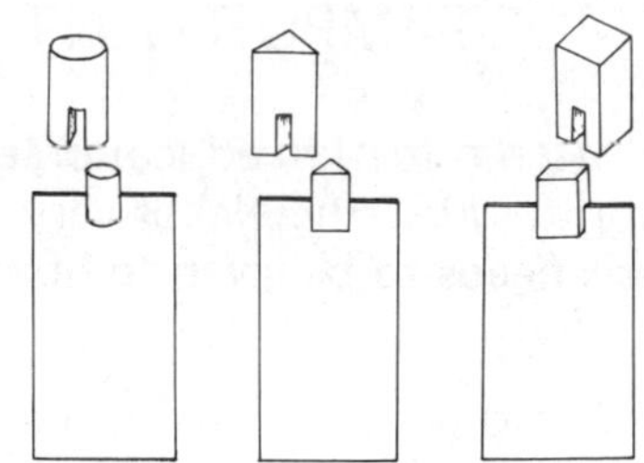

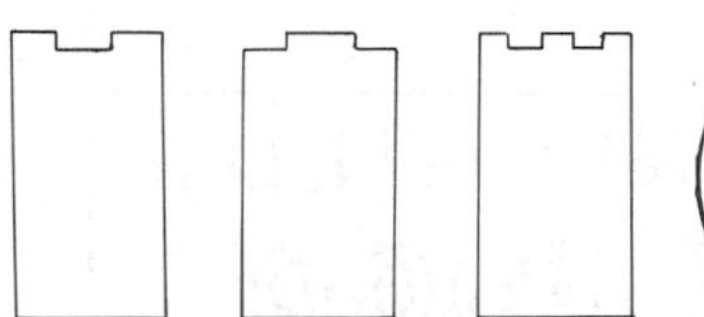

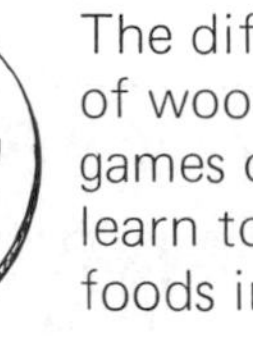

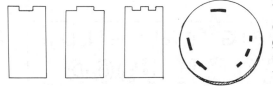

The different-shaped tabs or pieces of wood can be used in matching games or puzzles to help students learn to use all 3 kinds of helper foods in addition to the main food.

By practicing putting the stool together using different choices of 'legs', the students come to understand that **the main food forms the base** that holds the child up. They also learn that **all 3 groups of helper foods are needed** to keep a balance and to prevent the child from 'falling' (falling ill).

Students can use this teaching aid to practice forming balanced meals based on the main food. Give each student a few food cards, and let them take turns building meals for babies, children, and adults with the foods that are available at different times of year.

This way students learn that certain helper foods can be used in either one or both of 2 different positions. For example, groundnuts serve both as GROW FOODS (because they have protein) and as GO FOODS (because they are rich in oil). (To show this, make 2 cards for a food like groundnuts. And make 2 different tabs or wood pieces, to fit into both positions in the stool.)

You can adapt the 3-legged stool idea for use on a flannel-board.

If people in your area do not use stools, maybe the group can think of a way to adapt this teaching aid to build on local traditions.

In Haiti, for example, people traditionally use 3 rocks to hold up the cooking pot.

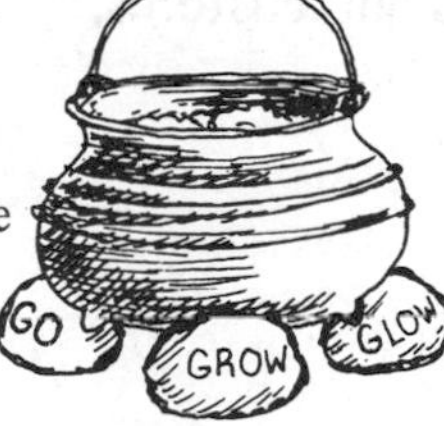

The pot can represent the main food.

The three rocks can represent the helper foods.

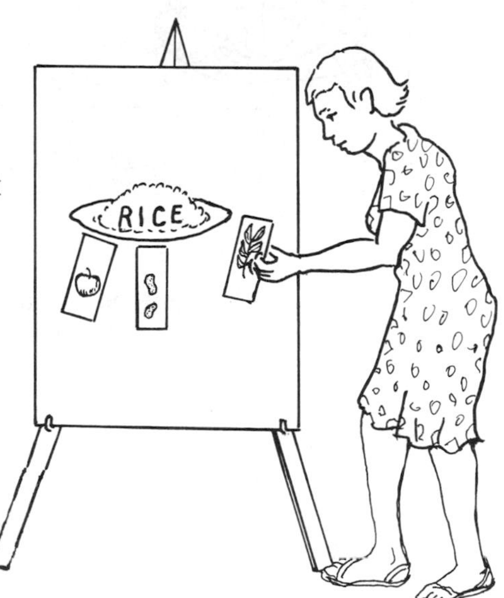

THE MOST IMPORTANT FOOD LESSON: *EATING ENOUGH!*

Too often nutrition education emphasizes diet *quality* and pays too little attention to *quantity.* Needs vary from place to place, but in general **far more emphasis needs to be given to how much a child eats, and how often.**

Some field workers suggest that, in places where regular child-weighing programs are being carried out, one main nutrition message should be emphasized:

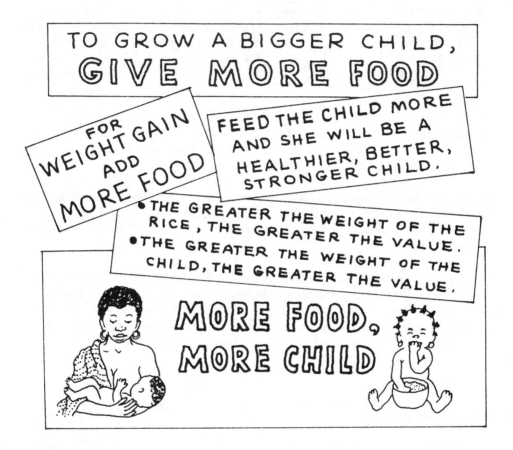

But before you accept any outsider's advice (including ours), be sure to question if it is true for your situation.

Adapt your message to people's beliefs and customs.

Looking at How Human Relations Affect Health

CHAPTER 26

Health, says the World Health Organization, ***is a state of complete physical, mental, and social well-being, and not merely the absence of disease or infirmity.*** We agree.

Throughout this book, we have pointed to the importance of the human factor in determining health and well-being. By the 'human factor' we mean ***how persons help or harm each other.*** We have seen how poverty lies behind the ills of most people. And in Chapters 23 and 25, we argued that hunger in the world is not primarily due to population growth or shortage of land and resources. Rather, it results from unfair distribution—of land, resources, and decision-making power. We conclude that:

Health depends less on technical than on social factors. The healthy person, family, community, or nation is one that is relatively self-reliant—one that can relate to others in a helpful, friendly way, as an equal.

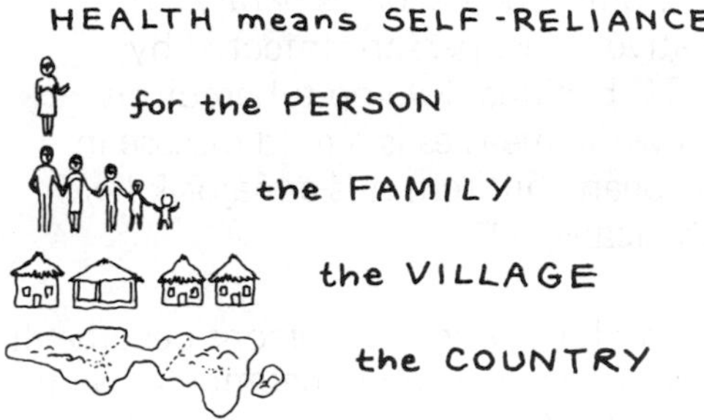
HEALTH means SELF-RELIANCE
for the PERSON
the FAMILY
the VILLAGE
the COUNTRY

The health worker's primary job is to help people gain greater control over their health and their lives. But this is easier said than done.

In this chapter, we look at ways of helping groups of people to become more aware of the social factors that affect their well-being, and to discover their own ability to change and improve their situation. The methods and activities we describe have been used effectively with groups of health workers-in-training. They have also been used by health workers to help community groups develop greater social awareness, self-confidence, and cooperative action.

First, we discuss a method used in Mexico to help groups observe how a variety of factors, both physical and human, combine to cause sickness and death. This is done by first telling or reading a story, then having the group analyze it by playing the question game, ***"But why . . . ?"***

Next, we explore group dialogue approaches for helping develop social awareness. We discuss the educational approach of the Brazilian educator, Paulo Freire, and look at ways that ***conscientization*** or 'awareness raising' has been adapted to health and nutrition work in villages and communities.

Finally, we look at strengths and weaknesses of different approaches to awareness raising. And we give examples of how people's increased understanding of their problems and their rights has led to organization and changes that contribute to better health.

ANALYZING THE CAUSES OF SICKNESS

One of the weaknesses of modern medicine is that it has led people to look at illness in terms of single causes. On the death certificate, the doctor writes as the cause of death 'typhoid' or 'polio' or 'tuberculosis' or 'measles'. He thinks of the cause of death in terms of a particular 'disease agent'—in these cases, either bacteria or virus.

However, **not all people who are infected with a disease agent become ill.** We know that many persons infected with typhoid bacteria never develop signs of the disease. Out of 400 children infected by the polio virus, only one becomes paralyzed. Relatively few persons infected by the TB bacillus develop tuberculosis. And while measles is a mild disease in European children, it is a major killer in Africa.

Different persons have different explanations for illness.

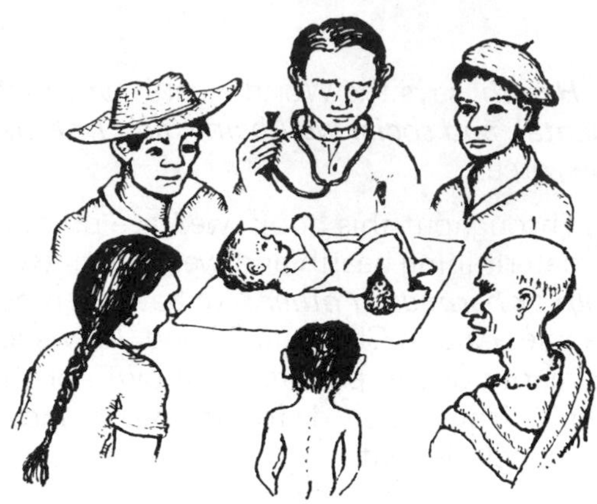

A good way to start a discussion about the causes of illness is to consider local beliefs and compare them with the explanations of doctors, educators, sanitary officers, social reformers, and others. (See *WTND*, p. 17.)

If we look at which persons become ill or die from diseases like tuberculosis, measles, diarrhea, and pneumonia, we find that many of them are poorly nourished. Or they live in crowded, unsanitary conditions. So in addition to the particular 'disease agent', we must also consider 'poor nutrition' or 'poor sanitation' as part of the cause of illness and death. But people usually do not eat poorly or live in unclean surroundings by choice. So poverty must also be included as an underlying cause of many illnesses. And so must the causes of poverty.

Sickness usually results from a combination of causes.

It is essential that health workers learn to look at illnesses and related problems in terms of their different causes: medical, physical, and human.

The following 'STORY OF LUIS' has been used in Mexico (and also Central America, Africa, and the Philippines) to help student health workers analyze the complex chain of causes that led to a boy's death. Tell the story to your group, or have students take turns reading it aloud, a paragraph at a time. Ask everyone to listen carefully and to try to notice all the factors that may have contributed to the boy's death.

Note: You may want to use a story that takes place in your own area. Perhaps your students can analyze the events leading to the death of someone they knew.

THE STORY OF LUIS

Consider Luis, a 7-year-old boy who died of tetanus. Luis lived with his family in the small village of Platanar, 11 km. by dirt road from the town of San Ignacio. In San Ignacio there is a health center staffed by a doctor and several nurses. The health center conducts a vaccination program and has a Jeep. But the vaccination program only occasionally reaches nearby villages. One year the health team began to vaccinate in Platanar, but after giving the first vaccination of the series, they never returned. Perhaps they grew discouraged because many parents and children refused to cooperate. Also, the road to Platanar is very dusty and hot.

When the staff of the health center failed to return to Platanar, a midwife from the village went to San Ignacio and offered to take the vaccine to the village and complete the vaccination series. She explained that she knew how to inject. But the doctor said no. He said that unless the vaccines were given by persons with formal training, it would be putting the children's lives in danger.

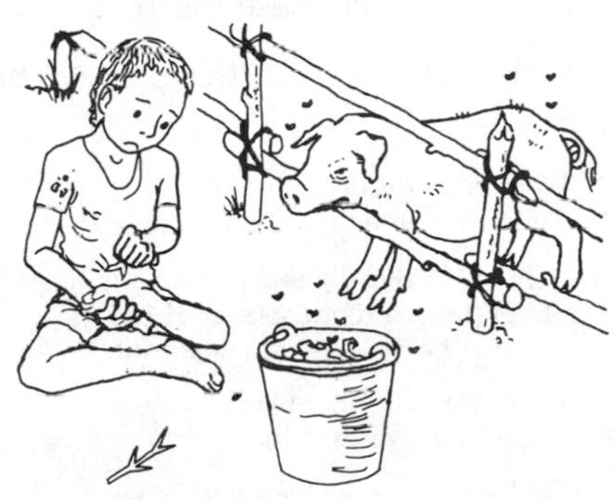

Three years later, the boy Luis took a bucket of food scraps to the pen where his family kept a mother pig and her piglets. On the way, he stepped on a long thorn with his bare foot. Normally Luis wore sandals, but his sandals had broken 3 days before and were too worn out to repair. Luis's father was a sharecropper who had to pay half his maize harvest as rent for the land he farmed. He was too poor to buy new sandals for his son. So Luis went barefoot. The boy pulled the thorn from his foot and limped back to the house.

Nine days later, the muscles in Luis's leg grew stiff and he had trouble opening his mouth. The following day, he began to have spasms in which all the muscles in his body suddenly tightened and his back and neck bent backwards.

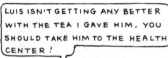

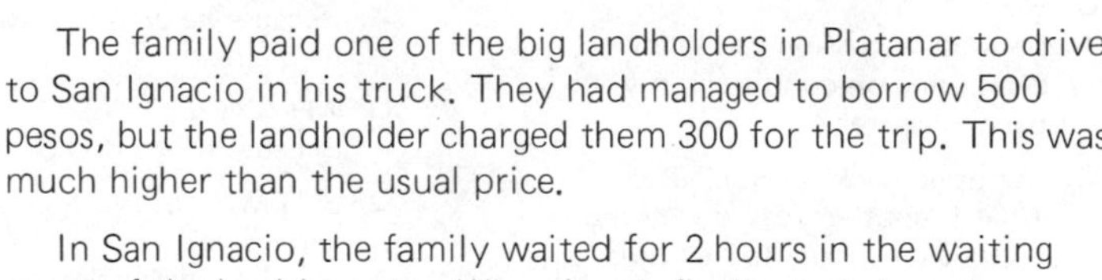

LUIS ISN'T GETTING ANY BETTER WITH THE TEA I GAVE HIM. YOU SHOULD TAKE HIM TO THE HEALTH CENTER!

The village midwife at first called his illness *congestion (WTND,* p. 23) and recommended an herbal tea. But when the spasms got worse, she suggested that Luis's parents take him to the health center in San Ignacio.

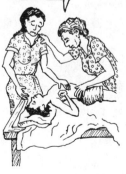

The family paid one of the big landholders in Platanar to drive to San Ignacio in his truck. They had managed to borrow 500 pesos, but the landholder charged them 300 for the trip. This was much higher than the usual price.

In San Ignacio, the family waited for 2 hours in the waiting room of the health center. When it was finally their turn to see the doctor, he at once diagnosed the illness as tetanus. He explained that Luis was in grave danger and needed injections of tetanus antitoxin. He said these were very expensive and, in any case, he did not have them. They would need to take Luis to the city of Mazatlan, 100 km. away.

The parents despaired. They had barely enough money left to pay the bus fare to Mazatlan. If their son died, how would they get his body back to the family graveyard in Platanar?

So they thanked the doctor, paid his modest fee, and took the afternoon bus back to Platanar. Two days later, after great suffering, Luis died.

What caused Luis's death? This is a key question to start discussion after reading or telling the story. The question can be approached in many ways. Here is one possibility.

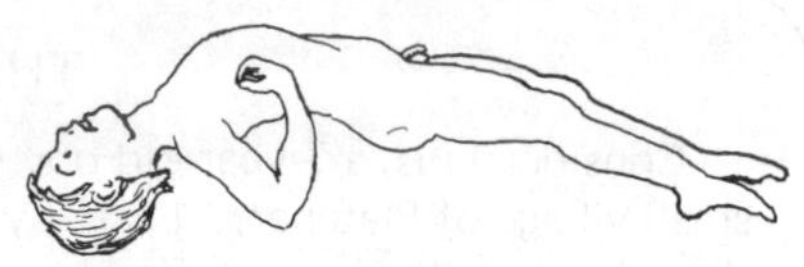

The question game: *"But why . . . ?"*

To help the group recognize the complex chain of causes that led to Luis's death, play the game, *"But why . . . ?"* Everyone tries to point out different causes. Each time an answer is given, ask the question *"But why . . . ?"* This way, everyone keeps looking for still other causes. If the group examines only one area of causes, but others exist, the discussion leader may need to go back to earlier questions, and rephrase them so that the group explores in new directions.

For the STORY OF LUIS, the *"But why . . . ?"* question game might develop like this:

Q: What caused Luis's illness?
A: Tetanus—the tetanus bacterium.

Q: BUT WHY did the tetanus bacteria attack Luis and not someone else?
A: Because he got a thorn in his foot.

Q: BUT WHY did that happen?
A: Because he was barefoot.

Q: BUT WHY was he barefoot?
A: Because he was not wearing sandals.

Q: BUT WHY not?
A: Because they broke and his father was too poor to buy him new ones.

Q: BUT WHY is his father so poor?
A: Because he is a sharecropper.

Q: BUT WHY does that make him poor?
A: Because he has to give half his harvest to the landholder.

Q: BUT WHY?
A: (A long discussion can follow, depending on conditions in your particular area.)

Q: Let us go back for a minute. What is another reason why the tetanus bacteria attacked Luis and not someone else?
A: Because he was not vaccinated.

Q: BUT WHY was he not vaccinated?
A: Because his village was not well covered by the vaccination team from the larger town.

Q: BUT WHY was the village not covered?
A: Because the villagers did not cooperate enough with the team when it did come to vaccinate.

Q: What is another reason?
A: The doctor refused to let the midwife give vaccinations.

Q: BUT WHY did he refuse?
A: Because he did not trust her. Because he thought it would be dangerous for the children.

Q: WHY did he think that way? Was he right?
A: (Again a whole discussion.)

Q: BUT not all children who get tetanus die. WHY did Luis die while others live?
A: Perhaps it was God's will.

Q: BUT WHY Luis?
A: Because he was not treated adequately.

Q: WHY NOT?
A: Because the midwife tried first to treat him with a tea.

Q: WHY ELSE?
A: Because the doctor in San Ignacio could not treat him. He wanted to send Luis to Mazatlan for treatment.

Q: BUT WHY?
A: Because he did not have the right medicine.

Q: WHY NOT?
A: Because it is too expensive.

Q: BUT WHY is this life-saving medicine so expensive?
A: (A whole discussion can follow. Depending on the group, this might include comments on the power and high profits of international drug companies, etc.)

Q: BUT WHY did Luis's parents not take him to Mazatlan?
A: They did not have enough money.

Q: WHY NOT?
A: Because the landholder charged them so much to drive them to San Ignacio.

Q: WHY did he do that? (A whole discussion on exploitation and greed can follow.)
A: Because they were so poor.
Q: BUT WHY are they so poor? (This question will keep coming up.)

Biological, physical, and social causes of illness

To analyze the causes of ill health and how they are related, it may help to group them as follows:

Symbols like these, adapted to your area, may help people understand and remember the different groups.

- *Biological:* caused by a living organism, such as a virus, bacterium, parasite, or fungus.
- *Physical:* caused by some condition in the physical environment, such as a thorn, lack of sufficient water, or crowded living conditions.
- *Social:* caused by human factors—the way people relate to or treat each other. These social causes can be divided into 3 sub-groups:
  - ***cultural:*** having to do with people's attitudes, customs, beliefs, and schooling (or lack of schooling).
  - ***economic:*** having to do with money, land, and resources—who has them and who does not.
  - ***political:*** having to do with power—who controls whom and how.

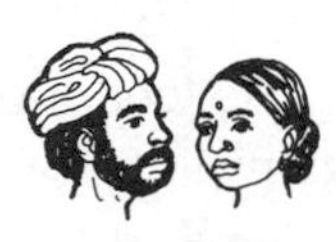

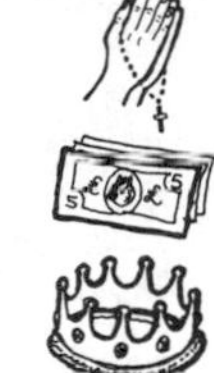

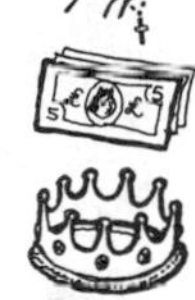

Ask the discussion group to list the various causes of a particular illness in columns under the headings ***biological, physical,*** and ***social.*** For example:

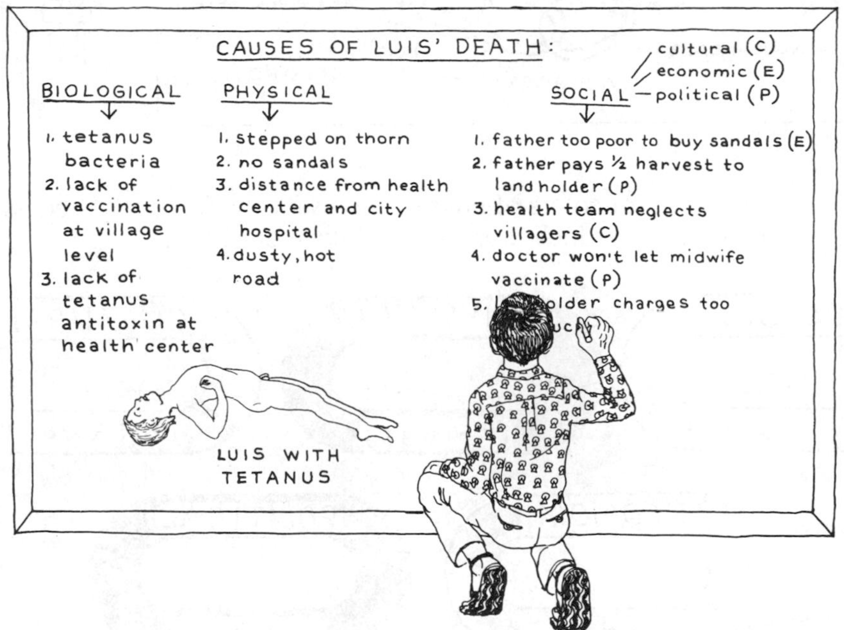

CAUSES OF LUIS' DEATH:
BIOLOGICAL
PHYSICAL
SOCIAL
cultural (C)
economic (E)
political (P)
1. tetanus bacteria
2. lack of vaccination at village level
3. lack of tetanus antitoxin at health center
1. stepped on thorn
2. no sandals
3. distance from health center and city hospital
4. dusty, hot road
1. father too poor to buy sandals (E)
2. father pays ½ harvest to land holder (P)
3. health team neglects villagers (C)
4. doctor won't let midwife vaccinate (P)
5. older charges too
LUIS WITH TETANUS

As the students draw up the list, they will soon realize that **social causes usually lie behind and are more numerous than the biological and physical causes.** It is very important that the group recognize and discuss these social causes, because . . .

- the social causes are often ignored or overlooked by professionals and authorities, and
- only after the underlying social causes of ill health have been dealt with, can there be a lasting improvement in the health of the poor.

The chain of causes

To help the group get a better idea of the chain or network of causes leading to illness and death, an actual chain can be formed. Each time another cause is mentioned, a new link is added to the chain.

Draw the chain on a blackboard or a large sheet of paper. Or cut out cardboard links, and drawings of Luis and a grave. These can be hung on a wall or fixed for use on a flannel-board.

The 'chain of causes' leading to Luis's death from tetanus might begin something like this:

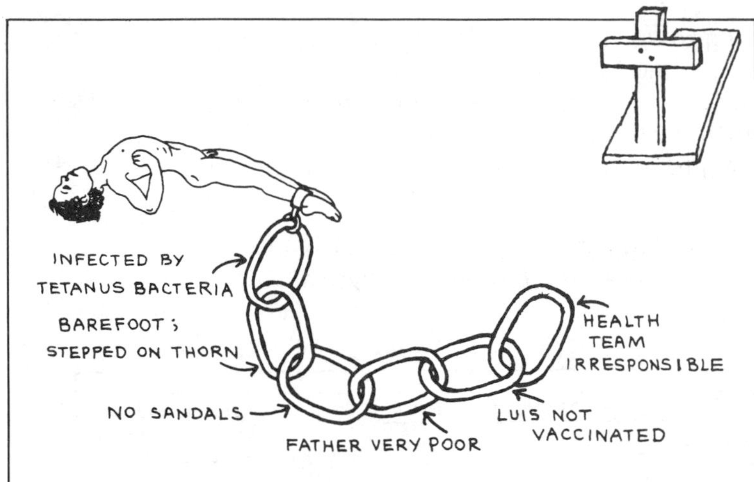

Be sure to use the symbol for the grave or death that is understood in your area.

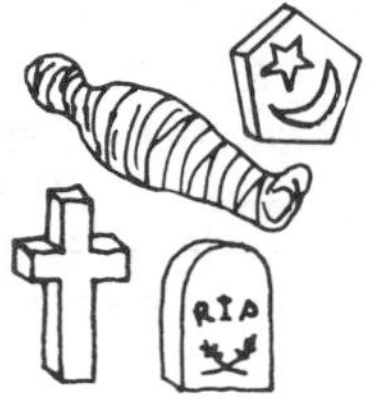

You can use 5 different colors of links to represent the 5 kinds of causes. Students can help make cardboard or flannel links themselves.

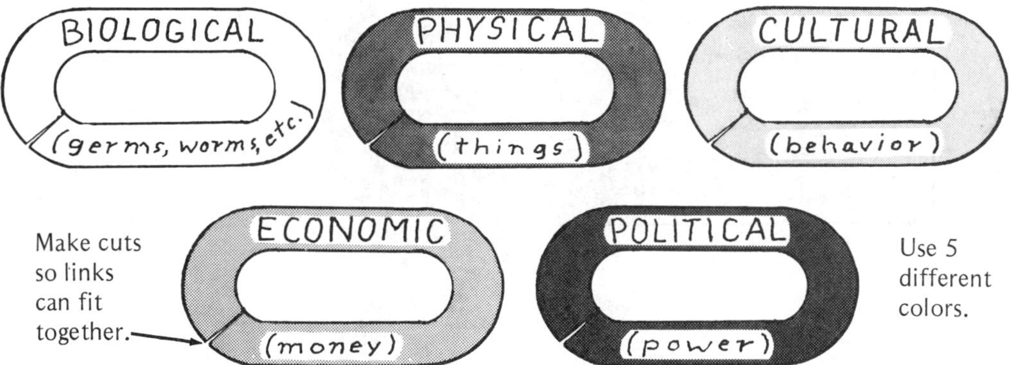

The group can form the 'chain of causes' as they play the game *"But why . . .?"* or as a review afterward. Give each student a few links. Then, each time a new cause is mentioned, everyone considers whether it is biological, physical, cultural, economic, or political. Whoever has the right link for a particular cause, comes forward and adds the link to the chain.

Link by link, the chain grows until it reaches the grave.

In this photo, students have pieced together the 'chain of causes' that led to the death of Luis.

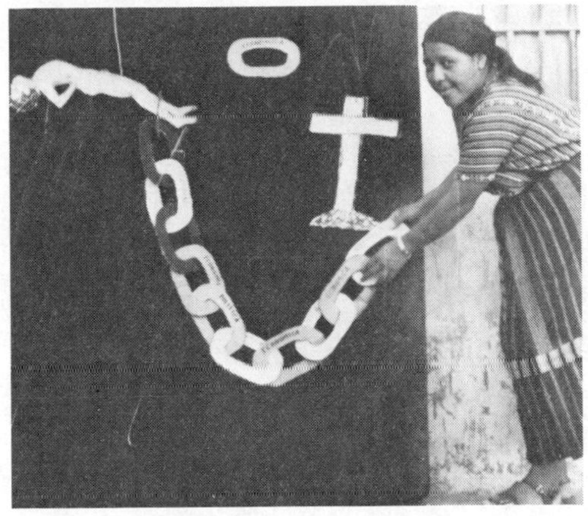

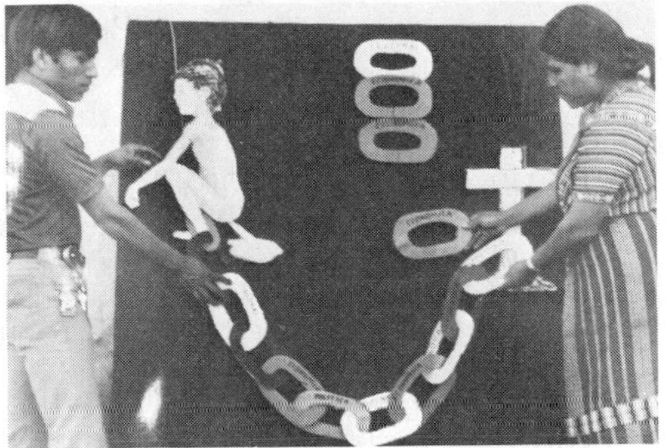

Here students build a chain based on a story about a child who died of diarrhea.

These teaching aids are useful early in a training course. They help increase the health workers' awareness about the different causes of health problems and the way they relate to each other. However, the aids can also be used by health workers to teach groups in their communities.

When playing the 'chain of causes' game with persons who cannot read, use local symbols on the links instead of (or as well as) words. Be sure to use symbols the people in your area will understand.

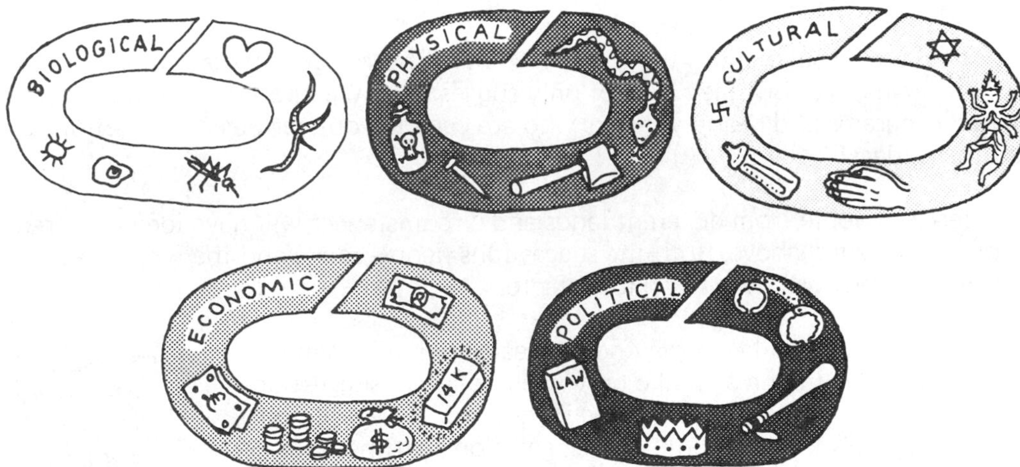

Note: You may be wise to avoid using big words like ***biological, physical,*** and ***social.*** Look for simpler terms people already use. For example, for ***cultural, economic,*** and ***political*** you might simply speak of causes related to ***beliefs, money,*** and ***power.***

BUT WHAT CAN WE DO?

After analyzing the causes of Luis's death, the next step is to ask the question, "What can we do?" **It is often easier for people to think of possibilities and discuss them openly if they first consider what other people might do.** So ask:

"What could the villagers of Platanar do to help prevent the death of other children like Luis?" Members of the discussion group may have a wide range of suggestions, some more realistic than others:

"Organize the community to insist that nurses from the health center come to vaccinate the children."

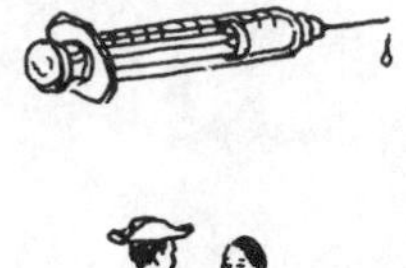

"Hold raffles and dances to collect an emergency fund for poor families that need medical treatment in the city."

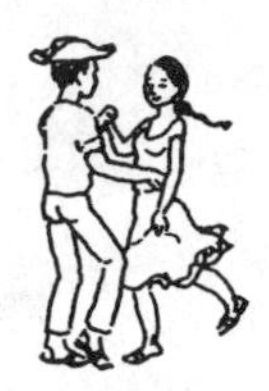

"Arrange to have someone from the village trained as a health worker."

"Start a cooperative, so people will not have to spend so much on food, and can afford sandals and other basic needs."

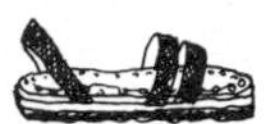

"Try to get the authorities to enforce laws calling for the redistribution of large landholdings."

"Organize the poor farmers to take over the land they now work as sharecroppers."

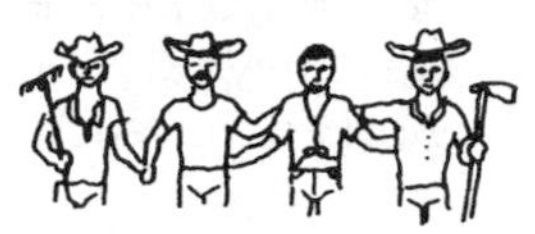

"Arrange for loans to groups of small farmers, so they can buy land they now farm as tenants."

"Unite with poor farmers' and workers' organizations to work for the changes that will put an end to sharecropping and other causes of poverty."

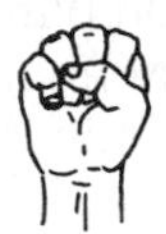

These are all suggestions that have been made by villagers in discussion groups in Latin America. But they are not only suggestions. We know of community-based programs and health workers who are carrying out various combinations of all these ideas!

Clearly, people from different lands and circumstances will have ideas different from those listed above. Both the suggestions people make and the ways they carry them out will depend on local factors.

In some places, villagers may not be ready to make many suggestions. Or they may make only 'well-behaved' suggestions such as, "Talk to the nurses and see if they would be willing to come vaccinate the children!" Any suggestion that the poor people organize, insist on their rights, or take action to resist the abuses of those in power may seem strange or fearful to them.

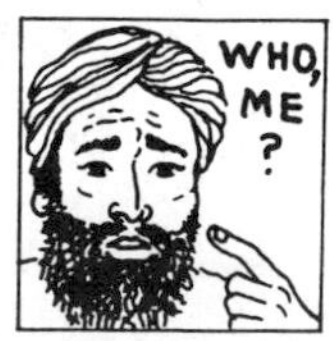

Even in places where more and more people are awakening to their own possibilities, **most of the poor still feel there is very little they can do to change their situation.**

For this reason, many community-based programs make the development of critical awareness a primary concern. Through special educational methods and 'group dialogues', they try to help people look at their situation more closely, realize their possibilities for changing it, and gain the self-confidence to take positive, cooperative action. This process of building social and self-awareness is the main theme of this chapter.

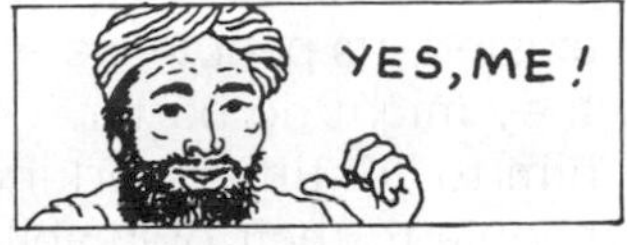
YES, ME!

Social change, through which the poor gain more control over the conditions that affect their well-being, is the key to "health for all."

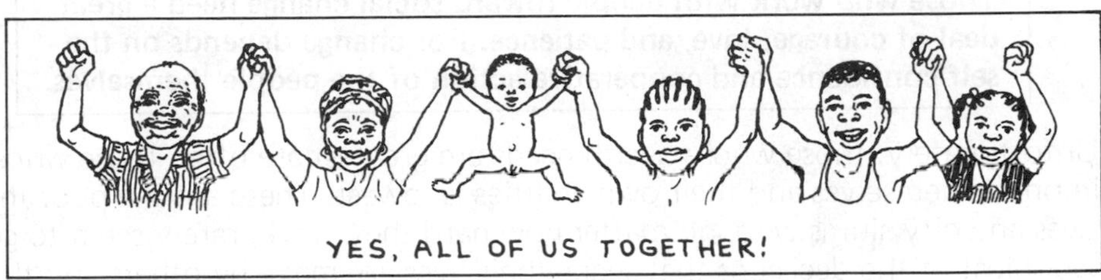
YES, ALL OF US TOGETHER!

DIFFICULTIES IN WORKING WITH PEOPLE TO IMPROVE THEIR SITUATION

Often health workers are eager to involve people in community action when they return to their villages after training. But many quickly grow discouraged.

We recently got a letter from a young man who had trained as a 'barefoot doctor' in a community-based program in Nuevo Leon, Mexico. His training, which had a strong political focus, had inspired him to try to organize people to work toward a fairer and healthier social order. In his letter to us, the health worker wrote of his frustration and sense of failure 6 months after returning to his own village:

"The people just don't seem to care!" he lamented. "I explain to them that in other communities farm workers have joined together to start cooperatives, taken action to regain land that is legally theirs, and replaced corrupt local officials with persons who represent their interests. But they just shrug their shoulders and admit they are exploited by the authorities, the shopkeepers, the landholders, and the money lenders. No one is willing to open his mouth in a village meeting or raise a finger to do anything about it. Nobody tries to look ahead; nobody even seems to care that much. When things are too bad, the men get drunk and beat their wives or children instead of coming together to solve their problems. The people in my village are hopeless! I give up!"

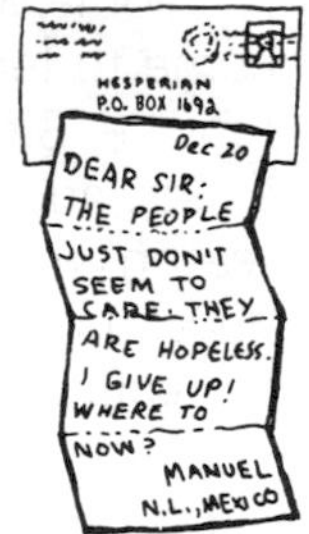
HESPERIAN
P.O. BOX 1692
Dec 20
DEAR SIR:
THE PEOPLE JUST DON'T SEEM TO CARE. THEY ARE HOPELESS. I GIVE UP! WHERE TO NOW?
MANUEL
N.L., MEXICO

He went on to ask if we could suggest a different village where he could work, where people would be more willing to work toward overcoming their problems.

We wrote back to the young health worker, saying that if such a community existed, its people were probably already working toward social change. And if so, they might do better without the help of an 'outsider' like himself. We encouraged him to continue working in his own village, and to look for ways of awakening people to their own ability to change things that affect their lives.

We pointed out that, for 16 years, the village health team that we helped get started has been trying to get poor farmers in their villages to work together against the abuses of local authorities and landholders. But it has been only in the last 3 or 4 years that any significant, if small, advances have been made.

Those who work with people toward social change need a great deal of courage, love, and patience. For change depends on the self-confidence and cooperative action of the people themselves.

Unfortunately, those whose health needs are greatest are often those whose opinion of themselves and their own abilities is lowest. These are the poor in villages and city slums who, no matter how hard they work, rarely seem to get ahead. Most of the decisions that shape their lives are made by others—by those who control the land, the wages, the rents, the prices, and the laws.

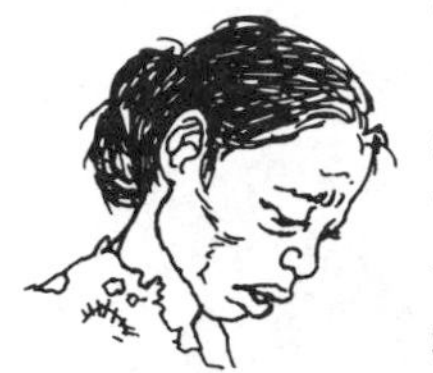

Because the poor are denied enough land or wages to adequately care for their families, they are often hungry and in debt. For their health and survival they become increasingly dependent on the aid and 'good will' of those in control. They learn that it is safest to suffer in silence, without question. Even without anger.

In time, those on the bottom begin to see themselves as the rich see them—worthless and lazy. They believe they are incapable of learning new skills or dealing adequately with their own needs. What choice do they have but to silently accept their fate? They suffer exploitation without protest. They obediently serve those who make decisions for them. And they celebrate with explosive abandon when there is an opportunity to temporarily forget the burden of day-to-day subsistence.

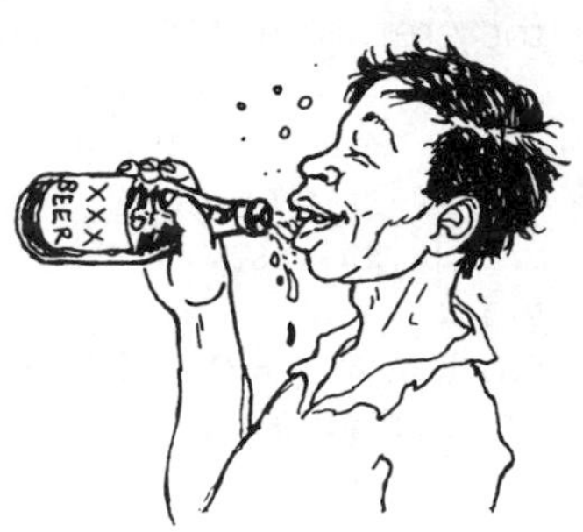

People who have long been on the bottom of the social order may also have come to fear the responsibilities that equality, social justice, and personal freedom require. Since childhood, they have been taught to defend the social order as it exists, and are suspicious of 'troublemakers' who seek to change it. For this reason, the health worker who speaks out against unfair or unhealthy doings in his community may find himself rejected even by those whose interests he is struggling to defend!

The biggest obstacle to change is the idea that change is impossible. The most important beginning moment in working toward change is when people achieve some success, no matter how small, in improving something they had never considered could be changed. On pages **26**-36 through **26**-38 are some examples of such successes.

THE NEED TO START WHERE PEOPLE ARE, AND WORK FROM THERE

Too often, those of us committed to social change have our heads in the clouds. We dream of the day when our country, or even the world, will be a place where . . .

- all people are treated as equals,
- all people have similar opportunities to work,
- all people have a right to a fair share of what the earth provides, and
- the many are no longer controlled and exploited by the few.

Such high and distant dreams have their place. For some of us, they provide a long-range vision and sense of direction—a sort of compass by which we can check our course.

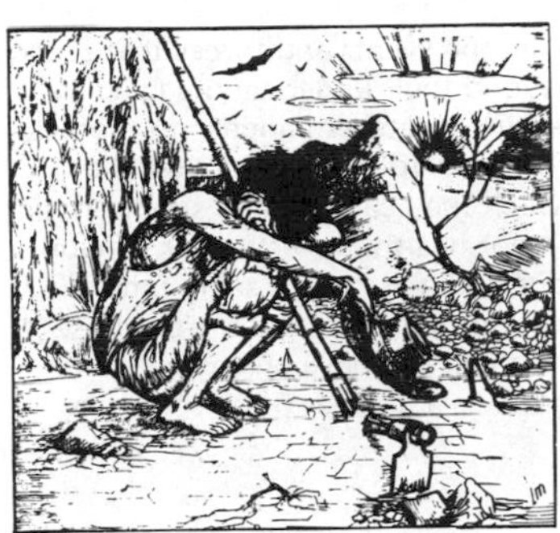

But for those among us who lack sufficient land to plant or who must worry about how to feed their children, their dreams are closer to home. Often they have little concern about national or international affairs, even those that affect their lives. Their concerns are here and now: "my village, my children, my struggle to keep my loved ones alive." Life is too uncertain right now to worry much about what happens far away or far in the future. Their concern is not for some vague and distant dream of 'social justice'. It is to feed and care for their families.

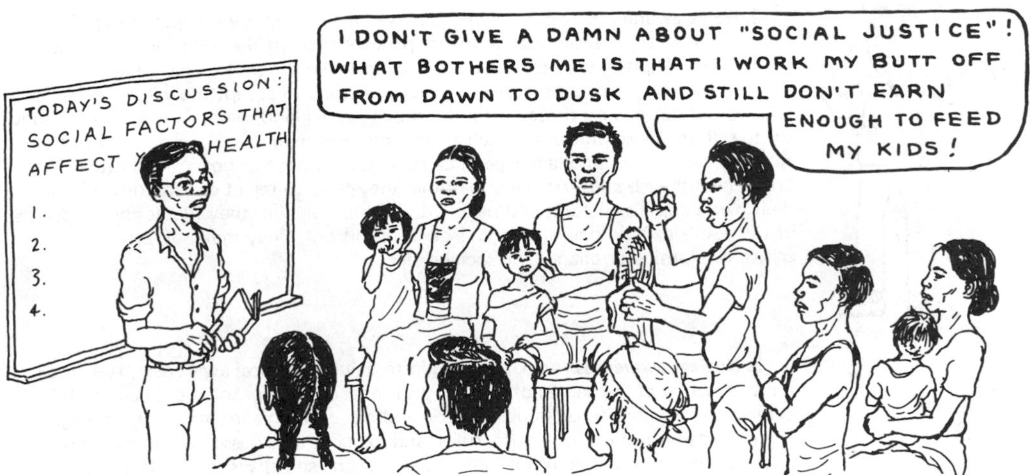
TODAY'S DISCUSSION:
SOCIAL FACTORS THAT
AFFECT
HEALTH
1.
2.
3.
4.
I DON'T GIVE A DAMN ABOUT "SOCIAL JUSTICE"! WHAT BOTHERS ME IS THAT I WORK MY BUTT OFF FROM DAWN TO DUSK AND STILL DON'T EARN ENOUGH TO FEED MY KIDS!

Discussion leaders sometimes fail to communicate because they talk in general terms or use unfamiliar expressions. Try to build discussion around people's specific, immediate concerns—in familiar, everyday words.

To be effective, the health worker needs to begin with the day-to-day concerns of the people, and work from there. As people begin to solve some of their most immediate problems, they will find courage to look further ahead. In time, they may become more concerned with how things at the national, or even international, level affect their lives. But start where the people are!

DIFFERENT LEVELS OR STAGES OF AWARENESS

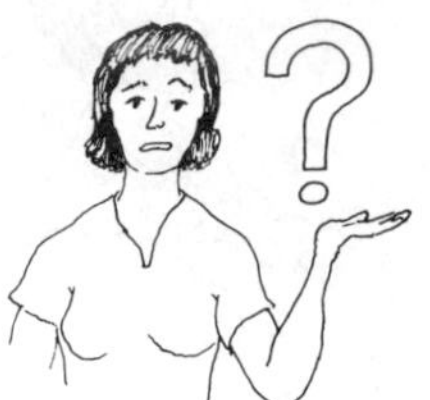

Why is it that so many people "just don't seem to care" about changing or improving their situation?

What can I do to help people awaken to their own possibilities?

To help health workers answer these questions, it may be useful to discuss the following 'stages of awareness'. These are based on the ideas of Paulo Freire, the Brazilian educator. Freire's methods for the development of 'critical awareness' became widely used in Brazil as a part of literacy programs (for learning to read and write). After the military coup in 1964, however, Freire was jailed and later thrown out of the country. Freire describes 3 main stages of awareness:

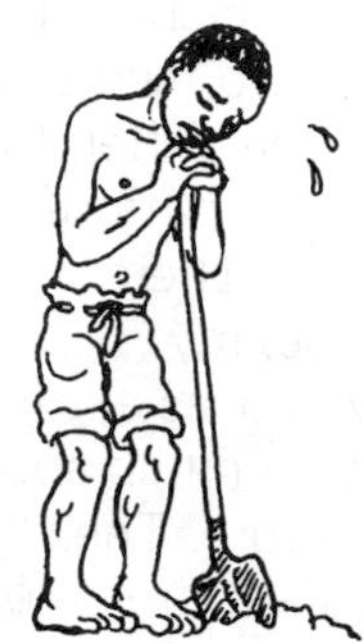

1. Magic awareness. At this stage, people explain the events and forces that shape their lives in terms of myths, magic, or powers beyond their understanding and control. They tend to be ***fatalistic,*** passively accepting whatever happens to them as fate or 'God's will'. Usually they blame no one for the hardships and abuses they suffer. They endure these as facts of life about which they cannot (and should not) do anything. Although their problems are great—poor health, poverty, lack of work, etc.—they commonly deny them. They are exploited, but are at the same time dependent upon those with authority or power, whom they fear and try to please. They conform to the image of themselves given to them by those on top. They consider themselves inferior, unable to master the skills and ideas of persons they believe are 'better' than themselves.

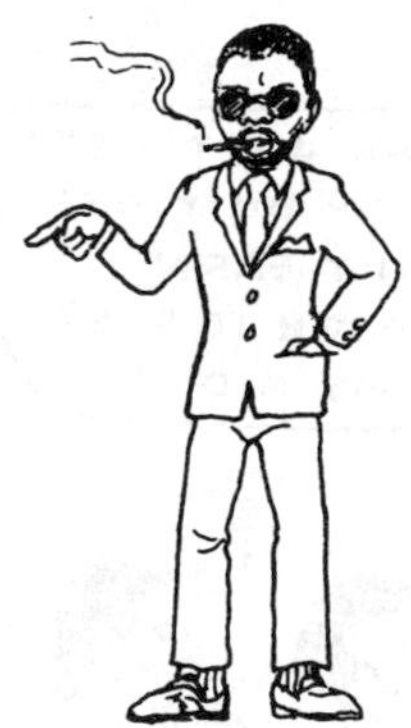

2. Naive awareness. A person who is ***naive*** has incomplete understanding. Persons at the naive stage of awareness no longer passively accept the hardships of being 'on the bottom'. Rather, they try to adapt so as to make the best of the situation in which they find themselves. However, they continue to accept the values, rules, and social order defined by those on top (authorities, big landholders, etc.). In fact, they try to imitate those on top as much as possible. For example, they may adopt the clothing, hair styles, and language of outsiders, or choose to bottle feed rather than breast feed their babies. At the same time, they tend to reject or look down upon their own people's customs and beliefs. Like those on top, they blame the hardships of the poor on their ignorance and 'lack of ambition'. They make no attempt to critically examine or change the social order.

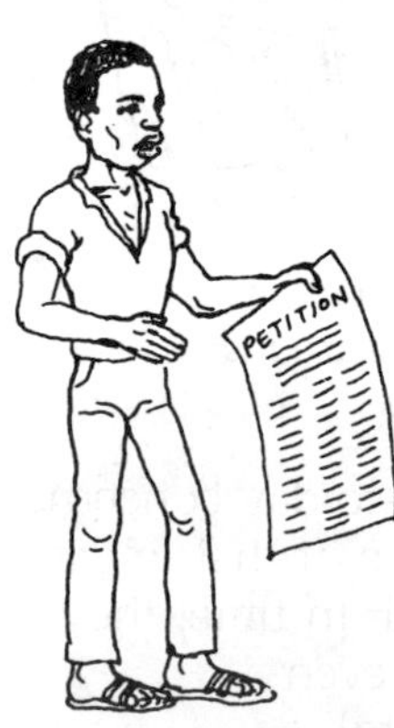

3. Critical awareness. As persons begin to develop critical awareness, they look more carefully at the causes of poverty and other human problems. They try to explain things more through observation and reason than through myth or magic. They start to question the values, rules, and expectations passed down by those in control. They discover that not individuals, but the social system itself, is responsible for inequality, injustice, and suffering. They find that it is set up to favor the few at the expense of the many, yet they see that those in power are in some ways also weak, and are also 'dehumanized' by the system. Critically aware persons come to realize that only by changing the norms and procedures of organized society can the most serious ills of both the rich and the poor be corrected.

As their awareness deepens, these persons also begin to feel better about themselves. They take new pride in their origins and traditions. Yet they are self-critical and flexible. They do not reject either the old or the new, but try to preserve from each what is of value. As their self-confidence grows, they begin to work with others to change what is unhealthy in the social system. Their observations and critical reasoning lead them to positive action.

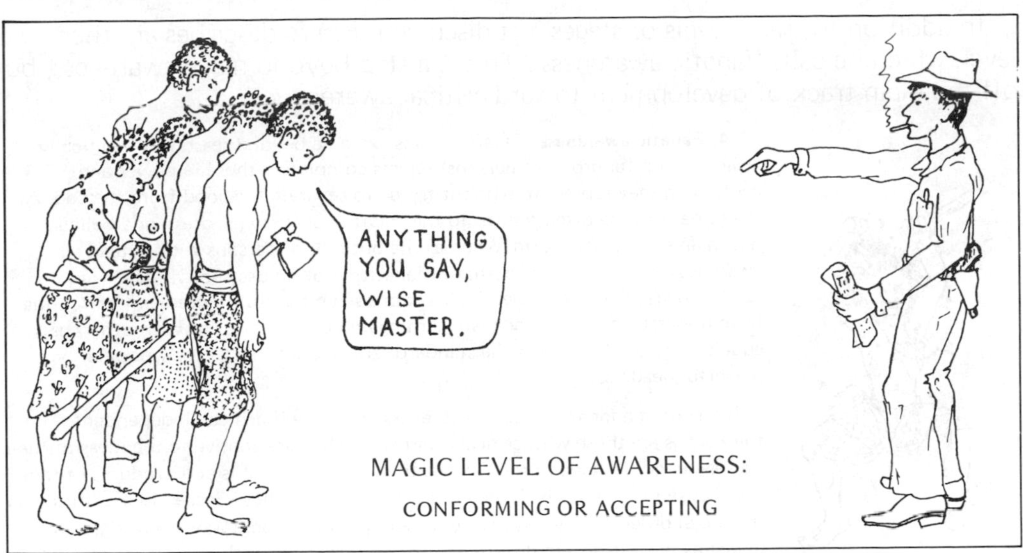
ANYTHING YOU SAY, WISE MASTER.
MAGIC LEVEL OF AWARENESS:
CONFORMING OR ACCEPTING

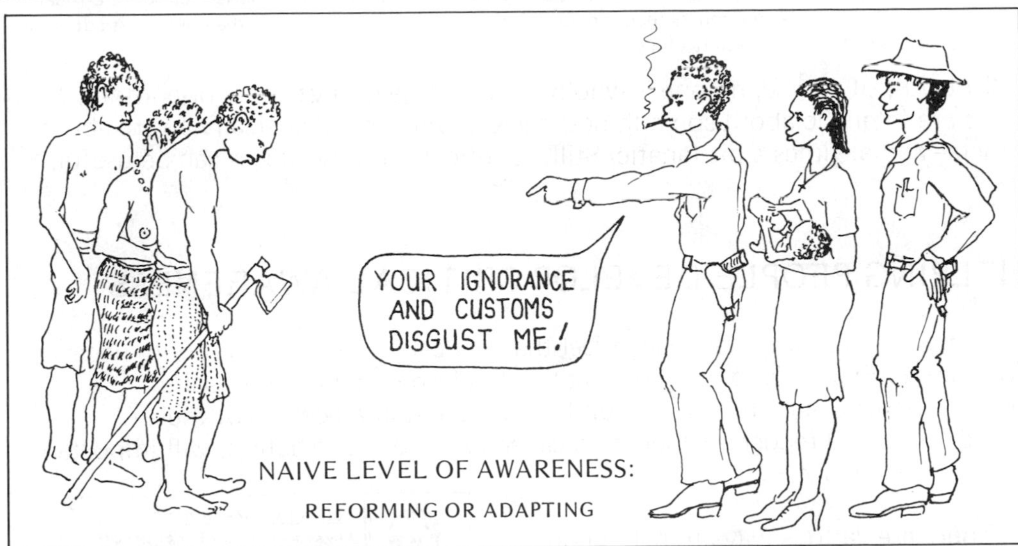
YOUR IGNORANCE AND CUSTOMS DISGUST ME!
NAIVE LEVEL OF AWARENESS:
REFORMING OR ADAPTING

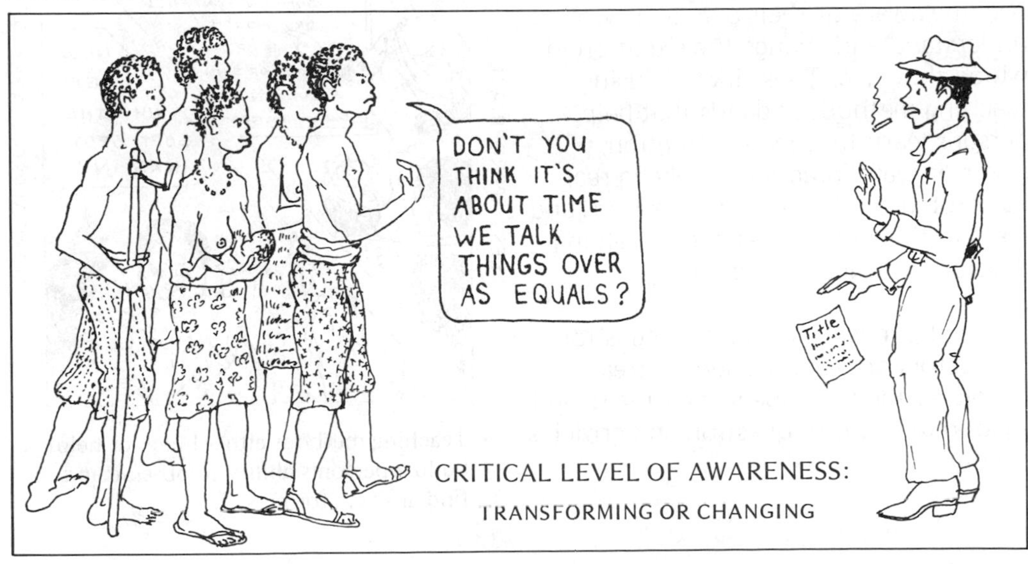
DON'T YOU THINK IT'S ABOUT TIME WE TALK THINGS OVER AS EQUALS?
Title
CRITICAL LEVEL OF AWARENESS:
TRANSFORMING OR CHANGING

In addition to the 3 levels or stages just discussed, Freire describes another level, which he calls 'fanatic awareness'. This is a step beyond naive awareness, but off the main track of development toward critical awareness.

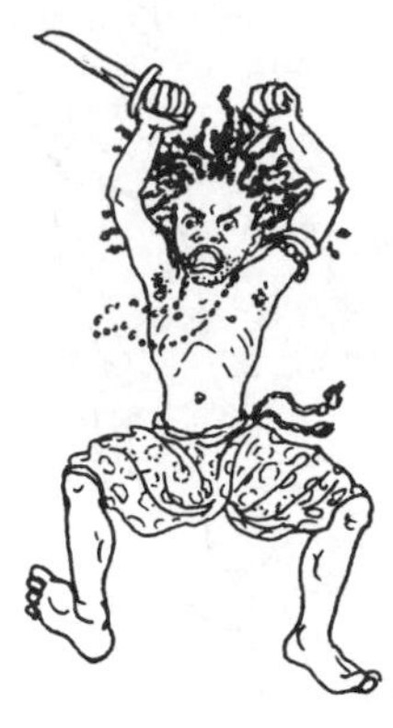

4. Fanatic awareness. *Fanatic* means extreme beyond reason. A fanatically aware person (or group of persons) rejects completely those in power and everything they represent, without trying to separate the good from the bad. At the same time, he often returns to the traditional customs, dress, and beliefs, but in an exaggerated form. Whereas the outlook of persons with critical awareness is mostly positive, that of fanatics is often destructive. Their opinions tend to be rigid, not flexible. Their actions seem to result more from hatred than from understanding. Rather than learning and communicating with others as equals, they tend to repeat the standard radical doctrines of their popular, yet powerful, leaders.

Persons at a fanatic level of awareness are not self-critical, independent thinkers as are those with critical awareness. They are captive to the ideas of their power-hungry leaders. In some ways, they are still servants and products of the social system against which they rebel. If and when they succeed in overthrowing the social order, the new system they set up may in some ways be as rigid and unjust as the old system it replaces. For all this, the fanatic is closer to critical awareness than someone in the naive stage and, if given the right short cut, may reach it sooner.

In truth, of course, no one is wholly at one stage of awareness or another. Many of us are fatalistic about some things, naive about others, critically aware about others—and at times a bit fanatic. Still, to reflect on these stages can be useful.

HELPING PEOPLE DEVELOP CRITICAL AWARENESS

Many leaders for social change feel that critical awareness is not only necessary for community development, but that it should be the primary goal of development. Only when people understand the human causes of their misfortunes and recognize their own capacity for positive action, will important changes take place.

There are various ways to help people become aware of their own ability to understand and change the situation in which they live. These include using teaching methods and aids that help persons learn through exploration, discovery, and practice in solving real-life problems. (Most of the methods and ideas in this book are aimed at helping develop critical awareness.)

But the most important thing is for instructors or group leaders to treat people as equals, respect their ideas, and encourage them to question and criticize openly.

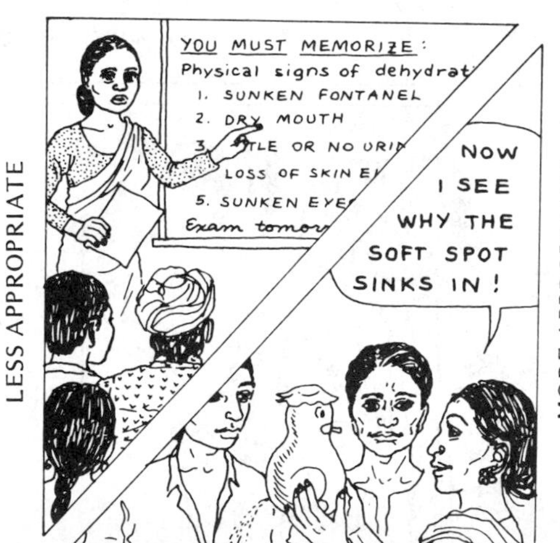
LESS APPROPRIATE
YOU MUST MEMORIZE:
1. SUNKEN FONTANEL
2. DRY MOUTH
NOW I SEE WHY THE SOFT SPOT SINKS IN!
MORE APPROPRIATE

Teaching methods either block or help build a person's ability to observe and find answers for herself.

To have critical awareness means to question—to doubt things that are often simply accepted. Development of such awareness in yourself and others is an important step in working toward a healthier situation for the poor.

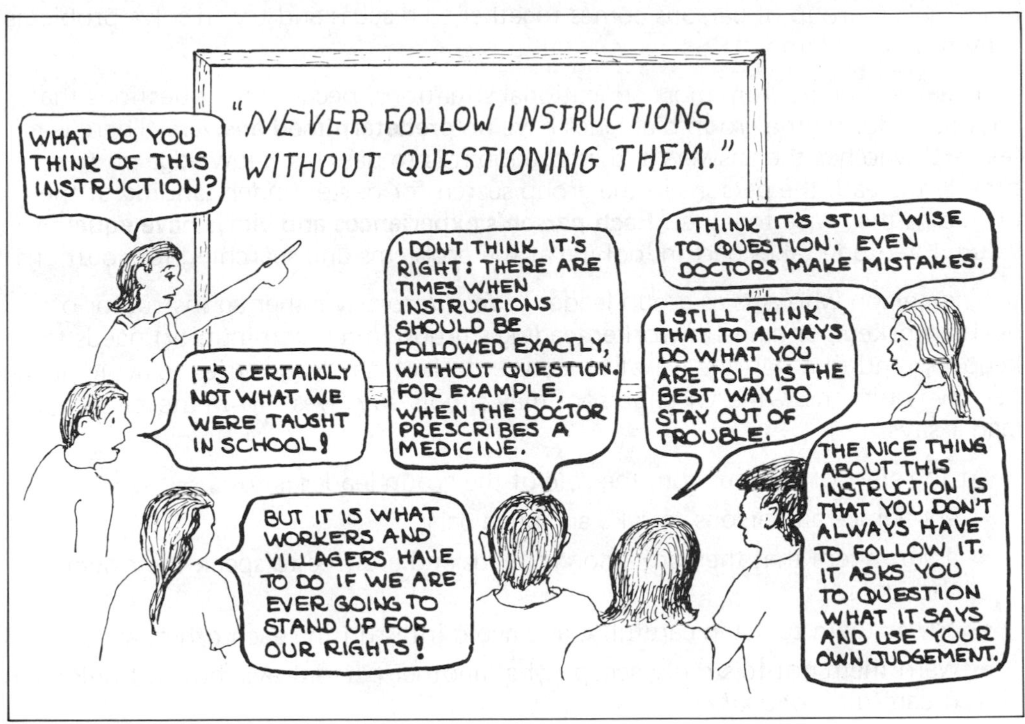
"NEVER FOLLOW INSTRUCTIONS WITHOUT QUESTIONING THEM."
WHAT DO YOU THINK OF THIS INSTRUCTION?
IT'S CERTAINLY NOT WHAT WE WERE TAUGHT IN SCHOOL!
BUT IT IS WHAT WORKERS AND VILLAGERS HAVE TO DO IF WE ARE EVER GOING TO STAND UP FOR OUR RIGHTS!
I DON'T THINK IT'S RIGHT: THERE ARE TIMES WHEN INSTRUCTIONS SHOULD BE FOLLOWED EXACTLY, WITHOUT QUESTION. FOR EXAMPLE, WHEN THE DOCTOR PRESCRIBES A MEDICINE.
I THINK IT'S STILL WISE TO QUESTION. EVEN DOCTORS MAKE MISTAKES.
I STILL THINK THAT TO ALWAYS DO WHAT YOU ARE TOLD IS THE BEST WAY TO STAY OUT OF TROUBLE.
THE NICE THING ABOUT THIS INSTRUCTION IS THAT YOU DON'T ALWAYS HAVE TO FOLLOW IT. IT ASKS YOU TO QUESTION WHAT IT SAYS AND USE YOUR OWN JUDGEMENT.

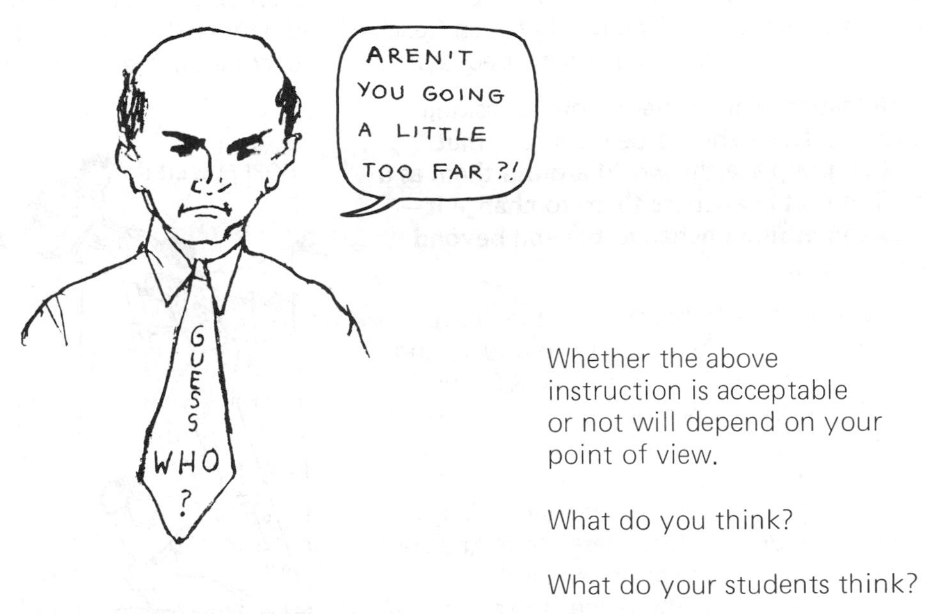
AREN'T YOU GOING A LITTLE TOO FAR?!
GUESS WHO?

Whether the above instruction is acceptable or not will depend on your point of view.

What do you think?

What do your students think?

PAULO FREIRE'S METHOD OF CONSCIENTIZATION

Awareness raising—or ***conscientization,*** as Freire calls the development of critical awareness—is an open-ended learning process carried out through 'group dialogue'. A group of persons comes together to discuss and try to solve problems they have in common.

This is different from most educational situations, because the questions that are raised during the group dialogues have **no predetermined answers.** There is **no 'expert'** who has the answers and whose job it is to pass his knowledge on to others. Instead, the persons in the group search for better understanding of the problems they face together. **Each person's experiences and views have equal value.** Everyone takes part in looking at the problems and searching for solutions.

The person who acts as group leader or ***facilitator*** (whether an instructor of health workers, or a health worker leading a group in her community) needs to keep in mind that her role is not to lecture. In fact, the leader tries to avoid giving her own opinions. Otherwise, persons may simply say "yes" to whatever the leader says.

At the start of a discussion, the role of the group leader is to . . .

- encourage all persons to take an active part,
- assure them that they are among friends and are free to speak their own thoughts,
- advise them to listen carefully, and avoid interrupting each other, and
- warn them not to simply accept what another person says, but to think about it carefully, or ***analyze*** it.

It is essential that the group leader genuinely feel that all persons in the group have their own knowledge and valid points of view. That way, everyone can learn from each other. The line between 'teacher' and 'student' is broken. The leader becomes a 'teacher/learner'. Each participant becomes a 'learner/teacher'.

The leader's role is mainly one of asking questions. These should be questions that help the group see the world around them as a situation that challenges them to change it—not as something unchangeable and beyond their control.

Helping people to realize that they have within themselves the capacity to understand and change their situation is not easy. This is especially true with persons who have learned to silently endure their misfortune and who accept society's view of themselves as powerless, ignorant, and hopeless (see Magic awareness, p. **26**-12). But these are the persons for whom a more critical understanding of their situation can be the ladder toward a healthier life.

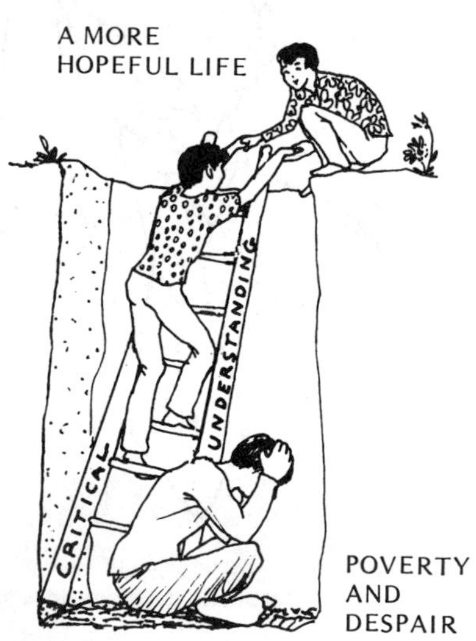

The group discussion has 3 objectives, each opening the way to the next:

1. To help awaken people to their **personal worth** and potential **group strength;** to help them gain confidence in themselves as thinking, active, capable human beings.
2. To help people **examine, analyze,** and **take action** to change their situation.
3. To help them obtain the tools and skills they need in order to take charge of their health and lives.

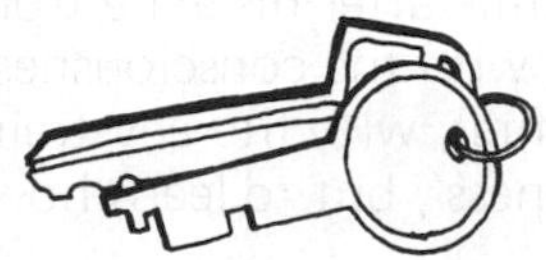

The use of key words and pictures

In order to help persons look more closely at themselves and their world, Freire found it useful to **start each discussion by having everyone look carefully at a specific word, thing, or situation.** Careful study needs to be done in advance to choose words, pictures, objects, or stories that have key significance to the particular group.

The key word or picture is used to 'spark' the members of the group to discuss themselves, their situation, their abilities, and their problems. Often a single word or picture will touch off a 1- or 2-hour discussion.

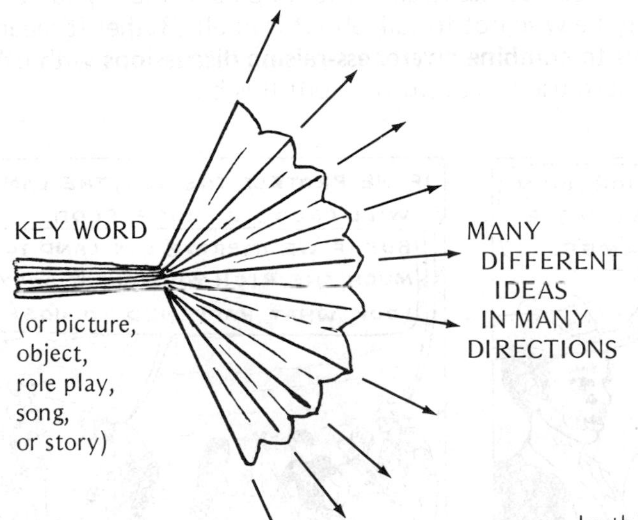

The key word or picture is like a fan, because it opens the way to discussion in many new directions.

It produces many new words, new pictures, and new observations in people's minds.

The group leader does not know ahead of time where the discussion will lead.

In this chapter we often speak of key words, objects, or stories as *discussion starters.*

Awareness-raising discussions sparked by key words, pictures, or stories can be used when teaching almost any basic skill: literacy, health, nutrition, agriculture, etc. The number of key words or pictures used and the number of times the group meets will depend in part on what skill is being learned.

Linking awareness development to the learning of practical skills

Paulo Freire first developed his methods of 'conscientization' as part of an effort to help Brazilian farm people learn how to read and write. Thus, education for the development of critical awareness was linked from the first with the learning of skills that made the poor more equal to the rich.

This linkage may be a key to success in the use of Freire's methods. In fact, many people who have tried to separate consciousness raising from the learning of practical skills have had serious difficulties. Freire himself, when he began to work in Chile after his exile from Brazil, found that people quickly grew impatient with the consciousness-raising dialogues unless they were combined, from the first, with literacy training. People had not come to 'raise their consciousness', but to learn how to read and write!

To be most effective, educational methods that increase self-confidence and social awareness should be built into all aspects of training programs and community activities.

Unfortunately, some training programs separate the development of awareness from the learning of practical skills. Instructors may hold special 'consciousness-raising' sessions based on group dialogue, but use conventional lectures for teaching about health. This is a big mistake. It would be more effective to forget the special sessions but to use awareness-building methods throughout all aspects of training.

This does not mean that 'consciousness raising' should be continually talked about. In some places, it may be wise not to talk about it at all. Rather it means that we should **look for ways to combine awareness-raising discussions with other study and activity.** This we have tried to do throughout this book.

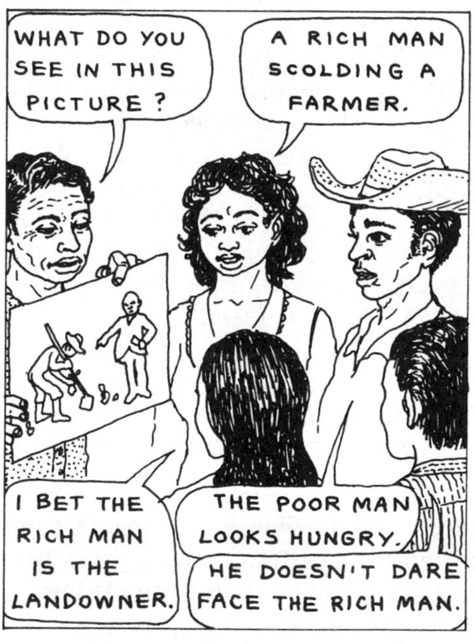
WHAT DO YOU SEE IN THIS PICTURE?
A RICH MAN SCOLDING A FARMER.
I BET THE RICH MAN IS THE LANDOWNER.
THE POOR MAN LOOKS HUNGRY.
HE DOESN'T DARE FACE THE RICH MAN.

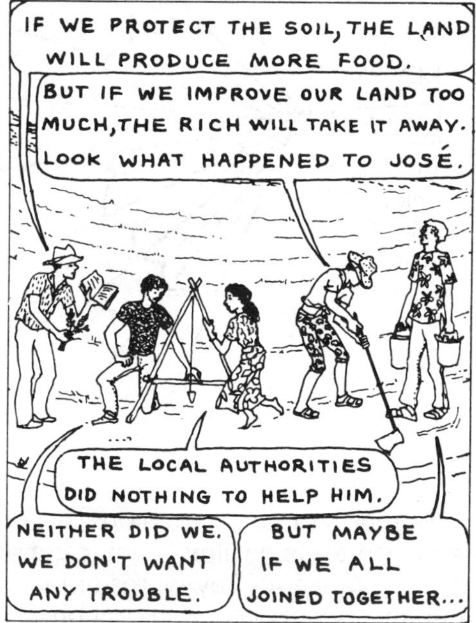
IF WE PROTECT THE SOIL, THE LAND WILL PRODUCE MORE FOOD.
BUT IF WE IMPROVE OUR LAND TOO MUCH, THE RICH WILL TAKE IT AWAY. LOOK WHAT HAPPENED TO JOSÉ.
THE LOCAL AUTHORITIES DID NOTHING TO HELP HIM.
NEITHER DID WE. WE DON'T WANT ANY TROUBLE.
BUT MAYBE IF WE ALL JOINED TOGETHER...

Development of critical awareness is more 'down to earth' when combined with learning practical skills, or working.

FREIRE'S METHOD IN LITERACY PROGRAMS

In the 1960's, Paulo Freire's program in Brazil became famous because of its quick results: people were learning to read and write in just 6 weeks! Freire's main contribution to literacy training is not speed, however. People learned quickly to read and write, but more important, they discovered their own ability to change the conditions that keep them poor.

We have warned against separating 'consciousness raising' from skills training, but the reverse is also true. Some programs have attempted to use Freire's literacy technique without discussing poverty or injustice. But in such programs, the students do not learn to read and write nearly as well. Freire was aware that the difficult task for his students was not learning the alphabet or recognizing words, but **overcoming the feeling that they were too ignorant to learn.** For these poor farmers, written words were part of the rich man's world, something beyond their reach.

This is Freire's starting point: getting people to take possession of words. Before the first class meeting, the instructors visit the village, getting to know the people and their way of life. Then, together with a small group of local people who will be in the class, they choose a short list of words that are central to the lives of the villagers. Words like ***hunger, school, landlord,*** and ***vote*** may be chosen for their ability to spark discussions in many directions (see the fan on page **26**-17). The words are also chosen so that every letter in the alphabet is included.

Usually a drawing or a photograph representing a word is shown before people see the word itself. The group discusses each word for a long time before they ever see how it is written. The drawings and photos are carefully chosen to represent a setting similar to, but not exactly the same as, the learners' village. That way, the people can safely discuss the problems of this 'nearby village' without feeling too threatened by criticism of their own lives. Later, when the consciousness of the group is greater, they will feel more secure about discussing their own problems, because they will know that they can change much of what they do not like.

When the learners finally see a word in print, it is not frightening, because **it has become their word.** In this way, the words on a page do not dominate the reader. Readers take control and put words in the order they choose. The action of writing sentences of their own creation is an important part of the conscientization process.

In conscientization, people do not simply discuss their lives. They think and then act to make changes where they are needed. Thus, **reading and writing become tools they can use, instead of weapons to be used against them.**

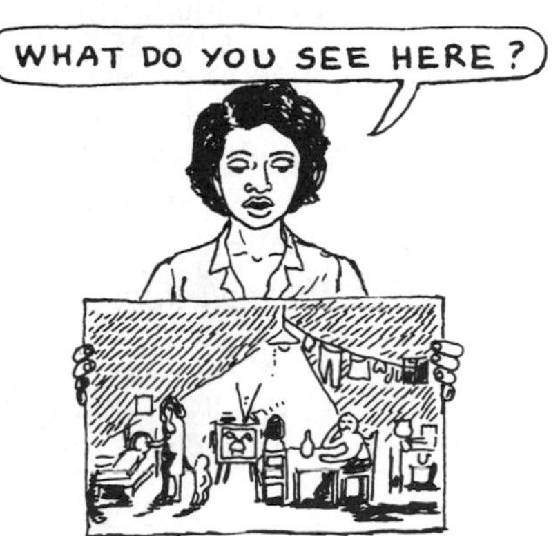

One literacy program using Freire's methods is based in Netzahualcoyotl, a huge slum near Mexico City. Twenty key words, and pictures representing each word, are used as discussion starters. On the next pages are 2 examples.

TELE (local slang for television)

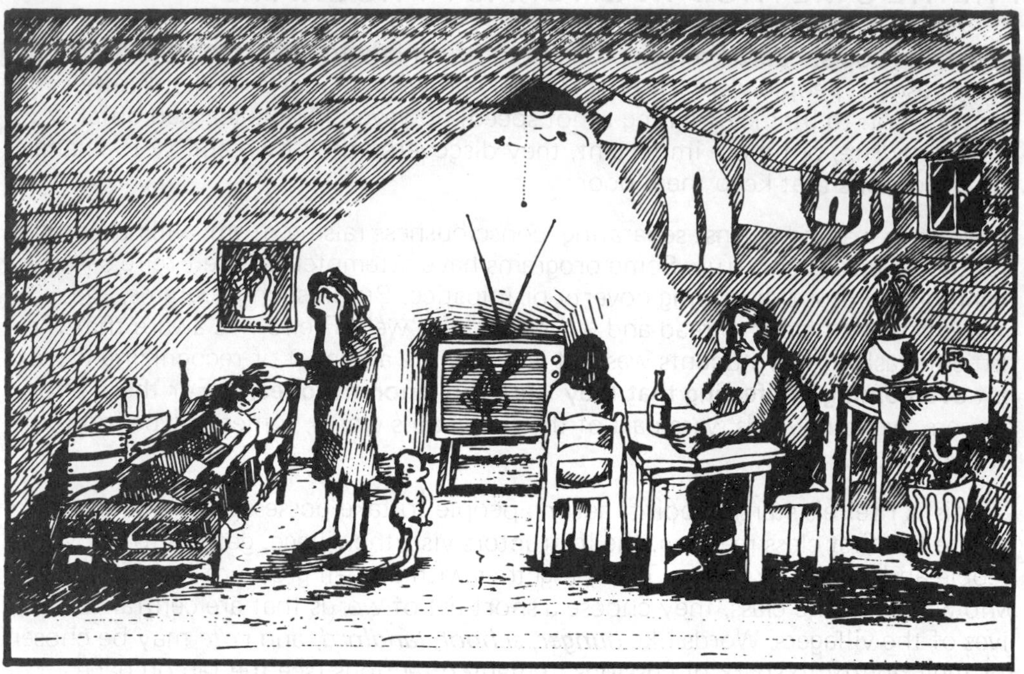

The group leader guides the discussion through 4 main areas of questions:

1. *Naming the problem*

What do you see in the picture? How does this family live? What do they have in their house? How does the television compare with the other objects in the house? What are the people doing? What problems do they have? What sort of things do they see on T.V.?

2. *Effects* on the discussion group

Does your family have a T.V.? How many families in the neighborhood have one? How much time do they spend watching it? Which programs do they prefer? Who watches most, young people or adults? In a half-hour program, how many minutes are spent on advertising?

3. *Causes* of the problem

What do people learn from T.V.? How does it affect children who watch it a lot? Who pays for the programs? Who benefits from television? Does it help people solve their problems? Does it provide an escape from problems? In what way? What larger problems relate to what we see in this picture?

4. *Possible solutions*

Would it be possible for T.V. to serve the people better? How? Is this likely to happen? Would it be possible to live without T.V.? Would this be better? What might this family do? What might we all do?

HUNGER

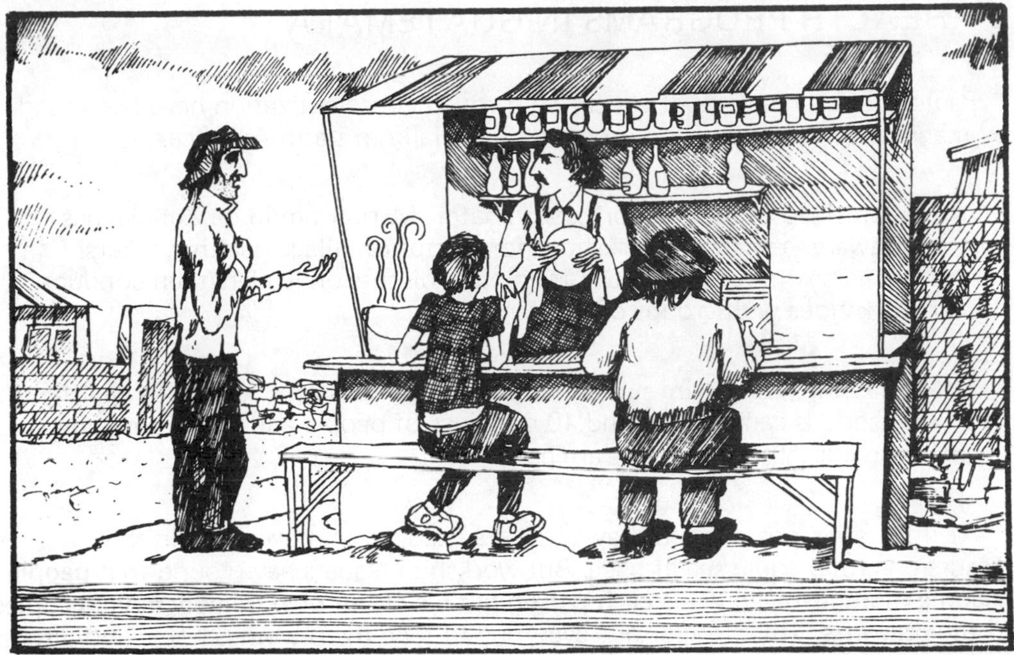

The group leader asks similar questions about this picture and the word HUNGER. The discussion eventually leads to questions like, ***Why is there hunger?*** and ***Can we do something at the family level to improve nutrition? What? What can we do at the community level?***

Each of the key words, along with its picture, serves as the starting point for a 2-hour session. The first hour is spent discussing what the word means to the members of the group, as we have described. The second hour is spent learning how to write the word, sound out the letters, and use those same letters to form other sounds and words. Because the group explores the meaning of each word before learning how to write it and use the letters it contains, becoming literate takes on immediate personal and social importance.

The first 4 weeks of this literacy program in Netzahualcoyotl are spent analyzing the key words and the pictures that go with them. During the 5th and 6th weeks, the students practice reading and writing. For this, simple illustrated stories are used that help the group analyze problems that are important in their lives. Since some words and phrases in the stories are left blank, the readers fill them in according to their own experience. So **students actually participate in writing their own stories.**

By the end of 6 weeks, the students not only have learned to read newspapers and announcements, but have gained confidence in their own ability to master new skills and to begin to change their situation.

The Netzahualcoyotl literacy materials are available from SEPAC, p. **Back**-4.

ADAPTATION OF FREIRE'S METHOD BY HEALTH PROGRAMS IN GUATEMALA

Paulo Freire's methods of education through conscientization have been used by many health and nutrition programs, especially in Latin America.

In Guatemala, a health network coordinator, Maria Hamlin de Zuñiga, has organized awareness-raising workshops for groups of village health workers. Health workers who receive special training as discussion leaders then conduct similar workshops with groups of villagers.

The workshops use Freire's methods to explore questions related to health. Each workshop is centered around 10 drawings of people and situations typical of the area where the workshops are held.

At first, large, poster-sized drawings were used, so that everyone in the discussion group could see at once. But workshop leaders have found that **people become more involved when each person has his or her own mimeographed copies of the drawings.** This also permits everyone to take the drawings home and discuss them with their families and friends.

Here are 9 of the 10 basic drawings (the other one is shown on p. **26**-26).

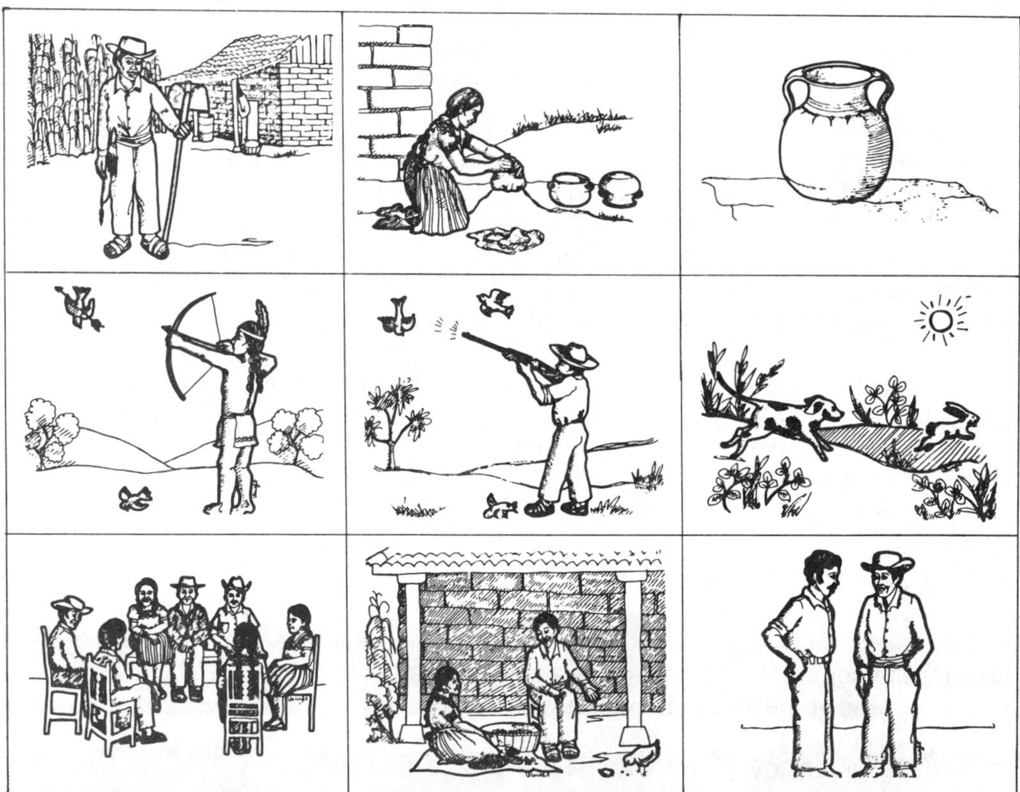

Care has been taken to make sure that these drawings look familiar to the people and are typical of their area. In fact, for several of the drawings, there are alternative versions that can be matched with the particular dress and customs of the village where the workshop is held.

For example, here are 3 alternatives for the man in the first drawing.

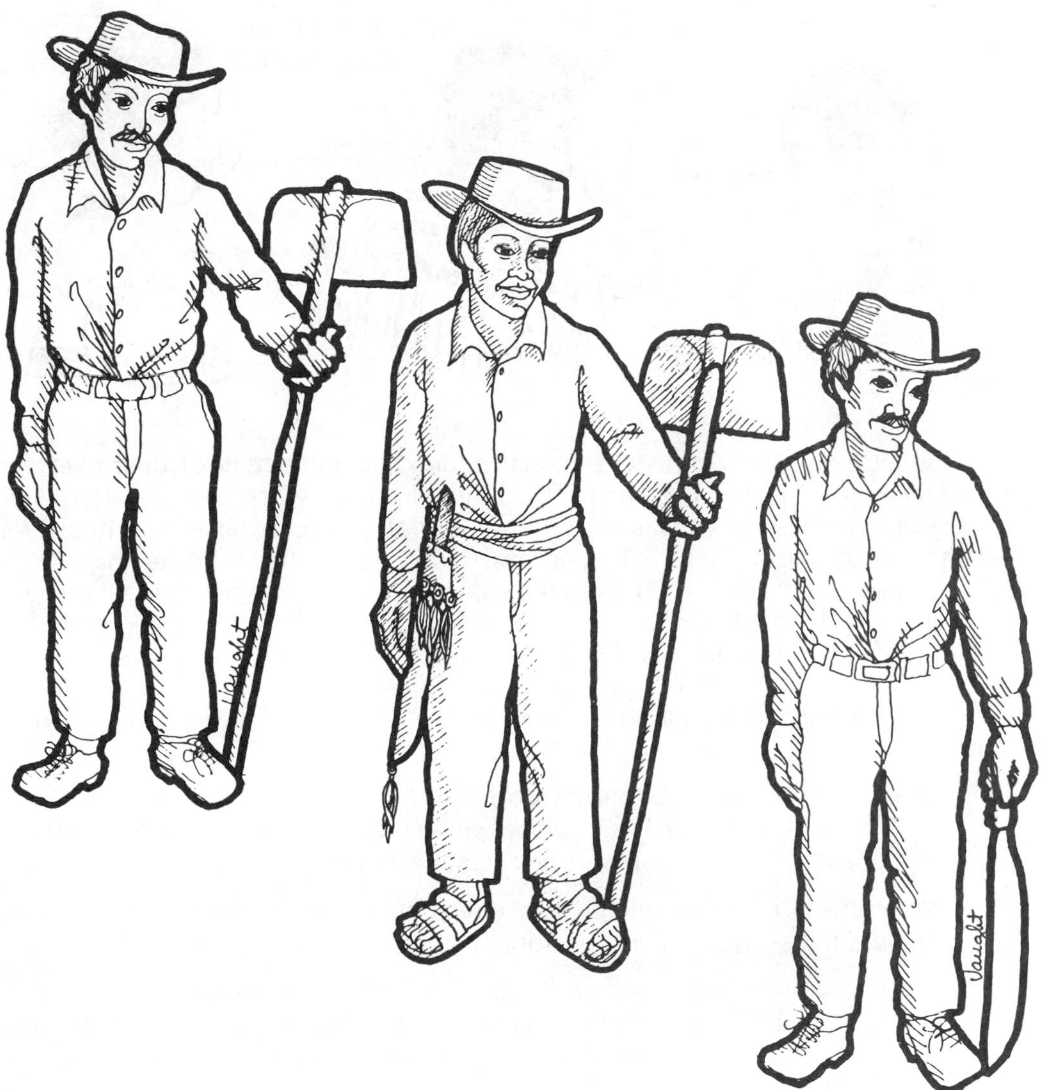

The first few drawings in the series are intended to help members of the group realize how **they change their surroundings through their daily activities.** They recognize how 'the farmer in the picture' is able to change a brush patch or strip of forest into a maize or bean field. By cultivating it, he changes or transforms a part of the 'world of nature' into the 'world of culture'. In a similar way, the woman in the second picture transforms 'nature' into 'culture' by shaping clay into a pot.

By asking questions that bring ideas like these out of the members of the group, the leader helps them realize that . . .

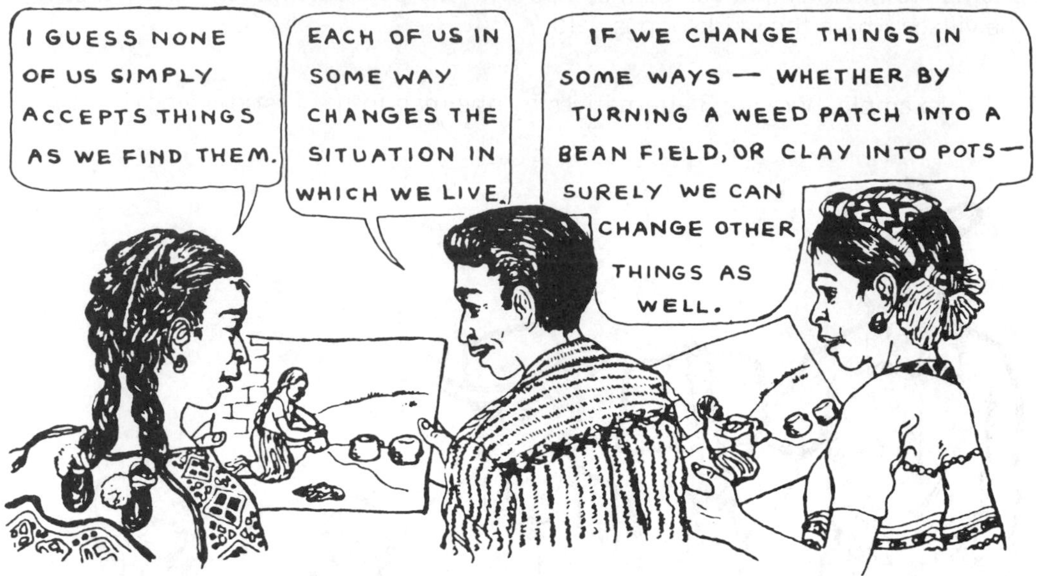

I GUESS NONE OF US SIMPLY ACCEPTS THINGS AS WE FIND THEM.
EACH OF US IN SOME WAY CHANGES THE SITUATION IN WHICH WE LIVE.
IF WE CHANGE THINGS IN SOME WAYS — WHETHER BY TURNING A WEED PATCH INTO A BEAN FIELD, OR CLAY INTO POTS— SURELY WE CAN CHANGE OTHER THINGS AS WELL.

These pictures also help people recognize the **value and extent of their own knowledge.** Because they have had little or no schooling, village people often consider themselves ignorant or even stupid. But after discussing all the things that 'the person in the picture' knows how to do, they realize that they have a special culture of their own. To help the group reflect on how much they already know and can do, the leader can ask other questions that help them find even wider meanings in the pictures. For example:

"Does the school teacher here in our village know how to find and prepare the clay to make pots or roof tiles?"

"Does the agricultural extension worker know how to make a wooden plow? Does he know what kind of local wood will make an axe handle that will not break, or fence posts that will not be eaten by termites?"

"When the nurse from the city runs out of medicines, does she know which wild plants to use to get rid of intestinal worms or to control bleeding?"

"If a doctor or lawyer moved onto this land with no more money or tools than the people in this picture have, could he farm the land as well? Would the people here help him or give him advice? How much would (or should) they charge him for their advice?"

"Who grows the food that doctors, lawyers, and businessmen eat? Which is more important to health—food or medicine? Which is worth more, the knowledge of the doctor or the knowledge of the farm people? Why? Why do doctors, lawyers, and businessmen earn so much more for their work than the people who grow the food? How does this affect people's health? Can people do anything to become less dependent on doctors, lawyers, and businessmen? What? How?"

By considering questions like these, people gain new respect for their own abilities and knowledge. They awaken to the possibilities for change and for making things better. They feel more equal to others, more self-confident, more fully human!

That, at least, is the theory. Whether or not the discussions actually produce this sort of 'awakening' will depend on the skill, attitude, and understanding of the discussion leader, as well as on the characteristics of the particular group.

Maria de Zuñiga points out some of the difficulties that may arise:

"At the start, particularly in the first session, some groups will react somewhat negatively, due to the fact that they are not used to this type of participation, but rather to simply listening to speeches or 'health talks'. Some persons may ask the leader to 'just tell us' how things are, insisting that they themselves 'know nothing'. Others will see it as a waste of time. Some may become bored or annoyed, and possibly walk out. Others may try to turn things into a joke. In any case, one has to sort his way through these situations, little by little helping the group to adopt the method and participate. If this happens, halfway through the series of pictures people will grow enthusiastic.

"Some groups will not begin to take part as quickly as others; some will become involved slowly, others rapidly. The leader will need to guide the discussion to match the rhythm and speed of the group, in order that they fully grasp the points that come out.

"Do not expect, during the discussion period, to touch upon all the themes that could relate to the picture, for this is impossible. In any case, a sign of success is to see that members of the group continue discussing on their own, in small groups, once the session is over.

"Finally, remember that people only fully grasp new ideas when they act on them—when dialogue leads them to act, observe, reflect, and once again act."

How many ways do you see that these people have changed things around them to better meet their needs?

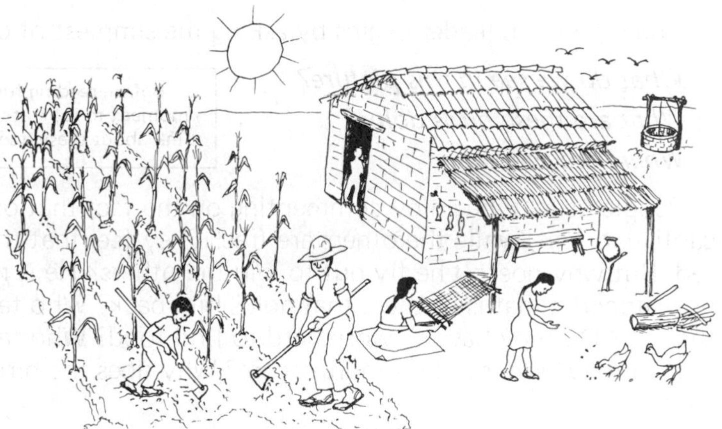

Group discussions with pictures and questions like this help build people's confidence in themselves and their ability to change things for the better. (From *Where There Is No Doctor,* p. w26.)

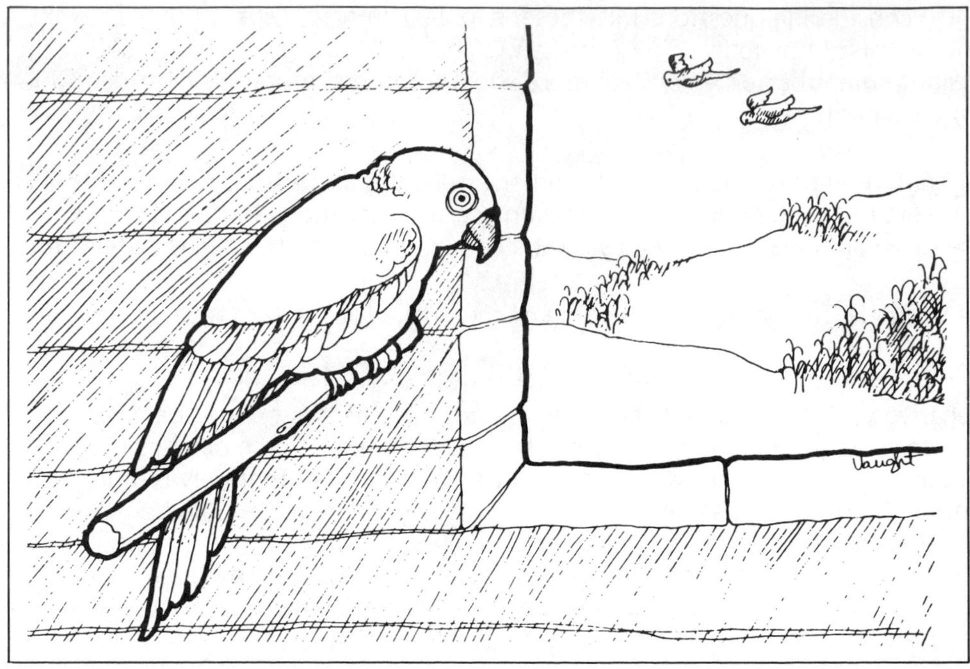

This is the seventh in the series of pictures used in the Guatemalan workshops. (It is the one we left out of the series on page **26**-22.)

At first glance, the picture does not seem very interesting—hardly a discussion starter for helping develop greater critical awareness. But we have seen this picture used with several groups of villagers, health workers, and instructors, and have been amazed by the amount and depth of discussion it can spark. Perhaps because the group looks first at birds and not at people, they find it easier to talk openly in a way that leads to soul-searching personal discussion.

The discussion leader begins by asking the simplest of questions:

What do we see in this picture?

What are these birds doing?

Where are they?

Before reading further, take a moment to look at the picture and think about these questions yourself.

People usually begin by commenting on the fact that one of the birds is a captive, or pet, while the others are free. They feel that the captive bird looks sad. But why doesn't he fly out to join the others? He is not tied; his wings are not clipped. What is it, then, that holds him back? Who takes care of the birds that fly? Do they have to work hard to find food? Who takes care of the bird in the window? Whose life is more secure? Why does the bird in the window look so sad?

From the discussion about the birds, the members of the group begin to reflect on their own lives and experiences. They ask themselves: ***In what ways are we people in our village free? In what ways are we captive? Is a person who is hungry free? Are all people equally free to provide for their families with their own hard work? Why or why not? Who has to think and work more—those who are free or those who are captive? How could we become more free, or live more according to our human nature? What stops us? Why are the free birds flying together?***

ALTERNATIVES TO PICTURES AS DISCUSSION STARTERS:

Usually key words, together with drawings or photographs, are used to spark discussions. But songs, role plays, or objects can also be used. Make sure that what you use is something familiar that can lead to eye-opening discussions in many directions.

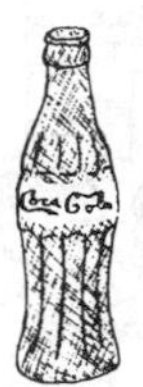

We have seen a group leader start a lively discussion by passing around a bottle of *Coca-Cola* and asking, "What does this mean to you?" The people's first reaction is to quote the advertisements:

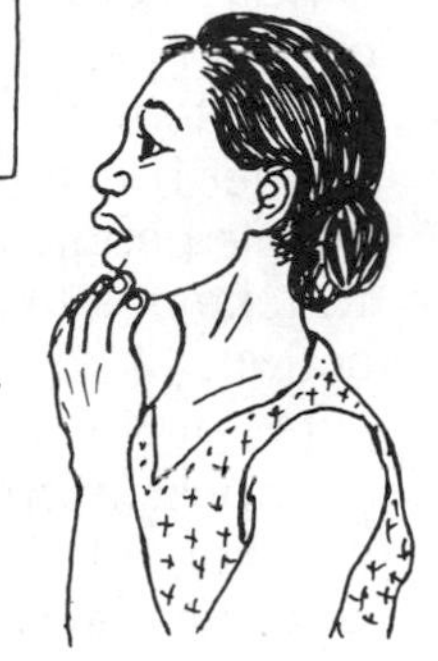

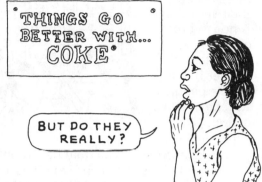

"The drink that refreshes!"
"The real thing!"
"Things go better with *Coke!*"

"But do they really go better?" asks the group leader.

And so the discussion begins. It may range from looking at 'junk foods' as a cause of malnutrition, tooth decay, stomach ulcers, and heart disease, to exploring how advertising influences people's thinking and idealizes foreign values. Depending on the sophistication of the group, they may also discuss the role of huge international corporations in the national and world-wide power structures.

In the Central American country where the discussion about ***'Coke'*** was held, some persons were aware that several union organizers had recently been shot to death in a ***Coca-Cola*** bottling plant. They had been trying to get fairer working conditions.

The group concluded that ***things might go better without Coke.***

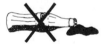

Even a toothbrush can serve as a discussion starter to help people look at things in new ways:

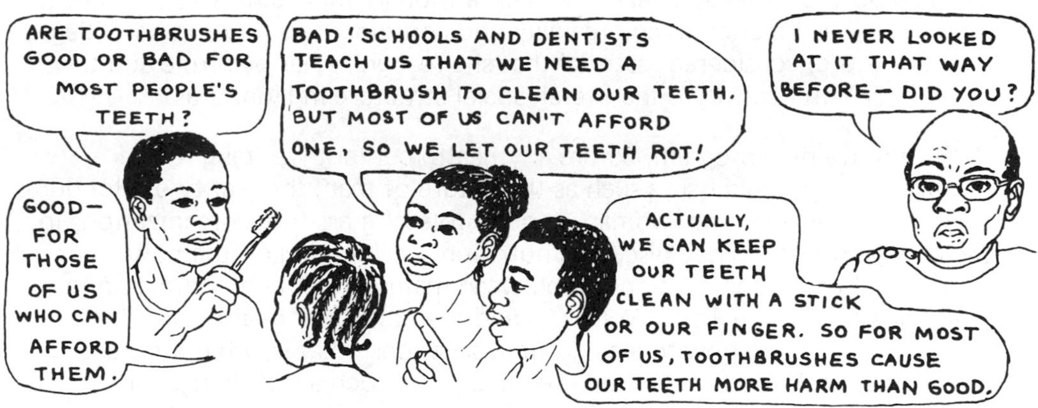

Similar consciousness-raising dialogues can be sparked by such things as baby bottles, cans of infant formula, plastic-wrapped 'junk food', or packages of refined sugar or flour. On page **15**-7, we show how ears of native and hybrid maize can be used to start a discussion.

FROM AWARENESS TO ACTION

The purpose of helping people become more aware of their situation is not to breed anger or discontent. Rather it is to enable people to take positive action.

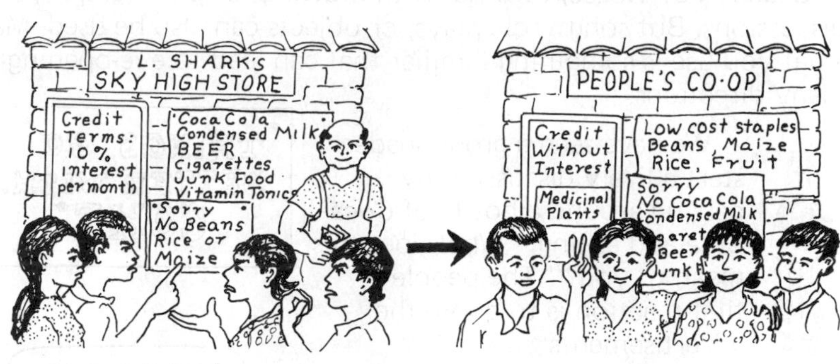
L. SHARK'S
SKY HIGH STORE
Credit Terms: 10% interest per month
Coca Cola
Condensed Milk
BEER
Cigarettes
Junk Food
Vitamin Tonics
Sorry
No Beans
Rice or
Maize
PEOPLE'S CO-OP
Credit Without Interest
Low cost staples
Beans, Maize
Rice, Fruit
Medicinal Plants
Sorry
No Coca Cola
Condensed Milk

'Consciousness raising' that begins only with talk and is not linked to practical skills or activities, often ends as it began—in just talk. But **when the development of critical awareness is linked to meeting specific local needs, it can help people find the spirit, energy, and sense of direction required for effective action.**

Consider the following example from Honduras:*

In Olancho, Honduras, rural health workers had been active for years, giving standard health talks and telling women how they should "change their behavior for better health." But almost no one paid any attention. Being talked at and told what to do did not convince anyone to change much of anything.

But when a new, community-based approach to meeting health needs was begun, things began to change. Women ***promotoras*** were trained with a strong emphasis on self-care and critical awareness of social conditions. Women were chosen rather than men because women were "viewed as the most stable and potentially most powerful element in the society—as well as the most oppressed."

The ***promotora's*** role as a health worker, although important, was seen as secondary to her function as an organizer and consciousness raiser in her village. It was, therefore, considered essential that she recognize her own role and the place of health in relation to the overall social structure in Honduras:

> "In the training program, before any health content was taught, the ***promotoras*** discussed issues such as the nature of man, the reality of Honduras, the role of the Honduran woman, and the role of grass-roots organizations in the change process. They discussed nutrition . . . focusing on the politics of food distribution, the relationship between malnutrition and oppression in Honduras and all the Third World . . . and the politics of health care. The women also learned how to lead group discussions—that is, what kind of questions to ask and how to lead the dialogue in such a way that their comrades would begin to critically analyze their reality, looking at root causes and consequences of problems, and searching for solutions that would bring about radical change rather than mere reform."

---

*This report, with language slightly simplified, is taken from "Creating Critical Consciousness in Health: Applications of Freire's Philosophy and Methods to the Health Care Setting," by Meredith Minkler. We also have visited and worked with ***promotoras*** from this program in Olancho, Honduras.

The results of the ***promotoras'*** work over the past few years have been impressive. The first big change occurred in the ***promotoras*** themselves. Early discussions of the role of Honduran women had shown a very low 'self-image' among the ***promotoras,*** who spoke of themselves as 'breeders', not much different from their farm animals in terms of function and role.

But in the process of group dialogue, the ***promotoras*** began to question their inferior position in relation to men, and their role as little more than 'breeders'. Their self-confidence also grew as they experienced success in their work.

With few exceptions, the women saw their role as one of service to their fellow women, and of helping to bring about a more just social order. Their training through group dialogue had helped them to see themselves as 'teacher/learners' and to relate to other women as friends and equals, rather than bossing them about as had many of the health workers before them. As a result, a spirit of cooperation and concern developed among the women they worked with.

Some of the accomplishments of the ***promotoras*** have been outstanding. It is reported that in every village where there is a ***promotora,*** members of the ***Club de Amas de Casa*** (housewives' club) now boil drinking water as a preventive health measure.* This is particularly impressive when it is considered that health workers before them had been trying for 25 years to get the women to boil their water, without success.

The ***promotoras*** also have been successful in organizing the women in activities beyond the area of health. When the men in one village failed to finish building a school, the women abandoned their typical sex role, walked down the mountain, and returned carrying lumber on their backs. They completed the school themselves.

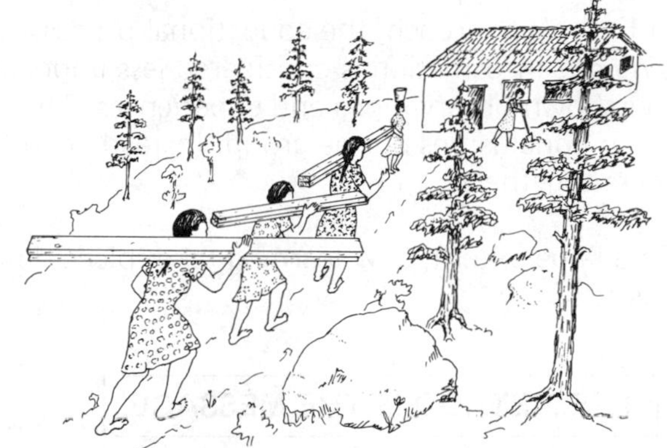

They completed the school themselves.

The ***promotoras*** have become active in land reform as well, helping to organize the people and make them aware of their legal rights. In Honduras, large parcels of land are held by persons who started out with smaller plots, but little by little moved their fences to include more and more land. (This has given rise to the popular saying, ***The fence posts walk at night.)*** The ***campesinos*** (poor farm people) in Olancho have begun to take back the illegally held land. Although at first some violence resulted, most of the ***campesinos*** have been able to keep the land they reclaimed.

The ***promotoras*** of Olancho have done far more for the long-term health of their people than have the regional health programs with their large budgets and government support. The ***promotoras'*** success has resulted from their ability to awaken their fellow women to their own capacity to combat the underlying social causes of their problems.

---

*See the discussion of 'to boil or not to boil' on page **15**-3.

THE DIFFERENCE BETWEEN CONSCIOUSNESS RAISING AND BRAINWASHING

Many 'experts' in health and development place great emphasis on **changing the attitudes and behavior of 'the people'** (by whom they mean the poor). They appear not to realize that it is just as important to people's health to **change the attitudes and behavior of the rich**—of those in control (see p. 1-29).

Freire's approach to critical awareness is refreshing because—in theory, at least—it does not involve imposing the ideas and attitudes of 'those who know' upon 'those whose behavior needs to be changed'.

Conventional instruction passes

from TEACHER
↓
to STUDENT.

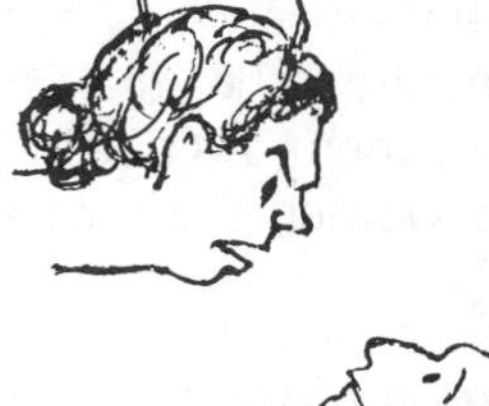

But with Freire's method, learning goes both ways.

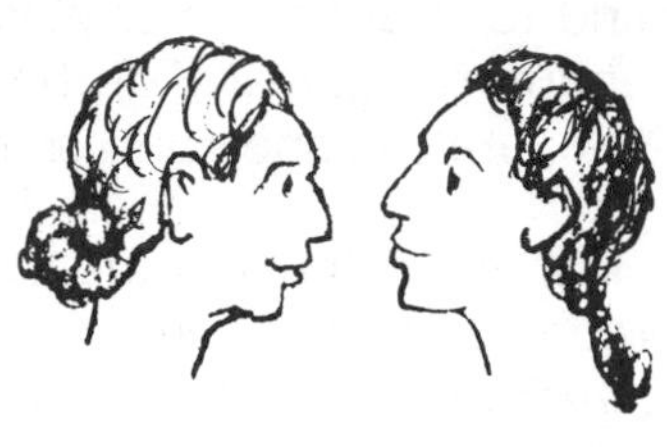

TEACHER ⟷ STUDENT

In Freire's approach, the educational process is open-ended and adventurous. *Passing out* information is considered less important than *putting together* the learners' own observations and experiences. The leader avoids imposing her own views or conclusions on the group. Instead, learning is based on looking for answers together.

To a large extent, ***how*** learning takes place determines ***what*** is learned. In other words . . .

THE METHOD IS THE MESSAGE.

Such, at least, is the theory. Unfortunately, in practice, 'consciousness raising' is full of contradictions and *pitfalls.*

Freire himself stresses how important it is for the discussion leader to **ask questions that do not already have the answers built in. The leader must be prepared to have the group come up with answers and ideas completely different from what she had expected.** She must be ready to learn from the group, not just about their culture, but about her own culture and herself. She, too, must be prepared to see things in a new way . . . to change.

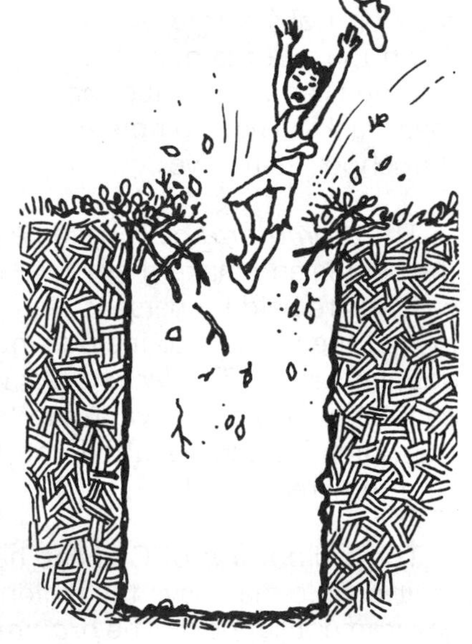

A *pitfall* is an unexpected difficulty.

But all this is more easily said than done. In spite of our good intentions, those of us who are attracted to Freire's method often have strong ideas of our own. We see the world in a certain way and want others to see it as we do. Frequently, there are deep contradictions within ourselves that we have never resolved. For example, we may believe that each individual needs to find his own truth for himself. Yet we feel the need to impose our own beliefs on others. And so we use—and often misuse—the process of conscientization.

Even in the leadership and writings of the famous teachers of awareness raising, the questions asked often have built-in answers. Look back at some of the questions we have given as examples in this chapter. You will see how the opinions and politics of the askers are often built into their questions. (We, the authors, often fall into the same trap ourselves.)

Pictures, like questions, can also be politically loaded. For example, a literacy worker in Netzahualcoyotl may hold up the two drawings shown below and simply say, "What do you see here?" But the drawings themselves make the leader's own viewpoint obvious.

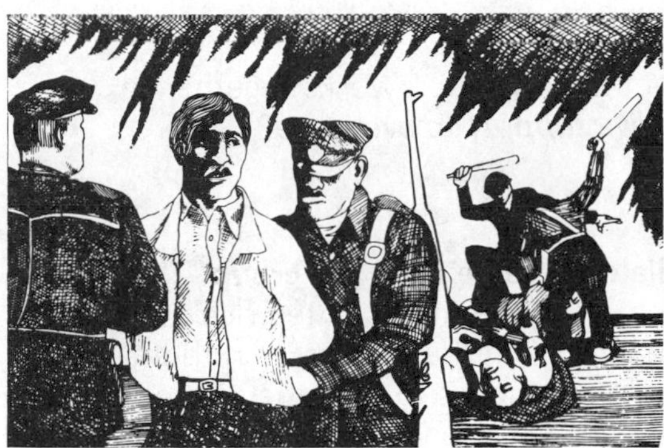

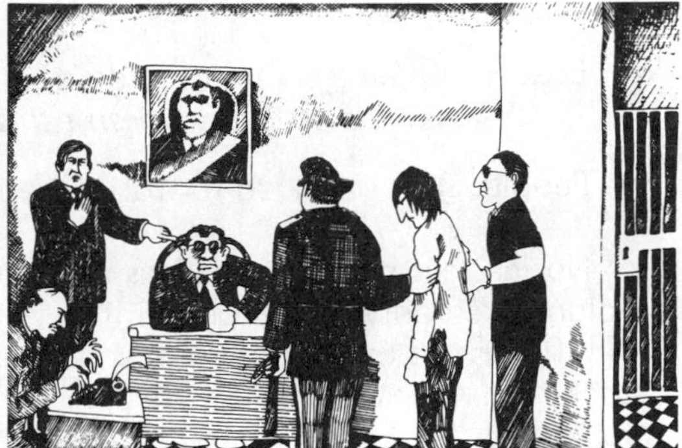

We are not saying that the events shown in these pictures do not happen. In Netzahualcoyotl they happen only too often. But the drawings make a strong, one-sided political statement. Pictures like these tend to put ideas into people's heads rather than drawing them out. The members of the learning group are ***indoctrinated*** with the social and political beliefs of the leader.

The beliefs may be true ones. But if people are to develop a more critical, independent way of looking at things, we need to let them reach their own conclusions and think their own thoughts—not ours!

The challenge for the group leader is to help persons make their own observations and arrive at their own answers.

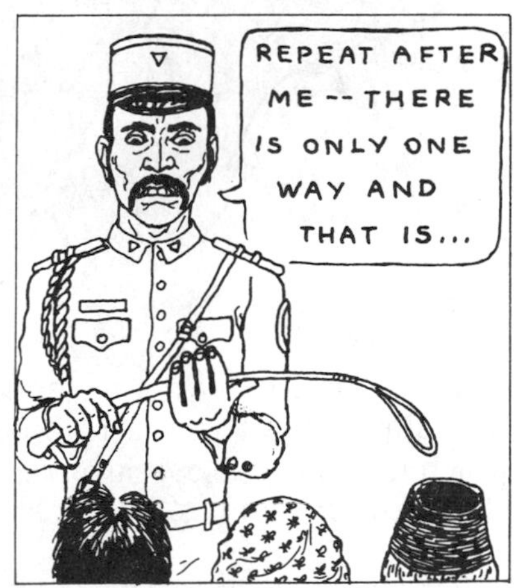
REPEAT AFTER ME -- THERE IS ONLY ONE WAY AND THAT IS...

Indoctrination is the process of putting ideas into people's heads.

As we have pointed out, when leading discussions it is very easy to impose our own ideas on other people—in spite of our sincere desires not to. An example of this is a well-known attempt to adapt Freire's methods to nutrition education in northeast Brazil. The leader of the project was very familiar with the methods, and gave an excellent summary of Freire's writings in her project report.* But when she tried to practice the methods in the field, like many of us, she fell into the trap of putting her own ideas, observations, and conclusions into people's mouths. The following is an excerpt from her tape-recorded dialogues:

Leader: You were . . . listening . . . to the radio program on how to grow community gardens . . . ***weren't you?***

People: *Yes*—that is right.

Leader: In order to make children and adults strong, ***right?***

People: *Yes*—that is what they said.

Leader: Have you ever done any planting together as a community?

People: *Yes,* we planted rice together last year.

Leader: When a community does something together, works together to solve a problem, ***doesn't this give support to everyone?***

People: *Yes,* it's good to work together . . .

Notice that **none of the ideas in this dialogue came from the group.** They volunteered only one piece of information: that they had planted rice together. All the rest of the information and ideas came from the leader. Even though she spoke only in questions, the people were given clues as to how they were expected to answer.

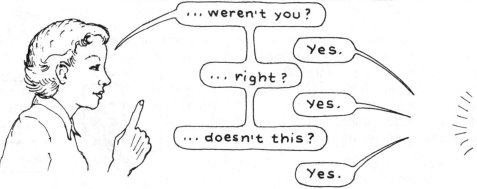

In this way, groups in 3 very different villages were led through a dialogue that was, to a large extent, pre-planned. It is no surprise that all 3 villages came up with almost the same nutrition plan: (1) to examine the children to find out which ones needed special care, and (2) to elect 'coordinators of health' for every 10 houses or families.

But whose ideas and plans were they?

---

*"Using the Method of Paulo Freire in Nutrition Education: An Experimental Plan for Community Action in Northeast Brazil," by Therese Drummond, Cornell University, 1975.

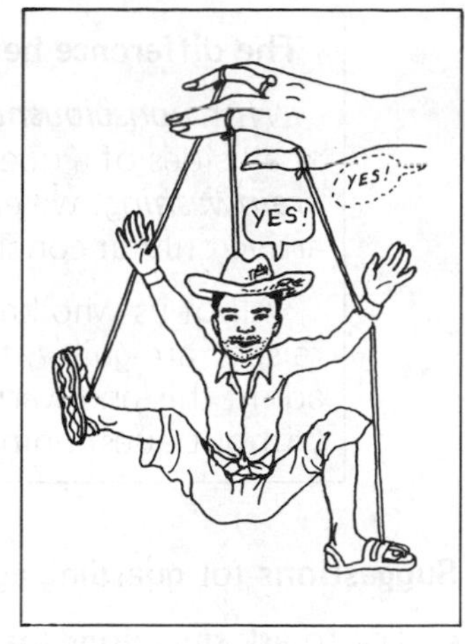

Manipulation is when someone tries to have a hand in the decisions somebody else is making.

The nutrition plan was clearly the invention of the group leader, not the people. Typical of plans designed by outsiders, it starts by wanting to collect data on things the local people mostly already know. Yet the ideas for the plan were consistently put into the people's mouths. In other words, the group dialogue was used to ***manipulate*** people into thinking the leader's ideas were their own. Although the leader had the highest regard for Freire's approach, in actual practice **her message overpowered the method.**

In fairness to the leader of this Brazilian project, we should add that much of the dialogue was far more open-ended than the part we quoted here. Some of it resulted in genuine participation, and at times unexpected viewpoints were expressed by the people. For example, in response to the nutrition plan the group leader was trying to promote, a young father burst out in anger:

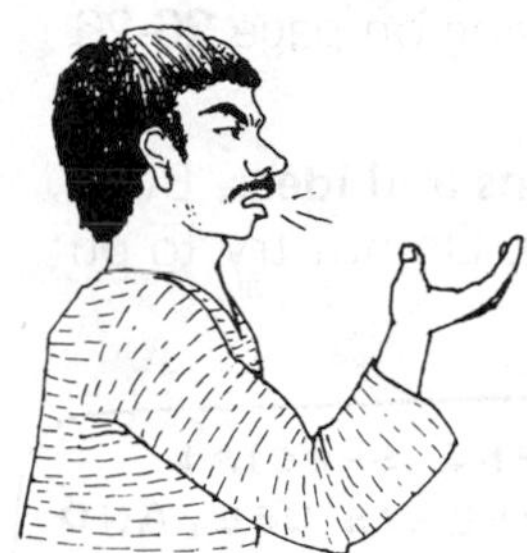

"You say you'll examine the children and tell us which ones are weak. Do you think we don't know that? . . . So you tell us to take them to a doctor. We could walk the day's journey to Alcantara in the burning sun. If the child lives long enough, we may even get to the end of the line at the clinic and see a doctor. So, what does he do? He gives us a piece of paper that says what medicine we should buy. And who gives us the money to buy that medicine? Will ***you*** buy that medicine?"

This outburst, completely unplanned, unexpected, and perhaps frustrating to the leader, was really the start of a sincere two-way dialogue. Here the people did, in fact, look critically at their social reality, and even found the courage to speak out against an outsider's nutrition plan that they considered inappropriate.

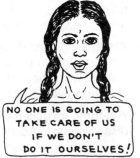

NO ONE IS GOING TO TAKE CARE OF US IF WE DON'T DO IT OURSELVES!

Facing up to the reality that "no one is going to take care of us if we don't do it ourselves" finally brought the people to exploring new possibilities. They began to realize that by working together and learning more about the nutritional needs of their children, they could prevent many from becoming weak and sick. So in the end, and in spite of the leader's pre-decided plan, the discussion served an awareness-raising purpose—at least in part.

In short, this community nutrition project in Brazil had both weaknesses and strengths. The group leader herself recognizes many of the problems. She states, "In listening to the tapes afterwards, I noted my mistakes, which often seemed glaring."*

May we all have the same courage to admit and learn from our own mistakes!

---

*Since writing this critique, we have discussed it with Therese Drummond. She agrees with it and tells us she is worried that her report is being used by so many programs as a model. Nevertheless, her report is an excellent discussion starter for critically considering the possibilities and pitfalls of the conscientization process.

The difference between consciousness raising and brainwashing:

With ***consciousness raising,*** we encourage other people to look at all sides of a question and draw their own conclusions. With ***brainwashing,*** we encourage others to look only at our side and to arrive only at conclusions we agree with.

All of us who have been discussion leaders and 'consciousness raisers' are guilty, to some degree, of brainwashing. We should admit this and warn our students against accepting anything we say without questioning it.

Suggestions for guarding against brainwashing when leading a group dialogue:

- Try to **ask questions that are truly open ended** and that do not let the group know what reply you prefer or expect.
- For 'discussion starters' use words, pictures, or objects that are familiar and will spark ideas. But leave the related social and political problems for the group to figure out from their own experiences. Avoid pictures or stories that take sides or spell everything out. (Compare the bird drawing on page **26**-26 with the police and law drawings on page **26**-31.)
- As much as possible, **try to avoid stating your own opinions and ideas.** But when you do state them, make it clear that they are yours. Do not try to put your thoughts into other people's mouths.
- Be prepared for the discussion to go in directions you never expected. Be ready to accept the opinions and conclusions of the group—even when you disagree.
- Alert the group to your own tendency to impose your ideas on them. Warn them to doubt and question everything you say.
- **Welcome criticism and disagreement.** Accept a sincere attack on your own ideas as a sign of successful leadership.
- **Keep your language simple.** Use the same words the people use to talk about their own experiences. Avoid like poison the *jargon* and *clichés* of public health, social science, and leftist politics. Also avoid the unusual and confusing language of 'consciousness raising' (see the next page). **Never use a word you cannot explain clearly and quickly to the people you are talking with.** Insist that others interrupt you whenever you use a word or expression they do not understand.

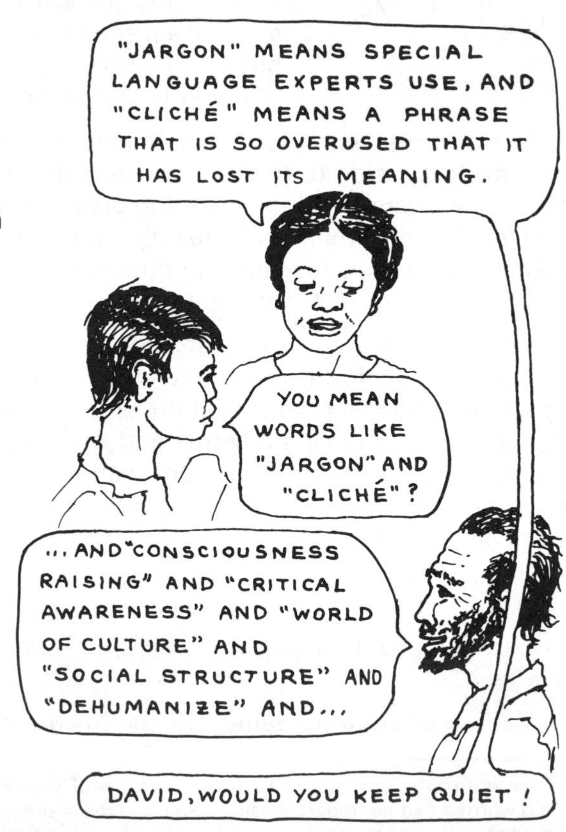
"JARGON" MEANS SPECIAL LANGUAGE EXPERTS USE, AND "CLICHÉ" MEANS A PHRASE THAT IS SO OVERUSED THAT IT HAS LOST ITS MEANING.
YOU MEAN WORDS LIKE "JARGON" AND "CLICHÉ"?
... AND "CONSCIOUSNESS RAISING" AND "CRITICAL AWARENESS" AND "WORLD OF CULTURE" AND "SOCIAL STRUCTURE" AND "DEHUMANIZE" AND...
DAVID, WOULD YOU KEEP QUIET!

THE SPECIAL LANGUAGE OF 'CONSCIENTIZATION'— A TOOL OR A TRAP?

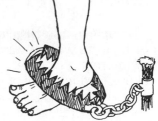

Education for critical awareness requires clear communication between persons as equals. Yet it has become one of the fields most muddied by language few people can understand.

This contradiction between method and language goes back to Paulo Freire himself. A frustrated health worker in Africa who had tried to read Freire's ***Pedagogy* of the Oppressed*** recently protested, "How can anyone who thinks so clearly write so badly?"

Unfortunately, the language that surrounds Freire's ideas prevents many community leaders with limited schooling from being able to learn from and use his methods. It also has led to a sort of 'cult' in which the use of terms like 'dehumanization', 'thematic universe', 'transforming the world', and even 'liberation' actually prevents others from understanding the ideas.

In ***Pedagogy of the Oppressed,*** Freire states that, "Many participants during these debates affirm happily and self-confidently that they are not being shown anything new, just remembering . . ." He gives this example:

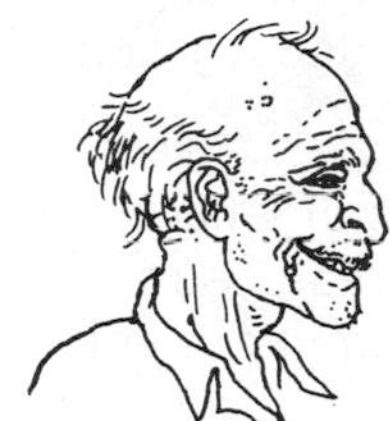

" 'I know that I am cultured,' an elderly peasant said emphatically. And when he was asked how it was that he knew himself to be cultured, he answered with the same emphasis, 'Because I work, and working, I transform the world.' "

Frankly, we would be more convinced that the old peasant was 'just remembering' if he had expressed his new feeling of self-worth in his own words and not in Freire's. After all, the purpose of conscientization is not to transform peasants into parrots!

And yet it seems to have turned many highly educated 'followers' into parrots as well. We have seen educators who have been completely unable to communicate with groups of villagers. Why? Because they were more concerned with getting across concepts such as 'the world of culture' than with helping people explore their own situation in their own words.

For example, one educator carried out a study on the 'level of consciousness' of highland Indians in Ecuador. One question he asked them was, "What are the most dehumanizing problems in your life now?" He reported that persons at the 'magic' level of consciousness often responded with 'problem denial'—meaning they either said nothing or denied that they had any problems. It does not seem to have occurred to the educator that the persons may not have understood the concept of 'dehumanization'. Or if they did, they may not have liked having the term applied to themselves. 'Problem denial' may, at least in part, be a problem of communication—or, in this case, well-justified distrust.

In any case, the tendency of educators to impose their 'mysterious language' on people has further blurred the distinction between consciousness raising and brainwashing. We encourage anyone who uses Freire's methods to look at them critically. Learn from Freire's wisdom. But, for everyone's sake, avoid his language!

Pedagogy: educational method

COMBATTING EXPLOITATION AT THE VILLAGE LEVEL

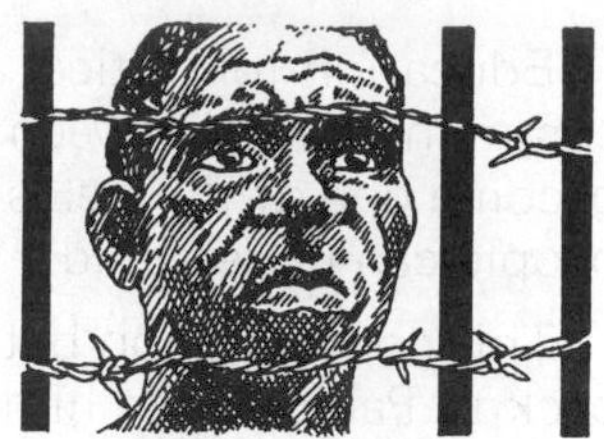

People in a small village or community will find it difficult to work toward social change at the national or international level. Attempts to protest or resist abuses and injustice originating outside the community can be frustrating, and sometimes dangerous. The forces 'outside' are so large and difficult to combat that one hardly knows where to begin.

However, within most villages or communities there exist important, sometimes crushing, forms of exploitation and abuse of those who are poorest or weakest. A health worker, health committee, or other local group may be able to help people work together to overcome some of these problems. It often makes sense to **combat injustices in one's own community before taking on the giant problems outside.** First groups of villagers, then groups of villages, can begin to help the poor gain more control over their health and their lives. A process of social *evolution* (gradual change) begins, which may prepare the way for social *revolution* (complete structural change of the whole society).

There are no simple formulas or instructions for overcoming exploitation at the village level. It is never easy, and rarely without some risk. Each local group must work out its own plan of action.

In this book we give many examples of ways in which groups of villagers have joined together to overcome forms of exploitation that have threatened their health and well-being. Sometimes it is a question of the poor coming together, finding strength in their numbers, and demanding their rights. Other times it means helping people gain awareness about the laws of their country. Then they can organize and demand that the laws no longer be broken at the expense of the poor.

AN EXAMPLE FROM INDIA*

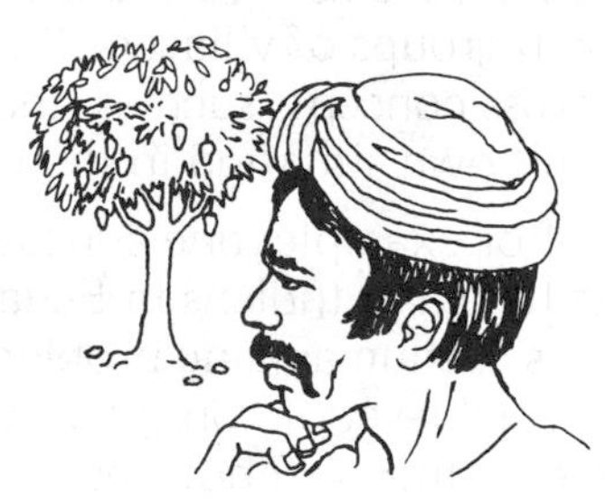

"In a cluster of 30 tribal villages, many families had fruit trees mortgaged to money lenders. Years ago, they had taken small loans for purposes of subsistence, or for getting their sons or daughters married. A widow had mortgaged 2 trees for a loan of 20 rupees 12 years ago. Others had lost the right to the fruit of 10 or more trees. Instead of paying interest, these persons had to bring the fruit of their trees to the doorstep of the money lender.

"A group of committed young volunteers had come to stay with these people one year ago. Being very realistic in their approach with people, they were able to assist them through a process of awakening, learning, planning, and acting, which enabled them to free themselves from this cruel bondage. This process of conscientization helped them discover with awe that all these years they had paid interest in kind to the tune of 100% to 300%!

*Taken from ***Moving Closer to the Rural Poor,*** by the Mobile Orientation and Training Team, Indian Social Institute, Lodi Road, New Delhi 110003 India.

"They learned that there are laws that make money lending of this type illegal. With the support of the voluntary team, the people succeeded in getting back their rights to the fruit trees. Through this action, the people brought about a small change in the structure of ownership, of very great significance to them. This action also made a small dent in the local power structure and helped the people realize better the need to build up their organizational strength."

Success stories such as this one from India can be important teaching tools. Health workers can use them to help villagers look at their own situation and find courage to take similar action. A health worker can tell a story to a group in his village, or perhaps a group can present the story to the whole village in the form of a sociodrama or farmworkers' theater.

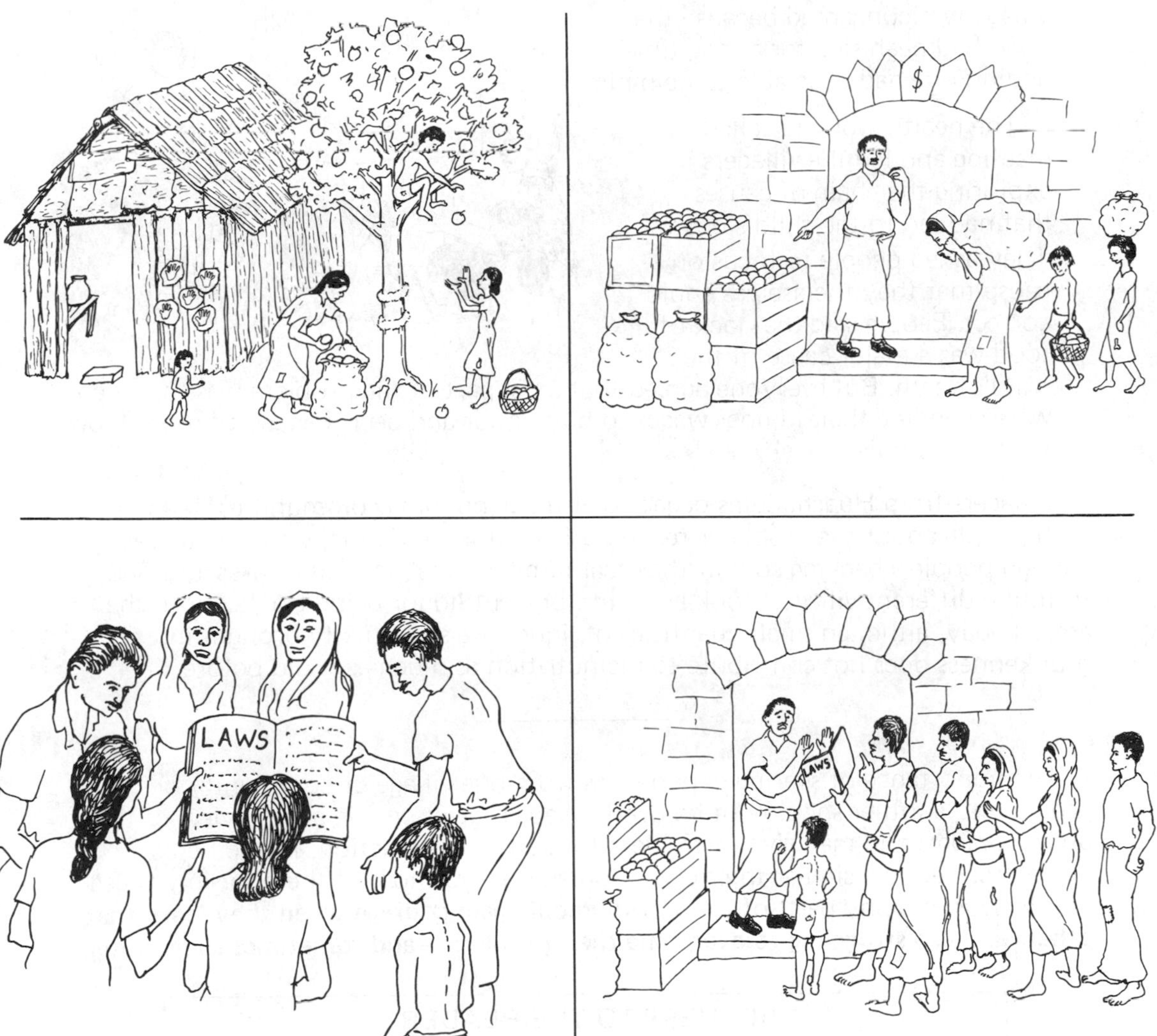

Pictures like these may add life to the story from India, when it is told or read to a group. Or the pictures can be used after the story is told, to help start a discussion.

SHARING IDEAS AND EXPERIENCES AMONG PROGRAMS

Growing communications between health programs in neighboring and distant locations have led to valuable sharing of ideas and experiences. Here is an example of how a teaching story from this book, shared by the health team in Ajoya, Mexico, helped health workers from another area to solve a community problem:

Health workers from Huachimetas, a lumbering area in Mexico, took part in an 'educational exchange' of training methods in Ajoya. Together with health workers from other countries, they read the STORY OF LUIS and analyzed the chain of causes that led to his death (see p. **26**-3 to **26**-7).

A few weeks after they returned to Huachimetas, a young, very thin child died of diarrhea. Everyone in the village was concerned because the child had been sick for a long time and no one had been able to help him.

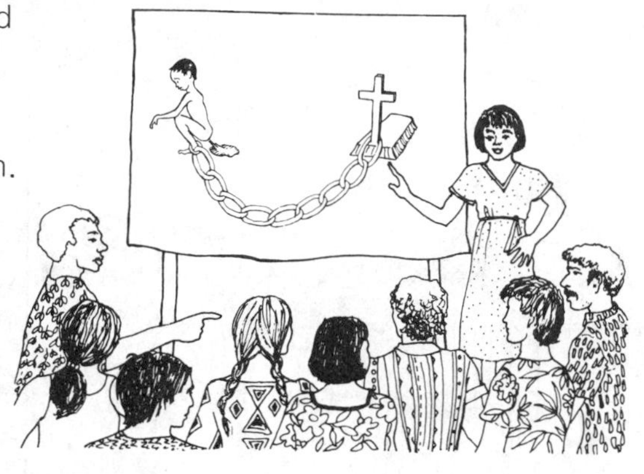

The health workers called a meeting and led the villagers in exploring the chain of causes that had led to the child's death. They asked people to focus on a cause that they themselves could correct. People said that lack of food was a major cause of the child's death. But everyone agreed that a big part of the problem was that men were spending their lumber wages to buy liquor and beer, instead of more food for their families.

Villagers from Huachimetas began to visit surrounding communities, talking with people about the problems resulting from drinking. Finally they gathered enough people's backing so that the local farmworkers' council (representatives from the different villages) took action to prevent liquor being trucked into the area. Today, although small quantities of liquor are still quietly brought in, drunkenness does not contribute to malnutrition as much as it did before.

The importance of sharing experiences from one village or community or program to another should not be overlooked. It gives people a fresh view of their own problems and may give them ideas for constructive action. It also helps people realize how similar their own problems are to those of the poor in villages and *barrios* in many parts of the world. **People gain courage when they learn that others are also struggling to overcome their problems—and sometimes succeeding.**

REQUEST TO THE READER

We hope you will send us your own examples of ways in which villagers and health workers in your area have acted to overcome difficult social problems that have affected people's health. We would like to make a collection of these stories so that everyone can learn and get ideas from the experiences of others.

Ways to Get People Thinking and Acting: Village Theater and Puppet Shows

CHAPTER 27

Role playing, sociodramas, people's theater, and puppet shows are all forms of action-packed story telling by a group. Each can be used to explore problems or situations by acting them out. At best, they are an excellent learning process for both actors and watchers, based on participation and discovery.

The difference between these dramatic forms is one of methods and subject:

ROLE PLAYING is the simplest form, often used as a learning game in class. Several students, or the whole group, act out a problem or situation. Each student pretends, or 'plays the role' of a particular person—for example a sick child, the child's mother or older sister, or the health worker. Usually role playing is done with little or no practice ahead of time, and no memorizing of parts. The story's details are developed by the group as they act it out.

Because role playing is such an excellent classroom method for bringing problems to life, we have discussed it already in Chapter 14. And there are more examples in other parts of this book. For instance, in Chapter 1 we use two role plays to compare 'the bossy teacher' with 'the good group leader' (see pages **1**-17 to **1**-20).

SOCIODRAMAS—or social dramas—are used to explore people's attitudes, feelings, and behavior. They often focus on social or political concerns: how some people affect the lives of others. Their main purpose is to **increase people's awareness** of underlying human problems, and to **explore possibilities for action and change.**

Sociodramas can be developed in class as spontaneous (unpracticed) role playing. Or they can be presented in public, perhaps before the whole village, with or without much practice and preparation.

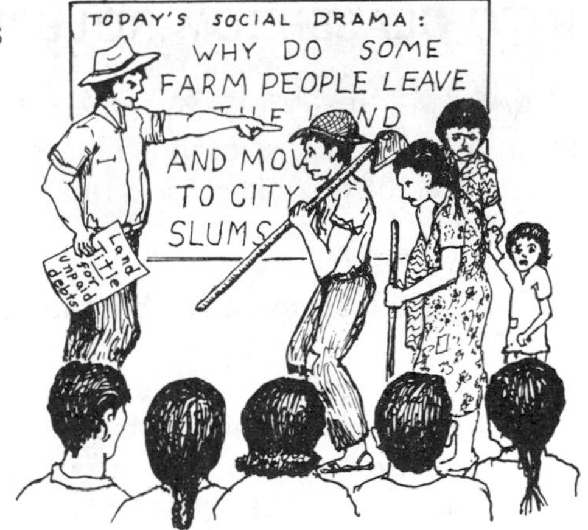
TODAY'S SOCIAL DRAMA:
WHY DO SOME FARM PEOPLE LEAVE
AND MO
TO CIT
SLUMS
Land Title for unpaid debts

THEATER is a form of public play acting. The story or 'play' is usually planned and practiced in advance. Parts may be memorized, but it is often more effective and a better learning process if participants understand their roles and speak in their own words.

Health-related theater is a good way to bring people together, including many who do not go to meetings or health talks. Theater can communicate messages, ideas, or concerns in a way that holds people's attention and makes them think—and act! **Make-believe action on stage can lead to real action in the community.**

PUPPET SHOWS are a form of play acting using small models (puppets or marionettes), or sometimes masks or 'giant heads' to act out stories or messages.

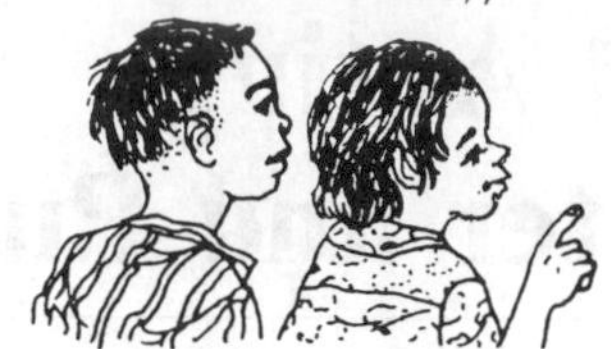

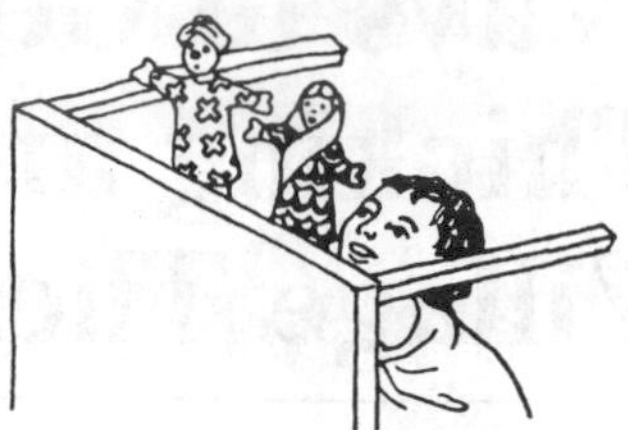

Puppets are especially fun for children. Children can make the puppets, as well as take part in creating and putting on the show.

However, puppets can also be used with adults, especially for exploring difficult social issues. A puppet can often make social criticisms or point out conflicting interests without causing personal offense. (If a 'real person' were to say the same things publicly, some people might be angry or hurt.) **Puppets add a sense of pretending and humor that can make the feared parts of our daily life easier to look at.**

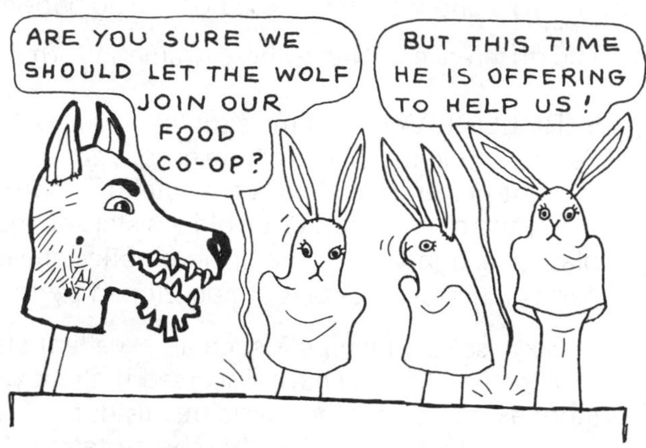
ARE YOU SURE WE SHOULD LET THE WOLF JOIN OUR FOOD CO-OP?
BUT THIS TIME HE IS OFFERING TO HELP US!

COMBINED FORMS OF DRAMA. In actual practice, there need be no sharp divisions between role playing, sociodrama, theater, and puppet shows. These different forms can be mixed, or one can lead to another.

WORKING SOCIAL DRAMA INTO CLASSROOM ROLE PLAYS

Any form of role playing, drama, or 'make believe' becomes more real and meaningful if it consciously includes social factors that relate to the situation. This is true even of role plays (or 'simulation exercises') to practice diagnosis and treatment.

Example: **A sociodrama about measles**

Suppose a group of student health workers acts out a scene in which a mother brings in a child with signs of measles. A student acting the role of health worker tries to diagnose the problem and advise the mother. This role play can be made far more real and useful if local social factors that commonly relate to the problem are acted out. Social factors can include those that relate to local traditions ***(cultural factors),*** those that relate to money or its lack ***(economic factors),*** and those that relate to who has power over whom ***(political factors).***

Here are some possibilities (based on social factors in Mexico):

CULTURAL FACTORS: The 'mother' insists that her child with measles should be given a purge or enema of kapok bark to bring out his rash (see *Where There Is No Doctor,* p. 11). She also believes it is dangerous to feed her child while he has a fever. ***Can the health worker help the mother change her views without making her feel stupid or ashamed, or showing disrespect for her traditions?***

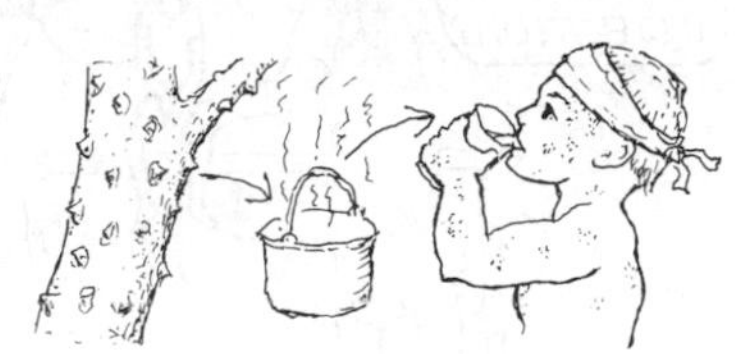

ECONOMIC FACTORS: The mother has several other small children who do not yet have measles, but who are poorly nourished. The father has no land and most of the time no work. The health worker reads in the book that measles is especially dangerous for malnourished children. ***What can the health worker do for this particular family?***

POLITICAL AND CULTURAL FACTORS: Let us suppose the mother lacks confidence in the health worker. This is partly because the health worker is from a poor family, and partly because the doctor on his weekly visits orders him around like a servant. The mother insists on giving her child a purge unless the health worker gives him an injection—which she believes the doctor would do. ***Can the health worker convince her, in a friendly way, that both purge and injection are unnecessary and might be harmful?***

Acting out these kinds of social factors that arise from the local reality can make the role play—or 'sociodrama'—a far more useful learning experience. It helps prepare health workers to handle the human problems that are bound to arise when they work in a community.

CLASSROOM ROLE PLAYS THAT LEAD TO COMMUNITY THEATER PRODUCTIONS

Some of the best village theater presentations we have seen have grown out of role plays and sociodramas that first took place in the classroom.

Example: **A skit about sensible treatment of the common cold**

A common difficulty for health workers is trying to convince people that injections and antibiotics are not needed for the common cold. Some health workers in Mexico used role playing to explore this problem. They acted out such a powerful skit that they decided to develop it into a short play and present it to the whole village. In its final form it included the following scenes:

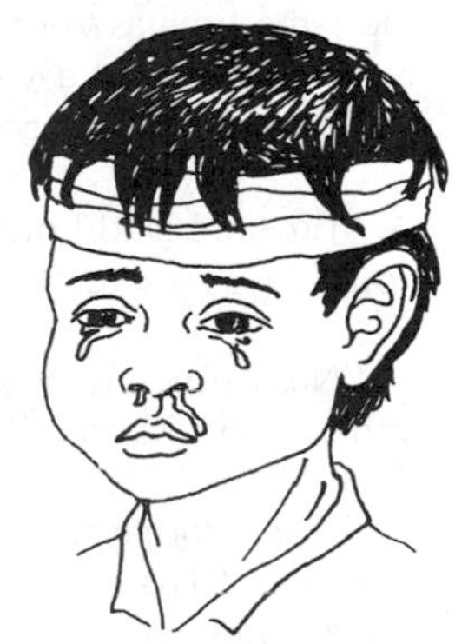

Scene 1. A mother, Marta, arrives at the health post with her small son, Ringo, who has a bad cold. She asks the health worker to give him an injection. The health worker examines the boy and finds only signs of a common cold.

He gives the appropriate advice:

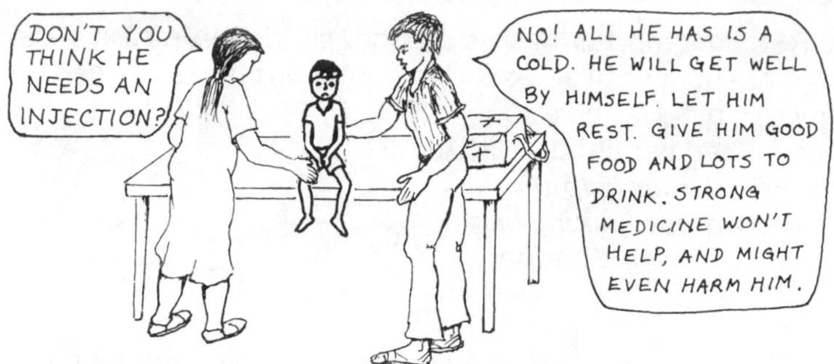
DON'T YOU THINK HE NEEDS AN INJECTION?
NO! ALL HE HAS IS A COLD. HE WILL GET WELL BY HIMSELF. LET HIM REST. GIVE HIM GOOD FOOD AND LOTS TO DRINK. STRONG MEDICINE WON'T HELP, AND MIGHT EVEN HARM HIM.

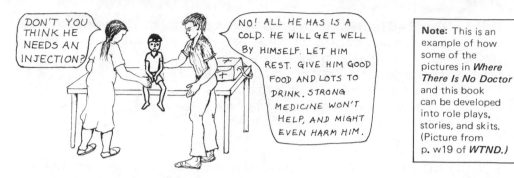

Note: This is an example of how some of the pictures in ***Where There Is No Doctor*** and this book can be developed into role plays, stories, and skits. (Picture from p. w19 of ***WTND.)***

But Marta insists that her son needs an injection of ***Respicil.*** (This is an antibiotic containing penicillin and streptomycin, commonly used in Mexico for colds, by doctors and by people in general.) The health worker explains as best he can why antibiotics are of no help for colds and may be harmful, but Marta looks doubtful. She thanks the health worker and leaves.

Scene 2. Another mother, Gloria, arrives with her daughter, Ana, who has a bad cold, too. Gloria also wants her child to be injected. But she listens to the health worker's advice and decides to try treating Ana with fruit juice, aspirin, and good food. For the cough, she agrees to give her daughter lots of water, and to have her breathe hot water vapors. The health worker shows Gloria how.

Scene 3. Marta, on leaving the health post, goes to the home of an ***inyectadora*** (a woman who injects). Much to Ringo's protests, the woman injects him. He screams in pain. Then, limping and crying, Ringo is led away by his mother.

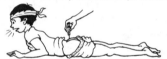

Scene 4. (Several days later.) Marta brings Ringo to the health worker. The boy limps in with the aid of a stick. He has a high fever, and an abscess on his backside where he was injected. The health worker recommends hot soaks and other appropriate treatment. He reminds Marta not to inject any of her children the next time they have a cold.

Scene 5. On their way home, Marta and Ringo meet Gloria and Ana on the street. Gloria asks Marta why her boy is limping. Marta explains, but adds, "At least the injection cured him of his cold!"

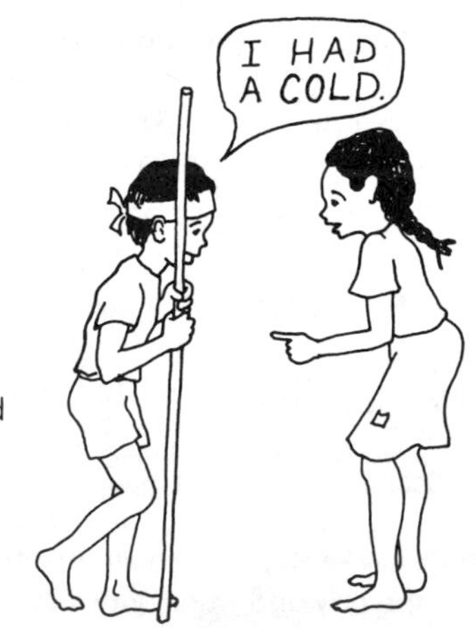
I HAD A COLD.

"Maybe not," says Gloria. "My Ana had a bad cold at the same time as your son. But I followed the health worker's advice. I gave her lots of fruit juices and aspirin and good food. She got over her cold in no time!"

"I'm sure glad I didn't get an injection and end up like you," says Ana to Ringo.

"Next time my boy has a cold, I won't have him injected either," says Marta. "I'll just give him aspirin!"

"Don't forget fruit juice, lots of water, and good food," says Ana. "They help fight off the cold. Next time Ringo will get well again as fast as I did!"

IDEAS FOR USING DRAMA TO TEACH ABOUT HEALTH

1. The value of homemade, open-ended drama

In this chapter we describe in detail some 'skits' that have been performed by health workers and villagers. But it is not our hope that any of these will be repeated as such. They are examples of how groups of health workers, mothers, and children can create their own performances.

Those who present a play or skit will learn twice as much if they also take part in creating or writing it. The story can be developed from the actual ideas and experiences of the participants. The group must invent the story and figure out how to present local problems in a convincing way. This helps them develop skills in planning, thinking, problem solving, organizing, and communicating. All these extra benefits are lost when students simply memorize a script written by someone else.

2. Encouraging people to speak in their own words (not memorize parts)

Speaking in public is not easy for many health workers and villagers. Often the poor are used to remaining silent in village meetings, while a select few do the talking and make the decisions. At first, health workers-in-training may be embarrassed to speak or play act in front of a group. Too shy to say things in their own words, they will often prefer to memorize the words of someone else. This takes more work, but seems safer. They feel less exposed.

However, the ability to stand up and state one's own thoughts with confidence is an extremely important skill—especially for those who would speak for the 'voiceless poor'. So encourage health workers to use their own words in role plays rather than simply parroting lines they have memorized.

But go slowly. Help people gain confidence little by little. Start with role plays in the classroom or with a small group in which everyone takes part. This way there is no audience. Or rather, all are actors and audience at the same time. As the students become more confident, they can begin to do presentations for larger groups.

BEFORE

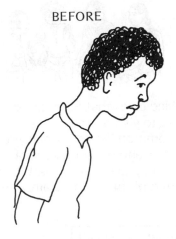

Taking part in role playing and people's theater helps the 'voiceless poor' gain confidence, courage, and skill to speak their thoughts.

AFTER

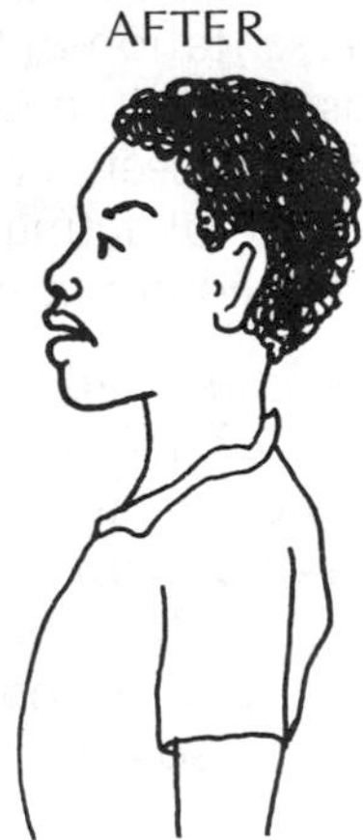

With practice, it is amazing how fast people's self-confidence can grow. We have seen a student group of village health workers who at first were so shy they would blush in confusion when asked a question in class. By the end of the two-month course, they enthusiastically presented a half-hour social drama for visiting instructors from several countries, speaking loud and clear in their own words. Their increase in confidence made the effort more than worth it!

3. **Involving mothers and children—Be sure the drama is important to them**

Health workers may be able to interest women or children in putting on skits or puppet shows for the community. People are more likely to take part if the subject of the drama is important to them.

For example, in Ajoya, Mexico most of the women refused in principle to be seen 'on stage'. But when they learned that a play was being planned on the problem of drunkenness, even some of the most reserved elderly women were eager to take part. (See p. **27**-19.)

4. **Entertainment is more powerful than preaching**

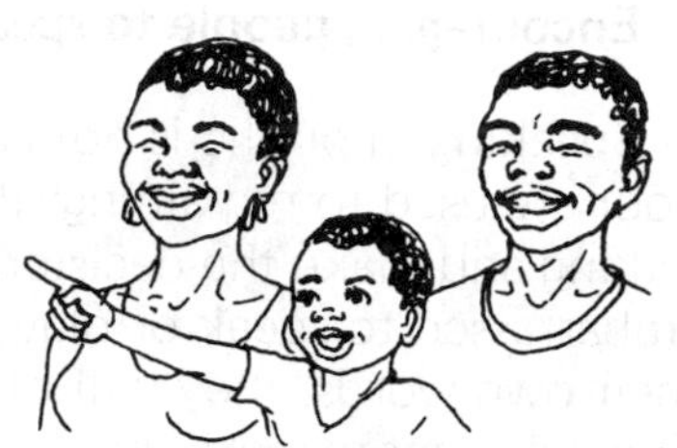

If popular theater is to reach many people, especially those who are most difficult to reach, it needs above all to be entertaining.

Theater can be used for health education. It can help get people thinking about specific problems and possibilities for action. It can contain a strong social message. But if it is to hold an audience and convince people to come back for more, **care must be taken not to preach.** Few people enjoy being told what they should or should not do, especially when they have come to have a good time.

It is more effective if the message is built into the story. The positive or negative results of the actors' actions can be made obvious. But let the people in the audience be free to draw their own conclusions. Respect their judgement and their intelligence!

5. **Leaving time for discussion afterwards**

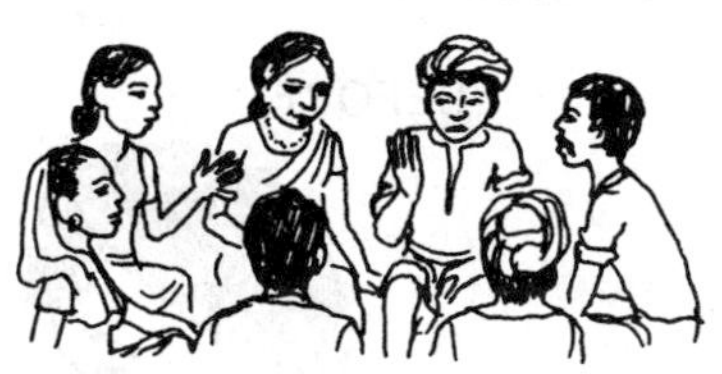

Whether it is a role play in the classroom or a theater presentation in the village, a discussion afterwards will help people relate personally to what they have seen. A follow-up discussion can help turn playful acting on the stage into positive action in the community.

For example, following a village skit on "Useless Medicines that Sometimes Kill" (see p. **27**-14), the audience formed a committee to visit all the stores in town. The committee asked storekeepers not to sell common useless or dangerous medicines, or at least to warn people about their dangers and proper use. As a result, some of the shopkeepers actually stopped selling certain medicines. When customers asked for those medicines, the shopkeepers took time to explain why they no longer sold them.

Follow-up discussions get people personally involved!

TECHNIQUES FOR EFFECTIVE, ENTERTAINING THEATER

1. The place and the stage

Popular theater can be performed almost anywhere. Sometimes a group of actors may simply begin to perform on the street. Little by little, people gather around to watch. Sometimes children or other persons from the crowd are encouraged to join in the spontaneous performance. The stage is life itself.

More often, however, a fixed area is used—either indoors, or outdoors in a large courtyard or enclosure.

Some sort of stage or platform lets the audience see better. You can build one from wood or blocks of adobe (mud brick). But this is expensive.

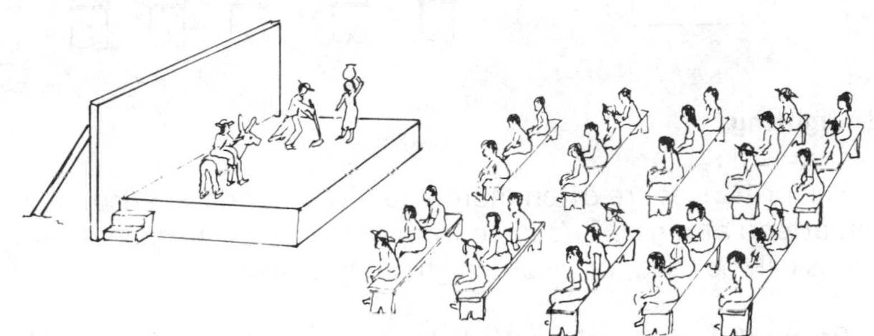

Your town may have a natural stage: a small hill in front of a slope where people can sit. If the school children and other villagers help with picks and shovels, the area can soon be made into a natural theater, or 'amphitheater'.

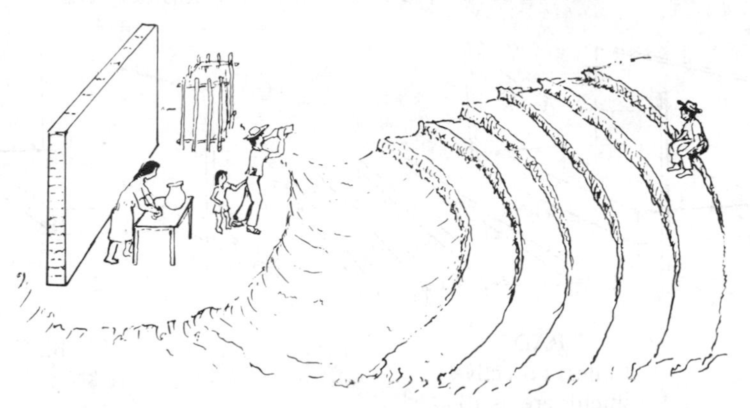

2. The crowd and being heard

In popular theater, one of the biggest difficulties the actors have is trying to be heard. When a whole village attends, mothers will be there with babies who begin to cry. Children of all ages will shout, laugh, play, and fight. There is almost always some sort of noise.

In villages that have electricity or a generator, microphones with loudspeakers may be available. But commonly they do not work. They buzz and squeak, or distort voices so much that it is hard to understand what is being said.

Usually the best solution is for the actors to shout. **They should try to speak so that the people farthest away can hear them.** When practicing, it helps if someone stands far away and interrupts every time he cannot understand what is said. Speaking slowly and clearly also helps. And never speak with your back to the audience.

If you think that the crowd will be too big, it may help to put on 2 or 3 performances. Invite part of the village one time, and the rest another time.

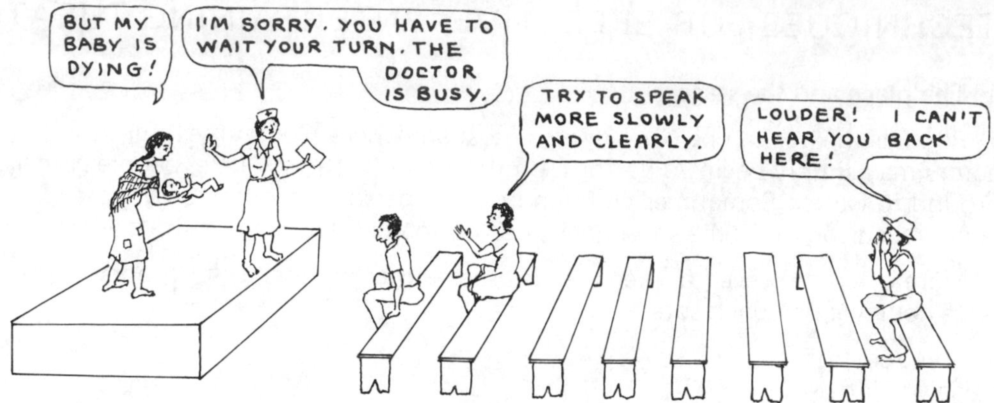
BUT MY BABY IS DYING!
I'M SORRY. YOU HAVE TO WAIT YOUR TURN. THE DOCTOR IS BUSY.
TRY TO SPEAK MORE SLOWLY AND CLEARLY.
LOUDER! I CAN'T HEAR YOU BACK HERE!

3. **Lighting**

Performances are often more effective after dark. Also, more working people can attend at night. But some form of lighting is needed. Gasoline or kerosene lamps can be used, or electric lights if available.

Be careful not to place the lights between the audience and the actors, unless the lights are covered so they do not shine in people's eyes.

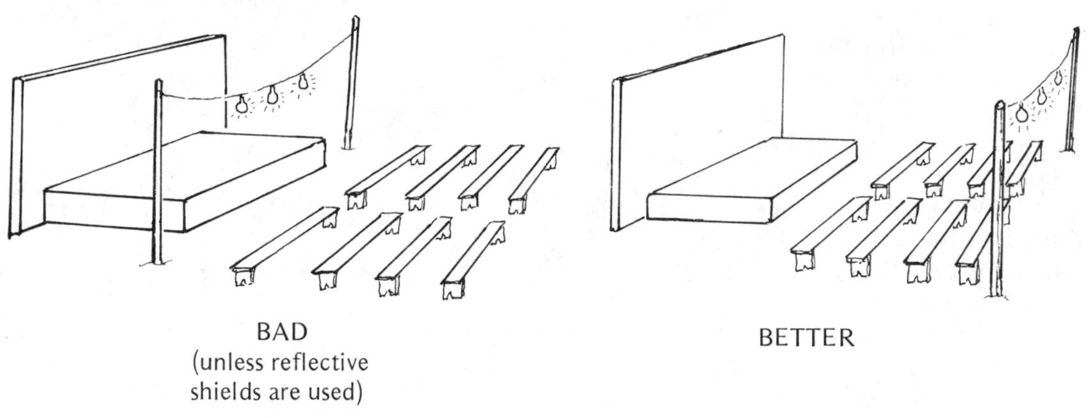

BAD (unless reflective shields are used)

BETTER

If possible, use a **reflective shield** to direct light toward the stage.

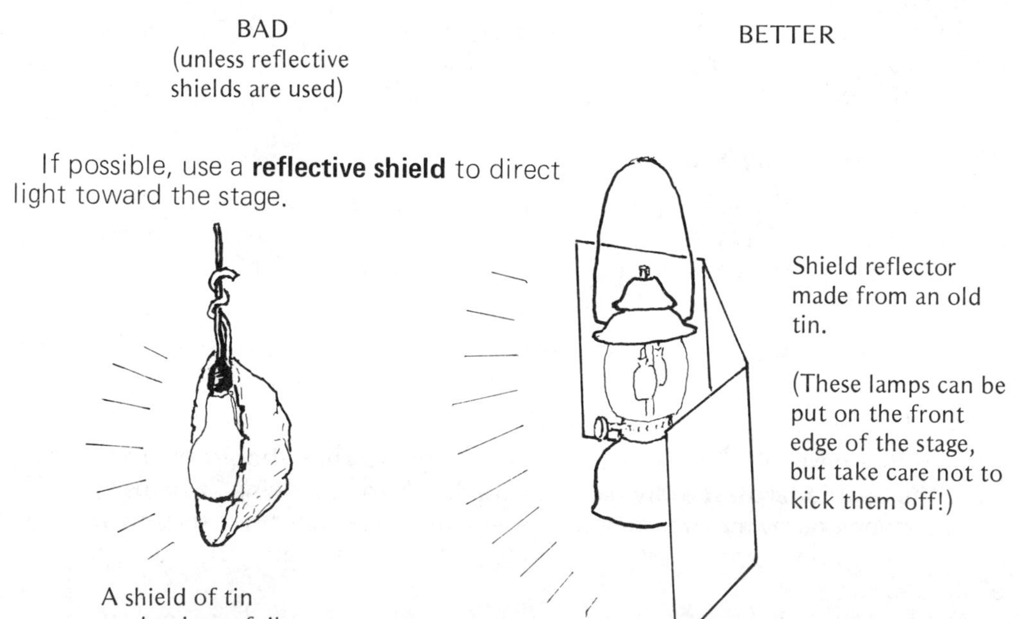

A shield of tin or aluminum foil.

Shield reflector made from an old tin.

(These lamps can be put on the front edge of the stage, but take care not to kick them off!)

4. Props and costumes

Props are objects such as tables, chairs, and tools, that are used on stage to add a sense of reality to a play.

A few simple props can be helpful, especially if they are colorful or imaginative. Here are some ideas:

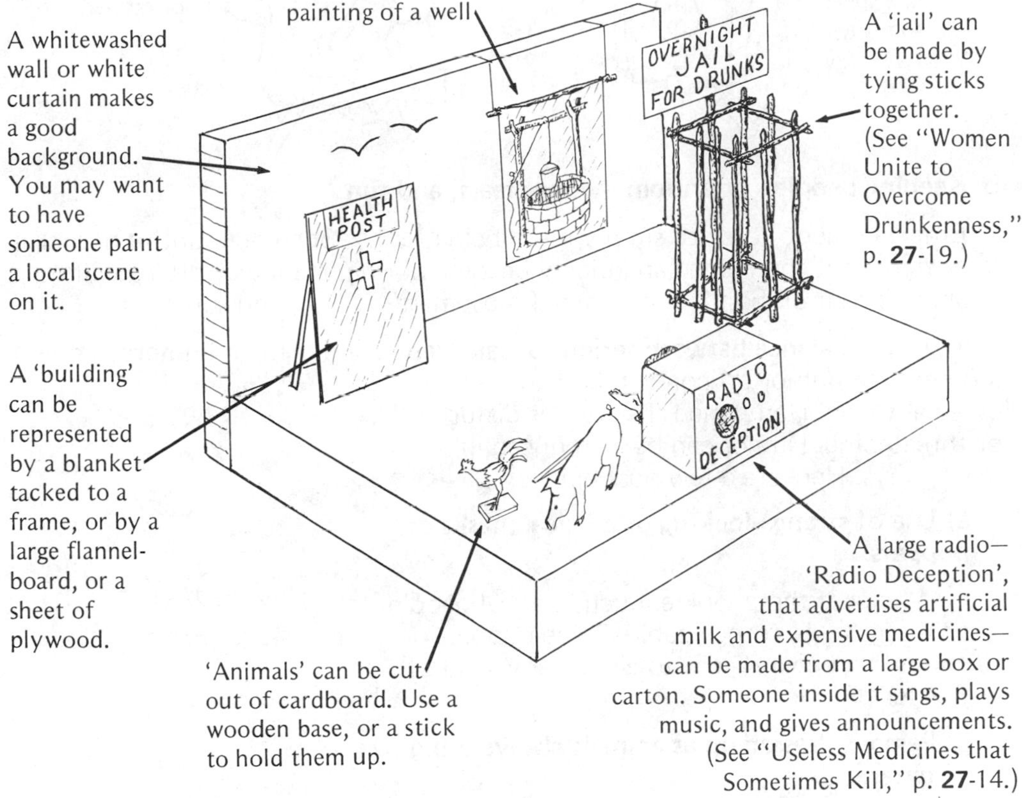

painting of a well
A whitewashed wall or white curtain makes a good background. You may want to have someone paint a local scene on it.

A 'building' can be represented by a blanket tacked to a frame, or by a large flannel-board, or a sheet of plywood.

A large radio—'Radio Deception', that advertises artificial milk and expensive medicines—can be made from a large box or carton. Someone inside it sings, plays music, and gives announcements. (See "Useless Medicines that Sometimes Kill," p. 27-14.)
'Animals' can be cut out of cardboard. Use a wooden base, or a stick to hold them up.

A few good, simple props are usually all that are needed. Many things, like walls and doors, can be imagined. The actors can help the audience imagine things are there, and this adds to the fun. For example, if the scene is inside a house, someone can pretend to knock on an unseen door:

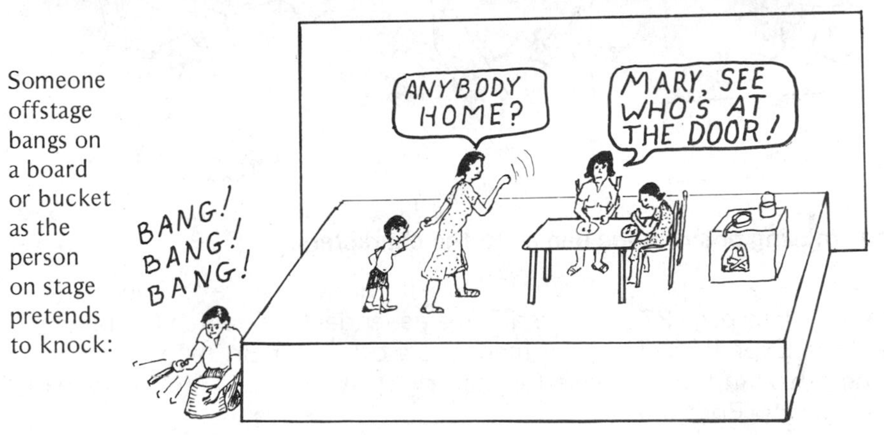
Someone offstage bangs on a board or bucket as the person on stage pretends to knock:
BANG! BANG! BANG!
ANYBODY HOME?
MARY, SEE WHO'S AT THE DOOR!
Then someone inside the 'house' pretends to open the door, and invites the visitor in.

Costumes, like props, can usually be kept simple. Easy-to-understand symbols help get ideas across. For example:

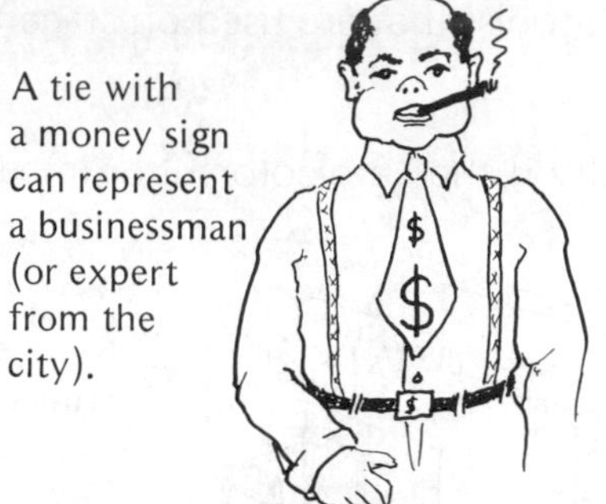

A tie with a money sign can represent a businessman (or expert from the city).

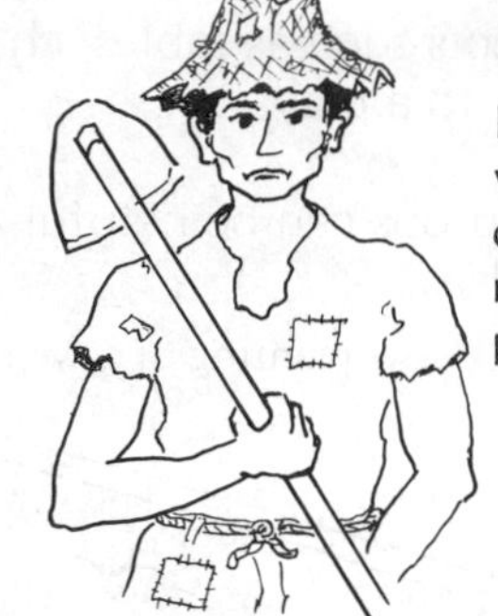

Ragged clothes with brightly colored patches represent the poor farmer.

5. **Keeping people's attention: Action, tears, and fun**

Entertainment does not simply mean being funny. Some amount of humor is important, but too much can quickly become boring. A play or drama will hold people's attention best if it has lots of movement, action, and surprises.

Try for a **balance between serious or sad events, and light or humorous ones.** Moments of humor or 'comic relief' are especially important when the story is disturbing or threatening. Humor can be introduced in many ways. Here are a few possibilities:

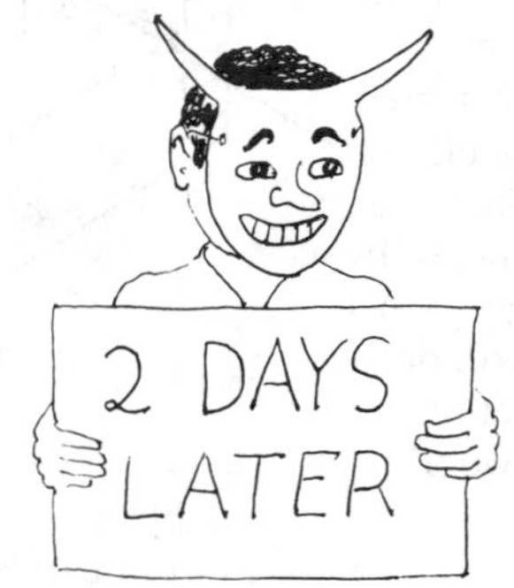

a) **Use of strange-looking or comical masks or puppets.**

It helps if these look enough like real people or things to be recognizable. Some puppets or masks can be worked into almost any kind of theater production.

b) **Persons dressed up as animals always bring laughter.**

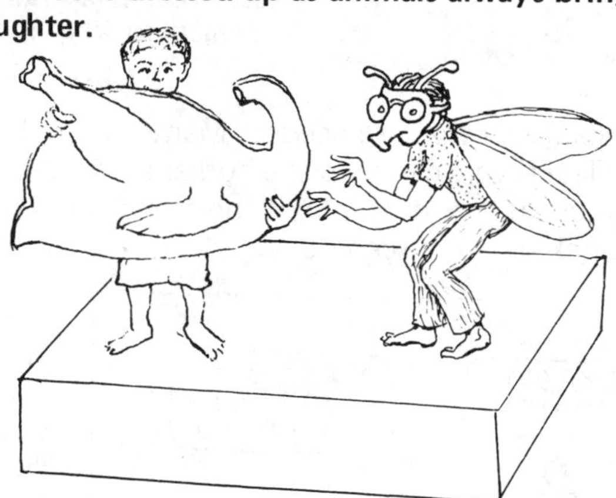

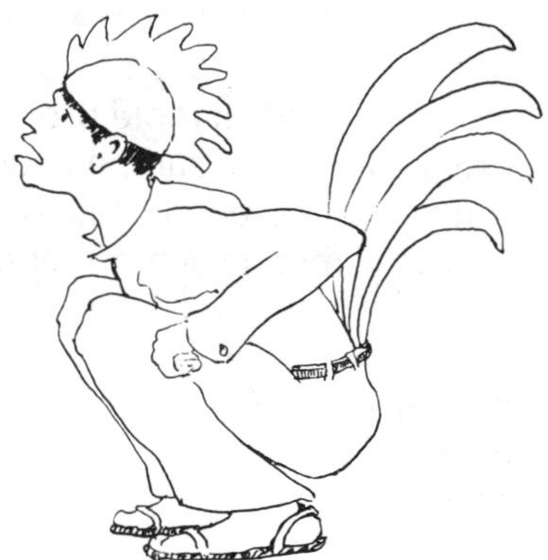

c) **Giving amusing or symbolic names to the characters.**

For example, in the play in Spanish, "Small Farmers Unite to Overcome Exploitation" (see page **27**-27), the rich maize-lender was named Brutelio, and his wife Doña Exploitiva. The poor man who worked for Brutelio rather than joining the others in their struggle for their rights was called Lamberino, which in Spanish means 'Boot-licker'.

d) **'Comic relief'**

A play called "Farmworkers Unite to Overcome Hunger" was put on by student health workers to get people thinking about how they might recover land held illegally by the rich. If irrigated, this land could produce two harvests a year and help landless farmworkers to feed their families. This serious play was made lighter at moments by the use of a papier mache donkey with two people inside it.

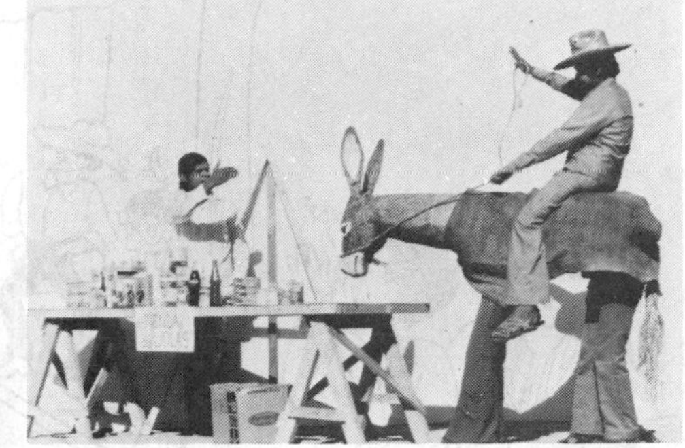

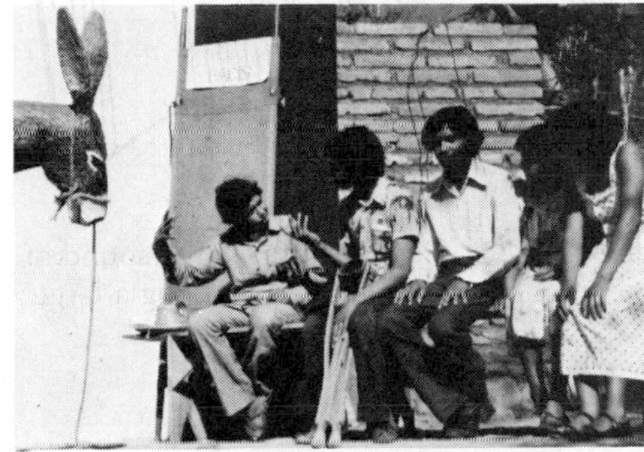

During one of the most serious scenes, 'comic relief' was provided by the donkey. It would nod its head in agreement with the farmworkers' decisions to take over the land.

e) **Use of songs, dance, and music**

Songs and music make a drama more entertaining. The play mentioned above opened with the singing of popular songs for which the health workers had written new words. And one scene showed a 'work festival' in which people dug an irrigation ditch to the rhythm of songs and music by the village musicians. The play finished with a celebration and dance—in which even the donkey began to dance!

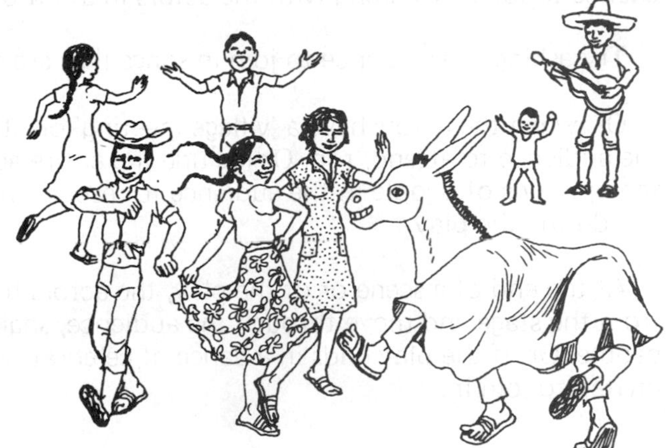

Songs with health messages can be introduced through popular theater. If the songs are clever enough, people may pick them up and continue singing them. This happened in Africa with a song about preventing eye disease, called "Brush the Flies from Baby's Eyes."

You might try giving a group of health workers, mothers, or school children a line like "Brush the flies from baby's eyes . . ." and see who can come up with the best song. Then perhaps it could be presented in a skit or puppet show. (See also the songs on pages **1**-27 and **15**-15.)

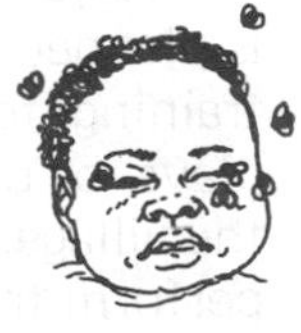

f) **Sound effects**

Sound effects, or artificial noises can be produced in many ways. Children can also help with sound effects for a play.

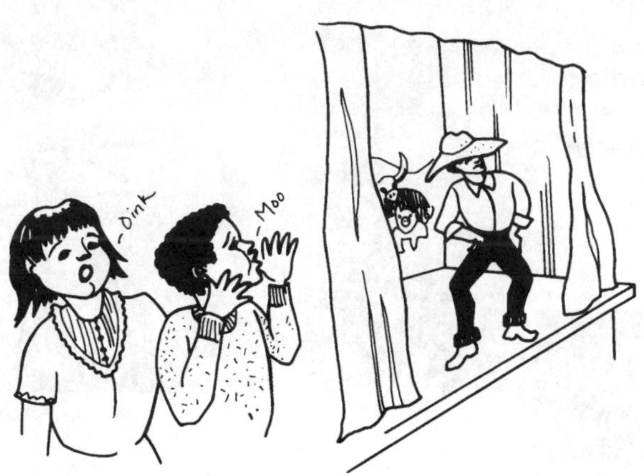

Children can make animal noises at the right moment while they are hidden from the audience.

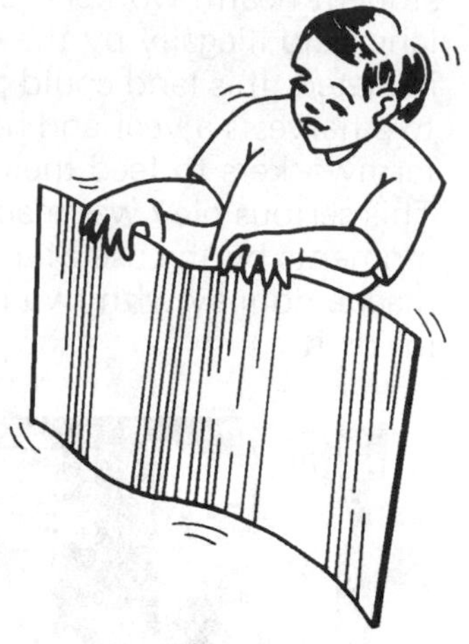

You can make the sound of thunder by shaking a large piece of sheet metal.

g) **Including the audience in the act**

People in the audience will become more interested and involved if they have a chance to take part along with the actors in a skit or play.

Try asking the audience to join in songs that are sung as a part of the drama.

Or, when the actors have a 'village meeting' on stage, invite a few persons from the audience to attend, too. Or include the entire audience in the 'meeting'. Ask the opinions of people in the audience to resolve arguments that are being acted out during the play.

At the end of a scene or of the play, the actors (or puppets) can come down from the stage and move through the audience, shaking hands and greeting people. Or, if the play ends in a dance of celebration, the whole audience can be invited to join in.

HEALTH FESTIVALS AND CIRCUSES

Some community programs organize periodic 'health festivals', or evenings of theater and entertainment.

In Ajoya, Mexico, such an evening of entertainment and farmworkers' theater is planned for the end of each 2-month training course. The health workers-in-training, together with mothers' groups and school children, put on several skits, plays, or puppet shows. These focus on important health and social concerns in the village. Between shows, the village musicians play and sing, or young people perform traditional dances.

In the "Hospital without Walls" Program in San Ramon, Costa Rica, the health team conducts a traveling 'health circus' with music, skits, and games. One of the biggest attractions is the 'magic show' in which Don Valeriano, a local magician, performs tricks that help teach aspects of health care. Here are 3 of his tricks:*

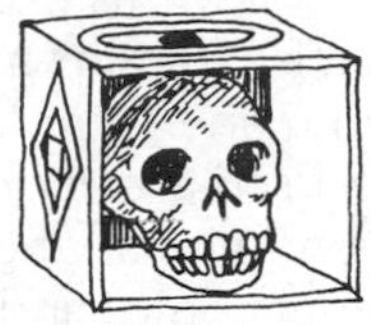

First he 'magically' changes several glassfuls of water into ***guaro*** (a cheap alcoholic drink). He then takes an empty box, covers it with a cloth, and asks children from the audience to guard it. He says a few magic words, pulls away the cloth, and the skull of a man who died from alcoholism appears inside the box. The skull starts to tell the audience about the dangers of drinking.

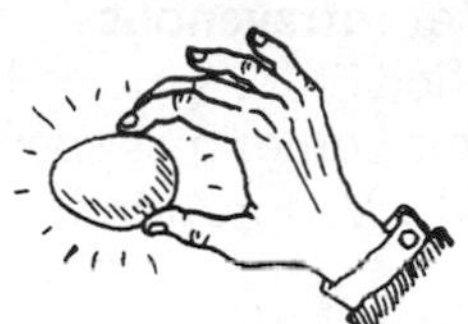

Don Valeriano waves a handkerchief over his hand, blows on it, says some magic words, and an egg appears in his hand. He then explains the importance of eggs in good nutrition.

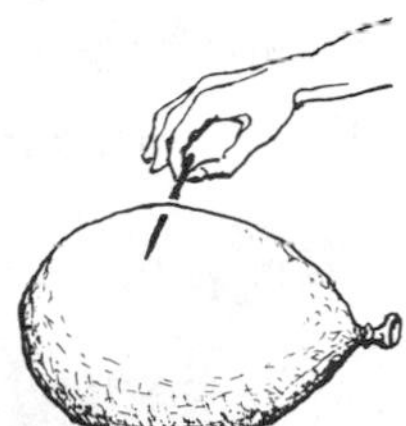

He blows up a white balloon, which represents a bottle-fed, malnourished baby who has not been vaccinated. He then takes a needle, stating that it is a disease, and pricks the balloon. The balloon pops, which means the child dies. He then blows up a red balloon, representing a healthy, breast-fed, vaccinated baby. When he tries to prick this balloon, it does not pop. The needle appears to pass right through it!

Having local entertainers help people learn about health can be exciting and effective. But beware of giving the idea that health care is 'magic', and therefore outside people's control.

EXAMPLES OF SOCIODRAMAS AND FARMPEOPLE'S THEATER

To follow are 4 examples of plays that have been put on by groups of mothers, children, and health workers in Ajoya, Mexico. These were all performed toward the end of 2-month training programs. The student health workers worked together with the mothers and children to plan and present the plays. In this way the students gain practical experience that helps them organize similar activities in their own villages.

Notice that each of these plays deals with an important social issue affecting people's health. Less dramatic forms of health education often are not effective in dealing with these issues because of people's strong attitudes, fears, and beliefs. But when people actually see (on stage) the harm or suffering that can result from certain practices, they are far more likely to take the message to heart.

Color slides and filmstrips of these 4 plays, and the puppet show on p. **27**-37, may be ordered from the Hesperian Foundation.

---

*Adapted from ***Salubritas,*** American Public Health Association, vol. 3, number 2, April, 1979.

VILLAGE THEATER

EXAMPLE 1: USELESS MEDICINES THAT SOMETIMES KILL

Overuse and misuse of medicines is a problem in many countries (see Ch. 18). In Mexico, this problem is made worse by international drug companies that advertise **'patent medicines'** by radio. They do this during the hours before dawn, when many farm families listen to popular country music. The medicines advertised are very expensive and of little use, yet many people are convinced by the smooth-talking voice in the radio. So they waste their limited money on vitamin tonics and other 'wonder drugs'.

Also, many rural people in Mexico and elsewhere believe that **intravenous solution** has tremendous healing powers. Villagers call it "artificial life." Instead of buying nutritious food, older people who are weak or anemic sometimes spend their last pesos to have a nurse or 'modern healer' put a liter of I.V. solution into their veins.

The following play tries to show the dangers of this kind of misuse of medicines. It was put on for the village of Ajoya by the team of local health workers, as part of a training program.

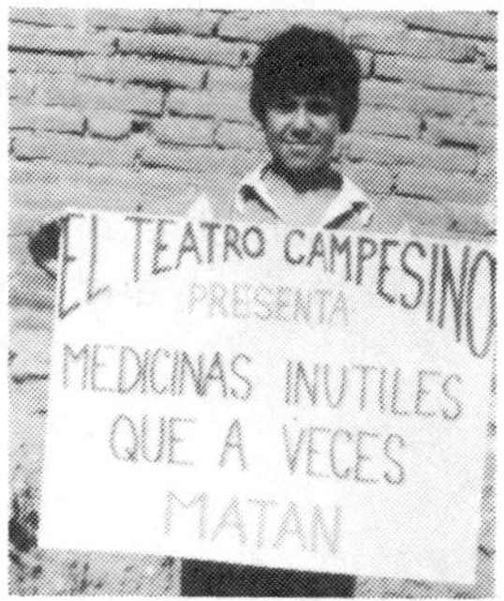
EL TEATRO CAMPESINO
PRESENTA
MEDICINAS INUTILES
QUE A VECES
MATAN

1) 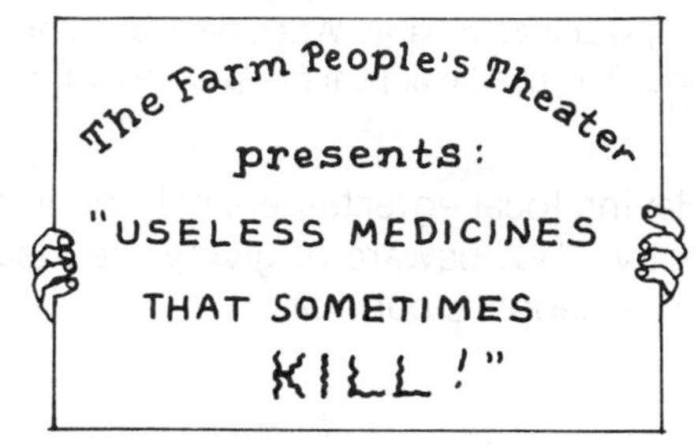

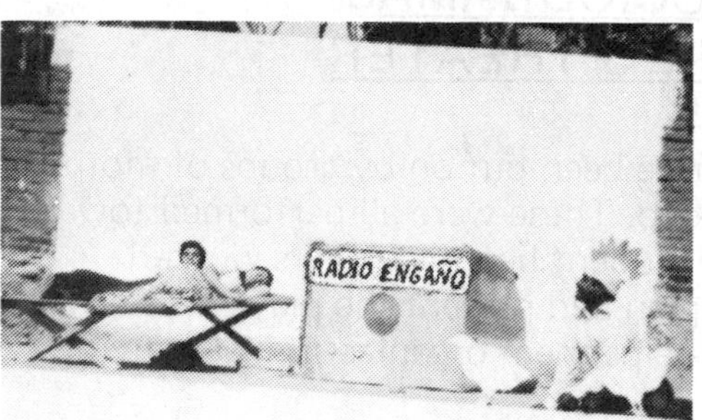
RADIO ENGAÑO

2) It is nearly dawn. The rooster crows, "Cock-a-doodle-doo." (The rooster is actually a health worker in costume; see p. 27-10.) The old man and his wife stir in bed, as they usually wake up early in the morning. Beside the bed is an enormous 'radio' with a sign that reads "RADIO DECEPTION." Hidden inside the radio is an actor.

RADIO DECEPTION

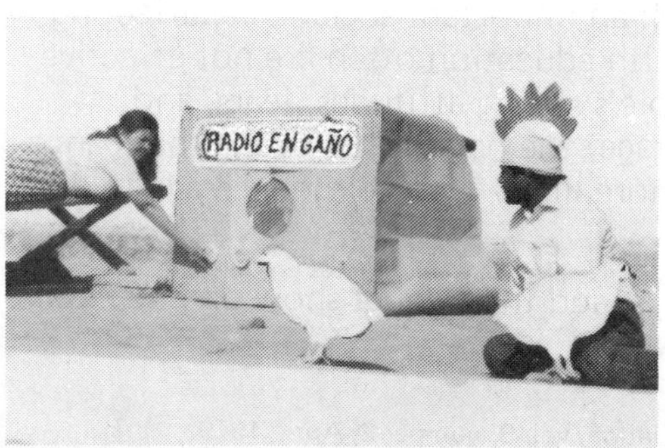
RADIO ENGAÑO

3) Old Doña Luisa turns on the radio. There are the sounds of country music. Then the voice from the radio says, "Good morning to you all. The last song was dedicated to Juanita Torres in Ajoya, Sinaloa. And now, before we play more country favorites, a word from Meyerhov Drug Company: Are you feeling weak and tired? Do you find it hard to wake up in the morning? You may be suffering from 'tired blood'. What you need are the new VITA-MEYERHOV vitamin pills. You'll wake up every morning feeling like dancing! Remember, VITA-MEYERHOV!"

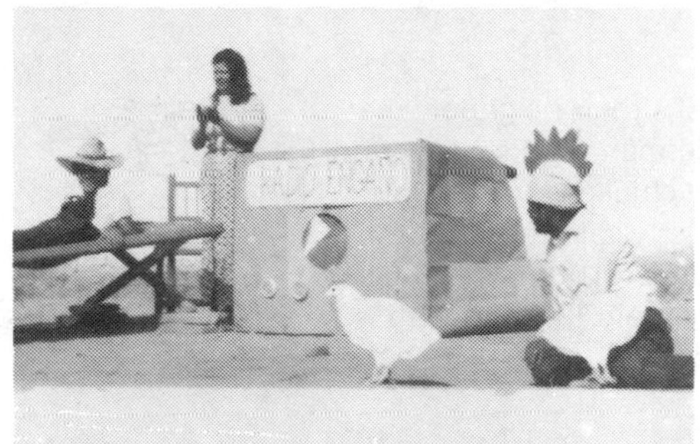

4) As Doña Luisa gets up and begins to make maize tortillas for breakfast, the music and advertisements continue. But look! Her husband, Don Lino, is still in bed! He feels too weak to get up.

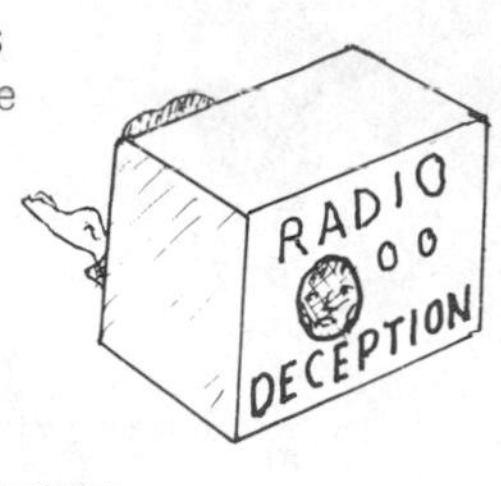

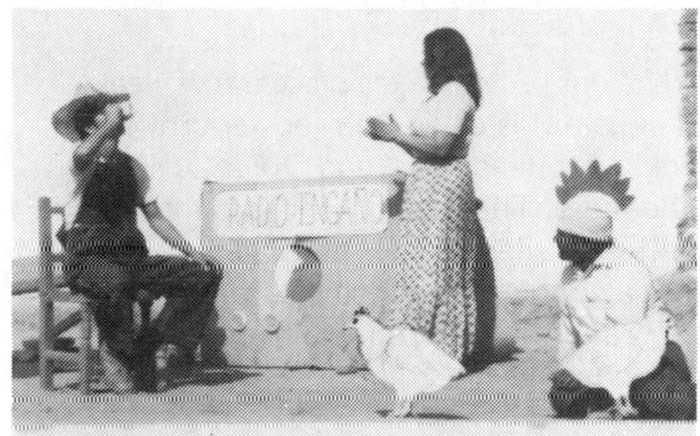

5) Finally Doña Luisa coaxes him out of bed and gives him a cup of coffee. He asks what there is for breakfast. She answers, "Just tortillas. You know that's all we have."

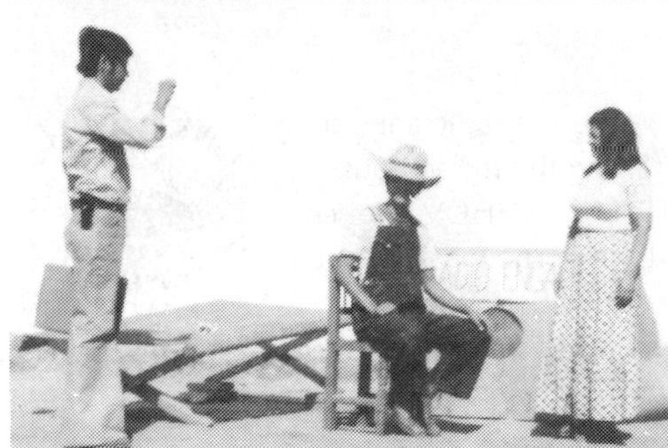

6) Just then, they hear a knock on the door. (Bang, bang, bang.) It is their neighbor, who makes his living by selling medicines that he buys in the city.

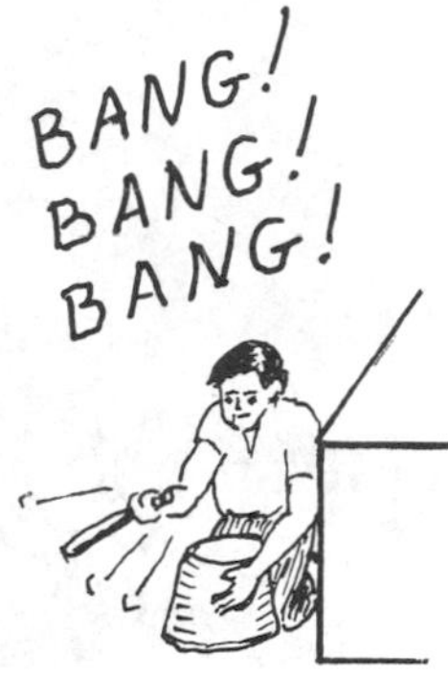

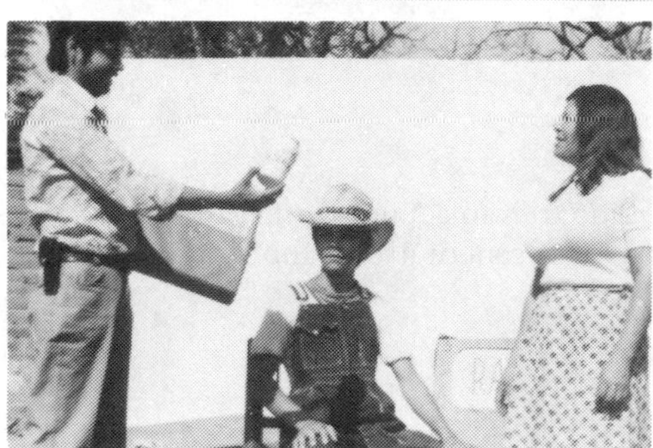

7) Today he is selling VITA-MEYERHOV. Old Luisa is excited because she just heard about VITA-MEYERHOV on the radio. She is sure that it will make her husband wake up strong and eager to work, like before. The salesman tells them the bottle is worth 300 pesos. But since they are such good friends, he will let them have it for only 150 pesos.

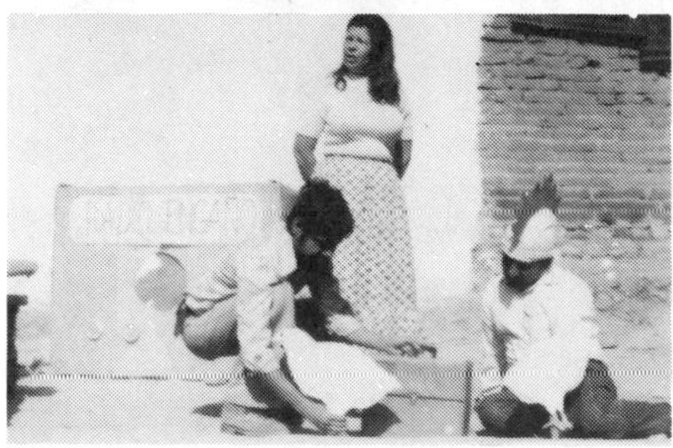

8) But the old couple only has 50 pesos. So they have to sell their 2 chickens, at 50 pesos each, in order to pay for the vitamins.

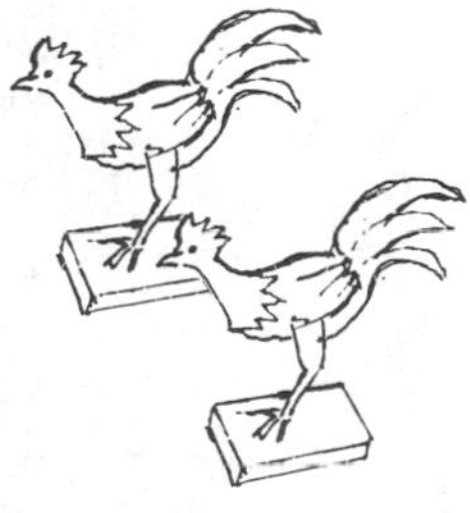

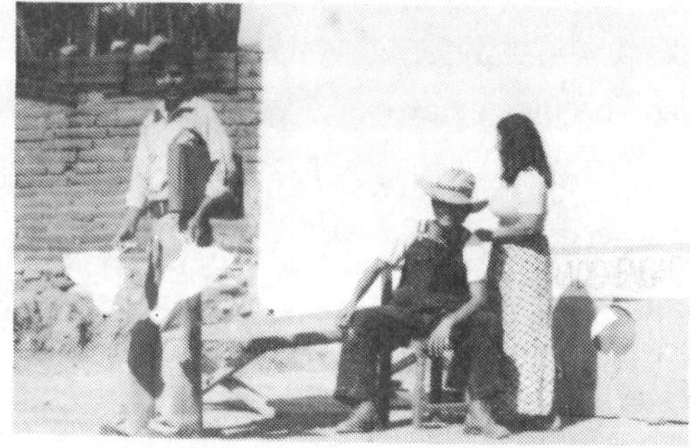

9) As their neighbor, the salesman, walks away with the chickens, the couple eagerly talks about how wonderful things will be when old Lino's health is restored.

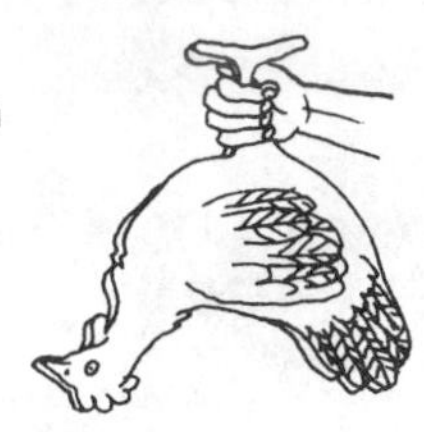

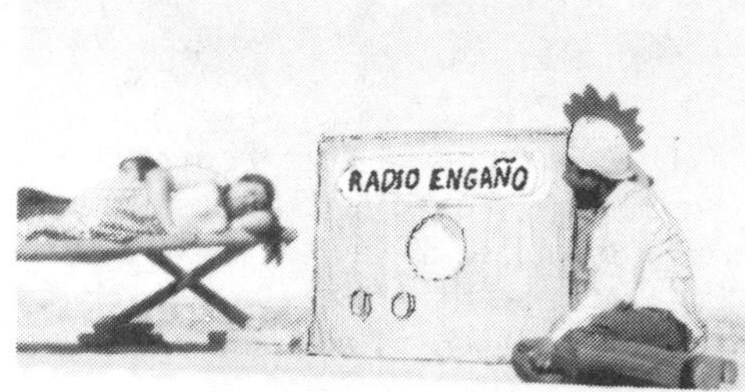

10) The next scene takes place a few weeks later. Again it is dawn, the rooster crows, "Cock-a-doodle-dooo," and Doña Luisa turns on the radio. The beat of ranchero music drifts out into the silent dawn. The radio announcer wishes a good morning to all, and goes on with more praise for the products from Meyerhov Drug Company.

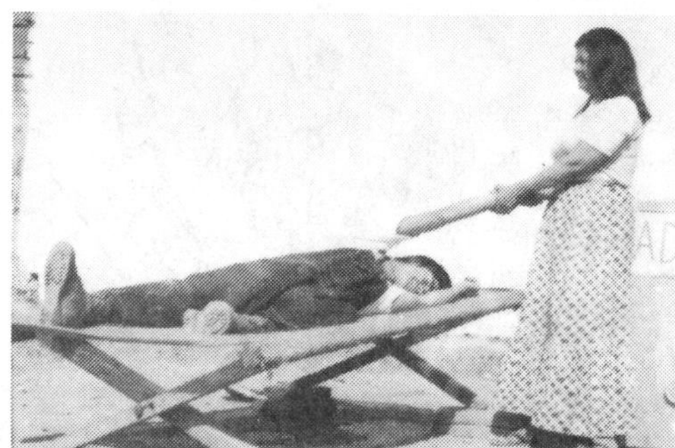

11) While the radio announcer is praising the miraculous VITA-MEYERHOV, we see old Lino is too weak to get out of bed by himself. His wife tries to pull him out.

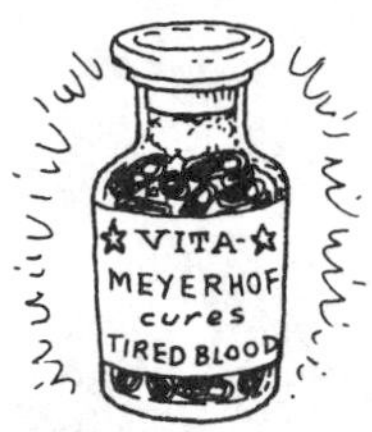

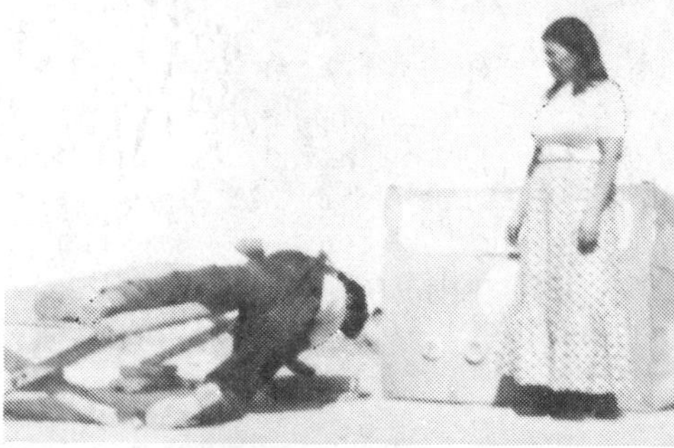

12) Lino tries to get up, but falls to the ground. Doña Luisa cannot lift him up by herself.

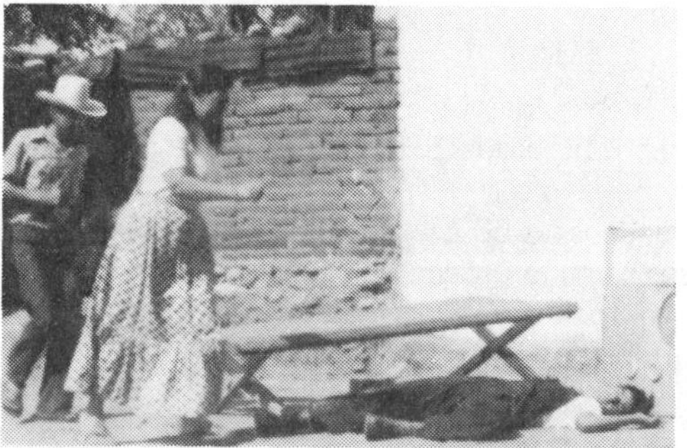

13) Frightened, she runs out to get help from the village health worker. The health worker comes running.

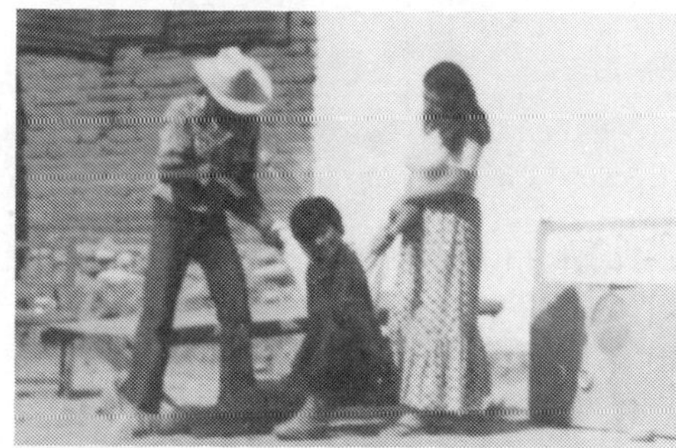

14) Between them, Doña Luisa and the health worker lift Lino back onto the bed. The health worker figures out that his weakness comes from not eating well. The family has barely enough maize to make tortillas, and none to trade for beans. They sold their last 2 chickens to buy the VITA-MEYERHOV vitamins.

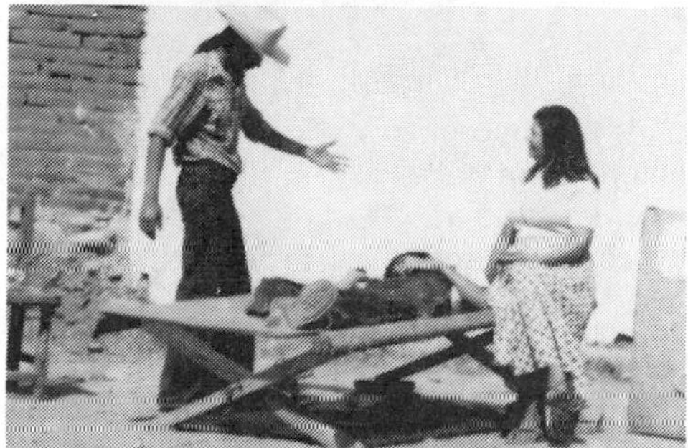

15) The health worker explains that the eggs from those chickens would have helped Lino much more than the vitamin pills. But Doña Luisa is not convinced. She thinks that her husband should be given 'artificial life' (I.V. solution). The health worker tells her that this is just sugar water; it would be safer and cheaper for Lino simply to mix sugar and water, and drink it. But what the old man really needs is more and better food. Maybe their neighbors can get together and help them out with the food problem. He will speak to them.

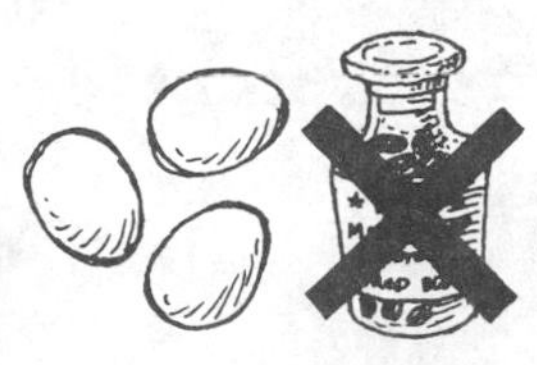

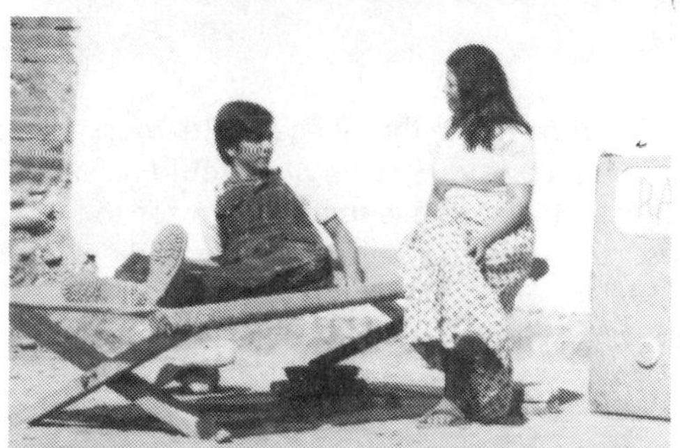

16) After the village health worker leaves, the old man and his wife talk things over. They are not sure they trust the young health worker. "What does he know? He is just a villager like us! We saw him when he was born. An ugly baby at that!" They decide to get Miss Ivy, the nurse, to give Lino an I.V.

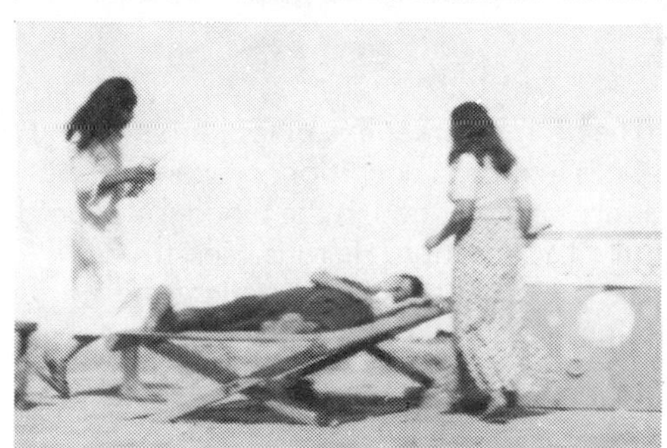

17) So that afternoon, Miss Ivy comes to the house. (To make the play more entertaining, the role of Miss Ivy is played by the same young man who plays the health worker. He has to change costumes quickly!)

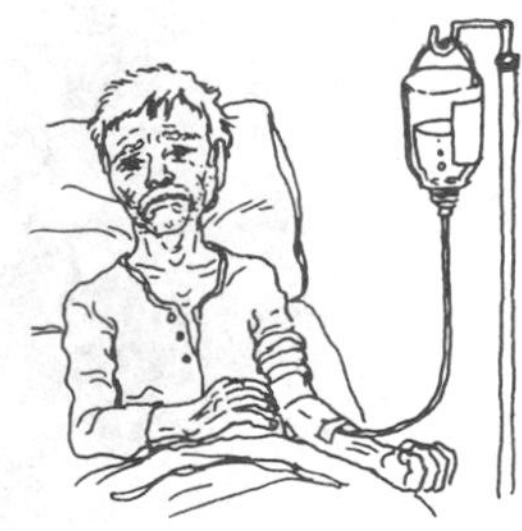

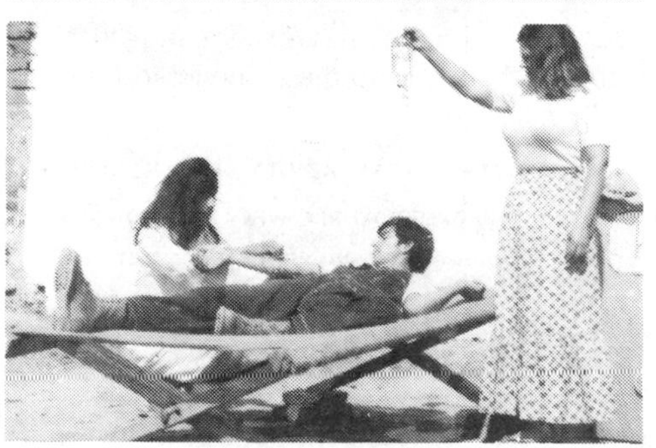

18) Nurse Ivy gives Lino an intravenous solution. He says he feels a little stronger already.

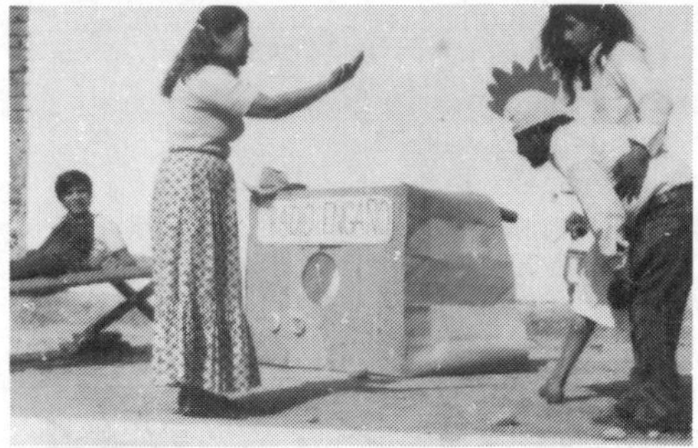

19) Because they do not have much money, the old couple gives the nurse their prize rooster as partial payment for her services. But they will still owe her money.

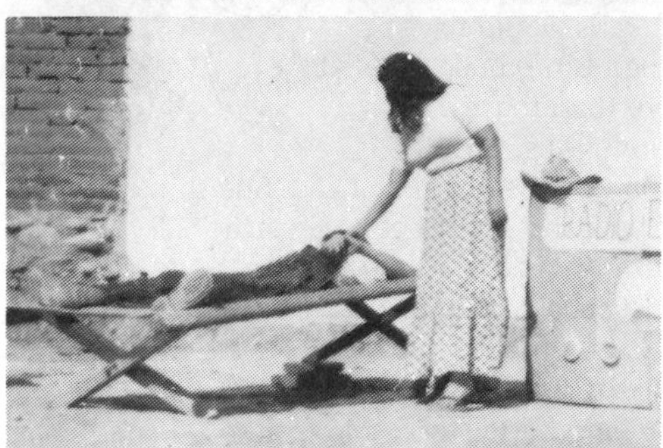

20) The next morning when old Luisa wakes up, she notices that Lino has a fever and seems very ill. She cannot waken him.

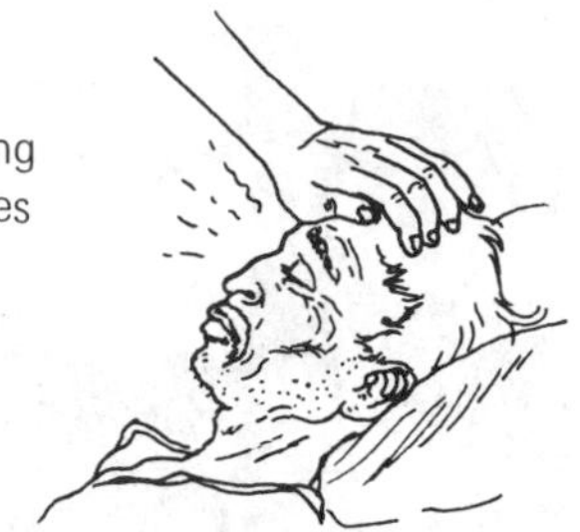

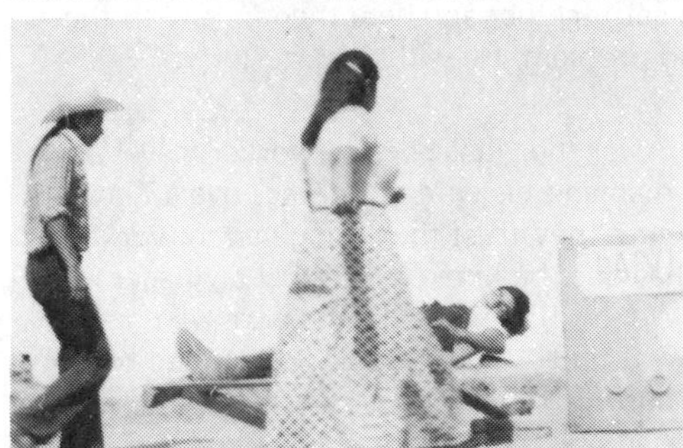

21) She runs to get the village health worker. He comes right away. He asks what could have happened to cause this sudden turn for the worse. Doña Luisa admits that they did not follow his advice and instead gave Lino I.V. solution.

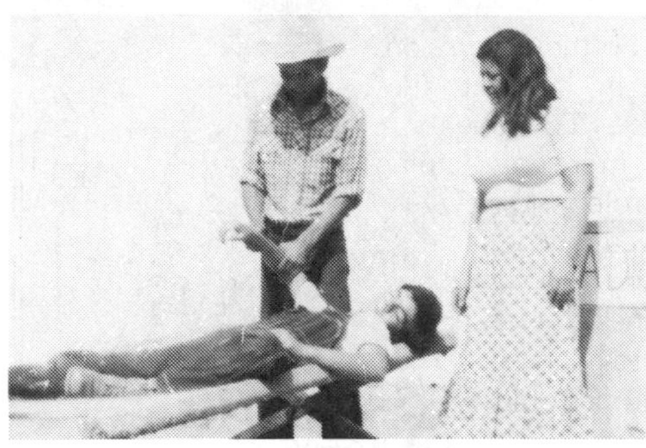

22) The health worker examines Lino and finds that he is in critical condition, probably because of an infection in the blood introduced with the I.V. solution. He runs back to the health post to get antibiotics to fight the infection.

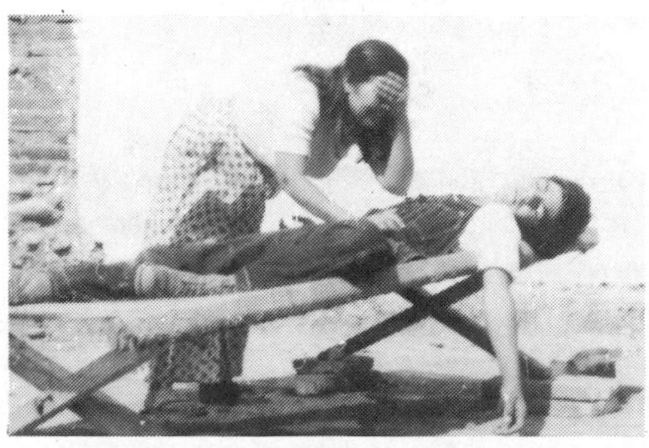

23) But before the health worker can return with the medicine, Lino dies. The lesson is painfully clear:

FOOD, NOT MEDICINE, IS THE KEY TO GOOD HEALTH--
ESPECIALLY FOR PEOPLE WHO ARE WEAK AND HUNGRY.
DO NOT WASTE YOUR MONEY ON VITAMINS OR OTHER
MEDICINES ADVERTISED ON THE RADIO.

BUY FOOD--NOT VITAMINS!

AND DO NOT USE I.V. SOLUTIONS TO GAIN STRENGTH.

VILLAGE THEATER

EXAMPLE 2: THE WOMEN JOIN TOGETHER TO OVERCOME DRUNKENNESS

In many parts of the world, the drinking of alcohol is one of the biggest problems affecting family health. It is also one of the most difficult problems for health workers, mothers, or other concerned persons to do anything about.

The idea for this play came from a collectively run squatter community on the outskirts of Monterrey, Mexico. Alarmed by the abuses of drunken men, the women of the community joined together to put a stop to drinking. They convinced the community leaders to make a special jail, so that men who became abusive when drunk could be locked up until they became sober. They also went with the leaders to all the local bars and whorehouses, taking away their beer, wine, and liquor. The women thought of handing it over to the health authorities, but feared it would be sold back to illegal bars. So they held a public 'bottle-smashing festival', in which they destroyed all the confiscated alcohol.

In Ajoya (200 miles away), the village women learned about the action taken by the courageous women in Monterrey. They decided to put on a play, to show everyone what a group of women could do. Many women, including some grandmothers who would normally refuse to be seen on stage, eagerly took part when they found the play was about the problem of drinking.

The men in the play were given funny names related to drinking. Also, there were many jokes and puns in Spanish. Many of them have been lost in this translation. But if you decide to try a similar play, be sure to make it entertaining by including plenty of jokes and funny names. These provide 'comic relief' (see p. **27**-11).

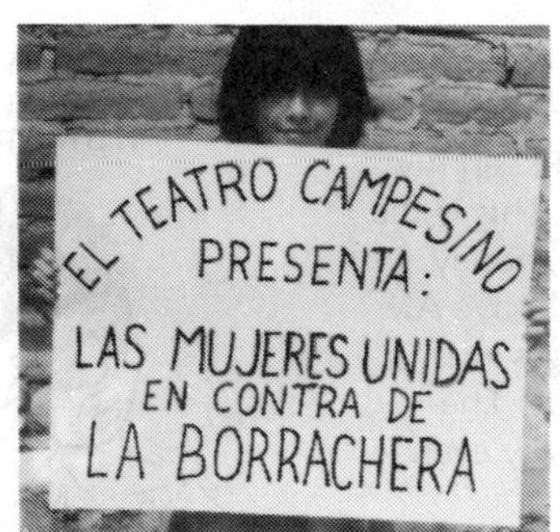
EL TEATRO CAMPESINO
PRESENTA:
LAS MUJERES UNIDAS
EN CONTRA DE
LA BORRACHERA

1)

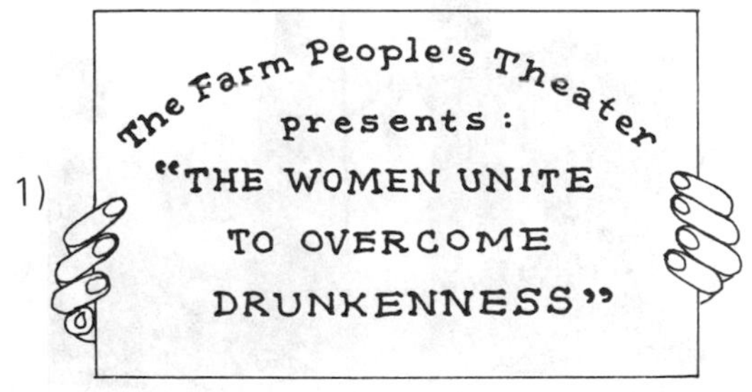

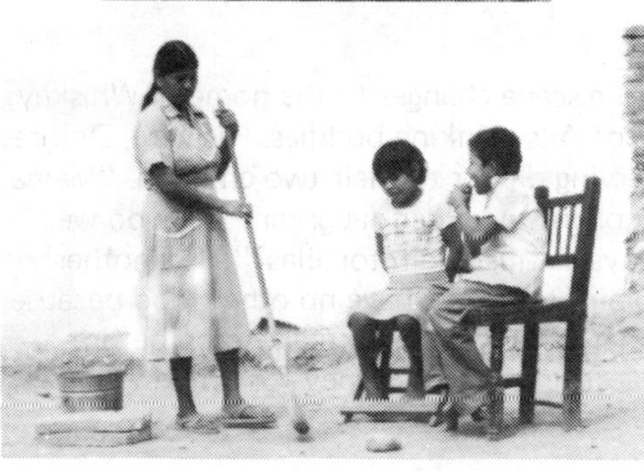

2) "Mama, I'm hungry!" With these words, the play begins. The scene is the home of Al Cole and his wife, Tristina. (*Triste* means 'sad' in Spanish.) Tristina is sweeping while her children cry with hunger. She explains that their father left an hour ago with the family's last money, to buy food at the village store. He should be back any minute. In fact, he is late. Tristina does not know what could be taking him so long. The children are hungry, and continue to cry and complain.

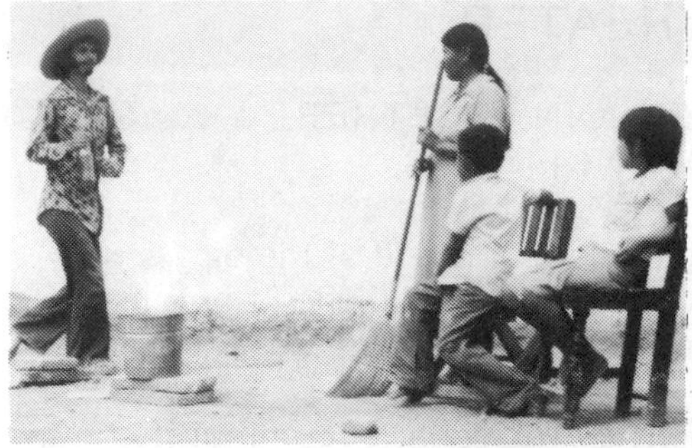

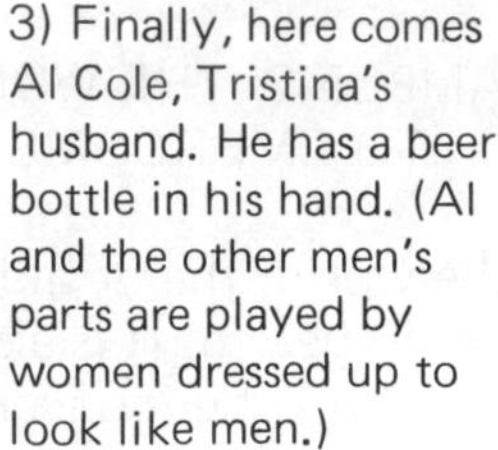

3) Finally, here comes Al Cole, Tristina's husband. He has a beer bottle in his hand. (Al and the other men's parts are played by women dressed up to look like men.)

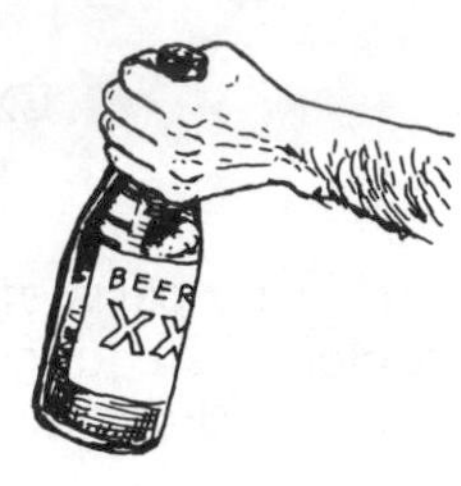

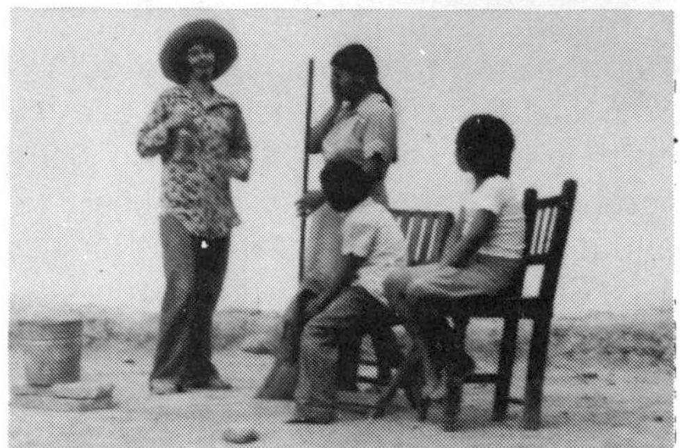

4) Tristina asks, "Where is the food you went to buy for dinner?" Al admits that he forgot. He tries to explain that he met some friends at the store. They gave him one drink, and then another and another. "And little by little, my judgement left me!" he says. "I felt I had to buy them drinks in return. So the money is gone. I'm sorry, Tristina. Really sorry!" The children begin to cry again from hunger, louder than before. Al feels ashamed and promises never to drink again.

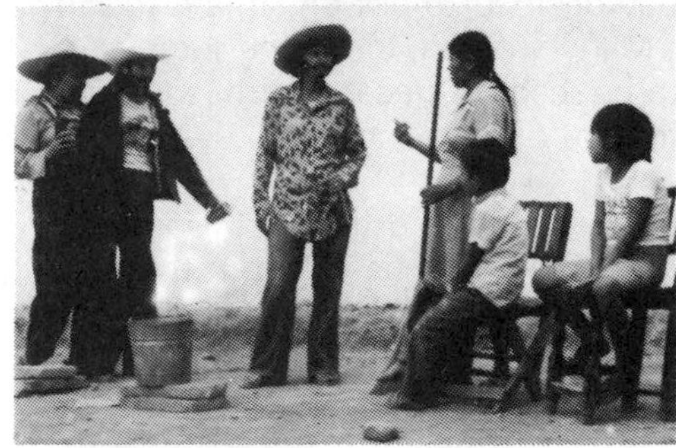

5) At that moment, Al's drinking buddies come along, singing loudly. (One could be named Mr. Whisk, and his friends could call him Whiskey. The other could be called Lee Core.) They shout for Al to join them. "The night is young. We just bought more beer."

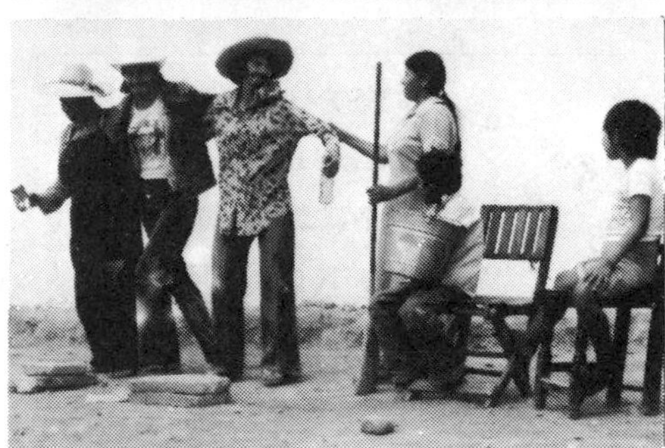

6) Tristina begs Al not to go. "You promised!" she cries. "And I'll keep my promise. This is the last time, honey. I swear it!" says Al, as he leaves with his friends. The children cry even harder.

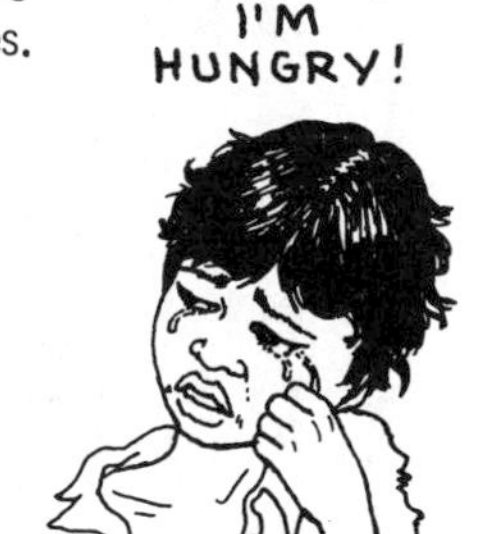

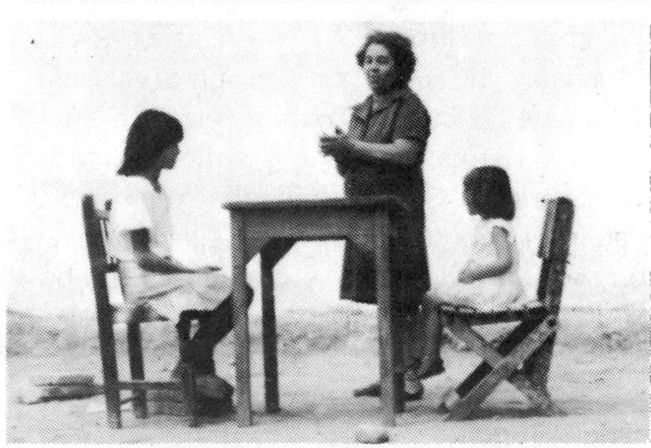

7) The scene changes to the home of Whiskey, one of Al's drinking buddies. His wife, Dolores, is serving dinner to their two children. "Mama," complains the older daughter, "Why do we always eat just plain tortillas?" Her mother explains that they have no other food because Father already sold the maize crop before harvest time to get money for drinking.

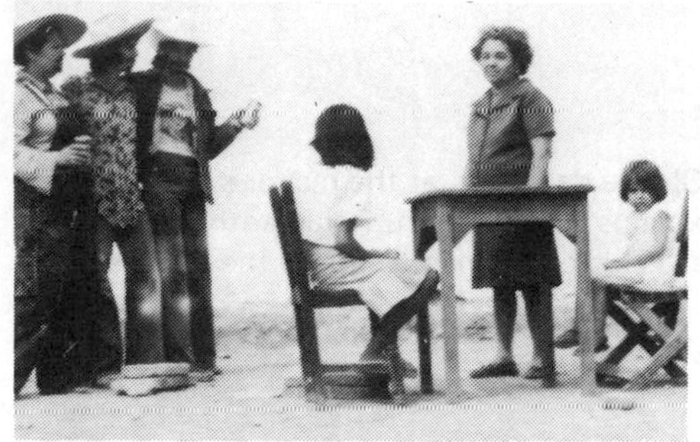

8) Here comes Whiskey now, with Al Cole and Lee Core. All 3 are drunk. Whiskey demands that Dolores feed them dinner. She answers that there is nothing but plain tortillas. He gets angry. He shouts that she is a useless wife because she cannot prepare a decent dinner.

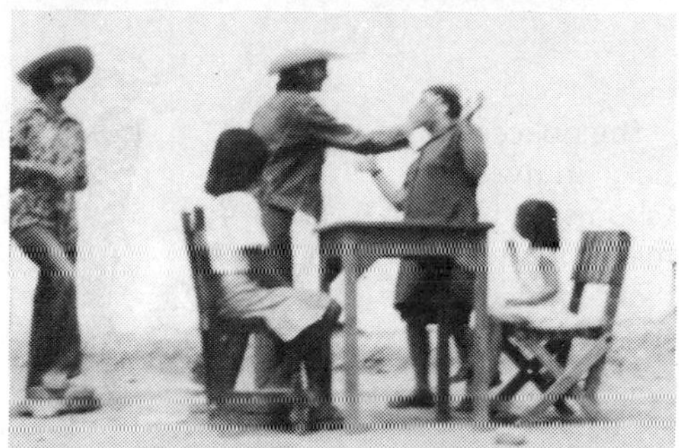

9) Dolores shouts back, "That's because you already sold the maize crop and wasted all the money on drink! How can I feed you if you don't provide the food?" Whiskey hits her. She screams and the children begin to cry.

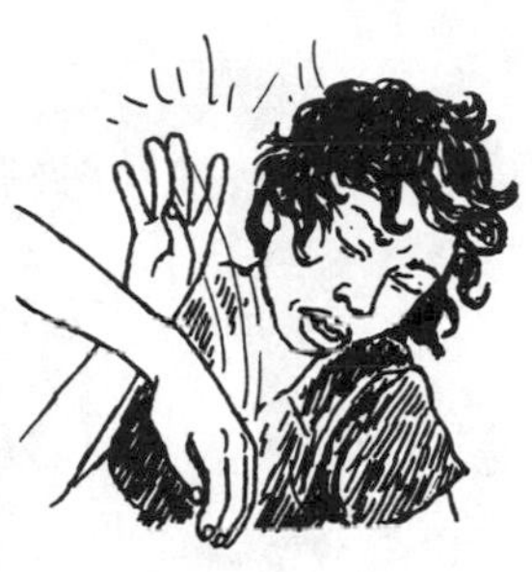

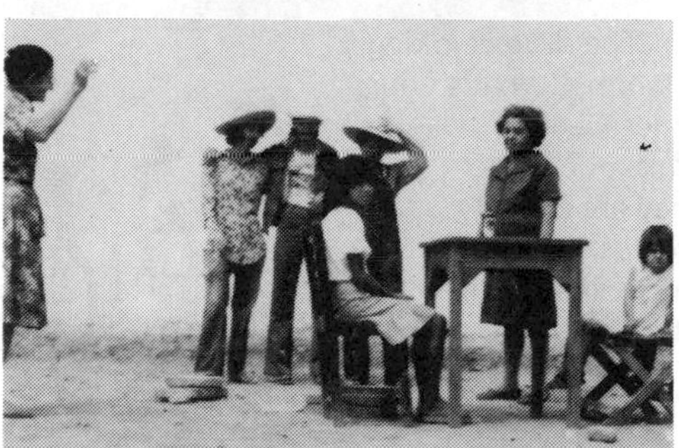

10) At this moment, there is a knock on the door. It is Whiskey's mother. She has heard the crying and come to see what it is all about.

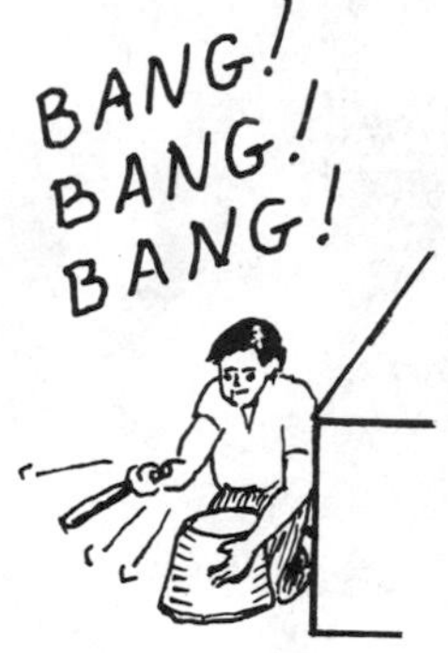

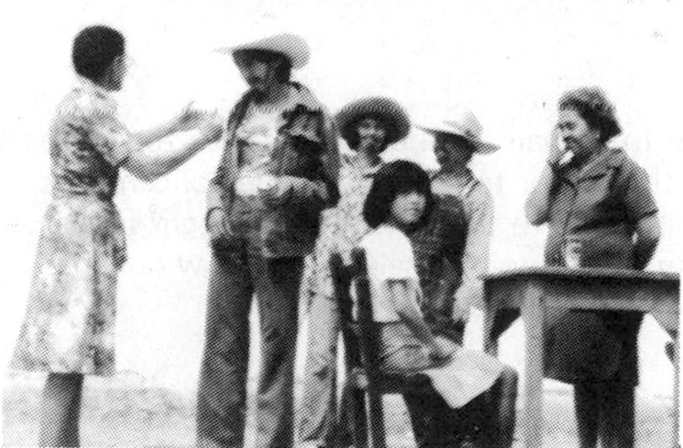

11) While Dolores and the children keep sobbing, the grandmother pleads with her son to stop drinking. "Can't you see the suffering you cause your wife and children?" Whiskey turns his back on her. He and his buddies begin to sing a drunken song.

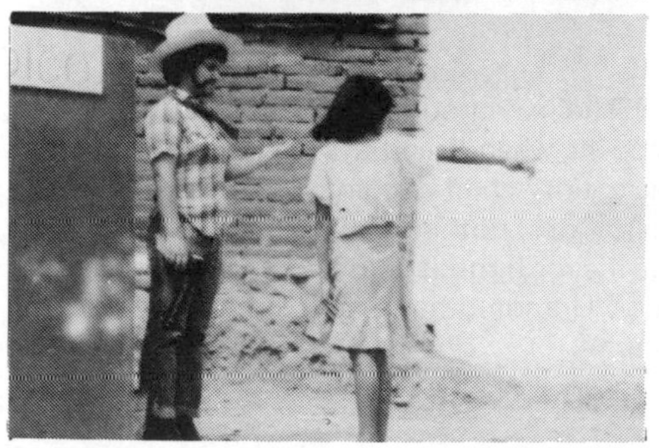

12) The grandmother sends the older daughter to tell the mayor that Whiskey has beaten his wife and that the police should come to put the drunkards out of the house.

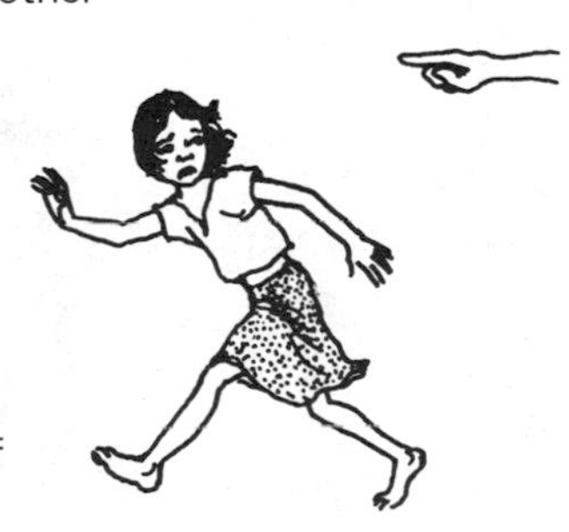

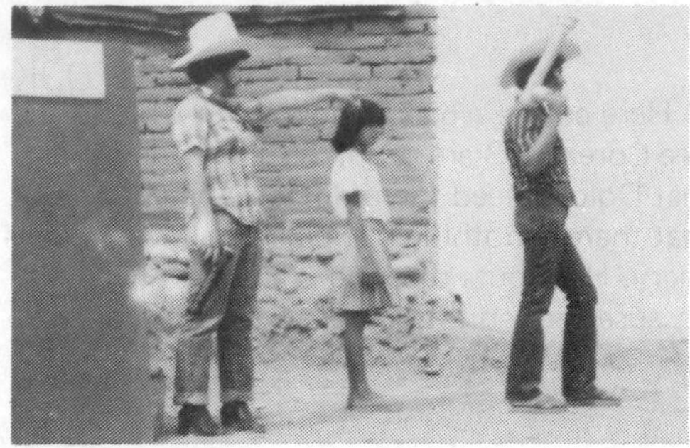

13) The daughter, at the mayor's house, explains the situation. Reluctantly, the mayor sends his policeman to throw the drunks out.

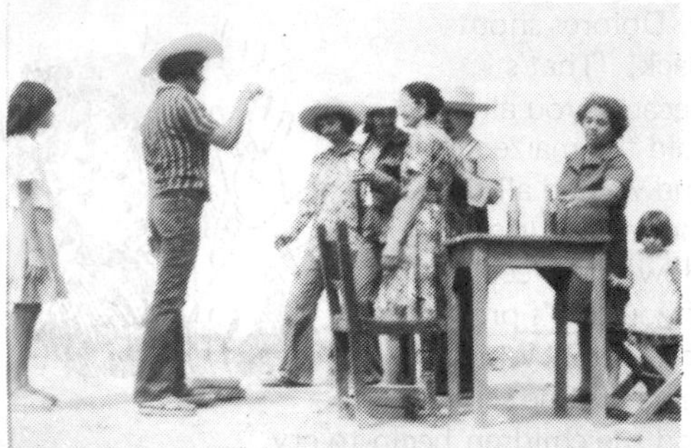

14) The policeman knocks on the door. He shouts, "I have come to bring law and order into this house."

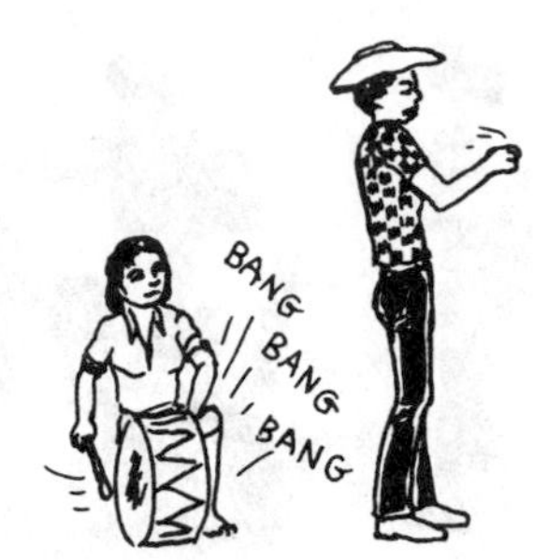

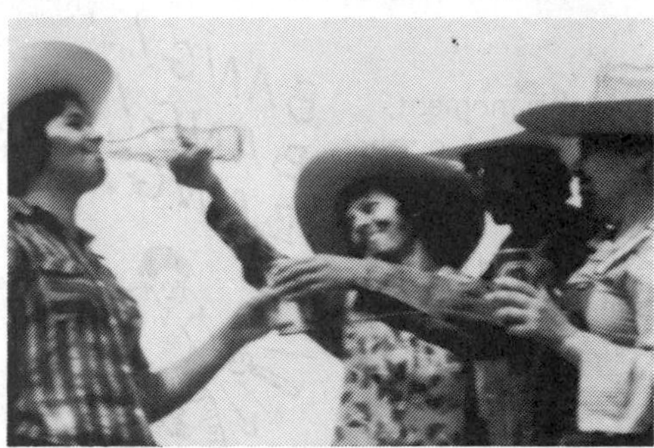

15) The drunks jokingly ask him, "What's your order, beer or whiskey?" Since they are all old friends, the policeman joins in the drinking.

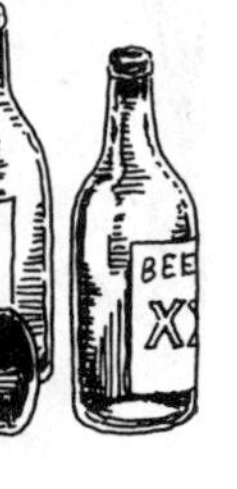

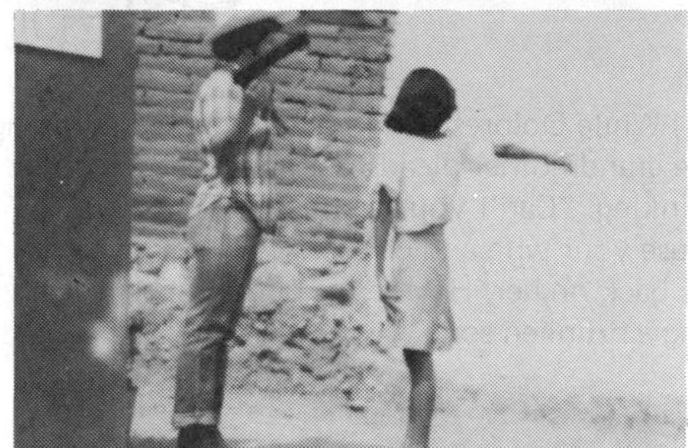

16) In despair, Grandmother sends the girl back to the mayor to report that the policeman is drinking with the other men. The girl insists that the mayor himself go to throw out the drunks.

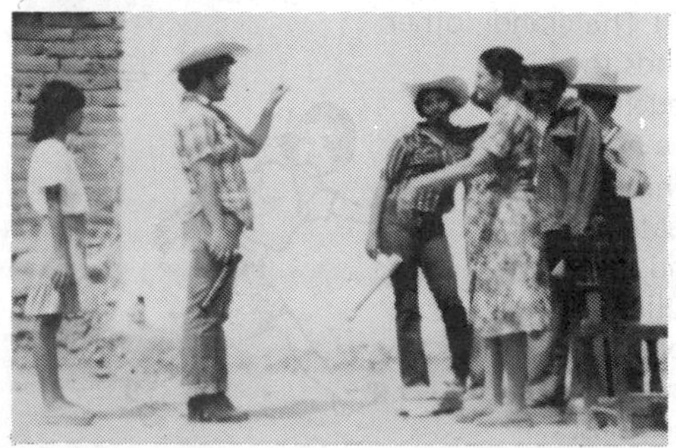

17) The mayor admits, "The same thing always happens when I send the policeman. But since the county chief appoints only his relatives to police jobs, nothing can be done about it." So the mayor himself goes and knocks on the door. Grandmother explains the situation to him.

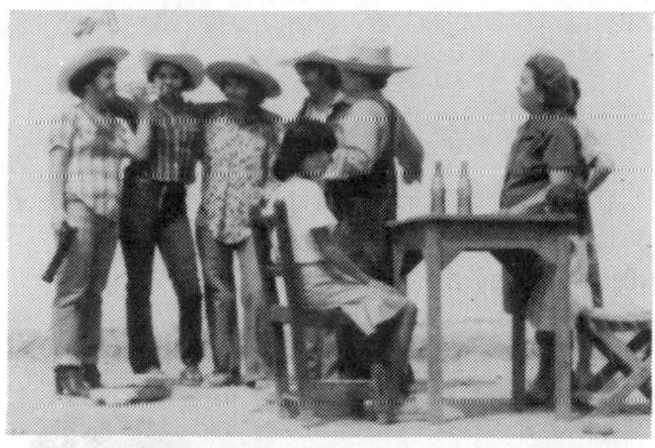

18) But in no time the men convince the mayor, too, to join them in a drink.

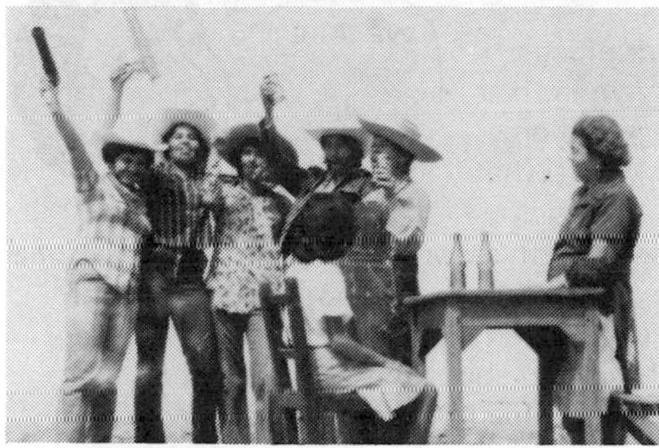

19) Soon all the men, including the mayor, are shouting and shooting 'joy shots' into the air with their guns. (In the play, firecrackers were exploded inside the pretend guns.)

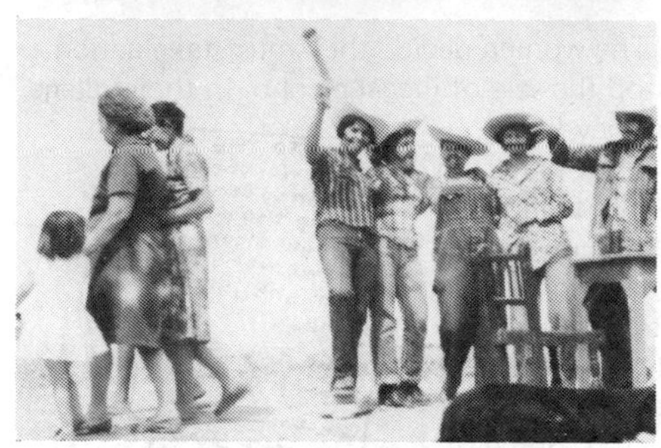

20) The women decide it is too dangerous to stay at home, and they leave with the children. The drunks laugh and say they are glad to get rid of them. "We can have a better time by ourselves!" they roar.

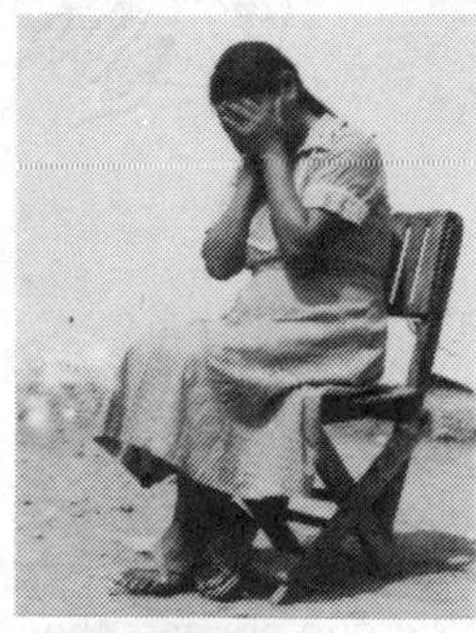

21) The scene changes back to Al Cole's house. By now, the children have cried themselves to sleep. Tristina sits alone, weeping. "How hard life is for a woman whose man drinks. What can a woman alone do when the men have all the power?" Just then, the women and children who were driven out of Whiskey's home knock on the door. They ask if they can stay with Tristina.

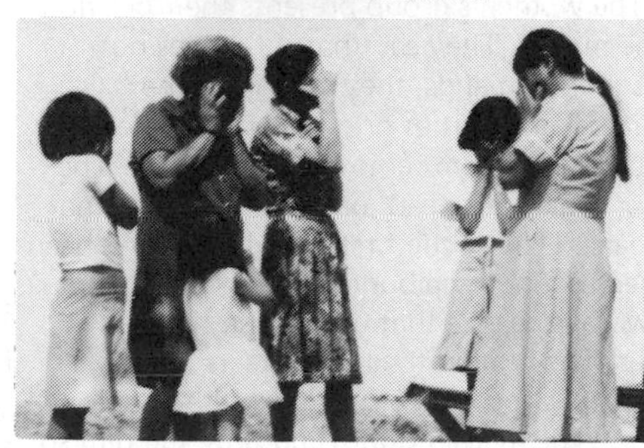

22) Tristina, still weeping, explains her sad story, and the others realize that it is their sad story, too. They all cry together.

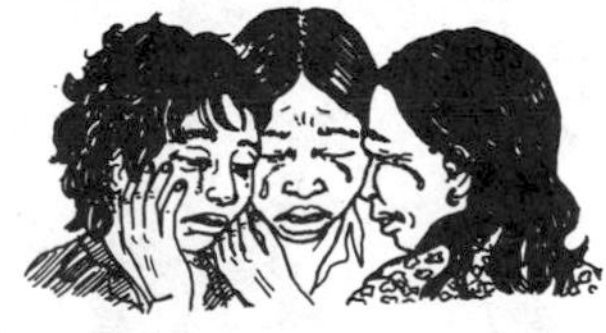

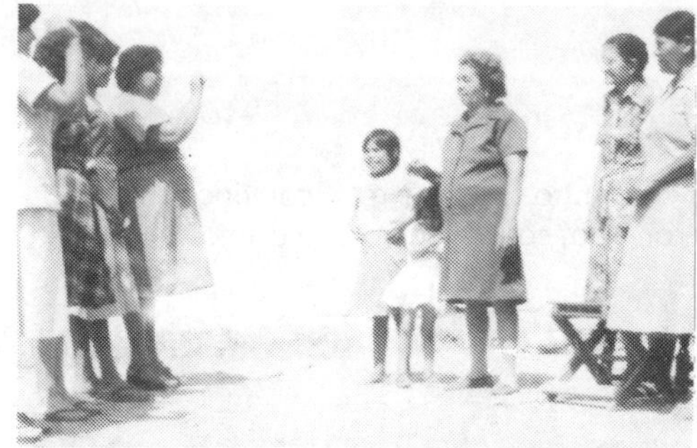

23) Other women in the neighborhood hear the loud crying and come over to see what the trouble is. They ask if they can help.

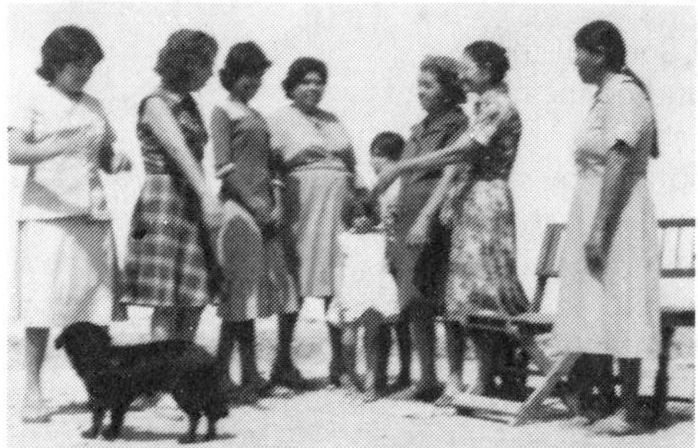

24) Together, the women discuss the drinking problem in their village. Dolores cries, "But what can a woman alone do in this world of men?" Another woman says, "Right now, we're not alone! There are lots of us here together!" She tells the others she has heard about the way women in Monterrey organized to fight drunkenness.

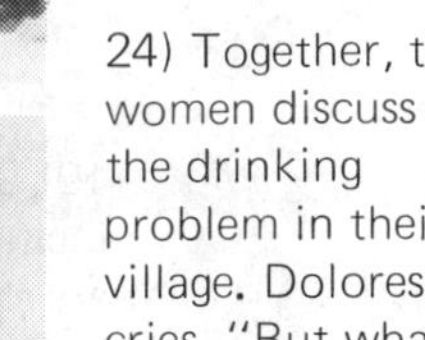

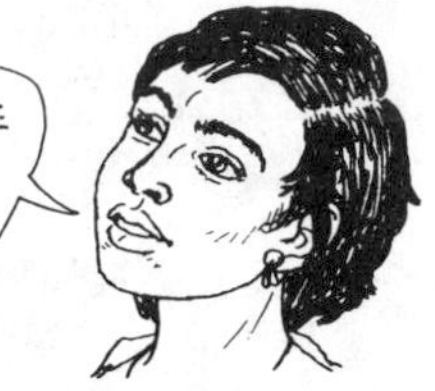

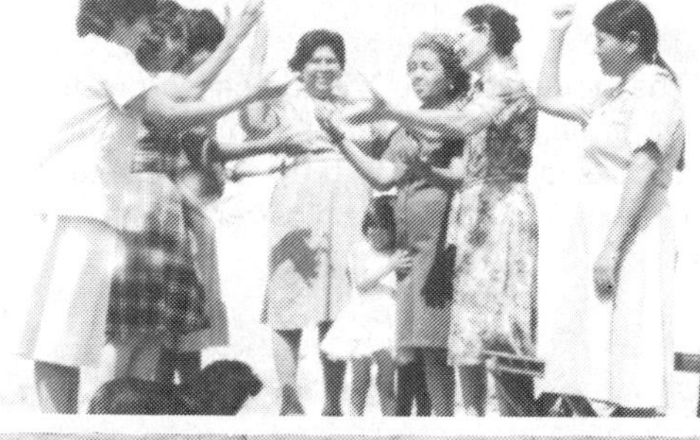

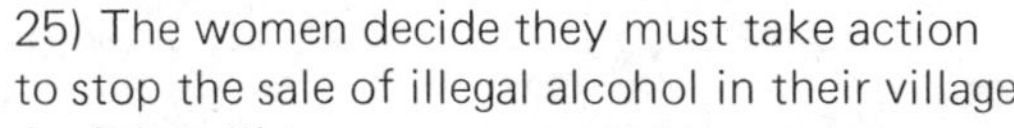

25) The women decide they must take action to stop the sale of illegal alcohol in their village. And they like the idea of an overnight jail for sobering up the drunks! So they write a petition and get all the women in town to sign it. Some of the men sign it, too.

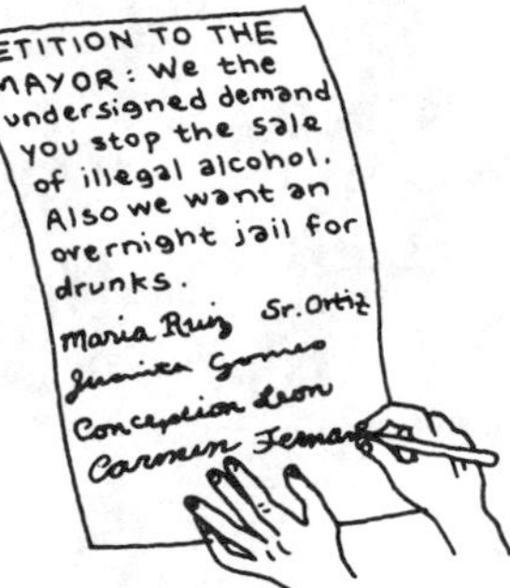
PETITION TO THE MAYOR: We the undersigned demand you stop the sale of illegal alcohol. Also we want an overnight jail for drunks.
Maria Ruiz
Sr. Ortiz
Juanita Gomes
Concepcion Leon
Carmen

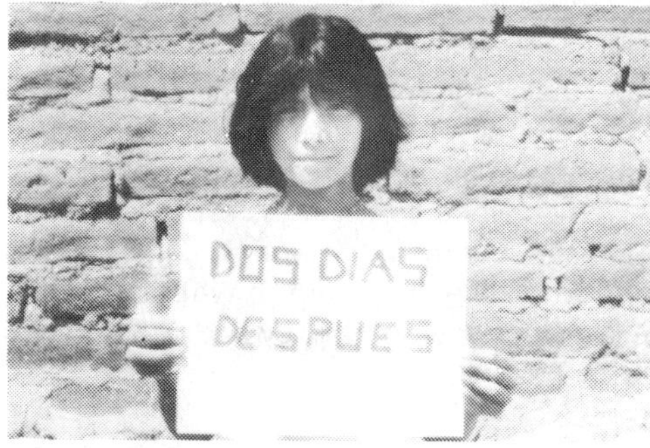
DOS DIAS
DESPUES

26) Two days later.

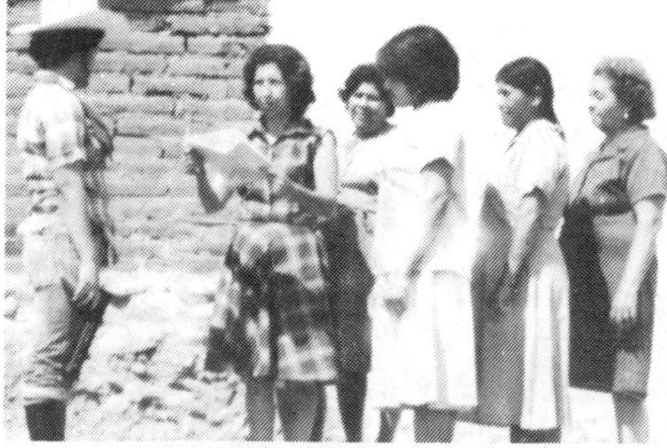

27) The women's group presents their petition to the mayor. They say that if he does not meet their demands, they will go to the municipal authorities or even to the state capital to have him removed from office. The mayor shakes his head, unable to believe what he hears. "This is the first time I have ever been pushed around by a bunch of old hens!" But the women realize that united they have power. They know the mayor fears being caught for accepting bribes from the people who sell the illegal liquor—and they tell him so.

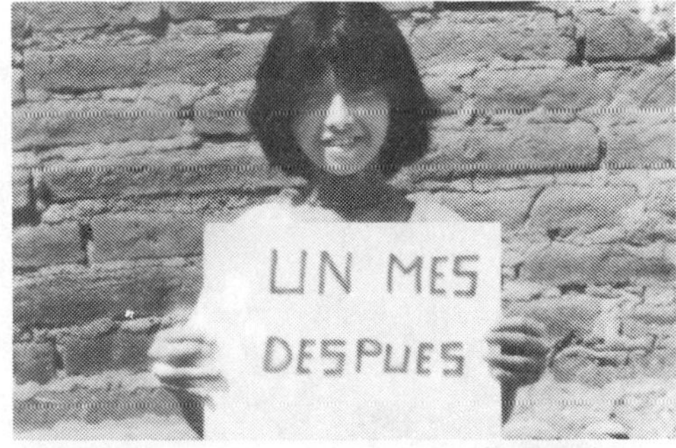

28) One month later.

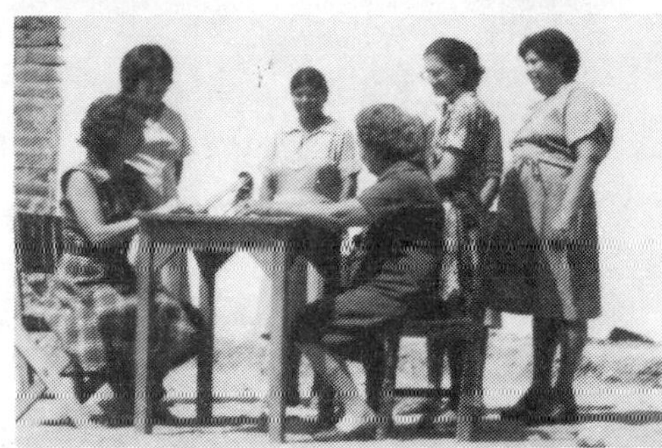

29) Here, the women's group meets in the home of Dolores. They discuss how life in the village has improved now that there is an overnight jail for drunks and less selling of illegal liquor. With their new-found strength and unity, the women are discussing other local problems and what they can do about them.

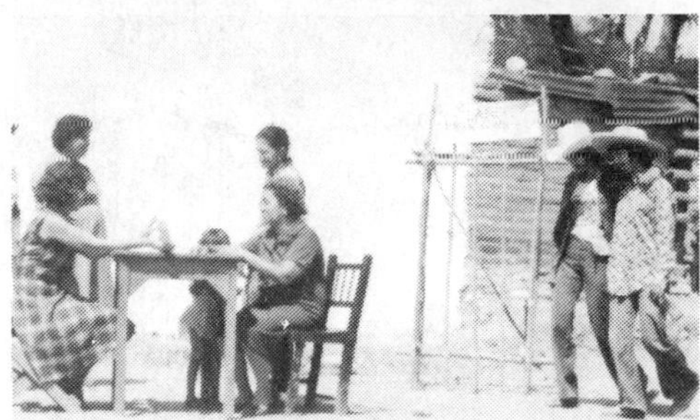

30) Just as they are commenting on how few drunks there have been lately, along come two men, singing loudly. They are Al Cole and Whiskey, drunk again.

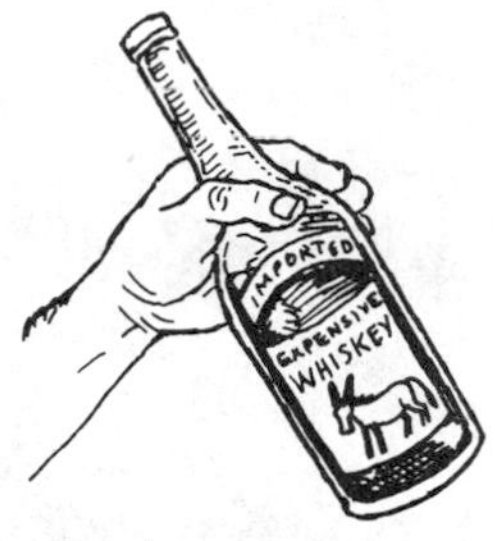

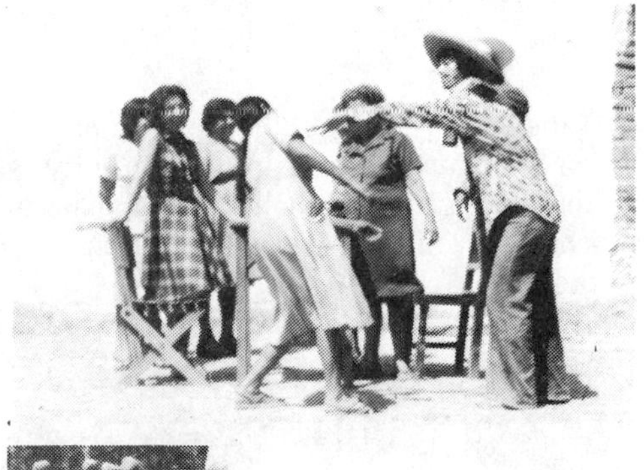

31) They stagger into the women's meeting, interrupting with loud, rude insults. They knock Tristina down because they are angry about how hard it is to buy alcohol now.

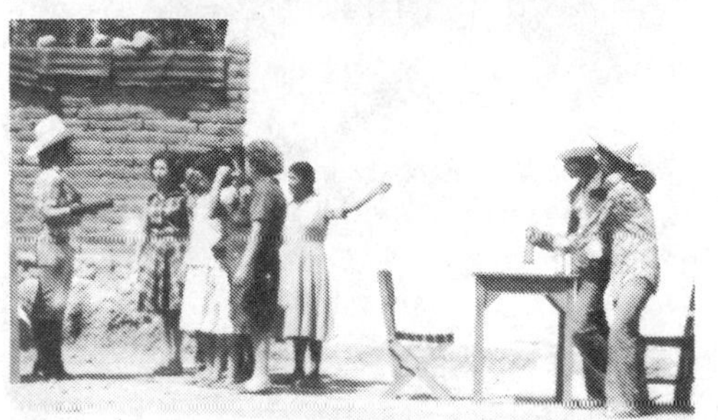

32) The women's group goes at once to the mayor and demands that the two drunks be thrown into jail until they sober up. The mayor protests, saying that they are his buddies. But the women remind him of their agreement and their threat to have him removed from office.

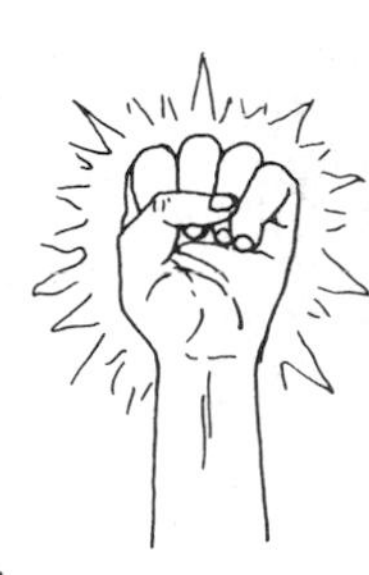

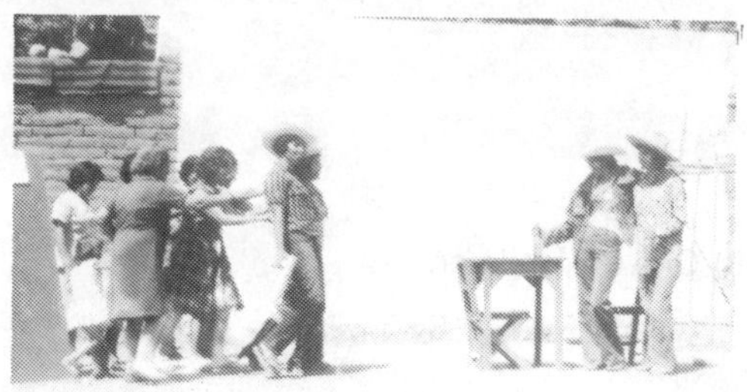

33) So, under pressure, the mayor and policeman go with the women.

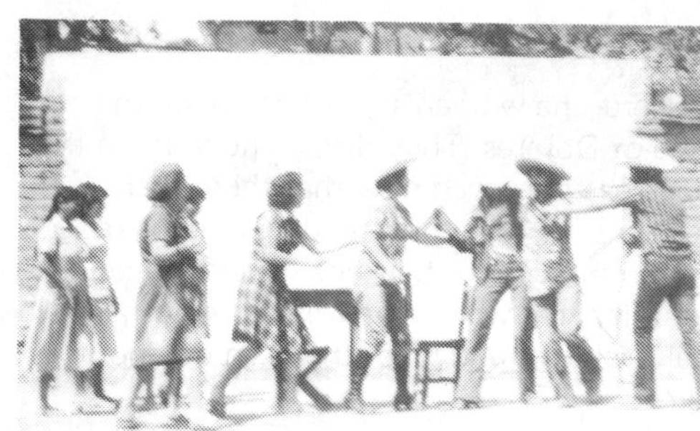

34) After a short struggle, the mayor and policeman arrest Al Cole and Whiskey.

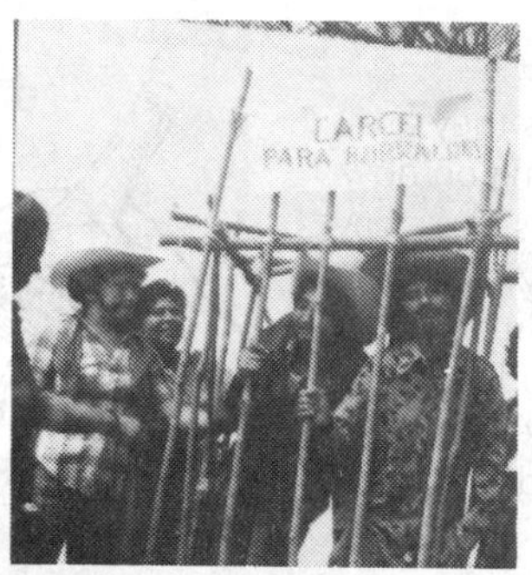

35) They throw the two drunks into jail to sober up. Here are Al and Whiskey begging to be let out. The angry women tell them they will not be released until the next morning, when they are sober.

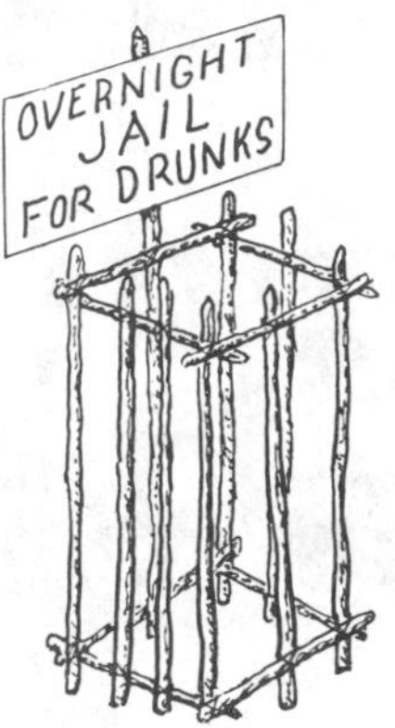

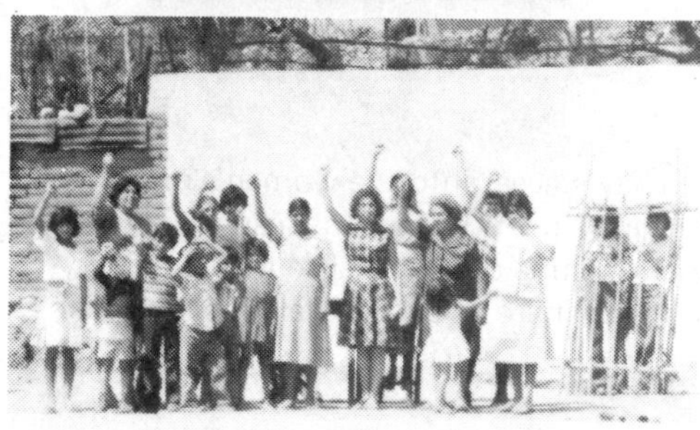

36) At the end of the play, the women and children celebrate the strength of their unity and their efforts to improve life in their village. They cheer, "Women united will never be overcome!"

THE ACTION THAT FOLLOWED THE PLAY

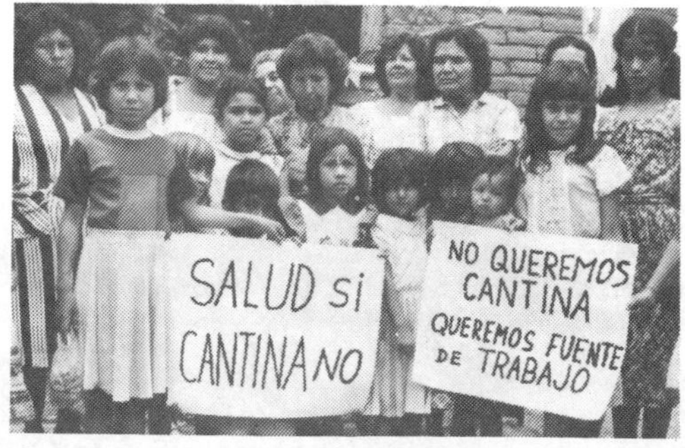

HEALTH YES, PUB NO!

Although a lively discussion followed this skit, nothing clearly came of it until 2 years later. At that time, local officials tried to open a public bar in the village for personal profit. The community protested, and officials jailed several local health workers for being 'agitators'. The village women collected signatures for a petition against the unfair jailings and the public bar. They took their protest to the state capital, where they gained the support of newspapers, which printed this photo. As a result of the villagers' action, state officials have had no choice but to prohibit the bar from opening.

VILLAGE THEATER

EXAMPLE 3: SMALL FARMERS JOIN TOGETHER TO OVERCOME EXPLOITATION

Poor nutrition is a common and serious problem in most areas, yet its causes are complicated, often rooted in social injustice.

In the Project Piaxtla Clinic in Ajoya, Mexico, health workers give advice about eating well, but often the people say, "What can we do? We don't have any land. We have already borrowed maize and gone into debt. After paying the high interest rates, we never have enough left to feed and care for our families well—no matter how hard we work!"

In this part of Mexico, poor farmers often borrow maize from the rich landholders at planting time. In return, the landholders demand 2½ to 3 times as much after the harvest. That is 150 to 200% interest in five months! This high-interest loan system is one of the main causes of malnutrition in the area. Because of this, the village health team formed a cooperative maize bank, to loan maize to poor farmers at much lower interest.

After the cooperative maize bank had been operating successfully for more than 2 years, the health workers put on this play. The play helped make everyone in the village aware of why the maize bank had been started.

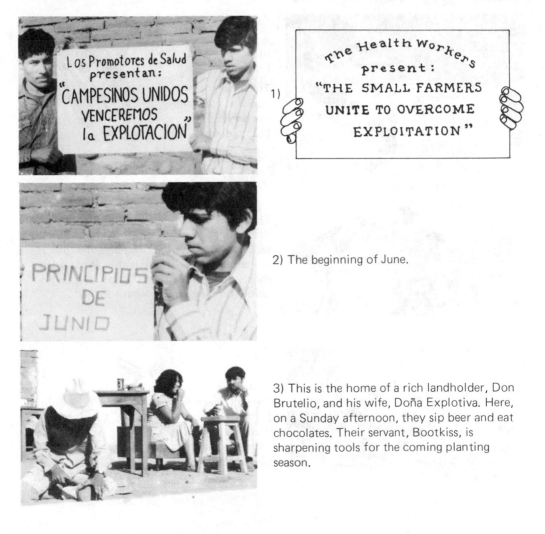

1)

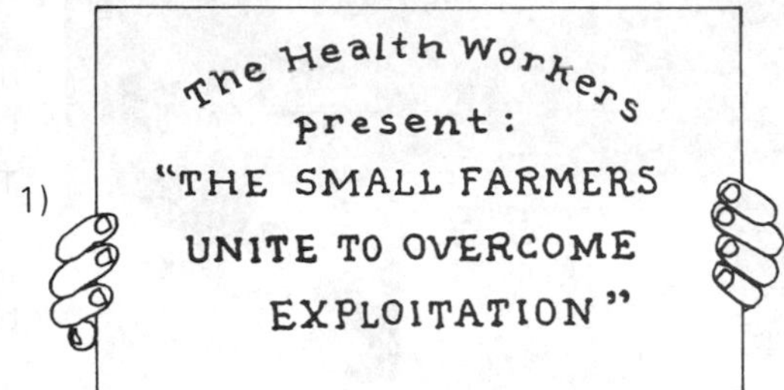

The Health Workers
present:
"THE SMALL FARMERS
UNITE TO OVERCOME
EXPLOITATION"

2) The beginning of June.

3) This is the home of a rich landholder, Don Brutelio, and his wife, Doña Explotiva. Here, on a Sunday afternoon, they sip beer and eat chocolates. Their servant, Bootkiss, is sharpening tools for the coming planting season.

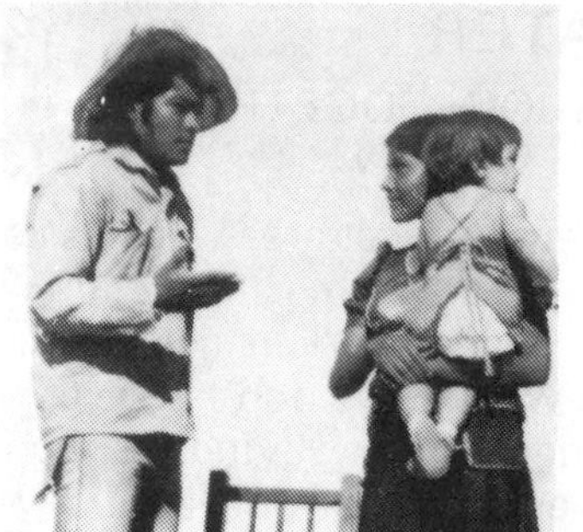

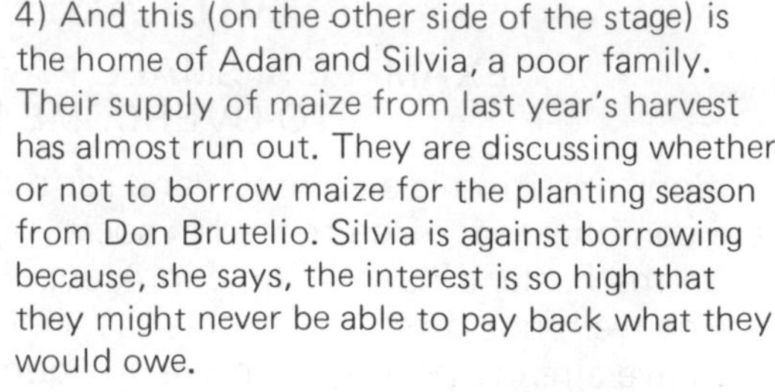

4) And this (on the other side of the stage) is the home of Adan and Silvia, a poor family. Their supply of maize from last year's harvest has almost run out. They are discussing whether or not to borrow maize for the planting season from Don Brutelio. Silvia is against borrowing because, she says, the interest is so high that they might never be able to pay back what they would owe.

But they both know they have no other choice.

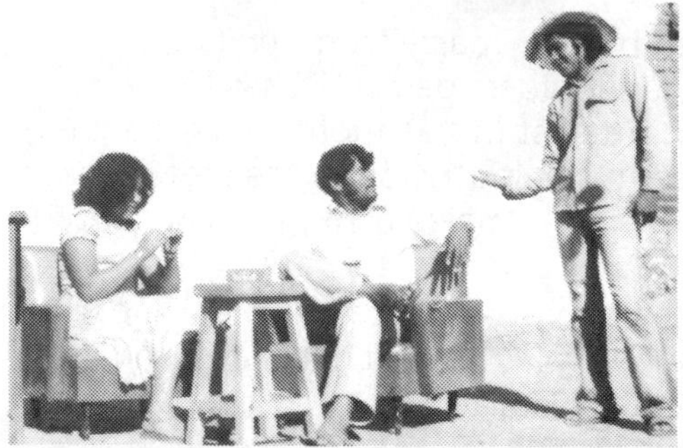

5) So Adan visits Brutelio to ask him for a loan, and Brutelio agrees to lend him 3 bags of maize. In December Adan will have to pay back 9 bags of maize for the 3 bags he borrowed.

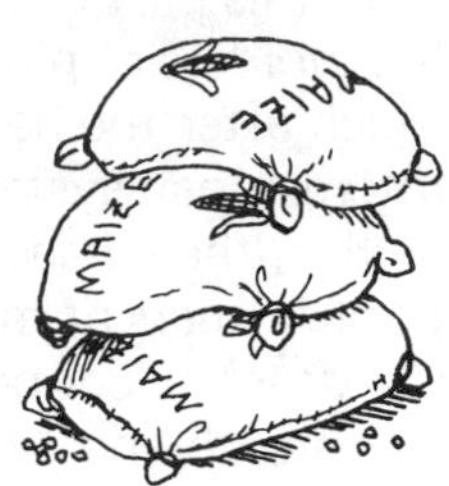

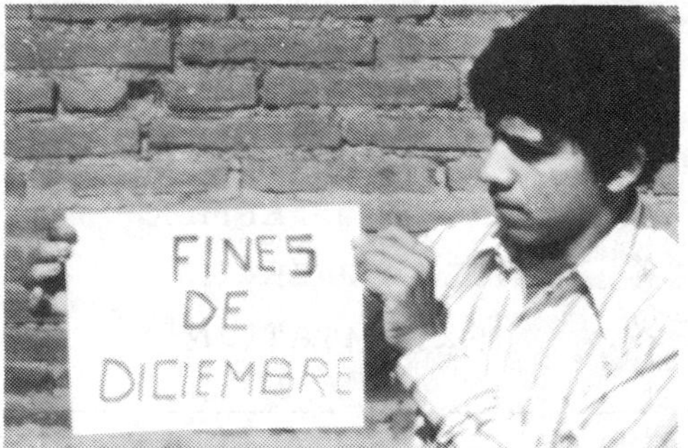

6) Near the end of December.

The growing season is over and the harvest has been picked.

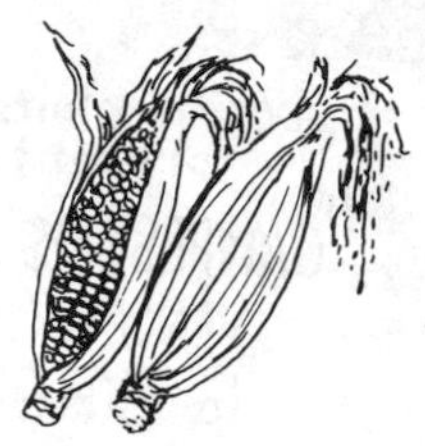

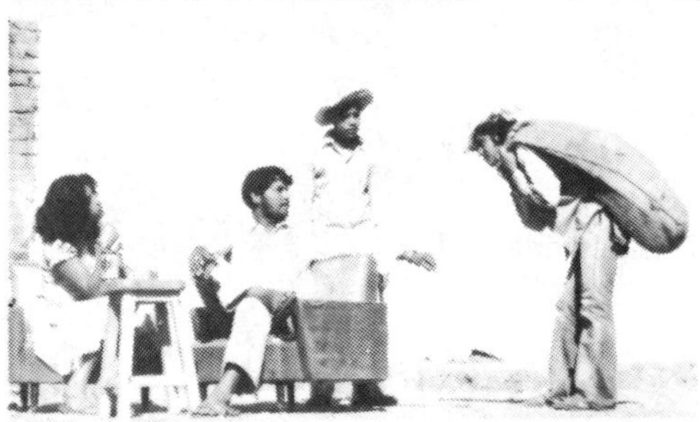

7) Adan is delivering the last of the 9 bags of maize that he owes. Don Brutelio has Bootkiss, his servant, measure it. He tells Adan that it is not enough; some maize is still owed. Adan insists that he measured it carefully at home before bringing it. But what can he do?

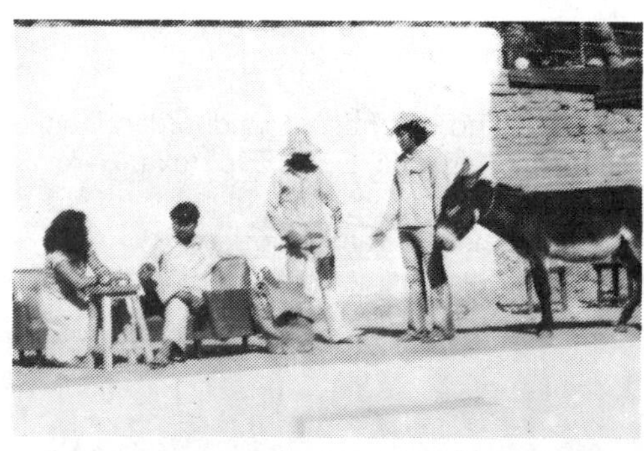

8) Adan is forced to give Brutelio his only donkey to complete the payment.

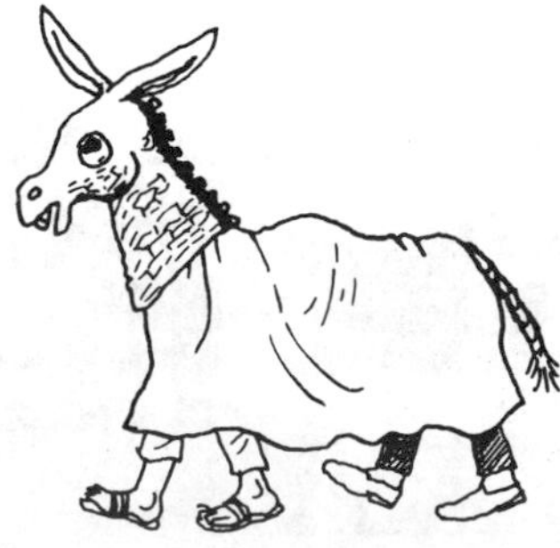

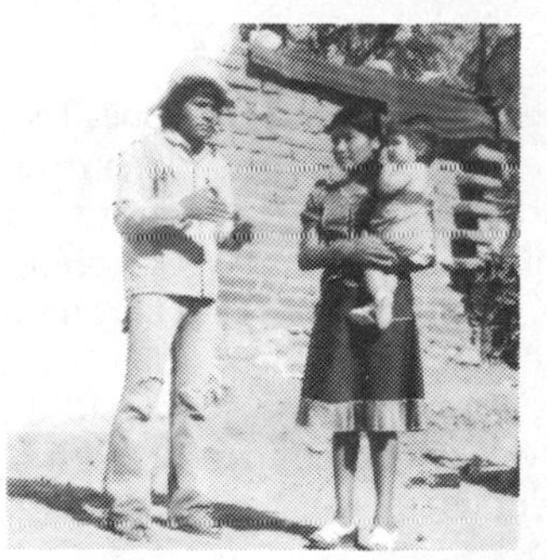

9) Adan returns home and tells Silvia the sad story. Now, without the donkey, it will be much harder to carry firewood and water to their house. They have only two bags of maize left to last them till the next harvest. Adan and Silvia suspect that Brutelio cheats them by using one scale when he lends the maize, and another when he is paid back.

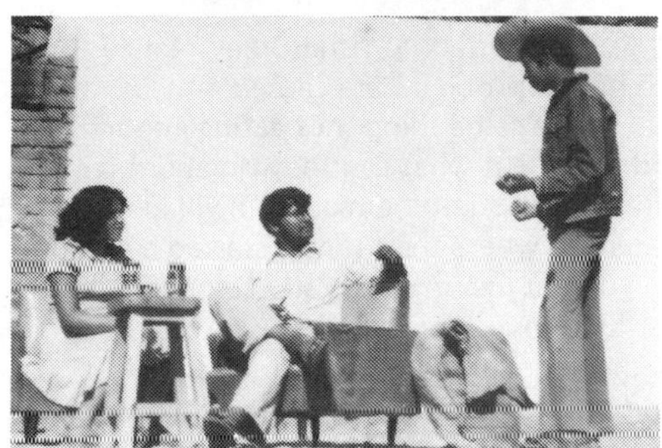

10) Because it did not rain enough during the growing season, other families are also having trouble paying their debts. This man, Carlos, explains to Brutelio that if he pays all the maize he owes him, he will have nothing left for his family. He asks for an extension of the loan.

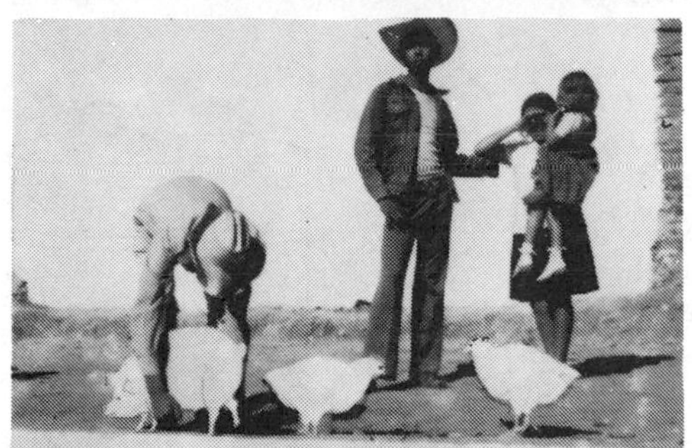

11) Brutelio refuses to extend the loan. Instead, he sends Bootkiss to take away all the family's animals. They have only one pig and two chickens. As Bootkiss takes the animals, Carlos tries to comfort his wife, who is weeping. With nothing left, they may have to move to the slums of the city.

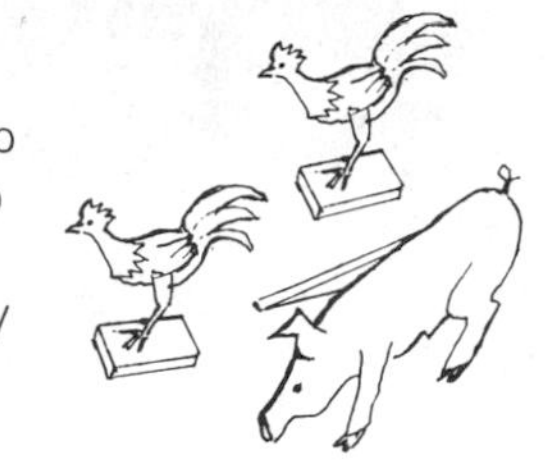

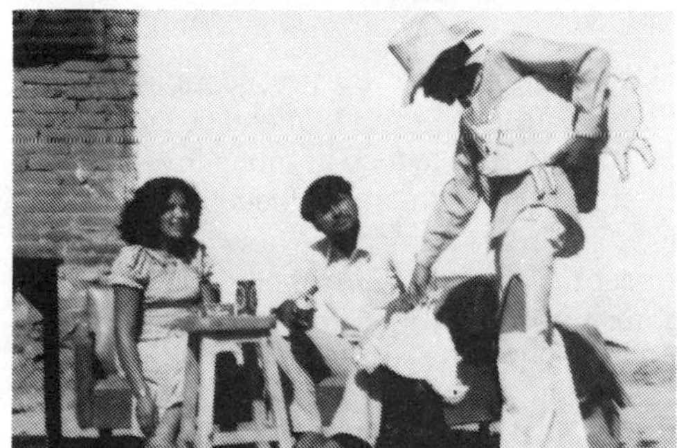

12) When Bootkiss returns with the animals, Brutelio and Explotiva sit drinking beer and eating chocolates, as usual.

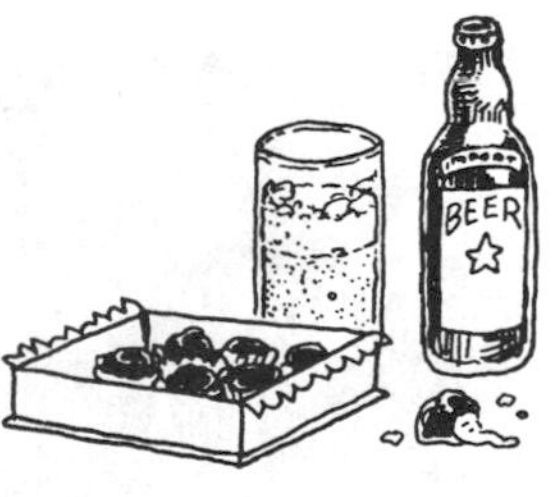

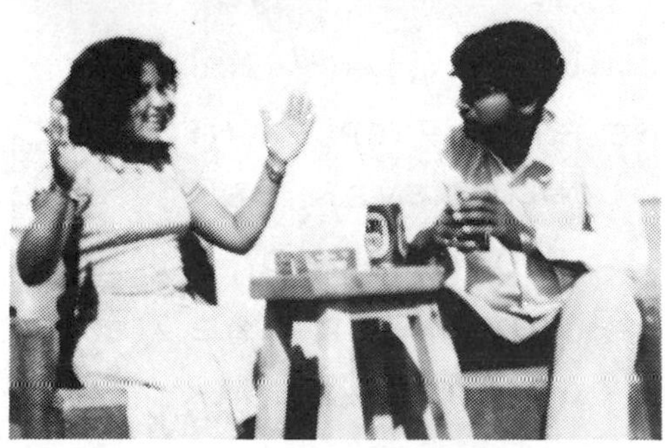

13) Doña Explotiva is overjoyed. "With what we have collected in interest this year, we can buy a color television set—this big!"

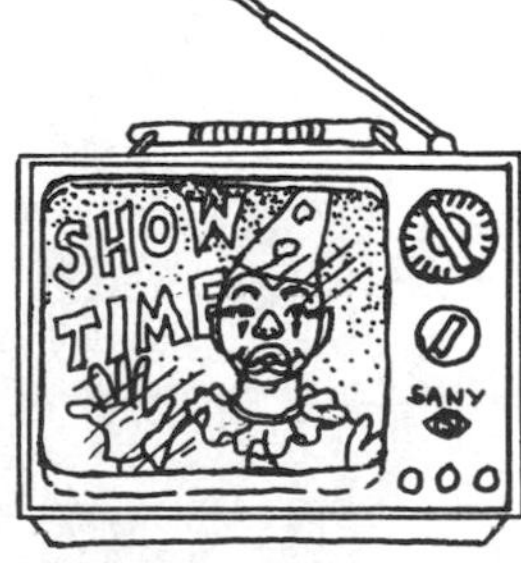

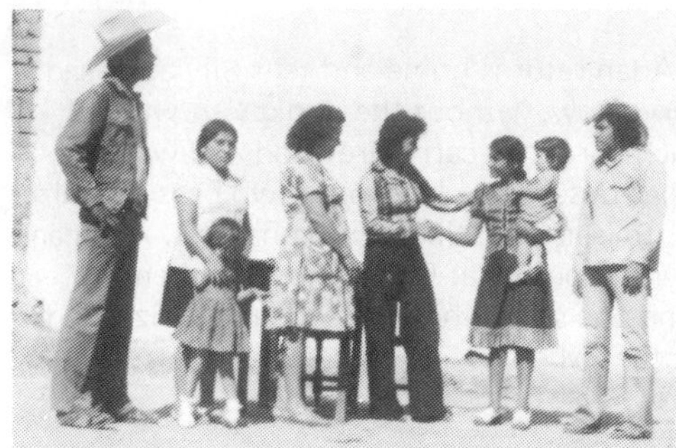

14) The next months are hard ones for the poor families in the area. Carlos and his wife, Juanita, bring their sick daughter to the two village health workers in the local clinic. The girl has chronic diarrhea and is getting very thin. While they are talking, Adan and Silvia arrive. Their daughter has a bad cold that has lasted for weeks without getting better. At night her coughing keeps everyone awake.

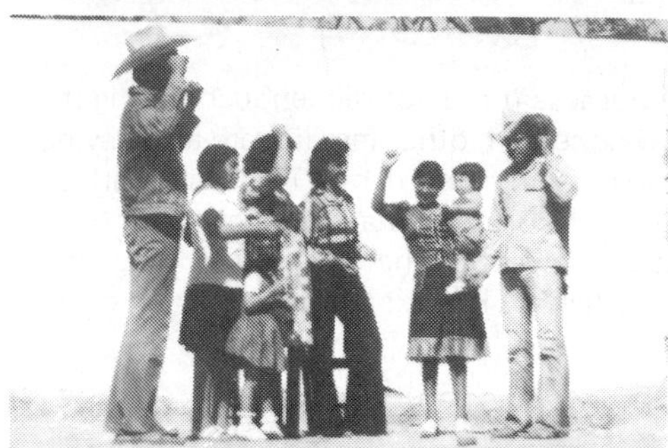

15) As they all talk together, they realize that both health problems are caused, at least in part, by the same thing: **not eating enough good food.** But what can they do about it? The health workers tell them about a village in Guatemala where the farmers started a co-op to loan grain at low interest rates to people in the area. Everyone agrees that, by working together, they may be able to solve their common problem. Eagerly they begin to make plans.

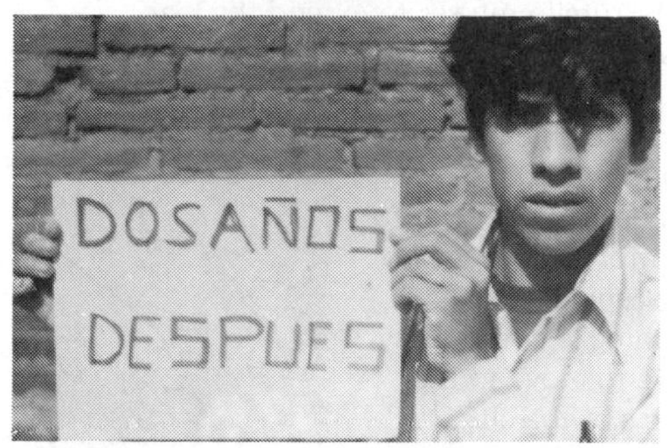

16) Two years later. What has been accomplished?

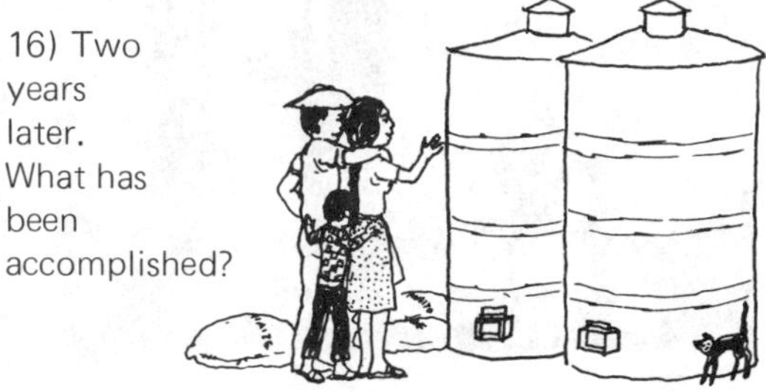

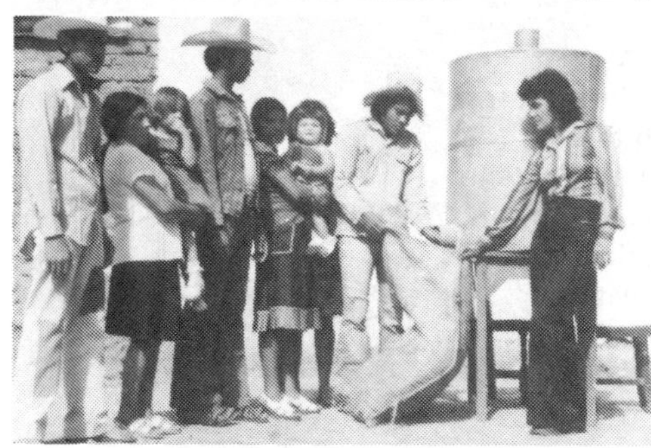

17) Here are the same villagers, scooping maize out of one of the co-op's homemade storage bins. This maize is loaned at much lower interest than the rich landholders used to charge. The poor farmers are now almost free from debt. They have built themselves a brighter future. Never again will they have to turn over their harvests to the rich while their children go hungry!

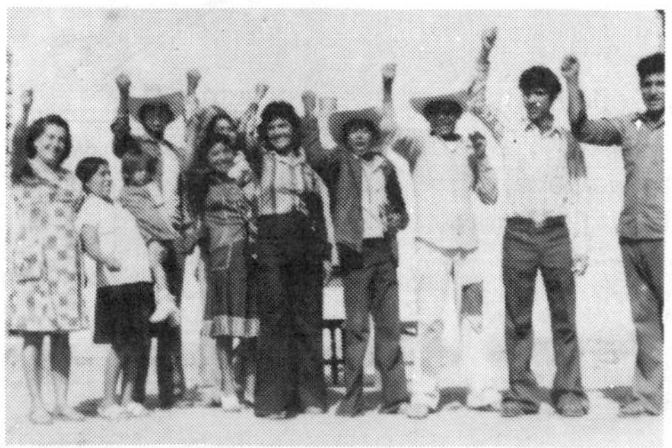

18) The play ends as everyone shouts,

WE FARM PEOPLE UNITED
WILL NEVER BE
DEFEATED!
HURRAH FOR THE
CO-OP MAIZE BANK!

VILLAGE THEATER

EXAMPLE 4: THE IMPORTANCE OF BREAST FEEDING

As part of the CHILD-to-child Program in Ajoya, Mexico, school children conducted a 'diarrhea survey' in their own homes. (This is described on page **24**-17.) From the survey the children learned that, in their village, **diarrhea is 5 times more common in bottle-fed babies than in breast-fed babies.** They also found that over 70% of the mothers were bottle feeding their babies!

Some of the women in Ajoya were very disturbed by the children's findings. A group of them decided to put on this play, to make the whole community aware of the importance of breast feeding. The health workers helped the women plan and organize the play.

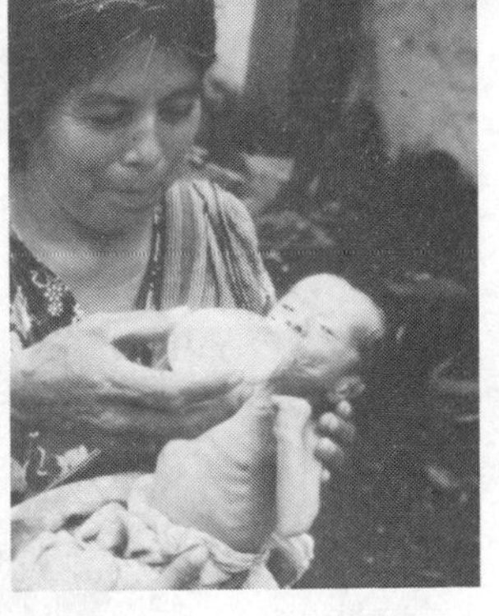

This bottle-fed baby, malnourished and with diarrhea, was brought to village health workers in Ajoya for treatment.

Note: The 'babies' used in this play were made from cardboard, carefully colored to make them look real. To show the 3 babies at different ages and states of health, 8 different cardboard figures were used.

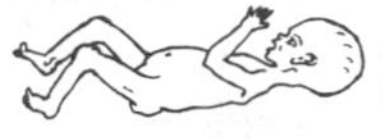

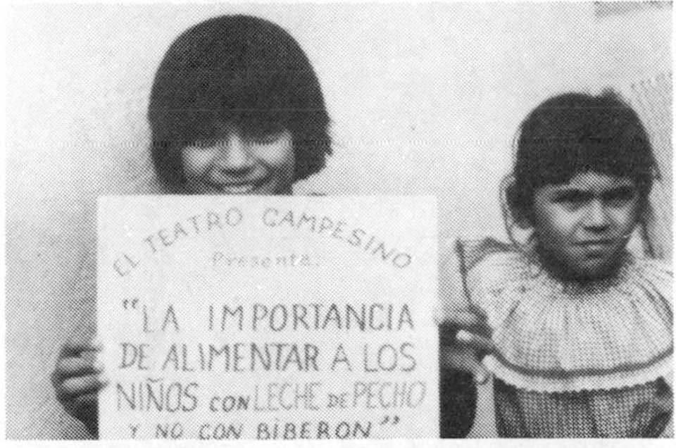

1)

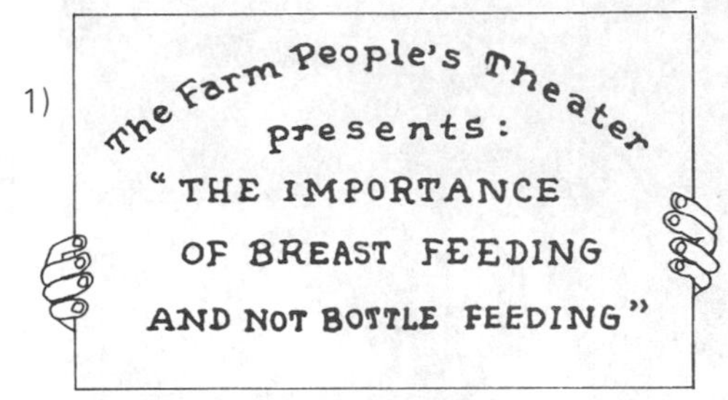

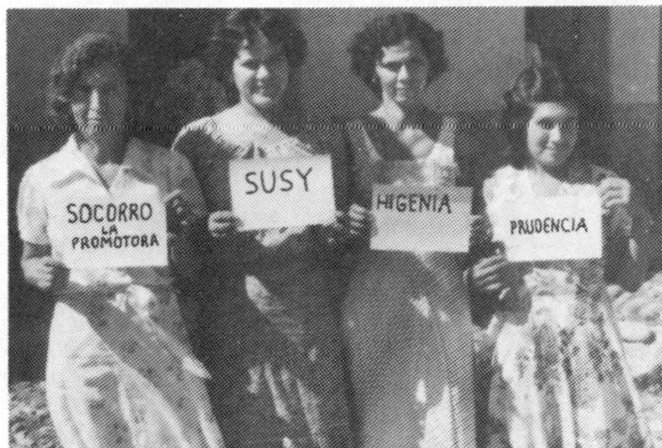

2) First, the main characters introduce themselves. Their names are symbolic. Adapted for this translation, they are:

CHARITY:	the village health worker
VANITY:	a rich woman, but vain (overly proud)
MODESTY:	a poor woman, but modest
PRUDENCE:	a poor woman, but prudent (wise)

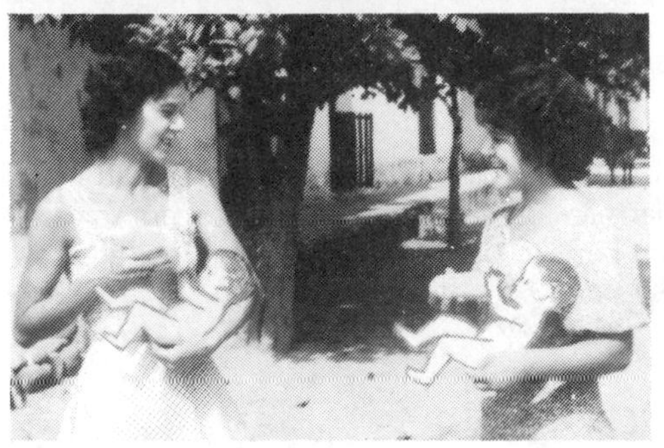

3) One day Modesty and Vanity meet in the street. They stop to chat about their babies. Both babies were born during the same week, and both look beautiful and healthy.

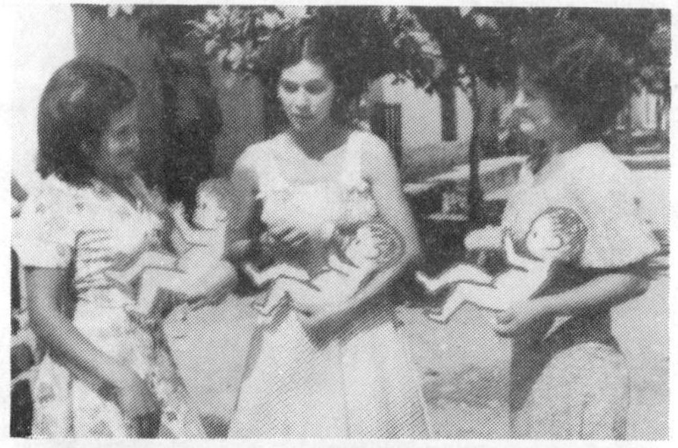

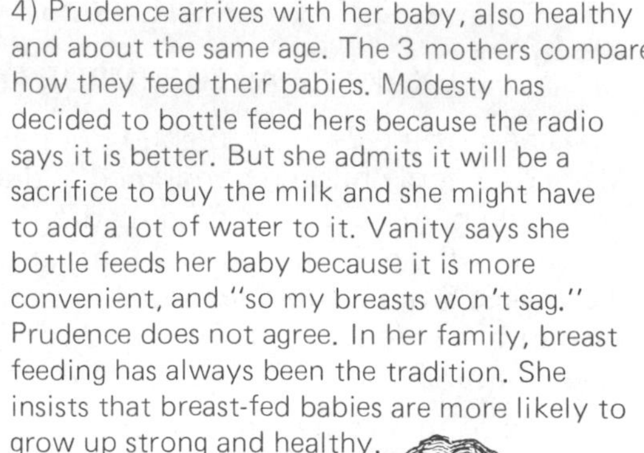

4) Prudence arrives with her baby, also healthy and about the same age. The 3 mothers compare how they feed their babies. Modesty has decided to bottle feed hers because the radio says it is better. But she admits it will be a sacrifice to buy the milk and she might have to add a lot of water to it. Vanity says she bottle feeds her baby because it is more convenient, and "so my breasts won't sag." Prudence does not agree. In her family, breast feeding has always been the tradition. She insists that breast-fed babies are more likely to grow up strong and healthy.

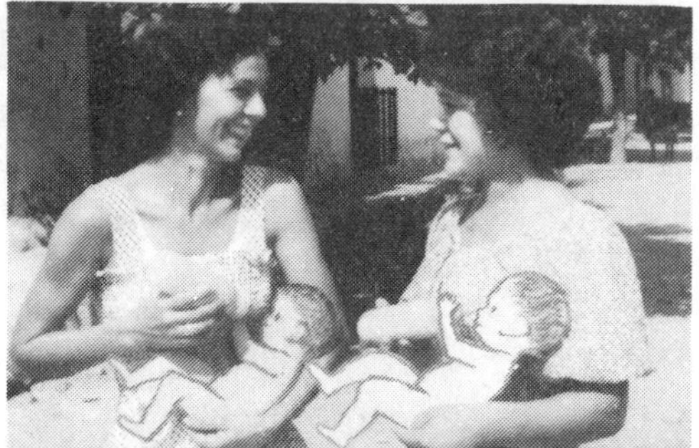

5) Modesty and Vanity laugh at Prudence. They say she is old fashioned because she does not bottle feed her baby.

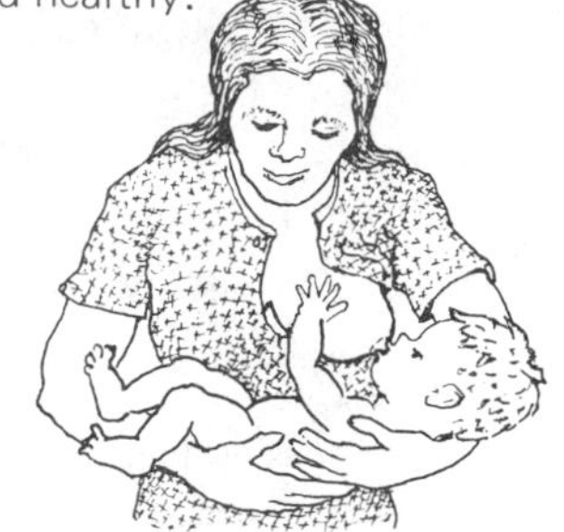

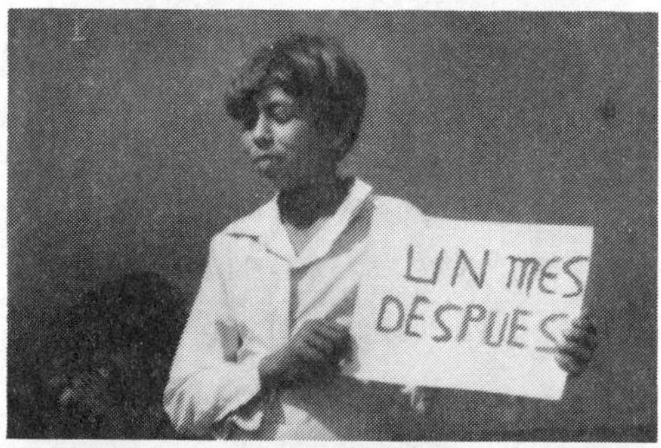

6) But let us look at the babies ONE MONTH LATER.

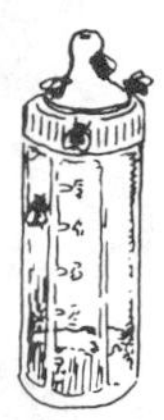

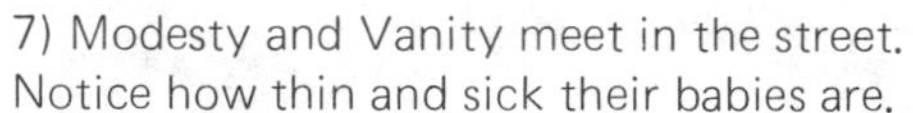

7) Modesty and Vanity meet in the street. Notice how thin and sick their babies are.

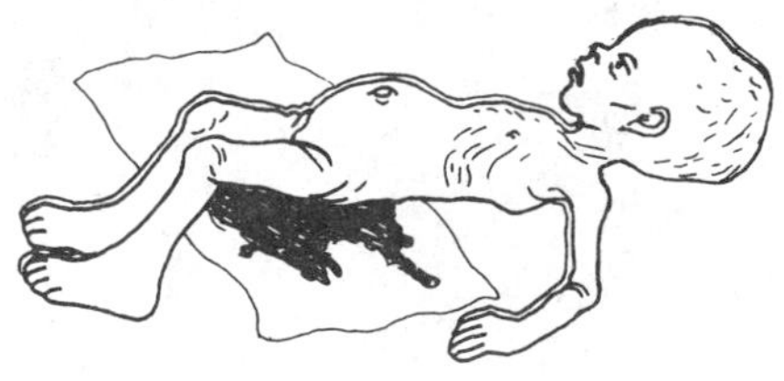

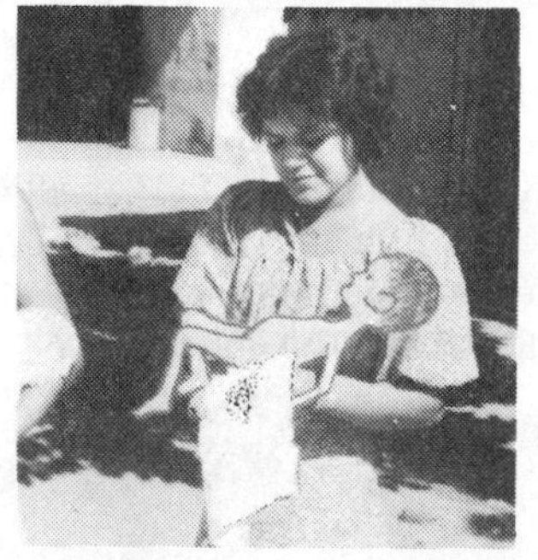

8) Vanity explains that her baby has had diarrhea for weeks, and does not seem to get any better. Right now the baby poops again. (She shows the dirty nappy.)

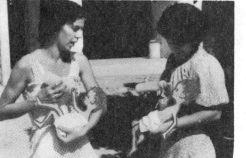

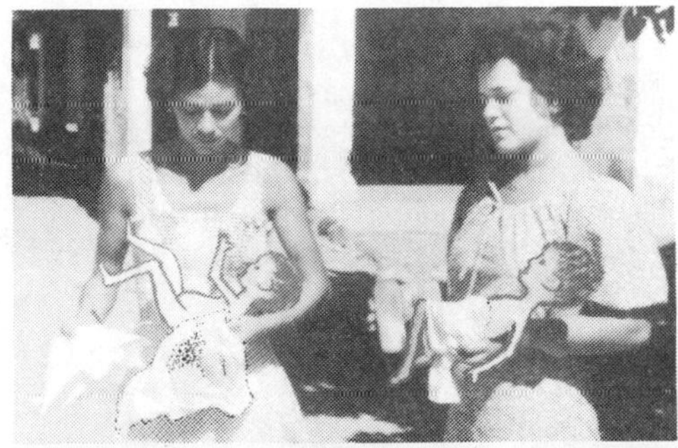

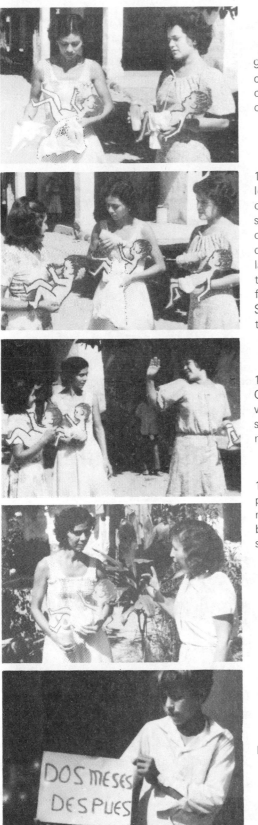

9) Modesty says that her baby also has a lot of diarrhea. Right then her baby poops, too! What can the mothers do with their skinny, sick children?

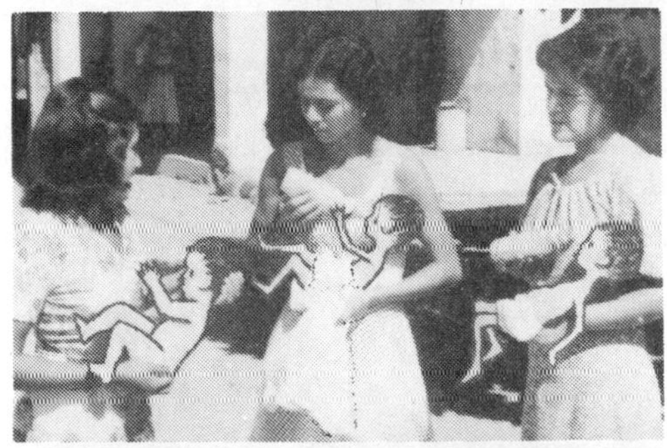

10) Just then Prudence comes by. Her baby looks strong and healthy. It has grown a lot. The other two mothers look at it jealously. Modesty suddenly realizes that bottle feeding may be the cause of her baby's diarrhea. She wishes she could breast feed her child, but says it is too late. Her breasts have dried up. But Prudence tells her about an aunt who started to breast feed her baby again after her milk was gone. She suggests that Modesty speak with Charity, the health worker, to see if she has any advice.

11) Modesty is eager to talk with Charity. She asks Vanity if she wants to go with her. But Vanity says, "Not me!" and leaves to buy medicine for her baby's diarrhea.

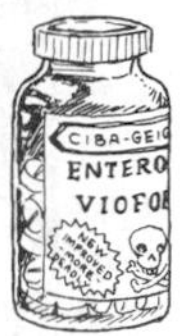

12) Modesty visits Charity and explains her problem. Charity tells her that, in many cases, mothers can get their milk back after their breasts have dried up. She gives her 4 suggestions from ***Where There Is No Doctor:***

1. Drink lots of liquid—water, juice, tea, or any other drink.
2. Eat as well as possible—especially milk, milk products, and foods rich in protein, such as beans, nuts, dark green leafy vegetables, eggs, chicken, meat, and fish.
3. Get plenty of sleep, and try to avoid getting tired or upset.
4. Nurse the baby often. Put him on the breast each time he is hungry, before you feed him other food.

Modesty is eager to try the suggestions.

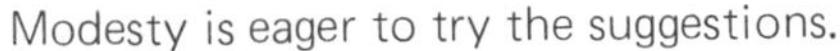

13) Let us see the results TWO MONTHS LATER.

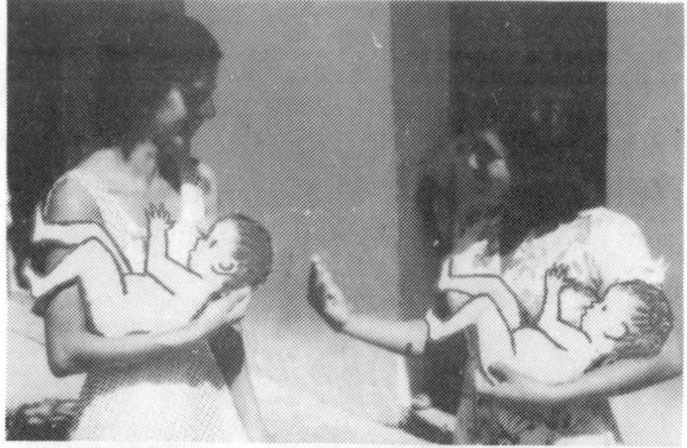

14) Modesty and Prudence meet in the street. Notice that Modesty's baby is now as fat and healthy as Prudence's baby. The 2 mothers are happy to see their children so healthy. They realize that it is because they are breast fed.

But what about Vanity's baby?

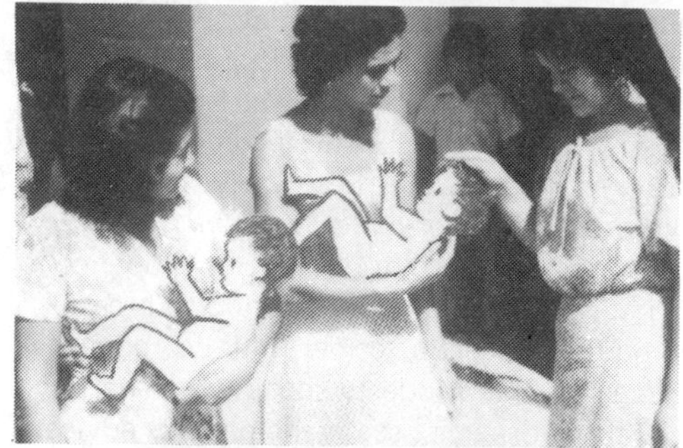

15) Just then Vanity arrives. By the black veil she is wearing, we can tell that her baby has died. With sad eyes she looks at Modesty's child. "How vain and foolish I was not to breast feed my baby. It cost his life to teach me that breast is best. If I have another baby, I'll breast feed him, believe me!"

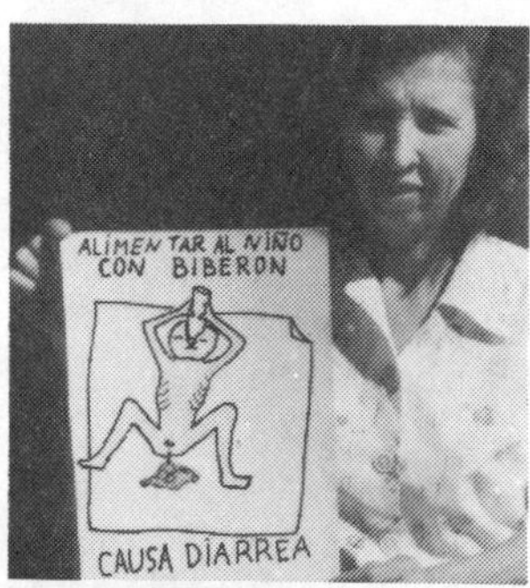

16) At the end of the skit, the health worker comes out with two posters made by the children of Ajoya. She gives a summary of what the children found out in their survey.

BOTTLE FEEDING CAUSES DIARRHEA.

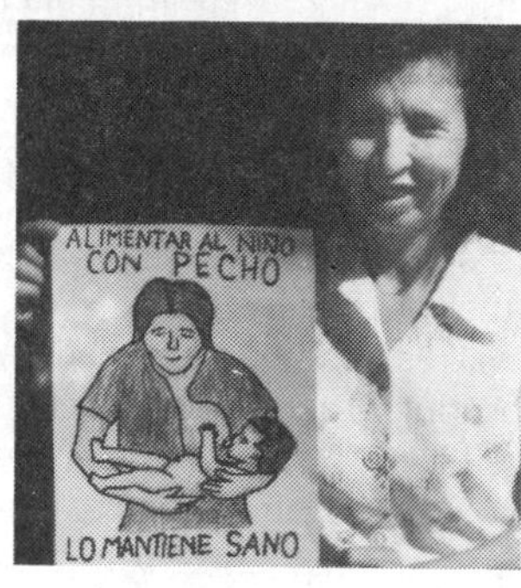

17) **BREAST FEEDING KEEPS BABY HEALTHY!**

Questions to ask health workers or people from the community after presenting this play (or the color slides or filmstrip):

- Does this problem exist in our community?
- Could the children or families here make a similar survey?
- What do you think of this idea for presenting the results of the survey in a short skit for the entire community?
- What else can we do to help solve the problem?

PUPPET SHOWS

Using puppets is a fun way to help children learn about health. Some health workers who have had trouble holding children's attention or getting them to speak their ideas, have found simple hand puppets especially useful. Children who are afraid to speak or argue with an adult will often talk freely to puppets.

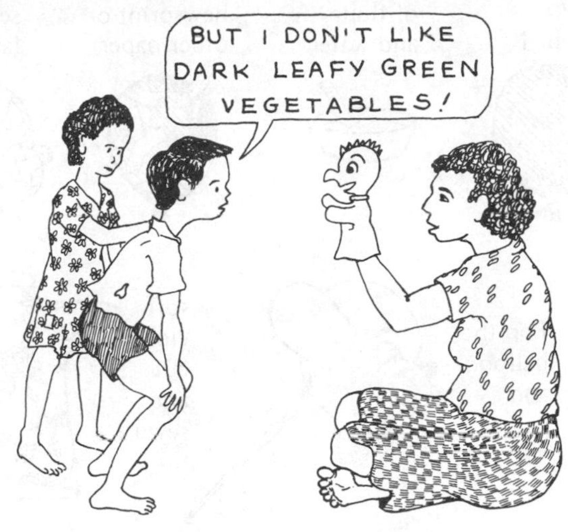

BUT I DON'T LIKE DARK LEAFY GREEN VEGETABLES!

Children are more likely to say what they think when talking with puppets.

HOW CHILDREN CAN MAKE PUPPETS

Puppets that open their mouths:

These work especially well for health skits about the mouth, throat, or teeth.

They are easy to make from a paper bag with the bottom folded over:

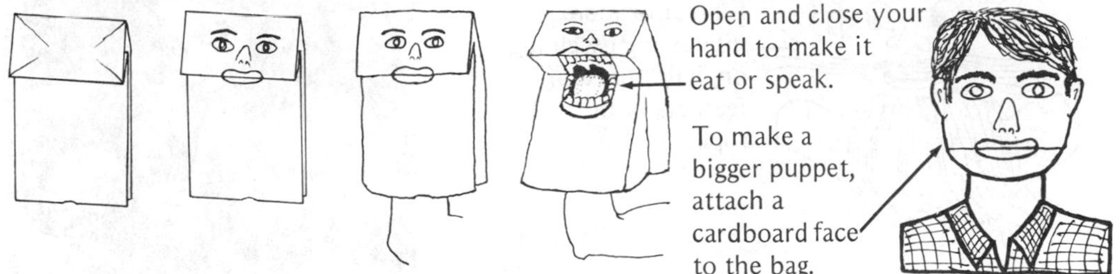

Open and close your hand to make it eat or speak.
To make a bigger puppet, attach a cardboard face to the bag.

Puppets that change faces:

On page **24**-8 we show how 'stick puppets' can be made to change the expression on their faces. However, in the way shown, only 2 different expressions are possible. The puppet below can have 4 different expressions—happy, angry, worried, and sad. Glue 2 pairs of faces back-to-back and attach them to 2 sticks as shown here:

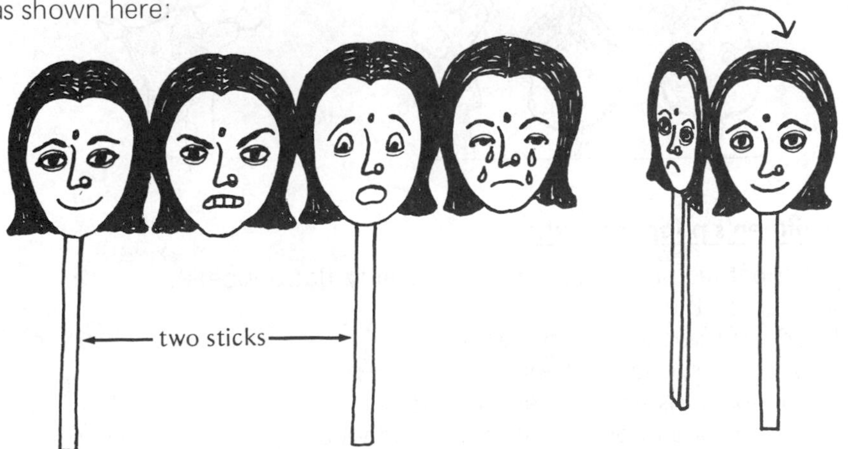

The expression can be changed by turning the sticks like pages of a book.

Making hand puppets out of papier mache (one of many ways):

balloon or gourd

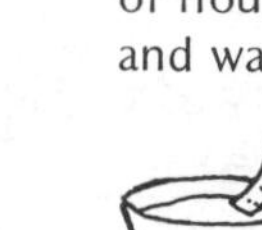

paste made of flour and water

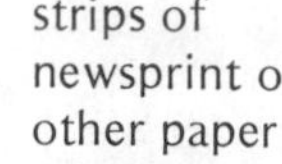

strips of newsprint or other paper

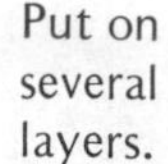

Put on several layers.

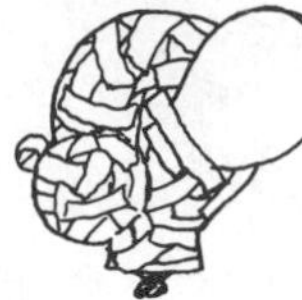

Let it dry. Pop the balloon and paint it.

soft cloth cut and sewn

Puppets can be made funnier or more interesting by gluing on 'hair' made of feathers or unraveled rope.

David Walker, World Education Reports

A local artist from Nepal makes a papier mache puppet.

Vegetable puppets:

Carve faces on squash, turnips, potatoes, etc.

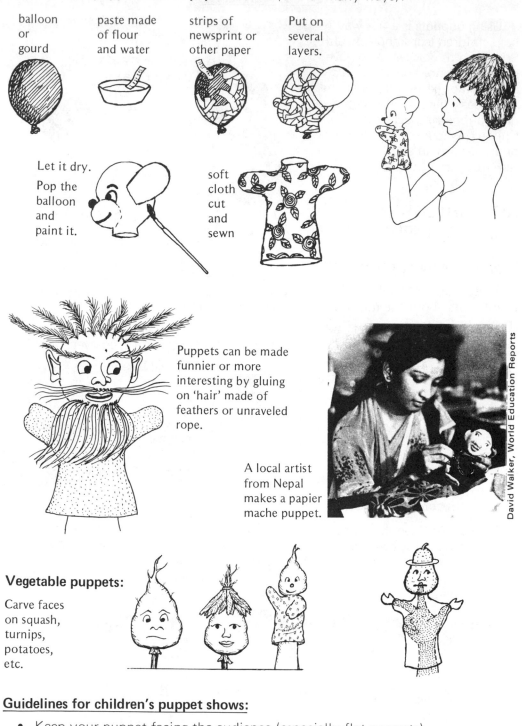

<u>**Guidelines for children's puppet shows:**</u>

- Keep your puppet facing the audience (especially flat puppets).
- Stay hidden behind the curtain.
- Move and nod your puppet when it speaks.
- Speak loudly, so everyone can hear.
- Use your own words instead of memorizing.
- Practice until everyone knows what to say and when.

PUPPET SHOWS—AN EXAMPLE

HOW TO CARE FOR THE TEETH

Preparations with the children

The Ajoya training course for health workers usually ends with an evening of skits and plays for the public. These usually deal with the causes of health problems in the town.

One year the school children also wanted to take part in the 'cultural festival'. So with the help of the health workers-in-training, a group of children planned and prepared their own skit. The health workers encouraged the children to make most of the decisions themselves. The children decided:

Where to meet and practice (the school, since it was empty in the evenings).

How to present the skit. They decided to use puppets (because they had seen puppets in another festival and liked them a lot).

What idea to present. They decided on prevention of tooth cavities because many of them suffered from this problem. (Children often insult each other by saying, "You have rotten teeth!")

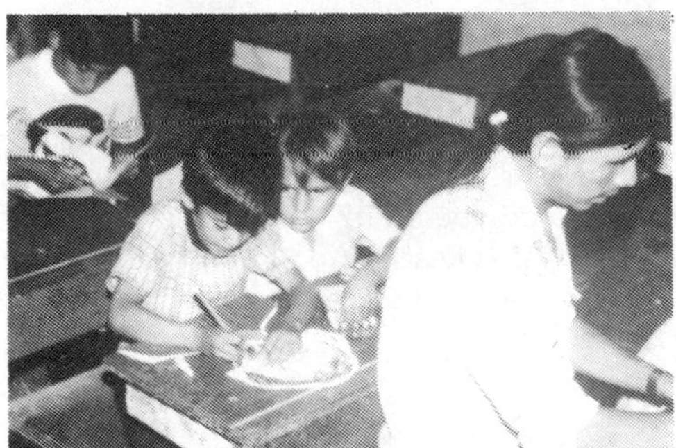

1) At the beginning, the children thought they could not make puppets themselves. But some of the health workers knew an easy way to make puppets out of paper bags. Because these puppets can open their mouths, they are particularly good for showing teeth. Here we see the children and one of the health workers making the puppets.

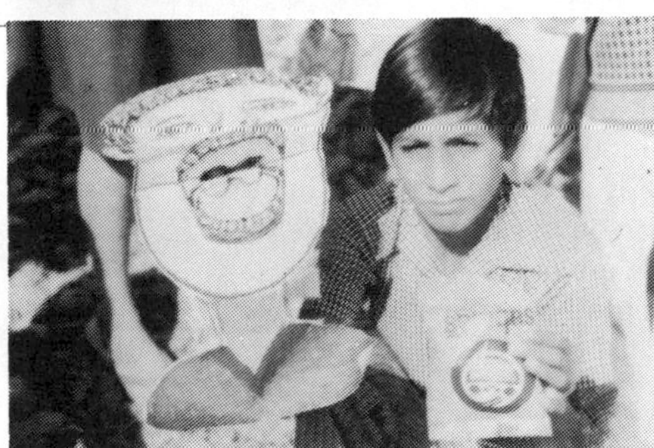

2) Each child gave his puppet a name. This boy named his puppet Sweet Tooth. It became one of the main characters. Puppets with good teeth were given names like Whitey, Pearl, and Sparkie. Puppets with bad teeth were named Candy, Sweetie, Sugar, Lolly, and Pop.

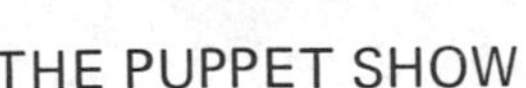

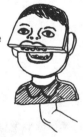

THE PUPPET SHOW

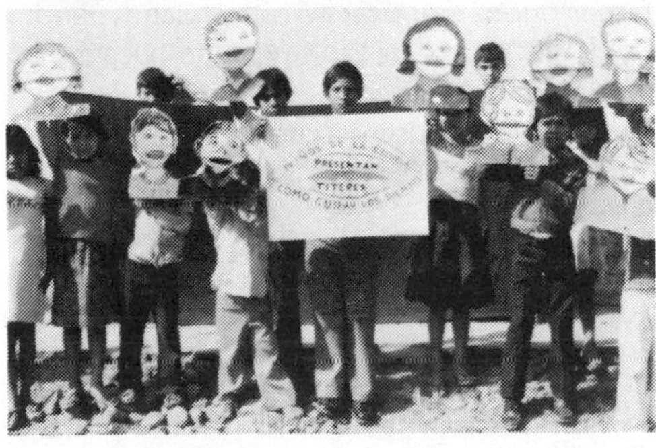

3) Here we see the children showing their puppets before going behind the curtain to present the show. The sign reads:

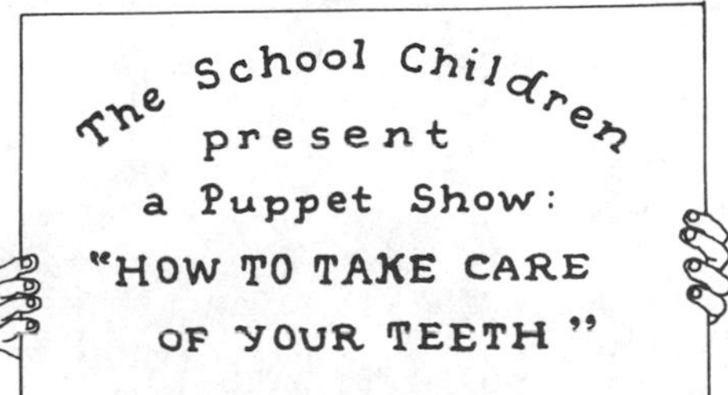

The School Children
present
a Puppet Show:
"HOW TO TAKE CARE
OF YOUR TEETH"

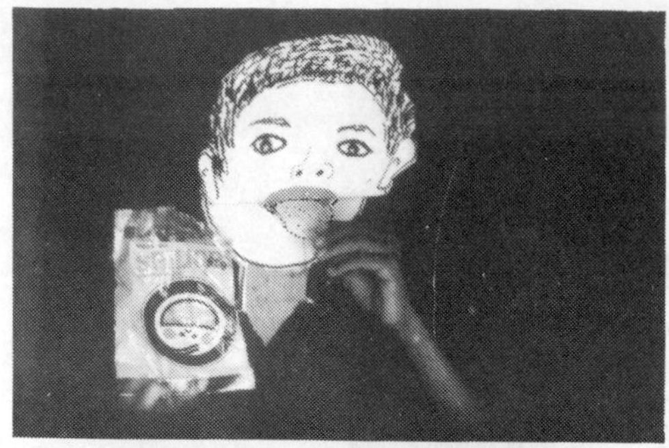

4) The show opens with Sweet Tooth alone, eating candy. The child working the puppet puts candies in Sweet Tooth's mouth, and he chews them. Crunch, crunch, crunch. "Ahhhh, I like candy so much! I could spend all day eating sweets!"

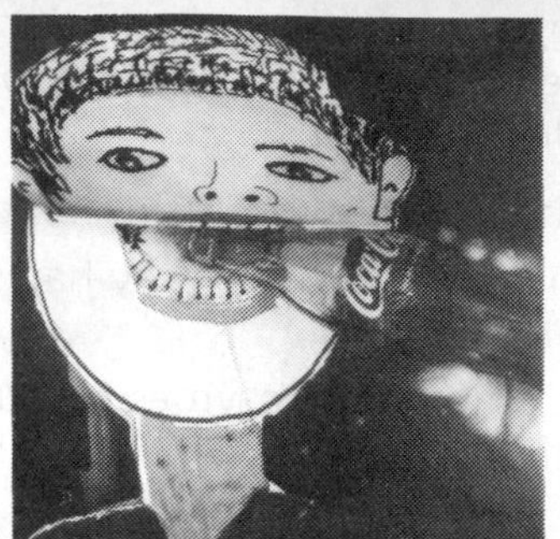

5) "Boy, that made me thirsty. I think I'll wash down the sweets with a Coke." The child lifts a Coke to the puppet's mouth. "Gulp, gulp, gulp."

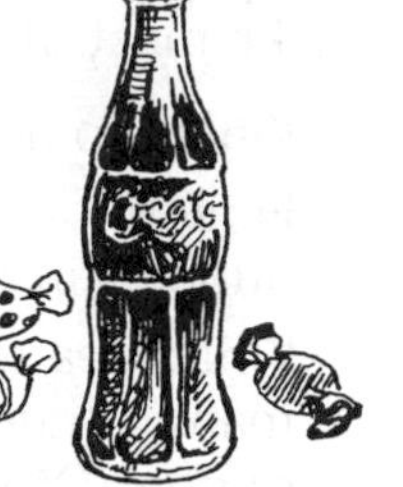

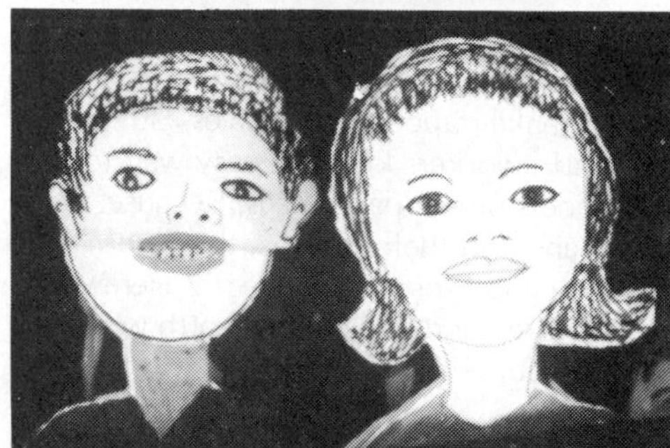

6) Sweet Tooth's friend, Pearl, appears. "Hello Pearl," he says. "My, you have such pretty teeth! How do you do it?" "I brush my teeth every day," says Pearl. "And I don't eat a lot of sweets like you do. Let's see your teeth, Sweet Tooth."

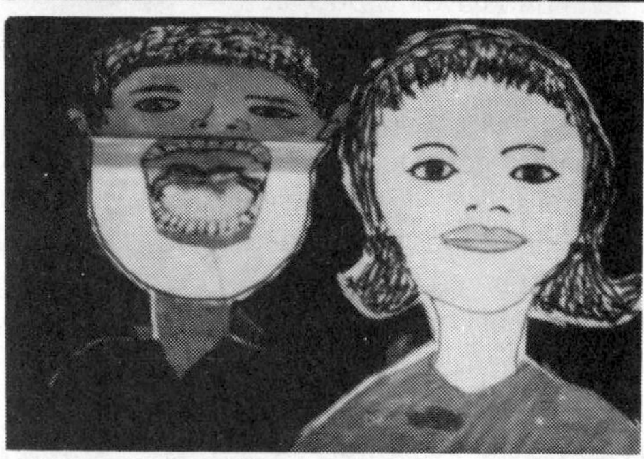

7) Sweet Tooth opens his mouth very wide. All his teeth are rotten. "Do you mean my teeth are like this because I eat so many sweets?"

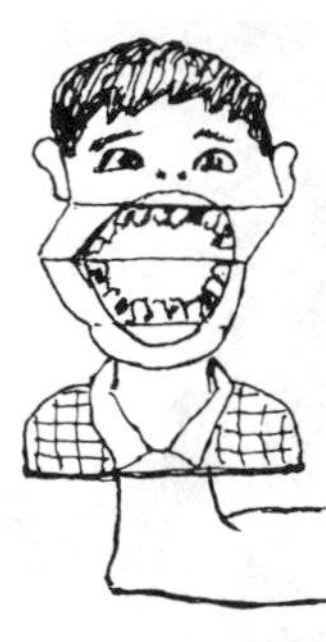

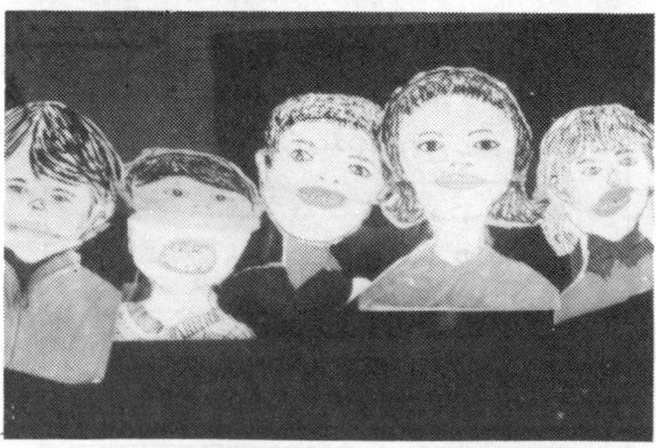

8) Other puppets appear: Whitey, Candy, and Lolly. "Yes," answers Whitey, "and because you drink a lot of sweet, fizzy drinks like Coke." "And because you don't brush your teeth," adds Pearl.

"But some of us can't afford toothbrushes and toothpaste," says Candy. "Like Lolly and me!" Candy and Lolly open their mouths wide to show their rotten teeth.

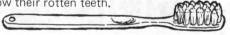

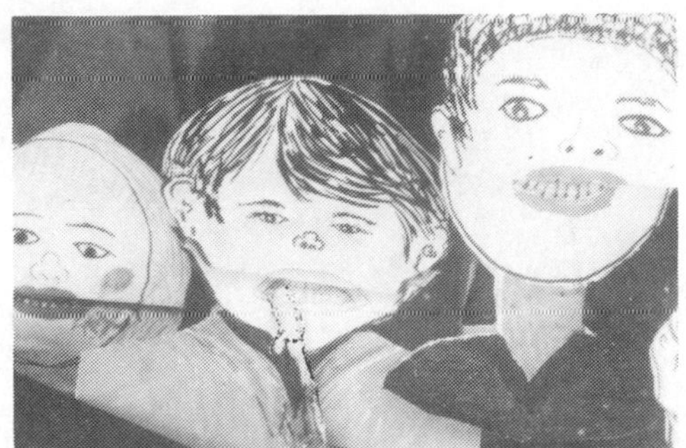

9) "But you don't need a toothbrush or toothpaste to keep your teeth clean," says Whitey. "Just look at mine!" He opens his mouth and shows his sparkling white teeth. "In our family, we clean our teeth like this, with a piece of rough cloth wrapped around a stick. Instead of toothpaste, we dip the stick in a mixture of salt and baking soda. It works great!" The child rubs the puppet's teeth with a stick wrapped in cloth.

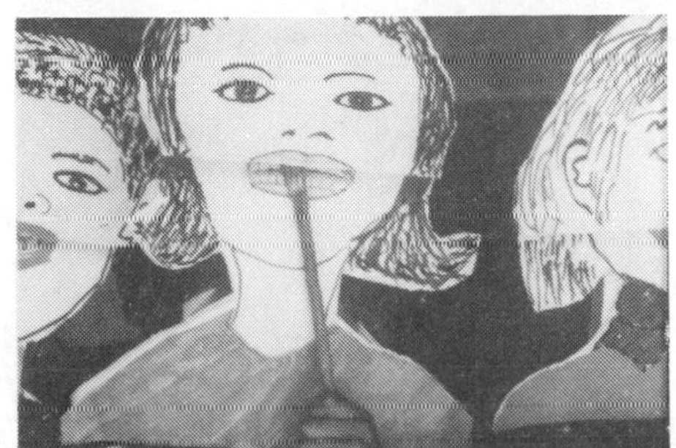

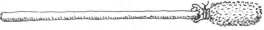

"Maybe you're right," says Lolly. "My grandfather still has perfect teeth and he has never had a toothbrush. He cleans his teeth with a powder made of burnt tortilla, on his finger! He also doesn't eat sweet things."

10) Pearl explains, "In our family, we don't have toothbrushes either. Instead, we use a stick like this." (She shows it.)

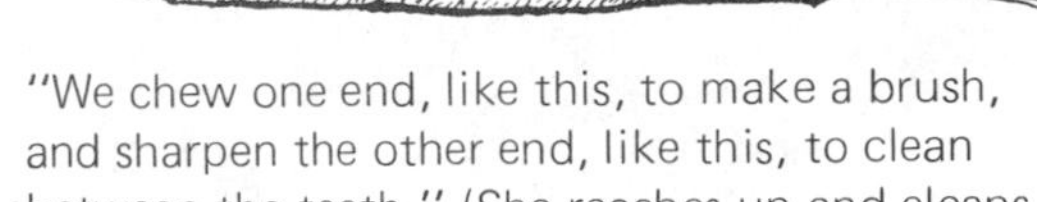

"We chew one end, like this, to make a brush, and sharpen the other end, like this, to clean between the teeth." (She reaches up and cleans her teeth.)

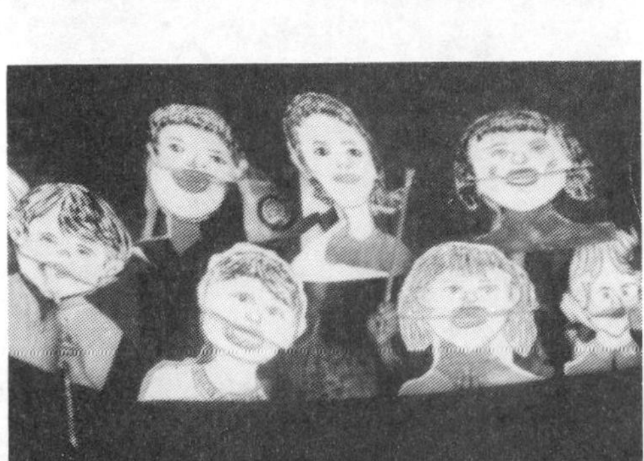

11) "Hurray!" shout the puppets. "Now we know how to clean our teeth without spending money on toothbrushes and toothpaste!" "And don't forget what my grandfather says," adds Lolly. "If you want to keep your teeth strong and healthy like his, don't eat a lot of sweet things or drink sweet, fizzy drinks!"

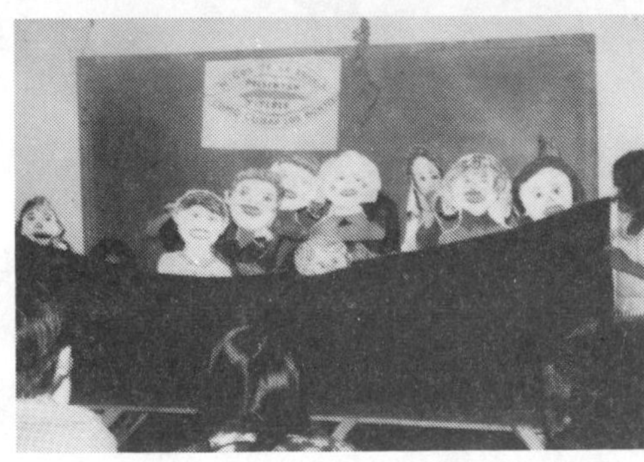

12) Everyone shouts together:

"LEARNING TOGETHER
WE LEARN A LOT:
CANDY IS DANDY,
BUT ROT IS NOT!

WE'VE FOUND A WAY
TO FIGHT TOOTH DECAY.

WE ALL HELP EACH OTHER
STAY HEALTHY, HURRAY!

A CALL FOR COURAGE AND CAUTION

For health workers to stand up for the interests of the poor and to work toward changing the social causes of poverty, hunger, and poor health clearly involves a certain risk. The degree of risk will vary from country to country, and even from village to village.

For this reason, the openness with which health workers work toward social awakening and change, and the methods they use, need to be adapted to each local situation. For example, some of the village theater productions led by the Project Piaxtla team in Mexico (see Ch. 27) have resulted in attempts by local authorities to close down the villager-run health program. But in certain other countries in Latin America, health workers have been tortured and killed for doing less.

Unfortunately, countries where the health needs of the poor are greatest are usually the same countries where repression and violation of rights by those in control is most severe. These are the countries where leaders of the poor and those who work for social change are in greatest danger.

We urge planners and instructors of health workers, as well as health workers themselves, to move forward with their eyes wide open. Evaluate the possible benefits and risks of any approach or activity you consider, especially if it involves confrontation or conflict of interests. The risks of taking any particular step toward change need to be weighed against the risks of not taking that step: "How many people may suffer from repression if we take a stand on this issue? How many children will continue to die of hunger-related diseases if we don't?"

Before training health workers in a people-centered approach, be sure that both you and they carefully consider the range of possible consequences.

We have had to struggle with these same questions in making the decision in this book to speak openly about social issues affecting health. We know we are taking a chance—both for ourselves and for others who care about people as we do. We hope and believe that in the long run the benefits will outweigh the costs. But each person needs to consider the balance and make his or her own informed decisions.

We urge those planners and officials who share the vision of a healthier, more self-reliant future for the poor to welcome criticism and suggestions from those working at the village and community level. If you are involved in a nationwide program to train health workers, help to defend and preserve those small, independent, community-based efforts that already exist. Learn from their strengths and weaknesses, criticize them and seek their advice and evaluation of your own program. Variety is essential for comparison and improvement.

At the same time, we urge those working at the community level, whether in government or independent programs, to look for ways to help the 'voiceless poor' be heard and take part in decision making at the central level.

If those of us who share the vision of a more fully human future join hands and work together, perhaps 'health for all' will, in fact, someday be possible.

LIST OF ADDRESSES FOR TEACHING MATERIALS

To obtain a more complete list of addresses for ordering health education materials, write to the Hesperian Foundation or to TALC. Explain which health subjects, countries, and languages you are interested in.

For other publications mentioned in this book, see pages **5**-2, **11**-28, **12**-4, **12**-15, **13**-1, **13**-9, **16**-3, **16**-13, **18**-2, **Part Three**-8, **22**-20, **25**-20, **25**-25, **25**-29, **26**-32, and **26**-36.

The Hesperian Foundation.
1919 Addison Street, Suite 304
Berkeley, California 94704 USA
Health books in basic language, ***Where There Is No Doctor***, ***Where Women Have No Doctor***, ***Disabled Village Children,*** and others, in English and Spanish. Also ***Hesperian Foundation News*** and ***Women's Health Exchange*** 4 times yearly.

APHA / Clearinghouse
1015 15th Street, N.W.
Washington D.C. 20005 USA
Mothers and Children, a quarterly health information newsletter in English, Spanish, and French.

World Neighbors / 4127 NW 122 Street
Oklahoma City, OK 73120-8869 USA
Soundings, a newsletter on rural development communications; many filmstrips and teaching aids in English and Spanish.

PAHO / 525 23rd Street, N.W.
Washington D.C. 20037 USA
Various materials in English and Spanish.

Save the Children Fund
54 Wilton Road, Westport, CT 06880 USA
Teaching materials in English and other languages.

International Women's Health Coalition
24 East 21st Street, 5th Floor
New York, NY 10010
Training course, teaching materials, and slides.

Teaching Aids at Low Cost (TALC)
P.O. Box 49, St. Albans
Herts., AL1 4AX, UK
Slide sets, weight charts, aids for weight charts (flannel-boards, etc.), free list of materials in English, French, and Spanish.

AHRTAG / 1 London Bridge Street
London SE1 9SG, England
Diarrhoea Dialogue, a newsletter about prevention and treatment of diarrhea. Other teaching aids about rehabilitation.

WHO / 1211 Geneva 27, Switzerland
Health Learning Materials newsletter, and other materials in English, French, and Spanish.

World Council of Churches \ CMC-Churches' Action for Health
150, route de Ferney, C.P. 2100
1211 Geneva 2, Switzerland
Contact, a newsletter concerned with appropriate health care in English, French, Spanish, and Portuguese, and selected issues also available in Kiswahili and Arabic.

Freedom from Hunger Campaign
FAO/Action for Development
00100 Rome, Italy
Ideas & Action, a newsletter exploring problems and solutions found by rural development programs working at the local level. In English, French, and Spanish.

Kahayag Foundation /121 University Avenue
Juna Subd., Matina
Davao City 8000, Philippines
Slide shows and information about health and development problems; **Mushawarah,** a women's newsletter in local Muslim language.

Voluntary Health Association of India (VHAI)
Tong Swasthya Bhavan
40 Institutional Area, near Quatab Hotel
New Delhi 110016, India
Flannel-board sets, books, flip charts; ***Where There Is No Doctor*** adapted for India, in English and local languages. List available.

Yayasan Indonesia Sejahtera
Unit PPSDM: P.O. Box 242
Jl. Tanjung No. 96, Karangasem Laweyan
Solo 57145, Indonesia
Vibro newsletter, in English.

Community Health and Integration Project
Dept. of Health Services,
Kathmandu, Nepal
Illustrated book, ***Community Health Leader Training-cum-working Manual,*** available in local language and English translation.

Centre pour le Promotion de la Sante
c/o Dr. J. Courtejoie
Kangu Majumbe, Republique du Zaire
Excellent materials for village use in French; also some in English and local languages.

Atelier de Material Didactique
Busiga, B.P. 18, Ngozi, Burundi
Good flip charts and teaching plans in French and local languages.

ENI Communication Centre
Box 2361, Addis Ababa, Ethiopia
Educational packages and visual aids about child health and nutrition.

ENDA - COORCOM
54, reu Carnot, B.P. 3370,
Dakar, Senegal
Where There Is No Doctor in French.

Rotary Club of Dar Es Salaam
P.O. Box 1533, Dar Es Salaam, Tanzania
Where There Is No Doctor in Swahili.

African Medical & Research Foundation
Box 30125, Nairobi, Kenya
The Defender, a newsletter with ideas for health education methods, and an excellent series of rural health books in English.

Editorial Pax-Mexico
Av. Cuauhtemoc, 1434
Mexico 13, D.F., Mexico
Donde No Hay Doctor; other books and photonovels on nutrition, midwifery, family planning, in Spanish.

SEPAC
Apartado 57, Cd. Netzahualcoyotl,
Edo. Mexico, Mexico
Books and pamphlets on literacy, awareness raising, health, cooperatives, etc. In Spanish.

CIDHAL, A.C.
Apartado 579, Cuernavaca, Morelos, Mexico
Pamphlets in Spanish on basic nutrition, growing and cooking soybeans, women's health, sexuality, and menopause.

Maria, Liberacion del Pueblo
Apartado 128, CIVAC, Jiutepec, Morelos,
CP62500, Mexico
Monthly newsletter in Spanish written by local women. Topics include local and international politics, nutrition, recipes, women's rights.

ASECSA
Apartado 27, Chimaltenango, Guatemala
El Informador newsletter, pamphlets, posters, books, and filmstrips on health subjects and teaching methods in Spanish.

CEMAT
Apartado 1160, Guatemala, Guatemala
Pamphlets on many health subjects, latrines, medicinal herbs, acupuncture, in Spanish.

CISAS
Apartado 3267, Managua, Nicaragua
All types of excellent educational materials about health.

Centro Amazonico Limoncocha
Casilla 5080, Quito, Ecuador
Pamphlets on literacy, education, health, and agriculture, in local Indian languages.

Centro Andino de Comunicaciones
Casilla 2774, Cochabamba, Bolivia
Posters, flip charts, and books ***(Guia de la Madre, Huertos Familiares)*** in Spanish and Quechua.

Instituto de Estudios Andinos
Apartado Postal 289, Huancayo, Peru
Fine books on family gardens and nutrition.

Instituto Linguistico de Verano
Casilla 2492, Lima 100, Peru
Excellent books, pamphlets, posters, flip charts in local languages.

INCUPO / Rivadavia 1275, 3560 Reconquista,
Santa Fe, Argentina
Accion newsletter and various pamphlets on first aid, nutrition, and diarrhea, in Spanish.

Paulus Editora / Rua Francisco Cruz, 229
04117-091 São Paulo, SP, Brazil
Where There Is No Doctor in Portuguese.

Caribbean Food and Nutrition Institute
U.W.I. Campus, P.O. Box 140
Kingston 7, Jamaica, West Indies
Cajanus, a nutrition bulletin; other materials in English for the Caribbean.

INDEX

D

E

F

G

H

I

J

K

L

M

N

O

P

Q

R

S

T

U

V

W

Y

Z

About Project Piaxtla and the authors:

Many of the ideas in this book came from a small community based health program in the mountains of rural Mexico called Project Piaxtla. This health program has been run and controlled by local villagers, some of whom have worked with the program since it began in 1966. The project has served over 100 small villages, some of which are 2 days by muleback from the training and referral center in the village of Ajoya. This mud-brick center has been run by a team of the more experienced local health workers, who trained and provided support for workers from the more remote villages. This book discusses details of selection, training, follow-up, and referral of the 2-month training course developed in Ajoya (see the Index).

Project Piaxtla began in an unlikely but very natural way. In 1964, David Werner, a biologist by training and a school teacher by trade, was wandering through the Sierra Madre observing birds and plants. He was impressed by the friendliness and self-reliance of the mountain people, but also by the severity of their health problems. Although he had no medical training, he felt that his scientific background and the people's resourcefulness and skills might be combined to meet health needs better. So, after apprenticing briefly in a hospital emergency room in the U.S., and painting bird pictures to raise money, he returned. David stayed for 10 years, until he was no longer needed. It seemed that the most helpful thing he and the other outsiders could do to allow the program to evolve further was to leave. So in 1976, the program changed and was run entirely by the local villagers, with no ongoing presence of outsiders or professionals.

In its focus of action, Project Piaxtla evolved through 3 stages: curative, preventive, and social. It began with curative care, which is what people wanted. In time, the central team gained a high degree of medical ability. Although most of the group had little formal schooling, they were able to effectively attend (or help the people attend) about 98% of the health problems they saw. Because of the difficulties in getting good care for persons they referred to city hospitals, the team made efforts to master a wide range of medical skills. These included minor surgery (including superficial eye surgery), delivery of babies, and treatment of serious diseases such as typhoid, TB, leprosy, and tetanus. (With the help of village mothers, who give the babies breast milk through a nose-to-stomach tube, they have been able to save 70% of the newborns with tetanus.) For severe problems beyond their capacity, the team slowly developed an effective referral system in the nearest city (see page **10**-18).

The health team, having been trained by a visiting radiologist, was also able to take X-rays using an old donated unit. A basic clinical laboratory for stool, urine, and blood analysis was run by Rosa Salcido, who had never been to school. Several village 'dentics', headed by Jesus Vega, would clean teeth, extract, drill and fill cavities, and make dentures—at a fraction of what these services cost in the cities.

Even as curative needs were being met, however, the same illnesses appeared again and again. So people became more concerned with prevention. The team began programs of vaccinations, latrine building, nutrition classes, child spacing, and community gardens. But in time the people began to realize that even these measures did not solve the root causes of poor health—those relating to land ownership, high interest rates on loans, and other ways that the strong profit from the weak. So little by little, the focus of the health team became more social, even political. Examples of actions they took are discussed in the introductory section (Why This Book Is So Political) and elsewhere in this book.

The health team came to feel that its first job was to help the poor gain self-confidence, knowledge and skills to defend their just interests. But this was not easy. Among other things, the health workers had to re-evaluate their own approaches to teaching and working with people, to develop new methods that help persons value their own experience and to weigh critically for themselves what they are taught and told. Many of the learning methods and materials discussed in this book have been developed by the team and student health workers through this process.

Project Piaxtla's relationship with the government was mixed. When the village team became increasingly effective in helping people deal with illegal land holdings, high interest rates, corruption of local officials, and abuses by health professionals, local authorities made repeated attempts to weaken the program or close it down.

But Piaxtla also had its strong supporters—even within the government. Although the Health Ministry, in many ways, opposed the villager-run program, those in other ministries appreciated its value. The Ministry of Agrarian Reform contracted with the village team to train its first group of community health workers. The Ministry of Education—which has considered making 'Health' a full-time school subject—sought the advice of Martin Reyes, the Project Piaxtla coordinator. CONAFE, a government program that set up basic skills libraries in villages throughout the country, employed Pablo Chavez to help train village 'cultural promoters' in the use of ***Where There Is No Doctor.*** (Pablo is the health worker who helped illustrate this book.)

Also within the Ministry of Health, Project Piaxtla had its friends. For years, the malaria control and vaccination programs cooperated with the village team. At first, things were more difficult with the tuberculosis program. The district chief refused to provide the health team with medications for those living too far away to make regular trips to the city health center. So a leader of the village team, Roberto Fajardo, went to Mexico City and convinced the head of the national program to give an order to the district chief to supply the team with medicine for proven cases of TB. In this way, the Project Piaxtla team began to affect government policy, making it more responsive to the needs of the rural poor.

The Ajoya team valued economic self-sufficiency. The part-time health workers from outlying villages also achieved this in their work. They earned most of their living by farming, and charged a small fee for services. Self-sufficiency proved more difficult for the team of coordinators in the training and referral center. However, they experimented with a number of income-producing activities: hog raising, chicken raising, vegetable gardening, fruit orchards, and bee keeping. These activities not only brought in funds, but helped improve local nutrition and provided examples of improved small-scale production. The team also charged a modest fee for services. Persons unable to pay could send a family member to help with the farming instead.

The village team came to feel that health workers from different programs and countries have much to share and learn from each other. The team was active in a regional Committee for Promoting Community Health in Central America. The committee's third international meeting was held in Ajoya. In this meeting, the number of professionals and outsiders was strictly limited, so that the health workers themselves could lead discussions and participate more easily. The Ajoya team also conducted a series of 'educational exchanges', inviting village-level instructors from health programs in Mexico and Central America to meet together and explore educational methods and materials. These 'exchanges' were valuable for gathering and testing many of the ideas in this book.

Project Piaxtla has evolved through trial and error, learning from both mistakes and successes. It struggled through many difficulties, many of which grew more severe as the team became active in defending the rights of the poor. The future of the project is as uncertain as is the future of the poor in Latin America.

Bill Bower, a North American who grew up in Venezuela, joined Project Piaxtla in 1974, just before outside volunteers were phased out from ongoing participation. Bill has a degree in human biology. He received training in community health in a special course taught by former Piaxtla volunteers, and also attended an alternative health training program in Mexico City. He helped the Ajoya team plan and organize health worker training courses and educational exchanges between programs. He played a leading part in preparing both the English version of ***Where There Is No Doctor,*** and the revised Spanish edition.

OTHER BOOKS FROM THE HESPERIAN FOUNDATION

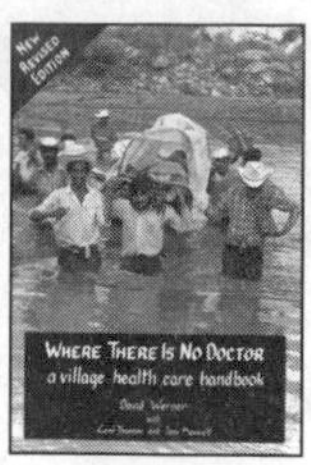

Where There Is No Doctor, by David Werner with Carol Thuman and Jane Maxwell. Perhaps the most widely used health care manual in the world, this book provides vital, easily understood information on how to diagnose, treat, and prevent common diseases. Emphasis is placed on prevention, including cleanliness, diet, and vaccinations, as well as the active role people must take in their own health care. 512 pages.

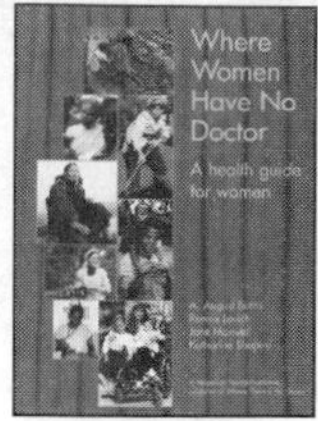

Where Women Have No Doctor, by A. August Burns, Ronnie Lovich, Jane Maxwell, and Katharine Shapiro, combines self-help medical information with an understanding of the ways poverty, discrimination, and cultural beliefs limit women's health and access to care. An essential resource on the problems that affect women or that affect women differently from men. 584 pages.

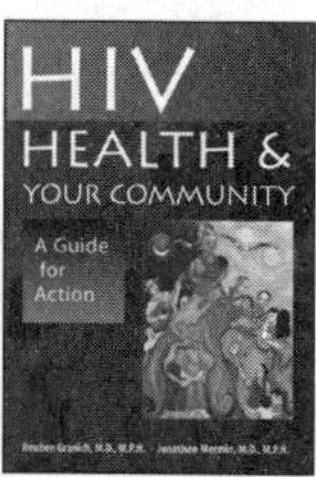

HIV, Health, and Your Community: A Guide for Action by Reuben Granich and Jonathan Mermin is an essential resource for community health workers and others confronting HIV/AIDS. This clearly written guide emphasizes prevention and also covers virus biology, epidemiology, and ideas for designing HIV prevention and treatment programs. Contains an appendix of common health problems and treatments for people with HIV/AIDS. 245 pages.

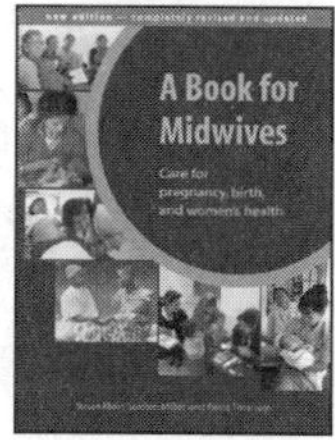

A Book for Midwives, by Susan Klein, Suellen Miller, and Fiona Thomson, completely revised in 2004, is for midwives, community health workers and anyone concerned about the health of women and babies in pregnancy, birth and beyond. An invaluable tool for training as well as a practical reference, it covers helping pregnant women stay healthy, care during and after birth, handling obstetric complications, breastfeeding, and includes expanded information for women's reproductive health care. 544 pages

Helping Children Who Are Deaf, by Sandy Neimann, Devorah Greenstein and Darlena David, helps parents and other caregivers build the communication skills of young children with difficulty hearing. Covers language development and how to foster communication through both sign and oral approaches, how to assess hearing loss, causes of deafness, and more. 250 pages.

Disabled Village Children, by David Werner, covers most common disabilities of children. It gives suggestions for rehabilitation and explains how to make a variety of low-cost aids. Emphasis is placed on how to help disabled children find a role and be accepted in the community. 672 pages.

Helping Children Who Are Blind, by Sandy Niemann and Namita Jacob, aids parents and other caregivers in helping blind children develop all their capabilities. Topics include: assessing what a child can see, preventing blindness, moving around safely, teaching common activities, and more. 192 pages.

Where There Is No Dentist, by Murray Dickson, shows how to care for teeth and gums, and prevent tooth and gum problems through hygiene, nutrition, and education. Includes detailed, well illustrated information on using dental equipment, placing fillings, taking out teeth, and more, and material on HIV/AIDS and oral health. 237 pages.

All titles are available from Hesperian in both English and Spanish. For information regarding other language editions, prices and ordering, or for a brochure about the Foundation's work, please contact us.

The Hesperian Foundation
Box 11577, Berkeley, California 94712-2577 USA
Telephone: (510) 845-4507, Fax (510) 845-0539
e-mail: bookorders@hesperian.org
visit our website: www.hesperian.org